Comprehensive Cleft Care

Editors

Joseph E. Losee, MD, FAAP, FACS
Chief, Pediatric Plastic Surgery
Director, Cleft-Craniofacial Center
Children's Hospital of Pittsburgh
University of Pittsburgh
Pittsburgh, Pennsylvania

Richard E. Kirschner, MD, FAAP, FACS
Mary Downs Chair in Craniofacial Treatment and Research
Director, Cleft Lip and Palate Program
The Children's Hospital of Philadelphia
University of Pennsylvania
Philadelphia, Pennsylvania

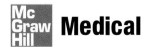

New York   Chicago   San Francisco   Lisbon   London   Madrid   Mexico City   Milan
New Delhi   San Juan   Seoul   Singapore   Sydney   Toronto

Comprehensive Cleft Care

1 2 3 4 5 6 7 8 9 0   CTP/CTP   12 11 10 9 8

ISBN 978-0-07-148180-9
MHID 0-07-148180-X

Notice

Medicine is an ever-changing science. As new research and clinical experience broaden our knowledge, changes in treatment and drug therapy are required. The authors and the publisher of this work have checked with sources believed to be reliable in their efforts to provide information that is complete and generally in accord with the standards accepted at the time of publication. However, in view of the possibility of human error and changes in medical sciences, neither the editors nor the publisher nor any other party who has been involved in the preparation or publication of this work warrants that the information contained herein is in every respect accurate or complete, and they disclaim all responsibility for any errors or omissions or for the results obtained from use of the information contained in this work. Readers are encouraged to confirm the information contained herein with other sources. For example and in particular, readers are advised to check the product information sheet included in the package of each drug they plan to administer to be certain that the information contained in this work is accurate and that changes have not been made in the recommended dose or in the contraindications for administration. This recommendation is of particular importance in connection with new or infrequently used drugs.

This book was set in Minion by Aptara®, Inc.
The editors were Marsha Loeb and Karen Edmonson.
The production supervisor was Phil Galea.
Project management was provided by Satvinder Kaur, Aptara®, Inc.
The designer was Janice Bielawa; the cover designer was Eve Siegel.
The indexer was Mayank Bahadur.
China Translation & Printing Services, Ltd. was printer and binder.
Front cover Image—Tucker Tillia By: Portraits Plus James Nocera photojim@gmail.com

This book is printed on acid-free paper.

Library of Congress Cataloging-in-Publication Data

Comprehensive cleft care / [edited by] Joseph E. Losee, Richard E. Kirschner.
      p. ; cm.
  Includes bibliographical references.
  ISBN 978-0-07-148180-9 (alk. paper)
 1. Cleft lip.   2. Cleft palate.   3. Cleft lip–Surgery.   4. Cleft palate–Surgery.   I. Losee, Joseph E.   II. Kirschner, Richard E.
  [DNLM: 1. Cleft Lip–therapy.   2. Cleft Palate–therapy.   3. Oral Surgical Procedures–methods. 4.   Reconstructive Surgical Procedures–methods.   WV 440 C737 2008]
  RD524.C66 2008
  617.5′22–dc22

          2008027183

"At times our own light goes out and is rekindled by a spark from another person.
Each of us has cause to think with deep gratitude of those who have lighted the flame within us."

Albert Schweitzer

For Nancy and Joe, who provided me with the tools to succeed in life.
For Joe, Lee, Scott, Don, and Linton, who taught me the trade.
And, for Franklyn, who has given meaning to it all.

Joseph E. Losee

For my patients, who teach me about Purpose.
For Alex, Justin, and Jessica, who teach me about Life.
And for LoriAnn, who has taught me about Love.

Richard E. Kirschner

Contents

Contents

Contributors

Ahmed M. Afifi, MD
Fellow
Pediatric Plastic and Craniofacial Surgery
Division of Pediatric Plastic Surgery
Children's Hospital of Pittsburgh
University of Pittsburgh
Pittsburgh, PA
Chapter 33, Post-Palatoplasty Fistulae: Diagnosis, Treatment
    and Prevention

Stephen B. Baker, MD, DDS, FACS
Associate Professor
Section Chief Craniofacial Surgery
Department of Plastic Surgery
Georgetown University Hospital
Washington, DC
Co-Director, Craniofacial Program
Inova Fairfax Hospital for Children
Falls Church, VA
Chapter 60, Cleft Orthognathic Surgery

Joan Barzilai, RN, MSN
Clinical Nurse Specialist
St. Louis Children's Hospital
St. Louis, Missouri
Chapter 10, Nursing Care of the Patient with
    Cleft Lip and Palate

Craig Birgfeld, MD
Assistant Professor
The University of Washington
Seattle, Washington
Chapter 55, Gingivoperiosteoplasty

Charles D. Bluestone, MD
Professor of Otolaryngology
University of Pittsburgh School of Medicine
Pittsburgh, Pennsylvania
Chapter 50, Cleft Palate and Middle Ear Disease

Vincent Boyd, MD
Resident
Baylor College of Medicine
Houston, Texas
Chapter 31, Correction of Secondary Bilateral Cleft Lip
    and Nose Deformities

Lawrence E. Brecht, DDS
Clinical Assistant Professor of Surgery (Maxillofacial
    Prosthetics) and Clinical Associate Professor
    of Prosthodontics
New York University School of Medicine
    Institute of Reconstructive Plastic Surgery and
    New York University College of Dentistry
New York, New York
Chapter 43, Prosthetic Management of Velopharyngeal
    Insufficiency
Chapter 45, Presurgical Orthopedics
Chapter 49, Prosthodontic Management of the Cleft Patient

Mary Breen, MS, RN
Clinical Nurse Specialist
Dell Children's Craniofacial and Reconstructive
    Plastic Surgery Center
Austin, Texas
Chapter 10, Nursing Care of the Patient with
    Cleft Lip and Palate

Terrence W. Bruner, MD, MBA
Senior Resident
Division of Plastic Surgery
Baylor College of Medicine
Houston, Texas
Chapter 31, Correction of Secondary Bilateral Cleft Lip
    and Nose Deformities

Contributors

Gary C. Burget, MD
Clinical Associate Professor
Section of Plastic and Reconstructive Surgery
The University of Chicago
Chicago, Illinois
Chapter 32, Open Rhinoplasty for the Cleft Lip Patient

H. Steve Byrd, MD
Professor
Department of Plastic Surgery
University of Texas Southwestern Medical Center
  at Dallas
Dallas, Texas
Chapter 30, Correction of Secondary Unilateral Cleft
  Lip and Nose Deformities

Michael H. Carstens, MD
Associate Professor of Plastic Surgery
Division of Plastic Surgery
St. Louis University
St. Louis, Missouri
Chapter 15, Developmental Field Reassignment (DFR)
  in Unilateral Cleft Lip: Reconstruction of the
  Premaxilla

James Brett Chafin, MD
Assistant Professor
Department of Pediatrics
Joan C. Edwards School of Medicine
Marshall University
Huntington, West Virginia
Chapter 50, Cleft Palate and Middle Ear Disease

Philip Kuo-Ting Chen, MD
Associate Professor
Chang Gung University, College of Medicine
Taiwan
Chapter 20, Bilateral Cleft Lip and Nose Repair
Chapter 61, Segmental Maxillary Osteotomies

Yu-Ray Chen, MD
Professor
Chang Gung University, College of Medicine
Taiwan
Chapter 61, Segmental Maxillary Osteotomies

Ming-Shiaw Cheng, FRCS (Edin), FCSHK,
  FHKAM (surg)
Associate Consultant
Department of Surgery
Kwong Wah Hospital
Hong Kong SAR, China
Chapter 19, Unilateral Cleft Lip and Nose Repair

Patricia D. Chibbaro, RN, MS, CPNP
Pediatric Nurse Practitioner
Institute of Reconstructive Plastic Surgery,
NYU Langone Medical Center
New York, New York
Chapter 10, Nursing Care of the Patient with Cleft Lip
  and Palate

Franklyn P. Cladis, MD
Assistant Professor of Anesthesiology
Division of Pediatric Anesthesia, Children's Hospital of
  Pittsburgh,
University of Pittsburgh Medical Center
Pittsburgh, Pennsylvania
Chapter 13, Anesthesia for Cleft Patients

Marilyn A. Cohen, BA
Administrative Director and Patient Care
  Coordinator Regional Cleft-Craniofacial Program
Moorestown, New Jersey
Cooper University Hospital
Camden, New Jersey
Chapter 67, Fundamentals of Team Care

Shelley R. Cohen, MA, CCC-SLP
Speech-Language Pathologist
New York University Medical Center
New York, New York
Chapter 43, Prosthetic Management of VPD

Gale Norman Coston, EdD, FASHA
Distinguished Professor Emeritus
Department of Communication Sciences and Disorders
School of Public Health
University of South Carolina
Columbia, South Carolina
Chapter 53, Nasal Airway Considerations

Michael L. Cunningham, MD, PhD
Professor of Pediatrics
Departments of Pediatrics, Oral Biology, Biological
  Structure, and Pediatric Dentistry
    Seattle Children's Hospital, Craniofacial Center
University of Washington
Seattle, Washington
Chapter 11, Pediatric Assessment and Management of
  Children with Cleft Lip and Palate

Court Cutting, MD
Professor
Division of Plastic Surgery
New York University Medical Center
New York, New York
Chapter 18, The Extended Mohler Unilateral Cleft Lip Repair

Diane V. Dado, MD
Professor of Surgery and Pediatrics
Division of Plastic Surgery
Loyola University Medical Center
Maywood, Illinois
Chapter 54, The Functional Cleft Lip Repair,
    Maxillary Orthopedic Segment Alignment, and Primary
    Osteoplasty

Daniela Damian, MD
Visiting Instructor
Division of Pediatric Anesthesia, Children's Hospital
    of Pittsburgh
University of Pittsburgh Medical Center
Pittsburgh, Pennsylvania
Chapter 13, Anesthesia for Cleft Patients

Linda L. D'Antonio, PhD
Professor
Department of Surgery
Loma Linda University
Loma Linda, California
Chapter 35, Communication Disorders
    Associated with Cleft Palate

Tron A. Darvann, MSc, PhD
Research Engineer
3D Craniofacial Image Research Laboratory
Copenhagen University Hospital
University of Copenhagen, Technical University of Denmark
Copenhagen N, Denmark
Chapter 48, Facial Growth and Development in
    Cleft Children

Scott Deacon, BDS, MSc, MFDS.RECPS, MOrth,
FDS(Orth).RCPS
Lead Consultant Orthodontist
South West Cleft Unit
United Kingdom,
Department of Child Dental Health, University of Bristol,
United Kingdom
Chapter 70, Assessment of Orthodontic Outcomes in Patients
with Clefts

Arlen D. Denny, MD, FACS, FAAP
Professor
Department of Plastic Surgery and Neurosurgery
Medical College of Wisconsin
Milwaukee, Wisconsin
Chapter 63, Mandibular Distraction for Infants with
    Pierre Robin Sequence

Deborah A. Driscoll, MD
Professor and Chair
Department of Obstetrics and Gynecology
University of Pennsylvania School of Medicine
Philadelphia, Pennsylvania
Chapter 5, Prenatal and Genetic Counseling

Kusai ElMusa, MD
Private Practice
Aesthetic and Craniofacial Plastic and Reconstructive
    Surgeon
Springfield Gardens, New York
Chapter 30, Correction of Secondary Unilateral Cleft
    Lip and Nose Deformities

Alvaro A. Figueroa, DDS, MS
Co-Director
Rush University Medical Center
Chicago, Illinois
Chapter 58, Treatment Planning for Cleft
    Orthagnathic Surgery
Chapter 62, Maxillary Distraction Osteogenesis

Matthew D. Ford, MS, CCC-SLP
Clinical Instructor of Surgery and Field Instructor
    for Communication Disorders
Department of Communication Disorders
Coordinator, Cleft-Cramiofacial Center
Children's Hospital of Pittsburgh
University of Pittsburgh School of Medicine
Pittsburgh, Pennsylvania
Chapter 33, Post-Palatoplasty Fistulae: Diagnosis, Treatment,
and Prevention

Christopher R. Forrest, MD, MSC, FRCS, FACS
Professor
Division of Plastic Surgery
Department of Surgery
University of Toronto
Toronto, Ontario, Canada
Chapter 41, Posterior Pharyngeal Flaps

Hans Friede, DDS, PhD
Professor Emeritus
Department of Orthodontics
Sahlgrenska Academy at University of Gothenburg, Sweden
Chapter 26, Two Stage Palate Repair

Harold Ira Friedman, MD, PhD
Professor of Surgery
University of South Carolina School of Medicine
Columbia, South Carolina
Chapter 53, Nasal Airway Considerations

Leonard T. Furlow Jr., MD
Clinical Professor
University of Florida College of Medicine
Chapter 23, Double Opposing Z-Plasty Palatal Repair
Chapter 40, Double Opposing Z-Plasty for
    Velpharyngeal Insufficiency

Contributors

Rebecca Ann Gaither, PhD
Pediatric Psychologist, Shriner's Hospitals for Children
Chicago, Illinois
Chapter 65, Psychological and Behavioral Aspects
of Clefting

Judah S. Garfinkle, DMD, MS
Director of Craniofacial Orthodontics
Assistant Professor of Plastic Surgery, Assistant
Professor of Orthodontics
Oregon Health and Science University
Portland, Oregon
Chapter 46, Nasoalveolar Molding and Columella Elongation
in Preparation for the Primary Repair of Unilateral and
Bilateral Cleft Lip and Palate

Edward R. Genecov, DDS
Adjunct Professor
Texas A and M University Health Science Center
Baylor College of Dentistry
Dallas, Texas
Chapter 19, Unilateral Cleft Lip and Nose Repair

Arun K. Gosain, MD
DeWayne Richey Professor and Vice Chair
Dept. of Plastic Surgery Chief
Division of Pediatric Plastic Surgery
Rainbow Babies and Children's Hospital
Case School of Medicine
Cleveland, Ohio
Chapter 22, Submucous Cleft Palate

Lynn Marty Grames, MA, CCC-SLP
Speech-Language Pathologist
St. Louis Children's Hospital
St. Louis, Missouri
Chapter 38, Speech Therapy for the Child with
Cleft Palate

Barry H. Grayson, DDS
Associate Professor of Surgery
Orthodontics
New York University Medical Center
Institute of Reconstructive Plastic Surgery
New York, New York
Chapter 46, Nasoalveolar Molding and Columella
Elongation in Preparation for the Primary Repair of
Unilateral and Bilateral Cleft Lip and Palate

Robert M. Greene, PhD
Professor
Department of Molecular Cellular and Craniofacial Biology
Director
Birth Defects Center
University of Louisville
Louisville, Kentucky
Chapter 73, Perspectives in Orofacial Cleft Research II:
Molecular Mechanisms

Andrew J. Haas, DDS, MS
Professor of Orthodontics
University of Illinois and Orthodontic Arts
Akron, Ohio
Chapter 59, Surgical Assisted Rapid Palatal Expansion

Carrie L. Heike, MD, MS, FAAP
Assistant Professor of Pediatrics
Division of Craniofacial Medicine Seattle Children's Hospital
University of Washington
Seattle, Washington
Chapter 11, Pediatric Assessment and Management of
Children with Cleft Lip and Palate

Nuno V. Hermann, DDS, PhD
Associate Professor
Department of Pediatric Dentistry and Clinical Genetics
School of Dentistry
University of Copenhagen
Copenhagen N, Denmark
Chapter 48, Facial Growth and Development in
Cleft Children

Patrick C. Hettinger, MD
Resident in Plastic Surgery
Medical College of Wisconsin
Milwaukee, Wisconsin
Chapter 22, Submucous Cleft Palate

Virginia A. Hinton, MA, PhD
Associate Professor
Communication Sciences and Disorders
The University of North Carolina at Greensboro
Greensboro, North Carolina
Chapter 37, Instrumental Measures of Velopharyngeal
Function

Nicholas Hogg, MD, DDS
Former Craniofacial Surgery Fellow
Charleston Area Medical Center
London, Ontario, Canada
Chapter 57, Alveolar Transport Distraction Osteogenesis

Larry H. Hollier, Jr., MD, FACS
Associate Professor, Residency Program Director
Division of Plastic Surgery
Baylor College of Medicine
Houston, Texas
Chapter 31, Correction of Secondary Bilateral Cleft Lip
and Nose Deformities

Richard Hopper, MD, MS, FRCSC, FACS
Chief, Pediatric Plastic Surgery, Seattle Children's Hospital
Associate Professor
The University of Washington
Seattle, Washington
Chapter 55, Gingivoperiosteoplasty

Bruce B. Horswell, MD, DDS, MS, FACS
Associate Clinical Professor of Surgery
Department of Surgery
West Virginia University
Charleston, West Virginia
Chapter 57, Alveolar Transport Distraction Osteogenesis

Martin H. S. Huang, MBBS, M.Med. Surg.,
    FRCS, FAMS
Private Practice, Consultant Plastic Surgeon
The Cosmetic Surgery Clinic
Singapore
Chapter 14, Anatomy of Cleft Lip and Palate

Donald V. Huebener, DDS, MS, MAEd
Professor, Plastic and Reconstructive Surgery
Department of Surgery
School of Medicine
Washington University
St. Louis, Missouri
Chapter 44, Pediatric Dentistry

Oksana Jackson, MD
Attending Surgeon
The Children's Hospital of Philadelphia
Assistant Professor
Division of Plastic Surgery
University of Pennsylvania School of Medicine
Philadelphia, Pennsylvania
Chapter 12, History of Cleft Surgery

Shao Jiang, MD
Assistant Professor of Surgery
Division of Pediatric Plastic Surgery
Children's Hospital of Pittsburgh
University of Pittsburgh Medical Center
Pittsburgh, Pennsylvania
Chapter 16, Lip Adhesion

Kenneth Lyons Jones, MD
Professor of Pediatrics
University of California at San Diego
La Jolla, California
Chapter 8, Syndromes of Orofacial Clefting

Marilyn C. Jones, MD
Professor of Pediatrics
University of California at San Diego
San Diego, California
Chapter 8, Syndromes of Orofacial Clefting

Kathleen A. Kapp-Simon, PhD
Pediatric Psychologist, Cleft-Craniofacial Clinic, Shriner's
    Hospitals for Children
Associate Professor
Department of Surgery
Feinberg School of Medicine
Northwestern University
Chicago, Illinois
Chapter 65, Psychological and Behavioral Aspects
    of Clefting

Alison E. Kaye, MD
Fellow, Pediatric Plastic Surgery
The Children's Hospital of Philadelphia
Philadelphia, Pennsylvania
Chapter 52, Pierre Robin Sequence

Richard E. Kirschner, MD, FAAP, FACS
Mary Downs Chair in Craniofacial Treatment and Research
Director, Cleft Lip and Palate Program
The Children's Hospital of Philadelphia
University of Pennsylvania
Philadelphia, Pennsylvania
Chapter 16, Lip Adhesion
Chapter 24, The Children's Hospital Modification of the
    Furlow Double-Opposing Z-Palatoplasty
Chapter 52, Pierre Robin Sequence

Paula G. Klaiman, MCl.Sc, CAGS
Instructor
Faculty of Medicine
University of Toronto
Toronto, Ontario, Canada
Chapter 41, Posterior Pharyngeal Flaps

Sven Kreiborg, DDS, PhD, DrOdont
Professor
Department of Pediatric Dentistry and Clinical Genetics
School of Dentistry
University of Copenhagen
Copenhagen, Denmark
Chapter 48, Facial Growth and Development in
    Cleft Children

David P. Kuehn, PhD
Professor
Department of Speech and Hearing Science
University of Illinois at Urbana-Champaign
Champaign, Illinois
Chapter 34, Anatomy and Physiology of the Velopharynx

Contributors

Ann W. Kummer, PhD, CCC-SLP, ASHA-F
Senior Director, Division of Speech Pathology
Cincinnati Children's Hospital Medical Center
Professor of Clinical Pediatrics
University of Cincinnati Medical Center
Cincinnati, Ohio
Chapter 36, Assessment of Velopharyngeal Function

Don LaRossa, MD
Professor of Surgery Emeritus
Division of Plastic Surgery
University of Pennsylvania School of Medicine
Philadelphia, Pennsylvania
Chapter 24, The Children's Hospital Modification of the
   Furlow Double-Opposing Z-Palatoplasty

Seng-Teik Lee, MBBS, FRCS, FAMS
Emeritus Consultant, Senior Consultant
Department of Plastic, Reconstructive and Aesthetic
   Surgery
Singapore General Hospital
Singapore
Chapter 14, Anatomy of Cleft Lip and Palate

Shu-Jin Lee, MD
National University of Singapore
Singapore
Chapter 14, Anatomy of Cleft Lip and Palate

James A. Lehman, Jr., MD
Professor of Plastic Surgery
Northeast Ohio Universities College of Medicine
Akron, Ohio
Chapter 59, Surgically Assisted Rapid Palatal
   Expansion

Jean-Marc Levaillant, MD
Department of Gynecology and Obstetrics
Centre Hospitalier Antoine-Beclere
Clamart, France
Chapter 4, Fetal Diagnosis

Wai-Yee Li, MB, ChB, MRCS
Resident
Department of Surgery
Division of Plastic and Reconstructive Surgery
University of Southern California
Los Angeles, California
Chapter 29, Complications of Cleft Lip and Palate Surgery

Andrew C. Lidral, DDS, PhD
Associate Professor
Department of Orthodontics
University of Iowa
Iowa City, Iowa
Chapter 7, Genetics of Nonsyndromic Clefting II:
   Results from Gene Mapping Studies

Eric J.W. Liou, DDS, MS
Associate Professor
Graduate School of Craniofacial Medicine
Chang Gung University
Taipei, Taiwan
Chapter 61, Segmental Maxillary Osteotomies

Ross E. Long, Jr., DMD, MS, PhD
Director
Lancaster Cleft Palate Clinic
Lancaster, Pennsylvania
Chapter 70, Assessment of Orthodontic Outcomes
   in Patients with Clefts

Joseph E. Losee, MD, FACS, FAAP
Chief, Pediatric Plastic Surgery
Director, Cleft-Craniofacial Center
Division of Pediatric Plastic Surgery
Children's Hospital of Pittsburgh
Pittsburgh, Pennsylvania
Chapter 16, Lip Adhesion
Chapter 28, Lateral Facial Clefts of Macrostomia
Chapter 33, Post-Palatoplasty Fistulae: Diagnosis, Treatment,
   and Prevention

David W. Low, MD
Attending Surgeon
The Children's Hospital of Philadelphia
Associate Professor
Division of Plastic Surgery
University of Pennsylvania
Chapter 24, The Children's Hospital Modification of the
   Furlow Double-Opposing Z-Palatoplasty

William P. Magee, Jr., DDS, MD, FACS
Professor of Plastic Surgery
University of Southern California
Associate Professor of Plastic Surgery
Eastern Virginia Medical School
Co-Founder & CEO
Operation Smile
President, Magee-Rosenblum Plastic Surgery
Director, Craniofacial Surgery
Children's Hospital of the King's Daughters
Norfolk, Virginia
Chapter 68, International Missions-Cleft Care

Mary L. Marazita, PhD, FACMG
Associate Dean, Research; Chair and Professor, Oral Biology;
   Professor, Human Genetics; Professor, Psychiatry
University of Pittsburgh
Pittsburgh, Pennsylvania
Chapter 6, Genetics of Nonsyndromic Clefting I:
   Family Patterns and Methods of Analysis
Chapter 7, Genetics of Nonsyndromic Clefting II:
   Results from Gene Mapping Studies

Alexander C. Marchac, MD
Medical Doctor
University Paris V
Paris, France
Chapter 19, Unilateral Cleft Lip and Nose Repair

Jeffrey Lowell Marsh, MD
Clinical Professor of Plastic Surgery
St. Louis University School of Medicine
St. Louis, Missouri
Chapter 42, Sphincter Pharyngoplasty

W. Jason Martin, MD
Rush University Medical Center
Chicago, Illiniois
Chapter 62, Maxillary Distraction Osteogenesis

Aaron Corde Mason, MD
Assistant Professor of Pediatrics
University of Texas Health Science Center
San Antonio, Texas
Chapter 41, Posterior Pharyngeal Flaps

Martha S. Matthews, MD
Associate Professor of Surgery
UMDNJ/Robert Wood Johnson Medical School
Camden, New Jersey
Chapter 5, Prenatal and Genetic Counseling

Mohammad Mazaheri, MMD, DDS, MSc
Lancaster Cleft Palate Clinic, Director of Medical and
    Dental Services
Hershey Medical Center, Professor of Surgery
Lancaster, Pennsylvania
Chapter 43, 45, 49, Prosthetic Management of
    Velopharyngeal Insufficiency, Presurgical Orthopedics,
    Prosthodontic Management of the Cleft Patient

Donna M. McDonald-McGinn, MS, CGC
Associate Director, Clinical Genetics Center
Program Director, The "22Q and You" Center
The Children's Hospital of Pittsburgh
University of Pennsylvania School of Medicine
Philadelphia, Pennsylvania
Chapter 5, Prenatal and Genetic Counseling
Chapter 9, The 22Q11.2 Deletion Syndrome

Nathan Menon, MD
Resident
Department of Plastic Surgery
Georgetown University Hospital,
Washington, DC
Chapter 60, Cleft Orthognathic Surgery

Ana Maria Mercado, DMD, MS, PhD
Clinical Assistant Professor
The Ohio State University
Columbus, Ohio
Chapter 47, Orthodontic Principles in the Management of
    Orofacial Clefts

Joseph Michienzi DMD, MD
Former Craniofacial Fellow of the International Institute of
Craniofacial and Cleft Surgery
Staff, Miami Children's Hospital and Private Practice
Miami, Florida
Chapter 19, Unilateral Cleft Lip and Nose Repair

Laura E. Mitchell, PhD
Associate Professor
Institute of Biosciences and Technology
Texas A&M University, Health Science Center
Houston, Texas
Chapter 3, Epidemiology of Cleft Lip and Palate

Mark P. Mooney, PhD
Professor
Departments of Oral Biology, Anthropology, Surgery-Plastic
    and Reconstructive Surgery and Orthodontics
University of Pittsburgh
Pittsburgh, Pennsylvania
Chapter 2, Classification of Orofacial Clefts

Lina Maria Moreno Uribe, DDS, PhD
Assistant Professor
Department of Orthodontics
College of Dentistry
University of Iowa
Iowa City, Iowa
Chapter 7, Genetics of Nonsyndromic Clefting II:
    Results from Gene Mapping Studies

John B. Mulliken, MD, FACS
Professor of Surgery Children's Hospital of Boston,
    Department of Plastic Surgery
Harvard Medical School
Boston, Massachusetts
Chapter 17, The Microform Cleft Lip
Chapter 21, Mulliken Bilateral Cleft Nasolabial Repair

Pauline Anne Nelson, BA Mons.
University of Manchester, UK, School of Dentistry
Manchester, England
Chapter 69, Clinical Outcomes Research and Evidence
    Based Practice

M. Samuel Noordhoff, MD, FACS
Emeritus Professor of Surgery
Chang Gung University, College of Medicine
Naples, Florida
Chapter 20, Bilateral Cleft Lip and Nose Repair

Contributors

Peg Nopoulos, MD
Professor of Psychiatry, Pediatrics and Neuroscience
University of Iowa, Carver College of Medicine
Iowa City, Iowa
Chapter 64, Neuropsychological and Neuroimaging
    Aspects of Clefting

Fernando Ortiz-Monasterio, MD
Professor Emeritus
Universidad National Autonoma de Mexico
Mexico D.F.
Chapter 27, Rare Craniofacial Clefts

Robert J. Paresi, Jr., MD, MPH
Plastic Surgery Fellow
Department of Plastic and Reconstructive Surgery
Rush University Medical Center
Chicago, Illinois
Chapter 62, Maxillary Distraction Osteogenesis

Jamie L. Perry, PhD
Assistant Professor
Illinois State University
Normal, Illinois
Chapter 34, Anatomy and Physiology of the Velopharynx

Sally J. Peterson-Falzone, PhD
Clinical Professor Emeritus
University of California-San Francisco
San Francisco, California
Chapter 71, Assessment of Speech Outcomes in
    Cleft Palate Surgery

M. Michele Pisano, PhD
Professor
Department of Molecular, Cellular and Craniofacial Biology
    and Birth Defects Center
University of Louisville
School of Dentistry
Louisville, Kentucky
Chapter 73, Perspectives in Orofacial Cleft Research II:
    Molecular Mechanisms

John W. Polley, MD
Professor and Chairman
Rush University Medical Center
Chicago, Illinois
Chapter 58, Treatment Planning for Cleft
    Orthagnathic Surgery
Chapter 62, Maxillary Distraction Osteogenesis

Gretchen Probst, MAT
Coordinator, Diagnostic Audiology Services
Children's Hospital of Pittsburgh
Pittsburgh, Pennsylvania
Chapter 51, Otologic, Audiologic, and Airway
    Assessment and Management

Barry L. Ramsey, BS
Research Associate
University of North Carolina at Chapel Hill
Chapel Hill, North Carolina
Chapter 66, Social, Cultural, and Ethical Issues in
    Cleft Care

Peter Randall, MD
Emeritus Professor of Plastic Surgery
The Children's Hospital of Philadelphia
The University of Pennsylvania
Philadelphia, Pennsylvania
Chapter 12, History of Cleft Surgery

John F. Reinisch, MD, FACS
Chief
Division of Plastic Surgery
Children's Hospital Los Angeles, Keck School of Medicine
University of Southern California
Los Angeles, California
Chapter 29, Complications of Cleft Lip and Palate Surgery

Lynn C. Richman, PhD
Professor and Director
Division of Pediatric Psychology
Children's Hospital, University of Iowa
Iowa City, Iowa
Chapter 64, Neuropsychological and Neuroimaging
    Aspects of Clefting

Sheldon W. Rosenstein, DDS, MSD
Clinical Professor, Orthodontics
Center for Advanced Dental Education
Graduate Department of Orthodontics
St. Louis University
Chicago, Illinois
Chapter 54, The Functional Cleft Lip Repair, Maxillary
    Orthopedic Segment Alignment, and Primary Osteoplasty

Daniel Rotten, MD
Chairman
Department of Gynecology and Obstetrics
Centre Hospitalier Delafontaine
Saint-Denis, France
Chapter 4, Fetal Diagnosis

Ramon L. Ruiz, DDS, MD
University of North Carolina
Chapel Hill, North Carolina
Chapter 56, Bone Graft Construction of the
    Cleft Maxilla and Palate

Diane L. Sabo, PhD
Associate Professor
Department of Communication Science and
    Disorders
School of Health and Rehabilitation Sciences,
    University of Pittsburgh
Pittsburgh, Pennsylvania
Chapter 51, Otologic, Audiologic, and Airway
    Assessment and Management

Kenneth E. Salyer, MD
Founder and Chairman of World Craniofacial
    Foundation
Dallas, Texas
Chapter 19, Unilateral Cleft Lip and Nose
    Repair

Nancy J. Scherer, PhD
Professor, Communicative Disorders
East Tennessee State University
Johnston City, Tennessee
Chapter 35, Communication Disorders Associated
    with Cleft Palate

Randy Sherman, MD F.A.C.S.
The Audrey Skirball Kenis
Professor & Chair
Division of Plastic Surgery
Keck School of Medicine
University of Southern California
Los Angeles, California
Chapter 68, International Missions-Cleft Care

Gunvor Semb, DDS, Dr. Odont.
Senior Lecturer, Adjunct Professor
University of Manchester, UK
University of Oslo, Norway
Manchester, England
Chapter 69, Strategies for Improving Cleft Care

William Shaw, FDS, PhD, Dr. Odont., MsCd
Professor
University of Manchester
Manchester, England
Chapter 69, Strategies for Improving Cleft Care

Darren M. Smith, MD
Resident
Division of Plastic Surgery
University of Pittsburgh
Pittsburgh, Pennsylvania
Chapter 33, Surgical Management of Palatal
    Fistulae

Brian C. Sommerlad, MB BS, FRCSEng, FRCSEd.(Hon)
Consultant Plastic Surgeon
Great Ormond Street Hospital for Children, London
St. Andrew's Centre for Plastic Surgery, Broomfield Hospital,
    Chelmsford, United Kingdom
Chapter 25, Cleft Palate Repair

Geoffrey H. Sperber, BDS, MS, PhD, FICD, Dr. Med.
    Dent (h.c), Hon FRSSAf
Professor Emeritus
University of Alberta, Edmonton
Edmonton, Alberta
Chapter 1, Embryology of Orofacial Clefting

Steven M. Sperber, MS, PhD
Department of Health and Human Services
Laboratory of Molecular Genetics
National Institute of Child Health and Human
    Development
Bethesda, Maryland
Chapter 1, Embryology of Orofacial Clefting

Samuel Stal, MD, FACS
Professor
Division Plastic Surgery
Baylor College of Medicine
Houston, Texas
Chapter 31, Correction of Secondary Bilateral Cleft Lip
    and Nose Deformities

Ronald P. Strauss, DMD, PhD
Dental Friends Distinguished Professor and Chair,
    Department of Dental Ecology, School of Dentistry
Professor, Department of Social Medicine,
    School of Medicine
University of North Carolina at Chapel Hill
Chapel Hill, North Carolina
Chapter 66, Social, Cultural, and Ethical Issues in
    Cleft Care

Peter J. Taub, MD, FACS, FAAP
Associate Professor, Surgery and Pediatrics
Mount Sinai Medical Center, Kravis Children's Hospital
New York, New York
Chapter 28, Lateral Facial Clefts of Macrostomia

Jesse A. Taylor, MD
Assistant Professor of Plastic and Reconstructive Surgery
Cincinnati Children's Hospital Medical Center
Cincinnati, Ohio
Chapter 27, Rare Craniofacial Clefts

Contributors

Paul S. Tiwana, DDS, MD, MS
Assistant Professor, Oral and Maxillofacial Surgery
School of Dentistry, The University of Louisville
Louisville, Kentucky
Chapter 56, Bone Graft Construction of the Cleft
    Maxilla and Palate

Timothy A. Turvey, DDS
Professor and Chairman
Department Oral and Maxillofacial Surgery
University of North Carolina
Chapel Hill, North Carolina
Chapter 56, Bone Graft Construction of the Cleft
    Maxilla and Palate

Mark M. Urata, MD, DDS
Assistant Professor of Plastic Surgery, Division of Plastic
    and Maxillofacial Surgery
Children's Hospital Los Angeles
Keck School of Medicine, University of Southern
    California
University of Southern California School of Dentistry
Los Angeles, California
Chapter 29, Complications of Cleft Lip and Palate
    Surgery

Michael VanLue, PhD
Associate Professor
Department of Rehabilitation Science
Medical University of South Carolina
Charleston, South Carolina
Chapter 53, Nasal Airway Considerations

Lisa Vecchione, DMD, MDS
Assistant Clinical Professor of Surgery Director, Craniofacial
    Orthodontics
Division of Pediatric Plastic Surgery
Children's Hospital of Pittsburgh
University of Pittsburgh School of Medicine
Pittsburgh, Pennsylvania
Chapter 28, Lateral Facial Clefts of Macrostomia
Chapter 33, Post-Palatoplasty Fistulae: Diagnosis, Treatment,
and Prevention

Katherine Winter Leta Vig, BDS, MS, D. Orth.,
    FDS, RCS
Professor Emeritus, Former Head of Orthodontics
The Ohio State University, College of Dentistry
Columbus, Ohio
Chapter 47, Orthodontic Principles in the Management
    of Orofacial Clefts

Jeffrey Weinzweig, MD, FACS
Chairman
Department of Plastic Surgery
Lahey Clinic Medical Center
Burlington, Massachusetts, Director, Craniofacial Anomalies
    Program, Floating Hospital for Children, Tufts Medical
    Center, Boston, Massachusetts
Chapter 72, Perspectives in Orofacial Cleft Research I:
    Animal Models

Peter D. Witt, MD
Clinical Associate Professor
UCSF Fresno
Children's Hospital of Central California
Madera, California
Chapter 39, Velopharyngeal Dysfunction:
    A Conceptual Approach

Arjang Yazdani, MD, FRCS
Assistant Professor
Division of Plastic Surgery
The University of Western Ontario
Ontario, Canada
Chapter 30, Correction of Secondary Unilateral Cleft Lip
    and Nose Deformity

Elaine H. Zackai, MD
Professor
Department of Pediatrics, Obstetrics and Gynecology
Genetics Director
Clinical Genetics Center
The Children's Hospital of Philadelphia
University of Pennsylvania School of Medicine
Philadelphia, Pennsylvania
Chapter 9, The 22Q11.2 Deletion Syndrome

Joshua S. Zukerman, BA
Student
Graduate of the University of North Carolina at Chapel Hill
Chapel Hill, North Carolina
Chapter 66, Social, Cultural, and Ethical Issues in
    Cleft Care

Foreword

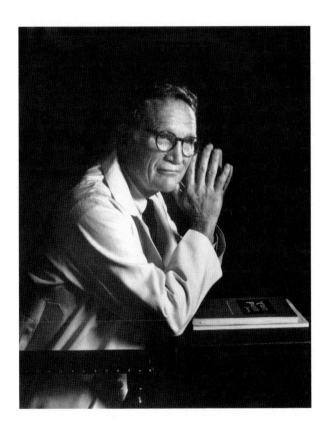

A multi-authored text not only brings authorities in many areas together, but also allows for the expression of differences of opinion. Such a publication has occurred in the field of cleft lip and palate only occasionally, but when it has been achieved, it usually has been very well received.

The selection of authors for this text by Dr. Joseph E. Losee and Dr. Richard E. Kirschner has been outstanding. They present a rare array of experience and talent and with an interesting international touch. Further, the willingness of so many exceptional authors to put together these chapters also shows their high regard for the two editors.

I have found the references selected by each author to be very interesting, noting those writings that have influenced the development of their own ideas.

The text should provide students at various levels and in many fields a great many fresh ideas and hopefully some inspiration for further improvement in the way they treat this exceptional group of patients. The general field of cleft lip and palate care can take pride in having established and developed the "team approach" to the overall care of these complicated problems. If we become more international in our interchange of plans and ideas, the standardization of evaluations, the establishment of longitudinal records and the greater use of prospective randomized trials of new techniques, we should be able to do even better.

We should also say a word about the character of this rare group of patients. From the time of their birth, they have faced hardships. Many parents have gone through pregnancy not expecting their newborn "bundle of joy" to have a cleft. More often than not, though they have most likely heard of cleft lip or palate and may have even known someone with these anomalies, few have ever seen an infant with an unrepaired cleft. After months of expectation, this can be very shocking. Ultrasonography, in many cases, has allowed for the accurate in utero diagnosis, which does help to prepare the way, but the real thing is still disrupting and adds potential difficulty to maternal bonding. Add to this the problems of infant suckling, in some cases difficulty in breathing, and in syndromic infants other clinical difficulties. One can see that many of these children have a tough time from the very beginning.

With the added trials of surgery in infancy, numerous trips to the hospital, facial incisions, and difficulty with hearing, the troubles are seen to go on and on. School age can be particularly difficult with teasing, taunting, and lack of acceptance. Yet after all of this, we usually find an individual who has learned the valuable ability to rise above the problem. These children have learned that they can face adversity and come through in spite of it. They have learned how to "take it," to be goal oriented, to "stick with it", and usually to emerge with a smile on their face. These are valuable character traits that are hard to learn from a textbook. Fortunately, all the fields involved in cleft care are improving and able to deliver a better result, while learning more about the character of the patient.

With encouragement from their parents and teachers, *and* from us, these children should do well. Part of our task is to see that they do well in all parameters. I feel that it has been a true privilege to have been associated with so many of these exceptional young people, their parents, and the clinicians devoted to their care.

Peter Randall, MD, FACS
The Children's Hospital of Philadelphia,
Philadelphia, Pennsylvania

Foreword

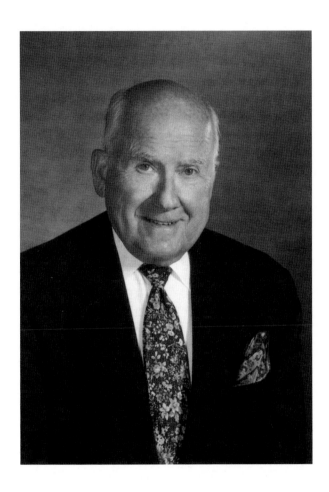

Since experience may not always be available in the hands of the neophyte cleft surgeon, it is essential that he or she have a reference point that covers all of the bases. Without wishing to sound sacrilegious, what I would refer to would be a scientific "bible." Giving birth to such a publication is a grand and noble effort made by this brave and intrepid duo of Editors. Both just on the sunny side of forty, they have already made their mark in the scientific world with this 73-chapter publication with greater than 120 authors from many parts of the world. The Editors have cast their net far and wide with some eight countries represented in the index of authors. The Editors have been perceptive enough to include authors who perhaps one might refer to allegorically as writing the Old Testament - such as the revered cleft notables Mazaheri, Randall, Furlow, Salyer, and Lehman. Anyone attempting to create a surgical, clinical, and psychological publication, such as this, has to make sure they "cover all the bases." In my opinion, after perusing the table of contents, the Editors have done exactly that.

There is an old and perhaps clichéd quotation from Don Quixote, "the proof of the pudding is in the eating." In my experience, when it comes to cleft palate treatment, whether this be surgical or prosthetic, lengthening or pharyngoplasty, the proof is found in the single word: *speech!* - non-nasal speech, reproducible outside the speech therapist's office. In my opinion, if pharyngeal competence is achieved, the speech therapist's game-plan can concentrate on articulation. All of this is assuming that the cleft patients' hearing has been adequately attained. It is a rare person, other than our friends in pediatric dentistry and otolaryngology, who actually look into people's mouths as intently as do the people who care for clefts.

I congratulate these brilliant young pediatric plastic and craniofacial surgeons. It is fascinating that the original foundation of the American Cleft Palate Association was by a group of prosthodontists in 1943, in mid-Pennsylvania, organizing the American Academy for Cleft Palate Rehabilitation, for forerunner of the current American Cleft Palate-Craniofacial Association. In 1969, I was honored to be the President of this formidable association, and in Houston, Texas we hosted the first International Congress with Professor Duane

While an old Pennsylvania Dutch expression asserts, "we grow too soon old and too late smart," some long forgotten sage wrote along the same line, "experience comes with age, which is the time it does you the least good." In almost all areas of endeavor, experience can, and frequently does, compensate for talent, book knowledge, or specialized training-whether it be for football lettermen, a 747 pilot, a gourmet chef, or even a plastic surgeon.

Spriestersbach from Iowa City as the first President and Chair of the International Cleft Group. This International Organization, as other international societies, now meets regularly, and thus, actually shares their special knowledge in many, many ways. This tradition of interdisciplinary scholarship is exemplified by this text, whose author list contains those who have remained active contributors to the American Cleft Palate-Craniofacial Association.

Ross H. Musgrave, MD
University of Pittsburgh School of Medicine,
Pittsburgh, Pennsylvania

Preface

Fill your paper with the breathings of your heart.
William Wordsworth

Why write yet another volume dedicated to the care of children with orofacial clefts? The library shelves already groan wearily under the burden of so many books on cleft surgery, orthodontics, and speech. Why, then, clutter the stacks with yet another tome?

Surely, it is not for the sake of vainglory, for, with rare exception, history rightfully ensures the obscurity of most of its medical writers. One need only select a dusty first edition at random from the library shelves to appreciate this truth. A writer should know his place. No, a book must serve a greater purpose. In order to justify its place, a book must fill a small gap in the world.

We conceived *Comprehensive Cleft Care* in the operating room one day as we contemplated such a gap. Although similar texts had already been penned, there remained no single contemporary and truly comprehensive multidisciplinary reference for the cleft care provider. We acknowledge those editors and writers who have come before us, for each has in some way filled a separate gap. We now hope that this volume will complement the outstanding works of our predecessors.

Our intention is that this text will be used as a resource by cleft care professionals both to enhance their knowledge in their respective disciplines and to gain a useful understanding of related fields. In the pages that follow, the reader will find a comprehensive discourse on topics in cleft embryology and genetics, nursing and primary care, surgical management, speech, dentistry and orthodontics, neuropsychosocial issues, and research. We expect that the critical reader will find some unintended oversights, and for this we offer our apologies and an earnest promise to correct any such omissions in subsequent editions. Inevitably, the reader will discover some thematic overlap between the book's chapters, an intended occurrence that will provide some insight into variations in patient care that may simply represent differences in style or belief and that help to make this text a "living" document. As is

often the case in the field of cleft care, these differences reflect the ongoing need for rigorous scientific inquiry to shed light on the best evidence-based practice, ideally balanced against the associated burden of care, for the children that we care for.

As must be the care of our patients, the production of this volume is necessarily the result of an extraordinary team effort, its whole being something much more than simply the sum of its parts. Each may have his own beliefs regarding the relative importance or contribution of any given discipline to the field, but such reductionism has little place in the care of the cleft-affected child. Take away the function of just one major organ system, no matter how small, and life as we know it cannot be sustained; the function of each system is critically dependent upon that of the others, and each is essential to the essence of the whole. And so it is for cleft care.

We gratefully acknowledge the contributions of the many authors of this work. We are genuinely humbled by their expertise and by their dedication both to this project and to the greater field of cleft care. This book is truly a collective effort . . . it is at once the product of each author's work and of all of the authors' work. Their contributions to cleft care have enhanced the lives of so many over so many years. It is now our wish that this collaboration will benefit many more for many years to come.

Why write another book on cleft care? The answer is simple: it is precisely to serve those whose lives will be bettered by its existence.

And indeed, this book belongs to them.

Joseph E. Losee
Richard E. Kirschner

Acknowledgments

Special thanks to Ms. Robin Rice for all of her tireless organizational efforts and administrative talents.

Embryology, Classification, Epidemiology, and Genetics

Embryology of Orofacial Clefting

Geoffrey H. Sperber, BDS, MS, PhD, FICD, Dr. Med Dent (h.c) • Steven M. Sperber, MSc, PhD

■ INTRODUCTION

Nature is nowhere more accustomed openly to display her secret mysteries than in cases where she shows traces of her working apart from the beaten path.

Harvey, 1657[1]

"The basis for most congenital malformations must be found, I think, in hampered development, that is, in arrest at different periods of development. In order to provide evidence for this, it was necessary to complement the pictures of malformations with illustrations of the normal development of the embryo" (Fig. 1–1).[2]

Thus did Vrolik, more than 150 years ago, lay the foundation for understanding the causes of orofacial clefts. The challenge for modern molecular medicine is to translate the clinically observed clefting defects, the phenotype, back through the intricate developmental phenomena that created them, to the coding genotype. The identification of the genetic predisposition to clefts and the environmental factors that determine and alter the varying threshold of normal versus dysmorphic development are among the central challenges for developmental biologists to decipher. Variations of gene expression (epigenetics) and variable environments may cause differing expressions of genetic traits (polyphenisms), among which are clefting syndromes. The prenatal diagnostic capabilities of chorionic villus sampling, amniocentesis, fetoscopy, and ultrasonography have vaulted gestational developmental phenomena into the field of concern to the clinician.[3] The maldeveloped intrauterine fetus has now become a potential patient[4] (Fig. 1–2).

The potential for clefting will ideally be diminished from its initial pathogenetic determination by prevention

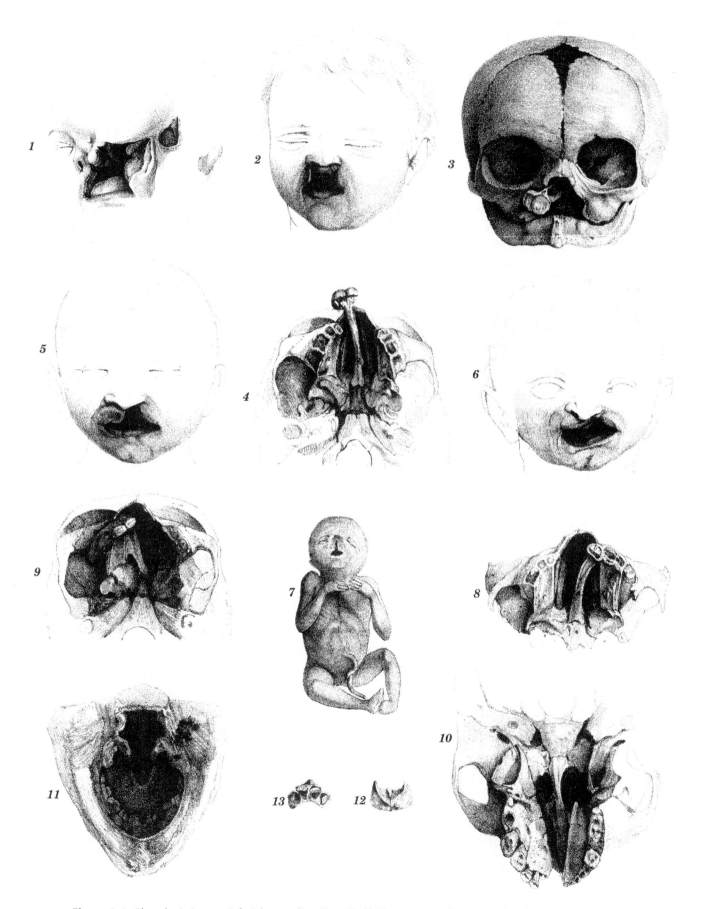

Figure 1–1. Plate depicting craniofacial anomalies. (*From Vrolik: The Human Embryo, Considered in its Normal and Ab-normal Development. By kind permission of Greenwood Genetic Center.*)

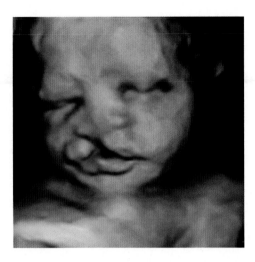

Figure 1–2. 3-dimensional sonographic image of an intrauterine fetus with unilateral cleft. (*Courtesy of Dr. Eileen Wang, University of Pennsylvania*)

rather than by post hoc treatment. Preimplantation genetic diagnosis (PGD) is becoming an adjunctive procedure to in vitro fertilization (IVF) to prevent genetically defective embryos being implanted. The basics of biology and molecular medicine will be translated from the laboratory bench to the bedside in the clinical practice of the future.

GENETICS

The mélange of molecular mechanisms involved in the cascading events of embryogenesis are predicated by the expression patterns of specific genes contained in the human genome, constrained by impacting environmental factors. Gene expression patterns are revealing regions of the emerging embryo that have been previously observed histologically and anatomically, but not heretofore realized as genetically distinct entities during development. Herein is the marriage of genetics with developmental biology becoming of potential clinical significance.

Current investigations are delineating a complete molecular embryology of development. Specific defects in molecular pathways and networks may provide insights into the etiology of clefting. While embryologists focus on the mechanisms of malformation, deformation, disruption, and dysplasia, clinicians focus on the etiology, diagnosis, treatment, prognosis, and prevention of clefting. The combination of basic and clinical sciences should provide the ideal goal of comprehensive cleft care.

In establishing etiology, it is useful to have available the gene expression patterns and flow of biochemical actions underlying morphologic events. Understanding the local regulation of cellular behaviors and misregulation of any step in these processes provides insights into clefting consequences. Recognition of the molecular and tissue elements responsible for normal labiopalatogenesis will allow prognostication of clefting defects in their deficiencies. The therapeutic

application of growth factors has the potential for biomimetic preventive and healing regimens.

Of the estimated 25,000 protein-coding[5] genes in the human genome, some 17,000 genes have been identified as contributing to craniofacial development. Databases of human genes are available containing information on more than 21,000 genes pooled from six collections of human complementary DNAs.[6] The complexity of contributions of the hundreds of genes to facial formation may now be elucidated by identifying each gene's individual expression pattern for each stage of development. The ever-constant identification of gene expression profiles of embryonic craniofacial and oral structures has led to the development of a consortium named COGENE (Craniofacial and Oral Gene Expression NEtwork) that can be accessed online at[7]: http://hg.wustl.edu/COGENE/. Therein is contained a list of all identified genes, that include growth factors, and signals involved in the expression profiles of structures between 4 and 8.5 weeks of human development. It is in the mutation or silencing of genes or the misappropriation of growth factors and signals that the source of some developmental defects is revealed. The intricacies of RNA editing, complex regulatory networks, crisscrossing molecular pathways, together with overlapping and redundancies of gene expression patterns make unraveling the skein of individual influences particularly difficult.

Some of the more significant genes implicated in craniofacial development are listed in Table 1–1. Ascribing specific functions to each of these genes is still a daunting challenge, but it is the realization of the biology encoded within each gene that will provide comprehension of developmental phenomena and their aberrations. Elucidation of gene expression patterns during development by serial analysis of gene expression (SAGE) libraries and microarray identification of regional targets has revealed 6927 genes expressed in the embryonic first pharyngeal arch during the fourth and fifth weeks postconception.[8] Human genetics can lead to insights of phenotypic synthesis, and provide understanding of the relationships of components of molecular circuitry that will improve the ability of genotypic information to predict the phenotype of complex clefting traits.

The genes associated with orofacial clefting that have been identified are those for nonsyndromic cleft lip/palate MSX1, which is located on chromosome 4p16.1 (OMIM: 142983), and TBX22, which is located on chromosome Xq12-q21 (OMIM: 300307). Cleft palate genes have been located on chromosome 14 on its short arm, p14-p16 and on its long arm, q31-q35. A genetic locus for cleft lip (IRF6) has been identified on chromosome 1q32-q41.[9]

The exact functions of relatively few genes have been established. Before a link between a gene and its expressed phenotype is recognized, there must be extensive characterization of the gene's products. The topographical areas and timing of gene expression need to be known for specific regions of orofacial development. Examining the expression of single genes can be complicated by genetic heterogeneity or by the fact that single gene effects are often too subtle to detect

Table 1–1.

Genes Implicated in Human Craniofacial Development*

Gene		Gene ID	Chromosome	Location
BARX1	Bar-like homeobox	56033	9	9q12
BMP4	Bone morphogenetic protein 4	652	14	14q22–q23
CD44	CD44 molecule	960	11	11p13
CFDP1	Craniofacial development protein	10428	16	16q22.2–q22.3
CHUK	Conserved helix-loop-helix ubiquitous kinase	1147	10	10q24–q25
DLX1	Distal-less homeobox 1	1745	2	2q32
DLX2	Distal-less homeobox 2	1746	2	2q32
DLX4	Distal-less homeobox 4	1748	17	17q21.33
DLX6	Distal-less homeobox 6	1750	7	7q22
FGF8	Fibroblast growth factor 8	2253	10	10q24
FGF10	Fibroblast growth factor receptor 10	2255	5	5p13–p12
FGFR2	Fibroblast growth factor receptor 2	2263	10	10q26
FGFR4	Fibroblast growth factor receptor 4	2264	5	5q35.1-qter
GSC	Goosecoid	145258	14	14q32.1
GSC2	Goosecoid 2	2928	22	22q11.21
GTF2IRD1	GTF2I repeat domain containing 1	9569	7	7q11.23
JAG2	Jagged2	3714	14	14q32
HOXA1	Homeobox A1	3198	7	7p15.3
IRF6	Interferon Regulatory Factor 6	3664	1	1q32.3–q41
LHX6	Lim homeobox protein 6	26468	9	9q33.2
MEOX2	Mesenchyme homeobox 2	4223	7	7p22.1–p21.3
MSX1	Muscle segment homeobox 1	4487	4	4p16.1
MSX2	Muscle segment homeobox 2	4488	5	5q34–q35
NHS	Nance-Horan syndrome	4810	X	Xp22.13
OTX1	Orthodenticle homeobox 1	5013	2	2p13
OTX2	Orthodenticle homeobox 2	5015	14	14q21–q22
PAX7	Paired box gene 7	5081	1	1p36.2–p36.12
PDGFB	Platelet-derived growth factor beta	5155	22	22q13.1
SHH	Sonic hedgehog	6469	7	7q36
SATB2	SATB Family member 2	23314	2	2q33
TBX22	T-box 22	50945	X	Xq21.1

(continued)

Table 1–1.

(*Continued*)

Gene		Gene ID	Chromosome	Location
TCOF1	Treacher Collins-Franceschetti syndrome I	6949	5	5q32–q33.1
TFAP2A	Transcription factor AP-2 α	7020	6	6p24
TGFBR1	Transforming growth factor, beta receptor I	7046	9	9q22
TGFBR2	Transforming growth factor, beta receptor II	7048	3	3p22
TGFB3	Transforming growth factor beta 3	7043	14	14q24
YPEL1	Yippee-like 1 (DiGeorge syndrome)	29799	22	22q.11.2

*www.ncbi.nlm.nih.gov/entrez/query.fcgi?db=gene.

with currently available metrics. Further, genetic redundancy and regulatory compensation due to plasticity of the genetic pathway complicates the tracing of gene expression patterns.

Interruption of components of the genetic–metabolic machinery responsible for normal embryonic development can lead to malformations. Disharmonic growth between embryonic components occasioned by subtle differences in the number of cell divisions or in the onset or offset times or rates of cellular activities may variously contribute to dysplasias. The biochemical basis of development and growth changes with time during different stages of development.

In a clinically oriented text, consideration of the very early stages of embryogenesis involving molecular biologic mechanisms, induction by signaling factors, tissue differentiation, histogenesis, organ morphogenesis and growth, each of which constitute enormous fields of study, must be greatly condensed. Appreciation of these underlying developmental phenomena is necessary to understand the series of cascading events leading from the initial zygote formed by the union of parental gametes to the fully fledged infant (Fig. 1–3). Aberrations or variations from the normal morphogenetic patterns, whether of genetic, epistatic, or environmental origin, are responsible for many of the congenital anomalies that constitute clinical syndromes. Currently, there are no specific tests available for genetic susceptibility to orofacial clefts. The revelation of associated congenital anomalies with cleft lip and palate may further identify the interrelationships of diverse embryonic developments with genetic mutations held in common.

EARLY EMBRYOLOGY

The relevance of embryologic understanding of facial development is becoming increasingly significant not only for seeking the etiology of orofacial anomalies, but also for the application of the molecular mechanisms of normal embryo-

genesis to the emerging fields of genetic engineering and tissue regeneration. The exploding field of stem cell research for tissue repair and organ replacement demands an understanding of the morphogenetic mechanisms occurring during facial formation. The recipe for differentiation of stem cells in therapeutic cloning is similar to that of the pathways taken by the multilineage pluripotential cells of the early embryo. The same genes, growth factors, and signaling pathways that operate in the embryo are replicated in directed stem cell differentiation for therapeutic tissue replacement. Fundamental insights into pathophysiology, diseases, and dysmorphology have been revealed by advances in molecular biology (Fig. 1–4).

The field of craniofacial embryology is currently undergoing a paradigmatic period of readjustment and discovery. The last decade has revealed a host of previously unknown factors in embryogenesis. During development, cells are monitored by genetically determined pathways and adjust their rates of accumulation, apoptosis, and hyperplasia to produce organs of predetermined size.[10] The precise control of growth is of inestimable importance for, if each cell in our face were to undergo just one more cell division, we would be horribly malformed.[11]

It is the brain underlying the future face that is a key component of cephalogenesis. The prior presence of the brain determines the subsequent development of the craniofacies. The rostral parts of the brain, the prosencephalon and mesencephalon, are specified by the orthodenticle homologues OTX1 and OTX2, while the HOX genes specify the rhombencephalon and establish spatial identity of prospective craniofacial compartments.

ORGANIZING CENTERS

Development of the head depends upon the inductive activities of the prosencephalic and rhombencephalic organizing

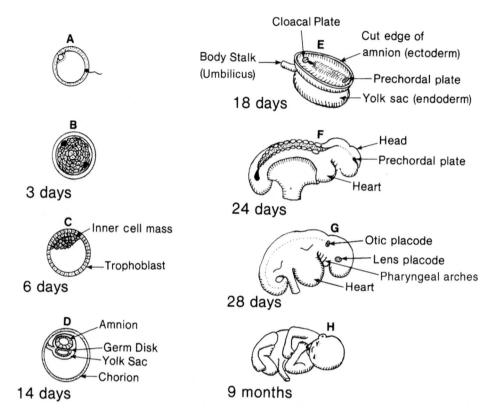

Figure 1–3. Diagrammatic synopsis of embryogenesis.

centers, which are regulated by the expression of the sonic hedgehog (SHH) gene as a signaling protein in the neural floor plate cells.[12,13] These organizing centers are the sites of origin of signaling factors that diffuse into surrounding areas to create "fate maps" that predetermine the details of differentiation of adjacent cells to form particular facial elements. Thus, the rostral prosencephalic center, derived from prechordal mesoderm, located at the rostral end of the notochord, induces the visual and inner-ear apparatus and upper third of the face (the neurocranium). The caudal rhombencephalic center induces the middle and lower thirds of the face, the viscerofacial skeleton (Fig. 1–5). The gradients of chemical and physical properties emanating from the organizing centers regulate craniofacial patterning by inducing a range of responses from uncommitted populations of neural crest tissue.[14]

NEURAL CREST TISSUE

The major contributor to facial formation is the peculiarly derived mesenchymal tissue that arises from the crests of the ectodermal neural folds that create the brain. Specification of the neural crest by the transcription factor Pax7 occurs very early in embryonic development, even before the neural plate appears.[15] Transition of the ectoderm into mesenchyme is a key factor in creating ectomesenchyme that provides a

lineage of pluripotential cells that gives rise to diverse tissues (Table 1–2). Facial morphogenesis is controlled by reciprocal epithiomesenchymal interactions with additional influences from the endoderm directing the regionalization of cell populations to specific fates.

The cranial neural crest cells migrate from their initial dorsal location above the rhombomeres of the brain to ventral destinations that are either predetermined by homeobox transcription factor (HOX) genes that constrain their distribution or influenced by local cues from overlying or underlying epithelia.[14,16–19]

Segmentation of the rhombencephalon into eight rhombomeres delineates the stepwise sequence of cascading streams of migrating ectomesenchyme to create six pharyngeal arches and five facial prominences (Fig. 1–6). Neural crest mesenchyme migrates in the median plane over the prosencephalon to create the frontonasal prominence. Neural crest tissue from the first two rhombomeres migrates ventrally on either side of the rhombencephalon into the first pharyngeal arch that will give rise to both the maxillary and mandibular arches and their derived skeletal elements.

Crest tissue from the fourth rhombomere contributes to forming the second pharyngeal arch, whereas rhombomeres 6 and 7 contribute to the third, fourth, and sixth arches. The neural crest overlying rhombomeres 3 and 5 suffers an apoptopic fate before migrating and therefore does not contribute to the arches.

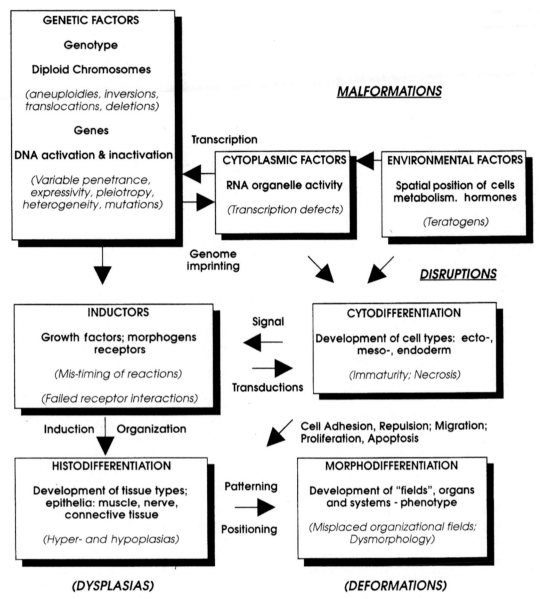

Figure 1–4. Schema of embryogenesis.

Inadequate neural crest mesenchymal proliferation, migration, or excessive apoptosis would result in deficiencies of tissues, causing clefts, among other hypoplasias.[18–20]

FACIAL FORMATION

The orofacial region is identified at the 28th day postconception by the appearance of the prechordal plate in the embryonic trilaminar germ disk. This disk is composed of the three primary germ layers, ecto-, meso-, and endoderm. The *prechordal plate* is characterized by lack of the intermediate mesoderm. The contiguous ectoderm and endoderm at the site of the prechordal plate combine to form a tenuous and temporary bilaminar oropharyngeal membrane that de-

marcates the location of the future mouth. The ectoderm will form the mucosa of the future oral cavity, whereas the endoderm will coat the pharyngeal walls. The oropharyngeal membrane identifies the topographic center of facial development by lining a central depression, the stomodeum, the primitive mouth around which five facial prominences swell during the fourth week of embryogenesis (Fig. 1–7). The prescient mouth is bordered rostrally by the developing median frontonasal prominence, laterally by the maxillary prominences, and caudally by the mandibular prominences, the latter two derived from the first pharyngeal arches (Fig. 1–8).

The tissues that constitute the frontonasal, maxillary, and mandibular prominences are composed of cells of different lineages that have migrated, relocated, and been displaced by epithelial–mesenchymal interactions. Neural crest

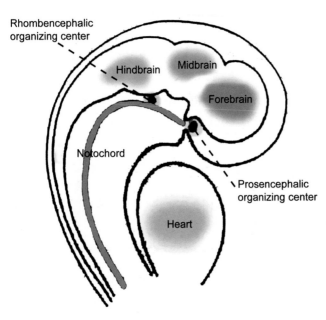

Figure 1–5. Schematic depiction of prosencephalic and rhombencephalic organizing centers.

Table 1–2.

Neural Crest Derivatives

Connective Tissues
Ectomesenchyme of facial prominences and
pharyngeal arches
Bones and cartilages of skull and face
Dermis of face
Stroma of salivary, thymus, thyroid, parathyroid, and
pituitary glands
Dental papilla, dentin, periodontal ligament,
cementum

Muscle Tissues
Ciliary muscles
Perimysium, epimysium, endomysium of pharyngeal
arch muscles (masticatory, facial, faucial, laryngeal)

Nervous Tissues
Supporting tissues
Leptomeninges of prosencephelon and part of
mesencephalon
Glia
Schwann sheath cells

Sensory ganglia
Autonomic ganglia
Sensory ganglia of trigeminal, facial, glossopharyngeal
and vagal nerves
Parasympathetic ganglia (ciliary, ethmoid,
spheno-palatine, submandibular, enteric system)

Pigment cells
Melanocytes in all tissues
Melanophores of iris

mesenchyme contributes the major tissue type that combines with core mesoderm and is covered by surface epithelia. The neural crest tissues give rise to the facial skeleton, whereas the mesoderm will form the facial muscles. Five key secreted growth factors control facial development by regulation of cell proliferation, survival, and apoptosis (cell death). These factors include endothelins, fibroblast growth factors (FGFs), sonic hedgehog (SHH), wingless (WNTs), and bone morphogenetic proteins (BMPs) (Fig. 1–9).[21,22]

These morphogens direct signaling pathways that interact coordinately and interdependently to regulate the growth, patterning, and shaping of the developing face.[23] Mutations of genes or misregulation of the signaling pathways result in misappropriated tissue interactions that are the source of facial maldevelopment. The molecular basis for variable expressivity of these genes and factors has not been fully elucidated, but is responsible for the epigenetic spectrum of phenotypic facial malformations. Developmental instability and teratogenic disruption of genetic signaling are other sources of dysmorphic development.[24] Moreover, mechanical pressures must operate within the confines of the epithelial constraints placed upon the expanding mesenchymal components of the facial prominences, influencing their architecture and developing facial features.[25] A precise mechanistic understanding of the numerous steps involved in signal transductions and migrations is as yet ill-defined.

The mesodermal core of the first pharyngeal arch condenses into myogenic elements that become innervated by the motor branch of the trigeminal nerve. These muscles migrate to their disparate destinations to perform masticatory and swallowing activities. Similarly, second pharyngeal arch mesodermal myogenic elements, innervated by the facial nerve branches, viz. the occipital, temporal, zygomatic, mandibular, and cervical, migrate through the mesenchymal milieu of the facial prominences to establish all the mimetic muscles of the face.[26] All these dispersed muscles retain their initially established nerve supply. The lingual musculature is derived from migration and elongation of the hypoglossal cord of somatic mesodermal origin, retaining its original hypoglossal (cranial nerve XII) innervation. Appropriate distribution of all these elements of tissue components will formulate a face of normal physiognomy. Deficiencies of the peri-oral muscles have been demonstrated in microforms and in full-fledged clefts of the upper lip.[27]

The frontonasal prominence, innervated by the frontal branch of the trigeminal nerve, contributes to the forehead and the nose. Some 173 genes have been identified in expressing their influence in early frontonasal development. On the inferolateral corners of the frontonasal prominence develops bilateral nasal placodes that differentiate into the olfactory epithelium and induce the underlying olfactory nerves. Defective or absent nasal placodal development not only will result in anosmia, but has a devastating effect on nasal and central facial development.

The sinking of the nasal placodes to form nasal pits is the result of the development of the elevated horseshoe-shaped

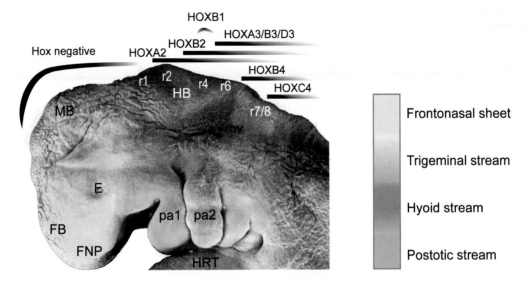

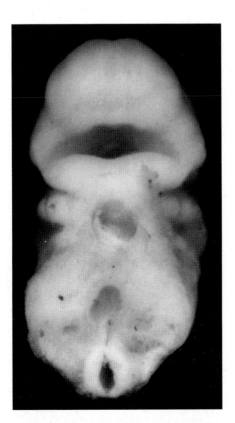

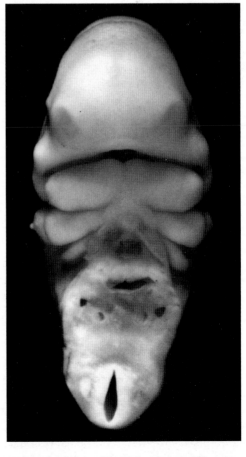

Figure 1–6. A stage 15, 33-day-old human embryo upon which are depicted the neural crest streams emanating from the rhombomeres (r1-8), influenced by the homeobox (HOX) gene expression patterns. FNP: frontonasal prominence; FB: forebrain; E: eye; MB: midbrain; HB: hindbrain; OV: otic vesicle; HRT: heart; pa1/2: pharyngeal arches 1/2. (*SEM by Prof Steding, Gottingen. By permission of Springer Verlag.*)

Figure 1–7. Frontal view of face of a 24-day-old human embryo (×36). (*Courtesy of Prof. Nishimura, Kyoto Collection.*)

Figure 1–8. Frontal view of face of a 32-day-old human embryo (×22). (*Courtesy of Prof. Nishimura. Kyoto Collection.*)

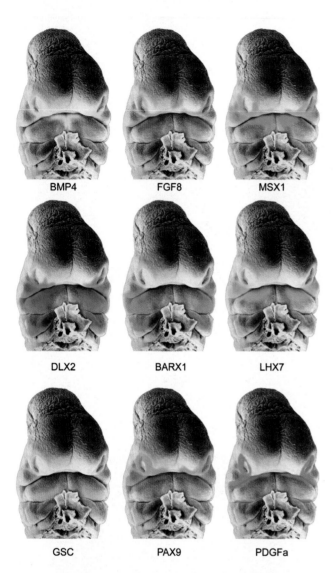

Figure 1–9. Scanning electron micrographs of the face of a Stage 15, 33-day-old human embryo depicting the gene expression patterns derived from mouse embryos. (*Faces from Hinrichsen. By kind permission of Springer Verlag.*)

medial and lateral nasal prominences (Fig. 1–10). The posterior aspect of each nasal pit, initially in communication with the stomodeum, becomes separated from the oral cavity by the transient oronasal membrane. This membrane normally disintegrates by the end of the fifth week postconception to open the posterior choanae connecting the nostrils to the posterior oral cavity. Failure of membrane disintegration leads to choanal atresia, a potentially fatal asphyxiating neonatal congenital anomaly.

Elevation of the lateral nasal prominences creates the alae of the nose. The expression patterns of 36 genes are manifested in the medial nasal prominences, and those of some 45 genes in the lateral nasal prominences. The location of these genes can be identified on the Gene Resource Locator (http://grl.gi.k.u-tokyo.ac.jp). Defects of medial nasal prominence development may result in arhinia, or a bifid nose, varying from a simple depression to complete separation of both nostrils. Other nasal malformations include degrees of aplasia of the alae, as well as atresia of the nasal fossa(e).

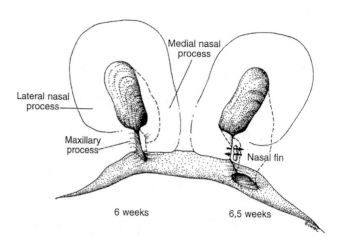

Figure 1–10. Formation of nostrils. Arrows indicate disintegration of the nasal fin between the medial nasal and maxillary prominences. (*Courtesy of J. Avery and Oxford University Press.*)

UPPER LIP DEVELOPMENT

Formation of the upper lip is a complex process involving WNT, SHH, FGF, and BMP signaling pathways that pattern cell proliferation and tissue configuration. The upper and lateral boundaries of the primitive oral cavity are formed by the freely projecting maxillary, medial nasal, and lateral nasal prominences. Initial fusion between the lower edges of the horseshoe-shaped medial and lateral nasal prominences completes the large rotund nostril openings. Maxillary prominence growth pushes the widely spaced nostrils medially and converts them into slits. Upper lip completion requires fusion of the bilateral maxillary and the two medial nasal prominences, with the lateral nasal prominences excluded but wedged in between (Fig. 1–11).

The medial tip of each maxillary prominence is initially separated from the inferolateral aspect of each medial nasal prominence by an intervening epithelial "nasal fin" that degenerates, allowing mesenchymal migration across the former boundaries, and sealing the initial cleft. Development of

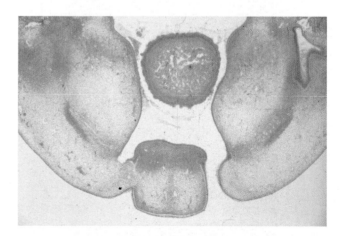

Figure 1–11. Horizontal section of human embryonic lip showing clefting on one side and fusion on the other side. Note the central tongue and unfused palatal shelves on each side. (*Figure courtesy of Dr. V. Diewert, University of British Columbia.*)

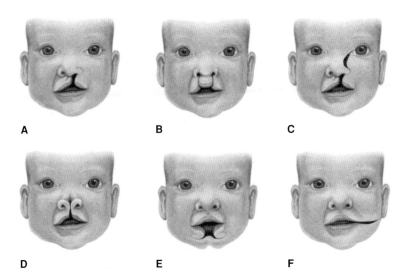

A   B   C

D   E   F

Figure 1–12. Facial clefts. A: Unilateral cleft lip; B: Bilateral cleft lip; C: Oblique facial cleft and cleft lip; D: Median cleft lip; E: Median mandibular cleft; F: Unilateral macrostomia. (*Courtesy of G. H. Sperber "Craniofacial Development" BC Decker Inc.*)

the fusing tissues is the result of cell proliferation, vascular invasion, extracellular matrix production, and fluid accumulation, all of which are subject to variations that may predispose to clefting conditions. Persistence of the nasal fin may contribute to clefting of the upper lip and anterior palate (see Fig. 1–10). Although the lateral nasal prominences do not contribute to the upper lip, failure of their initial fusion with the medial nasal prominences is implicated where clefts of the upper lip extend into the nostril.[28]

All these fusions involve programmed cell death (apoptosis) of the periderm of surface epithelia, epithelial–mesenchymal transformations, and filopodial and adhering interactions. Epithelial filopodia project and anchor into the opposing prominences, followed by mesenchymal fusion. These phenomena are all exquisitely timed and precisely geometrically coordinated to effect the fusions. Inexact contacts by topographic divergences of the prominences or delayed sequences of hierarchical cascading events will inevitably result in clefting of the upper lip.

The initially widely separated median nasal prominences merge in the midline to form an intervening intermaxillary segment, from which is derived the tip of the nose, the columella, the philtrum, the labial tuberculum of the upper lip, the frenulum, and the entire primary palate. The central intermaxillary segment provides continuity to the upper lip, accounting for its maxillary nerve innervation. The philtrum and cupid's bow shape of the upper lip form between the third and fourth intrauterine months (i.e., much later than the melding of the maxillary prominences) as a result of collagen condensation in the midline to produce the philtral groove. The philtrum may be congenitally absent when the upper lip lacks a cupid's bow outline, as in the fetal alcohol syndrome.

Clefting of the upper lip (cheiloschisis) is one of the most frequent of all congenital anomalies; its unilateral incidence (usually on the left) varies among different racial groupings, indicating its inherited character: it is highest in frequency among Asian people, intermediate in incidence among whites, and least frequent in blacks (varying from

1:500 to 1:2000 births). The anomaly appears more commonly in males and has been ascribed to inadequate neural crest tissue migration to the lip area. The degree of clefting varies enormously; the anomaly is rarely median, a characteristic of a major holoprosencephaly syndrome. Lip clefts may be associated with cleft palate, which in isolation has a separate inheritance pattern and a different etiopathogenic pathway (see "Palatogenesis"). However, failure of upper lip fusion may impact the much later-occurring secondary palate conjunctions, accounting for combined cleft lip and cleft palate defects.

The primitive wide stomodeal aperture is reduced by migrating mesenchyme fusing the maxillary and mandibular prominences to form the "corners" of the definitive mouth.

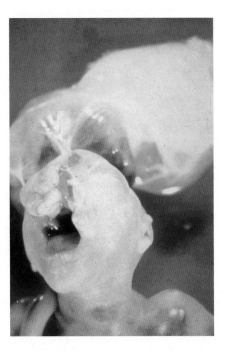

Figure 1–13. Amniotic band disruption clefts in the face of a fetus. (*Courtesy of G.A. Machin.*)

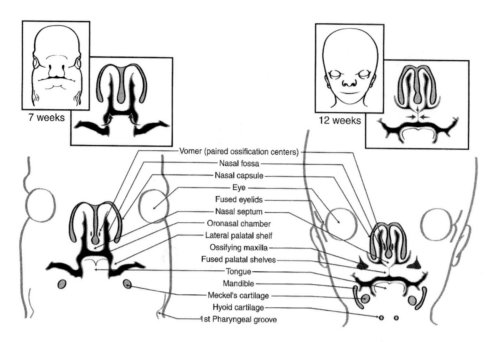

Vomer (paired ossification centers)
Nasal fossa
Nasal capsule
Eye
Fused eyelids
Nasal septum
Oronasal chamber
Lateral palatal shelf
Ossifying maxilla
Fused palatal shelves
Tongue
Mandible
Meckel's cartilage
Hyoid cartilage
1st Pharyngeal groove

Figure 1–14. Schematic depiction of midcoronal sections of heads at 7 and 12 weeks depicting palatal lifting. (*Figure courtesy of G.H. Sperber.*)

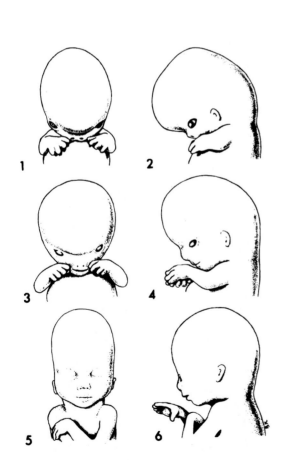

Figure 1–15. Schematic depiction of fetal head movements from frontal and lateral perspectives at (1, 2) 8 weeks; (3, 4) 10 weeks and (5, 6) 12 weeks. (*Figure courtesy of Dr. V. Diewert and Oxford University Press.*)

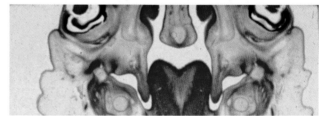

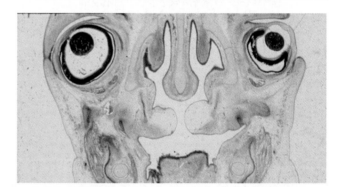

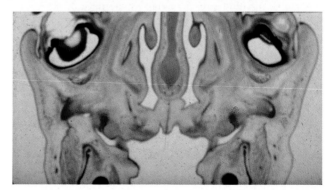

Figure 1–16. Coronal sections of embryos at 7.5 (top), 8 (middle), and 9 (bottom) weeks depicting palatal shelf elevation and fusion. (*Figure courtesy of Dr. Virginia Diewert and Carnegie Embryo Collection.*)

Inadequate ectomesenchyme results in macrostomia (unilateral or bilateral), a form of facial clefting, while excessive fusion produces microstomia or astomia (Fig. 1–12), usually associated with other congenital anomalies (e.g., agnathia and synotia). Fusion of the bilateral mandibular prominences in the midline creates the continuity of the lower lip. The lower lip is rarely defective, but if so, it is clefted in the midline, contrasting with the more usual unilateral clefting of the upper lip.

The rare persistence of the lines of fusion between the maxillary and lateral nasal prominences leads to potential oblique facial cleft(s) in the line of the nasolacrimal canal.

Amniotic bands constitute another potential source of orofacial clefting. Such connective tissue bands may detach from the amniotic sac in utero and may be swallowed by the fetus, tethering the fetal face to the amnion and tearing through the face to form congenital disruption clefts that are unrelated to embryonic fusion lines (Fig. 1–13).

PALATOGENESIS

The development of the intact palate separating the respiratory and masticatory chambers is an evolutionary advance

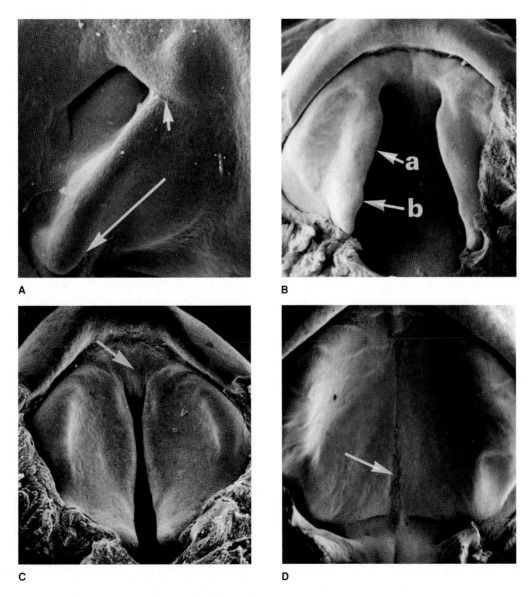

Figure 1–17. (A) View of the right half of a 6-week-old human embryo showing early vertical palatal shelf and lip forming from the maxillary prominence (SEM ×30). (B) Palatal shelves of a 7-week-old human embryo showing anterior end of right shelf (a) becoming horizontal, while the posterior end (b) remains vertical (SEM ×11). (C) Palatal shelves of an 8-week-old human embryo showing the horizontal shelves approaching each other and the anterior primary palate (arrow) (SEM ×11). (D) The nearly fused palatal shelves of a 9-week-old human fetus. The soft palate region (arrowed) is still unfused (SEM ×8). (*Scanning electron micrographs. In Shaw, Sweeney, et al. (eds). Textbook of Oral Biology. Philadelphia: W.B. Saunders Co., 1978.*)

over the common oronasal chamber that occurs in reptilian and avian antecedents. The mammalian secondary palate is initially developed as a bilaterally separated structure, and the persistence of the clefted condition may a priori be considered an atavistic phenomenon. Clefts of the palate are the norm in reptiles and birds. Separation of the respiratory chamber (the nasal fossae) from the food ingestion chamber (the mouth) has enabled the development of speech and of leisurely mastication with its accompanying epicurean enjoyment, and hence the "palatability," of food. Paradoxically, the hard palate contains no taste buds, although the soft palate does. In contrast to mammalian mastication, birds and reptiles characteristically gulp their food to minimize airway impedance.

The intact palate is composed of three embryological elements derived respectively from the median frontonasal prominence, the primary palate, and the two lateral palatal shelves of the maxillary prominences. These elements are initially widely separated in the confining stomodeal chamber by the intrusive developing tongue. The continually growing lateral palatal shelves are deflected down vertically on either side of the tongue prior to the eighth week of development (Fig. 1–14). As a result of growth of the stomodeum at the beginning of the fetal period (eighth week), and the occurrence of mouth opening reflexes, the tongue is withdrawn from between the vertical shelves. The mechanical withdrawal of the tongue requires functioning of the hyoglossus muscle, necessitating neuromuscular and jaw joint activity (Fig. 1–15). All of these factors are critically dependent upon the temporal sequencing of both genetic and environmental factors, which, if perturbed, disrupts the precision of palatal fusion.

In a short period, the palatal shelves flow into the horizontal plane, enabling them to establish contact with each other in the midline, with the primary palate anteriorly, and with the lower edge of the perpendicular nasal septum. Thereby, the single stomodeal chamber is subdivided into the upper nasal fossae and the lower oral cavity (Figs. 1–16 and 1–17). The conjunction of the shelves with the nasal septum may be unilateral, leading to asymmetrical cleft palate, with only one nasal fossa opening into the mouth.

The palatal shelves are not homogeneous along their dorsoventral axis. They exhibit heterogeneous patterns that divide the fetal palate into several discrete molecular and morphologic regions. The dorsal or future nasal surface becomes lined with ciliated columnar respiratory epithelium; the ventral oral side develops stratified squamous epithelium, while the intermediate medial edge epithelium undergoes transformation. Anteroposterior genetic and molecular specification within the shelves is differentially heterogeneous, accounting for variations in the morphogenetic mechanisms of palatogenesis.[29] Manifestations of abnormal development are evident in fetal cleft palates exhibiting arrested maxillary dimensions.[30]

Palatal shelf elevation occurs by a number of mechanisms, including biochemical transformations of the physical consistency of the connective tissue of the shelves, blood flow into the shelves increasing tissue turgor and differential proliferation of mesenchyme, creating mechanical elevating forces. The increase in tissue turgor depends on a critical role played by hyaluronic acid, a molecule that interacts with several extracellular matrix proteins. The gene CD44, the major hyaluronan receptor of the hyaladherin family, is transiently and dynamically expressed during secondary palate development.[31] Recent evidence has indicated that platelet derived growth factor (PDGFC) signaling regulates palatogenesis by the lifting of the palatal shelves and by promoting their fusion. The PDGFC gene region located on chromosome 4 shows strong linkage association with cleft lip and palate.[32]

Outgrowth of the palatal shelves is stimulated by the activity of FGF10, a growth factor in the mesenchyme that stimulates a receptor, FGFR2b, in the surface epithelium. The epithelium, in turn, increases sonic hedgehog (SHH) signaling back to the mesenchyme.[33] The expression of Interferon Regulatory Factor 6 and Lim Homeobox protein 6 in the facial primordia plays a key part in primary palatogenesis.[34] When the palatal shelves meet in the midline, the surface periderm of the medial edge epithelial cells undergoes apoptosis[35] and an epithelial–mesenchymal transformation occurs.[36] Transforming growth factor $\beta3$ (TGF$\beta3$) and its receptor (TGFβR3) are essential growth factors in promoting epithelial–mesenchymal transformation during palatal fusion.[37,38]

During palate closure, the mandible becomes more prognathic and the vertical dimension of the stomodeal chamber increases, but the lateral maxillary width remains stable, allowing shelf contacts to occur. The medial edge epithelium of the palatal shelves is of particular significance in establishing fusion. The fusion seam initially forms in the midpalatal region of the hard palate proceeding both anteriorly and posteriorly, with MSX1 expression restricted to the anterior mesenchyme. Thus, palatal fusion is a two-stage process involving cell proliferation and migration and seam coalescence, dictated by different signaling mechanisms. Posterior palate fusion proceeds caudally to complete merging of the shelves in the soft palate region. A combination

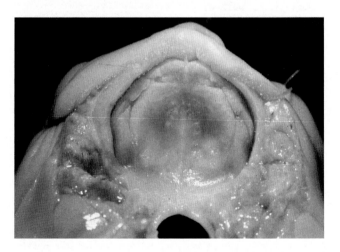

Figure 1–18. Palate and upper lip of a 22-week-old fetus. Note the developing rugae in the hard palate and the extensive soft palate posteriorly.

of apoptopic surface epithelial cells and a surface-coat of glycoproteins and desmosomes facilitates epithelial adherence between the contacting palatal shelves.[39] Epithelial–mesenchymal transformation of the underlying basal epithelial cells may be a factor for mesenchymal coalescence of the shelves.[40] Failure of glycoprotein adhesiveness and transformation of epithelial cells into mesenchyme, allowing epithelial persistence, are factors contributing to palatal clefting.

Ossification of the palate commences in the eighth week postconception from primary centers in the maxillae and palatine bones and spreading centrifugally to create the hard palate, with the intervening sagittal midpalatal and the coronal transverse maxillo-palatine sutures. Ossification does not occur in the most posterior part of the palate, giving rise to the region of the soft palate. Myogenic mesenchymal tissue of the first and fourth pharyngeal arches migrates into this

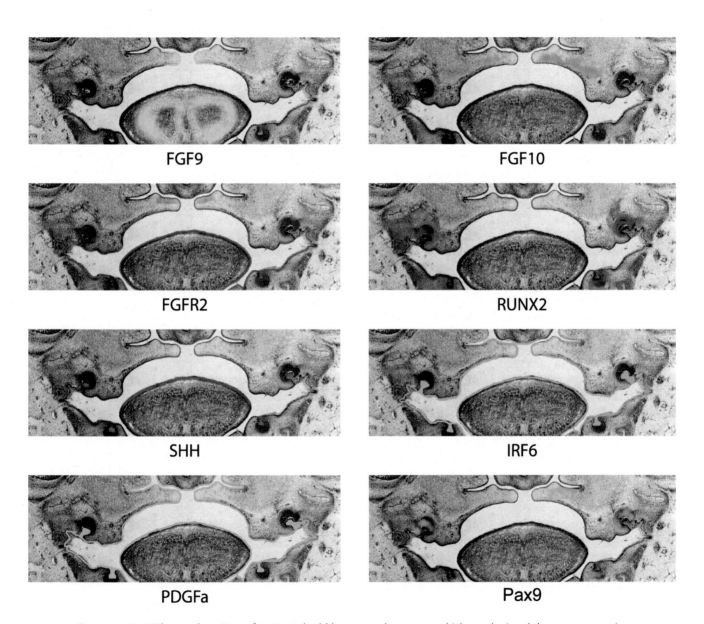

FGF9

FGF10

FGFR2

RUNX2

SHH

IRF6

PDGFa

Pax9

Figure 1–19. Midcoronal sections of an 8-week-old human embryo upon which are depicted the gene expression patterns derived from mouse embryos. Gene expression patterns are as follows: *FGF9* (yellow) is expressed in the ectoderm of the palatal shelves, enamel knot, and myoblasts of the tongue; *FGF10* (purple) is initially expressed in the anterior palatal mesenchyme beneath the medial edge epithelium (MEE) on the oral side and gradually displaced ventrolaterally, the tongue, and floor of the mouth; *FGFR2* (red) is expressed in the oral epithelium and the medial nasal palatal mesenchyme; *RUNX2* (blue) is expressed in the MEE and the chondrogenic condensations; *SHH* (green) is expressed in the MEE and oral side of the palatal epithelium and tongue dorsal epithelium. *IRF6* (cyan) is expressed in the tooth germs, and initially in the tips of the palatal shelves and then in the oral epithelium, and the base of the nasal septum; *PDGFa* (orange) is expressed in the epithelium of the pharynx; *Pax9* (light green) is expressed in the palatal shelf, tooth mesenchyme, and medial nasal mesenchyme, and myoblasts of the tongue. (*SEMs from Hinrichsen:Human-Embryologie. By kind permission of Springer Verlag.*)

faucial region, supplying the musculature of the soft palate and fauces. The tensor veli palatini is derived from the first arch (trigeminal nerve) and the levator palatini, uvular and faucial pillar muscles are derived from the fourth arch (vagus nerve) (Fig. 1–18).

PALATOSCHISIS

Failure of fusion of the palatal shelves on either side of the midline results in cleft palate. The vulnerability of the palate to clefting is indicative of its relatively recent evolution, and the process is susceptible to a variety of environmental influences acting on a background of genetic predispositions to clefting. Such predisposition is inherent in the shape and size of the face, and particularly the maxillae, from which the palatal shelves arise.[41] Evidence of impending palatal clefting is detectable by a peculiar abnormal trapezoid pattern in the maxillary primary growth centers of fetuses.[30] The risk for orofacial clefting is increased with maternal smoking and specific detoxification gene variants.[42] The timing of potential teratogenic agent's activities is crucial in labiopalatal clefting.[43]

Clefting of the palate is a consequence of several factors impeding the fusion of the three palatal elements. These include absence or deficiency of the hyoglossus muscle, a HOX gene mutation effect, allowing continued impedance of shelf elevation by the tongue.[44] The tongue normally flattens, but remains highly arched in cleft palate cases. Failure of elevation has been attributed to a number of genetic mutations, notably those of Msx1 and Jagged 2.[45,46] Complex antagonistic interactions between MSX1 and DLX5 have been further implicated in clefting syndromes, as has haploinsufficiency of the SUMO1 gene.[47] The Fgf10/Fghr2b signal loop is critical for palatogenesis,[48] and impaired FGF signaling contributes to clefting of the lip and palate.[49] Even if the shelves are elevated, persistence of the epithelial seam between them creates conditions for clefting, and may leave remnants of epithelial "pearls" that may become cysts. The complex interactions of numerous genes, transcription factors, and signaling transductions are revealed in several recent reports on the phenomena of palatogenesis (Figs. 1–19 and 1–20).[50–55] Identification of the regulatory roles of specific proteins, such as glycogen synthase kinase-3B (GSK-3B) and their genetic determinants in the complex interactions of palatal fusion will allow prospective preventive interventions of potential clefting.[56]

The shape of the cleft in the palate is indicative of its etiology. V-shaped clefts are the consequence of inadequate tissues in the shelves to complete closure. U-shaped clefts are usually associated with micrognathia and glossoptosis (Pierre Robin sequence) resulting from the tongue obtruding between the shelves, preventing their elevations.[57] The least severe form of cleft palate is the bifid uvula, of relatively common occurrence but one that is seldom clinically significant. Increasingly severe clefts always involve posterior involvement, the cleft advancing anteriorly in contradistinction

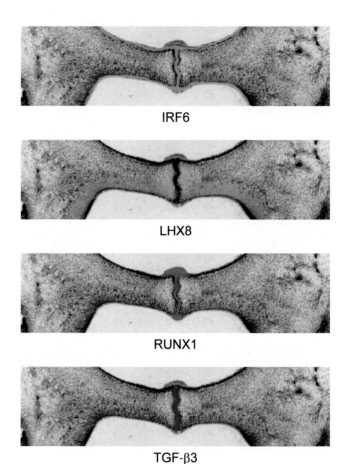

Figure 1–20. Midpalatal fusion gene expression patterns derived from mouse embryos. Gene expression patterns of *IRF6* (cyan) in the medial edge epithelium; *LHX8* (green) expression is restricted to the oral palatal mesenchyme; *RUNX1* (blue) is expressed in the epithelial tips of the palatal shelves; *TGF-β3* (red) is expressed in the medial edge epithelium. (*SEMs from Hinrichsen: Human-Embryologie. By kind permission of Springer Verlag.*)

to the direction of normal fusion (Fig. 1–21). Deficient fusion posterior to the incisive foramen derives from the secondary, rather than the primary palate, whereas anterior clefts involve primary palate deficiencies. Secondary postfusion clefting or congenital fenestration of the palate may develop prenatally as a confounding etiological phenomenon.[58,59] Clefts may be submucous in nature, involving muscle discontinuity, yet with an intact overlying mucosa. The consequences of palatal clefting are multifarious, including oronasal food regurgitation, speech impediments, dental malocclusion, facial growth impedance, and social isolation.

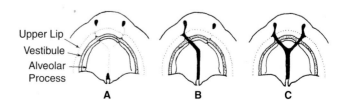

Figure 1–21. Schematic depiction of degrees of palatal clefting. A: Bifid uvula; B: Unilateral cleft palate and cleft lip; C: Bilateral cleft palate and cleft lip.

CONCLUSION

The preceding insights into orofacial development provide clinicians with a rationale for understanding the occurrence of clefts as deviations of normal morphogenesis. With the recent identification of chromosomes, genes, and growth factors responsible for development of the orognathofacial complex, clinical geneticists, speech pathologists, and surgeons are in a better position to predict, prognose, and diagnose clefts of the face, lips, and palate. The anticipation of biomimetic intervention by genetic engineering and molecular growth factors in producing scarless healing of cleft surgical repair is becoming ever more realistic. The current explosion of molecular biology encompassing genomics, proteomics, metabolomics, and pharmacogenomics for targeted drug therapy will have a profound impact upon the prognostication, treatment modalities, and prevention of labiopalatal clefting. The rapid advances in our understanding of cellular behavior during embryonic development leading to differentiation and morphogenesis provide opportunities to exploit this knowledge in preventive, curative, and regenerative healing applications. The current cornucopia of cognitive diagnostic capabilities provided by genetics, immunohistochemistry, computers, obstetrical ultrasonography, CAT scanning, magnetic resonance (MR) scanning, 3D computer stereology, and polymerase chain reaction (PCR) technology provide the potential for prenatal diagnosis and possible therapeutic intervention in preventing palatofacial clefting. Nonetheless, much remains to be done for these techniques to be translated into clinical practice, and such is the central challenge of laboratory bench-to-bedside transition technology.

WEBSITES

1. www.ncbi.nlm.nih.gov/entrez/query.fcgi?db=gene
2. www.ncbi.nlm.nih.gov/entrez/query.fcgi?db=OMIM
3. www.genepaint.org/
4. www.cmbi.ru.nl/GeneSeeker/
5. http://hg.wustl.edu/COGENE/
6. http://grl.gi.k.u-tokyo.ac.jp

References

1. Harvey W. *The Works of William Harvey: Translated from the Latin with a Life of the Author by R. Willis.* London: Sydeham Society, 1847.
2. Vrolik W. Tabulae. *Illustrating Normal and Abnormal Development in Man and Mammals.* Amsterdam: Keys Printing, Greenwood Genetic Centre, Greenwood SC, 2004, p. 184.
3. Stoll C, Clementi M. The Euroscan Study Group. Prenatal diagnosis of dysmorphic syndromes by routine fetal ultrasound examination across Europe. *Ultrasound Obstet Gynecol* 21:543–551, 2003.
4. Jones MC. Prenatal diagnosis of cleft lip and palate: Detection rates, accuracy of ultrasonography, associated anomalies, and strategies for counseling. *Cleft Palate Craniofac J* 39:169–173, 2002.
5. Human Genome Sequencing Consortium I. Finishing the euchromatic sequence of the human genome. *Nature* 431:931–945, 2004.
6. Imanishi T, Itoh T, Suzuki Y, et al. Integrative annotation of 21,037 human genes validated by full-length cDNA clones. *PLoS Biol* 2(6):e162, 2004.
7. COGENE. COGENE: The Craniofacial and Oral Gene Expression Network [Web Page]. Available at http://hg.wustl.edu/COGENE/ (Accessed 17 April 2006).
8. Cai J, Ash D, Kotch LE, et al. Gene expression in pharyngeal arch 1 during human embryonic development. *Hum Mol Genet* 14:903–912, 2005.
9. Scapoli L, Palmieri A, Martinelli M, et al. Strong evidence of linkage disequilibrium between polymorphisms at the IRF6 locus and nonsyndromic cleft lip with or without cleft palate, in an Italian population. *Am J Hum Genet* 76:180–183, 2005.
10. Lien WH, Klezovitch O, Fernandez TE, et al. alphaE-catenin controls cerebral cortical size by regulating the hedgehog signaling pathway. *Science* 311:1609–1612, 2006.
11. Gilbert S. *Developmental Biology*, 8th edn. Sunderland, MA: Sinauer Associates, 2006, p. 5.
12. De Robertis EM, Morita EA, Cho KW. Gradient fields and homeobox genes. *Development* 112:669–678, 1991.
13. Opitz JM. The developmental field concept. *Am J Med Genet* 21:1–11, 1985.
14. Hu D, Marcucio RS, Helms JA. A zone of frontonasal ectoderm regulates patterning and growth in the face. *Development* 130:1749–1758, 2003.
15. Basch ML, Bronner-Fraser M, Garcia-Castro MI. Specification of the neural crest occurs during gastrulation and requires Pax7. *Nature* 441:218–222, 2006.
16. Eberhart JK, Swartz ME, Crump JG, et al. Early Hedgehog signaling from neural to oral epithelium organizes anterior craniofacial development. *Development* 133:1069–1077, 2006.
17. Le Douarin NM, Creuzet S, Couly G, et al. Neural crest cell plasticity and its limits. *Development* 131:4637–4650, 2004.
18. Helms JA, Cordero D, Tapadia MD. New insights into craniofacial morphogenesis. *Development* 132:851–861, 2005.
19. Noden DM, Trainor PA. Relations and interactions between cranial mesoderm and neural crest populations. *J Anat* 207:575–601, 2005.
20. Wilkie AO, Morriss-Kay GM. Genetics of craniofacial development and malformation. *Nat Rev Genet* 2:458–468, 2001.
21. Francis-West PH, Robson L, Evans DJ. Craniofacial development: The tissue and molecular interactions that control development of the head. *Adv Anat Embryol Cell Biol* 169:III–VI, 1–138, 2003.
22. Spears R, Svoboda KKH. Growth factors and signaling proteins in craniofacial development. *Semin Orthod* 11:184–198, 2005.
23. Tapadia MD, Cordero DR, Helms JA. It's all in your head: New insights into craniofacial development and deformation. *J Anat* 207:461–477, 2005.
24. Sperber GH. New insights in facial development. *Semin Orthod* 12:4–10, 2006.
25. Radlanski RJ, Renz H. Genes, forces, and forms: Mechanical aspects of prenatal craniofacial development. *Dev Dyn* 235:1219–1229, 2006.
26. Noden DM, Francis-West P. The differentiation and morphogenesis of craniofacial muscles. *Dev Dyn* 235:1194–1218, 2006.
27. Landes CA, Weichert F, Geis P, et al. Evaluation of two 3D virtual computer reconstructions for comparison of cleft lip and palate to normal fetal microanatomy. *Anat Rec A Discov Mol Cell Evol Biol* 288:248–262, 2006.
28. Jiang R, Bush JO, Lidral AC. Development of the upper lip: Morphogenetic and molecular mechanisms. *Dev Dyn* 235:1152–1166, 2006.
29. Okano J, Suzuki S, Shiota K. Regional heterogeneity in the developing palate: Morphological and molecular evidence for normal and abnormal palatogenesis. *Congenit Anom (Kyoto)* 46:49–54, 2006.
30. Kim S, Lee Y, Lee S, Kim Y, et al. Abnormal maxillary trapezoid pattern in human fetal cleft lip and palate. *Cleft Palate Craniofac J* 45:131–140, 2008.
31. Hudson LM, Moxham BJ. Expression of CD44 splice variants during development of the rat secondary palate. *J Anat* 208: 412, 2006.

32. Ding H, Wu X, Bostrom H, et al. A specific requirement for PDGF-C in palate formation and PDGFR-alpha signaling. *Nat Genet* 36:1111–1116, 2004.

33. Ito Y, Yeo JY, Chytil A, et al. Conditional inactivation of Tgfbr2 in cranial neural crest causes cleft palate and calvaria defects. *Development* 130:5269–5280, 2003.

34. Washbourne BJ, Cox TC. Expression profiles of cIRF6, cLHX6 and cLHX7 in the facial primordia suggest specific roles during primary palatogenesis. *BMC Dev Biol* 6:18, 2006.

35. Hay ED. The mesenchymal cell, its role in the embryo, and the remarkable signaling mechanisms that create it. *Dev Dyn* 233:706–720, 2005.

36. Kang P, Svoboda KK. Epithelial-mesenchymal transformation during craniofacial development. *J Dent Res* 84:678–690, 2005.

37. Cui XM, Chai Y, Chen J, et al. TGF-beta3-dependent SMAD2 phosphorylation and inhibition of MEE proliferation during palatal fusion. *Dev Dyn* 227:387–394, 2003.

38. Nakajima A, Ito Y, Asano M, et al. Functional role of transforming growth factor-beta type III receptor during palatal fusion. *Dev Dyn* 236:791–801, 2007.

39. Cuervo R, Covarrubias L. Death is the major fate of medial edge epithelial cells and the cause of basal lamina degradation during palatogenesis. *Development* 131:15–24, 2004.

40. Sani FV, Hallberg K, Harfe BD, et al. Fate-mapping of the epithelial seam during palatal fusion rules out epithelial—mesenchymal transformation. *Dev Biol* 285:490–495, 2005.

41. Young N, Wat S, Diewert V, Browder L, Hallgrimsson B. Comparative morphometrics of embryonic facial morphogenesis: Implications for cleft lip etiology. *Anat Rec* 290:123–139, 2007.

42. Shi M, Christensen K, Weinberg CR, et al. Orofacial cleft risk is increased with maternal smoking and specific detoxification-gene variants. *Am J Hum Genet* 80:76–90, 2007.

43. Yamada T, Mishima K, Fujiwara K, Imura H, Sugahara T. Cleft lip and palate in mice treated with 2,3,7,8-tetrachlorodibenzo-p-dioxin: A morphological in vivo study. *Congenit Anom (Kyoto)* 46(1):21–25, 2006.

44. Barrow JR, Capecchi MR. Compensatory defects associated with mutations in Hoxa1 restore normal palatogenesis to Hoxa2 mutants. *Development* 126:5011–5026, 1999.

45. Alappat SR, Zhang Z, Suzuki K, et al. The cellular and molecular etiology of the cleft secondary palate in Fgf10 mutant mice. *Dev Biol* 277:102–113, 2005.

46. Zhang Z, Song Y, Zhao X, et al. Rescue of cleft palate in Msx1-deficient mice by transgenic Bmp4 reveals a network of BMP and Shh signaling in the regulation of mammalian palatogenesis. *Development* 129:4135–4146, 2002.

47. Alkuraya FS, Saadi I, Lund JJ, Turbe-Doan A, Morton CC, Maas RL. SUMO1 haploinsufficiency leads to cleft lip and palate. *Science* 313:1751, 2006.

48. Riley BM, Mansilla MA, Ma J, et al. Impaired FGF signaling contributes to cleft lip and palate. *Proc Natl Acad Sci U S A* 104:4512–4517, 2007.

49. Nie X, Luukko K, Kettunen P. FGF signalling in craniofacial development and developmental disorders. *Oral Dis* 12:102–111, 2006.

50. Yu L, Gu S, Alappat S, et al. Shox2-deficient mice exhibit a rare type of incomplete clefting of the secondary palate. *Development* 132:4397–4406, 2005.

51. Liu W, Sun X, Braut A, et al. Distinct functions for Bmp signaling in lip and palate fusion in mice. *Development* 132:1453–1461, 2005.

52. Sasaki Y, Tanaka S, Hamachi T, et al. Deficient cell proliferation in palatal shelf mesenchyme of CL/Fr mouse embryos. *J Dent Res* 83:797–801, 2004.

53. Lan Y, Ovitt CE, Cho ES, et al. Odd-skipped related 2 (Osr2) encodes a key intrinsic regulator of secondary palate growth and morphogenesis. *Development* 131:3207–3216, 2004.

54. Rice R, Spencer-Dene B, Connor EC, et al. Disruption of Fgf10/Fgfr2b-coordinated epithelial-mesenchymal interactions causes cleft palate. *J Clin Invest* 113:1692–1700, 2004.

55. Stanier P, Moore GE. Genetics of cleft lip and palate: Syndromic genes contribute to the incidence of non-syndromic clefts. *Hum Mol Genet* 13(Spec No 1):R73–R81, 2004.

56. Liu KJ, Arron JR, Stankunas K, Crabtree GR, Longaker MT. Chemical rescue of cleft palate and midline defects in conditional GSK-3beta mice. *Nature* 446:79–82, 2007.

57. Hanson JW, Smith DW. U-shaped palatal defect in the Robin anomalad: Developmental and clinical relevance. *J Pediatr* 87:30–33, 1975.

58. Arnold WH, Rezwani T, Baric I. Location and distribution of epithelial pearls and tooth buds in human fetuses with cleft lip and palate. *Cleft Palate Craniofac J* 35:359–365, 1998.

59. Rogers GF, Murthy A, Mulliken JB. Congenital fenestration of the palate: A case of embryologic syzygy. *Cleft Palate Craniofac J* 43:363–366, 2006.

2

Classification of Orofacial Clefting

Mark P. Mooney, PhD

INTRODUCTION

Orofacial clefts (OFCs) for this discussion will include the isolated cleft lip (CL), cleft lip with and without cleft palate (CL/P), isolated cleft palate (CP), and facial clefts (FCs). A recent comprehensive study on birth defects by the Centers for Disease Control and Prevention (CDCP)[1] reported that OFCs are the most common birth defect in the United States with a birth prevalence of 16.87/10,000 live births. The prevalence of OFCs varies by population, gender, and socioeconomic status (SES). Amerindian and Asian-derived populations have the highest birth prevalence for CL/P (15.0–36.0/10,000), followed by European-derived populations with the next highest birth prevalence for CL/P (10.0/10,000), while African-derived populations have the lowest birth prevalence for CL/P (5.0/10,000).[2–6] There is an approximate 2:1 ratio of males:females for CL/P, although slightly more females than males (3:2) have CP.[4,7] Within unilateral clefts, the ratio of left-sided to right-sided clefts is also about 2:1.[6] Also individuals born in rural areas with a lower SES have a higher risk for CL/P compared to ethnically similar groups born in more urban areas with a higher SES.[4]

OFCs are very heterogeneous and their etiologies are complex and multifactorial, thus making them difficult to classify.[4,7–15] They can occur as part of Mendelian syndromes, as part of the phenotype resulting from chromosomal anomalies, or as the result of prenatal exposure to certain teratogens and environmental insults. Much progress has been made in recent years in delineating Mendelian disorders and in gene discovery of such disorders; and one can refer to the Online Mendelian Inheritance in Man [OMIM] database available on the National Center for Biotechnology Information (NCBI) web site [http://www.ncbi.nlm.nih.gov] for a catalog of such disorders. The OMIM database lists 174 Mendelian disorders associated with CL/P and 312 disorders associated with CP.[4] The London Dysmorphology Database, which also includes other nongenetic and teratogenic disorders, lists 205 disorders associated with CL/P and 441 disorders associated with CP.[4,16] However, only a small portion of individuals with orofacial clefts has a known etiology.[4,8,9,12,17] While there are over

300 syndromes identified in which orofacial clefts are part of the phenotype, and about half of those are due to Mendelian inheritance of alleles at a single genetic locus, the majority of orofacial clefts are isolated and nonsyndromic (approximately 75% of CL/P and 50% of CP)[4] and are considered complex traits.[6] Cohen[8] also reported that CP is associated more frequently with other congenital malformations (13–50%) than CL (7–13%) or CL/P (2–11%); however, some studies have suggested that associated anomalies occur with a frequency as high as 44% to 64% in patients with OFCs.[8]

As suggested by Saal,[4] it is important to distinguish between syndromic and nonsyndromic OFCs to help determine clinical and surgical management, assess recurrence risk rates for patients and families, and more accurately describe the phenotypes to facilitate genetic analysis. Although it is not universally accepted,[4] nonsyndromic or isolated OFCs have been defined as those with no or one major anomaly or two or fewer minor anomalies.[17] Major anomalies are defined as those of functional or cosmetic significance needing some degree of medical intervention.[4,18] Minor anomalies are defined as those of minimal or no cosmetic or functional significance, which occur in less than 5% of the population.[4,18,19] Cohen[8] defines a syndrome as a pattern of multiple anomalies thought to be pathogenetically related and not representing a sequence (i.e., a pattern of multiple anomalies derived from a single prior anomaly or mechanical factor). Syndromes are composed of multiple malformations with variable expression (e.g., bifid uvula vs. median facial cleft which may appear in different individuals with the same syndrome). Malformation syndromes are characterized by embryonic pleiotropy where a developmentally unrelated pattern of malformations occurs, but have a common cause and are thought to be pathogenetically related (i.e., cranial base and digit dysmorphologies in the various Craniofacial Dysostoses Syndromes).[8] Saal[4] has further suggested that for practical purposes, syndromic OFCs should be defined as those with three or more minor anomalies, which are strongly associated with the presence of a major anomaly.[4,20,21]

As presented above, there are complex, myriad facets of OF clefting. This has affected the development of a classification system of OFCs, which is widely accepted and useful across disciplines and in all situations.[4,6,13–15] It has been suggested that there is a need to develop a consistent and biologically accurate OFC classification system, based, in part, on our increasing knowledge of embryonic development and craniofacial genetics.[4,13] The word "cleft," once attached to an anomaly, becomes equated with any failure of fusion in the orofacial complex. Palatal clefts, posterior to the incisive foramen (secondary palate) often occur together with clefts of the lip and maxillary alveolus anterior to the incisive foramen (primary palate). However, while these two different types of clefts have quite disparate etiopathogeneses, it has been the tendency for clinicians and researchers to deal with them equivocally. In addition, with the recent identification and increasing understanding of the specific genes involved with syndromic and nonsyndromic orofacial clefting, both these factors (i.e., embryonic dysmorphogenesis and specific gene mutations) may be useful in developing a more accurate classification system of OF clefting, based in part, on specific genetic mutations and timing of craniofacial development, rather than solely on postnatal craniofacial morphology and anatomy.[4,8,13]

OROFACIAL CLEFT CLASSIFICATION SYSTEMS

The importance of categorizing OFCs stems from the fact that orofaacial clefting is multifactorial and etiologically heterogeneous.[6,9,11–13] Surgical and clinical management, genetic counseling, and research data are dependent on an accurate classification of individual cases. However, these different disciplines require or utilize different information concerning OFCs which have prevented the development of a universally acceptable and usable classification system to date. Craniofacial surgeons need specific information regarding anatomical deficiencies and pathogenesis for presurgical planning of functional and esthetic OFC repair.[14,15,22,23,25,26,61] In contrast, clinicians and genetic councilors draw conclusions about treatment outcomes and recurrent risk rates based on the primary diagnosis, not the cleft type.[4,5,8,13,27] However, within each individual diagnosis, it would be possible to draw conclusions about the effects of cleft type, especially for those syndromes that have both clefts of the secondary palate alone and clefts of both the primary and secondary palate combined.[13]

Historically, classification of OFCs was descriptive and based on categorizing the morphology or anatomy of defects. These classification systems were very useful for practical applications such as surgical management and orthodontic treatment, given that the classification systems were accurate and specific enough.[22,25–37] However, morphological or anatomically based classification systems can not (1) explain the etiopathogenesis of the OFC, (2) delineate the broad spectrum of other medical conditions often seen with OFCs, or (3) give sufficient information regarding possible recurrence risks.

Once our knowledge and understanding of developmental and craniofacial biology increased, classification systems, based on early pathogenesis and embryogenesis, were developed. Many of these classification systems correlate clinical features of OFCs with embryogenic events in an attempt to facilitate surgical reconstruction.[14,34,36,38–41] However, even though pathogenic- or embryogenic-based classification systems may suggest a pathogenic causal mechanism, such systems still can not (1) explain the etiology of the OFC, (2) elucidate the high degree of anatomic variability of OFCs, (3) delineate the broad spectrum of other non-craniofacial medical conditions often seen with OFCs, or (4) give sufficient information regarding possible recurrence risks.

In recent years, much progress has been made in delineating Mendelian disorders and in gene discovery of such disorders causing OFCs, and are specifically discussed elsewhere in this volume. Classification systems based on known etiologies from chromosomal analysis, gene mapping, and gene linkage and association studies may be developed and combined with morphologically and pathogenically based systems.[4,5,8,9,13,27]

The following sections present short reviews of historically and currently utilized OFC classification systems by emphasis, and address common characteristics that make such classification systems useful (or not) to specific disciplines.

Morphologically Based Classification Systems

As reviewed by Sphrintzen,[13] early OFC classifications coincided with the "modern" era of surgery following World War I when reconstructive surgeons began applying procedures developed to treat battle trauma for facial reconstruction to children with OFCs. At the time, little was known about the etiology of OF clefting, and categorizations were primarily a tool for descriptive purposes. Davis and Ritchie[62] devised a classification system based on observed morphology with three groups of cleft types.

> Group 1: Clefts of the lip (without inclusion of the maxillary alveolus)
>
> Group 2: Clefts inclusive of all defects of the palate from the incisive foramen posterior (submucous clefts were not mentioned)
>
> Group 3: Complete clefts of the lip and palate (unilateral or bilateral)

Later, Veau[29] presented a widely accepted (at the time) system for classifying oral clefts (OCs) that divided cleft anomalies into four subgroups, but they were different than those offered by Davis and Ritchie.[62] By describing Veau cleft types, surgeons were presumably able to communicate with another about the anatomic nature of the defect in their patient. This type of classification system also allowed researchers to classify OCs according to an operational definition that permitted the grouping together of classes of patients for clinical studies. The Veau classification divided clefts into four subtypes.

> Type I: Clefts of the soft palate
>
> Type II: Clefts of the soft and hard palate, posterior to the incisive foramen
>
> Type III: Complete unilateral cleft lip and cleft palate
>
> Type IV: Complete bilateral cleft lip and cleft palate

In an effort to improve on Veau's OC classification system, Fogh-Andersen[30,31] divided OCs into three main groups based on affected anatomy:

> 1) Cleft Lip (CL) Group: Clefts of the primary palate, including lip, alveolus, and incisive foramen
>
> 2) Cleft Lip and Palate (CLP) Group: Unilateral and bilateral clefts of the lip (complete or incomplete) that extend into the hard palate (Figs. 2–1 and 2–2)

> 3) Cleft Palate (CP) Group: Midline clefts of the secondary palate, posterior to the incisive foramen (Fig. 2–3A,B).

These early classification systems were based purely on anatomy and were used sporadically by clinicians and researchers.[13,34] They were designed by surgeons to try and specify particular cleft types for management and research, but it failed to do this well.[13,34]

In an attempt to be anatomically more precise, Kernahan[33] suggested a pictorial representation using a "striped Y" schematic diagram that represents the lip, palate, and maxillary alveolus. Kriens[35] suggested a labeling system he called LAHSHAL (a palindromic acronym for Lip, Alveolus, Hard palate, Soft palate, Hard palate, Alveolus, Lip). The LAHSHAL classification system assigned a letter to each portion of orofacial anatomy that connoted the location of the cleft, moving from the patient's right to left. The use of upper and lower case letters would connote if the cleft were complete or incomplete (upper case for complete, lower case for incomplete). As an example, LAs would connote a complete cleft of the right lip, complete cleft of the right alveolus, and incomplete cleft of the soft palate. SHAL would connote a complete left-sided unilateral cleft lip and palate. The LAHSHAL system was devised to allow easy retrieval of data regarding cleft type to allow the proper grouping of patients. It has been suggested that the LAHSHAL classification system is reliable and reproducible, and that it can be utilized for insurance coding purposes and intensive epidemiological studies that require numerous subgroups with information about laterality and OC severity.[37] The LAHSHAL classification system has been proposed for usage by the Interdisciplinary Cleft Palate and Craniofacial Anomalies Committee of the German Associations for Cranio-Maxillofacial Surgery, Orthodontics, Phoniatrics, Pedaudiology, and ENT.[37] The LAHSHAL system was also selected for cross-institutional use to standardize cleft classification by the large, NIDCR funded, multicenter Cleft-Craniofacial Center Outcomes Registry project, and also by the Pittsburgh Oral-Facial Cleft Study at our center.[46]

However, Sphrintzen[13] suggests that the morphologically based classification systems of Veau,[29] Kernahan,[33] and Kriens[35] are only of limited descriptive value. Ross and Johnston,[34] as well as Sphrintzen,[13] pointed out that (1) very few clinicians utilize these cumbersome classification systems, (2) they have a limited presence in the scientific literature, (3) they do not recognize a number of important factors related to OFCs that are of critical importance in their diagnosis and management such as the etiologic heterogeneity of OF clefting, and (4) some of these morphologically based classification categories collapse the high degree of anatomic variability seen among patients with OCs into "homogeneous" types, which have little relevance to surgical management.

A number of studies have also attempted to classify rare facial clefts (FCs) based on anatomical and morphological characteristics.[32,47–50] Tessier[22] proposed an anatomic and

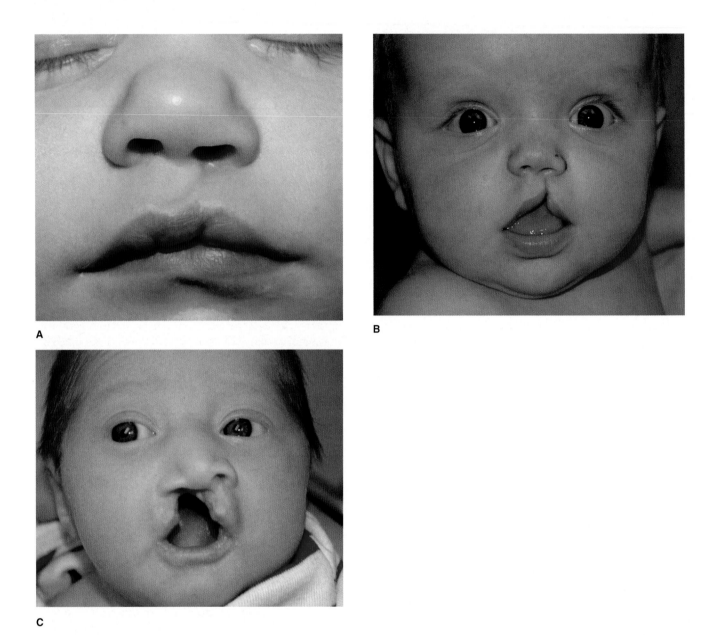

Figure 2–1. Variability in unilateral orofacial clefts: (A) microform cleft lip, (B) incomplete cleft lip, and (C) complete cleft lip.

descriptive classification system in which the various types of bony and soft tissue defects are located on definitive axes on the face with numbers assigned to the cleft site relative to the facial midline (Figs. 2–4 and 2–5).[8] Cleft numbered lines may be either superior (cranial) or inferior (facial) to the orbital margin. Cranial numbered lines have facial numbered counterparts, although these are not related and may be etiologically different. The Tessier classification includes numbered clefts from 0 (a midline cleft of the lip and nose) to 30 (a mandibular cleft)[8,15,25,26] (Figs. 2–4 and 2–5). Tessier clefts numbered 1–3 are through the upper lip, clefts numbered 4–6 are oro-ocular clefts (although cleft number 6 does not start in the oral cavity), clefts numbered 7–9 are lateral facial clefts (although only cleft number 7 starts in the oral cavity), and the remaining clefts are above the palpebral fissure (Fig. 2–4). Additional anatomically based systems have also

been proposed to classify congenital nasal[25] and mandibular[51] anomalies associated in part with FCs.

While the Tessier classification permits accurate anatomical description of both the location and extent of unusual FCs and is widely used,[8,14] it is still inadequate for classifying OCs,[15] describing the extent and type of affected tissues,[26,36] as well as delineating the etiology of OFCs.[8] To better evaluate affected tissues and the severity of rare FCs, Zhou et al.[26] recently proposed the **S**kin, **T**issue (soft), **O**sseous, (**STO**) classification system as an adjunct to the Tessier classification of FCs. In a reclassification of 81 cases of Tessier FCs using the STO classification, Zhou et al.[26] reported that typically, defects from the midline to the infraorbital foramen are predominantly soft tissue, while defects from the infraorbital foramen to the temporal bone are predominantly osseous. He concluded that the STO classification

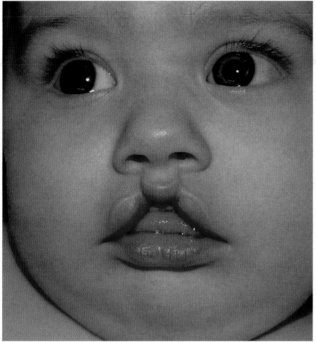

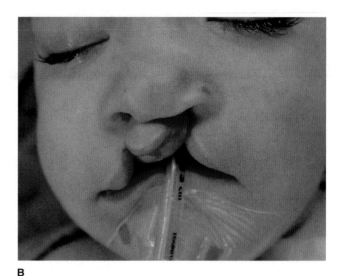

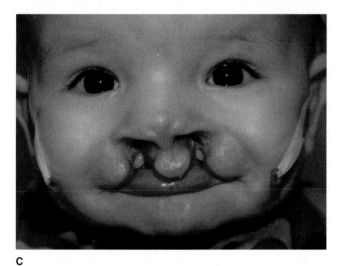

Figure 2–2. Variability in bilateral orofacial clefts: (A) incomplete bilateral cleft lip, (B) incomplete and complete cleft lip, and (C) bilateral complete cleft lip.

system could add important information to the Tessier classification system.

A number of these morphologically based classification systems have been widely used by surgeons (Fogh-Andersen[30,31] and Tessier[22] systems) as a convenient method of classifying OFCs and promoting meaningful research and communication between interested basic scientists and clinicians.[4,8,13,34] However, these morphologically or anatomically based classification systems do not explain the etiopathogenesis of the OFC; delineate the broad spectrum of other medical conditions often seen with OFCs, or give sufficient information regarding possible recurrence risks.[4,8,13,34] Thus, many different clinical problems addressed by Ortho-

dontists, Speech Pathologists, Genetic Counselors, and other Health Care Specialists may make these classification systems less useful to the nonsurgical specialists.[4,8,13,34]

Pathogenically Based Classification Systems

Once our knowledge and understanding of developmental and craniofacial biology increased, classification systems based on early pathogenesis and embryogenesis were developed. Many of these classification systems attempted to correlate clinical features of OFCs with embryogenic events in an attempt to facilitate surgical reconstruction.[4,14,23,24,34,38–41,61]

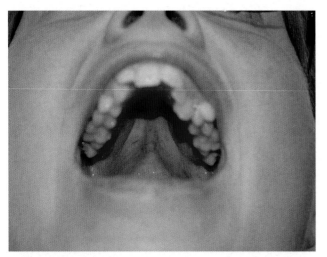

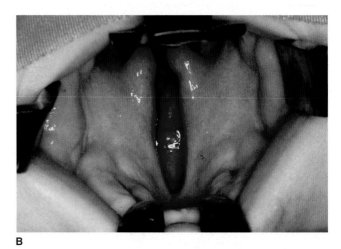

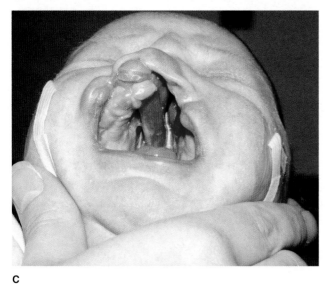

Figure 2–3. Variability in palatal clefts: (A) submucous cleft palate, (B) partial cleft of the palate, and (C) complete cleft of the hard and soft palate.

Noting the limitations of anatomically or morphologically based classification systems in use at the time, the International Confederation for Plastic and Reconstructive Surgery, at their 1967 congress, developed a classification system of OCs based on the embryology of the developing structures. They identified three major groups of OCs[4,38]:

Group 1. Clefts of the primary palate

a. Lip

b. Alveolus

Group 2. Clefts of the primary and secondary palate

a. Lip

b. Alveolus

c. Hard palate (secondary palate)

Group 3. Clefts of the secondary palate

a. Hard palate

b. Soft palate

Ross and Johnston[34] proposed an etiological and developmentally based classification system based on two major groupings or events (i.e., primary or secondary palatogenesis). The first group includes those clefts of the lip and anterior maxilla, regardless of whether the cleft involves portions of the remaining hard and soft palate. The second major group of OCs includes those involving the hard and soft palate only. They proposed this classification scheme:

Primary palatal defects

- CL—Clefts involving the lip (and alveolus)
- CLP—Clefts involving the lip and palate

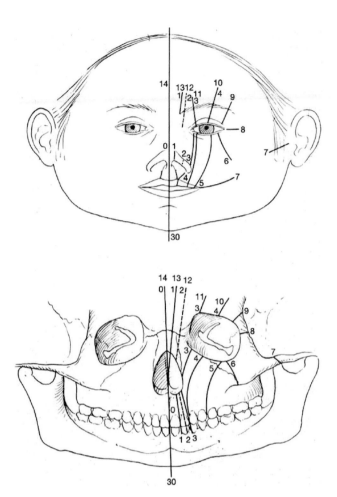

Figure 2–4. Tessier orofacial cleft classification. (*With permission from Eppley BL, van Aalst JA, Robey A, et al. The spectrum of orofacial clefting. Plast Reconstr Surg 115:101, 2005.*)

- CL (P)—Clefts involving the lip with or without cleft palate

Secondary Palatal Defects

- CP—Clefts involving the hard and soft palate only

Ross and Johnston[34] did recognize the simplistic nature of this classification system and suggested that another classification system will have to be used for intensive epidemiological studies that require precise data and numerous subgroups related to laterality and cleft severity in each anatomic region.

van der Meulen et al.[39,40] attempted to correlate clinical features of FCs with embryological events. Based on the locations of the Tessier clefts (Fig. 2–4), they described the bilateral craniofacial skeleton as being formed by two-reversed letter "Ss."[14] The top of the "S" would be at approximately Tessier cleft number 9, it would extend medially, curve around the orbit, continue laterally below the orbit, curve around the TMJ, continue medially on the mandible, and end at the mandibular symphysis at Tessier cleft site number 30. The authors collectively use the term "Focal Fetal Dysplasias," instead of FCs, to describe malformations, deformations, and/or disruptions

in skin, muscle, and bone of the craniofacial skeleton. However, a distinction is made between transformation defects and developmental arrests that occur before primary palatogenesis. van der Meulen et al.[39] named the specific craniofacial dysplastic anomaly on the basis of the anatomical areas involved. For example, the deformity produced by medial and lateral nasomaxillary dysplasia is an oblique facial cleft and corresponds to a Tessier cleft number 3, while the deformity produced by a zygotemporoauromandibular dysplasia is the craniofacial phenotype produced by Treacher-Collins Syndrome and corresponds to Tessier clefts number 6, 7, and 8.[14] Other variations on this theme have also been reported.[36,41]

Recently, Carstens[23,24,61] has proposed that OFCs can be understood and classified by which developmental field (i.e., neuromeric-induced, segmented migratory pattern) was disrupted in the craniofacial region. Carstens[23,24,61] further proposes a Functional Matrix Cleft Repair technique, which is based on these surgically useful fate maps of developmental fields, and the neuromeric origins of the various tissue types. Although not a true classification system, it is nevertheless based on an understanding (or classification) of the embryogenic patterns of craniofacial development and dysmorphogenesis. It also has potential application for the presurgical planning of OFC correction and the explanation of relapse after some traditional approaches. Briefly, Carstens[23,24,61] draws on the well-described neuromeric model of developmental fields to understand OFC formation, and is more specifically discussed in a separate chapter in this volume. The neuromeric model proposes that the early development of the embryonic craniofacial skeleton is under the inductive direction of the developing central nervous system segments (the neuromeres). In the human craniofacial region around the 4th week of embryonic development, the neuromeres induce the neural crest cells to migrate into the pharyngeal arches in a segmented pattern, forming what is referred to as a developmental field. Detailed neuromeric and neural crest cell fate maps have been created to describe these segmented, developmental fields in the craniofacial skeleton. Uneventful developmental interactions and migrations will lead to normal craniofacial morphogenesis and normal primary and secondary palatogenesis. Interruptions in (1) the number or composition of the cells of the neuromeres, (2) cell–cell signaling, and/or (3) migratory patterns will lead to predictable patterns of dysmorphogenesis in the craniofacial complex, depending on the particular developmental field or segment involved. Carstens[23,24,61] proposes that a knowledge of (1) the migratory patterns of the various developmental fields, (2) the end tissue types that are formed by these fields, and (3) the predictable pattern of dysmorphogenesis found during field disruption, can all be used for effective presurgical planning, the development of new surgical techniques, and to explain relapses found in traditional surgical techniques.

As can be seen, classification systems based on pathogenesis or embryogenesis can give additional information about the causal mechanisms producing OFCs compared to anatomically or morphologically based classification systems.

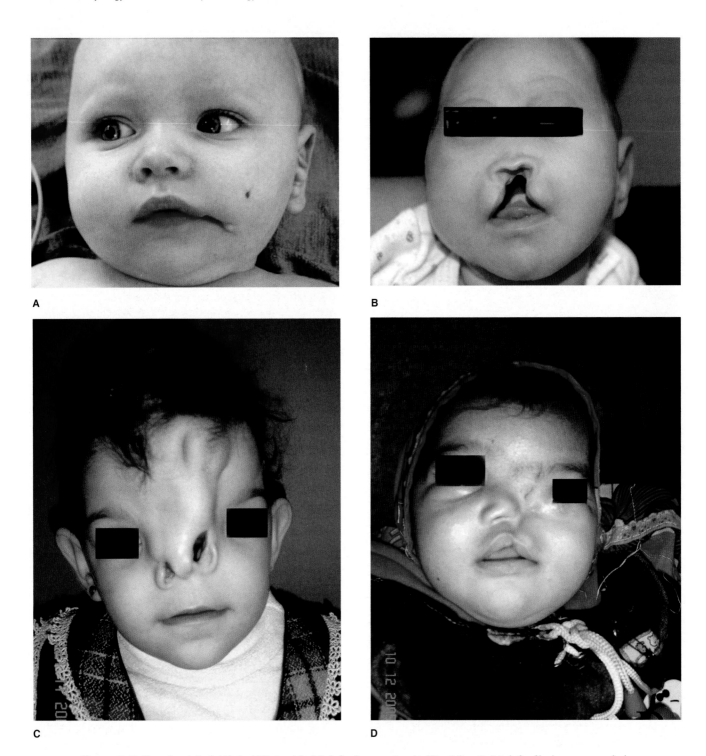

Figure 2–5. Rare Craniofacial Clefts (A) lateral facial cleft of macrostomia, (B) midline 0–14 cleft of holoprosencephaly, (C) bilateral 2–12 craniofacial clefts, and (D) left sided 3–11 craniofacial cleft.

However, there are still a number of deficiencies associated with these classification systems. Pathogenically based classification systems still do not (1) explain the etiology of the OFC, (2) elucidate the high degree of anatomic variability of OFCs having little relevance to surgical management, (3) delineate the broad spectrum of other non-craniofacial medical conditions often seen with OFCs, or (4) give sufficient information regarding possible recurrence risks.

Etiologically Based Classification Systems

OFCs are extremely heterogeneous and their etiology is complex and multifactorial, thus making them difficult to classify.[4,6,9–15,52,63] OFCs can be caused in part by hundreds of genetic, chromosomal, or teratogenic diseases, or even by extrinsic factors that cause disruptions, as seen in the amniotic disruption sequence. As described earlier in this chapter and later in this volume, the extreme variability in OFCs comes from multiple sources: anatomic variation and etiologic variation. Such extreme variability has stimulated the need for simple classification systems that help make "sense" of this condition for surgical and clinical management, as well as research. Both clinical management and research data are dependent on an accurate classification of individual cases. When collecting clinical data, it is important to draw conclusions about treatment outcomes based both on the primary diagnosis, as well as on the OFC type. Within each individual diagnosis, it is be possible to draw outcome conclusions with respect to the effects of cleft type, especially for those syndromes having both clefts of the secondary palate alone and clefts of both the primary and secondary palate.

However, the degree of variability among the population of individuals with OFCs is so great that it is impossible to simplify something that is very complex.[4,13] Although many clefts are treated similarly, regardless of etiology, this may represent a current lack of sophistication in treating each case individually, and in the most efficient manner related to cause or structure.[13] In some cases, a few variations that demand different modes of management have been appreciated. Operations that are often utilized in routine cases of clefting can be less effective in syndromic cases. For example, pharyngeal flaps are highly effective in treating post-operative velopharyngeal insufficiency that can occur after repair of cleft palate; however, pharyngeal flaps may be contraindicated in patients with Treacher Collins syndrome because of the high potential for upper airway obstruction.[53] As well, primary repair of the palate alone in Velocardiofacial syndrome (22q11.2 del) is less likely to result in a successful speech outcome. Thus, in theory, clinical and surgical management should be tailored to the individual diagnosis based, in part, on the etiologic classification, and not exclusively on the morphologic or pathogenic classification type.[4,8,13]

Until recently, this was not possible. However, great strides have been made in delineating Mendelian disorders, and in gene discovery of such disorders causing nonsyndromic and syndromic OFCs. The details of which are further discussed later in this volume. OFC classification, based on known etiologies from chromosomal analysis, gene mapping, and gene linkage and association studies, is being developed and combined with morphologically and pathogenically based systems (Tables 2–1 and 2–2).[4–6,8–10,13,27,52,54,63] Thus, as our understanding of the myriad etiologies of OFCs improves, our ability to diagnose, classify, and manage these conditions also improves.

A number of authors have proposed OFC classifications that combine morphologic, pathogenic, and/or etiologic data in an attempt to better understand the mechanism of inheritance and the etiology of OFCs.[4–6,8,13,27,32,34,56–59,63] Such classification systems should lead to a faster identification of causative factors and more accurate counseling of at-risk families.[4,5,8,13] The Iowa system of OFC classification for research data collection and genetic analysis,[52] divides OFCs into five distinct categories, and is similar to the pathogenically based classification system proposed by Ross and Johnston[34]:

Group 1: Cleft of the lip only

Group 2: Secondary palatal clefts

Group 3: Clefts of the lip, alveolus, and palate (complete cleft lip and palate)

Group 4: Primary cleft palate and lip

Group 4: Miscellaneous

Tolarova and Cervenka[27] proposed a simple clinical classification system for genetic analysis studies that divides OFCs into two categories based on the relative position of the cleft. A "typical cleft" includes a unilateral or bilateral cleft lip and palate and cleft palate. An "atypical cleft" includes median cleft lip and unilateral or bilateral transverse, oblique, or other types of Tessier OFCs. Both typical and atypical clefts could be associated with other malformations. Recently, Farina et al.[5] combined morphologic and etiologic data in an attempt to classify the phenotypes of patients with nonsyndromic OFCs. Categorical data from a series of individuals with CL/P and isolated CP were analyzed, and the frequency distribution of cases linked to markers on chromosomes 6 and 2 were estimated. They reported that three reliable groups were identified based on laterality and the presence of a cleft. A single right-sided pattern displayed a statistically different distribution of linkage to chromosome 6 when compared with the homologous left side. Farina et al.[5] concluded that nonsyndromic CL/P can be classified according to laterality, which developmentally may be under genetic control. They proposed a clinical classification system based on this data, which is similar to the Iowa[52] and Ross and Johnston[34] classification systems, with the inclusion of laterality data as an important adjunct:

Class 1: Any CL with or without right or bilateral cleft of the primary palate.

Class 2: Cleft of secondary palate with or without right or bilateral CL or cleft of the primary palate.

Class 3: Left cleft of the primary palate with left or bilateral CL with or without cleft of the secondary palate.

Johnston and Bronsky[59] and Marazita and Mooney[6] classified OFCs based on the developmental timing of gene expression or mutations in various gene classes. Johnston and Bronsky[59] classified OFCs as belonging to the holoprosencephalies, otocephalies, or neurocristopathies, and discussed etiologic mechanisms and pathogenesis in each class. Marazita and Mooney[6] grouped OFC syndromes by functional gene class. They noted that, of the total 150 Mendelian clefting syndromes, more than 30 genes have been cloned[44,54,60] (Table 2–2). These genes fall into various classes, including transcription factors (GLI3, 7p13; PAX3, 2q35—Waardenburg syndrome; SIX3, 2p21—holoprosencephaly 2; and SOX9, 17q24.3-q25.1—Campomelic dysplasia), extracellular matrix proteins (COL2A1, 12q13.1-q13.2—Stickler syndrome type I; COL11A2, 1p21—Stickler syndrome type II, and GPC3, Xp22—Simpson–Golabi–Behmel syndrome), and cell signaling molecules (FGFR2, 10q26, Apert–Crouzon syndrome; PTCH, 9q22.3—Basal cell nevus syndrome; and

Table 2–1.

Classification of Nonsyndromic OFCs by Suspected Chromosomal Regions and Candidate Genes

| Chromosomal Region | Candidate Genes* | | Genome Scan† |
	Animal Models‡	Candidate Gene (L/A)§	L/A/M
1p36-31	SKI1, LHX8: K/O, E	MTHFR (L,A)	L
1q32	IRF6: E	IRF6 (A)	M
2p13	TGFA: E	TGFA (A)	L, M
2q35			L, M
3p25			A
3q26	TP63: K/O, E		L
4p16	MSX1: K/O, E	MSX1 (L,A)	A
4q31			L
5p15			L, A
6p23	TFAP2A: K/O, E	F13A1 (L,A)	L, M
6q25			L
7p13			A, M
7q21			L, A, M
8p21			L
8q23			L
9q21			L
10q25			L
11p12			L, A
12p11			L, A
14q12	TGFB3: K/O, E	TGFB3 (A)	L
15q22			L
16q			L
17p11			L
17q12	KCNJ2: K/O	RARA (A)	M
18q23			
19q13		APOC2/BCL3 (L,A)	L
20p12			L, A
Xq21	TBX22: E		L

*Candidate genes: genes potentially involved in orofacial clefting with evidence from animal models and/or human linkage and association studies.

†Genome scan: regions with positive linkage (L) or association (A) results with anonymous markers spaced ≤10 cM apart throughout the genome (one or more genome scans); M = positive meta-analysis results over all genome scans.

‡Animal models: genes investigated in animal models with phenotypes that include clefting. K/O = knockout, E = expression studies.

§Candidate genes/regions: genes and regions with at least two positive reports of linkage (L) or association (A) in the literature.

Data taken from Marazita ML, Mooney MP. Current concepts in the embryology and genetics of cleft lip and cleft palate. *Clin Plast Surg* 31:125, 2004.

Table 2–2.

Classification of Syndromic Craniofacial Anomalies with OFCs by Suspected Chromosomal Regions and Candidate Genes

Syndrome	Chromosomal Region	Candidate Gene
van der Woude	1q32-41	
Ectrodactyly ectodermal dysplasia	3q27	P63
Margarita Island ectodermal dysplasisa	11q23	
Aicardi	Xp22	
Craniofrontonasal dysplasia	Xp22	
Hypertelorism-microtia-clefting	1q, 7p	
Kallman	Xp22	KAL1
Gorlin	9q22-31	LMX1B
del(22q11.2)	22q11.2	UFD1L/CDC45L/HIRA
Treacher Collins	5q32-q33.1	Treacle
X-linked cleft palate with or	Xq21.3-q22	
Without ankyloglossia	Xq13-q21.31	
Waardenburg	7p13	GLI3
Waardenburg	2q35	PAX3
Holoprosencephaly 2	2p21	SIX3
Campomelic dysplasia	17q24.3-q25.1	SOX9
Stickler syndrome type I	12q13.1-q13.2	COL2A1
Simpson-Golabi-Behmel	Xp22	GPC3
Apert-Crouzon	10q26	FGFR2
Basal cell nevus	9q22.3	PTCH
Orofacial clefting or high arched palate	deletion 1p36, 18q23, 8p23, or 22q13	
Holoprosencephaly 3	7q36	SHH

Data taken from Cohen MM, Jr. Syndromes with orofacial clefting. In Wysznyski D (ed). Cleft Lip and Palate: From Origin to Treatment. New York: Oxford University Press, 2002, p. 53; Eppley BL, van Aalst JA, Robey A, et al. The spectrum of orofacial clefting. Plast Reconstr Surg 115:101, 2005; Schutte BC, Murray JC. The many faces and factors of orofacial clefts. Hum Molec Genet 8:1853, 1999; Marazita ML. Genetic etiologies of facial clefting. In Mooney MP, Siegel MI (eds). Understanding Craniofacial Anomalies: The Etiopathogenesis of Craniosynostosis and Facial Clefting. New York: Wiley, 2002, p. 147.

SHH, 7q36, holoprosencephaly 3). Classification of OFCs by functional gene class may provide a framework to elucidate developmental causal mechanisms, explain phenotypic variability, and facilitate surgical and clinical management.

These etiologically based classification systems are obviously in their infancy. However, as our knowledge of causative factors that produce OFCs increases, and our ability to detect and diagnose gene mutations in individuals with OFCs improves, such etiologically based classification systems should develop as a natural consequence.

CONCLUSIONS

A myriad of classification systems of OFCs have been proposed and utilized over the years. These systems are based on detailed descriptions of the morphology, pathogenesis, and etiology of OFCs. However, the majority of these classification systems are discipline dependent and do not translate well. In theory, a classification system combining information on the morphology, pathogenesis, and etiology of OFCs, while addressing the needs of the clinician and researcher, would be most useful; but such a unifying classification system has yet to be developed. The development of a unifying classification system of OFCs is dependant on a number of factors: (1) Further advances in the development of molecular technologies for the identification and diagnosis of OFCs, (2) a more thorough understanding of genotype–phenotype interactions responsible for craniofacial embryogenesis, (3) a better appreciation of the gene–environment interactions that are responsible in part for producing phenotypic variability in individuals with OFCs, and (4) a change in our mind set concerning OFCs. As Shprintzen[13] suggested, OFC should be viewed merely as a symptom of an interruption of an embryologic process rather than an anatomic category. Thus, by focusing our attention on the cleft as a disease, rather than the cleft as a symptom, we may not be seeing the forest for the trees.

Clinical pictures kindly provided by Joseph E. Losee, MD, Children's Hospital of Pittsburgh.

References

1. Canfield MA, Ramadhani TA, Yuskiv N, et al. Improved national prevalence estimates for 18 selected major birth defects—United States, 1999–2001. *CDC Morbid Mort Wk Rep* 54:1301, 2006.
2. Vanderas AP. Incidence of cleft lip, cleft palate, and cleft lip and palate among races: A review. *Cleft Pal J* 24:216, 1987.
3. Croen LA SG, Wasserman CR, Tolarova MM. Racial and ethnic variations in the prevalence of orofacial clefts in California, 1983–1992. *Am J of Med Genet* 79:42, 1998.
4. Saal HM. Classification and description of nonsyndromic clefts. In Wysznyski D (ed). *Cleft Lip and Palate: From Origin to Treatment.* New York: Oxford University Press, 2002, p. 47.
5. Farina A, Wyszynski DF, Pezzetti F, et al. Classification of oral clefts by affection site and laterality: A genotype-phenotype correlation study. *Orthod Craniofac Res* 5:185, 2002.
6. Marazita ML, Mooney MP. Current concepts in the embryology and genetics of cleft lip and cleft palate. *Clin Plast Surg* 31:125, 2004.
7. Cohen MM, Jr. Etiology and pathogenesis of orofacial clefting. *Oral Maxillofac Clin North Amer* 12:379, 2000.
8. Cohen MM, Jr. Syndromes with orofacial clefting. In Wysznyski D (ed). *Cleft Lip and Palate: From Origin to Treatment.* New York: Oxford University Press, 2002, p. 53.
9. Murray JC. Invited editorial—Face facts: Genes, environment, and clefts. *Amer J Med Genet* 57:227, 1995.
10. Murray JC. Gene/environment causes of cleft lip and/or palate. *Clin Genet* 61:248, 2002.
11. Berk NW, Marazita ML. The costs of cleft lip and palate: Personal and societal implications. In Wysznyski D (ed). *Cleft Lip and Palate: From Origin to Treatment.* New York: Oxford University Press, 2002, p. 458.
12. Shashi V, Hart TC. Environmental etiologies of orofacial clefting and craniosynostosis. In Mooney MP, Siegel MI (eds). *Understanding Craniofacial Anomalies: The Etiopathogenesis of Craniosynostosis and Facial Clefting.* New York: Wiley, 2002, p. 163.
13. Shprintzen RJ. Terminology and classification of facial clefting. In Mooney MP, Siegel MI (eds). *Understanding Craniofacial Anoma-*
lies: The Etiopathogenesis of Craniosynostosis and Facial Clefting. New York: Wiley, 2002, p. 17.
14. Hunt JA, Hobar PC. Common craniofacial anomalies: Facial clefts and encephaloceles. *Plast Reconstr Surg* 112:606, 2003.
15. Eppley BL, van Aalst JA, Robey A, et al. The spectrum of orofacial clefting. *Plast Reconstr Surg* 115:101, 2005.
16. Winter RM, Baraitser M. *London Dysmorphology Database.* London: Oxford University Press, 1996.
17. Jones MC. Etiology of facial clefts: Prospective evaluation of 428 patients. *Cleft Pal J* 25:16, 1988.
18. Spranger JW, Benirschke K, Hall JG, et al. Errors of morphogenesis: Concepts and terms. *J Pediatr* 100:160, 1982.
19. Jones KL: *Smith's Recognizable Patterns of Human Malformations.* Philadelphia: WB Saunders, 1997.
20. Leppig KA, Werler MM, Cann CI, et al. Minor malformations: Significant or insignificant. *Amer J Dis Child* 142:127, 1988.
21. Leppig KA, Werler MM, Cann CI, et al. Predictive value of minor anomalies. I. Association with major malformations. *J Pediatr* 110:531, 1987.
22. Tessier P. Anatomical classification facial, cranio-facial and latero-facial clefts. *J Maxillofac Surg* 4:69, 1976.
23. Carstens MH. Development of the facial midline. *J Craniofac Surg* 13:129, 2002.
24. Carstens MH. Functional matrix cleft repair: Principles and techniques. *Clin Plast Surg* 31:159, 2004.
25. Losee JE, Kirschner RE, Whitaker LA, et al. Congenital nasal anomalies: A classification scheme. *Plast Reconstr Surg* 113:676, 2004.
26. Zhou YQ, Ji J, Mu XZ, et al. Diagnosis and classification of congenital craniofacial cleft deformities. *J Craniofac Surg* 17:198, 2006.
27. Tolarova MM, Cervenka J. Classification and birth prevalence of orofacial clefts. *Amer J Med Genet* 75:126, 1998.
28. Harkins CS, Berlin A, Harding RL, et al. A classification of cleft lip and cleft palate. *Plast Reconstr Surg* 29:31, 1962.
29. Veau V. *Division Palatine.* Paris: Masson, 1931.
30. Fogh-Andersen P. *Inheritance of Harelip and Cleft Palate.* Copenhagen: Nyt Nordisk Forlag, Arnold Busck, 1942.
31. Fogh-Andersen P. Epidemiology and etiology of clefts. In Bergsma D (ed). *Third Conference on the Clinical Delineation of Birth Defects.* Baltimore: Williams and Wilkins, 1971, p. 50.
32. Cohen MM, Jr., Sedano HO, Gorlin RJ, et al. Frontonasal dysplasia (median cleft face syndrome): comments on etiology and pathogenesis. *Birth Defects Orig Artic Ser* 7:117, 1971.
33. Kernahan DA. The striped Y—A symbolic classification for cleft lips and palates. *Plast Reconstr Surg* 47:469, 1971.
34. Ross RB, Johnston MC. *Cleft Lip and Palate.* New York: R. Krieger, 1979.
35. Kriens O. LAHSHAL. A concise documentation system for cleft lip, alveolus, and palate diagnoses. In Kriens O (ed). *What is a Cleft Lip and Palate? A Multidisciplinary Update.* Stuttgart: Thieme, 1989, p. 30.
36. Zhang DS, Mu XZ, Chen YR. Classification of craniofacial deformities. In Wang W. (ed). *Plastic Surgery.* Hangzhou: Zhejiang Science and Technology Press, 1999, p. 701.
37. Koch J, Koch H, Grzonka M, et al. Facial clefts and their coding with LAHS nomenclature. *Mund Kiefer Gesichtschir* 7:339, 2003.
38. Millard DR, Jr. *Cleft Craft, Vol 1,* 1st edn. Boston: Little Brown, 1976.
39. van der Meulen JCH, Mazzola R, Vermey-Keers C, Stricker M, Raphael B. A morphogenetic classification of craniofacial malformations. *Plast Reconstr Surg* 71:560, 1983.
40. van der Meulen JCH. Oblique facial clefts: Pathology, etiology, and reconstruction. *Plast Reconstr Surg* 76:212, 1985.
41. Pfeifer G. Craniofacial anomalies: The key to a surgical classification of human malformations. In Pfeifer G (ed). *Craniofacial Abnormalities and Clefts of the Lip, Alveolus, and Palate.* New York: Thieme Medical Publishers, 1991, p. 27.
42. Moreno LM, Lidral AC. Genetics of nonsyndromic clefting II: Results from gene mapping studies. In Losee JE, Kirschner RE (eds).

Comprehensive Cleft Care. New York: McGraw-Hill Publishing, 2007, pp. 89–106.

43. Marazita ML, Lidral AC. Genetics of nonsyndromic clefting I: Family pattern and methods of analysis. In Losee JE, Kirschner RE (eds). *Comprehensive Cleft Care.* New York: McGraw-Hill Publishing, 2007, pp. 83–88.

44. Jones MC, Jones KL. Syndromes of orofacial clefting. In Losee JE, Kirschner RE (eds). *Comprehensive Cleft Care.* New York: McGraw-Hill Publishing, 2007, pp. 107–128.

45. McDonald-McGinn D, Zackai EH. 22q11.2 deletion syndrome. In Losee JE, Kirschner RE (eds). *Comprehensive Cleft Care.* New York: McGraw-Hill Publishing, 2007, pp. 129–146.

46. Weinberg SM, Neiswanger K, Martin R, et al. The Pittsburgh oral-facial cleft (POFC) study: Expanding the cleft phenotype. Part 1. Justification and study design. *Cleft Pal-Craniofac J* 43:7, 2006.

47. Karfik V. Proposed classification of rare congenital cleft malformations in the face. *Acta Chir Plast* 8:63, 1966.

48. Pruzansky S. Anomalies of the face and brain. *Birth Def Orig Art Ser* 11:183, 1975.

49. Whitaker LA, Pashayan H, Reichman J. A proposed new classification system of craniofacial anomalies. *Cleft Pal J* 18:161, 1981.

50. Farag MM, Ragaie A, el-Oteify MA. Rare midline congenital anomalies of the face. *J Laryngol Otol* 102:1040, 1998.

51. Singh DJ, Bartlett SP. Congenital mandibular hypoplasia: Analysis and classification. *J Craniofac Surg* 16:29, 2005.

52. Hanson JW, Murray JC. Genetic aspects of cleft lip and palate. In Morris HL, Bardach J (eds). *The Multi Disciplinary Management of Cleft Lip and Palate.* Philadelphia: W.B. Saunders, pp. 121–124.

53. Shprintzen RJ, Singer L, Sidoti EJ, et al. Pharyngeal flap surgery: Postoperative complications. *Int Anesthesiol Clin* 30:115, 1992.

54. Schutte BC, Murray JC. The many faces and factors of orofacial clefts. *Hum Molec Genet* 8:1853, 1999.

55. Cohen MM, Jr. Syndromes with cleft lip and cleft palate. *Cleft Pal J* 15:306, 1978.

56. Gorlin RJ, Cohen MM, Jr., Hennekam RC. *Syndromes of the Head and Neck*, 4th edn. New York: Oxford Monographs on Medical Genetics No. 42, Oxford University Press, 2001.

57. Chong SS, Cheah FSH, Jabs EW. Genes implicated in lip and palate development. In Wysznyski D (ed). *Cleft Lip and Palate: From Origin to Treatment.* New York: Oxford University Press, 2002, p. 25.

58. Melnick M, Jaskoll T. Molecular studies of facial clefting: From mouse to man. In Mooney MP, Siegel MI (eds). *Understanding Craniofacial Anomalies: The Etiopathogenesis of Craniosynostosis and Facial Clefting.* New York: Wiley, 2002, p 519.

59. Johnston MC, Bronsky PT. Craniofacial embryogenesis: Abnormal developmental mechanisms. In Mooney MP, Siegel MI (eds). *Understanding Craniofacial Anomalies: The Etiopathogenesis of Craniosynostosis and Facial Clefting.* New York: Wiley, 2002, p. 61.

60. National Center for Biotechnology Information (NCBI), http://www.ncbi.nlm.nih.gov.

61. Carstens MH. Neuromeric theory of clefts: Developmental field repair. In Losee JE, Kirschner RE (eds). *Comprehensive Cleft Care.* New York: McGraw-Hill Publishing, 2007.

62. Davis JS, Ritchie HP. Classification of congenital clefts of the lip and palate. *J Amer Med Assoc* 79:1323, 1922.

63. Marazita ML. Genetic etiologies of facial clefting. In Mooney MP, Siegel MI (eds). *Understanding Craniofacial Anomalies: The Etiopathogenesis of Craniosynostosis and Facial Clefting.* New York: Wiley, 2002, p. 147.

3

Epidemiology of Cleft Lip and Palate

Laura E. Mitchell, PhD

INTRODUCTION

The epidemiological studies of orofacial clefts often include both cleft lip, with or without cleft palate (CL ± P), and cleft palate only (CPO). This is attributable, at least in part, to the phenotypic overlap between these conditions, which results in similarities in the treatment and health care needs of affected individuals and which thus facilitates the ascertainment of study subjects with either condition from the same source. Other forms of orofacial clefts (e.g., midline, oblique) are generally not included with CL ± P and CPO in epidemiological investigations. This is likely to be due to the relative rarity of these other malformations.

Despite the phenotypic overlap between CL ± P and CPO, it is generally believed that there are etiological differ-

ences between these two malformations. This belief is largely based on family studies that have demonstrated that CL ± P and CPO aggregate within families but usually do not cosegregate within the same family. That is, compared to the general population, the relatives of individuals with CL ± P are at increased risk for CL ± P but not for CPO and the relatives of individuals with CPO are at increased risk for CPO but not for CL ± P.

Given the familial aggregation patterns for CL ± P and CPO and the differences in the embryological processes involved in the development of the lip and palate as discussed in Chapter 1, there is a general consensus that the optimal design for epidemiological studies of orofacial clefts should allow for separate statistical analyses of data for CL ± P and CPO. Nonetheless, data for these two conditions are often combined in a single analysis, usually because the number of cases in one or both groups is too small to allow for meaningful analysis and interpretation. Whether such "lumping" of data for CL ± P and CPO is appropriate is a topic of debate. If CL ± P and CPO are etiologically distinct, lumping these conditions will increase the within-group heterogeneity and reduce study power. However, if CL ± P and CPO share risk factors, lumping will increase the sample size and may increase study power for at least some hypotheses.

Although it is generally thought that CL ± P and CPO are etiologically distinct conditions, there is a growing literature that indicates that these two conditions may share some common genetic underpinnings. The classic example of this is the Van der Woude's syndrome, an autosomal dominant disorder caused by mutations in the IRF6 gene, for which the phenotype can include lip pits, CL ± P, and/or CPO in the affected members of a single family.[1] Because Van der Woude's syndrome is relatively uncommon, it was believed to represent a rare exception to the general rule that CL ± P and CPO do not cosegregate within families. However, there is now evidence that a common variant in the IRF6 gene is associated with the risk of both CL ± P and CPO.[1] In addition, common variants of other genes (e.g., MSX1) have been associated with the risk of both CL ± P and CPO.[2] Hence, the extent to which CL ± P and CPO share risk factors may be larger than previously believed, suggesting that analyses based on combined data for these two conditions may be appropriate in at least some situations.

Considering whether data for CL ± P and CPO should be lumped or split represents just the first of such considerations in epidemiological investigations of these conditions. An additional consideration is whether or not data from all cases of CL ± P and/or CPO should be included in any given analysis. Specific subgroups that can be included, excluded, or analyzed separately can be defined by the presence/absence of a known syndrome or additional, nonsecondary malformations. Most, although not all, epidemiological studies of CL ± P and CPO exclude data from cases with an identified syndrome of chromosomal, single gene, teratogenic, or unknown etiology. The remaining group is often referred to as being "nonsyndromic" and may be further divided into cases with no additional malformations (i.e., isolated clefts) and cases that have additional, nonsecondary malformations (i.e., multiple or associated clefts). Such exclusions and subdivisions are likely to reduce the within-group heterogeneity and should increase the power to detect true associations. However, because the number of identifiable malformation syndromes including orofacial clefts is continuously increasing, because syndromes can be difficult to diagnose, and because the definition of what constitutes an associated malformation is somewhat arbitrary, the composition of these subgroups (i.e., syndromic, multiple, isolated) can be quite different across studies[3] (see below for additional details regarding these subgroups).

Additional considerations in epidemiological investigations of orofacial clefts are the specific phenotypes that will be included in a study and the subphenotypes that will be analyzed. For example, although clefts of the palate may be overt or submucosal, most epidemiological studies include only overt clefts in the CPO category. In addition, CL ± P can be subdivided based on the presence or absence of cleft palate, the extent of the lip defect (i.e., unilateral or bilateral), or (in cases of unilateral cleft lip) by the side of the lip that is involved. Analyses are often performed within subgroups defined by these phenotypic features.

While general guidelines for studies of CL ± P and CPO have been developed,[4] there is no "gold standard" for defining or subgrouping CL ± P and CPO in epidemiological studies. The lack of such a standard reflects the current level of understanding regarding the etiology of these conditions. It remains unclear to what extent CL ± P and CPO share common underpinnings and to what extent the various subgroups within these conditions differ with respect to their underlying etiology. As our understanding of the causes of CL ± P and CPO continues to evolve, it may well be prudent to caste our nets widely. Studies that lump cases as well as split them in a variety of ways are likely to provide the greatest insights with respect to shared and unique etiological mechanisms. Such studies should be widely inclusive in order to ensure appropriate sample sizes within all subgroups and also to retain adequate power in the face of multiple comparisons.

DESCRIPTIVE EPIDEMIOLOGY

The epidemiology of orofacial clefts has been extensively studied for several decades. The literature on this topic can be difficult to synthesize, given the lack of a common standard for defining and subgrouping cases. Nonetheless, much is known about the general characteristics of these conditions.

Prevalence

Within a given location and time, the prevalence of CL ± P tends to be higher than that of CPO. The reported prevalence of CL ± P ranges from approximately 0.2 to 2.3 per 1000 births, and for CPO it ranges from 0.1 to 1.1 per 1000 births.[5] To some extent, the variability in prevalence estimates across studies reflects differences in inclusion criteria (e.g., live births, fetal deaths, pregnancy terminations), case definition (e.g., syndromic, nonsyndromic), and ascertainment sources (e.g., hospital, registry). However, there is also evidence of both temporal and geographic differences in the prevalence of CL ± P and CPO.[5] In addition, the prevalence of both conditions varies by race and ethnicity. For example, based on a study conducted in Texas, it was reported that compared to the offspring of white women the prevalence of CL ± P is significantly lower in the offspring of black women and the prevalence of CPO is significantly lower in the offspring of both black and Hispanic women.[6] The prevalence of orofacial clefts also appears to be higher in Pacific Islanders and Asians as compared to whites, and there may be further differences in the prevalence of these conditions across Asian subgroups (e.g., Far East Asians and Filipinos).[7]

Sex Ratio

Studies of orofacial clefts have consistently identified an excess of males among individuals with CL ± P. The sex ratio (male/female) for CL ± P is approximately 1.5–2.0. The sex ratio for individuals with CPO is generally believed to be the opposite of that for CL ± P. However, the often quoted female predominance among cases with CPO may be restricted to specific subgroups of CPO. For example, in a Danish study with near complete ascertainment of CPO, the sex ratio for all cases of CPO was 1.1. A female excess (sex ratio: 0.90) was only observed among liveborn cases that were treated surgically.[8]

CLASSIFICATION

In clinical practice and in epidemiological investigations, it is important to distinguish between the syndromic, multiple, and isolated forms of orofacial clefts. Clinically, this distinction is important for establishing prognosis, determining recurrence risks, and evaluating options for prenatal diagnosis. In epidemiological studies, this distinction helps to identify relatively homogenous subgroups of cases.

Syndromic

The syndromic group includes cases with CL ± P or CPO who also have an identified syndrome of known or unknown origin. This subgroup is heterogenous and may include individuals with chromosomal abnormalities (e.g., trisomy 13 and 18), single gene, or Mendelian disorders (e.g., Van der Woude's and Rapp-Hodgkin syndromes), known teratogenic exposures (see below for additional details regarding teratogens that have been associated with orofacial clefts), and recognizable patterns of malformations for which the underlying etiology is unknown. The estimated proportion of cases that occur as part of a malformation syndrome varies across studies but may be as high as 30% for CL ± P and 50% for CPO.

Multiple

The multiple subgroup includes individuals with CL ± P or CPO who have other major malformations that do not form part of a recognizable syndrome. This subgroup is also heterogenous in that a variety of different malformations may occur in association with nonsyndromic CL ± P and CPO, including malformations of the eye, ear, head, neck, respiratory tract, gastrointestinal tract, and musculoskeletal system.[9,10] In addition, this subgroup is likely to include cases with unrecognized syndromes or undocumented teratogenic exposures, which if correctly classified would be included in the syndromic subgroup. In general, CPO is more likely to be

associated with additional malformations than is CL ± P, but estimates of the proportion of nonsyndromic cases with associated malformations vary dramatically across studies.[3]

Isolated

The isolated group includes cases that do not have an underlying syndrome or additional, nonsecondary malformations. Most epidemiological studies of orofacial clefts focus on this subgroup of cases, although many studies also include data from the multiple subgroup.

RISK FACTORS

Established and suspected risk factors for CL ± P and CPO include family history, maternal and nutritional factors, and exogenous exposures. Given that the development of the upper lip and the palate are completed by weeks 7 and 9 postconception, respectively, these risk factors must be present prior to these times in order to influence risk.

Family History

A family history of CL ± P is one of the strongest risk factors for this disorder. The risk of CL ± P in the first-degree relatives (i.e., parents, offspring, siblings) of individuals with nonsyndromic CL ± P is approximately 3% and is consistently reported to be higher than the risk in the general population. An increased risk of CL ± P has also been reported for identical twins and for second- and third-degree relatives of affected individuals.[11] Similarly, a positive family history is also one of the strongest risk factors for CPO. The risk of CPO in the first-degree relatives of individuals with nonsyndromic CPO is approximately 3%, and increased risks have also been reported for identical twins and for second- and third-degree relatives of individuals with CPO.[12]

The patterns of familial risk observed for nonsyndromic CL ± P and CPO indicate that genes are involved in the etiology of these conditions. However, the observed familial aggregation patterns for these conditions are not consistent with single gene (i.e., Mendelian) inheritance. Rather, the observed familial aggregation patterns suggest that most cases of nonsyndromic CL ± P and CPO are determined by the effects of multiple genes that interact with each other and/or with exogenous factors to influence disease risk (see Chapters 6 and 7).

Maternal Use of Medications

Retinoids

Maternal use of isotretinoin, a retinoid (13-*cis*-retinoic acid) used to treat severe recalcitrant cystic acne, is associated with a marked increase in the risk (relative risk, ~26) of having a child with a congenital malformation including cleft palate.[13] Maternal use of etretinate or acitretin—oral retinoids used to treat severe psoriasis and disorders of keratinization—is also associated with an increased risk of congenital malformations in offspring.[14] However, an increased risk of orofacial clefts has not been demonstrated for these medications.[14,15]

Anticonvulsants

Women who have epilepsy are at increased risk of having a child with a congenital malformation compared to the general population. This risk appears to be primarily attributable to maternal use of anticonvulsant drugs.[16] In a population-based, case–control study, maternal use of anticonvulsants was found to be more common in infants with CL ± P (odds ratio: 7.8; 95% CI, 2.0–26.0) and CPO (OR = 3.6; 95% CI, 0.1–26.5) than in control infants.[17]

The overall risk of having a child with a congenital malformation and the risks for specific categories of malformations (e.g., orofacial clefts) are related to the specific anticonvulsant drug or drug combination used by the mother.[16,18] Orofacial clefts have been reported in the offspring of women taking phenytoin, phenobarbital, valproic acid, or carbamazepine alone or in combination.[16,19,20] Women who use these drugs for indications other than epilepsy (e.g., bipolar disease, migraine, chronic pain) are also at increased risk of having a child with an orofacial cleft or other birth defect should they become pregnant while taking these drugs.

Folate Antagonists

The mechanism by which anticonvulsants increase the risk of having a child with congenital malformations, including orofacial clefts, has not been established. However, since valproic acid and carbamazepine both have antifolate properties, it is possible these drugs exert their effect on embryonic development via alterations in folate metabolism. Other drugs with antifolate properties, including the dihydrofolate reductase inhibitors—trimethoprim, triamterene, and sulfasalazine—have also been associated with an increase in the risk of congenital malformations, including orofacial clefts, relative to the risk in the general population.[21]

Benzodiazepines

Benzodiazepines are used to treat anxiety, insomnia, and epilepsy and have been associated with an increased risk of a range of malformations in the offspring of women who take these medications during pregnancy. However, not all studies have confirmed an association between maternal use of benzodiazepine and increased risk of malformation in offspring. No evidence of an association between benzodiazepine use and orofacial clefts was found in an analysis based on pooled data from the available cohort studies.[22] However, analyses based on pooled data from the available case–control studies provided evidence for an 1.8-fold increase in the risk of orofacial clefts among the offspring of women who used benzodiazepines as compared to those who did not.[22]

Corticosteroids

Several case–control studies have demonstrated that maternal systemic corticosteroid use is associated with an increased risk of orofacial clefts in offspring, and in at least one study nonsystemic use was also associated with an increased risk for orofacial clefts. The most recent case–control study reported that the risks of CL ± P (OR = 4.3; 95% CI, 1.1–17.2) and CPO (OR = 5.3; 95% CI, 1.1–26.5) were increased in the offspring of women who used corticosteroids for a number of different indications,[23] providing support for the teratogenic effect of the drug rather than of the underlying disease condition.

Maternal Diseases

Diabetes Mellitus

Women with pregestational diabetes are at increased risk of having a child with a range of congenital malformations (i.e., diabetic embryopathy) that includes orofacial clefts. In these women, the risk of having a child with CL ± P and/or CPO has been reported to be two- to seven-fold higher than the risk in the general population. The mechanism underlying the teratogenic effect of maternal diabetes has not been established, but is associated with the degree of maternal metabolic control during the period of embryogenesis.[24]

Gestational Diabetes

The risk of congenital malformations in the offspring of women who develop gestational diabetes is lower than that for women with pregestational diabetes, but may be higher than the risk in the general population.[25,26] However, the risk of orofacial clefts does not appear to be increased[26] or is only very modestly increased[25] in the offspring of women with gestational diabetes as compared to the general population.

Other

Several other disease states, when present during pregnancy, have been associated with an increased risk of CL ± P and/or CPO in offspring, including panic attack disorder, influenza, the common cold, orofacial herpes, gastroenteritis, sinusitis, bronchitis, and angina pectoris. However, the data supporting these associations are limited and additional studies are required to establish or refute an association between these maternal conditions and orofacial clefts.

Maternal Characteristics and Behaviors

Smoking

Maternal smoking is one of the leading, preventable causes of pregnancy complications including placental abruption, preterm delivery, and low infant birth weight.[27] In addition, epidemiological studies provide fairly convincing evidence that the risks of CL ± P and CPO are increased in the offspring of women who smoke. A meta-analysis based on data from 24 published studies indicates that the offspring of women who smoke during pregnancy are approximately 1.3 times more likely to have CL ± P (OR = 1.3; 95% CI,

1.2–1.4) and 1.2 times more likely to have CPO (OR = 1.2; 95% CI, 1.1–1.34) than the offspring of women who do not smoke.[28] Moreover, at least some of the published studies support a dose–response relationship between the risk for these conditions and the number of cigarettes smoked per day by the mother.[28]

The increased risk of CL ± P and CPO among the offspring of women who smoke is modest. However, in some populations the proportion of women who smoke during pregnancy is relatively high. For example, among women in the United States who were pregnant in 1999, approximately 13% reported that they smoked during pregnancy, and in some subgroups (e.g., American Indians/Alaskan natives and women with less than 12 years of education) this proportion was as high as 20%.[29] Hence, in some populations, maternal smoking during pregnancy may account for an appreciable proportion of the cases of CL ± P and CPO.

In order to obtain more precise estimates of the proportion of cases of CL ± P and CPO that may be attributable to maternal smoking during pregnancy, it will be necessary to obtain a better understanding of the mechanism underlying this association. Specifically, whether exposure to maternal cigarette smoke acts independently or interacts with other factors to influence the risk of CL ± P and CPO. Several genetic variants that might interact with maternal smoking to influence the risk of these conditions have been evaluated, including the transforming growth factor alpha (TGFA) Taq1 variant, variants of genes that produce enzymes that are involved in the detoxification of chemicals in cigarette smoke, and variants of genes that produce enzymes that are adversely influenced by cigarette smoke.

Genotype for the TGFA Taq1 variant has been associated with the risk of CL ± P and/or CPO in several although not all of the studies that have examined this association. Several studies have also evaluated whether the genotype for this variant might interact with exposure to maternal cigarette smoke to influence the risk of these conditions. A meta-analysis of these studies suggests that the risk of CPO, but not CL ± P, is influenced by an interaction involving maternal smoking and infant genotype for the TGFA Taq1 variant.[30]

There are relatively few published studies that have evaluated whether the relationship between CL ± P and CPO and maternal smoking is modified by variants of other genes. However, some interesting findings have been reported for variants of genes that produce enzymes influencing the biotransformation of chemicals in cigarette smoke (e.g., CYPA1, NAT1, NAT2, GSTT1, GSTM1)[31,32] and enzymes with a function impacted by cigarette smoke (e.g., NOS3).[33] The role of such potential interactions in the etiology of orofacial clefts remains to be confirmed in independent studies.

Alcohol Consumption

The offspring of women who consume excessive amounts of alcohol during pregnancy are at increased risk for a range of malformations (i.e., fetal alcohol syndrome). However, a relationship between more moderate alcohol consumption during pregnancy and increased risk for specific malformations has not been established. Epidemiological studies relating maternal alcohol consumption during pregnancy to the risk of orofacial clefts in offspring have provided inconsistent results, as have studies aimed at determining whether the association between maternal alcohol consumption and orofacial clefts may be modified by genetic factors.

Obesity

Maternal obesity (usually defined as a prepregnancy body mass index [BMI] greater than 29 kg/m^2) is associated with a range of pregnancy-related complications and appears to be related to the risk of having a child with a neural tube defect. Specifically, the offspring of obese women have a 1.5- to 3.5-fold higher risk of having a neural tube defect than the offspring of nonobese women. Given the observed association between maternal BMI and neural tube defect risk in offspring, there has been considerable interest in determining whether maternal obesity is associated with other congenital malformations including CL ± P and CPO.

Studies evaluating the association between maternal BMI and orofacial clefts have provided conflicting results. The largest of the published studies[34] suggests that maternal obesity is a risk factor for both CL ± P and CPO—women with BMI > 29 kg/m^2 have a 1.3 times higher risk of having a child with either birth defect than women with a lower BMI. Moreover, this study suggests that the association between maternal BMI and clefts may be stronger among cases that have associated malformations than among those with isolated defects. Additional research to clarify the relationship between maternal BMI and the risk of orofacial clefts is critical, given the current epidemic of obesity in children and young adults.

Stress

The occurrence of at least one stressful life event (e.g., death or major illness of someone close, separation/divorce, loss of job) during the periconceptional period has been associated with an increased risk of CL ± P and other defects of the cranial neural crest.[35] Stress during pregnancy could influence the risk of orofacial clefts through several mechanisms including the increased production of corticosteroids. This potential mechanism is of particular interest since maternal use of corticosteroids has also been associated with an increased risk of orofacial clefts (see above).

Other

Additional maternal characteristics including age, parity, and reproductive history have been associated with the risk of orofacial clefts. An association between the risk of orofacial clefts and paternal age, independent of the effect of maternal age, has also been reported. However, in general, the evidence relating these characteristics to the risk of orofacial clefts is inconsistent.

Nutrition

Folic Acid

There has been a long-standing interest in the relationship between maternal nutrition and the risk of congenital malformations. The most significant outcome of epidemiological investigations of this relationship has been the demonstration that maternal periconceptional folic acid supplementation can reduce the risk of neural tube defects in offspring.[36] This has led to implementation of mandatory folic acid food fortification programs in several countries. Reports from countries that have implemented such programs indicate that the population prevalence of neural tube defects has declined significantly following fortification.[37−39] Hence, folic acid fortification of the food supply appears to be the first successful, population-based strategy for the primary prevention of a common congenital malformation.

Given the well-established relationship between maternal periconceptional use of folic acid and neural tube defects, it is not surprising that there is considerable interest in the relationships between folic acid and other nutrients and congenital malformations, including CL ± P and CPO. Unfortunately, studies seeking to determine the relationship between folic acid and CL ± P and CPO have not been as consistent in identifying a protective effect as were the studies that evaluated the association between folic acid and neural tube defects.[40] Although several observational studies suggest that maternal periconceptional use of folic acid and/or multivitamins is associated with a reduced risk of CL ± P and/or CPO, other studies have not confirmed these associations. Moreover, even in the positive studies, the observed associations may not be directly attributable to folic acid, but rather may be the consequence of other vitamins or maternal behaviors that are associated with the use of folic acid. Such alternate explanations are difficult to rule out in observations studies, and there have been no published results from randomized clinical trials of folic acid supplementation for the prevention of CL ± P or CPO.

Some indirect evidence that maternal folic acid intake may be related to the risk of CL ± P and CPO is provided by estimates of the prevalence of these conditions in the United States prior to and after folic acid fortification of the food supply. Based on data reported by states to the National Birth Defects Prevention Network, it has been estimated that the prevalence of CPO in the United States decreased 12% (prevalence ratio: 0.9; 95% CI, 0.82–1.0) between the pre- and post-fortification eras. A reduction in the prevalence of CL ± P was also noted, but this decline was significant only in states that conducted prenatal surveillance for birth defects (prevalence ratio: 95% CI, 0.77–1.0).[41]

One potential explanation for the lack of consistent results regarding the relationship between folic acid and CL ± P and CPO is that this relationship may involve additional factors that vary in prevalence across populations. Failure to account for such factors in epidemiological analyses could give rise to biased results. In the Philippines, for example, the relationship between CL ± P and folate was found to vary across regions, and this variability was attributed to a statistical interaction between folate, vitamin B6, and case-/control status.[42] Interactions involving folic acid and other nutrients or genes that are involved in folate transport and metabolism might also influence the relationship between folic acid and CL ± P and CPO. However, only a few studies investigating such interactions have been reported, and there is currently no conclusive evidence that the risk of CL ± P or CPO is influenced by specific interactions involving folic acid.

Vitamin A

Maternal intake of very high doses of vitamin A from supplements (≥25,000 IU/day) has been associated with a pattern of malformations, including orofacial clefts, in offspring and is similar to that observed among infants exposed, in utero, to retinoic acid (see above). An increased risk of malformations in the offspring of women who consumed more than 10,000 IU/day of vitamin A from supplements and food sources has also been reported,[43] but has not been supported by other epidemiologic investigations.[44−46]

Other

Other nutrients that have been investigated for an association with CL ± P and/or CPO include B vitamins other than folic acid, zinc and other vitamins and minerals, micronutrients, and macronutrients. However, there is currently insufficient evidence to make dietary recommendations specifically for the purpose of reducing the risk of having a child with CL ± P or CPO. Women of reproductive age should be advised to take a multivitamin or eat a breakfast cereal that includes the recommended amount of folic acid on a daily basis (e.g., the Centers for Disease Control and Prevention in the United States recommends that all women who are capable of becoming pregnant consume 0.4 mg of folic acid per day[47]). This advice holds even in regions where folic acid fortification of the food supply has been implemented, since such programs do not guarantee that a given individual will receive an adequate level of folic acid on a daily basis. In addition, reproductive age women should be informed that excessive intake of vitamin A shortly before and during pregnancy may increase the risk of having a child with a congenital malformation.

Exogenous Exposures

Water Chlorination By-Products

Chlorine reacting with raw water that contains natural organic materials produces organochlorine by-products (i.e., chlorination disinfection by-products), including chloroform. Based on a meta-analysis of studies that have assessed the relationship between water chlorination and various birth defects, it was concluded that water chlorination is associated with the risk of neural tube and urinary system defects. The evidence for an association between water chlorination and orofacial clefts was inconclusive.[48]

Occupational Exposures

Occupational exposure to a number of different chemicals, including dyes and pigments, propellants, insecticides, glycol esters, and organic solvent mixtures has been associated with an increased risk of orofacial clefts. However, no specific exposure has been sufficiently studied as to provide conclusive evidence of an association.

Other

Numerous other exposures (e.g., lead, pesticides, hazardous waste) have been associated with the risk of orofacial clefts. Additional research is needed, however, to establish the extent to which such exposures truly influence the risk of orofacial clefting.

SUMMARY

CL ± P and CPO are common, serious birth defects. Hence, they are a high priority for epidemiological research, and there is an extensive body of literature describing the prevalence and characteristics of affected individuals and investigating potential risk factors. Although many potential risk factors have been identified, most of the reported associations have been weak and difficult to replicate. There are relatively few factors, therefore, that are established, or strongly suspected to be, risk factors for CL ± P and/or CPO.

Several factors undoubtedly contribute to the relative lack of success encountered in epidemiological investigations of CL ± P and CPO including (1) uncertainty regarding phenotypic classification and the resulting heterogeneity in case definition across studies, (2) difficulties related to the accurate assessment of exposure status, level, and timing, and (3) challenges related to the ascertainment of large samples for conditions with relatively low prevalence.

An additional factor that is likely to have contributed to the relative lack of success of past epidemiological studies of orofacial clefting was the inability to account for the etiologic complexity of these conditions. Based on the familial aggregation patterns exhibited by CL ± P and CPO, it has long been suspected that these conditions are multifactorial in nature, involving both genetic and environmental components. However, the tools required to study potential genetic risk factors for conditions like CL ± P and CPO within the context of an epidemiological investigation did not become available until the late 1980s.

Although still in their infancy, genetic epidemiological studies have begun to provide exciting new clues about the etiology of CL ± P and CPO. Evidence for several intriguing gene–environment interactions (e.g., maternal smoking and infant genotypes for both NAT1 and GSTT1[31,32]) that may influence the risk of these conditions has been reported, and future studies, utilizing more comprehensive strategies for assessing individual genes and ultimately the entire genome, offer the very real possibility of unraveling the complex etiology of these conditions. More than ever, this will require collabo-

ration between epidemiologists and geneticists. Indeed, in the future, it may be impossible to separate the discussion of the genetics and epidemiology of these conditions into separate textbook chapters.

References

1. Zucchero T, Cooper ME, Maher BS, et al. Interferon regulatory factor 6 (IRF6) gene variants and the risk of isolated cleft lip or palate. *N Engl J Med* 351(8):769–780, 2004.
2. van den Boogaard MH, Dorland M, Beemer FA, van Amstel HKP. MSX1 mutation is associated with orofacial clefting and tooth agenesis in humans. *Nat Genet* 24(4):342–343, 2000.
3. Wyszynski DF, Sarkozi A, Czeizel AE. Oral clefts with associated anomalies: Methodological issues. *Cleft Palate Craniofac J* 43(1):1–6, 2006.
4. Mitchell LE, Beaty TH, Lidral AC, et al. Guidelines for the design and analysis of studies on non-syndromic cleft lip and cleft palate in humans. Summary report from a workshop of the International Consortium for Oral Clefts Genetics, 2000. (Personal Communication.)
5. Mossey PA, Little J. Epidemiology of oral clefts: An international perspective. In Wyszynski DF (ed). *Cleft Lip and Palate. From Origin to Treatment.* New York: Oxford University Press, 2002, pp. 127–144.
6. Hashmi SS, Waller DK, Langlois P, Canfield M, Hecht JT. Prevalence of nonsyndromic oral clefts in Texas, 1995–1999. *Am J Med Genet* 134A:368–372, 2005.
7. Forrester MB, Merz RD. Descriptive epidemiology of oral clefts in a multiethnic population, Hawaii, 1986–2000. *Cleft Palate Craniofac J* 41(6):622–628, 2004.
8. Christensen K, Holm NV, Olsen J, Kock K, Fogh-Andersen P. Selection bias in genetic–epidemiologic studies of cleft lip and palate. *Am J Hum Genet* 51:654–659, 1992.
9. Shaw GM, Carmichael SL, Yang W, Harris JA, Lammer EJ. Congenital malformations in births with orofacial clefts among 3.6 million California births, 1983–1997. *Am J Med Genet* 125A:250–256, 2004.
10. Forrester MB, Merz RD. Structural birth defects associated with oral clefts in Hawaii, 1986 to 2001. *Cleft Palate Craniofac J* 43(3):356–362, 2006.
11. Mitchell LE, Christensen K. Analysis of the recurrence patterns for nonsyndromic cleft lip with or without cleft palate in the families of 3, 073 Danish probands. *Am J Med Genet* 61:371–376, 1996.
12. Christensen K, Mitchell LE. Familial recurrence-pattern analysis of nonsyndromic isolated cleft palate—a Danish registry study. *Am J Hum Genet* 58:182–190, 1996.
13. Lammer EJ, Chen DT, Hoar RM, et al. Retinoic acid embryopathy. *N Engl J Med* 313(14):837–841, 1985.
14. Chan A, Hanna M, Abbott M, Keane RJ. Oral retinoids and pregnancy. *Med J Aust* 165:164–167, 1996.
15. Barbero P, Lotersztein V, Bronberg R, Perez M, Alba L. Acitretin embryopathy: A case report. *Birth Defects Res (Part A)* 70:831–833, 2004.
16. Matalon S, Schechtman S, Goldzweig G, Ornoy A. The teratogenic effect of carbamazepine: A meta-analysis of 1255 exposures. *Reprod Toxicol* 16:9–17, 2002.
17. Abrishamchian ARR, Khoury MJ, Calle EE. The contribution of maternal epilepsy and its treatment to the etiology of oral clefts: A population based case–control study. *Genet Epidemiol* 11:343–351, 1994.
18. Artama M, Auvinen A, Raudaskoski T, Isojarvi I, Isojarvi J. Antiepileptic drug use in women with epilepsy and congenital malformations in offspring. *Neurology* 64:1874–1978, 2005.
19. Kozma C. Valproic acid embryopathy: Report of two siblings with further expansion of the phenotypic abnormalities and a review of the literature. *Am J Med Genet* 98:168–175, 2001.
20. Wide K, Windbladh B, Kallen B. Major malformtions in infants exposed to antiepileptic drugs in utero, with emphasis on

carbamazepine and valproic acid: A nation-wide, population-based register study. *Acta Genet Med Gemellol* 93:174–176, 2004.

21. Hernandez-Diaz S, Werler MM, Walker AH, Mitchell AA. Folic acid antagonists during pregnancy and the risk of birth defects. *N Engl J Med* 343:1608–1614, 2000.

22. Dolovich LR, Addis A, Vaillancourt JMR, Power JDB, Koren G, Einarson TR. Benzodiazepine use in pregnancy and major malformations or oral cleft: Meta-analysis of cohort and case–control studies. *Br Med J* 317:839–843, 1998.

23. Carmichael SL, Shaw GM. Maternal corticosteroid use and risk of selected congenital anomalies. *Am J Med Genet* 86:242–244, 1999.

24. McLeod L, Ray JG. Prevention and detection of diabetic embryopathy. *Community Genet* 5:33–39, 2002.

25. Janssen PA, Rothman I, Schwartz SM. Congenital malformations in newborns of women with established and gestational diabetes in Washington state, 1984–1991. *Paediatr Perinat Epidemiol* 10:52–63, 1996.

26. Aberg A, Westbom L, Kallen B. Congenital malformations among infants whose mothers had gestational diabetes or preexisting diabetes. *Early Hum Dev* 61:85–95, 2001.

27. Zdravkovic T, Genbacev O, McMaster MT, Fisher SJ. The adverse effects of maternal smoking on the human placenta: A review. *Placenta* 26(Suppl A):S70–S75, 2005.

28. Little J, Cardy A, Munger RG. Tobacco smoking and oral clefts: A meta-analysis. *Bull World Health Organ* 82:213–218, 2004.

29. Nishimura BK, Adams EK, Melvin CL, Merritt RKTPJ, Stuart G, Rivera CC. *Prenatal Smoking Data Book*. Centers for Disease Control and Prevention, 2006.

30. Zeiger JS, Beaty TH, Liang KY. Oral clefts, maternal smoking, and TGFA: A meta-analysis of gene-environment interaction. *Cleft Palate Craniofac J* 42(1):58–63, 2005.

31. Lammer EJ, Shaw GM, Iovannisci DM, Finnell RF. Maternal smoking during pregnancy: Genetic variation of Glutathione-S-Transferases and risk for orofacial clefts. *Epidemiology* (in press).

32. Lammer EJ, Shaw GM, Iovannisci DM, van Waes J, Finnell RF. Maternal smoking during pregnancy: Genetic variation of acetyl-N-transferase (NAT) 1 and 2 and risk of orofacial clefts. *Epidemiology* 15:1–7, 2004.

33. Shaw GM, Iovannisci DM, Yang W, et al. Endothelial nitric oxide synthase (NOS3) genetic variants, maternal smoking, vitamin use, and risk of human orofacial clefting. *Am J Epidemiology* 192(12):1207–1214, 2005.

34. Cedergren M, Kallen B. Maternal obesity and the risk of orofacial clefts in offspring. *Cleft Palate Craniofac J* 42(2):367–371, 2005.

35. Carmichael SL, Shaw GM. Maternal life event stress and congenital anomalies. *Epidemiology* 11:30–35, 2000.

36. MRC. Prevention of neural tube defects. *Lancet* 338:131–137, 1991.

37. Ray JG, Meier C, Vermeulen MJ, Boss S, Wyatt PR, Cole DE. Association of neural tube defects and folic acid food fortification in Canada. *Lancet* 360(9350):2047–2048, 2002.

38. Castilla EE, Orioli IM, Lopez-Camelo JS, da Graca Dutra M, Nazer-Herrera J. Preliminary data on changes in neural tube defect prevalence rates after folic acid fortification in South America. *Am J Med Genet* 123A:123–128, 2003.

39. Mersereau P, Kilker K, Carter H, et al. Spina bifida and anencephaly before and after folic acid mandate—United States, 1995–1996 and 1999–2000. *Morb Mortal Wkly Rep* 53(17):362–365, 2004.

40. Bailey LB, Berry RJ. Folic acid supplementation and the occurrence of congenital heart defects, orofacial clefts, multiple births, and miscarriage. *Am J Clin Nutr* 81(suppl):1213S–1217S, 2005.

41. Canfield MA, Collins JS, Botto LD, et al. Changes in the birth prevalence of selected birth defects after grain fortification with folic acid in the United States: Findings from a multi-state population-based study. *Birth Defects Res A Clin Mol Teratol* 73:679–689, 2005.

42. Munger RG, Sauberlich HE, Corcoran C, Nepomuceno B, Daack-Hirsch S, Solon FS. Maternal vitamin B-6 and folate status and risk of oral cleft birth defects in the Philippines. *Birth Defects Res (Part A)* 70:464–471, 2004.

43. Rothman KJ, Moore LL, Singer MR, Nguyen US, Mannino S, Milunsky A. Teratogenicity of high vitamin A intake. *N Engl J Med* 333(21):1369–1373, 1995.

44. Shaw GM, Wasserman CR, Block G, Lammer EJ. High maternal vitamin A intake and risk of anomalies of structures with a cranial neural crest cell contribution. *Lancet* 347:899–900, 1996.

45. Mills JL, Simpson JL, Cunningham GC, Conley MR, Ricci R. Vitamin A and birth defects. *Am J Public Health* 177:31–36, 1997.

46. Mastroiacovo P, Mazzone T, Aderem A, et al. High vitamin A intake in early pregnancy and major malformations: A multicenter prospective controlled study. *Teratology* 59:7–11, 1999.

47. CDC. Recommendations for the use of folic acid to reduce the number of cases of spina bifida and other neural tube defects. *Morb Mortal Wkly Rep* 41:1–7, 1992.

48. Hwang B-F, Jaakkola JJK. Water chlorination and birth defects: A systematic review and meta-analysis. *Arch Environ Health* 58:83–91, 2003.

4

Prenatal Diagnosis of Facial Clefts

Daniel Rotten, MD • Jean-Marc Levaillant, MD

INTRODUCTION

Different techniques have been proposed to prenatally detect and diagnose facial clefts. Fetoscopy allows direct visualization of the fetal face, but it is highly invasive, scars the uterus, and presents the risk of inducing a spontaneous abortion. Its use may be appropriate in the exceptional cases when an integumental biopsy is necessary to ascertain a diagnosis.[1] Detection of enzymatic anomalies in the amniotic fluid was proposed by Raposio et al.,[2] as they found increased lactate dehydrogenase and creatine phosphokinase levels (×4 and ×2.4, respectively); however, their study was limited to three cases of cleft lip (CL) and was neither extended nor repeated. Computed tomography and magnetic resonance imaging (MRI) have been proposed in recent publications and have specific indications. However, ultrasonography, because of its noninvasive, widespread use in pregnancy, has become the technique of choice for prenatal diagnosis of orofacial clefting.

The first meaningful publications about the analysis of the fetal face and the search for clefts with ultrasound appeared in the literature in the early 80s coincident with the advent of real-time ultrasonography.[3–6] However, 20 years later, the exact role of fetal face examination with ultrasound, during low-risk pregnancy, remains debated. At the present time in many countries, the routine surveillance of pregnancy includes repeated sonographic examinations, including one midpregnancy "anatomic" examination at 20–22 weeks. When face analysis is included in the study protocol, it is possible to detect the principal anomalies when present. In the case of orofacial clefts, precise anatomical (type of cleft) and etiopathogenic (isolated/associated) delineation of the defect is possible.

It is generally accepted that prenatal recognition of facial anomalies in utero has many benefits. It allows for a more comprehensive, diagnostic work-up that may include additional imaging and when necessary, invasive testing. In addition, it facilitates the delivery of more information to the parents. In the case of anomalies amenable to medical or surgical treatment, knowledge of a particular diagnosis

may help physicians organize special plans for the child's birth. The medical team is often able to prepare the parents for the morphological anomaly and explain various treatments and interventions, as well as a long-term prognosis. In the case of complex malformations accompanying syndromes or chromosomal anomalies, the parents can be educated and made to take an informed decision to continue or terminate the pregnancy. In all cases, the parents are provided psychological support during the continuation of the pregnancy or, when necessary, during the process of its termination.

However, controversy exists regarding prenatal diagnosis of orofacial clefting[7] and includes the following arguments: the condition is rarely life-threatening; in most instances, it does not involve cognitive decline; in some centers, termination is rarely offered to the parents; in utero, surgery is not an option at the present time; and finally, postnatal surgery is generally favorable. Therefore, it is the opinion of some that the major consequence of presenting this information to parents is increased anxiety. This position, in our opinion, is marginally maintained.

This chapter will focus on the prenatal imaging of orofacial clefts; both screening and precise delineation of the defect will be addressed. The embryology and genetics of these anomalies are addressed in other chapters dedicated to these topics and the imaging of associated anomalies is beyond the scope of this chapter.

TERMINOLOGY

Anatomic Classification

The common cleft of the lip and nose is anterolateral; while other types include median, oblique, transverse, and complex (Table 4–1a). Anterolateral clefts can include the following structures: (1) the upper lip; (2) the primary palate (the bony palate anterior to the incisive foramen including the alveolar ridge or alveolus and the anterior maxilla or premaxilla); and (3) the secondary palate (the posterior hard palate and soft palate or velum).

Table 4–1a.

Anatomic Classifications

Type of Cleft		Denomination and Anatomic Structure Involved	
Facial, typical	Cleft lip ± cleft palate	Cleft lip	Unilateral or bilateral
		Cleft lip and alveolus	Complete or incomplete
		Cleft lip + alveolus + posterior palate	
	Cleft palate only	Cleft of the posterior palate only	
Facial, atypical	Median, transverse, oblique		
Craniofacial	Various Tessier's types		

Table 4–1b.

Etiopathogenic Classification

Isolated

Part of a sequence of etiopathogenetically anomalies
    related to a simple primary defect

Associated (part of multiple congenital anomalies)
    Related to a chromosomal aberration
    Nonchromosomal
        Syndromic (part of a known association)
        Part of a complex (not characterized) association

A CL can be complete, with no tissue connection between the alar base and the medial labial element, or incomplete, when the cleft of the lip does not extend through the nasal sill or floor of the nostrils. In addition, clefts of the lip can be unilateral or bilateral. An anterolateral cleft can involve the lip(s) only, CL; extend into the primary palate (cleft of the lip and alveolus or cleft lip and alveolus, CLA, or labioalveolar cleft); or extend into the posterior palate (cleft of the lip, alveolus, and posterior palate, CLAPP). All these forms of anterolateral clefts constitute an entity united under the term "cleft lip with or without cleft palate" (CL ± P or CL(P)).

In the sonographic literature, the term "cleft lip with cleft palate" has long referred to clefts extending at least to the alveolus with no delineation about the integrity of the secondary palate. In particular, this was seen in the publications prior to 2000 as the secondary palate was impossible to visualize with sonography because of technical limitations. Present-day sonographic studies often allow for the description of the anterolateral cleft's extension into the "palate," differentiating lesions of the primary and secondary palate. Clefts of the secondary/posterior palate, with no anterior involvement, constitute a different nosographic entity, and are usually referred to as "CP only" or "CP alone."

Etiopathogenic Classification

A cleft can be isolated with no other fetal anomaly recognized or it can be associated as one of the multiple congenital anomalies, either morphologic and/or chromosomal (Table 4–1b). More than 350 named syndromes are known including orofacial clefting (see the corresponding Chapter 8).

IN UTERO RECOGNITION RATE FOR FACE ANOMALIES

Published rates for prenatal sonographic recognition of face anomalies are highly variable. It is recognized that several factors influence the reported results and these include study methodologies and the specific details of cleft imaging. In particular, there is an intricate relationship between the prevalence of the defect in the population and the sonographic examination protocol (Fig. 4–1).

Prevalence in the Population and Conditions of Ultrasound Examination

In a multicenter study published in 2001, Shaikh et al.[7] reported a global sonographic detection rate for CL(P) of 23/130 (17.7%). While most of the participating centers did routine screening, one locale was a tertiary center that participated in both routine screening as well as the evaluation of patients referred with a suspected fetal anomaly. The detection rate in this center was 14/20 (70%).[8] This greater rate of anomaly detection is attributed to the higher prevalence of the defect in the examined population and the likely greater expertise of the ultrasonographers in referral centers. Vial et al.[9] analyzed the prenatal recognition rate of facial clefts in the Swiss Canton of Vaud from January 1994 to December 1998. In this county, routine anatomic ultrasound screening is offered to all women during pregnancy. Out of a total of 42 facial clefts (type unspecified) that occurred during the study period, 21/42 (50%) were prenatally diagnosed. Routine screening was more efficient when performed in the tertiary center and approached the efficiency obtained in patients referred with a suspected fetal anomaly (Table 4–2).

Differences in Examination Protocol

Differences in the sonographic examination protocol is likely responsible in part for the lower recognition rate observed in populations with low prevalence of the defect. Routine ultrasound examination of pregnant women has become a common practice, in particular in Europe.[10] This practice has been challenged[11] and is not generalized in the United States. In addition, the sonographic examination protocol is highly variable with respect to visualization of the face. Some protocols given to ultrasonographers completely ignore visualization of the face,[12] some recommend only selected views, and few include a comprehensive examination. The importance of analyzing the face along the three orthogonal sonographic planes has received experimental confirmation by Babcook et al.[13] with studies performed in vitro and in utero. Reported rates of prenatal recognition of fetal face anomalies range between 20% and 30% when only one or two planes are examined. The rates of recognition rise to nearly 90% when all the three planes, sagittal, coronal, and axial, are systematically analyzed. This latter recognition rate is close to rates obtained in referral centers when complete fetal facial examination is part of the work-up of a high-risk patient or a patient referred for a suspected fetal anomaly.

Anatomic Form of the Defect

The recognition rate increases with the severity of the defect as shown in the series by Hanikeri et al.[14] Table 4–3 depicts

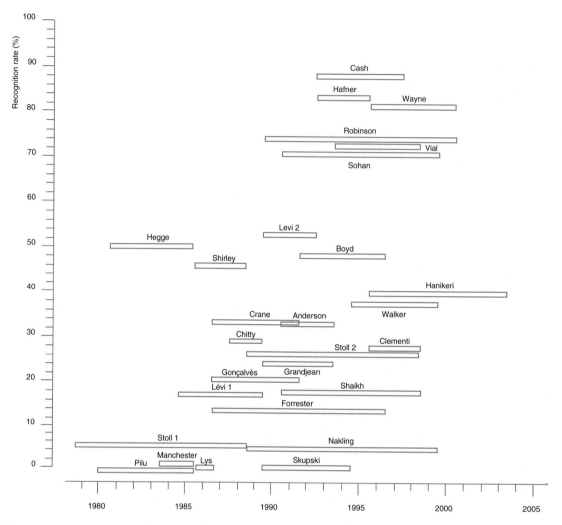

Figure 4–1. Recognition rate of CL(P) according to different published series. The width of the rectangles indicates the years of cases accrual. CP only has been excluded from the computation when possible. Arabic numbers after the name of the first author of the publication indicate following time periods within the same study.

the number of prenatally diagnosed cases for each category of cleft (Table 4–2). For example, the "forme fruste" CL had a poor recognition rate, when compared with other types of CL(P)s, whose ultrasonographic detection was superior to 40%.

Isolated or Associated Clefts

The recognition rates of isolated clefts have been shown to be lower than when associated with other anomalies. Stoll et al.[15] reported the results observed in a series of 309 CL(P)s collected over 20 years (1979–1998) in a congenital

Table 4–2.

Prenatal Recognition Rate of Facial Clefts According to Conditions of Ultrasound Examination

Location Where Sonography was Performed	Type of Examination	Number of Clefts Prenatally Diagnosed/ Total Number per Category (%)
General practice office and/or center	Routine screening	14/34*(41.2)
Referral center	Routine screening	7/8* (87.5)
Referral center	Referred patients	11/15 (73.3)

* $p = 0.04$.
Data from the study by Vial Y, Tran C, Addor MC, Hohlfeld P. Screening for fetal malformations: Performance of routine ultrasonography in the population of the Swiss Canton of Vaud. Swiss Med Wkly 131:490–494, 2001.

Table 4–3.

Recognition Rate of Facial Clefts According to the Anatomical Type c

Anatomic Form of the Cleft	"Form Fruste" CL	Unilateral CL(P)	Bilateral CL(P)	CP Only
Number prenatally diagnosed/ total number per category (%)	1/7 (14.3)	39/96 (40.6)	8/18 (44.0)	0/95 (0)

CL: cleft lip; CL(P): cleft lip with or without cleft palate; CP only: cleft palate only.
Data from the study by Hanikeri M, Savundra J, Gillett D, Walters M, McBain W. Antenatal transabdominal ultrasound detection of cleft lip and palate in Western Australia from 1996 to 2003. Cleft Palate Craniofac J 43:61–66, 2006.

malformation registry. Sonographic screening was offered to all women in the corresponding population. CP only is excluded from the computations. For the first time period (1979–1988), the recognition rate was 1/87 (1.1%) for isolated CL(P), and 6/45 (13.3%) for CL(P) with associated clefts. This difference persisted during the second time period (1989–1998), with recognition rates of 19/121 (15.7%) and 28/56 (50%), respectively. The data by Clementi et al.,[10] corresponding to study years 1996–1998 are confirmatory (Table 4–4). The global recognition rate for CL(P) in that series was 148/553 (26.8%). This rate increased from 65/366 (17.8%) for isolated CL(P), to 83/187 (44.4%) for CL(P) with associated anomalies.

Inclusion/Exclusion of CP Only in the Calculations

CP alone has long been deemed impossible to image with ultrasound. In the series by Shaikh et al.,[8] all 140 CP only anomalies were unable to be diagnosed prenatally by ultra-

sound. This was also found in the series reported by Sohan et al.[7] of eight CP alone anomalies. The current state of ultrasound diagnosis has only marginally changed, with some cases of CP only, now diagnosed by ultrasound. Thus, when cases of CP only are included in the calculations, the prenatal recognition rate of facial clefts is obviously lower. For example, in the series reported by Clementi et al.,[10] including CP only in the calculations would decrease the prenatal recognition rate of clefts from 26.8% (148/553) to 21.4% (161/751) (Table 4–4). Similarly, in the report by Shaikh et al.,[8] the recognition rate of facial clefts would fall from 23/130 (17.7%) to 23/270 (8.5%).

Time Trend

Over the time, increases in ultrasonographic recognition rates of orofacial clefts have been apparent in published series. Levi et al.[16] reported a prenatal recognition rate for facial anomalies of 13/44 (29.5%) over the period 1984–1992. A more precise analysis of this data demonstrates an increase from 5/29

Table 4–4.

Diagnostic Rate of CL(P) and CP Only in Absence/Presence of Associated Anomalies

		Number of Prenatally Diagnosed Clefts/Total Number per Category (%)	
		CL(P)	**CP Only**
All clefts	Total	148/553 (26.8)	13/198 (6.6)
	Isolated	65/366 (17.8)	1/109 (0.9)
	Associated	83/187 (44.4)	12/89 (13.5)
Clefts associated with other anomalies	Total	83/187 (44.4)	12/89 (13.5)
	Chromosomal	32/62 (51.6)	4/14 (28.6)
	Multiple anomalies	29/89 (32.6)	5/38 (13.2)
	Syndromic	22/36 (61.1)	3/37 (8.1)

CL(P): cleft lip with or without cleft palate; CP only: cleft palate only.
Data from the study by Clementi M, Tenconi R, Bianchi F, Stoll C and. EUROSCAN study group. Evaluation of prenatal diagnosis of cleft lip with or without cleft palate and cleft palate by ultrasound: Experience from 20 European registries. Prenat Diagn 2000;20:870–875, 2000.

Table 4–5.

Prenatal Screening for Fetal Face Anomalies

Imaged Plane	Visualized Facial Features	Type of Anomalies Diagnosed
Coronal	Orbits and eyes	Anomalies in position (symmetry, cyclopia), spacing (hypotelorism, hypertelorism), size (absent/small orbits and eyes, microphthalmia, anophthalmia), and content (congenital cataracts)
	Eyelids and adnexa	Eyelid anomalies (fusion) and nasolacrimal cysts
	Nose and nares	Anomalies in shape (deformities, asymmetry, saddle nose) or development (hypoplasia) and anomalies in nares direction
	Nasal bones	Morphologic anomalies and disjunction between both bones
	Philtrum	Length and (un)evenness
Sagittal	Front	Frontal bossing
	Nasal bones	Biometric anomalies
	Chin	Retrognathia, micrognathia, and mandible agenesia
	Facial angles	Open superior facial angle and closed inferior facial angle
Parasagittal	Ears	Anomalies in form, size, and position
Axial	Orbits and eyes	(See above)
	Tongue	Macroglossia
	Mandible	(See above)

(17.2%) in the years 1984–1989 to 8/15 (53.3%) % in the years 1990–1992. Similarly, Stoll et al.[15] reported an increase in the rate of prenatal recognition of facial clefts from 7/132 (5.3%) to 47/177 (26.6%) over the two time periods 1979–1988 and 1989–1998, respectively. This increase has been attributed to the improved technical expertise of the ultrasonographer and physician, as well as the regular improvements in the sono-graphic equipment and software. In particular, the use of 3D ultrasonography has improved the analysis of the fetal face.

However, this trend is absent in the series by Robinson et al.[17] who observed no difference in sonographic recognition rates of CL(P) between two 5-year periods: 1990–1995, 23/32 (72%) and 18/24 (76%) in the time period 1996–2000 ($p = 0.79$). The authors list some proposed explanations

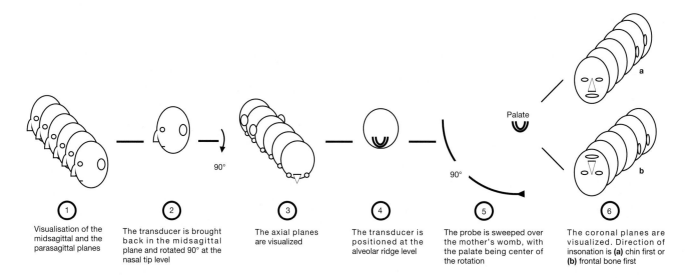

1. Visualisation of the midsagittal and the parasagittal planes

2. The transducer is brought back in the midsagittal plane and rotated 90° at the nasal tip level

3. The axial planes are visualized

4. The transducer is positioned at the alveolar ridge level

5. The probe is swept over the mother's womb, with the palate being center of the rotation

6. The coronal planes are visualized. Direction of insonation is **(a)** chin first or **(b)** frontal bone first

Figure 4–2. Technique of sonographic examination of the face.

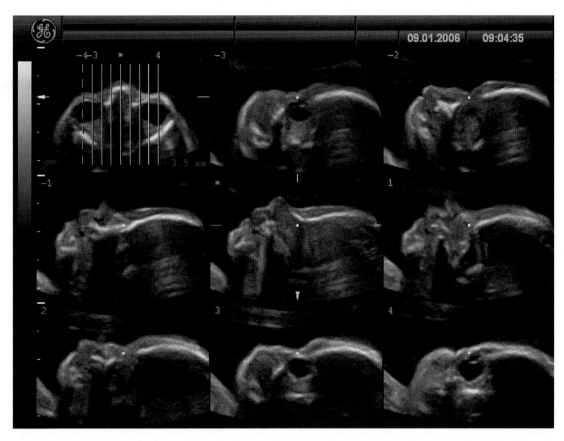

Figure 4–3. Normal face (GA: 22 weeks). Sagittal/parasagittal views: 3D multiplanar reconstruction. The following section planes are 3.9-mm spaced. They span from the right eye to the left eye level. The level of each section is shown on the axial view (upper left view).

including a high-risk population, a single center study, and all exams being performed by both a technician and a physician.

Gestational Age at Sonography

Most data addressing age at sonography and the incidence of ultrasonographic diagnosis of orofacial clefting surround the midtrimester anatomic scan, usually performed at 20–24 weeks gestation. Within this time period, the detection rate is better with advancing gestational age. For example, Robinson et al.[17] demonstrated a significant difference in the ability to detect clefts before 20 weeks of pregnancy, when compared to after that time point: 12/21 (57%) and 29/35 (83%), respectively ($p = 0.035$). The sonographic evaluation of facial clefts in the late first trimester to early second trimester is addressed later in the chapter.

FETAL FACE ANOMALIES: THE SCREENING PARADIGM

When screening for orofacial clefts, the ultrasonographer usually follows the following guidelines: (1) detect the defect, (2) precisely characterize its extent, and (3) determine if it is associated with other abnormalities, in particular other facial anomalies. In general, complete facial analysis is performed

with the same methodology as for cleft analysis, and each of the three orthogonal sonographic planes (sagittal, coronal, axial) allow for the preferential examination of the different facial organs (eyes, nose, ears) and features. The type of cleft and other facial defects (if any) direct the ultrasonographer toward specific chromosomal or syndromic associations.[18]

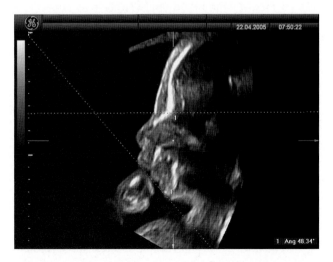

Figure 4–4. Robin sequence (GA: 24 weeks). Midsagittal 2D view: The retrognathism is readily apparent with an IFA angle = 48°.

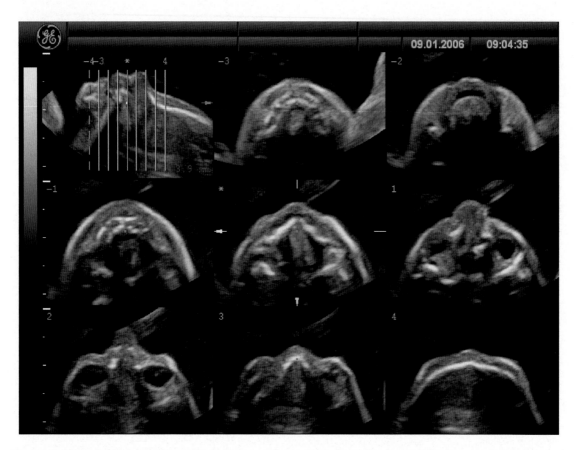

Figure 4–5. Normal face. Axial views: 3D multiplanar reconstruction. The following section planes are 3.9-mm spaced. They span from the mandible to the front level. The level of each section is shown on the sagittal view (upper left view).

The following paradigm is thus presented: (1) detection of a cleft, (2) analysis of cleft features, (3) complete facial analysis, and (4) preferential orientation toward associated pathologies. Table 4–6 lists some anomalies of the face that can lead in turn to specific diagnoses.

ULTRASOUND EXAMINATION

Using the 2D modality, a standardized technique of performing an ultrasound examination of the face is described.[19] The transducer is positioned to visualize the midsagittal plane (Fig. 4–2), and the midsagittal and sagittal planes are examined. The transducer is brought back to the midsagittal plane and rotated 90° around its axis at the level of the nasal tip (the nose being a central landmark of the face). The transducer is now along an axial plane and the axial planes are serially examined from forehead to chin. Remaining in the axial plane, the transducer is then positioned at the level of the alveolar ridge (the palate is a central landmark for facial examination). The probe is now rotated a further 90° by sweeping the transducer in an arch over the woman's abdomen until the coronal view is obtained. During the sweeping process, the fetal palate is used as the reference mark for the rotation. Usually, the probe is moved in order to identify the chin first. However, depending on the fetal position, it is sometimes easier to invert

the direction of the sweep so that the junction of the nasal bones with the frontal bone is identified first. Serial coronal planes are imaged from front (skin level) to back (bony structures).

The 3D ultrasound modality allows for a major simplification of the procedure. The 2D midsagittal view is obtained and a 3D volume data set is acquired. The 3D volume data set is displayed on the screen, using the standard multiplanar reconstruction mode. The volume data set is rotated in order to display the three reference planes (sagittal, axial, coronal). Each family of planes is then analyzed following the same systematic examination protocol as that used with 2D sonography. By scrolling through the volume, the examiner is able to move forward and backward visualizing successive parallel planes.

Three dimensional imaging offers other specific examination modalities. By using various filter settings, it is possible to preferentially image the soft or bony tissue of the examined structure. The 3D surface rendering mode provides a soft tissue rendering, thus showing surface features of the fetal face and mainly the lips. The transparency mode provides bony tissue rendering, thus showing the bony component of the examined structures and mainly the palate.

Real-time 3D, the so-called 4D modality, combines the possibility of continuous (real-time) inspection of a given structure and the adjustment of filter settings. The

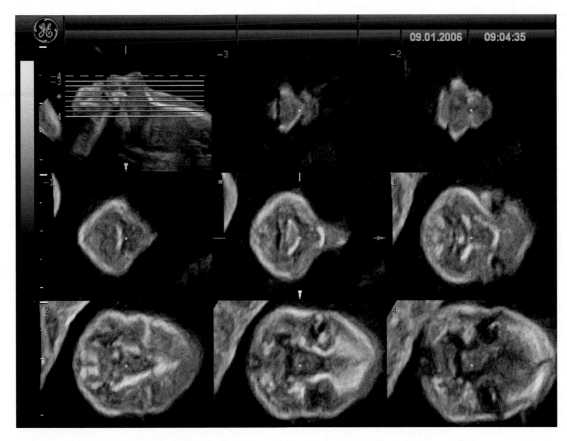

Figure 4–6. Normal face. Coronal views: 3D multiplanar reconstruction. The following section planes are 2-mm spaced. They span from the anterior "nose–mouth" view to the secondary palate level. The level of each section is shown on the sagittal view (upper left view).

3D examination begins by visual inspection of the face with real-time 3D, both with surface rendering and transparency mode. Then, the standard 3D mode is switched on. A 3D volume data set block is recorded. By using the multiplanar reconstruction mode, the different groups of planes are displayed and analyzed as explained earlier. In general, the best multiplanar reconstructions are obtained when the 3D volume data set is acquired when starting from a strict midsagittal plane.

ECHOANATOMY OF THE NORMAL FACE

Sagittal Planes

The forehead presents first as a smooth bend, then almost linear until the junction with the nasal bones. There is no prefrontal edema. The nasal bones are oblique along the frontocaudal direction. Their length is approximately one half of the total length of the nose. The columella is oblique or horizontal but should not be vertical. The philtrum is almost linear. It should not show any anterior bulging. Its length is approximately that of the columella. The secondary palate is visible behind the alveolus. It presents as a thick echoic line, beginning at the alveolar level, and extending horizontally

backward. A notch marks the middle of the secondary palate mostly visible on the superior edge. It corresponds to the transverse palatal suture. The tongue occupies the oral cavity. It is almost horizontal, its direction being slightly obliquely upward with a 10°–15° angle. The tip of the tongue lies

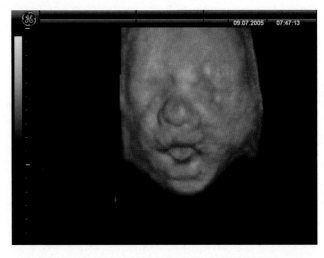

Figure 4–7. Normal face (GA: 22 weeks). Coronal view: 3D surface rendering mode. This mode focuses on the surface of the skin of the fetal face.

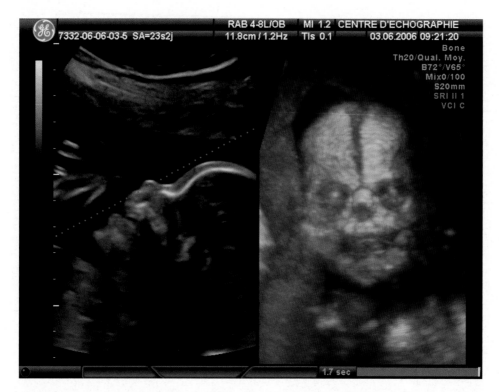

Figure 4–8. Normal face (GA: 22 weeks). Coronal view: 3D transparency mode. This mode focuses on the bony content of the fetal face. 2D sagittal view: The dotted line indicates the plane along which the 3D reconstruction is made.

Table 4–6.

Sonography of Cleft Lip, Unilateral or Bilateral

Section Planes	Unilateral Cleft	Bilateral Cleft
Sagittal and parasagittal	No direct image of the cleft can be seen on the midsagittal view. However, the modifications caused by the cleft are visible: A columella distorted and out of direction, loss of lip regularity. The parasagittal view shows the cleft of the upper lip as a defect between two thickened zones with visible asymmetry between both sides of the defect. The lips seem to end into the nostril on the pathologic side. The narinal alae is always complete but there is a flattened narinal bend (Fig. 4–9).	The normal image of the lip is replaced by a protruding soft tissue mass, the premaxillary prolabium, that projects anteriorly. The prolabium is stuck to the nose, which is consequently flattened. The columella cannot be analyzed (Fig. 4–10).
Axial	This view confirms the loss of continuity of the labial arch. The nostrils are asymmetric and distorted but the nasal alae are always present constituting a bridge over the cleft. There is flaring of the nostril on the pathologic side (Figs. 4–11 to 4–12).	The protruding prolabium is separated, on each side, from the remaining upper lip extremities by the clefts. Both nostrils are flattened but complete (Figs. 4–13 to 4–14).
Coronal	This view is the major view for the diagnosis of CL. The loss of lip continuity is clearly apparent. Clefting of the lip can extend into the nostril (Figs. 4–15 to 4–17).	The defects in lip continuity are clearly apparent (Figs. 4–18 to 4–19).

Adapted from Rotten D, Levaillant JM. Two and three dimensional sonographic assessement of the fetal face. 2. Analysis of cleft lip, alveolus, and palate. Ultrasound Obstet Gynecol 24:402–411, 2004, with modifications.

Table 4–7.

Sonography of Cleft Alveolus, Unilateral or Bilateral

Section Planes	Unilateral Cleft	Bilateral Cleft
Sagittal and parasagittal	The central parasagittal view shows, behind the slanted lip, an anechoic defect and the alveolar ridge is absent. The defect in the alveolar ridge is of variable importance: from a slight indentation in the anterior edge of the alveolar to a complete cleft (Fig. 4–9).	A mass, the premaxilla, projects anteriorly. It is clearly apparent and bulges under the nose. Careful analysis shows that the mass is of mixed structure and contains both soft and bony tissue. At the back end of the bulging mass, the absent part of the alveolar ridge is replaced by an hypoechoic zone. On both sides, this hypoechoic zone is flanked by normal alveolae (Fig. 4–10).
Axial	This view is the major view for the diagnosis of the alveolar cleft. The alveolar defect ranges from a simple slant to a cleft involving the alveolus and premaxilla. Clefts involving the alveolus present as a defect in alveolar continuity: –a simple irregularity in the alveolar lining signals an alveolar slant; –a defect in the alveolar ridge signals a total alveolar cleft; –a defect in alveolar regularity with anteroposterior shift between the two hemimaxillae signals; a cleft involving the alveolus and pre-maxilla*. (Figs. 4–11 to 4–12)	The premaxilla is protruded together with the prolabium. The premaxillary mass can be precisely analyzed (size, soft tissue, and bone content)[†]. The external parts of both alveolae are symmetrical (Figs. 4–13 to 4–14).
Coronal	There is a defect in alveolar continuity with missing buds (Fig. 4–15).	There is a median defect in alveolar continuity. This contrasts with an intact hard palate (Fig. 4–18).

*Although the clefting is complete, the shift can be limited if a cutaneous band (Simonart's band) bridges the alveolar gap and keeps the maxillary segments in good alignment.[20]

[†] In case of an associated maxillar hypoplasia, there is no protruding mass, and misdiagnosis with a median cleft is possible.[21]

Adapted from Rotten D, Levaillant JM. Two and three dimensional sonographic assessement of the fetal face. 2. Analysis of cleft lip, alveolus, and palate. Ultrasound Obstet Gynecol 24:402–411, 2004, with modifications.

immediately behind the alveolar ridge. The tongue does not move upward during the swallowing movements. Both lips rest edge to edge and share the same axis. The inferior lip is slightly posterior to the superior lip. The chin should be at the level of a straight line traced on the prefrontal skin (esthetic vertical line of the face) (Fig. 4–3). The sagittal view allows for the measurement of the length of the nasal bones, the measurement of the superior facial angle (SFA) (angle between the vertical section of the frontal bone and the nasal bones), and the measurement of the inferior facial angle (IFA). The IFA is defined by the crossing of

- a line orthogonal to the vertical section of the forehead, drawn at the level of the junction with the fetal bones ("reference line")
- a line joining the tip of the chin and the anterior border of the more protrusive lip ("profile line"). These lines are shown in Fig. 4–4.

Parasagittal Section Planes (from Midline to Lateral Planes)

The upper lip has a slightly bulging appearance. The nasal base has a gentle curvature with a concavity directed downward. It presents no discontinuity. Both nares look downward. The nostril bends are identical on both sides. The parasagittal section planes also allow for the analysis of the ears (form, position, and morphometric analysis [length and width]), an essential additional step in complete facial analysis (Fig. 4–3).

The Axial Section Planes (from Top to Bottom)

The orbits are on the same level with an interorbital axis perpendicular to the sagittal axis. The nasal septum is perpendicular to the axial planes. The two malar arches are symmetrical

Table 4–8.

Sonography of Cleft of the Secondary Palate, Uni or Bilateral

Section Planes	Secondary Palate Cleft with a Unilateral CLA	Secondary Palate Cleft with a Bilateral CLA
Midsagittal and parasagittal	The successive view shows a defect in hard palate continuity. This defect is asymmetric, median, and slighty lateralized, usually toward the same side as the CLA cleft (Fig. 4–9).	An hyperechoic midline image is present in the midsagittal view. Care must be taken when interpreting this image; although a median line is present, it is not the palate but the vomer bone. The sagittal view, the parasagittal view show the hard palate defects (Fig. 4–10).
Axial	When looking for the palate caudally to the alveolus (remember that the alveolus are separated by a defect and a shift), one does not find it. The only apparent image is that of an oblique vomer bone (10–15°) toward the side opposite to the cleft (Figs. 4–11 to 4–12).	The anteroposterior hyperechoic line corresponding to the vomer bone is present. Anteriorly, it extends into the premaxilla and prolabium. On each side of this median structure, the cleft is readily apparent (Figs. 4–13 to 4–14).
Coronal	Medially, the palatal arch is interrupted by a wide defect. Actually, this defect is not symmetrical, but slighty lateralized on the same side as the CLA cleft. Thus the two half-arches are not symmetrical. The wider half is on the non-pathologic side. The vomer bone is deflected toward the half-arch situated on the pathological side, and rests on it (Fig. 4–15).	The hard palate cannot be imaged. The vomer appears as a suspended midline with no supportive structure to rest on. The palatal arch is reduced to two small lateral structures (Fig. 4–18).

Data from Rotten D, Levaillant JM. Two and three dimensional sonographic assessement of the fetal face. 2. Analysis of cleft lip, alveolus, and palate. Ultrasound Obstet Gynecol 24:402–411, 2004, with modifications.

with regard to the nasal septum. The upper lip presents no discontinuity. The maxilla appears as a regular, U-shaped echoic bend. The tooth buds appear as hypoechoic spots regularly positioned along the alveolar ridge. There is no shift between adjacent alveolar ridges. The hard palate is hypere-

choic. Its anterior part is semicircular and lies immediately behind the alveolar ridge. The posterior part has a rectangular shape with a notch at its distal side. The tongue occupies the totality of the oral cavity and lies immediately behind the alveolar ridge. Posteriorly, the tongue extends toward the

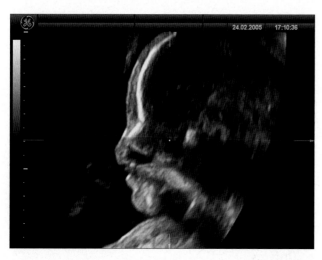

Figure 4–9. Right unilateral labioalveolar and secondary palate cleft (GA: 23 weeks). Midsagittal 2D view: There is a deformation of the columella; the superior lip is not well-defined, and the primary and secondary palate is absent.

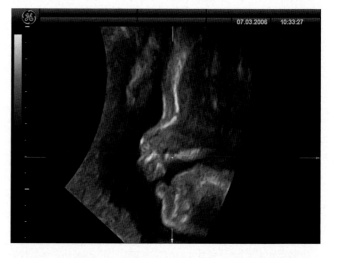

Figure 4–10. Bilateral labioalveolar and secondary palate cleft (GA: 23 weeks). Midsagittal 2D view: The prolabium–premaxilla is protruded under the nose, and the bony primary, and secondary palate are absent. The hyperechoic structure behind the protruding mass is not the palate but the vomer bone.

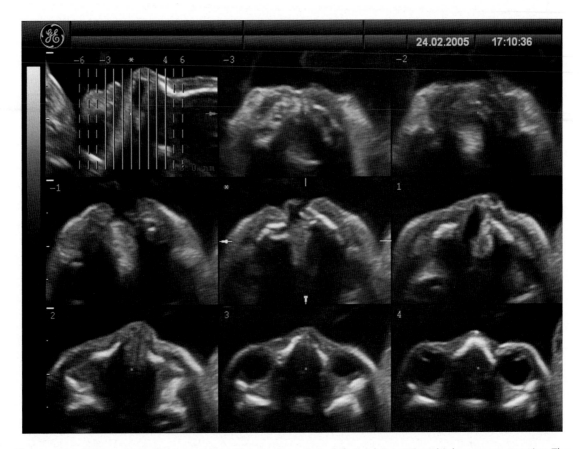

Figure 4–11. Right unilateral labioalveolar and secondary palate cleft. Axial view: 3D multiplanar reconstruction. The following section planes are 3-mm spaced. They span from the mandible to the orbit level. Level of the different sections is shown on the sagittal view (upper left view). The view at level 0 demonstrates the bipartition of the face, with an anteroposterior displacement of the two hemimaxillae.

oropharynx level. The mandible appears as an echoic image and is U-shaped (rather than the usual V-shaped description). The symphysis menti is clearly apparent. The tooth buds appear as regularly layered hypoechoic spots. The axial views allow for the measurement of the orbits (inter and outer interorbital lengths), the maxilla and mandible (maxillary width, mandibular width, and the calculated mandibular width/maxillary width ratio), and the tongue (width and length) (Fig. 4–5).

Coronal Section Planes (from Front to Back)

The anterior nose–mouth view demonstrates the soft tissues of the eyelids, the lips, and the nostrils (two little, symmetric hypoechoic areas). Both nasal alae are intact. The columella shows no discontinuity. The superior lip has a crescent shape and shows no discontinuity. The intermediate views demonstrate both orbits—the maxilla and the anterior portion of the mandible. The tooth buds appear as hypoechoic holes regularly layered along the hyperechoic alveolar ridge. The posterior view demonstrates the hard palate as bow-shaped with a symmetrical bend. On either side of midline, there is no discontinuity between the hard palate and the malar bone.

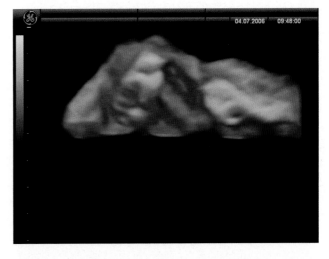

Figure 4–12. Right unilateral labioalveolar and secondary palate cleft (GA: 24 weeks). Axial view: 3D surface rendering reconstruction. The view shows the bipartition of the alveolus, primary and secondary palate, and the deviation of the vomer bone.

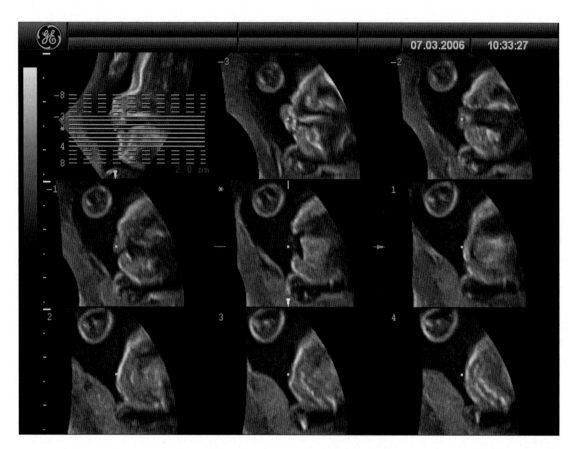

Figure 4–13. Bilateral labioalveolar and secondary palate cleft (GA: 23 wks). Axial view: 3D multiplanar reconstruction. The following section planes are 2-mm spaced. They span from the nose to the mandible. Level of the different sections is shown on the sagittal view (upper left view). The white hyperechoic line on level (−3) corresponds to the vomer bone.

In the retropalatal region, the vomer bone appears as a medial echoic spot, isolated in an empty space, with no supporting structure (Fig. 4–6 to 4–8).

SONOGRAPHIC APPEARANCE OF ANTEROLATERAL CLEFTS

Tables 4–6 to 4–8 summarize the ultrasonographic appearance of anterolateral clefts.

Can Ultrasonographic Examination Predict the Exact Extent of Anterolateral Clefts?

Minimal defects of either the soft or bony tissue are usually not amenable to sonographic diagnosis. Within these limitations, ultrasound can accurately describe unilateral or bilateral defects, as well as the extent of soft tissue clefting. The possibility of identifying palatal involvement is a recent phenomenon; and in early reports, mention of the palate referred to the alveolus. For example, Benacerraf and Mulliken reported in 1993 a series of 32 CL(P).[22] In none of the cases (two CLA, three CLAPP) was the palatal involvement diagnosed. In comparison, Nyberg et al. in 1995 reported on a series of 40 CL(P) cases,[21] where palatal involvement was recognized in the 35 cases when present. In this series, two cases were incorrectly

diagnosed. In one incorrectly diagnosed case, severe CL and CP were mistaken for a median facial cleft. This occurred because of associated hypoplasia of the primary palate that resulted in a flattened midface instead of the usual image of premaxillary protrusion. As shown in the Table 4–9,[7,8,21,23–25]

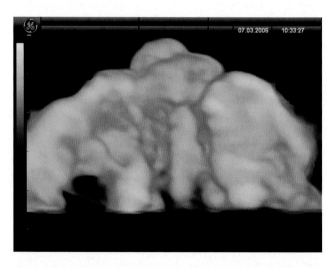

Figure 4–14. Bilateral labioalveolar and secondary palate cleft (GA: 23 wks). Axial view: 3D multiplanar reconstruction. The view shows the tripartition of the alveolus, and lips. The vomer bone is visible through the cleft palate.

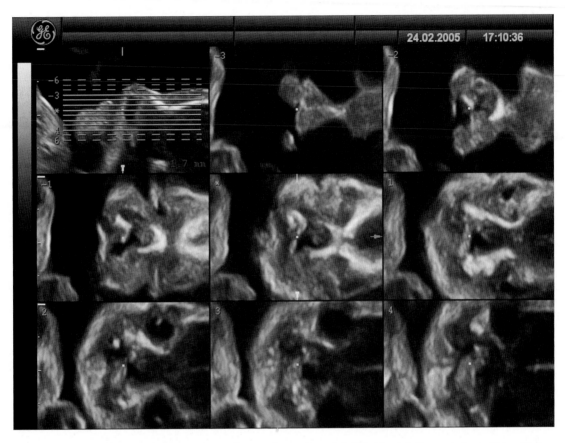

Figure 4–15. Right unilateral labioalveolar and secondary palate cleft (GA: 23 wks). Coronal views: 3D multiplanar reconstruction. The following section planes are 1.7-mm spaced. They span from the nose tip ("nose–mouth" view) to the oropharynx level. The level of the different sections is shown on the sagittal view (upper left view). The different views show the defect of the upper lip and the asymmetry of the nares. The view at level 1 demonstrates the absence of secondary palate.

palatal (alveolar) involvement can be missed but is rarely over-diagnosed.

Improvements in ultrasonographic equipment and greater expertise of the ultrasonographers have increased the likelihood of differentiating the extent of alveolar and posterior palatal clefting. Wayne et al.[26] reported on 26 cases of prenatally diagnosed CL(P), studied between 1996 and 2000. Three cases of CLA were misclassified (one for CL, two for CLAPP) and two cases of CLAPP were misclassified (one for CL and one for CLA). The other 21 cases were correctly

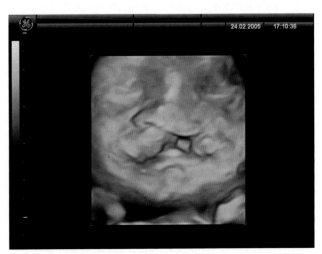

Figure 4–16. Right unilateral cleft lip (GA: 24 weeks). Coronal view: 3D surface rendering reconstruction. The view shows a small cleft lip.

Figure 4–17. Right unilateral labioalveolar and secondary palate cleft (GA: 23 wks). Coronal view: 3D surface rendering reconstruction. The view shows the wide labial cleft and the asymmetry of the nares. The cleft seems to enter into the nostril on the cleft side.

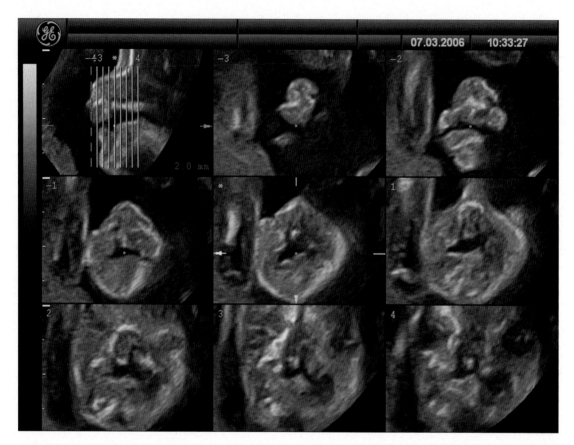

Figure 4–18. Bilateral labioalveolar and secondary palate cleft (GA: 23 wks). Coronal views: 3D multiplanar reconstruction. The following section planes are 2-mm spaced. They span from the nose tip ("nose–mouth" view) to the pharynx level. The level of the different sections is shown on the sagittal view (upper left view). The view at level 1 demonstrates the absence of the secondary palate. The median nasal cartilaginous wall appears with no structure to rely on.

diagnosed; however, the details were not given. In 2004, we published a series including 96 CL(P).[27] Only isolated clefts were included. The sonographic diagnosis was compared to the anatomic description as indicated on the operative report. This series has now been extended to include 131 CL(P) (unpublished results), as shown in Table 4–11.

The advantage of 3D ultrasonography for the exact diagnosis of cleft type has been analyzed by different investigators. Pretorius et al.[28] demonstrated that 3D technology simplifies the lip and alveolar analysis before 24 weeks of gestation. Chen et al.[29] found that the diagnosis of palatal involvement was uncertain in 15/21 (71.4%) cases utilizing 2D ultrasonography; however, with 3D technology, 21/21 cases were accurately diagnosed. Johnson et al.[30] studied 28 patients referred for suspected CL(P). The lip was incorrectly characterized in four cases with 2D (one false negative, three false positive); however, with 3D sonography it was always exact. The palate was incorrectly characterized in 15 cases with 2D (4 false negative, 10 equivocal, 1 false positive) and in 6 cases with 3D (5 equivocal, 1 false positive). However, Ghi et al.[25] reported correctly diagnosing palatal extension in 10/10 cases by using 2D ultrasonography. In addition, the authors stated that 3D technology failed to provide additional information and in one case, it was less informative than 2D technology. These authors went on to report that in the last years, they

were able to clearly image the involvement of the secondary palate when present.

The 2D–3D controversy is probably transient as 3D ultrasonography offers the additional ability of producing 2D-like images (multiplanar reconstruction) with the advantage

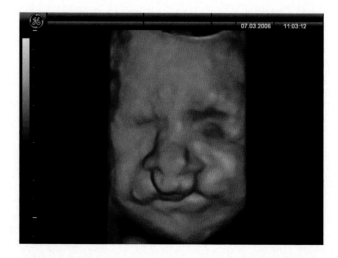

Figure 4–19. Bilateral labioalveolar and secondary palate cleft (GA: 23 wks). Coronal view: 3D surface rendering reconstruction. The bilateral cleft, with the protruding prolabium, is readily apparent.

Table 4–9.

Recognition Rate of "Palatal" (Alveolar) Involvement with Ultrasound

Study	Missed	Correctly Diagnosed	Unduly Diagnosed
Nyberg et al. (1995[21])	0	35*	0
Cash et al. [23]	0	12	1
Berge et al. [24]	2	50	0
Shaikh et al. [8]	6	8	0
Sohan et al. [7]	4	11	0
Ghi et al. [25]	0	10	0

One was misclassified as median cleft.

of easier systematization, as well as new modes of imaging (surface reconstruction, transparency mode).

ASSOCIATED ANOMALIES OF OROFACIAL CLEFTS

CL(P) may be an isolated defect or one component of a multiple defect sequence or genetic syndrome (Table 4–1a). It is important to prenatally diagnose associated anomalies, if present, as they may predict intrauterine fetal demise or severe morbidity or postnatal death, and in all cases, are likely to influence the parents' decision on continuation of the pregnancy.

The rate of associated anomalies in cases of orofacial clefting is highly variable. Milerad et al.[31] reported a series of 377 CL(P) with 302 (80.1%) isolated clefts and 75 (19.9%) having associated anomalies (CL(P), liveborn, malformation registry). Tolarova and Cervenka[32] reported 4433 CL(P) with 1935 (73.5%) isolated clefts and 699 (26.5%) having associated anomalies (CL(P), both liveborn and stillborns, malformation registry). Chmait et al.,[33] after reviewing the literature, reported the incidence of associated anomalies found in CL(P) to be 35–63%. Among the various reported series,

Table 4–10.

Concordance Between the Sonographic Description and the Anatomic Defect at Surgery

Anatomic Defect	Sonographic Result					
	CL-u	CL-b	CLA-u	CLA-b	CLAPP-u	CLAPP-b
CL-u	23				1	
CL-b						
CLA-u	2		15		4	
CLA-b				2		2
CLAPP-u	4		1		50	
CLAPP-b			1		4	22

CL-u: unilateral cleft lip; CL-b: bilateral cleft lip; CLA-u: unilateral cleft lip and alveolus; CLA-b: bilateral cleft lip and alveolus; CLAPP-u: unilateral cleft lip, alveolus, and posterior palate; CLAPP-b: bilateral cleft lip, alveolus, and posterior palate.
The darkened cells correspond to an exact sonographic diagnosis. The cells under the darkened cells correspond to an excess diagnosis with ultrasonography and the cells under to an insufficient diagnosis.

Table 4–11.			

Associated Morphologic and Chromosomal Anomalies According to the Type of Cleft

Type of Anomaly	Type of Cleft	CL(P) ($N = 57$) N (%)	CP Only ($N = 2$) N (%)	Median Cleft ($N = 11$) N (%)
Associated morphologic anomalies	Central nervous system	28 (49.1)	2 (100)	10 (90.9)
	Skeleton	23 (40.4)		6 (54.5)
	Heart	21 (36.8)	2 (100)	5 (45.5)
	Kidneys	9 (15.8)	2 (100)	5 (45.5)
	Abdomen	4 (7.0)	1 (50)	3 (27.3)
Chromosomal anomalies	Trisomy 13	18 (31.6)	2 (100)	8 (72.7)
	Trisomy 18	5 (8.8)	—	1 (9.1)
	Triploidy	1 (1.8)	—	—
	Marker chromosome	1 (1.8)	—	—

Data from Bergé SJ, Plath H, Van de Vondel PT, et al. Fetal cleft lip and palate: Sonographic diagnosis, chromosomal abnormalities, associated anomalies, and postnatal outcome in 70 fetuses. Ultrasound Obstet Gynecol 18:422–431, 2001.

anomalies differ and no specific frequency could be offered (Tables 4–11 and 4–12).[24,34] The variability among studies is due to multiple factors including the different populations analyzed[35] (malformation registries, birth certificates, postnatally referred patients).

In addition, the incidence of associated anomalies depends in part upon the anatomical type of cleft. In the series reported by Milerad et al.,[31] the overall rate of associated anomalies with CL(P) was 127/377 (33.7%). For CL only, it was 13/163 (8.0%); for unilateral CL(P), it was 35/143 (24.5%); and for bilateral CL(P), it was 25/71 (35.2%).

However, despite the significant incidence of associated anomalies, the prenatal recognition rate may be low. For instance, in the study by Chmait et al.,[33] 16 fetuses out of 45 postnatally diagnosed with CL(P) had an additional anomaly and only half of these were diagnosed prenatally.

In the study by Walker et al.,[34] the risk of an unidentified major abnormality at birth, when no anomaly was

Table 4–12.			

Associated Morphologic and Chromosomal Anomalies According to the Type of Cleft

	CL (u + b) ($N = 84$) N (%)	CLP (u + b) ($N = 179$) N (%)	CL(P) ($N = 263$) N (%)
Number prenatally diagnosed	19 (22.6)	79 (44.1)	98 (37.3)
Aneuploidy	1 (1.2)	14 (7.8)	15 (5.7)
Major associated anatomic anomalies	7 (8.3)	44 (24.6)	51 (19.4)
Sonographically detectable	1 (1.2)	23 (12.8)	24 (9.1)
Sonographically occult	6 (7.1)	21 (11.7)	27 (10.3)
Aneuploidy and major anatomic anomalies	1 (1.2)	14 (7.8)	15 (5.7)
Sonographically detectable	1 (1.2)	13 (7.3)	14 (5.3)
Sonographically occult	0 (0)	1 (0.6)	1 (0.4)

CL: cleft lip only; CLP: cleft lip and palate; u + b: unilateral + bilateral; CL(P): cleft lip with or without cleft palate.
Data from Walker SJ, Ball RH, Babcook CJ, Feldkamp MM. Prevalence of aneuploidy and additional anatomic abnormalities in fetuses and neonates with cleft lip with or without cleft palate. A population study based in Utah. J Ultrasound Med 20:1175–1180, 2001.

Table 4–13.

Isolated and Associated Clefts of the Secondary Palate

Study	CL(P)			CP Only		
	Isolated *N* (%)	Associated *N* (%)	Total	Isolated *N* (%)	Associated *N* (%)	Total
Milerad et al. [31]	302 (80.1)	75 (19.9)	377	187 (78.2)	52 (21.8)	239
Tolarova et al. [32]	1935 (73.5)	699 (26.5)	2634	784 (47.5)	867 (52.5)	1651
Clementi et al. [10]	366 (66.2)	187 (33.8)	553	109 (55.1)	89 (44.9)	198

identified prenatally with sonography, was 5/71 (7.0%). Of note, there is a strong association between anatomical and chromosomal anomalies. In the series by Walker et al.,[34] 263 CL(P) were associated with 51 major anatomical anomalies (19.4%) among which 24 (9.1%) were sonographically detectable. Fifteen fetuses were aneuploid (5.7%). Only one aneuploidy was present in a fetus with a nondetectable associated anatomical anomaly and none were present in a fetus with no associated anatomical anomaly (Table 4–12). Similarly, Nyberg et al.,[21] demonstrated a variable rate of chromosomal anomalies with cleft type. In CL alone, the incidence of a chromosomal anomaly approaches zero. This raises the question of routinely proposing to families the karyotyping of fetuses for this anomaly. This practice is not adopted by all centers. In other cases of clefting and associated anomalies, karyotyping appears indicated.

In short, presence of a CL(P) is an indication for the ultrasonographer to complete a thorough morphologic examination of the fetus. Indeed, as shown above, the type of cleft leads one to rule out potential anomalies (e.g., median cleft in brain). However, in all cases, even in the presence of a limited anomaly, the sonographic examination must be complete.

CLEFTS OF THE POSTERIOR PALATE "ONLY"

The diagnosis of CP only has long been deemed impossible at sonography. For instance, in the series reported by Clementi et al. in 2000,[10] the global antenatal recognition rate of CL(P) is 26.8% but only 6.6% for CP only. With

Table 4–14.

Sonographic Appearance of Posterior Clefts

Section Planes	Sonographic Appearance
Sagittal and parasagittal	The bony palate is evidenced in this view. Visually, it appears short with a length being usually less than 10 mm. However, this sign is conspicuous. Sagittal and parasagittal views are essential to visualize associated signs when present: retrognatism and abnormal ears (Figs. 4–4 and 4–20).
Axial	In theory, the horseshoe appearance of the bony palate should be readily apparent in this view. With present techniques, this image is almost impossible to obtain. The axial views are however of high interest to visualize associated signs: assess the integrity of the maxilla, visualize the maxilla and the mandible, analyze their shape, measure their width, and calculate the mandible width/maxilla width ratio (Ref. 19) (Fig. 4–21).
Coronal	The following level planes show a defect in the bony palatal structure. The defect appears immediately behind the alveolar arch, at a distance usually of 5–6 mm. The defect is difficult to image and the use of 3D multiplanar reconstructions is necessary (Fig. 4–22). The posterior palatal defect can also be directly imaged by combining 3D surface reconstruction and an "down to up" insonation angle. The ultrasound beam is directed in a vertex and posterior direction. The view is obtained when the fetus has an open mouth. The amniotic fluid present in the fetal oral cavity is used as a contrast liquid and the surface of the palate is imaged. The cleft palate has an horseshoe shape with a posteriorly open concavity. A technical example in a normal fetus is given in Fig. 4–23.

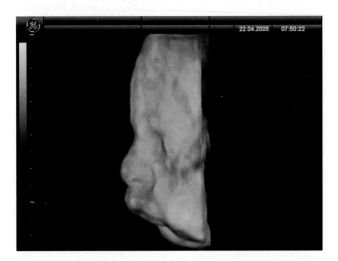

Figure 4–20. Robin sequence. 3D surface rendering mode (GA: 24 wks).

technical advances in sonographic equipment, particularly the 3D modalities, it is presently possible to image the posterior palate.[38] However, the diagnosis of CP only will probably remain sporadic as the secondary palate is routinely evaluated only in selected situation, such as the existence of specific risk factors (familial, exposure to teratogens, etc.), or the discovery of unique findings at screening sonography. When the screening ultrasound identifies malformations, an extensive search of associated malformations of the fetus, including a detailed examination of the face, is indicated. As shown in Table 4–13,[10,31,32] CP only is found to have associated anomalies in 25–50% of the cases. In addition, the recognition rate for CP only, with no other associated fetal anomalies, is particularly low when compared to CP only with associated anomalies.

During the fetal ultrasound, if an abnormal mandible if identified, this finding prompts one to examine the posterior palate, as an abnormal mandible is associated with numerous conditions that include posterior clefts. The mandible can be abnormal in shape (recessed chin or retrognathia) and/or insufficient in size (micrognathia).[36,37] The usual ultrasonographic descriptions are based on subjective (visual) descriptions: receding chin, posterior displacement of the mandible (retrognathia), and small chin, jaw, or mandible (micrognathia). Often it can be difficult to differentiate between these conditions, and the term retrognathia is sometimes used for both in the sonographic literature. However, a sonographic procedure allowing precise characterization of mandible anomalies has been described.[38] Retro/micrognathia can be

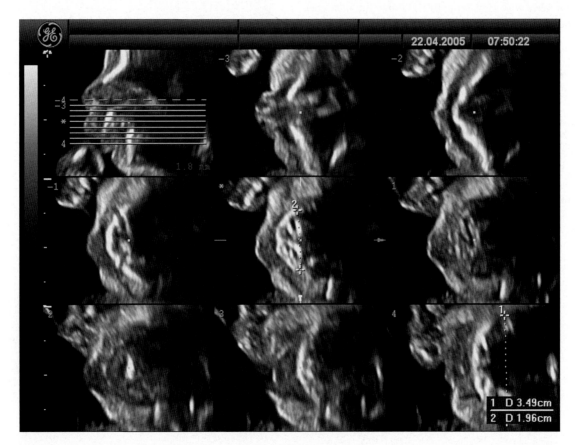

Figure 4–21. Robin sequence (GA: 24 wks). Axial views: 3D multiplanar reconstruction. The following sections are 1.8-mm spaced. They span from the malar bones (level -3) to the mandible (level +4). The level of the different sections is shown on the sagittal view (upper left view). Maxillary width is 3.49 cm (level 0). Mandibular width (measured 1 cm behind the tip of the dental arch) is 1.96 cm (level 4). Note the unusual form of the mandible, which is, in the present case, flat and wide (level 4 view).

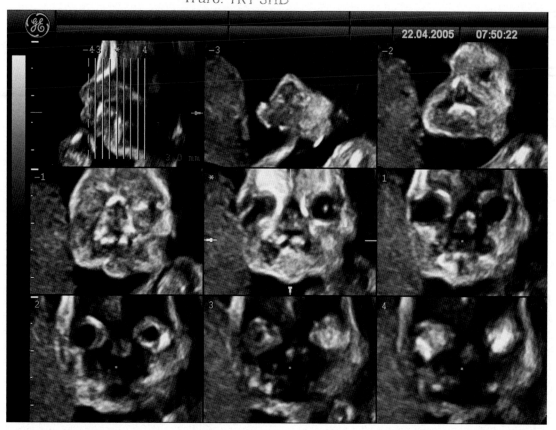

Figure 4–22. Robin sequence (GA: 24 wks). Coronal views: 3D multiplanar reconstruction. The following sections are 3-mm spaced. They span from the anterior "nose–mouth" view (nares, level -3) to the posterior end of the vomer bone (level 4). The level of each section is shown on the sagittal view (upper left view). The posterior cleft is readily apparent on levels -1 and 0.

isolated, part of a genetic or chromosomal syndrome, or part of a sequence such as *Pierre Robin sequence*. In this case, retro/micrognathia is associated with glossoptosis, an arched palate, frequently, a posterior cleft palate, and respiratory distress at birth. Some believe that retrognathia is specifically associated with Pierre Robin sequence and micrognathia with Pierre Robin "complexes"—part of a chromosomal syndrome. In rare cases, the mandible is flattened, "C" shaped, ending in a large mandible. Table 4–14 summarizes the ultrasonographic appearance of posterior clefts in Pierre Robin sequence. The situations when CP only is specifically looked for are summarized in Table 4–15.

LATE FIRST—EARLY SECOND TRIMESTER OF PREGNANCY RECOGNITION OF FACIAL CLEFTS

The embryologic development of the palate begins at the end of the sixth week of gestation, and the upper lip and the primary palate have usually fused by the seventh week of gestation. Formation of the secondary palate has occurred by fusion of the palatal shelves by the week 12 of gestation.

The soft tissues of the fetal face become distinct by the weeks 13–14 by transabdominal sonography and a little earlier by transvaginal sonography.[39] The alveolar ridge can be visualized as early as the week 14 of gestation, and the bony palate can be observed from the week 15 of gestation.[40,41]

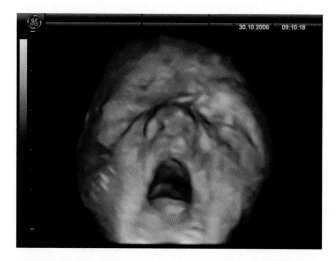

Figure 4–23. Normal fetus. Coronal 3D surface rendering mode: "down to up" angle. This view shows the technique of direct visualization of the posterior palate.

Table 4–15.

When to Search for CP Only

Anatomic anomaly discovered at screening sonography	→	Face examination?	→	CL and/or CP?	→ Cleft of the secondary palate?
Diagnosis of a CL	→	Cleft alveolus?	→	Cleft of the secondary palate?	→ Other associated malformations?
Detection of retrognathia or micrognathia	→	Cleft of the secondary palate?	→	Robin anomalad?	→ Other associated malformations?

An early prenatal diagnosis of facial clefts between weeks 10 and 17 of gestation is possible, and sporadic publications have been reported discussing the topic.[42,43] Salvedt et al.[44] published a comparative study between early and late second trimester screening. Their protocol included one coronal view of the face. The total population comprised 71 facial clefts. Recognition rates were 5/71 (7.0%) over the weeks 15–22 of gestation time range and 1/71 (1.4%) when evaluated at week 23 of gestation and greater. Bronshtein et al.[45] reported the result of systematic screening for fetal malformations with sonography in 14,988 women (1987–1993) during the late first or early second trimester of pregnancy (weeks 12–16 of gestation). The fetal face was systematically analyzed with one tangential coronal view and one sagittal paramedian view. In this series, 11/12 (91.7%) of orofacial clefts present in the population were detected. The earliest cleft diagnosis occurred at 13 weeks of gestation. The diagnosed clefts included classical and median clefts, both isolated or with associated anomalies. Although in most cases a cleft palate was present, the authors specify that only the lip malformation was detected at ultrasound. The protruding prolabium was the most characteristic sonographic sign. The cleft that was missed by ultrasound was a minimal unilateral CL. These results have been extended by Blumenfeld et al.[46] to the screening of nearly 30,000 women, over the years 1987–1999, with a detection rate of 24/25 (96.0%). According to Bronshtein et al. and Blumenfeld et al., the high efficiency of the screening is attributed to the use of the vaginal route for sonography. The fact that the face was systematically analyzed is obviously essential to the results obtained.

The studies by Bronshtein[45] and Blumenfeld[46] raise another important issue. These studies report that the number of couples who opted for termination of pregnancy, whether the cleft was isolated or associated with other anomalies, was unusually high: 23/24 (95.8%). However, these data are unique when compared to the numbers found in other studies.[40] The following questions are therefore raised: "Is the early detection of orofacial clefts responsible for this high rate of pregnancy termination?" "Or, does this unusually high rate of termination reflect the specific attitude of the population scanned?" Unfortunately at the present time, there is no definitive answer available for these questions.

In the recent years, there has been a dramatic increase in the number of sonographic examinations performed during the late first trimester (weeks 11–13 of gestation). The main goals of these early examinations are to determine the precise gestational age and to search for the presence of nuchal translucency, a sign highly indicative of aneuploidy. The increasing ability to analyze other organs, and in particular the face, at the same time will be an interesting subject of ongoing investigation and discussion. Souka et al.[47] reported the results of screening for major structural abnormalities at the 11–14-week gestation ultrasound scan. The face was examined with two views: orbits and lenses. The one CL present in the population was not diagnosed.

MEDIAN CLEFTS

Anterior midline clefts differ from anterolateral clefts in their presentation, associated chromosomal defects, associated anomalies, and ultimate outcome.[48–52] Midline clefting syndromes can be divided in two main groups:[53] the premaxillary agenesis-holoprosencephaly syndrome and the frontonasal dysplasia-median cleft syndrome.

The premaxillary agenesis-holoprosencephaly syndrome is a condition where facial anomalies are associated with brain anomalies. Facial anomalies range from minor forms such as a single maxillary central incisor to the more complete premaxillary agenesis/central clefting. Other facial anomalies can be identified, such as hypotelorism whose most severe form is seen with cyclopia. The typical brain anomaly found in this syndrome is holoprosencephaly but a variety of structural midline brain anomalies can exist, such as microcephaly or hypoplasia of the vermis.

The frontonasal dysplasias-median cleft syndrome is a condition associated with different facial anomalies such as hypertelorism and duplicated nasal structures. The antenatal diagnosis of midline clefts with sonography is usually deemed

Table 4–16.

Sonography of Median Cleft Lip (Premaxillary Agenesis-Holoprosencephaly Syndrome)

Section Planes	Ultrasonography
Midsagittal and parasagittal	The nose is flat, almost not prominent, the inferior lip is protruded. No distinct feature exists between the "tip" of the nose and the inferior lip.
Axial	The primary palate is totally absent. The secondary palate is present in the back.
Coronal	A defect is clearly apparent in the middle of the face corresponding to the absent upper lip and primary palate. The nose is absent or when present has an abnormal shape. The cleft appears as a hole in form of an uppercase "X," limited by the nose, the inferior lip, and the two defective jaws (Figs. 4–24 to 4–25).

"easy," with a central "hole" or defect in the middle of the fetal face (Table 4–16).

CONTRIBUTION OF OTHER IMAGING MODALITIES TO THE DIAGNOSIS OF FACIAL CLEFTS

MRI is noninvasive imaging tool and provides an excellent definition of soft tissues. Images obtained with MRI demonstrate sharper definition than sonography in selected fetal defects, such as those of the central nervous system. Preliminary studies have evaluated the possible contribution of MRI to the prenatal diagnosis of anterolateral facial clefts[54,55,56] with precise indications including the detection of clefts in high-risk patients and when an orofacial cleft was uncertain on ultrasonography. MRI has also been used to precisely delineate the severity of the cleft such as the presence or absence of secondary palatal defects. The studies used T2-weighted, single-shot, fast-spin echo, standard or real-time MRI. The image planes analyzed were similar to those described in the multiplanar sonographic reconstructions.

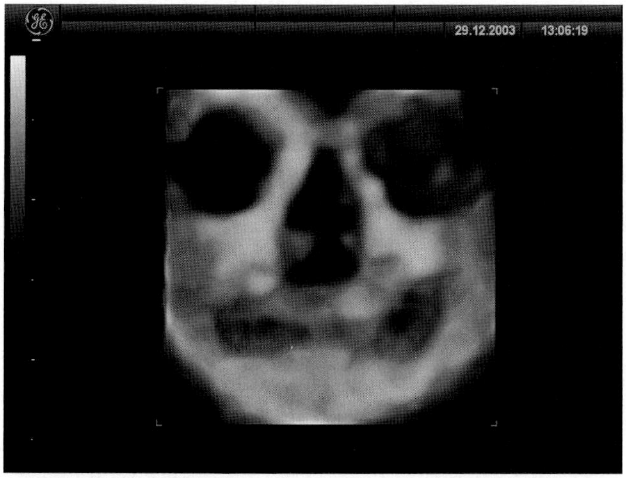

Normal Face

Sequential coronal views show the nose and lips symmetrical across midline. The axial views show the alveolus and nasal septum. Tooth buds follow a smooth and regular alignment along the maxillary arch. In the sagittal view, a hypointense strip separates the nasal fossae from the oral cavity and represents the bony palate. The bony palate extends from the upper lip anteriorly to the level of the choanae posteriorly where the nasopharynx and the oropharynx join together. The oropharynx is partially obliterated by the tongue. The soft palate is visible as a continuous arch extending posteriorly from the bony palate with a concavity inferiorly and soft tissue signal intensity. Small amounts of hyperintense fluid at the level of the pharynx may help identify the posterior limit of the soft palate.

Clefts

On coronal view, a unilateral CL is seen as a unilateral defect of the superficial soft tissue. In bilateral CLs, the protruding prolabium is clearly apparent on the sagittal view. Axial views reveal the disrupted maxillary arch with abnormal or missing tooth buds in the medial alveolar ridge. The nasal septum is deviated toward the cleft. In bilateral clefts, the protruding premaxilla is clearly apparent on midsagittal and axial views. Clefts of the secondary palate are seen on midsagittal images that demonstrate the absence of palatal tissue. Direct communication between the oropharynx and nasopharynx as well as a tongue positioned high in the oral cavity are indirect signs of a defect in soft palate continuity.

Ghi et al.[55] analyzed six fetuses with facial clefts (three CLA, three CLAPP). Ultrasound diagnosed CL(P) in all cases while MRI correctly defined two cases of CLA and two cases

Figure 4–24. Median cleft (GA: 20 weeks). Coronal view: 3D surface rendering, transparency mode. A central hole occupies most of the face. The first structure visible under the hole is the tongue.

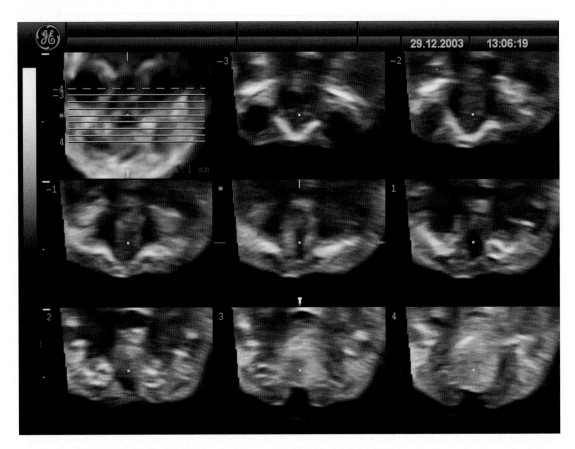

Figure 4–25. Median cleft (GA: 20 wks). Axial views, 3D multiplanar reconstruction. The following section planes are 1.1-mm spaced. The level of the different sections is shown on the coronal view (upper left view). The median cleft and the two hemimaxillae are apparent on views at levels 1, 2, and 3.

of CLAPP. In one case of CLA and one case of CLAPP, no clear sagittal view of the palatal region could be obtained with MRI and no precise definition of the defect was available. Kazan-Tannus et al.[57] investigated the use of MRI to diagnose CP only. They evaluated five fetuses at high risk of CP only. At birth, two infants had a normal palate, one had a complete posterior cleft (hard and soft palate), and two had a cleft of the soft palate only. MRI correctly diagnosed all prenatally. Despite preliminary studies and interest in MRI as an imaging modality, more studies are necessary to determine the exact role of MRI in the antenatal diagnosis of facial clefting.

MANAGEMENT OF PATIENTS WITH AN ANTENATAL DIAGNOSIS OF FETAL CLEFT PALATE

Once the prenatal diagnosis of orofacial clefting has been made, the parents should benefit from the expertise of an interdisciplinary team dedicated to the comprehensive care and rehabilitation of children with cleft-craniofacial anomalies.[58] Parental counseling is an essential component of the prenatal diagnosis and treatment program. The parent's choice to con-

tinue or terminate the pregnancy is a complicated personal decision process and they must receive thorough and honest information. This difficult decision-making process can be represented as an algorithm, as presented by Jones et al. in 2002[59] with the end question being: *"Is the defect amenable to a satisfactory correction, or does the severity of the defect and/or the associated anomalies make termination of pregnancy a legitimate option to consider?"* The questions raised by the initial steps of the algorithm may appear coldly scientific (Fig. 4–26) and include the following questions:

1. What is the reliability of the sonographic diagnosis? Is a cleft actually present?
2. What type of cleft is present, and what is the extent of the anomaly?
3. Have all the associated anomalies been visualized?
4. If associated anomalies have been found, are supplementary noninvasive and/or invasive examinations (for example, echocardiography or fetal karyotyping) available?

The final steps of the algorithm involve multiple factors such as parental beliefs, societal acceptance, legal issues, and insurance coverage. Clearly, the fallibility and uncertainty of medical science make this difficult decision one greatly

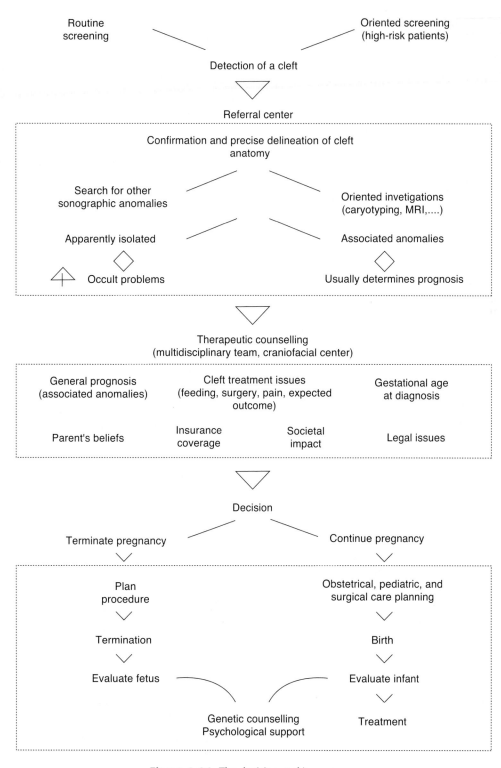

Figure 4–26. The decision-making process.

influenced by personal beliefs. The degree of risk parents are willing to accept for their unborn child's future is not a pure scientific issue.

Finally, a variety of other issues, many of them unlikely to affect all cases, may influence the decision process.[40,58–64] What follows is a brief summary of a few of these issues.

Medical Outcome of the Pregnancy

The natural history of pregnancies with orofacial clefting must be considered. Some fetuses with clefting will, in addition, have abnormal karyotypes with the potential for associated anomalies. Often, these pregnancies spontaneously abort without any medical intervention.[65,66]

Future Life of the Child and Family

The "philosophical line" between life-threatening or seriously impairing conditions and those conditions that are compatible with a normal quality of life is determined by cultural, social, and personal factors. These same factors play a role in defining what is an acceptable burden to be imposed on the child and family—prior to the end result of postnatal treatments. Some infants with orofacial clefting may experience early feeding problems and all will require several surgical procedures. Further therapy will likely involve preventive and restorative dental care, speech and language therapy, orthodonture, and otolaryngology intervention with bilateral myingotomy and tube placement along with care for repeated medial otitis.

Social Issues

Despite the advances in the comprehensive care of cleft patients, including surgical outcomes that often result in minimal postoperative stigmata of clefting, repeated visits with health care providers and recurrent hospitalizations, may extract a toll on the young patient. The question of how residual speech, dental, or physical stigmata of clefting will affect the child's psychosocial development and their peer's acceptance remains.

Regulatory and Legal Issues

The parental right to choose termination of a pregnancy varies among countries and jurisdictions and other factors, such as gestational age, play important roles. With respect to legal nuances, there have been cases documented where families have sued physicians for allegedly providing incorrect or incomplete information that did not enable them to seek for pregnancy termination ("wrongful birth suit"). Similarly, children or their representatives have sued the medical team with the allegation that their burden is too heavy to bear and that it would have been better not to be born at all ("wrongful life suit"). The question naturally arises, "*Will we see children with antenatally diagnosed anomalies suing their own parents for 'incorrect prenatal care' resulting in the inappropriate decision regarding their birth as they had the information but chose not to abort?*" On the contrary, families have considered the prenatal information provided too pessimistic and that this resulted in the inappropriate request for pregnancy termination.

Financial Issues

A multitude of questions addressing the financial ramifications of antenatally diagnosed fetal anomalies arise. Will there be insurance coverage to cover the costs of the child's treatment? Who will financially cover the potential special needs (medical care, orthodonture, speech therapy, assistance in daily life and school, etc) over the life of the child? A very critical question remains, "*Can an antenatally diagnosed anomaly be considered 'a preexisting condition' and result in exclusion from insurance benefits?*"

Conflict of Interest

Among the many issues raised regarding prenatal diagnosis and counseling of parents, some involve the medical team. Although counselors should only help the parents to arrive at a decision based on their own judgment, it has been shown that the doctor's own feelings and beliefs influence the parent's choice. Furthermore, a conflict of interest exists for the medical team, particularly the cleft-craniofacial team, as the parental decision to terminate pregnancy will eliminate a potential patient.

Fetal Surgery

At the present time, fetal surgery is not an option for orofacial clefting as the risk–benefit for the fetus and mother is felt to be too great. However, some of these same risk–benefit issues are common with postnatal appearance-related facial surgery.

Ethical Issues

In addition to the traditional ethical issues regarding the interruption of life that accompany prenatal diagnosis and treatment, a more universal ethical issue with regard to society as a whole exists. The elimination of diseased subjects raises both the question of tolerating human difference in a society and the potential reduction in the variability of the human genome.

References

1. Dommergues M, Lemerrer M, Couly G, Delezoide Al, Dumez Y. Prenatal diagnosis of cleft lip at 11 menstrual weeks using embryoscopy in the Van der Woude syndrome. *Prenat Diagn* 15:378–381, 1995.
2. Raposio E, Panarese P, Santi P. Fetal unilateral cleft lip and palate: Dectection of enzymic anomalies in the amniotic fluid. *Plast Reconstr Surg* 103:391–394, 1999.
3. Christ JE, Meininger MG. Ultrasound diagnosis of cleft lip and cleft palate before birth. *Plast Reconstr Surg* 68:854–859, 1981.
4. Savoldelli G, Schmid W, Schinzel A. Prenatal diagnosis of cleft lip and palate by ultrasound. *Prenat Diagn* 2:313–317, 1982.
5. Seeds JW, Cefalo RC. Technique of early sonographic diagnosis of bilateral cleft lip and palate. *Obstet Gynecol* 62(Suppl):2S–7S, 1983.
6. Benacerraf BR, Frigoletto FD, Jr., Bieber FR. The fetal face: Ultrasound examination. *Radiology* 153:495–497, 1984.
7. Shaikh D, Mercer NS, Sohan K, Kyle P, Soothill P. Prenatal diagnosis of cleft lip and palate. *Brit J Plast Surg* 54:288–289, 2001.
8. Sohan K, Freer M, Mercer N, Soothil P, Kyle P. Prenatal detection of facial clefts. *Fetal Diagn Therap* 16:196–199, 2001.
9. Vial Y, Tran C, Addor MC, Hohlfeld P. Screening for fetal malformations: Performance of routine ultrasonography in the population of the Swiss Canton of Vaud. *Swiss Med Wkly* 131:490–494, 2001.
10. Clementi M, Tenconi R, Bianchi F, Stoll C, and EUROSCAN study group. Evaluation of prenatal diagnosis of cleft lip with or without cleft palate and cleft palate by ultrasound: Experience from 20 European registries. *Prenat Diagn* 20:870–875, 2000.
11. Ewigman BG, Crane JP, Frigoletto FD, LeFevre ML, Bain RP, McNellis D. The RADIUS study group. Effect of prenatal ultrasound screening on prenatal outcome. *New Engl J Med* 329:821–827, 1993.

12. American Institute of Ultrasound in Medicine. AIUM practice guideline for the performance of an antepartum obstetric ultrasound examination. AUIM guidelines, 2003. *J Ultrasound Med* 22:1116–1125, 2003.

13. Babcook CJ, McGahan JP, Chong BW, Nemzek WR, Salamat MS. Evaluation of fetal midface anatomy related to facial clefts: Use of US. *Radiology* 201:113–118, 1996.

14. Hanikeri M, Savundra J, Gillett D, Walters M, McBain W. Antenatal transabdominal ultrasound detection of cleft lip and palate in Western Australia from 1996 to 2003. *Cleft Palate Craniofac J* 43:61–66, 2006.

15. Stoll C, Dott B, Alembik Y, Roth MP. Evaluation of prenatal diagnosis of cleft lip/palate by fetal ultrasonographic examination. *Ann Genet* 43:11–14, 2000.

16. Levi S, Schaaps JP, De Havay P, Coulon R, Defoort P. End-result of routine ultrasound screening for congenital anomalies: The Belgian multicentric study 1984–1992. *Ultrasound Obstet Gynecol* 5:366–371, 1995.

17. Robinson JN, McElrath TF, Benson CB, et al. Prenatal ultrasonography and the diagnosis of fetal cleft lip. *J Ultrasound Med* 20:1165–1170, 2001.

18. Pashayan HM. What else to look for in a child born with a cleft of the lip and/or palate. *Cleft Palate J* 20:54–82, 1983.

19. Rotten D, Levaillant JM. Two- and three-dimensional sonographic assessment of the fetal face. 1. A systematic analysis of the normal face. *Ultrasound Obstet Gynecol* 23:224–231, 2004.

20. Mulliken JB, Benacerraf BR. Prenatal diagnosis of cleft lip. What the sonologist needs to tell the surgeon. *J Ultrasound Med* 20:1159–1164, 2001.

21. Nyberg DA, Sickler GK, Hegge FN, Kramer DJ, Kropp RJ. Fetal cleft lip with and without cleft palate: US classification and correlation with outcome. *Radiology* 195:677–684, 1995.

22. Benacerraf BR, Mulliken JB. Fetal cleft lip and palate: Sonographic diagnosis and postnatal outcome. *Plast Reconstr Surg* 92:1045–1051, 1993.

23. Cash C, Set P, Coleman N. The accuracy of antenatal ultrasound in the detection of facial clefts in a low-risk screening population. *Ultrasound Obstet Gynecol* 18:432–436, 2001.

24. Bergé SJ, Plath H, Van de Vondel PT, et al. Fetal cleft lip and palate: Sonographic diagnosis, chromosomal abnormalities, associated anomalies, and postnatal outcome in 70 fetuses. *Ultrasound Obstet Gynecol* 18:422–431, 2001.

25. Ghi T, Perolo A, Banzi C, et al. Two-dimensional ultrasound is accurate in the diagnosis of fetal craniofacial malformation. *Ultrasound Obstet Gynecol* 19:543–551, 2002.

26. Wayne C, Cook K, Sairam S, Hollis B, Thilaganathan B. Sensitivity and accuracy of routine antenatal ultrasound screening for isolated facial clefts. *Brit J Radiol* 45:584–589, 2002.

27. Rotten D, Levaillant JM. Two and three dimensional sonographic assessement of the fetal face. 2. Analysis of cleft lip, alveolus, and palate. *Ultrasound Obstet Gynecol* 24:402–411, 2004.

28. Pretorius DH, House M, Nelson TR, Hollenbach KA. Evaluation of normal and abnormal lips in fetuses: Comparison between three- and two-dimensional sonography. *Am J Roentgenol* 165:1233–1237, 1995.

29. Chen ML, Chang CH, Yu CH, Cheng YC, Chang FM. Prenatal diagnosis of cleft palate by three-dimensional ultrasound. *Ultrasound Med Biol* 27:1017–1023, 2001.

30. Johnson DD, Pretorius DH, Budorick NE, et al. Three-dimensional ultrasound of the fetal lip and palate. *Radiology* 217:236–239, 2000.

31. Milerad J, Larson O, Hagberg C, Ideberg M. Associated malformations in infants with cleft lip and palate. A prospective, population-based study. *Pediatrics* 100:180–186, 1997.

32. Tolarova MM, Cervenka J. Classification and birth prevalence of orofacial clefts. *Am J Med Genet* 75:126–137, 1998.

33. Chmait R, Pretorius D, Moore T, et al. Prenatal detection of associated anomalies in fetuses diagnosed with cleft lip with or without cleft palate in utero. *Ultrasound Obstet Gynecol* 27:173–176, 2006.

34. Walker SJ, Ball RH, Babcook CJ, Feldkamp MM. Prevalence of aneuploidy and additional anatomic abnormalities in fetuses and neonates with cleft lip with or without cleft palate. A population study based in Utah. *J Ultrasound Med* 20:1175–1180, 2001.

35. Wyszynski DF, Sarkösi A, Czeizel AE. Oral clefts with associated anomalies: Methodological issues. *Cleft Palate Craniofac J* 43:1–6, 2006.

36. Cohen MM, Jr. Robin sequences and complexes: Causal heterogeneity and pathogenic/phenotypic variability. *Am J Med Gen* 84:311–315, 1999.

37. Cohen MM, Jr. Interface between Robin sequence and ordinary cleft palate. *Am J Med Genet* 101:288, 2001.

38. Rotten D, Levaillant JM, Martinez H, Ducou Le Pointe H, Vicaut E. The fetal mandible: A 2D and 3D sonographic approach to the diagnosis of retrognathia and micrognathia. *Ultrasound Obstet Gynecol* 19:122–130, 2002.

39. Cockell A, Lees M. Prenatal diagnosis and management of orofacial clefts. *Prenat Diagn* 20:149–151, 2000.

40. Johnson N, Sandy J. Prenatal diagnosis of cleft lip and palate. *Cleft Palate Craniofac J* 40:186–189, 2003.

41. Sherer DM, Sokolovski M, Abulafia O. Nomogram of ultrasonic measurements of the fetal hard palate width, length, and area throughout gestation. *Ultrasound Obstet Gynecol* 24:35–41, 2003.

42. Picone O, de Keersmaecker B, Ville Y. Ultrasonic features of orofacial clefts at first trimester of pregnancy: Report of two cases. *J Gynecol Obstet Biol Reprod* 32(Suppl 1):736–739, 2003.

43. Hafner E, Sterniste W, Scholler J, Schuchter K, Philipp K. Prenatal diagnosis of facial malformations. *Prenat Diagn* 17:51–58, 1997.

44. Saltvedt S, Almstrom H, Kublickas M, Valentin L, Grunewald C. Detection of malformations in chromosomally normal fetuses by routine ultrasound at 12 or 18 weeks of gestation. A randomised controlled trial in 39572 pregnancies. *Brit J Obstet Gynaecol* 113:664–674, 2006.

45. Bronshtein M, Blumenfeld I, Kohn J, Blumenfeld I. Detection of cleft lip by early second trimester transvaginal sonography. *Obstet Gynecol* 84:73–76, 1994.

46. Blumenfeld Z, Blumenfeld I, Bronshtein M. The early prenatal diagnosis of cleft and the decision-making process. *Cleft Palate Craniofac J* 36:105–107, 1999.

47. Souka AP, Pilalis A, Kavalakis I, et al. Screening for major structural abnormalities at the 11- to 14-week ultrasound scan. *Am J Obstet Gynecol* 194:393–396, 2006.

48. Nyberg DA, Mack LA, Bronstein A. Holoprosencephaly: Prenatal sonographic diagnosis. *AJR Am J Roentgenol* 149:1051–1058, 1987.

49. McGahan J, Nyberg DA, Mack LA. Sonography of facial features of alobar and semilobar holoprosencephaly. *AJR Am J Roentgenol* 154:143–148, 1990.

50. Benacerraf BR. Prenatal sonography of autosomal trisomies. *Ultrasound Obstet Gynecol* 1:66–75, 1991.

51. Nicolaides KH, Salvesen DR, Snijders RJM, Gosden CM. Fetal facial defects: Associated malformations and chromosomal anomalies. *Fetal Diagn Ther* 8:1–9, 1993.

52. Chen CP. Prenatal sonographic diagnosis of median facial cleft should alert holoprosencephaly with premaxillary agenesis and prompt genetic investigations. *Ultrasound Obstet Gynecol* 19:421–422, 2002.

53. Thorne CH. Craniofacial clefts. *Clin Plast Surg* 20:803–814, 1993.

54. Benacerraf BR, Sadow PM, Barnewolt CE, Estroff JA, Benson C. Cleft of the secondary palate without cleft lip diagnosed with three-dimensional ultrasound and magnetic resonance imaging in a fetus with Fryns' syndrome. *Ultrasound Obstet Gynecol* 27:566–570, 2006.

55. Ghi T, Tani G, Savelli L, Colleoni GG, Pilu G, Bovicelli L. Prenatal imaging of facial clefts by magnetic resonance imaging with emphasis on the posterior palate. *Prenat Diagn* 23:970–975, 2003.

56. Smith AS, Estroff JA, Barnewolt CE, Mulliken JB, Levine D. Prenatal diagnosis of cleft lip and cleft palate using MRI. *AJR Am J Roentgenol* 183:229–235, 2004.

57. Kazan-Tannus JF, Levine D, McKenzie C, et al. Real-time magnetic resonance imaging aids prenatal diagnosis of isolated cleft palate. *J Ultrasound Med* 24:1533–1540, 2005.

58. Elmendorf EN, III, D'Antonio LL, Hardesty RA. Assessment of the patient with cleft lip and palate. A developmental approach. *Clin Plast Surg* 20:607–621, 1993.

59. Jones MC. Prenatal diagnosis of cleft lip and palate: Detection rates, accuracy of ultrasonography, associated anomalies and strategies for counselling. *Cleft Palate Craniofac J* 39:169–173, 2002.

60. Moss A. Controversies in cleft lip and palate management. *Ultrasound Obstet Gynecol* 18:420–421, 2001.

61. Aspinall CL. Dealing with the prenatal diagnosis of clefting: A patient's perspective. *Cleft Palate Craniofac J* 39:183–187, 2002.

62. Strauss RP. Beyond easy answers: Prenatal diagnosis and counselling during pregnancy. *Cleft Palate Craniofac J* 39:164–168, 2002.

63. Saal HM. Prenatal diagnosis: When the clinician disagrees with the patient's decision. *Cleft Palate Craniofac J* 39:174–178, 2002.

64. Matthews MS. Beyond easy answers: The plastic surgeon and prenatal diagnosis. *Cleft Palate Craniofac J* 39:179–182, 2002.

65. Bergé SJ, Plath H, von Lindern JJ. Natural history of 70 fetuses with a prenatally diagnosed orofacial cleft. *Fetal Diagn Therapy* 17:247–251, 2002.

66. Kraus BS, Kitamura H. Malformations associated with cleft lip and palate in human embryos and fetuses. *Am J Obstet Gynecol* 86:321–327, 1963.

5

Prenatal and Genetic Counseling

Donna M. McDonald-McGinn, MS, CGC • Deborah Driscoll, MD • Martha Matthews, MD

Prenatal detection of a craniofacial anomaly such as cleft lip and/or cleft palate, regardless of the severity, may be devastating to the family that then mourns the loss of the expected "normal" child. However, the manner in which the information is delivered, the subsequent diagnostic evaluations, and the opportunity to speak with experienced professionals and support organizations can substantially reduce the burden on the family. In fact, some couples may consider the prenatal recognition of a cleft to be "a positive" in hindsight, since it offers the family and the medical staff the opportunity to prepare for the birth of the affected child or to consider alternative reproductive options.

In general, families come to the attention of a genetic counselor in one of two ways. They may present with a family history of orofacial clefting or following the detection of a cleft during routine prenatal ultrasonography. Once the diagnosis of a cleft is made, multiple concerns may arise for both patients and caregivers regarding the prognosis, etiology, recurrence risk, and potential prenatal and postnatal interventions. In order to provide any of this information, an accurate diagnosis is required. Thereafter, the following questions can be better answered: Is this problem genetic? If so, what is the cause (i.e., a chromosomal abnormality, a single gene disorder, a teratogen such as maternal alcohol exposure, a sporadic occurrence (50–75%), or a multifactorial problem)?[1] What is the prognosis? And, how complicated is the potential treatment?

Establishing a diagnosis, especially in the unborn patient, is complex and requires multiple components. These include a complete family history, further diagnostic testing, and at times, referrals to other subspecialists and a physical examination of the parents.

Specifically, the family history should include information regarding: relatives with clefts and/or other con-genital anomalies (congenital heart disease, for example, or later onset problems such as significant myopia, cataracts, glaucoma, hearing loss, psychiatric disease, etc.); spontaneous miscarriages or intrauterine fetal deaths; mental retardation, learning disabilities, or behavioral health issues; consanguinity; and prenatal teratogenic exposures such as alcohol and anticonvulsive agents. Whenever possible, the parents should be examined to obtain standard growth parameters, including height and head circumference, as well as more specific measures such as interpupillary distance; intraoral inspection with careful attention to abnormalities of the uvula, frenulum, and dentition; and evaluation for lip pits and general dysmorphology. In addition, some situations dictate parental evaluation by a subspecialist such as an ophthalmologist to rule out the presence of high myopia or retinal abnormalities associated with Stickler syndrome, while others require laboratory studies to exclude familial aneuploidy masquerading as an autosomal dominant disorder.[2]

Further evaluation of the fetal anatomy often includes a subsequent or serial high-level ultrasonography (Fig. 5–1) and/or 3D (Fig. 5–2) or 4D ultrasound, a fetal echocardiogram, and a fetal MRI. Laboratory studies most often performed via amniocentesis include chromosome analysis to rule out aneuploidy, fluorescence in situ hybridization (FISH), comparative genomic hybridization (CGH), biochemical studies, and direct mutational analysis.

Prenatal consultations with subspecialists are especially helpful to families in order to best understand the postnatal ramifications for their offspring. These frequently include discussions with plastic surgery, ENT, and genetics but may also include meetings with cardiology, neurology, neurosurgery, orthopedics, ophthalmology, etc., depending on the prenatal findings.

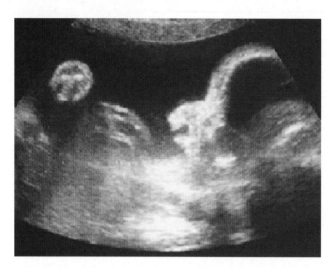

Figure 5–1. Prenatal ultrasonography frequently identifies cleft lip, as seen here on this fetal profile. (*Image courtesy of Natalie Blagowidow, MD.*)

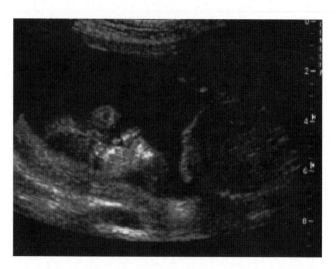

Figure 5–3. A midline cleft lip, as seen here on prenatal ultrasonography, led to the diagnosis of holoprosencephaly in this fetus. (*Image courtesy of Natalie Blagowidow, MD.*)

In addition to gathering the above information, the type of cleft is exceedingly important, as it too helps to narrow the differential diagnosis. It is generally accepted that "the face predicts the brain," and therefore a midline cleft (Fig. 5–3) is a clue to the potential diagnosis of holoprosencephaly, wherein there is failure of the developing forebrain to divide into two separate hemispheres. Importantly, holoprosencephaly encompasses a continuum of brain malformations including alobar, wherein there is a single ventricle and no separation of the cerebral hemispheres; semilobar, wherein the left and right frontal and parietal lobes are fused, and the

interhemispheric fissure is only present posteriorly; and lobar, wherein most of the right and left cerebral hemispheres and lateral ventricles are separated, but the most rostral aspect of the telencephalon, the frontal lobes, are fused, especially ventrally. Developmental delay is present in all patients, seizures are common, and severely affected children do not survive beyond early infancy; however, more mildly affected children generally survive past 12 months of age with varying degrees of disabilities. In addition, craniofacial findings vary widely among patients with holoprosencephaly, with cyclopia being the most severe presentation. Many patients present with a midline cleft (Fig. 5–4), whereas others will have a milder phenotype, including bilateral cleft lip and palate, unilateral cleft lip and palate, bifid uvula, or simple absence of the superior labial frenulum. Holoprosencephaly is also etiologically heterogeneous, with 25–50% of cases due to chromosomal abnormalities (trisomy 13, trisomy 18, and triploidy, for example), with trisomy 13 being the most commonly associated cytogenetic cause (Fig. 5–5). Other chromosomal

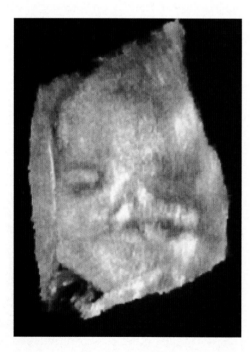

Figure 5–2. A unilateral cleft lip is seen here on a 3D ultrasound. Unlike the traditional ultrasound, 3D ultrasound waves are directed from multiple angles. These waves are reflected back, captured, and used to construct a three-dimensional image. When captured rapidly and animated, a 4D ultrasound is produced. (*Image courtesy of Natalie Blagowidow, MD.*)

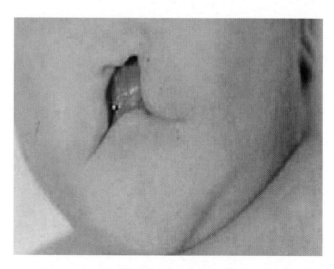

Figure 5–4. A midline cleft lip is seen here in a newborn with holoprosencephaly. (*Image courtesy of Elaine H. Zackai, MD.*)

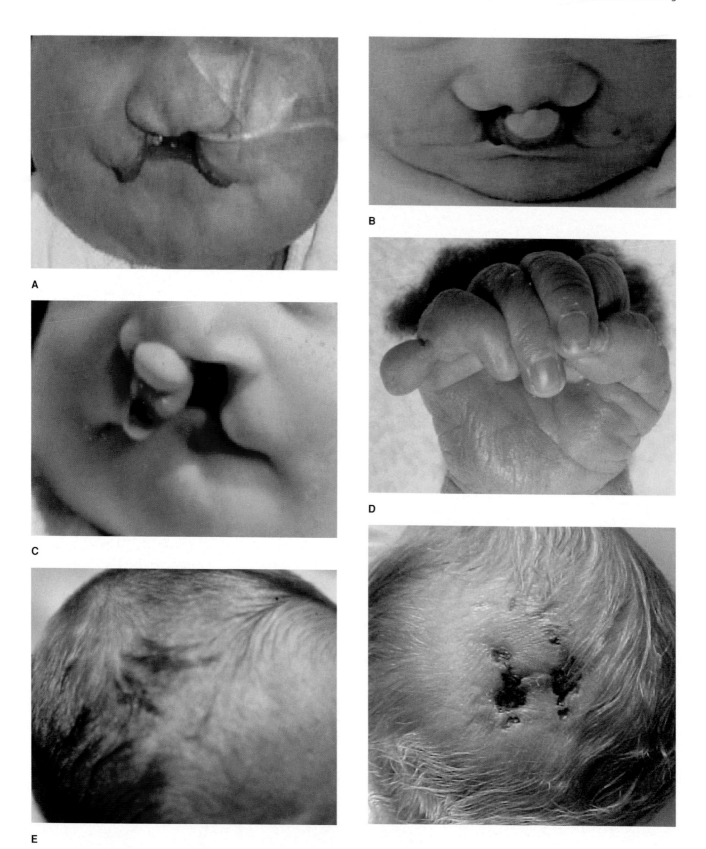

Figure 5–5. Three patients are shown here, each with trisomy 13 but demonstrating significant phenotypic variability: (A) With a midline cleft lip and palate; (B) with a bilateral cleft lip and palate; (C) with a unilateral cleft lip and palate. Additional features often associated with trisomy 13 include (D) postaxial polydactyly and (E) posterior scalp defects.

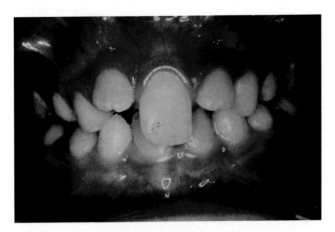

Figure 5–6. A single central maxillary incisor, as seen here, has been seen as a form fruste sign of autosomal dominant holoprosencephaly.

aneuploidies causing holoprosencephaly include deletions and duplications of 13q, deletions of 2p21, deletions of 7q36, deletions of 18p, deletions of 21q22.3, and duplications of 3p24-pter. Furthermore, with the advent of more sophisticated laboratory studies such as FISH, CGH, and whole genome array, submicroscopic chromosomal deletions which include genes that cause holoprosencephaly, such as sonic hedgehog (*SHH*) on chromosome 7q and *TGIF* on chromosome 18p11.3, have been identified in up to 5% of affected individuals. In addition, approximately 18–25% of patients with holoprosencephaly have a mutation in a single gene, and at least 25 separate conditions have been described where holoprosencephaly is an occasional finding. Genes associated with the autosomal dominant forms of holoprosencephaly include: *SHH*, *ZIC2*, *SIX3*, *TGIF*, and *PATCHED-1* (*PTCH*). Importantly, it is estimated that about one-third of individuals with a mutation causing an autosomal dominant form of

holoprosencephaly are asymptomatic and are normal intellectually. This data underscores the need to obtain a careful family history, as well as to examine parents for "forme fruste" signs of holoprosencephaly, such as a single central maxillary incisor (Fig. 5–6), short stature, anosmia, or growth hormone deficiency prior to providing recurrence risk counseling for such families. Lastly, holoprosencephaly can be seen as the result of a teratogenic exposure, such as maternal diabetes. In fact, infants of diabetic mothers have a 200-fold increase in their risk for holoprosencephaly. Additional teratogenic agents include alcohol, retinoic acid, and perhaps cholesterol lowering drugs such as statins. Thus, holoprosencephaly is an important cause of clefting and should always be considered in the prenatal differential diagnosis when a fetal cleft is appreciated. It is found in 1:250 embryos and in 1:10,000 to 1:20,000 live births.[3] It is important to note that midline clefts are also found in oral–facial–digital syndrome type I (Fig. 5–7), Ellis-van Creveld syndrome, and Majewski short-rib polydactyly syndrome type II, to name a few. However, these syndromes will generally have extracraniofacial findings, such as polydactyly, that may be observed using additional imaging studies.

Unilateral or bilateral cleft lip and/or palate (Fig. 5–8) are found in approximately 1:1000 Caucasian births[1] and can also be seen as part of multiple congenital anomaly syndromes with a variety of etiologies, including chromosomal abnormalities, single gene disorders, teratogens, and sporadic conditions.

Chromosomal aneuploidy associated with orofacial clefting includes the trisomies (in particular, trisomy 13), as well as Wolf-Hirschorn syndrome (deletion 4p), the 22q11.2 deletion, and numerous other numeric deletions or duplications that typically include additional anatomic structural abnormalities and cognitive deficits. These associations

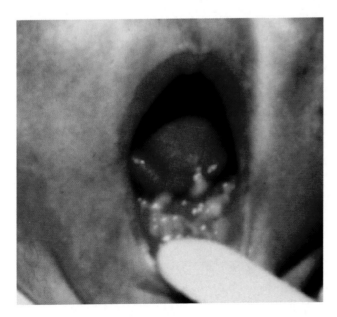

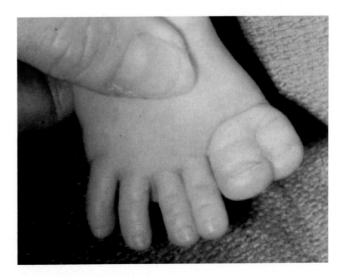

Figure 5–7. Patients with oral–facial–digital syndrome type I often present with a small midline cleft lip, lingual lumps, multiple frenula, and preaxial polydactyly as seen here.

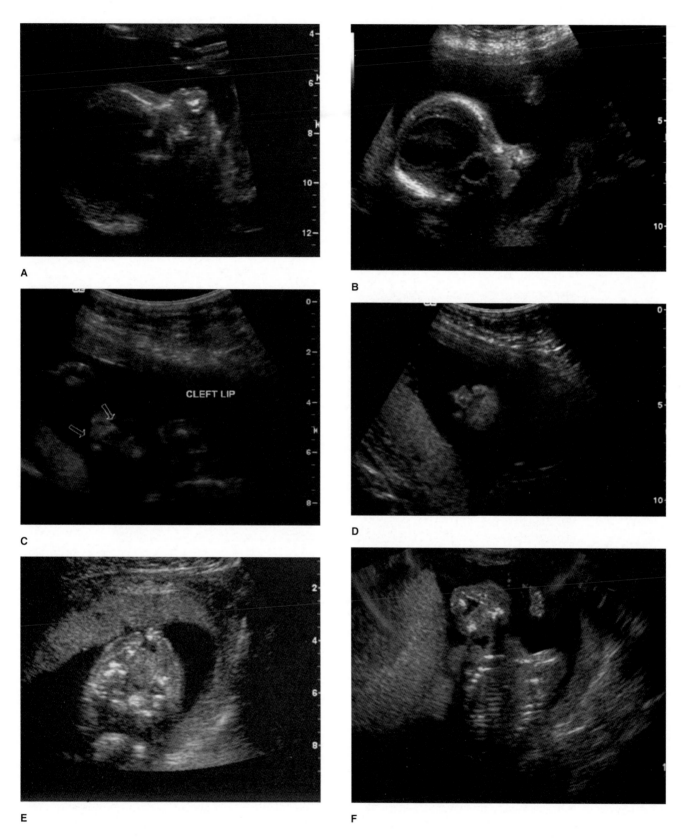

Figure 5–8. Utilizing prenatal ultrasonography, bilateral cleft lip and palate is appreciated here on both lateral (A, B) and transverse (C, D) views, whereas a unilateral cleft lip and palate is seen in two fetuses on a transverse view (E, F). (*Image courtesy of Natalie Blagowidow, MD.*)

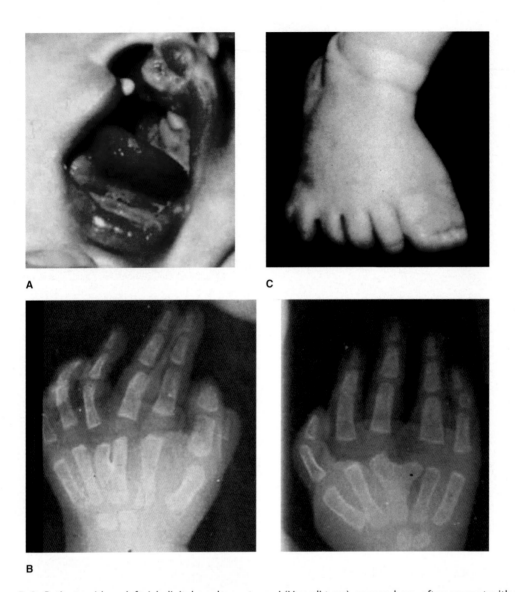

Figure 5–9. Patients with oral–facial–digital syndrome type vi (Varardi type), as seen here, often present with cleft lip and palate (A); pre- and postaxial polydactyly of the hands, as well as central polydactyly, which is characterized by a single Y-shaped metacarpal (B) and polysyndactyly of the feet (C).

support consideration of prenatal chromosome analysis, as well as additional imaging studies, when a cleft is identified.

Single gene cleft disorders, on the contrary, are more variable and include many well-described autosomal dominant conditions, such as Van der Woude and popliteal pterygium syndromes, due to mutations in *IRF6*, and Rapp Hodgkin ectodermal dysplasia and EEC syndromes, which are both due to mutations in *P63*. Oral–facial–digital syndrome type VI (Varardi type) (Fig. 5–9) is an autosomal recessive cause of cleft lip, whereas Opitz G/BBB syndrome (Fig. 5–10) is heterogeneous, with autosomal dominant and X-linked recessive inheritance having been described, as well as an association with 22q11.2 deletions.[4–7] Fetal Hydantoin/Dilantin exposure is a known teratogenic cause of clefting. Again, these associations support consideration of additional prenatal imaging studies when a cleft is identified, as well as a careful family/pregnancy history and parental examinations. Lastly, cleft lip and/or cleft palate are seen in sporadic condi-

tions such as Goldenhar/oculo-auriculo-vertebral spectrum, which may be due to an embryonic vascular disruption.

Cleft palate (Fig. 5–11), which is often more difficult to observe on prenatal ultrasound than cleft lip, is thought to be a separate entity from cleft lip and is also quite common, with a birth incidence of 1/2500.[1] It also has multiple causes, including chromosomal aneuploidy, such as trisomy 18, trisomy 8 mosaicism, and the 22q11.2 deletion; autosomal dominant conditions, such as Van der Woude syndrome (due to mutations in *IRF6*) and Stickler syndrome (due to mutations in *COL2A1* and *COL11A1*); autosomal recessive conditions, such as Smith-Lemli-Opitz syndrome (due to a defect in cholesterol biosynthesis) (Fig. 5–12); teratogens, as in fetal alcohol syndrome; and generally sporadic conditions with as yet unknown etiologies, such as Kabuki syndrome.

The well-recognized association of micrognathia and glossoptosis, with or without cleft palate, known as Pierre Robin sequence or anomalad, is also heterogeneous and is

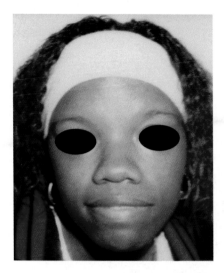
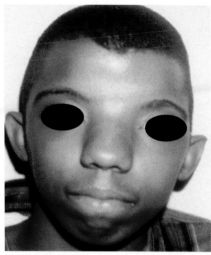
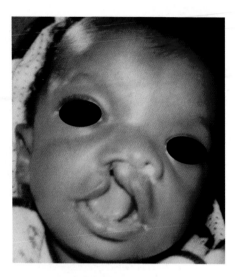

Figure 5–10. Cleft lip and palate is a variable manifestation of Opitz G/BBB syndrome as seen here in this child whose affected mother and uncle have hypertelorism due to a mutation in *MID1* on Xp22.3. It is a heterogeneous disorder with autosomal dominant and X-linked recessive inheritance, as well as, an association with the 22q11.2 deletion having been described. (*Photos courtesy of Elaine H. Zackai, MD.*)

frequently observed prenatally (Fig. 5–13). Associated chromosomal abnormalities include deletions of 4q, 6q, and 22q11.2 and duplications of 11q. Examples of associated single gene disorders include the autosomal dominant Stickler syndrome, Treacher Collins syndrome, and spondyloepiphyseal dysplasia congenital; the autosomal recessive diastrophic dysplasia; the X-linked otopalatodigital syndrome; and the heterogeneous cerebrocostomandibular, Nager and Larsen syndromes and skeletal dysplasia achondrogenesis (Fig. 5–14). Pierre Robin sequence has also been seen as a result of teratogen exposures including alcohol, dilantin, and trimethadione, as well as of fetal constraint due to oligohydramnios, in association with neurologic/neuromuscular disorders, and as the result of a disruption (such as an amniotic band) or a vas-

cular insult (as seen in the hypoglossia-hypodactylia/Hanhart syndrome) (Fig. 5–15). However, isolated occurrences are also common. With this in mind, the presentation of Pierre Robin sequence in the prenatal setting, like holoprosencephaly, elicits a broad differential diagnosis, with Stickler syndrome and the 22q11.2 deletion as the most common genetic causes. Such should therefore trigger consideration of adjunct imaging and laboratory studies. Equally important, this diagnosis, with its associated respiratory insufficiency, prompts careful planning in terms of medical management in both the delivery room and subsequent newborn period.

Having described many of the syndromic causes of clefting, it is important to note that the majority of clefts occur as an isolated finding or in combination with other malformations in a nonspecific manner more commonly than would be expected by chance alone.[8] Therefore, most families will receive guarded but relatively reassuring information regarding the prognosis for their child when a cleft is identified in the prenatal setting. Furthermore, isolated cleft lip/cleft lip and palate appears to be a separate entity from cleft palate alone in that a relative of an individual with an isolated cleft palate has no greater chance of having a child affected with a cleft lip and palate than someone from the general population. Exceptions to this rule have been observed, however, including both the 22q11.2 deletion and Van der Woude/popliteal pterygium syndrome. In these disorders, both cleft lip and/or palate and cleft palate alone may be observed.[9] Therefore, these diagnoses should be considered when a family history reveals both types of clefting.

Isolated clefting, like other common congenital malformations (including congenital heart disease, neural tube defects, and pyloric stenosis), is a "multifactorial or polygenic disorder" with a relatively low recurrence risk and a very good prognosis in terms of morbidity, mortality, and neurocognitive outcomes. Nonetheless, orofacial clefting comes with a

Figure 5–11. Cleft palate is generally more difficult to observe on prenatal ultrasonography as compared with cleft lip and palate; however, it is noted here by the arrow. (*Image courtesy of Natalie Blagowidow, MD.*)

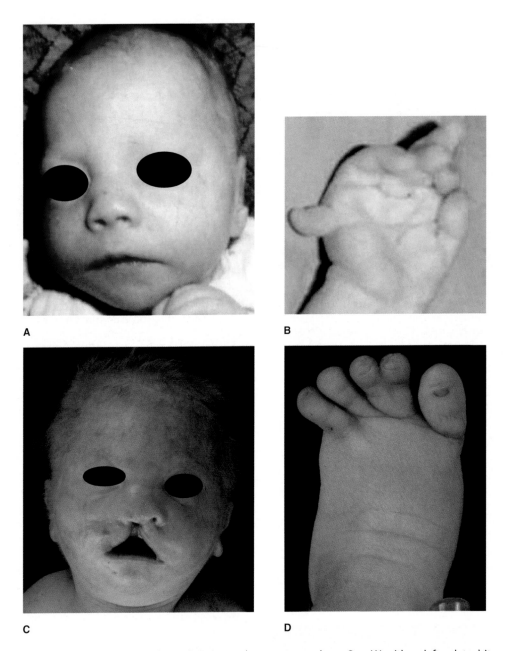

Figure 5–12. Two patients with Smith-Lemli-Opitz syndrome are seen here. One (A) with a cleft palate, bitemporal narrowing, micrognathia, and postaxial polydactyly (B); the other (C) with a unilateral cleft lip and palate and 2–3 syndactyly of the toes (D).

significant burden of care for both the patient and the family. With this in mind, it seems prudent that genetic counseling, both pre- and postnatal, become an integral component of general cleft care.

As described above, isolated cleft lip and/or palate is thought to have "multifactorial inheritance." This suggests that there are combinations of risk genes contributed by both parents that predispose the child to have a cleft; however, some nongenetic or "environmental" factor is also required in order for a certain threshold to be reached and subsequently for the cleft to occur (Fig. 5–16). Evidence for the genetic basis of this model includes well-documented familial occurrences. However, unlike single gene disorders, including autosomal recessive conditions where both parents contribute a non-

working gene and the recurrence risk is 25% (Fig. 5–17) or autosomal dominant conditions where only one causal gene is required and the recurrence risk is 50% (Fig. 5–18), the recurrence risks in multifactorial disorders are much smaller and may be influenced by sex, race, or the severity of the condition. For example, an individual with a bilateral cleft lip and palate is at an empirically higher chance of having a child with a cleft than is a person with a unilateral cleft. Evidence for the presence of nongenetic factors is also quite strong in that there are many instances of identical twins that are discordant for the presence of clefting. Therefore, recurrence risk counseling is based on empiric data and includes consideration of the sex of the affected individual/individuals, the severity of the defect (i.e., unilateral versus bilateral), the

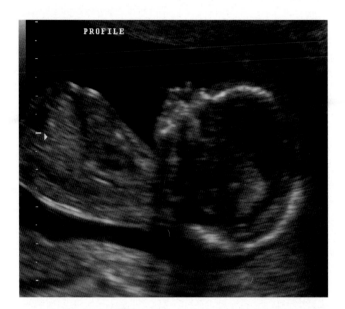

Figure 5–13. This ultrasound image demonstrates micrognathia in a fetus that was subsequently diagnosed with Pierre Robin anomalad postnatally as part of the skeletal dysplasia achondrogenesis. (*Image courtesy of Juan M. Gonzalez, MD and Michael T. Mennuti, MD.*)

racial and ethnic background of the family, and the number of affected persons in the family. When there are three or more affected individuals in a nuclear family, it is reasonable to consider a single gene disorder, even in the absence of salient clinical features (such as lip pits in the autosomal dominant Van der Woude syndrome). Table 5–1 lists the recurrence risks based on an adaptation of published European and American sources.[10]

In offering recurrence risk counseling to affected individuals or their relatives, it is imperative to distinguish isolated clefting from that which is associated with cytogenetic abnormalities, microdeletions, single gene disorders, teratogens, or "isolated associations." For example, a unilateral cleft lip and palate would most often be isolated but could be associated with trisomy 13 (which would be visible on a standard karyotype); Wolf–Hirschorn syndrome (requiring fluorescence in situ hybridization (FISH) studies using specific probes to the telomeric region of chromosome 4p for confirmation of the clinical diagnosis or comparative genomic hybridization); oral–facial–digital syndrome type VI (an autosomal recessive condition with no identifiable mutation to date); Rapp–Hodgkin ectodermal dysplasia (an autosomal

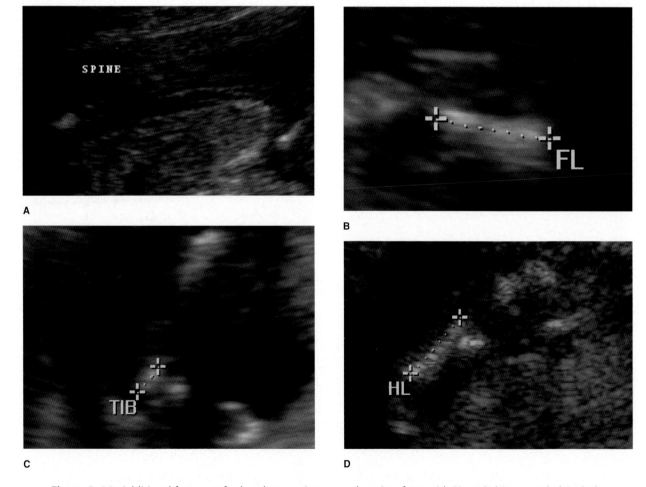

Figure 5–14. Additional features of achondrogenesis, as seen here in a fetus with Pierre Robin anomalad, include: severe under mineralization of the spine (A); moderate under mineralization of all bones with quadromicromelia as seen in the femur (B), tibia (C), and humerus (D). (*Images courtesy of Juan M. Gonzalez, MD and Michael T. Mennuti, MD.*)

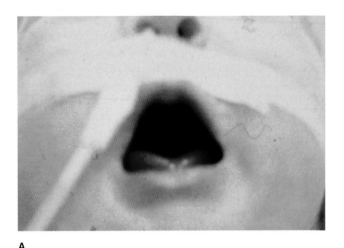

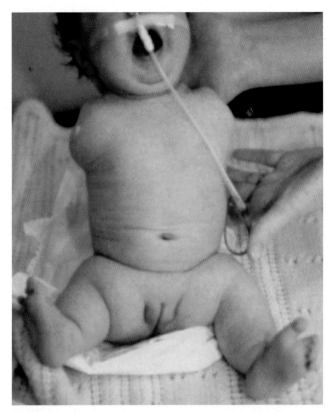

Figure 5–15. This patient with a V-shaped cleft palate (A) and micrognathia also has adacytlia of the upper extremities and hypodactylia of the lower extremities (B) as part of hypoglossia-hypodactylia/Hanhart/oromandibular-limb hypogenesis syndrome.

B

dominant condition with mutations in the *P63* gene); fetal alcohol syndrome (due to a maternal teratogenic exposure); or hemifacial microsomia (thought to be an isolated constellation of findings perhaps secondary to a vascular interruption during embryogenesis). Thus, genetic counseling for clefting must include either direct examination of the affected individual(s) or review of pertinent records and photographs by an experienced clinician whenever possible. Once a determination has been made regarding the etiology of the cleft,

appropriate recurrence risks (Figs. 5–17 to 5–19) may be given and the availability of prenatal testing offered.

For isolated clefting, preconception counseling may include a discussion of folic acid intake. Recent evidence for reduction of neural tube defects, such as anencephaly and spina bifida, by administration of dietary supplements of folic acid has produced studies that support the use of preconception folate intake to decrease the incidence of clefting, especially in families with an affected first-degree relative.[11–13]

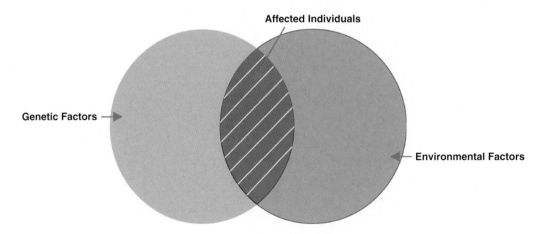

Figure 5–16. This diagram demonstrates the overlapping factors, which need to be present in order for a cleft to occur when due to multifactorial inheritance. These include a combination of genes contributed by both parents that predispose the child to having a cleft plus nongenetic or environmental factors, which cause the cleft to occur (affected individuals).

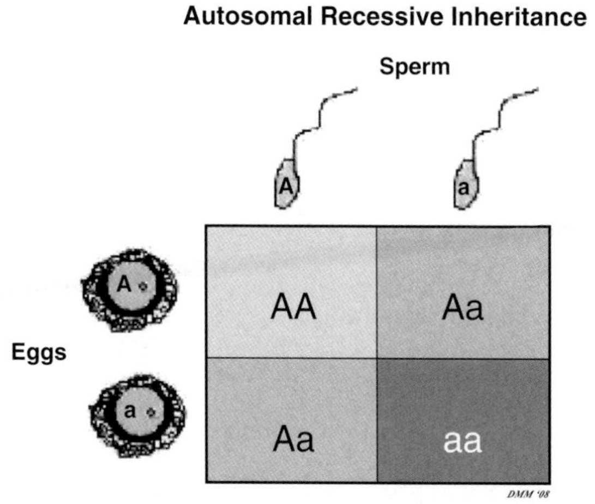

Autosomal Recessive Inheritance

Figure 5–17. This Punnett square demonstrates autosomal recessive inheritance where both parents are silent carriers of the condition and therefore each contributes a nonworking gene (a), in order for the problem to occur. The risk of having an affected child is therefore 25% (aa); whereas the remaining 75% of offspring will be unaffected (AA or Aa), although 2/3rds will be carriers for the nonworking gene (Aa).

Furthermore, the efficacy of prenatal imaging in a subsequent pregnancy may also be discussed. No additional genetic studies are currently available to detect isolated clefts.

For previously identified syndromic clefts, other prenatal modalities to be offered in addition to ultrasonography may include fetal echocardiography (when congenital heart disease is associated with the diagnosis) and amniocentesis or chorionic villus sampling (when cytogenetic, FISH studies, aneuploidies identified via CGH or direct mutational analysis is feasible). Preconception options may include donor gametes (artificial insemination by donor or donor egg) or preimplantation genetic diagnosis utilizing in

Table 5–1.

Recurrence Risk for Isolated Clefting

Relationship to Index Case	Cleft Lip +/− Cleft Palate	Cleft Palate Only
Sib (overall risk)	4.0%	1.8%
Sib (affected sibling with bilateral cleft lip/palate)	5.7%	—
Sib (affected sibling with unilateral cleft lip/palate)	4.2%	—
Sib (affected sib with cleft lip only)	2.5%	—
Child	4.3%	3.0%
Sib (2 affected sibs)	10.0%	8.0%
Sib (affected parent and sib)	10.0%	—

Adapted from Harper PS. Practical Genetic Counseling, 6th edn. London: Hodder Arnold, 2004.

vitro fertilization with single cell genetic analysis where applicable.

From the psychosocial perspective, the prenatal diagnosis of a cleft can have several advantages. Prenatal diagnosis can provide time for the family to adjust to the unexpected news and, in general, allow their health care providers

Autosomal Dominant Inheritance

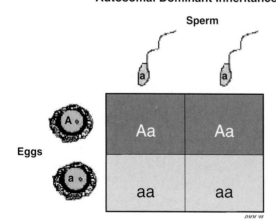

Figure 5–18. This Punnett square demonstrates autosomal dominant inheritance where an affected individual has only one gene, which causes the disorder to occur (A). The risk of having an affected child is therefore 50% (Aa) and an unaffected individual (aa) is at no increased risk over the general population of having an affected child.

X-Linked Recessive Inheritance

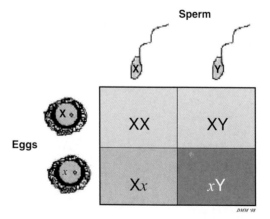

Figure 5–19. This Punnett square demonstrates X-linked recessive inheritance, such as in the X-linked form of Opitz G/BBB syndrome due to mutations in the *MID1* gene, where a carrier mother (X*x*) passes either the nonworking gene (*x*) or the working gene (X) to her offspring; however, in general, only males manifest the disorder (*x*Y). Thus the risk of having an affected child is 25% but the chance of having an affected son is 50%.

the opportunity to consider a more complex diagnosis. Furthermore, in certain situations, prenatal diagnosis allows the family and the health care team the opportunity to consider alternative plans for delivery, such as the use of a tertiary care facility when needed (in the presence of severe Pierre Robin sequence, for instance). In addition, having the information in the prenatal setting allows time for the family to become educated regarding the potential surgical, speech, and feeding needs of their child, as well as regarding the available resources in their area. Lastly, prenatal diagnosis allows the family the opportunity to meet with the cleft palate/craniofacial team and to initiate the long-term relationship that will ultimately benefit the well being of their child.

It is important to remember that the diagnosis of a cleft in the prenatal setting can also have a negative impact on the family. For example, without the opportunity to yet bond with their baby, the family will likely become anxious about the diagnosis of a cleft and the potential associated problems. This anxiety can produce multiple concerns about prognosis and remediation, which may not be completely answered until after the birth of the child. In addition, many families feel a sense of guilt and blame when told that their child has an anomaly. Thus, genetic counseling not only addresses the diagnostic needs of the patient, but also the psychosocial concerns of the family. It should be noted, however, that there are times when families need additional support, in which case a referral to an adjunct health care provider, such as a psychologist/psychiatrist with experience in this area, should be considered.

The same parental issues and concerns may arise in the postnatal period as well, and the recommendations are identical. Furthermore, as children with clefts reach adulthood, it is imperative to consider genetic counseling for them, both from a diagnostic/recurrence risk perspective, as well as from the psychosocial standpoint. Although, it has been found that the majority of children and adults with cleft lip and/or palate do not experience significant psychosocial problems, there are specific problems that often arise, such as teasing over their appearance.[14] With this in mind, caregivers must anticipate the need to support patients and their families around concerns in these areas. Finally, it is important to counsel teenagers with clefts, as well as their siblings, about their own recurrence risk prior to discharge from the cleft palate/craniofacial clinic.

References

1. Gorlin RJ, Cohen MM, Hennekam RCM. *Syndromes of the Head and Neck*, 4th edn. New York: Oxford University Press, 2001.
2. McDonald DM, Emanuel BS, Driscoll DA, et al. Chromosomal aneuploidy masquerading as autosomal dominant inheritance. *Am J Hum Genet* 43A:169, 1988.
3. Muenke M, Gropman A. Holoprosencephaly overview. *Gene Reviews* 2005. www.geneclinics.org
4. Optiz JM. G syndrome (hypertelorism with esophageal abnormality and hypospadias or hypospadias-dysphagia, or "Optiz-Frias" or "Optiz-G" syndrome). *Am J Hum Genet* 28:275–285, 1987.
5. McDonald-McGinn DM, Driscoll DA, Bason L, et al. Autosomal dominant "Opitz" GBBB syndrome due to a 22q11.2 deletion. *Am J Hum Genet* 59(1):103–113, 1995.
6. LaCassie Y, Arriaza MI. Letter to the editor: Opitz GBBB syndrome and the 22q11.2 deletion syndrome. *Am J Med Genet* 62:318, 1996.
7. Fryburg JS, Lin KY, Golden EF. Chromosome 22q11.2 deletion in a boy with Opitz oculo-genito-laryngeal syndrome. *Am J Med Genet* 62:274–275, 1996.
8. Harper PS. *Practical Genetic Counseling*, 3rd edn. London: Wright, 1988.
9. Kondo S, Schutte BC, Richardson RJ, et al. Mutations in *IRF6* cause Van der Woude and popliteal pterygium syndromes. *Nat Genet* 32(2):285–259, 2002.
10. Harper PS. *Practical Genetic Counseling*, 6th edn. London: Hodder Arnold, 2004.
11. Tolarova M. Orofacial clefts in Czechoslovakia. Incidence, genetics and prevention of cleft lip and palate over a 19-year period. *Scand J Plast Reconstr Surg Hand Surg* 21(1):19–25, 1987.
12. Shaw GM, Lammer EJ, Wasserman CR, et al. Risks of orofacial clefts in children born to women using multivitamins containing folic acid periconceptionally. *Lancet* 346(8972):393–396, 1995.
13. Tolarova M, Harris J. Reduced recurrence of orofacial clefts after periconceptional supplementation with high-dose folic acid and multivitamins. *Teratology* 51(2):71–78, 1995.
14. Hunt O, Burden D, Hepper P, et al. The psychosocial effects of cleft lip and palate: A systematic review. *Eur J Orthodont* 27:274–285, 2005.

6

Genetics of Nonsyndromic Clefting I: Family Patterns

Mary L. Marazita, PhD

INTRODUCTION

The highest frequency orofacial clefts (OFCs) are cleft lip (CL) and cleft palate (CP), with CL with or without CP (CL/P) considered etiologically distinct from CP alone (see Chapters 1–3). CL/P and CP can occur as part of single-gene Mendelian syndromes, as part of chromosomal abnormalities, or as part of syndromes due to teratogenic exposures (see Chapters 1–3, 7, and 8). However, OFCs due to a known etiology comprise only a small portion of all individuals with a CL/P or CP, and thus a major current focus of a number of research groups is to develop an understanding of the family patterns and etiology of the more common isolated (also termed "nonsyndromic") forms of OFCs.

Family patterns in CL/P and CP, particularly familial aggregation of OFCs, and thereby the relevance of inheritance in the etiology of CL/P and CP has been reported in the scientific literature for more than 200 years. The first published description of a family with several affected members was in 1757.[1] Charles Darwin[2] pointed out a publication of "the transmission during a century of hare-lip with a cleft-palate" by Sproule,[3] describing the author's family. Rischbieth[4] summarized pre-1900 publications of familial cases of cleft lip ("hare-lip") and cleft palate (abridged facsimile of Rischbieth[4] and commentary putting Rischbieth's conclusions into historical perspective are provided by Melnick[5]); he epitomized the anti-Mendelian view of Pearson and the other members of the Galton Laboratory by concluding that the inheritance of CL/P and CP was an expression of general physical and racial degeneracy which could be traced to poor protoplasm.[5] Bateson, on the other hand, was a leading proponent of Mendel and included "hare-lip" as one of a group of "Dominant Hereditary Diseases and Malformations."[5,6]

The fundamental tenet first described by Mendel, i.e. unit inheritance, has since been demonstrated to be correct and has led to today's burgeoning field of genetics. In this chapter, we will review the evidence for particular family patterns in CL/P and CP, and also summarize the evidence that additional phenotypic features can enhance our understanding of such family patterns.

FAMILY PATTERNS IN CL/P AND CP

Statistical Methods for Assessing Family Patterns

There are two categories of inheritance in humans, autosomal inheritance and X-linked inheritance based on whether the gene for a particular trait is located on one of the autosomes (chromosomes 1–22) or on the X chromosome. In addition to a trait's chromosomal location, the pattern of dominance for the alleles at a particular gene influences the resulting family patterns for a trait. A trait is said to follow dominant inheritance if only one allele is necessary for phenotypic expression and recessive if two alleles are necessary. If a trait is due to autosomal dominant inheritance, the typical family pattern will include equal numbers of affected males and females. Approximately half of the offspring of an affected person will also be affected, and people in each generation will be affected. In contrast, for autosomal recessive inheritance, equal numbers of males and females are affected, but the parents of affected individuals are usually unaffected. Generally, fewer affected family members are clustered in the same generation. Most X-linked traits follow recessive inheritance, resulting in a much higher proportion of affected males than females. Affected males in a family will be related through females.

Fig. 6–1 depicts a typical OFC family. In this family, there are two affected individuals, but the family does not demonstrate the expected attributes of autosomal dominant, autosomal recessive, or X-linked recessive inheritance.

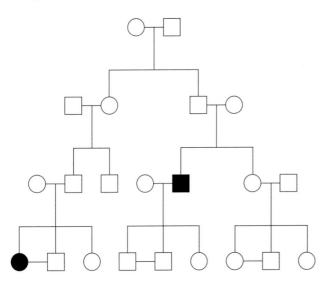

Figure 6–1. A typical OFC family. Circles are females; squares are males. The dark symbols are affected individuals.

Because OFC families do not clearly follow the expected Mendelian patterns but do show familial aggregation, they are often said to be part of the category of "complex" human traits. Many other human traits are also complex, including many common disorders such as cardiovascular disease and cancer. Therefore, a variety of approaches are necessary to understand the etiology of OFCs and other complex traits.

In assessing family patterns, statistical methods are necessary to correct for the inherent biases of most studies of human family data. In studies of animals, it is possible to design controlled matings that allow direct inference of the inheritance pattern of the trait of interest. The ideal human family study design would involve obtaining a large, random, population-based sample of families, taking a subset of the random families in which there are individuals with clefts, and then determining the genotypic mating type and offspring for each family. For a number of reasons, however, this ideal study design is not feasible for most human traits, including OFCs. The necessary fully informative matings are generally not available, and the genotypes of family members are usually unknown. A further difficulty in studying inheritance patterns in humans is that the traits most often under study are relatively rare. OFCs, for example, are a common birth defect but still occur in only 1 in 500 to 1 in 1000 births (see Chapter 2). Therefore, it is generally not possible to take a random sample of a population with any hope of obtaining the necessary numbers of families with cleft individuals. Families for study of human traits are most often ascertained through affected individuals, thus requiring appropriate statistical correction to eliminate potential biases introduced by the mode of ascertainment.

"Segregation analysis" refers to statistical methods that are used to determine the mode of inheritance of a trait. Segregation in this context is therefore derived from Mendel's laws regarding the segregation of alleles in the formation of gametes[7] (translated by Bateson[8,9]). The first statistical methods for segregation analysis were designed to assess Mendelian patterns of inheritance, i.e., to test whether family data were consistent with a single genetic locus. Today, the term is used more broadly to encompass tests of many types of transmission of traits, not limited to Mendelian patterns. Complex segregation analysis is sometimes used to describe statistical methods that incorporate two or more distinct, functionally independent parameters.

There are many different segregation analysis methods that have been applied to OFCs[9] in an effort to elucidate OFC family patterns. This chapter does not describe the methods in detail, but the next section will summarize the conclusions drawn from these methods for CL/P and CP. Each of the approaches defines an underlying general model with assumptions as to the probability distributions and parameters of interest. The hypotheses to be tested are each nested within the underlying general model. That is, each hypothesis corresponds to restrictions on the parameters of the underlying model. Likelihoods are calculated for each hypothesis, and parameters are estimated by maximum likelihood.[10] The likelihood ratio criterion is used to compare the likelihood of each restricted hypothesis to that of the most general, unrestricted model in order to determine statistical significance.

Family Studies of CL/P and CP: Descriptive

Most of the early studies of CL/P and CP family patterns were essentially descriptive. That is, they presented a hypothesis regarding the inheritance of OFCs and described how their data fit the hypothesis, without attempting any statistical tests. In Rischbieth's[4] summary of pre-1900 oral-facial cleft families, the hypothesis was that such families were the result of general physical degeneracy. Bateson,[6] on the other hand, attributed clefting in such families to dominantly inherited genes. Fogh-Anderson[11] was the first investigator to collect a systematic dataset of cleft families and to evaluate the observed inheritance patterns. He concluded that the inheritance patterns within CL/P families were consistent with segregation of alleles at a single genetic locus with variable penetrance and that those of CP families were consistent with autosomal dominant inheritance with greatly reduced penetrance.

In the 1960s and 1970s, there was a paradigm shift. A specific statistical model termed the multifactorial threshold model (MF/T) was described and was invoked to explain the familial patterns of oral-facial clefts.[12,13] Under the MF/T model, the occurrence of a cleft depends on a very large number of genes, each of equal, minor, and additive effect, plus environmental factors. An accumulation of these genes and environmental factors is tolerated by the developing fetus to a point, termed the threshold, beyond which there is the risk of malformation. This model has testable predictions, and, in theory, could explain many of the features observed for oral-facial clefts in families. The early proponents of the MF/T model published several large series of cleft families from a variety of populations, and each concluded that the data were consistent with the MF/T model.[14-18] None of these early studies, however, attempted any statistical tests of the model.

Family Studies of CL/P and CP: Test Predictions

The early OFC family descriptive studies were followed by studies that did test the predictions of the MF/T model.[19-21] In each of these studies, some or all of the predictions of the MF/T model could be rejected. However, statistical tests of the predictions of a model do not constitute a statistical test of that model. Other investigators then formulated and parameterized models to test the goodness-of-fit of the MF/T model; a number of investigators applied such models to oral-facial cleft family data.[20,22,23] The results of the goodness-of-fit studies were mostly inconclusive, with the MF/T model being rejected for some, but not all, portions of the parameter space in most studies.

Family Studies of CL/P and CP: Test Models

In the late 1970s and early 1980s, investigators began to apply formal segregation analysis methods to be able to contrast and statistically test the MF/T model and the major alternative of one or a few genes. Some of the first statistical analyses of OFCs were inconclusive[24,25] because the sample sizes were inadequate to distinguish between models. There were then studies of sufficient sample sizes.[9] In virtually every such study of CL/P, the MF/T model could be rejected in favor of either a mixed model (single locus plus multifactorial background[21,25]) or a major locus alone.[26-28] Most of such studies were conducted in Caucasian populations, although there were a few in Asian populations.[27] Given these segregation analysis results, gene mapping studies of CL/P were then considered feasible and are a current focus of intensive research (see Chapter 7).

There are many fewer segregation analyses of nonsyndromic CP than there are of CL/P. There are only three published studies, one in Hawaiian[24] and two in Caucasian populations.[25,29] Chung et al.[24] and Demenais et al.[25] could not distinguish between MF/T model and single gene models; Clementi et al.[29] concluded that a single recessive gene with reduced penetrance was sufficient to explain their data. There is also a significant subset of nonsyndromic CP families in which CP is X-linked, as evidenced by multiple descriptive and gene-mapping studies.[30-37]

EXTENDED PHENOTYPIC FEATURES IN CL/P AND CP FAMILIES

As summarized in the previous section, the results from numerous investigations of family patterns in CL/P and CP indicate that there are likely to be relatively few genes increasing cleft risk. The challenges facing etiologic research in CL/P and CP are to identify those genes, to investigate interactions between those genes and between those genes and environmental factors, and finally to investigate gene expression and function. A major difficulty in meeting these challenges and better understanding the complex CL/P and CP family patterns is phenotype definition. Misclassification of individuals due to inconsistent or inaccurate phenotyping can severely weaken one's ability to detect relevant disease genes[38,39] and is most crucial for complex traits such as OFC with a highly variable disease phenotype (see Chapters 1–3). Numerous lines of evidence suggest that OFC phenotypes are even more complex than typically assumed and are characterized by a variety of associated subclinical markers or endophenotypes.[40]

The concept of an expanded OFC phenotype is based primarily on the wide variety of subclinical morphological variations that have been associated with overt clefts and/or shown to be manifested more frequently in the unaffected relatives of cleft individuals compared to unaffected controls. The available evidence suggests that these associated traits can either be nonspecific in nature, probably reflecting increased developmental stress, or can be understood as cleft microforms.[40] In this section we summarize the morphologic variants that are considered to be informative in orofacial clefting.

Craniofacial

Face Shape Differences

More than 20 studies have investigated heritable aspects of facial shape; in general, each has found numerous differences between unaffected relatives of cleft cases and controls. The most consistent findings across studies are increased upper- and mid-facial widths.[41,42]

Elevated Directional Asymmetry

Several cephalometric studies have found significantly more directional asymmetry in unaffected parents of NS cleft cases than in controls.[43–45] There is also some evidence that excess soft tissue nasal asymmetry may represent a cleft microform.

Orbicularis Oris Muscle Defects

Using high resolution ultrasound, significantly more subclinical defects (e.g., gaps) in the orbicularis oris muscle have been identified in relatives of nonsyndromic CL/P than in controls.[46–48] Figs. 6–2 and 6–3 depict two families that have members with CL/P and other members with orbicularis oris discontinuities. As can be seen in the figures, the family patterns look more like autosomal dominant inheritance when the individuals with orbicularis defects are considered.

Dental

Developmental Anomalies

Numerous reports suggest that nonsyndromic cleft cases are characterized by an increased frequency of hypodontia, supernumerary teeth, asymmetric growth and eruption, enamel formation defects, delayed dental age, and tooth size reduction compared to controls. Evidence for elevated rates of such defects in unaffected family members has been inconsistent.[49,50]

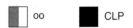

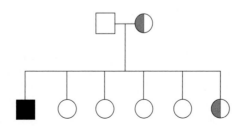

Figure 6–2. A family with an individual with CL/P (dark symbol) and two individuals with *Orbicularis Oris* muscle discontinuities visualized by ultrasound (red symbols).

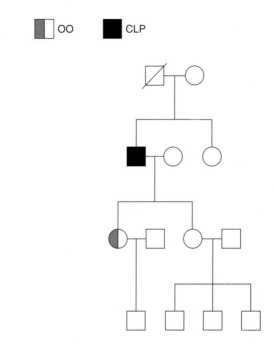

Figure 6–3. A family with an individual with CL/P (dark symbol) and one individual with *Orbicularis Oris* muscle discontinuities visualized by ultrasound (red symbols).

Elevated Fluctuating Asymmetry

Multiple studies to date have reported elevated dental fluctuating asymmetry in nonsyndromic CL/P cases compared to controls with a more pronounced effect in familial cases than in sporadic cases. Further, the asymmetry appears to be pervasive, affecting multiple teeth in both the deciduous and permanent dentition of the maxilla and mandible.[51,52]

Brain

Structural Differences

Recent neuroimaging studies suggest that the brains of adult men with NS clefting are characterized by significantly larger frontal and parietal lobes, smaller temporal and occipital lobes, decreased cerebellar volumes, and an increased frequency of midline brain anomalies than matched controls. Further, cases demonstrate significantly more posterior cerebral and cerebellar asymmetry than controls.[53,54]

Excess Non-Righthandedness (NRH)

Elevated rates of NRH in nonsyndromic CL/P cases compared to controls have been reported in several studies, but with no consistent findings related to cleft laterality. Studies have also reported increased NRH in unaffected parents of cleft cases.[55,56]

Atypical Hair Whorls

Recent data suggest that NS CL/P unaffected family members are characterized by an increased frequency of counterclockwise parietal hairwhorls.[57]

Dermatoglyphics

Pattern Type Differences

Assessed in several OFC populations to date. In general, cleft cases tend to possess a higher frequency of arches and ulnar loops and a lower frequency of whorls compared to controls. Similar trends are reported for unaffected relatives of cleft cases.[58–60]

Elevated Fluctuating Asymmetry

Increased levels of both metric and nonmetric dermatoglyphic FA have been reported in OFC cases compared to controls, with a more pronounced effect in familial cases than in sporadic cases. There is also some evidence for elevated dermatoglyphic FA in unaffected case relatives.[61,62]

FAMILY PATTERNS IN CL/P AND CP: SUMMARY

In summary, segregation analyses of CL/P and CP have consistently resulted in evidence for genes of major effect. Although such studies might seem to imply a single gene model, hypotheses of multiple interacting genes or genetic heterogeneity cannot be ruled out, and indeed, have not been explicitly tested in any of the published segregation analyses to date.[63] Furthermore, analyses of recurrence risk patterns[64–68] have been consistent with estimates ranging from 3 to 14 possibly interacting genes as responsible for CL/P.

Despite over 200 years of interest in the familial aggregation of oral-facial clefts, we still do not have a definitive understanding of the genetic component of the familiality. However, in the current golden age of genetics, ultimate confirmation of the existence of major genes for OFC is at hand (see Chapter 7 for progress to date). Segregation analyses have provided significant insights; the powerful statistical and molecular approaches available to geneticists today should continue to build upon that foundation. Finally, continued progress in identifying expanded phenotypic features that may represent mild (non-cleft) manifestations of cleft genes will improve the power of our gene-mapping research and also the ability to make reliable recurrence risk estimates in clinical settings.

References

1. Trew CJ. Sistens plura exempla palati deficientis. Nova Acta Physico-Medica Academiae Caesarae Leopoldin-Carolinae 1:445–447, 1757.
2. Darwin C. *The Variation of Animals and Plants under Domestication, Vol 5.* New York: Appelton, 1875, p. 466.
3. Sproule J. Hereditary nature of hare-lip. *Br Med J* 1:412, 1863.
4. Rischbieth H. Hare-lip and cleft palate. In Pearson K (ed). *Treasury of Human Inheritance. Part IV.* London: Dulau, 1910, pp. 79–123.
5. Melnick M. Cleft lip and palate etiology and its meaning in early 20th century England: Galton/Pearson vs. Bateson; polygenically poor protoplasm vs. Mendelism. *J Craniofac Genet Dev Biol* 17:65–79, 1997.
6. Bateson W. *Mendel's Principles of Hereditary.* Cambridge, England: Cambridge University Press, 1909.
7. Mendel G. Versuche über pflanzenhybriden. *Verhandlungen des Naturforschenden Vereines in Brunn* 4:3–17, 1866.
8. Bateson W. *Mendel's Principles of Heredity: A Defence.* Cambridge, England: Cambridge University Press, 1902.
9. Marazita ML. Segregation analysis. In Wyszynski DF (ed). *Cleft Lip and Palate: From Origin to Treatment.* Oxford: Oxford University Press, 2002, pp. 222–233.
10. Edwards AWF. *Likelihood, Expanded Edition.* Baltimore: Johns Hopkins University Press, 1992.
11. Fogh-Andersen P. *Inheritance of Harelip and Cleft Palate.* Copenhagen: Nyt Nordisk Forlag, Arnold Busck, 1942.
12. Carter CO. Genetics of common single malformations. *Br Med Bull* 32:21–26, 1976.
13. Fraser FC. The multifactorial threshold concept-uses and misuses. *Teratology* 14:267–280, 1976.
14. Woolf CM, Woolf RM, Broadbent TR. A genetic study of cleft lip and palate in Utah. *Am J Hum Genet* 15:209–215, 1963.
15. Woolf CM, Woolf RM, Broadbent TR. Cleft lip and heredity. *Plast Reconstr Surg* 34:11–14, 1963.
16. Carter CO, Evans K, Coffey R, et al. A family study of isolated cleft palate. *J Med Genet* 19:329–331, 1982.
17. Carter CO, Evans K, Coffey R, et al. A three generation family study of cleft lip with or without cleft palate. *J Med Genet* 19:246–261, 1982.
18. Hu DN, Li JH, Chen HY, et al. Genetics of cleft lip and cleft palate in China. *Am J Hum Genet* 34:999–1002, 1982.
19. Bear JC. A genetic study of facial clefting in Northern England. *Clin Genet* 9:277–284, 1976.
20. Melnick M, Bixler D, Fogh-Andersen P, et al. Cleft lip ± cleft palate: An overview of the literature and an analysis of Danish cases born between 1941 and 1968. *Am J Med Genet* 6:83–97, 1980.
21. Marazita ML, Spence MA, Melnick M. Genetic analysis of cleft lip with or without cleft palate in Danish kindreds. *Am J Hum Genet* 19:9–18, 1984.
22. Mendell NR, Spence MA, Gladstien K, et al. Multifactorial/threshold models and their application to cleft lip and cleft palate. In Melnick M, Bixler D, Shields ED (eds). *Etiology of Cleft Lip and Cleft Palate.* New York: Alan R. Liss, 1980, pp. 387–406.
23. Marazita ML, Spence MA, Melnick M. Major gene determination of liability to cleft lip with or without cleft palate: A multiracial view. *J Craniofac Genet Dev Biol* 2:89–97, 1986.
24. Chung CS, Ching GH, Morton NE. A genetic study of cleft lip and palate in Hawaii. II. Complex segregation analysis and genetic risks. *Am J Hum Genet* 26:177–188, 1974.
25. Chung CS, Bixler D, Watanabe, et al. Segregation analysis of cleft lip with or without cleft palate: A comparison of Danish and Japanese data. *Am J Hum Genet* 39:603–611, 1986.
26. Demenais F, Bonaiti-Pellie C, Briard ML, et al. An epidemiological and genetic study of facial clefting in France. II. Segregation analysis. *J Med Genet* 21:436–440, 1984.
27. Hecht JT, Yang P, Michels VV, et al. Complex segregation analysis of nonsyndromic cleft lip and palate. *Am J Hum Genet* 49:674–681, 1991.
28. Marazita ML, Hu DN, Spence MA, et al. Cleft lip with or without cleft palate in Shanghai, China: Evidence for autosomal major locus. *Am J Hum Genet* 51:648–653, 1992.
29. Nemana LJ, Marazita ML, Melnick M. Genetic analysis of cleft lip with or without cleft palate in Madras, India. *Am J Med Genet* 42:5–9, 1992.
30. Clementi M, Tenconi R, Forabosco P, et al. Inheritance of cleft palate in Italy. Evidence for a major autosomal recessive locus. *Hum Genet* 100:204–209, 1997.
31. Rushton AR. Sex-linked inheritance of cleft palate. *Hum Genet* 48:179–181, 1979.
32. Rollnick BR, Kaye CI. Mendelian inheritance of isolated nonsyndromic cleft palate. *Am J Med Genet* 24:465–473, 1986.
33. Moore GE, Ivens A, Chambers J, et al. Linkage of an X-chromosome cleft palate gene. *Nature* 326(5):91–92, 1987.

34. Moore GE, Williamson R, Jensson O, et al. Localization of a mutant gene for cleft palate and ankyloglossia in an x-linked Icelandic family. *J Craniofac Genet Dev Biol* 11:372–376, 1991.

35. Bjornsson A, Arnason A, Tippet P. X-linked cleft palate and ankyloglossia in an Icelandic family. *Cleft Palate J* 26(1):3–8, 1989.

36. Gorski SM, Adams KJ, Birch PH, et al. The gene responsible for X-linked cleft palate (CPX) in a British Columbia native kindred is localized between PGKI and DXYSI. *Am J Hum Genet* 50:1129–1136, 1992.

37. Forbes SA, Brennan L, Richardson M, et al. Refined mapping and YAC contig construction of the X-linked cleft palate and ankyloglossia locus (CPX) including the proximal X-Y homology breakpoint within Xq21.3. *Genomics* 31:36–43, 1996.

38. Haines JL, Pericak-Vance MA. Overview of mapping common and genetically complex human disease genes. In Haines JL, Pericak-Vance MA (eds). *Approaches to Gene Mapping in Complex Human Diseases.* New York: Wiley-Liss, Inc., 1998, pp. 1–16.

39. Rice JP, Saccone NL, Rasmussen E. Definition of the phenotype. In Rao DC, Province MA (eds). *Genetic Dissection of Complex Traits.* San Diego: Academic Press, 2001, pp. 69–76.

40. Weinberg SM, Neiswanger K, Martin RA, et al. The Pittsburgh oral-facial cleft (POFC) study: Expanding the cleft phenotype. Background and justification. *Cleft Palate Craniofac J* 43:7–20, 2006.

41. McIntyre GT, Mossey PA. The craniofacial morphology of the parents of children with orofacial clefting: A systematic review of cephalometric studies. *J Orthod* 29:23–29, 2002.

42. Ward RE, Moore ES, Hartsfield JK. Morphometric characteristics of subjects with oral facial clefts and their relatives. In Wyszynski DF (ed). *Cleft Lip and Palate: From Origin to Treatment.* Oxford: Oxford University Press, 2002, pp. 66–86.

43. Farkas LG, Cheung GC. Nostril asymmetry: Microform of cleft lip palate? An anthropometrical study of healthy North American Caucasians. *Cleft Palate J* 16:351–357, 1979.

44. McIntyre GT, Mossey PA. Asymmetry of the parental craniofacial skeleton in orofacial clefting. *J Orthod* 29:299–305, 2002.

45. Weinberg SM, Maher BS, Marazita ML. Parental craniofacial morphology in cleft lip with or without cleft palate as determined by cephalometry: A meta-analysis. *Orthod Craniofac Res* 9:18–30, 2006.

46. Martin RA, Hunter V, Neufeld-Kaiser W, et al. Ultrasonographic detection of orbicularis oris defects in first degree relatives of isolated cleft lip patients. *Am J Med Genet* 90:155–161, 2000.

47. Weinberg SM, Neiswanger K, Mooney MP, et al. Genome scan of cleft lip with or without cleft palate (CL/P): Part I. Broadening the phenotype to include lip muscle defects (Abstract). *Am J Hum Genet* 73(Suppl):291, 2003.

48. Neiswanger K, Weinberg SM, Rogers CR, et al. Orbicularis oris muscle discontinuities as an expanded phenotypic feature in nonsyndromic cleft lip with or without cleft palate. *Am J Med Genet* 2006 143:846–852, 2007.

49. Ranta R. A review of tooth formation in children with cleft lip/palate. *Am J Orthod Dentofacial Orthop* 90:11–18, 1986.

50. Harris EF. Dental development and anomalies in craniosynostoses and facial clefting. In Mooney MP, Siegel MI (eds). *Understanding Craniofacial Anomalies: The Etiopathogenesis and Craniosynostoses and Facial Clefting.* New York: Wiley-Liss, Inc., 2002, pp. 425–467.

51. Sofaer JA. Human tooth-size asymmetry in cleft lip with or without cleft palate. *Arch Oral Biol* 24:141–146, 1979.

52. Werner SP, Harris EF. Odontometrics of the permanent teeth in cleft lip and palate: Systemic size reduction and amplified asymmetry. *Cleft Palate J* 26:36–41, 1989.

53. Nopoulos P, Berg S, Canady J, et al. Abnormal brain morphology in patients with isolated cleft lip, cleft palate, or both: A preliminary analysis. *Cleft Palate Craniofac J* 37:441–446, 2000.

54. Nopoulos P, Berg S, Canady J, et al. Structural brain abnormalities in adult males with clefts of the lip and/or palate. *Genet Med* 4:1–9, 2002.

55. Rintala AE. Relationship between side of the cleft and handedness of the patient. *Cleft Palate J* 22:34–37, 1985.

56. Wentzlaff KA, Cooper ME, Yang P, et al. Association between non-right-handedness and cleft lip with or without cleft palate in a Chinese population. *J Craniofac Genet Dev Biol* 17:141–147, 1997.

57. Scott NM, Weinberg SM, Neiswanger K, et al. Hair whorls and handedness: Informative phenotypic markers in nonsyndromic cleft lip with or without cleft palate (NS CL/P) cases and their unaffected relatives. *Am J Med Genet (A)* 136A:158–161, 2005.

58. Balgir RS. Dermatoglyphics in cleft lip and cleft palate anomalies. *Indian Pediatr* 30:341–346, 1993.

59. Neiswanger K, Petiprin SS, Bardi KM, et al. Phenotypic variation in individuals with cleft lip with or without cleft palate and their unaffected family members (Abstract). *Am J Hum Genet* 69(Suppl):305, 2001.

60. Scott NM, Weinberg SM, Neiswanger K, et al. Dermatoglyphic phenotypic heterogeneity among individuals with nonsyndromic cleft lip with or without cleft palate (CL/P) and their unaffected relatives in China and the Philippines. *Hum Biol* 77(2):257–266, 2005.

61. Adams MS, Niswander JD. Developmental 'noise' and a congenital malformation. *Genet Res* 10:313–317, 1967.

62. Woolf CM, Gianas AD. A study of fluctuating asymmetry in the sibs and parents of cleft lip propositi. *Am J Hum Genet* 29:503–507, 1977.

63. Jarvik GP. Statistical Genetics '98. Complex segregation analyses: Uses and limitations. *Am J Hum Genet* 63:942–946, 1998.

64. Farrall M, Holder S. Familial recurrence-pattern analysis of cleft lip with or without cleft palate. *Am J Hum Genet* 50:270–277, 1992.

65. Mitchell LE, Risch N. Mode of inheritance of nonsyndromic cleft lip with or without cleft palate: A reanalysis. *Am J Hum Genet* 51:323–332, 1992.

66. FitzPatrick D, Farrall M. An estimation of the number of susceptibility loci for isolated cleft palate. *J Craniofac Dev Biol* 13:230–235, 1993.

67. Christensen K, Mitchell LE. Familial recurrence-pattern analysis of nonsyndromic isolated cleft palate—A Danish registry study. *Am J Hum Genet* 58:182–190, 1996.

68. Schliekelman P, Slatkin M. Multiplex relative risk and estimation of the number of loci underlying an inherited disease. *Am J Hum Genet* 71:1369–1385, 2002.

Genetics of Nonsyndromic Clefting II: Results from Gene Mapping Studies

Lina M. Moreno, DDS, PhD • Mary L. Marazita, PhD • Andrew C. Lidral, DDS, PhD

INTRODUCTION

Studies of orofacial clefting have shown that nonsyndromic cleft lip with or without cleft palate (CL/P) has complex inheritance patterns, and there is solid evidence that genetic factors have an etiologic role. Nevertheless, segregation analyses have not conclusively defined the mode of inheritance (see Chapter 6). Studies have estimated that 3–14 genes (most likely 3–6) interacting multiplicatively may be involved, indicating that CL/P is a heterogeneous disorder.[1] The purpose of this chapter is to summarize the genetic studies that have focused on identifying genes for CL/P.

GENETIC MAPPING

Human genetic mapping studies have used both linkage and association statistical genetic analyses to identify etiologic genes for CL/P. Linkage analyses are typically used first to provide the rough location of an etiologic gene; association analyses can then narrow the location further to implicate specific genes, which can then be screened for mutations.

Linkage

Linkage refers to genes that are close together on a chromosome; linkage analysis is a type of statistical test that exploits the cosegregation of alleles (e.g., DNA variations) at two or more genes during meiosis. In practice, marker genes, i.e., those with known chromosomal locations, are evaluated in families with two or more affected individuals. Statistical analyses then assess evidence for and against linkage between a putative disease gene and the marker gene(s), thereby narrowing the likely location of the disease gene.

Humans are diploid organisms with each cell containing 23 pairs of chromosomes. For each chromosome pair, there is one paternal and one maternal chromosome. Meiosis results in the formation of gametes (sperm or ova) that are haploid, meaning that each gamete contains only a single set of 23 chromosomes. During meiosis, there are two mechanisms that result in genetic diversity. One mechanism results from one of Mendel's original observations, i.e., the independent assortment of parental chromosomes, such that only one parental chromosome (maternal or paternal) for each of the 23 chromosomes enters a gamete. Given that there are pairs of each of the 23 chromosomes, one person can produce 2^{23} (8.4×10^6) different combinations of their parental chromosomes.[2] Recombination between parental chromosomes is the second mechanism underlying genetic diversity and is an exception to Mendel's law of independent assortment. During meiosis, the two parental chromosomes form pairs in a conformation that allows exchange (recombination) to occur between them. In this process, breaks in the chromosomes occur, and the ends of these breaks can join with an identical break in the other parental chromosome, resulting in recombined chromosomes that contain both maternal and paternal DNA. Therefore, the actual number of different gametes that one person can create is *much* larger than 2^{23}.

Assortment and recombination can be used to map disease genes. DNA variation is detected by a variety of laboratory techniques, and allows identification of which chromosome or allele came from each parent. DNA variations can be polymorphic genetic markers or the actual disease mutations. The frequency of recombination events between DNA variations is a function of the distance between them; hence recombination is more likely to occur between DNA variations that are far apart and less likely between DNA variations near each other. Observing which marker alleles (variations) co-segregate with a disease will identify which chromosome contains the etiologic DNA variant (which can be either a mutation or a polymorphic variant) and where on the chromosome the etiologic variant is likely to reside. DNA variations that cosegregate with each other more often than would be expected by chance (assuming independent assortment) are assumed to be genetically linked (Fig. 7–1). Linkage can be statistically detected over relatively large regions and therefore requires relatively few genetic markers to cover the entire genome (depending on informativeness, as few as 400 polymorphic markers).

Association

Association analysis is a statistical approach which identifies nonrandom correlations (i.e., associations) between alleles at

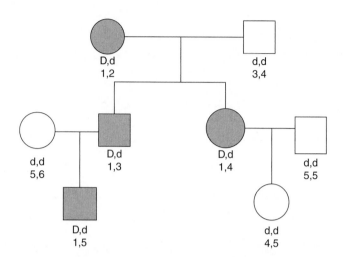

Figure 7–1. Linkage. Pedigree displaying an autosomal dominant trait (D = disease allele; d = normal allele) in linkage with a genotyped polymorphic marker containing six alleles. Affected individuals are shaded in gray. Notice that all individuals affected with the disease have the marker allele 1.

two or more genetic loci in a population. Conceptually, linkage and association are contrasting approaches in that linkage assesses correlation of alleles within families whereas association assesses allelic correlation across a population (Fig. 7–2). An implicit assumption underlying association gene mapping approaches is that affected individuals would have a shared ancestor on whose chromosomes the original etiologic DNA variation or mutation arose. This would result in shared alleles for markers near the etiologic variation among affected individuals, while recombination that has occurred throughout the entire history of the population would result in random

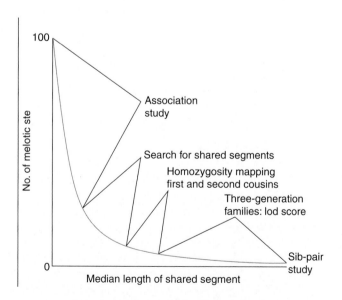

Figure 7–2. Genetic mapping strategies. Linkage and association strategies are at opposite ends of the spectrum. (*From Strachan T, Read AP. Human Molecular Genetics 2. New York: Wiley, 1999, Fig. 12.3.*)

segregation of the regions outside of the disease locus. Association approaches have great study power for genetically complex diseases.[3] However, because many more chances for recombination exist in a population, association can typically be observed only over short genetic distances. Hence, hundreds of thousands of different markers are necessary to cover the human genome for association approaches.

The use of association in disease gene mapping requires a carefully matched control group for comparison and if not appropriately matched, association can reflect an inherent but unknown difference between the case and control populations. Alternatively, family-based association tests, such as the transmission disequilibrium test (TDT), have been developed to reduce this potential bias. The TDT assesses the transmission of alleles from parents who are heterozygous (meaning the parent has two different alleles) at a given marker to their children.[4] Under Mendelian inheritance, there should be a 50:50 chance for the transmission of a given allele from a heterozygous parent to a child. For TDT association mapping, the transmission patterns would be observed in many families, and significant deviations from the expected 50:50 transmission ratio would indicate association between that marker and the disease.

CANDIDATE GENES AND REGIONS FOR NONSYNDROMIC CL/P

Past efforts to identify genes for nonsyndromic CL/P have generally relied on candidate gene approaches[5–8]. Candidate genes have been chosen based on their biologic function, expression patterns during facial development, and cleft phenotypes in mutant mice. Over 40 knockout (KO) or transgenic mice have been created whose phenotypes include orofacial clefts.[13] Remarkably, only five have clefts of the primary palate (CL), including mice chimeric for *Ap-2a* null alleles,[14] mice lacking *Egfr*,[15] *Ski* (midline cleft)[16] *Folbp1*[17] or compound *Rar* knockout mice[18] and a dominant negative *Rar* transgenic mouse model.[19] CL/P also occurs spontaneously in the "A" strain of mice,[20] including the A/WySn strain. With a CL/P prevalence of approximately 20–25%, the A/WySn strain has been the focus of genetic mapping efforts that have identified a strong maternal effect in addition to two loci: *Clf1*, which is caused by a retrotransposon insertion near the Wnt9b gene in a region syntenic to human 17q21.32, and *Clf2*, which maps to a 5.5 Mb region with synteny to human 5p15.[21] These genes and additional candidate genes have been evaluated for linkage and/or association with CL/P.

Multi-center collaborative projects utilizing linkage and association approaches applied to substantial numbers of multiplex families and triads have shown significant progress towards the identification of candidate regions containing plausible etiological loci for CL/P.[22–31] In addition, important contributions of environmental factors and their influence in CL/P risk have also been identified.[7] For instance, comprehensive environment and gene–environment interaction studies have shown that maternal smoking early in pregnancy increases the odds of CL/P by a factor of 1.29–1.62[32–34] and that this risk is modulated by variants in genes involved in cigarette detoxification pathways such as *GSTT1*[34,35] and *NAT2*.[34] The following is a summary of the human and mouse research studies performed in candidate gene/chromosomal regions that best support the role of transcription factors, growth factors, and signaling molecules as etiological factors in nonsyndromic CL/P.

1p36 Region (MTHFR, SKI)

Folic acid plays an important role in DNA synthesis and DNA methylation by participating in de novo synthesis of nucleotides and methylation of homocysteine to methionine, which is a source of methyl groups in cellular metabolism.[36] DNA synthesis and DNA methylation are required during cell division and regulation of gene expression,[37,38] both basic mechanisms in the development of an organism.

Methylenetetrahydrofolate reductase (MTHFR) is an important enzyme in folate metabolism. In a major public health discovery, maternal supplementation of folic acid has been shown to decrease the risk of neural tube defects.[39] Furthermore, some studies have shown a reduction in the risk of CL/P as well.[40–43] Hence, variants of proteins involved in folic acid metabolism may have a functional impact in the risk for CL/P.

There are two major functional MTHFR polymorphisms, A222V and E429A. The former codes for a thermolabile enzyme with reduced activity that is responsible for elevated plasma homocysteine levels and lowered plasma folate.[44] The latter results in reduction of MTHFR activity but not as significantly as A222V. However, in conditions of low folate intake or during periods of high folate requirements such as embryogenesis, the E429A polymorphism may have clinical relevance.[45] Results of several association studies of these polymorphisms and the risk of CL/P have been contradictory.[46–54] Linkage analyses have also been performed using markers near MTHFR in the 1p36 region, but only weakly positive results have been observed.[22,55] The lack of strong genetic evidence implicating this gene in CL/P may be due in part to the probability that this gene exerts small effects on the phenotype. Alternatively, assuming that MTHFR is not sufficient but necessary to cause CL/P, analytical methodologies that consider interactions between *MTHFR* and other genes involved in folate metabolism, such as *TCN1, TCN2, MTR, MTRR,*[56] *RFC1,*[52,57] and folate receptors,[17,58] or that take into account environmental covariates might be more powerful at detecting a relationship between genes in the folate pathway and CL/P.[59]

SKI is a nuclear protein that also maps to the human 1p36 region and that constitutes an important negative regulator of *TGFβ* and bone morphogenetic protein (BMPs) signaling. *Ski* null mice on a C57BL6/J background have a severe midline facial cleft.[16] Further studies revealed that *SKI* is deleted in patients with 1p36 deletion syndrome,[16] which includes orofacial clefting as part of the phenotype. The implication of *SKI* in orofacial clefting might be explained through its antagonistic effects on TGFβ and BMP activation of target genes during lip and palate development. Inactivation of *Tgfb3* in mice results in lack of palatal fusion.[60,61] In addition, members of the BMP pathway, *Bmp4* and *Bmpr1A*, are involved in lip and palate fusion.[62] Furthermore, overexpression of *Msx2*, a known BMP target,[63] results in craniofacial phenotypes similar to the ones present in the *Ski* null mouse (facial clefting and exencephaly).[64] Therefore, it is possible that in the absence of SKI, a lack of repression of TGFβ and BMP target genes is deleterious to craniofacial development.[65]

Human studies have revealed an association between SKI and CLP.[66] In addition, a few rare mutations resulting in amino acid substitutions have been identified.[67] These findings suggest that variants within SKI modify the risk for orofacial clefting, and therefore these variants warrant further studies.

1q32 (IRF6)

Mutations in IRF6 have been shown to be etiologic for two orofacial cleft syndromes, Van der Woude syndrome (VWS) and Popliteal Pterygium syndrome (PPS).[68] VWS is an autosomal dominant syndrome characterized by the presence of cleft lip with or without cleft palate, cleft palate, lower lip pits and hypodontia. PPS, also dominantly inherited, has an orofacial phenotype similar to VWS plus additional skin and genital anomalies.

IRF6 belongs to a family of nine transcription factors that contain a DNA binding domain and a protein–protein interaction domain (SMIR Smad-interferon regulatory factor-binding domain).[69] *IRF6* is expressed in the medial edge epithelium of the palatal shelves as well as in hair follicles, tooth buds, genitalia, and skin.[68] *Irf6* deficient mice have abnormal palatal development in addition to limb and skin anomalies.[70,71] The latter are caused by a primary defect in keratinocyte differentiation and proliferation.

The majority of mutations found in *IRF6* in patients with VWS are localized in the DNA-binding domain and in the SMIR protein–protein domain, suggesting functional importance of both these domains. PPS missense mutations were localized mainly within the DNA-binding domain. This difference in the location of mutations might suggest that VWS is caused by loss of function of the *IRF6* gene, whereas PPS seems to be caused by a dominant negative effect due to inactive transcription complexes that result when *IRF6* DNA-binding ability is compromised. Both these syndromes have significant phenotypic variability, suggesting that other genes modify *IRF6* mutations.

Given the similarity between the phenotypes observed for VWS and nonsyndromic CL/P, it was hypothesized that allelic variants of the *IRF6* gene might contribute to the etiology of the nonsyndromic forms. A common *IFR6* variant (V274I) was shown to be highly associated with nonsyndromic CL/P (p-value $<10^{-9}$) in a study of 10 populations with ancestry in Asia, Europe, and South America[26]). Several indepen-

dent studies have since replicated this initial association.[72–75] Interestingly, linkage studies revealed minimally positive results, underscoring the utility of implementing both linkage and association mapping strategies.[22,76] Nevertheless, a meta-analysis of 13 genome-scan studies revealed modest evidence of linkage to this region.[28] Research is actively ongoing to identify mutations that can be demonstrated to have an effect on *IRF6* expression or function.

The role of *IRF6* in nonsyndromic CL/P etiology constitutes one of the most exciting discoveries in cleft lip and palate research so far. It has been estimated that variants at the *IRF6* locus may contribute to 12% of the genetic etiology of CL/P.[26] Also, in families with multiple individuals with CL/P, the inheritance of the risk allele increased the recurrence amongst siblings to three times empiric recurrence risk. *IRF6* is known to be involved in skin development.[70,71] Evidence that the TGFβ signaling pathway regulates *IRF6* expression[77] and also has a role in skin wound healing and scar formation[78] raises the hypothesis that IRF6 is involved in scar formation as well. Anecdotal evidence suggesting that patients with VWS or PPS have more problems with scarring provides additional support for this hypothesis.

The successful identification of IRF6 as an etiologic factor for nonsyndromic CL/P underscores the importance of studying rare, syndromic forms of clefting (see Chapter 8 for a discussion of clefting syndromes) as models to understand the etiology of the more complex nonsyndromic forms.[5]

2p13 (TGFA)

Transforming growth factor alpha (TGFA) is a transmembrane glycoprotein that contains 160 amino acids.[79] It shows 40% sequence homology with epidermal growth factor, and both can bind to the EGF receptor (EGFR). *Tgfa* is expressed in the mesenchymal tissue of the palate in the midline seam at the time of secondary palatal fusion in mice.[80] However, *Tgfa* knockout mice do not present with a cleft palate. Instead, homozygous mutants display misalignment of hair follicles and eye abnormalities.[81] *Egfr* knockout mice, however, present narrow and elongated snouts, underdeveloped lower jaws, and CL/P and CP.[15] The palatal shelves are capable of fusing, but they often have residual epithelium.

Many studies in Caucasian populations have shown positive associations with *TGFA* and CL/P. The majority of these studies have used a case-control approach.[82–88] Some studies,[85,89] including a meta-analysis of all Caucasian association data,[90] have suggested a modifier role rather than a major role for *TGFA*gn the etiology of CL/P. Other studies have not been able to replicate positive associations between *TGFA* and nonsyndromic CL/P.[91–95] The lack of replication in results amongst different studies might be a reflection of different study designs, heterogeneity between samples, and lack of power needed to detect loci of minor effects.

Linkage analyses have also been performed; yet, results have been either negative[23,76,96,97] or weakly positive.[22,89,98–100] Recently, a meta-analysis of 13 genome-wide scan studies[28] revealed suggestive results in the 2p13 region, which corroborates the hypothesis that this gene is a modifier rather than necessary or sufficient to cause clefting.

Gene–environment studies have been performed to test interactions between alleles at the TGFA gene and environmental factors such as smoking and vitamin intake. For smoking, studies have found positive[101,102] and negative interaction results.[94,103–105] In terms of vitamin consumption, one study[102] has demonstrated signals of gene–environment interaction between a particular genotype of the *TGFA* gene and mothers who did not use vitamins (OR = 3.0; 95% CI 1.4–6.6). In addition, two-locus interaction signals between 6p23–p24 and 2p13 have been demonstrated in the Italian population.[99] Also, interactions between *TGFA* and *MSX1*[94] and TGFA and *MTHFR* have also been demonstrated for both CL/P and CP.[106]

An extensive search for causal *TGFA* mutations in 250 CL/P subjects revealed five rare variants in conserved regions of the gene,[107] and these variants were not found in 179 control individuals. *TGFA* sequencing of 93 Iowa and 91 Filipino individuals with CL/P identified another nine rare noncoding variants.[67] These variants might be rare causes of clefting and provide additional evidence supporting the role of this gene in this trait's etiology. A recent extensive review and meta-analysis of articles published from 1986 to 2005 concluded that *TGFA* has a minor, but nevertheless detectable, role in nonsyndromic clefting.[108]

2q11–2q37

Duplications and deletions in different regions throughout 2q11-q37 have been found in patients exhibiting CLP and CPO phenotypes, supporting the presence of a clefting susceptibility locus in the long arm of chromosome 2.[109–115] Evidence of linkage[25] and LD[88] of this region has been described for a variety of populations. Genes located within this region that are known to be involved in facial development include *DLX1*, *DLX2*,[116–118] and *SATB2*.[119] *DLX1* and *DLX2* belong to the distal-less family of homeobox-containing transcription factors. *DLX1* and *DLX2* are expressed in the epithelium and mesenchyme of the first branchial arches, and their expression is regulated by mechanisms involving *BMP4* and *FGF8*,[120] which are involved in facial development.[121] Homozygous null mice for *Dlx1* and *Dlx2* exhibit malformations of proximal first arch structures, including cleft palate and loss of maxillary molars.[116,117]

Two patients with CP and additional mild structural anomalies were found to have translocation breakpoints affecting the *SATB2* gene.[119] A *SATB2* mutation was found in one of 91 Filipino samples with nonsyndromic cleft lip and palate.[67] SATB2 is a transcriptional regulator and is expressed in the mesenchyme underlying the medial edge epithelium of the palatal shelves.

SUMO1 is another gene that maps to 2q33.1. A translocation disrupting *SUMO1* was observed in a patient with CL/P, and inactivation of *Sumo1* in mice results in CP.[122]

4p16 (MSX1)

MSX1 is a transcription factor that belongs to a family of homeobox-containing genes homologous to the Drosophila msh (Muscle segment homeobox). In mice three members have been identified and they share a highly conserved homeodomain. *Msx1* and *Msx2* are strongly expressed in the developing craniofacial region in an overlapping manner, while Msx3 is not expressed during facial development.[123] *Msx1* has a role in epithelial–mesenchymal interactions and is expressed in the anterior portion of the palatal mesenchyme as well as in the dental mesenchyme.[124] Mice lacking *Msx1* exhibit clefts of the secondary palate along with tooth agenesis.[125]

In humans, MSX1 mutations have been found in patients with an autosomal dominant form of selective tooth agenesis (second premolars and third molars).[126–128] The phenotype associated with MSX1 mutations was expanded to include CP and CL/P in a study of a Dutch family with tooth agenesis and various combinations of CP and CL/P.[129] MSX1 mutations are causal for the Witkop syndrome (tooth-nail syndrome), which is a rare autosomal condition that includes nail dysplasia and congenitally missing teeth (predominantly premolars, first and third molars).[130]

Many studies have attempted to elucidate the role of *MSX1* in nonsyndromic CL/P cases. Significant association results have been found by some authors[92,131,132] for Caucasian populations and by others[133] for Asian populations. Schultz et al.[100] found weakly positive association and linkage (recessive model) results for the *MSX1* CA in a Filipino population. Other studies, however, have failed to show significant results for this locus.[22,91,94,132] Jezewski et al.[134] found *MSX1* variants in 2% of patients with nonsyndromic orofacial clefting. These variants were located in conserved amino acid regions or in areas of high mouse homology. Recent studies have yielded similar findings in patients with CL/P from the Vietnamese and Thai populations, confirming the importance of the *MSX1* gene in lip and palate development.[133,135]

6p23–p25 Region

Several mouse studies have mapped the susceptibility to cortisone-induced cleft palate to the mouse H2 region that is the counterpart of the human *HLA* region on the short arm of chromosome 6 (i.e., 6p).[136] Based on this finding, human linkage and association studies have been performed to evaluate the role of the human *HLA* region in orofacial clefting (see Table 7-1).[137–141]

The first significant linkage finding for nonsyndromic CL/P was reported in a Denmark study in which 58 pedigrees with apparent autosomal dominant inheritance of CL/P (49) and CP (9) were tested for linkage to 42 protein polymorphisms. This study found the highest linkage result to be at the *F13A* locus at 6p25. As a result of this finding, the *F13A* locus received the denomination Orofacial Cleft 1 (*OFC1*), indicating that a gene involved in CL/P appears to be in this region. Since this report, positive evidence of linkage and association has been found within a 15–20 cM region (15.1–34.6 cM) that corresponds to 6p23–24.[22,141–145]

Table 7–1.

Chromosomal Rearrangements Involving the Region 6p23–24

Rearrangement	Phenotype	6p24 Location	9q22 Location	Reference
3 family members with balanced translocation t(6:9)(p24;q22.3)	CL/P and ectodermal dysplasia	Most 3′ exon of OFCC1. 930 Kb distal to 5′ end of *TFAP2A*	5 Kb interval between *EDAG-NEFIP*	[9,10]
1 case with a balanced translocation 46XY,t(6:7)(p24.3;q36)	CL/P and other malformations	Most 3′ exon of OFCC1. 830 Kb distal to 5′ end of *TFAP2A*		[10,11]
1 case with a balanced translocation 46,XX,t(6;9)(p24.3;p23)	CP and other malformations	*OFCC1* Intron 3. 375 Kb distal to 5′ end of *TFAP2A*		[10,12]
1 case with a deletion 46XX,del(6)p23;pter)	CL/P and other malformations			[11]

Two of these studies, performed in families from Northeastern Italy, obtained LOD scores above 3.0, the threshold for significance in genetic linkage analysis, for 6p at 30 cm and 27.8 cm respectively.[142,143] An interesting study attempting to model the complex genetics of CL/P found that families that map to 6p23 also had significant results at 2p13 near TGFα, indicating that in these families mutations at both loci are involved.[99] This interaction result is in agreement with data suggesting that two genes were involved in the etiology of CL/P in these families from Italy.[146]

Negative linkage results for markers in the 6p23–25 region have also been reported.[137,139,140,147] These results may reflect the underlying genetic heterogeneity of CL/P, in which the clefts in some families are caused by mutations at one locus while those in other families are caused by mutations at other loci. Recently, a meta-analysis of seven genome-wide scans found significant linkage at cM 68 (6p23).[28] In agreement with the Italian results, significant linkage (HLOD = 3.74) was obtained using a model that accounted for genetic heterogeneity, showing that 52% of the families mapped to 6p23. This result is above the threshold for genome-wide significance (≥ 3.2)[148] and therefore confirms the presence of a locus for CL/P in this region.

A number of patients with CL/P with chromosome anomalies in the 6p23–p25 region have also been described.[10–12,149–151]

Potential candidate genes localized in the short arm of chromosome 6 include FOXQ1 (12.5Mb), FOXF2 (13.3Mb), FOXC1 (15.5Mb) (Bone Morphogenic Protein 6 (*BMP6*) (12.62-14 cM), Orofacial Cleft Candidate 1 (*OFCC1*) (18 cM), Transcription Factor AP2 Alpha (*TFAP2A*, 18.22 cM), and Endothelin-1 (*EDN1*) (27 cM).

The FOX genes comprise a large family of transcription factors that contain the forkhead DNA-binding domain.

Foxq1, *Foxf2*, and *Foxc1* are all expressed in the embryonic facial mesenchyme.[152,153] Inactivation of *Foxf2* in mice results in cleft palate[154] and mutations in the *Foxc1* related gene, *Foxc2*, cause the lymphadema, distichiasis, cleft palate syndrome,[155] indicating these FOX genes may be involved in CL/P.

Bone morphogenic proteins (BMPs) are secreted signaling molecules that belong to the TGFβ family. These molecules are expressed during embryonic development.[156,157] BMPs are regulated by sonic hedgehog, MSX genes, and fibroblast growth factors[156] and these genes are also involved in facial development. In mice, *Bmp6* is expressed in the frontonasal process.[158] However, *Bmp6* null mice have delayed ossification that is confined to the sternum and no other obvious craniofacial or neural phenotypes, possibly due to compensation by other BMPs during development.[159] *OFCC1* is a novel gene that was identified by mapping the break points of three chromosomal translocations that occurred in patients having CL/P[11,12,149] (see Table 7–1). Expression of this gene occurs at 6 weeks in the human fetal hard palate. One translocation, 46,XX,t(6;9)(p24.3;p23), occurs in intron 3 of *OFCC1* and likely causes its inactivation.[10] Breakpoints in the other two cases map close to the last exon of the *OFCC1* gene.

TFAP2A is a transcription factor that is highly expressed in cranial neural crest cells, ectoderm, and nervous system. Disruption of *TFAP2A* causes multiple congenital anomalies, including body wall and neural tube closure phenotypes, and severe dysmorphogenesis of the face, skull, sensory organs, and cranial ganglia.[160] Chimeric mice composed of both wild type and TFAP2A null cells display an array of phenotypes. Two-thirds of the animals show craniofacial abnormalities independent of neural tube defects. Amongst these, cleft lip and palate and midline cleft of the primary palate have been described.[161] In addition, neural crest-specific disruption of

TFAP2A also results in neural tube defects and craniofacial abnormalities, including cleft palate as the most common manifestation.[162]

Endothelin-1 (EDN1) is a ligand in the endothelin pathway that includes two additional ligands, EDN2 and EDN3, and their receptors, Endothelin-A receptor (ETA) and Endothelin-B receptor (EDNRB). The endothelin pathway also includes two isoenzymes of the Endothelin-converting enzyme (ECE-1 and ECE-2).[157] *EDN1* is expressed in the epithelium and paraxial mesoderm core of pharyngeal arches, endothelium of the aortic arch, and cardiac outflow tracts. Mice deficient in EDN1, ETA, and ECE-1 all have malformations of pharyngeal arch-derived craniofacial structures and also cardiovascular abnormalities.[163–165] Recently, Ozeki et al.[166] re-examined the ET1 null mice phenotype and concluded that the craniofacial morphology and gene expression patterns observed in these mice are consistent with a homeotic-like transformation of the mandible into a maxillary arch, suggesting a role for the ET1/ETA pathway in dorsoventral mandibular patterning.

Three genes of the endothelin pathway (*ETA*, *ETB*, and *ECE1*) were tested for linkage in nine nonsyndromic CL/P families where the trait was not linked to 6p23, but no evidence of linkage to any of these genes was found.[167]

8p11–p23

Recent linkage and association studies performed in 276 extended CL/P Filipino families have found suggestive results in markers that map to the 8p11–p23 region, including SNPs within the *FGFR1* gene.[168] A variety of potentially causal genes map to this region, including *NAT1*, *EPHX2*, *BAG4*, and *FGFR1*.

It is well established that maternal exposure to tobacco smoke causes an increased risk for orofacial clefting.[33] NAT1 is an arylamine *n*-acetyltransferase involved in detoxifying xenobiotics, including constituents of tobacco smoke. Two recent studies have shown the risk for CL/P is associated with gene–environment interactions involving NAT1 polymorphisms. Certain *NAT1* alleles and maternal smoking resulted in a fourfold increased risk,[169] whereas the same *NAT1* alleles increased the risk by twofold in mothers who did not take periconceptional multivitamin supplements.[170]

Fibroblast growth factors (FGFs) and their receptors (FGFRs) constitute a large family of molecules with important functions during embryogenesis. So far, 23 FGFs and 4 FGFRs have been identified. FGF binding to FGFRs initiates a signaling cascade that ultimately activates transcription factors to regulate targeted genes.[171] *FGF3*, *FGF8*, *FGF9*, *FGF10*, *FGF17*, and *FGF18* all have partially overlapping ectodermal expression in the nasal processes,[172] and these patterns correlate with *FGFR1* and *FGFR2* ectodermal and mesenchymal expression. Mutations in FGFR1 are causal for Kallmann syndrome,[173] a genetically heterogeneous syndrome characterized by hypogonadism, dental anomalies, and anosmia and orofacial clefting. In families with Kallmann syndrome, some individuals can present with apparently isolated CL/P, raising

the possibility that some families with Kallmann syndrome are misdiagnosed.[31] Anosmia is a distinguishing feature of Kallmann syndrome; hence, screening all cleft patients for anosmia will help identify those families with the 50% recurrence risk of Kallmann syndrome vs. the 2–5% recurrence risk in isolated orofacial clefting.

Recently, a thorough evaluation of FGF signaling has identified a number of mutations in FGFR1, FGFR2, and FGF8 that likely alter their normal function.[31] Furthermore, association studies showed positive results for *FGF3*, *FGF7*, *FGF10*, *FGF18*, and *FGFR1*. These results are not unexpected given the plethora of biological data demonstrating the importance of this pathway in facial development.[174]

9q22–q33

Genome scans performed in Colombian and US CL/P families found positive evidence of linkage to the region 9q22–q33.[175] Furthermore, a meta-analysis of recent genome-wide linkage studies, revealed that the highest linkage results reported for CL/P occur at the 9q22–33 region, suggesting it is a major locus for CL/P (Fig. 7–3).[28]

Genes that map to this region and that are involved in craniofacial development include *ROR2*, *BARX1*, *PTCH*, *FOXE1*, *TGFBR1*, and *ZNF189*. ROR2 is a receptor tyrosine kinase expressed in the frontonasal process[176] and causal for Robinow syndrome, which includes facial anomalies including clefting.[177,178] PTCH is the receptor for Sonic hedgehog (SHH) gene that is known to be expressed in the frontonasal processes. Mutations in PTCH cause the autosomal dominant Gorlin syndrome,[179,180] in which 4% of the patients have orofacial clefting.[181] Recently, PTCH mutation searches in nonsyndromic cleft lip and palate patients identified two missense mutations likely to confer susceptibility to CLP.[182]

BARX1 is a homeobox-containing gene that is expressed in mice at day 10.5 in areas of the first and second branchial arches.[183] *Barx1* expression is regulated by *Fgf8* and *Bmp4*, which are important epithelial-mesenchymal regulators[124,184–186] acting under the control of *Shh* during facial development.[187,188] FOXE1 belongs to the large family of fork-head transcription factors. Mutations in FOXE1 are causal for the recessive Bamforth–Lazarus syndrome that is characterized by thyroid agenesis, spiky hair, and cleft palate.[189,190] In a large candidate gene mutation screen, two missense mutations (A207V and D285V) were identified in patients with CL/P.[67]

Tgfbr1 is expressed in the palatal shelves,[191] and activation of *Tgfbr1* in *Tgfb3* null mice rescues palatal fusion. Furthermore inactivation of the *Tgfbr1* in palatal epithelium prevents palate fusion.[192] Recently, mutations in TGFBR1 have been found in patients with the recently described autosomal dominant Loeys–Dietz syndrome, which includes bifid uvula and cleft palate.[193]

ZNF189 belongs to the Kruppel-associated, box-containing zinc finger proteins. These molecules are capable

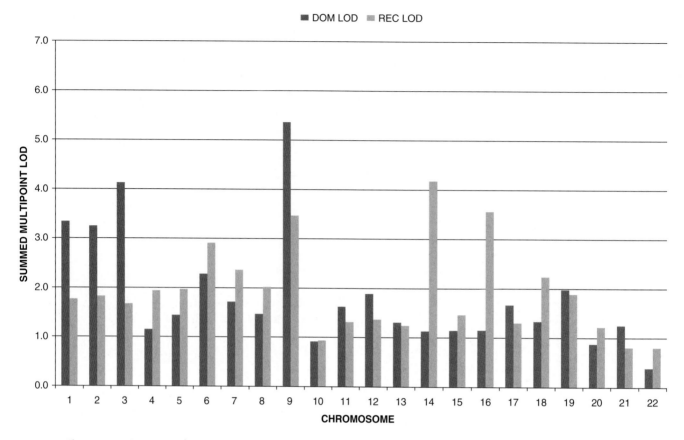

Figure 7–3. Summary of a genome-wide linkage meta-analysis of seven populations. The maximum summed multipoint HLOD for each chromosome, under both dominant (DOM) and recessive (REC) genetic models for CL/P.

of binding DNA and are thought to play important roles in development and differentiation.[194]

14q24 (TGFB3)

Human association and linkage studies have been performed to assess the genetic role of *TGFB3* in nonsyndromic CL/P, yielding inconsistent findings (Table 7–2). A recent genome scan meta-analysis for CL/P yielded a heterogeneity LOD score (HLOD) of 3.92 for this region, corroborating the evidence in favor of *TGFB3* as an orofacial clefting candidate gene.[28] Nevertheless only 15% of the families were linked to this region, which may partially explain the inconsistent results that have been observed among different studies.

Members of the TGFβ superfamily include the genes *TGFβ 1–5*, the more distantly related bone morphogenetic proteins, and the Activin/Inhibin family.[199] TGFβs are ligands that bind to two transmembrane serine/threonine-kinase receptors, which stimulate SMAD proteins to migrate from the cytoplasm to the nucleus, where they function as transcriptional regulators.[200]

Tgfb1, *2*, and *3* are expressed in the developing palate at different time points and regions.[201] *Tgfb3* is expressed in the medial edge epithelium of the palatal shelves before and during palatal shelf elevation, but its expression ceases around the time of palatal fusion. Inactivation of TGFB3 via antibodies, antisense RNA, or targeted deletion results in cleft palate both in vitro and in vivo.[60,61,202] Lack of palatal fusion in null embryos is due to impaired adhesion of the medial edge epithelia and to persistence of the midline epithelial seam.[203] In terms of lip fusion, in vitro experiments have shown that exogenous TGFB3 increases mesenchymal cell proliferation and angiogenesis while accelerating overall lip fusion.[204] In the secondary palate, *Tgfb3* is upstream of *Pax9*,[205] a pair-box containing transcription factor that, when inactivated, also results in cleft palate.[206] *PAX9* also maps near this region, and a missense mutation has been found in a small family with two individuals having CL/P.[207] *BMP4*, which is located between *PAX9* and *TGFB3*, is another candidate, given that its inactivation results in CL/P in mice.[62] Thus, it is plausible that the positive linkage results to this region may be due to any of these three genes.

17q21 (RARA, WNTs)

Vitamin A is an essential nutrient for normal cellular function. Animal models have shown that vitamin A deficiency and excess have teratogenic effects on embryonic development.[208,209] Furthermore, malformations have been observed in humans exposed to high vitamin A doses (25,000 IU/day)

Table 7–2.

Summary of Linkage and Association Results for *TGFB3*

Analysis	Sample	Results	Reference
TDT	Caucasian CL/P	D14S61* (allele 6) $p = 0.01$	[195]
Case-control	Philippines CL/P and CPO	No association for *TGFB2* or *TGFB3*	[91]
TDT	USA Caucasian CL/P and CPO	Significant association. Also found two rare TGFB3 variants in CPO patients	[92]
Case-control	USA Caucasian CL/P and CPO	G-E interactions† High risk for CL/P and CP if mothers smoke more than 10 cigarettes/day and infants are homozygous for specific alleles at *TGFB3*.	[105]
Case-control	European Caucasian CL/P and CPO	No evidence of **G-E interactions for CL/P. Positive association for CP and TGFB3	[196]
TDT	South American CL/P and CPO	*TGFB3* 5′ UTR (254bp allele) in CPO	[197]
Linkage	UK CL/P Caucasian	Exclusion	[22]
Linkage	Asian CL/P	Exclusion	[23]
Linkage	Philippines CL/P	Exclusion	[100]
TDT	Japanese	Significant association	[198]

D14S61 is a STRP marker located 450 Kb from the TGFB3 gene.
†*G-E: Gene-environment.*

from supplements.[210] The teratogenic effects of vitamin A are mediated through its conversion to retinoic acid (RA), a metabolic derivative of vitamin A.[209]

RA activity is mediated by members of the retinoic acid receptor (RAR) family, such as RARA, RARB, RARG, and Retinoic X receptors (RXRs). These receptors are transcriptionally active molecules containing centrally located DNA-binding domains as well as ligand-binding domains. There is a high degree of functional redundancy among RAR receptor family members. For instance, mice lacking RARa1 or RARab1 isoforms appear normal, and RARa1b2, RARab2, and RARb2g double mutants are indistinguishable from control mice. In contrast, RARag double mutants and mice expressing a dominant negative RAR present with a number of congenital malformations, including clefts of the primary and secondary palate.[18,19]

The first evidence of association between CL/P and markers near the *RARA* gene (17q12) was found by Chenevix-Trench et al.[211] in a sample of Caucasian (Australian) subjects. Since this report, various studies using linkage, association, and gene–environment approaches have been performed in different populations (Table 7–3). The first report of positive linkage to this region was obtained by Peanchitlertkajorn et al.[215] in 36 Chinese CL/P families.

More recently, a meta-analysis of 13 genome-wide scans for nonsyndromic CL/P found significant results for the re-

gion 17q12–21.[28] In addition to containing the *RARA* gene, this region is syntenic to the mouse *Clf1* locus, which is one of the loci causal for CL/P in the A/WySn mouse strain. The *Clf1* region encompasses 1.5 million base pairs and is 1–3 cM away from the *Rara* gene.[216] This mouse strain has a retrotransposon insertion 6.6 Kb from the 3′ end of the *Wnt9b* gene. A complementation test using a Wnt9b knockout strain confirmed that Wnt9b is affected by the *Clf1* mutation.[21] *WNT* genes have important roles in neural crest cell induction, specification of dorso-ventral patterning, and chondrocyte differentiation both in the limb and the face.[157,217,218] Interestingly, *WNT3* is within 35 kb of *WNT9B* and in humans a nonsense mutation in WNT3 causes tetra-amelia, a rare autosomal recessive syndrome, characterized by limb, craniofacial (cleft lip and palate), and urogenital malformations.[219] Association studies have shown more positive results for markers in *WNT3* than in *WNT9B*.[220] Since both genes have partially overlapping expression in the nasal and maxillary processes, it is possible that *WNT3* is the affected gene in humans.

19q13.1 (BCL3, CLPTM1, PVR PVRL2, TGFB1)

BCL3 is a proto-oncogene that is involved in cell proliferation, differentiation, and apoptosis.[221] Based on these characteristics, *BCL3* was tested for linkage and association, yielding positive results for both approaches.[222] This report was

Table 7–3.

Summary of Linkage and Association Studies Performed in the Region 17q12–21

Analysis	Sample	Results	Reference
Association	Australian Caucasian CL/P subjects	Positive	[211]
Linkage and association	8 British CL/P families and 61 unrelated cases	Negative	[98]
Linkage	14 Indian CL/P families	Negative	[212]
Linkage	92 UK Sibpairs	Negative	[22]
Linkage and association	38 CL/P Northeastern Italy families	Modest evidence of association	[213]
Association and sequencing of the RARA gene	48 CL/P Japanese triads	Negative. Also found two variants in the gene but no causality was determined for these variants	[214]
Association and G-E interaction	Danish case-control CL/P (222) and CP (80) samples	Only association between a *RARA* SNP and consumption of vitamin A and liver in women who had a child with CL/P	210
Linkage and association	36 CL/P Chinese families	Modest linkage and association findings	[215]

followed by a number of studies with both positive[23,195,223,224] as well as negative[22,76,92] linkage and association results for markers near the *BCL3* gene (Table 7–4). Yoshiura et al.[225] reported fine mapping of the 19q13.3 breakpoint of a chromosomal translocation t(2;19)(q11.2:q13.3) in five members of a three-generation family, two of whom presented with CL/P in addition to other abnormalities. The translocation breakpoint occurred within a novel gene, *CLPTM1*. This gene encodes a transmembrane protein that is expressed during craniofacial development. However, mutation searches performed in families that previously demonstrated linkage to the 19q region[222] as well as in other nonsyndromic CL/P cases did not identify CL/P causal variants in the *CLPTM1* gene.

Other potential candidate genes in the 19q13 region include PVR, *PVRL2*, and *TGFB1*. PVR and PVRL2 are transmembrane proteins that belong to the poliovirus receptor family. Mutations in a member of this family, *PVRL1*, which maps to 11q23–q24, are known to cause the autosomal recessive cleft lip/palate-ectodermal dysplasia syndrome (CLPED1).[226] Furthermore, heterozygotes for the W185X mutation in *PVRL1* are thought to have an increased risk of nonsyndromic CL/P.[227] *PVRL1* and *PVRL2* mutation searches in nonsyndromic families from Italy, Iowa, the Philippines, and South America have found a number of rare variants that may confer risk for CLP.[228–230] Among these, two missense mutations have been found near the V1 domain, which mediates cell–cell and cell–virus adhesion.[229]

GENES INVOLVED IN CL/P: SUMMARY

With the development of high-throughput instruments for genotyping and sequencing, significant steps forward have been made by studies applying these techniques to find genes for CL/P. It is now possible to screen a large number of candidate genes at once, perform genome-wide linkage studies,[28] and sequence a relatively large number of genes[67] to locate the position of CL/P genes and to identify potentially causal mutations in these genes. Results from these studies, together with evidence from research of human genes involved in clefting syndromes and of animal knockout models, provide a wealth of knowledge about both the genetic basis for CL/P in humans and the underlying biologic processes. The genetic basis for approximately 25% of CL/P has now been identified, including 12% by IRF6,[26] 2% by MSX1,[134] 6% by variants in FOXE1, GLI2, MSX2, SKI, and SPRY2,[67] PTCH,[182] PVRL1,[229] PVR and PVRL2,[230] and 5% by variants in the FGF signaling pathway.[168]

In general, the gene identification process for CL/P is still in its early stages, due in large measure to the genetic complexity of clefting. It is anticipated that there are additional genes involved in CL/P that have yet to be identified, and the functional effects of identified mutations have yet to be discerned. However, with the recent publication of genome-wide linkage scans and similar ongoing studies, the field is rapidly advancing toward a deeper understanding of

Table 7–4.

Summary of Linkage and Association Studies in the 19q13 Region

Analysis	Sample	Results	Reference
Linkage and association	38 USA Caucasian and 1 USA African American CL/P families	Positive linkage (HLOD = 7.0) and association ($p = 0.002$) for markers near the *BCL3* gene. (cen-D9S178-*BCL3*-*APOC2*-tel)	[222]
Linkage and association	30 USA and 11 Mexican CL/P families	*BCL3* marker, significant association: USA data ($p = 0.001$) Mexican data ($p = 0.018$) Combined data set ($p < 0.001$)	[223]
Association	110 USA CL/P triads	Significant association ($p < 0.01$) for marker D19S178 (68 cM).	[195]
Linkage and association	40 Caucasian families from Northeastern Italy	Positive nonparametric linkage ($p < 0.01$) and positive association ($p = 0.015$) for marker D19S574 (69 cM).	[224]
Association	133 CL/P cases	No association for the *BCL3* CA polymorphism	[92]
Linkage	19 Swedish CL/P families	No evidence of linkage for markers BCL3 (67 cM), D19S178 (68 cM), and D19S412 (70 cM).	[76]
Linkage	92 UK CL/P Sibpairs	No evidence of linkage to this region	[22]
Linkage and association	36 CL/P families from Shanghai	Positive nonparametric linkage D19S246 (78 cM) ($p = 0.007$)	[23]

the genetic and biologic processes involved in the etiology of CL/P. This knowledge, along with epidemiologic studies of environmental factors and gene–environment interactions also involved in CL/P, will lead to public health recommendations to decrease the prevalence of this common birth defect.

ABBREVIATION

Allele	A genetic variation for a given marker or locus
cM	Centimorgan. 1 cM is equal to 1% recombination and approximately 1 million base pairs
Exon	The DNA sequence for any protein coding portion of a gene
Gene	The DNA sequence encoding for a protein
Genome	The entire genetic material for a given organism. For humans this consists of 22 pairs of chromosomes plus two sex chromosomes either XX or XY.
Genotyping	A laboratory technique used to determine which alleles exist for a marker in a person
Haplotype	A combination of alleles for markers as they occur on a chromosome
Heterogeneity— Allelic	This describes the situation where two or more mutations in the same gene cause the same phenotype. This complicates association strategies which look for the presence of a given allele to be found more often in cases than controls. If more than one allele contributes to the disease risk, this may be difficult to detect in situations with inadequate study power.

Heterogeneity— Locus	A disease that can be caused by a mutation in 1 of 2 or more genes. This complicates linkage analysis, since positive signals by families linked at one locus can be cancelled out by negative signals from families linked at another locus.
Heterozygosity	The presence of two different alleles for a given marker
Homozygosity	The presence of the same alleles for a given marker
Intron	Noncoding regions of a gene that occur between Exons
Locus	A given region of the human genome
Marker	A region of the human genome that contains DNA variation within it. The variation is used as a marker to follow inheritance of the genetic material within the locus.
Mb	Megabase = 1 million base pairs
Mutations Silent	Mutations in the coding region of a gene that do not change the amino acid sequence of a protein
Neutral	Mutations in the coding region that cause the substitution of a biochemically similar amino acid. These may result in subtle functional changes to the protein, but not enough to cause drastic changes
Missense	Mutations in the coding region of a gene that results in an amino acid substitution. The effect of the substitution can vary from significantly affecting the protein function to not having any effect at all depending upon how chemically similar the substituted amino acid is to the original amino acid.
Nonsense	Mutations in the coding region of the gene that results in premature cessation during the translation of the gene
Penetrance	The frequency that the disease phenotype is expressed when the disease mutation is present
Polymorphism	Synonymous with genetic marker
SNP	Single nucleotide polymorphism— these have a lower mutation rate than repeat polymorphisms, thus more likely reflect historical mutation and recombination events.
STRP	Short Tandem Repeat Polymorphism—repetitive elements of di, tri, and tetranucleotides that vary in repeat number for a given locus.

References

1. Schliekelman P, Slatkin M. Multiplex relative risk and estimation of the number of loci underlying an inherited disease. *Am J Hum Genet* 71(6):1369–1385, 2002.
2. Strachan T, Read AP. *Human Molecular Genetics*, 3rd edn. New York: Wiley-Liss, 2003.
3. Risch N, Merikangas K. The future of genetic studies of complex human diseases. *Science* 273(5281):1516–1517, 1996.
4. Spielman RS, McGinnis RE, Warren JE. Transmission test for linkage disequilibrium: The insulin gene region and insulin-dependent Diabetes Mellitus (IDDM). *Am J Hum Genet* 52:506–516, 1993.
5. Schutte BC, Murray JC. The many faces and factors of orofacial clefts. *Hum Mol Genet* 8(10):1853–1859, 1999.
6. Spritz RA. The genetics and epigenetics of orofacial clefts. *Curr Opin Pediatr* 13(6):556–560, 2001.
7. Murray J. Gene/environment causes of cleft lip and/or palate. *Clin Genet* 61(4):248–256, 2002.
8. Carinci F, Pezzetti F, Scapoli L, et al. Recent developments in orofacial cleft genetics. *J Craniofac Surg* 14(2):130–143, 2003.
9. Donnai D, Heather LJ, Sinclair P, et al. Association of autosomal dominant cleft lip and palate and translocation 6p23; 9q22.3. *Clin Dysmorphol* 1:89–97, 1992.
10. Davies SJ, Wise C, Venkatesh B, et al. Mapping of three translocation breakpoints associated with orofacial clefting within 6p24 and identification of new transcripts within the region. *Cytogenet Genome Res* 105(1):47–53, 2004.
11. Davies AF, Stephens RJ, Olavesen MG, et al. Evidence of a locus for orofacial clefting on human chromosome 6p24 and STS content map of the region. *Hum Mol Genet* 4(1):121–128, 1995.
12. Davies AF, Imaizumi K, Mirza G, et al. Further evidence for the involvement of human chromosome 6p24 in the aetiology of orofacial clefting. *J Med Genet* 35(10):857–861, 1998.
13. Wilkie AO, Morriss-Kay GM. Genetics of craniofacial development and malformation. *Nat Rev Genet* 2(6):458–468, 2001.
14. Nottoli T, Hagopian-Donaldson S, Zhang J, et al. AP-2-null cells disrupt morphogenesis of the eye, face, and limbs in chimeric mice. *PNAS* 95(23):13714–13719, 1998.
15. Miettinen PJ, Chin JR, Shum L, et al. Epidermal growth factor receptor function is necessary for normal craniofacial development and palate closure. *Nat Genet* 22(1):69–73, 1999.
16. Colmenares C, Heilstedt HA, Shaffer LG, et al. Loss of the SKI protooncogene in individuals affected with 1p36 deletion syndrome is predicted by strain-dependent defects in Ski-/- mice. *Nat Genet* 30(1):106–109, 2002.
17. Tang LS, Finnell RH. Neural and craniofacial abnormalities secondary to altered gene expression in the folic acid-binding protein 1 (Folbp1) deficient mouse embryo. *Birth Defects Res Part A Clin Mol Teratol* 67(4):209–218, 2003.
18. Lohnes D, Mark M, Mendelsohn C, et al. Function of the retinoic acid receptors (RARs) during development: (I) Craniofacial and skeletal abnormalities in RAR double mutants. *Development* 120:2723–2748, 1994.
19. Damm K, Heyman RA, Umesono K, et al. Functional inhibition of retinoic acid response by dominant negative retinoic acid receptor mutants. *Proc Natl Acad Sci* 90:2989–2993, 1993.
20. Reed SC, Snell GD. Harelip. A new mutation in the house mouse. *Anat Rec* 51(1):43–50, 1931.
21. Juriloff DM, Harris MJ, McMahon AP, et al. Wnt9b is the mutated gene involved in multifactorial nonsyndromic cleft lip with or

without cleft palate in A/WySn mice, as confirmed by a genetic complementation test. *Birth Defects Res A Clin Mol Teratol* 76(8):574–579, 2006.

22. Prescott NJ, Lees MM, Winter RM, et al. Identification of susceptibility loci for nonsyndromic cleft lip with or without cleft palate in a two stage genome scan of affected sib-pairs. *Hum Genet* 106(3):345–350, 2000.

23. Marazita ML, Field LL, Cooper ME, et al. Genome scan for loci involved in cleft lip with or without cleft palate, in Chinese multiplex families. *Am J Hum Genet* 71(2):349–364, 2002.

24. Wyszynski DF, Albacha-Hejazi H, Aldirani M, et al. A genome-wide scan for loci predisposing to non-syndromic cleft lip with or without cleft palate in two large Syrian families. *Am J Med Genet* 123A(2):140–147, 2003.

25. Zeiger JS, Hetmanski JB, Beaty TH, et al. Evidence for linkage of nonsyndromic cleft lip with or without cleft palate to a region on chromosome 2. *Eur J Hum Genet* 11(11):835–839, 2003.

26. Zucchero TM, Cooper ME, Maher BS, et al. Interferon regulatory factor 6 (IRF6) gene variants and the risk of isolated cleft lip or palate. *N Engl J Med* 351(8):769–780, 2004.

27. Marazita ML, Field LL, Tuncbilek G, et al. Genome-scan for loci involved in cleft lip with or without cleft palate in consanguineous families from Turkey. *Am J Med Genet* 126A(2):111–122, 2004.

28. Marazita ML, Murray JC, Lidral AC, et al. Meta-analysis of 13 genome scans reveals multiple cleft lip/palate genes with novel loci on 9q21 and 2q32–35. *Am J Hum Genet* 75(2):161–173, 2004.

29. Field LL, Ray AK, Cooper ME, et al. Genome scan for loci involved in nonsyndromic cleft lip with or without cleft palate in families from West Bengal, India. *Am J Med Genet* 130A(3):265–271, 2004.

30. Moreno L. Cleft lip genome scan, 2007.

31. Riley BM, Schultz RE, Cooper ME, et al. A genome-wide linkage scan for cleft lip and cleft palate identifies a novel locus on 8p11–23. *Am J Med Genet A* 143(8):846–852, 2007.

32. Wyszynski DF, Duffy DL, Beaty TH. Maternal cigarette smoking and oral clefts: A meta-analysis. *Cleft Palate Craniofac J* 34(3):206–210, 1997.

33. Little J, Cardy A, Arslan MT, et al. Smoking and orofacial clefts: A United Kingdom-based case-control study. *Cleft Palate Craniofac J* 41(4):381–386, 2004.

34. Shi M, Christensen K, Weinberg CR, et al. Orofacial cleft risk is increased with maternal smoking and specific detoxification-gene variants. *Am J Hum Genet* 80(1):76–90, 2007.

35. van Rooij IA, Wegerif MJ, Roelofs HM, et al. Smoking, genetic polymorphisms in biotransformation enzymes, and nonsyndromic oral clefting: A gene-environment interaction. *Epidemiology* 12(5):502–507, 2001.

36. Voet D, Voet JG. *Biochemistry,* 2nd edn. New York: Wiley, 1995.

37. Razin A. CpG methylation, chromatin structure and gene silencing—A three-way connection. *Embo J* 17(17):4905–4908, 1998.

38. Razin A, Kantor B. DNA methylation in epigenetic control of gene expression. *Prog Mol Subcell Biol* 38:151–167, 2005.

39. MRC Vitamin Study Research Group. Prevention of neural tube defects: Results of the Medical Research Council Vitamin Study. *Lancet II* 338(8760):131–137, 1991.

40. Tolarova MM, Harris J. Reduced recurrence of orofacial clefts after periconceptional supplementation with high-dose folic acid and multivitamins. *Teratology* 51:71–78, 1995.

41. Shaw GM, Lammer EJ, Wasserman CR, et al. Risks of orofacial clefts in children born to women using multivitamins containing folic acid periconceptionally. *Lancet* 346(8972):393–396, 1995.

42. van Rooij IALM, Ocke MC, Straatman H, et al. Periconceptional folate intake by supplement and food reduces the risk of nonsyndromic cleft lip with or without cleft palate. *Prev Med* 39(4):689–694, 2004.

43. Wilcox AJ, Lie RT, Solvoll K, et al. Folic acid supplements and risk of facial clefts: National population based case-control study. *Bmj* 334(7591):464, 2007.

44. Frosst P, Blom HJ, Milos R, et al. A candidate genetic risk factor for vascular disease: A common mutation in methylenetetrahydrofolate reductase. *Nat Genet* 10(1):111–113, 1995.

45. Pezzetti F, Martinelli M, Scapoli L, et al. Maternal MTHFR variant forms increase the risk in offspring of isolated nonsyndromic cleft lip with or without cleft palate. *Hum Mutat* 24(1):104–105, 2004.

46. Shaw GM, Rozen R, Finnell RH, et al. Infant C677T mutation in MTHFR, maternal periconceptional vitamin use, and cleft lip. *Am J Med Genet* 80(3):196–198, 1998.

47. Mills JL. Folate and oral clefts: Where do we go from here? New directions in oral clefts research. *Teratology* 60(5):251–252, 1999.

48. Blanton SH, Kolle BS, Hecht JT, et al. No evidence supporting MTHFR as a risk factor in the development of familial NSCLP. *Am J Med Genet* 92(5):370–371, 2000.

49. Blanton SH, Patel S, Hecht JT, et al. MTHFR is not a risk factor in the development of isolated nonsyndromic cleft lip and palate. *Am J Med Genet* 110(4):404–405, 2002.

50. Prescott NJ, Winter RM, Malcolm S. Maternal MTHFR genotype contributes to the risk of non-syndromic cleft lip and palate. *J Med Genet* 39(5):368–369, 2002.

51. Jugessur A, Wilcox AJ, Lie RT, et al. Exploring the effects of methylenetetrahydrofolate reductase gene variants C677T and A1298C on the risk of orofacial clefts in 261 Norwegian case—Parent triads. *Am J Epidemiol* 157(12):1083–1091, 2003.

52. Vieira AR, Murray JC, Trembath D, et al. Studies of reduced folate carrier 1 (RFC1) A80G and 5,10-methylenetetrahydrofolate reductase (MTHFR) C677T polymorphisms with neural tube and orofacial cleft defects. *Am J Med Genet A* 135(2):220–223, 2005.

53. Zhu J, Ren A, Hao L, et al. Variable contribution of the MTHFR C677T polymorphism to non-syndromic cleft lip and palate risk in China. *Am J Med Genet A* 140(6):551–557, 2006.

54. Chevrier C, Perret C, Bahuau M, et al. Fetal and maternal MTHFR C677T genotype, maternal folate intake and the risk of nonsyndromic oral clefts. *Am J Med Genet A* 143(3):248–257, 2007.

55. Martinelli M, Scapoli L, Pezzetti F, et al. Linkage analysis of three candidate regions of chromosome 1 in nonsyndromic familial orofacial cleft. *Ann Hum Genet* 65(Pt 5):465–471, 2001.

56. Martinelli M, Scapoli L, Palmieri A, et al. Study of four genes belonging to the folate pathway: Transcobalamin 2 is involved in the onset of non-syndromic cleft lip with or without cleft palate. *Hum Mutat* 27(3):294, 2006.

57. Pei L, Zhu H, Zhu J, et al. Genetic variation of infant reduced folate carrier (A80G) and risk of orofacial defects and congenital heart defects in China. *Ann Epidemiol* 16(5):352–356, 2006.

58. Scapoli L, Marchesini J, Martinelli M, et al. Study of folate receptor genes in nonsyndromic familial and sporadic cleft lip with or without cleft palate cases. *Am J Med Genet A* 132(3):302–304, 2005.

59. Prescott NJ, Malcolm S. Folate and the face: Evaluating the evidence for the influence of folate genes on craniofacial development. *Cleft Palate Craniofac J* 39(3):327–331, 2002.

60. Kaartinen V, Voncken JW, Shuler C, et al. Abnormal lung development and cleft palate in mice lacking TGF-B3 indicates defects of epithelial—mesenchymal interaction. *Nat Genet* 11:415–421, 1995.

61. Proetzel G, Pawlowski SA, Wiles MV, et al. Transforming growth factor-B3 is required for secondary palate fusion. *Nat Genet* 11:409–414, 1995.

62. Liu W, Sun X, Braut A, et al. Distinct functions for Bmp signaling in lip and palate fusion in mice. *Development* 132(6):1453–1461, 2005:dev.01676.

63. Barlow AJ, Francis-West PH. Ectopic application of recombinant BMP-2 and BMP-4 can change patterning of developing chick facial primordia. *Development* 124(2):391–398, 1997.

64. Winograd J, Reilly M, Roe R, et al. Perinatal lethality and multiple craniofacial malformations in MSX2 transgenic mice. *Hum Mol Genet* 6(3):369–379, 1997.

65. Luo K. Ski and SnoN: Negative regulators of TGF-beta signaling. *Curr Opin Genet Dev* 14(1):65–70, 2004.

66. Lu W, Volcik K, Zhu H, et al. Genetic variation in the proto-oncogene SKI and risk for orofacial clefting. *Mol Genet Metab* 86(3):412–416, 2005.

67. Vieira AR, Avila JR, Daack-Hirsch S, et al. Medical sequencing of candidate genes for nonsyndromic cleft lip and palate. *PLoS Genet* 1(6):e64, 2005.

68. Kondo S, Schutte BC, Richardson RJ, et al. Mutations in IRF6 cause Van der Woude and popliteal pterygium syndromes. *Nat Genet* 32(2):285–289, 2002.

69. Taniguchi T, Ogasawara K, Takaoka A, et al. IRF family of transcription factors as regulators of host defense. *Annu Rev Immunol* 19:623–655, 2001.

70. Ingraham CR, Kinoshita A, Kondo S, et al. Abnormal skin, limb and craniofacial morphogenesis in mice deficient for interferon regulatory factor 6 (Irf6). *Nat Genet* 38(11):1335–1340, 2006.

71. Richardson RJ, Dixon J, Malhotra S, et al. Irf6 is a key determinant of the keratinocyte proliferation-differentiation switch. *Nat Genet* 38(11):1329–1334, 2006.

72. Houdayer C, Bonaiti-Pellie C, Erguy C, et al. Possible relationship between the van der Woude syndrome (VWS) locus and nonsyndromic cleft lip with or without cleft palate (NSCL/P). *Am J Med Genet* 104(1):86–92, 2001.

73. Ghassibe M, Bayet B, Revencu N, et al. Interferon regulatory factor-6: A gene predisposing to isolated cleft lip with or without cleft palate in the Belgian population. *Eur J Hum Genet* 13(11):1239–1242, 2005.

74. Scapoli L, Palmieri A, Martinelli M, et al. Strong evidence of linkage disequilibrium between polymorphisms at the IRF6 locus and nonsyndromic cleft lip with or without cleft palate, in an Italian population. *Am J Hum Genet* 76(1):180–183, 2005.

75. Srichomthong C, Siriwan P, Shotelersuk V. Significant association between IRF6 820G->A and non-syndromic cleft lip with or without cleft palate in the Thai population. *J Med Genet* 42(7):e46, 2005.

76. Wong FK, Hagberg C, Karsten A, et al. Linkage analysis of candidate regions in Swedish nonsyndromic cleft lip with or without cleft palate families. *Cleft Palate Craniofac J* 37(4):357–362, 2000.

77. Xu X, Han J, Ito Y, et al. Cell autonomous requirement for Tgfbr2 in the disappearance of medial edge epithelium during palatal fusion. *Dev Biol* 297(1):238–248, 2006.

78. Ferguson MW, O'Kane S. Scar-free healing: From embryonic mechanisms to adult therapeutic intervention. *Philos Trans R Soc Lond B Biol Sci* 359(1445):839–850, 2004.

79. Collin GB, Marshall JD, Naggert JK, et al. TGFA: Exon-intron structure and evaluation as a candidate gene for Alstrom syndrome. *Clin Genet* 55(1):61–62, 1999.

80. Dixon MJ, Garner J, Ferguson MW. Immunolocalization of epidermal growth factor (EGF), EGF receptor and transforming growth factor alpha (TGF alpha) during murine palatogenesis in vivo and in vitro. *Anat Embryol (Berl)* 184(1):83–91, 1991.

81. Luetteke NC, Qiu TH, Peiffer RL, et al. TGFalpha deficiency results in hair follicle and eye abnormalities in targeted and waved-1 mice. *Cell* 73:263–278, 1993.

82. Ardinger HH, Buetow KH, Bell GI, et al. Association of genetic variation of the transforming growth factor-alpha gene with cleft lip and palate. *Am J Hum Genet* 45(3):348–353, 1989.

83. Chenevix-Trench G, Jones K, Green A, et al. Further evidence for an association between genetic variation in transforming growth factor-alpha and cleft lip and palate. *Am J Hum Genet* 48:1012–1013, 1991.

84. Holder SE, Vintiner GM, Farren B, et al. Confirmation of an association between RFLPs and the transforming growth factor-alpha locus and non-syndromic cleft lip and palate. *J Med Genet* 29:390–392, 1992.

85. Stoll C, Qian JF, Feingold J, et al. Genetic variation in transforming growth factor alpha: Possible association of BamHI Polymorphism with bilateral sporadic cleft lip and palate. *Am J Hum Genet* 50:870–871, 1992.

86. Sassani R, Bartlett SP, Feng H, et al. Association between alleles of the transforming growth factor-alpha locus and the occurrence of cleft lip. *Am J Med Genet* 45:565–569, 1993.

87. Jara L, Blanco R, Chiffelle I, et al. Association between alleles of the transforming growth factor alpha locus and cleft lip and palate in the Chilean population. *Am J Med Genet* 57:548–551, 1995.

88. Beaty TH, Hetmanski JB, Fallin MD, et al. Analysis of candidate genes on chromosome 2 in oral cleft case—Parent trios from three populations. *Hum Genet* V120(4):501–518, 2006.

89. Field LL, Ray AK, Marazita ML. Transforming growth factor alpha: A modifying locus for nonsyndromic cleft lip with or without cleft palate? *Eur J Hum Genet* 57(2):159–165, 1994.

90. Mitchell LE. Transforming growth factor alpha locus and nonsyndromic cleft lip with or without cleft palate: A reappraisal. *Genet Epidemiol* 14(3):231–240, 1997.

91. Lidral AC, Murray JC, Buetow KH, et al. Studies of the candidate genes TGFB2, MSX1, TGFA, and TGFB3 in the etiology of cleft lip and palate in the Philippines. *Cleft Palate Craniofac J* 34(1):1–6, 1997.

92. Lidral AC, Romitti PA, Basart AM, et al. Association of MSX1 and TGFB3 with nonsyndromic clefting in humans. *Am J Hum Genet* 63(2):557–568, 1998.

93. Scapoli L, Pezzetti F, Carinci F, et al. Lack of linkage disequilibrium between transforming growth factor alpha Taq I polymorphism and cleft lip with or without cleft palate in families from Northeastern Italy. *Am J Med Genet* 75(2):203–206, 1998.

94. Jugessur A, Lie RT, Wilcox AJ, et al. Variants of developmental genes (TGFA, TGFB3, and MSX1) and their associations with orofacial clefts: A case-parent triad analysis. *Genet Epidemiol* 24(3):230–239, 2003.

95. Passos-Bueno MR, Gaspar DA, Kamiya T, et al. Transforming growth factor-alpha and nonsyndromic cleft lip with or without palate in Brazilian patients: Results of a large case-control study. *Cleft Palate Craniofac J* 41(4):387–391, 2004.

96. Hecht JT, Wang Y, Blanton SH, et al. Cleft lip and palate: No evidence of linkage to transforming growth factor alpha. *Am J Hum Genet* 49:682–686, 1991.

97. Wyszynski DF, Maestri N, Lewanda AF, et al. No evidence of linkage for cleft lip with or without cleft palate to a marker near the transforming growth factor alpha locus in two populations. *Hum Hered* 47(2):101–109, 1997.

98. Vintiner GM, Lo KK, Holder SE, et al. Exclusion of candidate genes from a role in cleft lip with or without cleft palate: Linkage and association studies. *J Med Genet* 30(9):773–778, 1993.

99. Pezzetti F, Scapoli L, Martinelli M, et al. A locus in 2p13–p14 (OFC2), in addition to that mapped in 6p23, is involved in nonsyndromic familial orofacial cleft malformation. *Genomics* 50(3):299–305, 1998.

100. Schultz RE, Cooper ME, Daack-Hirsch S, et al. Targeted scan of fifteen regions for nonsyndromic cleft lip and palate in Filipino families. *Am J Med Genet* 125A(1):17–22, 2004.

101. Hwang SJ, Beaty TH, Panny SR, et al. Association study of transforming growth factor alpha (TGFa) TaqI polymorphism and oral clefts: Indication of gene-environment interaction in a population based sample of infants with birth defects. *Am J Epidemiol* 141(7):629–636, 1995.

102. Shaw GM, Wasserman CR, Murray JC, et al. Infant TGF-alpha genotype, orofacial clefts, and maternal periconceptional multivitamin use. *Cleft Palate Craniofac J* 35(4):366–370, 1998.

103. Beaty TH, Maestri NE, Hetmanski JB, et al. Testing for interaction between maternal smoking and TGFA genotype among oral cleft cases born in Maryland 1992–1996. *Cleft Palate Craniofac J* 34(5):447–454, 1997.

104. Christensen K, Olsen J, Norgaard-Pedersen B, et al. Oral clefts, transforming growth factor alpha gene variants, and maternal smoking: A population-based case-control study in Denmark, 1991–1994. *Am J Epidemiol* 149(3):248–255, 1999.

105. Romitti PA, Lidral AC, Munger RG, et al. Candidate genes for non-syndromic cleft lip and palate and maternal cigarette smoking and alcohol consumption: Evaluation of genotype-environment interactions from a population-based case-control study of orofacial clefts. *Teratology* 59(1):39–50, 1999.

106. Jugessur A, Lie RT, Wilcox AJ, et al. Cleft palate, transforming growth factor alpha gene variants, and maternal exposures: Assessing gene-environment interactions in case-parent triads. *Genet Epidemiol* 25(4):367–374, 2003.

107. Machida J, Yoshiura K, Funkhauser CD, et al. Transforming growth factor-alpha (TGFA): Genomic structure, boundary sequences, and mutation analysis in nonsyndromic cleft lip/palate and cleft palate only. *Genomics* 61(3):237–242, 1999.

108. Vieira AR. Association between the transforming growth factor alpha gene and nonsyndromic oral clefts: A HuGE review. *Am J Epidemiol* 163(9):790–810, 2006.

109. Brewer C, Holloway S, Zawalnyski P, et al. A chromosomal deletion map of human malformations. *Am J Hum Genet* 63(4):1153–1159, 1998.

110. Brewer CM, Leek JP, Green AJ, et al. A locus for isolated cleft palate, located on human chromosome 2q32. *Am J Hum Genet* 65(2):387–396, 1999.

111. Bird LM, Mascarello JT. Chromosome 2q duplications: case report of a de novo interstitial duplication and review of the literature. *Am J Med Genet* 100(1):13–24, 2001.

112. Riegel M, Schinzel A. Duplication of (2)(q11.1–q13.2) in a boy with mental retardation and cleft lip and palate: Another clefting gene locus on proximal 2q? *Am J Med Genet* 111(1):76–80, 2002.

113. Ahn JM, Koo DH, Kwon KW, et al. Partial trisomy 2q(2q37.3–>qter) and monosomy 7q(7q34—>qter) due to paternal reciprocal translocation 2;7: A case report. *J Korean Med Sci* 18(1):112–113, 2003.

114. Casas KA, Mononen TK, Mikail CN, et al. Chromosome 2q terminal deletion: Report of 6 new patients and review of phenotype-breakpoint correlations in 66 individuals. *Am J Med Genet A* 130(4):331–339, 2004.

115. Ounap K, Ilus T, Laidre P, et al. A new case of 2q duplication supports either a locus for orofacial clefting between markers D2S1897 and D2S2023 or a locus for cleft palate only on chromosome 2q13–q21. *Am J Med Genet A* 137(3):323–327, 2005.

116. Qiu M, Bulfone A, Martinez S, et al. Null mutation of *Dlx-2* results in abnormal morphogenesis of proximal first and second branchial arch derivatives and abnormal differentiation in the forebrain. *Genes Develop* 9:2523–3538, 1995.

117. Qiu M, Bulfone A, Ghattas I, et al. Role of the Dlx homeobox genes in proximodistal patterning of the branchial arches: Mutations of Dlx-1, Dlx-2, and Dlx-1 and -2 alter morphogenesis of proximal skeletal and soft tissue structures derived from the first and second arches. *Dev Biol* 185(2):165–184, 1997.

118. Depew MJ, Lufkin T, Rubenstein JLR. Specification of jaw subdivisions by Dlx genes. *Science* 2002, DOI: 10.1126/science.1075703.

119. FitzPatrick DR, Carr IM, McLaren L, et al. Identification of SATB2 as the cleft palate gene on 2q32–q33. *Hum Mol Genet* 12(19):2491–2501, 2003.

120. Thomas BL, Liu JK, Rubenstein JL, et al. Independent regulation of Dlx2 expression in the epithelium and mesenchyme of the first branchial arch. *Development* 127(2):217–224, 2000.

121. Liu W, Sun X, Braut A, et al. Distinct functions for Bmp signaling in lip and palate fusion in mice. *Development* 132(6):1453–1461, 2005.

122. Alkuraya FS, Saadi I, Lund JJ, et al. SUMO1 haploinsufficiency leads to cleft lip and palate. *Science* 313(5794):1751, 2006.

123. Alappat S, Zhang ZY, Chen YP. Msx homeobox gene family and craniofacial development. *Cell Res* 13(6):429–442, 2003.

124. Zhang Z, Song Y, Zhao X, et al. Rescue of cleft palate in Msx1-deficient mice by transgenic Bmp4 reveals a network of BMP and Shh signaling in the regulation of mammalian palatogenesis. *Development* 129(17):4135–4146, 2002.

125. Satokata I, Maas R. *Msx1* deficient mice exhibit cleft palate and abnormalities of craniofacial and tooth development. *Nat Genet* 6:348–356, 1994.

126. Vastardis H, Karimbux N, Guthua SW, et al. A human MSX1 homeodomain missense mutation causes selective tooth agenesis [see comments]. *Nat Genet* 13(4):417–421, 1996.

127. Lidral AC, Reising BC. The role of MSX1 in human tooth agenesis. *J Dent Res* 81(4):274–278, 2002.

128. De Muynck S, Schollen E, Matthijs G, et al. A novel MSX1 mutation in hypodontia. *Am J Med Genet A* 128(4):401–403, 2004.

129. van den Boogaard MJ, Dorland M, Beemer FA, et al. MSX1 mutation is associated with orofacial clefting and tooth agenesis in humans [published erratum appears in *Nat Genet* 25(1):125, May 2000]. *Nat Genet* 24(4):342–343, 2000.

130. Jumlongras D, Bei M, Stimson JM, et al. A nonsense mutation in MSX1 causes Witkop syndrome. *Am J Hum Genet* 69(1):67–74, 2001.

131. Blanco R, Chakraborty R, Barton SA, et al. Evidence of a sex-dependent association between the MSX1 locus and nonsyndromic cleft lip with or without cleft palate in the Chilean population. *Hum Biol* 73(1):81–89, 2001.

132. Beaty TH, Hetmanski JB, Zeiger JS, et al. Testing candidate genes for non-syndromic oral clefts using a case—Parent trio design. *Genet Epidemiol* 22(1):1–11, 2002.

133. Suzuki Y, Jezewski PA, Machida J, et al. In a Vietnamese population, MSX1 variants contribute to cleft lip and palate. *Genet Med* 6(3):117–125, 2004.

134. Jezewski PA, Vieira AR, Nishimura C, et al. Complete sequencing shows a role for MSX1 in non-syndromic cleft lip and palate. *J Med Genet* 40(6):399–407, 2003.

135. Tongkobpetch S, Siriwan P, Shotelersuk V. MSX1 mutations contribute to nonsyndromic cleft lip in a Thai population. *J Hum Genet* 51(8):671–676, 2006.

136. Biddle FG, Fraser RC. Cortisone-induced cleft palate in the mouse. A search for the genetic control of the embryonic response trait. *Genetics* 85(2):289–302, 1977.

137. Van Dyke DC, Goldman AS, Spielman RS, et al. Segregation of HLA in sibs with cleft lip or cleft lip and cleft palate: Evidence against genetic linkage. *Cleft Palate J* 17(3):189–193, 1980.

138. Van Dyke DC, Goldman AS, Spielman RS, et al. Segregation of HLA in families with oral clefts: Evidence against linkage between isolated cleft palate and HLA. *Am J Med Genet* 15:85–88, 1983.

139. Watanabe T, Ohishi M, Tashiro H. Population and family studies of HLA in Japanese with cleft lip and cleft palate. *Cleft Palate J* 21:293–300, 1984.

140. Hecht JT, Wang Y, Connor B, et al. Nonsyndromic cleft lip and palate: No evidence of linkage to HLA or factor 13A. *Am J Hum Genet* 52:1230–1233, 1993.

141. Sakata Y, Tokunaga K, Yonehara Y, et al. Significant association of HLA-B and HLA-DRB1 alleles with cleft lip with or without cleft palate. *Tissue Antigens* 53(2):147–152, 1999.

142. Carinci F, Pezzetti F, Scapoli L, et al. Nonsyndromic cleft lip and palate: Evidence of linkage to a microsatellite marker on 6p23 [letter]. *Am J Hum Genet* 56(1):337–339, 1995.

143. Scapoli L, Pezzetti F, Carinci F, et al. Evidence of linkage to 6p23 and genetic heterogeneity in nonsyndromic cleft lip with or without cleft palate. *Genomics* 43(2):216–220, 1997.

144. Carreno H, Paredes M, Tellez G, et al. Association of non-syndromic cleft lip and cleft palate with microsatellite markers located in 6p. *Rev Med Chil* 127(10):1189–1198, 1999.

145. Blanco R, Suazo J, Santos JL, et al. Evaluation of the association between microsatellite markers located on 6p22–25 and no syndromic cleft lip palate using the case—Parents trio design in Chilean population. *Rev Med Chil* 131(7):765–772, 2003.

146. Clementi M, Tenconi R, Collins A, et al. Complex segregation analysis in a sample of consecutive newborns with cleft lip with or without cleft palate in Italy. *Human Heredity* 45:157–164, 1995.

147. Blanton SH, Crowder E, Malcom S, et al. Exclusion of linkage between cleft lip with or without cleft palate and markers on chromosome 4 and 6. *Am J Hum Genet* 58:239–241, 1996.

148. Lander E, Kruglyak L. Genetic dissection of complex traits: Guidelines for interpreting and reporting linkage results. *Nat Genet* 11(3):241–247, 1995.

149. Donnai D, Heather LJ, Sinclair P, et al. Association of autosomal dominant cleft lip and palate and translocation 6p23;9q22.3. *Clin Dysmorphol* 1(2):89–97, 1992.

150. Law CJ, Fisher AM, Temple IK. Distal 6p deletion syndrome: A report of a case with anterior chamber eye anomaly and review of published reports. *J Med Genet* 35(8):685–689, 1998.

151. Balci S, Aypar E, Son YA, et al. Balanced de novo translocation t(6;7)(p25;q31) and cleft palate as an isolated finding. *Genet Couns* 15(3):317–320, 2004.

152. Aitola M, Carlsson P, Mahlapuu M, et al. Forkhead transcription factor FoxF2 is expressed in mesodermal tissues involved in epithelio-mesenchymal interactions. *Dev Dyn* 218(1):136–149, 2000.

153. Choi VM, Harland RM, Khokha MK. Developmental expression of FoxJ1.2, FoxJ2, and FoxQ1 in Xenopus tropicalis. *Gene Expr Patterns* 6(5):443–447, 2006.

154. Wang T, Tamakoshi T, Uezato T, et al. Forkhead transcription factor Foxf2 (LUN)-deficient mice exhibit abnormal development of secondary palate. *Dev Biol* 259(1):83–94, 2003.

155. Erickson RP. Lymphedema-distichiasis and FOXC2 gene mutations. *Lymphology* 34(1):1, 2001.

156. Wozney JM, Rosen V. Bone morphogenetic protein and bone morphogenetic protein gene family in bone formation and repair. *Clin Orthop Relat Res* (346):26–37, 1998.

157. Mina M. Regulation of mandibular growth and morphogenesis. *Crit Rev Oral Biol Med* 12(4):276–300, 2001.

158. Furuta Y, Piston DW, Hogan BL. Bone morphogenetic proteins (BMPs) as regulators of dorsal forebrain development. *Development* 124(11):2203–2212, 1997.

159. Solloway MJ, Dudley AT, Bikoff EK, et al. Mice lacking Bmp6 function. *Dev Genet* 22(4):321–339, 1998.

160. Schorle H, Meier P, Buchert M, et al. Transcription factor AP-2 essential for cranial closure and craniofacial development. *Nature* 381(6579):235–238, 1996.

161. Nottoli T, Hagopian-Donaldson S, Zhang J, et al. AP-2-null cells disrupt morphogenesis of the eye, face, and limbs in chimeric mice. *Proc Natl Acad Sci U S A* 95(23):13714–13719, 1998.

162. Brewer S, Feng W, Huang J, et al. Wnt1-Cre-mediated deletion of AP-2[alpha] causes multiple neural crest-related defects. *Dev Biol* 267(1):135–152, 2004.

163. Kurihara Y, Kurihara H, Suzuki H, et al. Elevated blood pressure and craniofacial abnormalities in mice deficient in endothelin-1. *Nature* 368(6473):703–710, 1994.

164. Clouthier DE, Hosoda K, Richardson JA, et al. Cranial and cardiac neural crest defects in endothelin-A receptor-deficient mice. *Development* 125(5):813–824, 1998.

165. Yanagisawa H, Hammer RE, Richardson JA, et al. Role of Endothelin-1/Endothelin-A receptor-mediated signaling pathway in the aortic arch patterning in mice. *J Clin Invest* 102(1):22–33, 1998.

166. Ozeki H, Kurihara Y, Tonami K, et al. Endothelin-1 regulates the dorsoventral branchial arch patterning in mice. *Mech Dev* 121(4):387–395, 2004.

167. Pezzetti F, Scapoli L, Martinelli M, et al. Linkage analysis of candidate endothelin pathway genes in nonsyndromic familial orofacial cleft. *Ann Hum Genet* 64(Pt 4):341–347, 2000.

168. Riley BM, Mansilla MA, Ma J, et al. Impaired FGF signaling contributes to cleft lip and palate. *PNAS* 104(11):4512–4517, 2007.

169. Lammer EJ, Shaw GM, Iovannisci DM, et al. Maternal smoking and the risk of orofacial clefts: Susceptibility with NAT1 and NAT2 polymorphisms. *Epidemiology* 15(2):150–156, 2004.

170. Lammer EJ, Shaw GM, Iovannisci DM, et al. Periconceptional multivitamin intake during early pregnancy, genetic variation of acetyl-N-transferase 1 (NAT1), and risk for orofacial clefts. *Birth Defects Res A Clin Mol Teratol* 70(11):846–852, 2004.

171. Bottcher RT, Pollet N, Delius H, et al. The transmembrane protein XFLRT3 forms a complex with FGF receptors and promotes FGF signalling. *Nat Cell Biol* 6(1):38–44, 2004.

172. Bachler M, Neubuser A. Expression of members of the Fgf family and their receptors during midfacial development. *Mech Dev* 100(2):313–316, 2001.

173. Dode C, Levilliers J, Dupont JM, et al. Loss-of-function mutations in FGFR1 cause autosomal dominant Kallmann syndrome. *Nat Genet* 33(4):463–465, 2003.

174. Jiang R, Bush JO, Lidral AC. Development of the upper lip: Morphogenetic and molecular mechanisms. *Dev Dyn* 235(5):1152–1166, 2006.

175. Moreno. *Manuscript in preparation* 2007.

176. Matsuda T, Nomi M, Ikeya M, et al. Expression of the receptor tyrosine kinase genes, Ror1 and Ror2, during mouse development. *Mech Dev* 105(1–2):153–156, 2001.

177. Afzal AR, Rajab A, Fenske CD, et al. Recessive Robinow syndrome, allelic to dominant brachydactyly type B, is caused by mutation of ROR2. *Nat Genet* 25(4):419–422, 2000.

178. van Bokhoven H, Celli J, Kayserili H, et al. Mutation of the gene encoding the ROR2 tyrosine kinase causes autosomal recessive Robinow syndrome. *Nat Genet* 25(4):423–426, 2000.

179. Hahn H, Wicking C, Zaphiropoulous PG, et al. Mutations of the human homolog of Drosophila patched in the nevoid basal cell carcinoma syndrome. *Cell* 85(6):841–851, 1996.

180. Johnson RL, Rothman AL, Xie J, et al. Human homolog of patched, a candidate gene for the basal cell nevus syndrome. *Science* 272(5268):1668–1671, 1996.

181. Manfredi M, Vescovi P, Bonanini M, et al. Nevoid basal cell carcinoma syndrome: A review of the literature. *Int J Oral Maxillofac Surg* 33(2):117–124, 2004.

182. Mansilla MA, Cooper ME, Goldstein T, et al. Contributions of PTCH gene variants to isolated cleft lip and palate. *Cleft Palate Craniofac J* 43(1):21–29, 2006.

183. Tissier-Seta JP, Mucchielli ML, Mark M, et al. Barx1, a new mouse homeodomain transcription factor expressed in cranio-facial ectomesenchyme and the stomach. *Mech Dev* 51(1):3–15, 1995.

184. Trumpp A, Depew MJ, Rubenstein JL, et al. Cre-mediated gene inactivation demonstrates that FGF8 is required for cell survival and patterning of the first branchial arch. *Genes Dev* 13(23):3136–3148, 1999.

185. Abzhanov A, Protas M, Grant BR, et al. Bmp4 and morphological variation of beaks in Darwin's finches. *Science* 305(5689):1462–1465, 2004.

186. Wu P, Jiang T-X, Suksaweang S, et al. Molecular shaping of the beak. *Science* 305(5689):1465–1466, 2004.

187. Haworth KE, Wilson JM, Grevellec A, et al. Sonic hedgehog in the pharyngeal endoderm controls arch pattern via regulation of Fgf8 in head ectoderm. *Dev Biol* 303(1):244–258, 2007.

188. Yamagishi C, Yamagishi H, Maeda J, et al. Sonic hedgehog is essential for first pharyngeal arch development. *Pediatr Res* 59(3):349–354, 2006.

189. Clifton-Bligh RJ, Wentworth JM, Heinz P, et al. Mutation of the gene encoding human TTF-2 associated with thyroid agenesis, cleft palate and choanal atresia. *Nat Genet* 19(4):399–401, 1998.

190. De Felice M, Di Lauro R. Thyroid development and its disorders: Genetics and molecular mechanisms. *Endocr Rev* 25(5):722–746, 2004.

191. Cui XM, Shuler CF. The TGF-beta type III receptor is localized to the medial edge epithelium during palatal fusion. *Int J Dev Biol* 44(4):397–402, 2000.

192. Dudas M, Nagy A, Laping NJ, et al. Tgf-[beta]3-induced palatal fusion is mediated by Alk-5/Smad pathway. *Dev Biol* 266(1):96–108, 2004.

193. Loeys BL, Chen J, Neptune ER, et al. A syndrome of altered cardiovascular, craniofacial, neurocognitive and skeletal development caused by mutations in TGFBR1 or TGFBR2. *Nat Genet* 37(3):275–281, 2005.

194. Odeberg J, Rosok O, Gudmundsson GH, et al. Cloning and characterization of ZNF189, a novel HumanKruppel-like zinc finger gene localized to chromosome 9q22–q31. *Genomics* 50(2):213–221, 1998.

195. Maestri NE, Beaty TH, Hetmanski J, et al. Application of transmission disequilibrium tests to nonsyndromic oral clefts: Including candidate genes and environmental exposures in the models. *Am J Med Genet* 73(3):337–344, 1997.

196. Mitchell LE, Murray JC, O'Brien S, et al. Evaluation of two putative susceptibility loci for oral clefts in the Danish population. *Am J Epidemiol* 153(10):1007–1015, 2001.

197. Vieira AR, Orioli IM, Castilla EE, et al. MSX1 and TGFB3 contribute to clefting in South America. *J Dent Res* 82(4):289–292, 2003.

198. Ichikawa E, Watanabe A, Nakano Y, et al. PAX9 and TGFB3 are linked to susceptibility to nonsyndromic cleft lip with or without cleft palate in the Japanese: Population-based and family-based candidate gene analyses. *J Hum Genet* 51(1):38–46, 2006.

199. Chong SS, Cheah FSH, Jabs EW. Genes implicated in lip and palate development. In Wyszynski DF (ed). *Cleft Lip and Palate: From Origin to Treatment.* New York: Oxford University Press, 2002, pp. 25–39.

200. Stoll C, Mengsteab S, Stoll D, et al. Analysis of polymorphic TGFB1 codons 10, 25, and 263 in a German patient group with nonsyndromic cleft lip, alveolus, and palate compared with healthy adults. *BMC Med Genet* 5(1):15, 2004.

201. Fitzpatrick DR, Denhez F, Kondaiah P, et al. Differential expression of TGF beta isoforms in murine palatogenesis. *Development* 109:585–595, 1990.

202. Brunet CL, Sharpe PM, Ferguson MWJ. Inhibition of TGF-B3 (but not TGF-B1 or TGF-B2) activity prevents normal mouse embryonic palate fusion. *Int J Dev Biol* 39:345–355, 1995.

203. Taya Y, O'Kane S, Ferguson M. Pathogenesis of cleft palate in TGF-beta3 knockout mice. *Development* 126(17):3869–3879, 1999.

204. Muraoka N, Shum L, Fukumoto S, et al. Transforming growth factor-beta3 promotes mesenchymal cell proliferation and angiogenesis mediated by the enhancement of cyclin D1, Flk-1, and CD31 gene expression during CL/Fr mouse lip fusion. *Birth Defects Res A Clin Mol Teratol* 73(12):956–965, 2005.

205. Sasaki Y, O'Kane S, Dixon J, et al. Temporal and spatial expression of Pax9 and Sonic hedgehog during development of normal mouse palates and cleft palates in TGF-[beta]3 null embryos. *Archives of Oral Biology* 52(3):260–267, 2007.

206. Peters H, Neubuser A, Kratochwil K, et al. Pax9-deficient mice lack pharyngeal pouch derivatives and teeth and exhibit craniofacial and limb abnormalities. *Genes Dev* 12(17):2735–2747, 1998.

207. Ichikawa E, Watanabe A, Nakano Y, et al. PAX9 and TGFB3 are linked to susceptibility to nonsyndromic cleft lip with or without cleft palate in the Japanese: Population-based and family-based candidate gene analyses. *J Hum Genet* 51(1):38–46, 2006.

208. Brickell P, Thorogood P. Retinoic acid and retinoic acid receptors in craniofacial development. *Semin Cell Dev Biol* 8(4):437–443, 1997.

209. Finnell RH, Shaw GM, Lammer EJ, et al. Gene-nutrient interactions: Importance of folates and retinoids during early embryogenesis. *Toxicol Appl Pharmacol* 198(2):75–85, 2004.

210. Mitchell LE, Murray JC, O'Brien S, et al. Retinoic acid receptor alpha gene variants, multivitamin use, and liver intake as risk factors for oral clefts: A population-based case-control study in Denmark, 1991–1994. *Am J Epidemiol* 158(1):69–76, 2003.

211. Chenevix-Trench G, Jones K, Green AC, et al. Cleft lip with or without cleft palate: Associations with transforming growth factor alpha and retinoic acid receptor loci. *Am J Hum Genet* 51:1377–1385, 1992.

212. Shaw D, Ray A, Marazita M, et al. Further evidence of a relationship between the retinoic acid receptor alpha locus and nonsyndromic cleft lip with or without cleft palate. *Am J Hum Genet* 53:1156–1157, 1993.

213. Scapoli L, Martinelli M, Pezzetti F, et al. Linkage disequilibrium between GABRB3 gene and nonsyndromic familial cleft lip with or without cleft palate. *Hum Genet* 110(1):15–20, 2002.

214. Kanno K, Suzuki Y, Yang X, et al. Lack of evidence for a significant association between nonsyndromic cleft lip with or without cleft palate and the retinoic acid receptor alpha gene in the Japanese population. *J Hum Genet* 47(6):269–274, 2002.

215. Peanchitlertkajorn S, Cooper ME, Liu YE, et al. Chromosome 17: Gene mapping studies of cleft lip with or without cleft palate in Chinese families. *Cleft Palate Craniofac J* 40(1):71–79, 2003.

216. Juriloff DM, Harris MJ, Dewell SL, et al. Investigations of the genomic region that contains the clf1 mutation, a causal gene in multifactorial cleft lip and palate in mice. *Birth Defects Res A Clin Mol Teratol* 73(2):103–113, 2005.

217. Garcia-Castro MI, Marcelle C, Bronner-Fraser M. Ectodermal Wnt function as a neural crest inducer. *Science* 297(5582):848–851, 2002.

218. Basch ML, Garcia-Castro MI, Bronner-Fraser M. Molecular mechanisms of neural crest induction. *Birth Defects Res C Embryo Today* 72(2):109–123, 2004.

219. Niemann S, Zhao C, Pascu F, et al. Homozygous WNT3 mutation causes tetra-amelia in a large Consanguineous Family. *Am J Hum Genet* 74(3):558–563, 2004.

220. Mishima et al. The Role of WNT9b in primary palatogenesis. 2008.

221. Gaspar DA, Matioli SR, de Cassia Pavanello R, et al. Maternal MTHFR interacts with the offspring's BCL3 genotypes, but not with TGFA, in increasing risk to nonsyndromic cleft lip with or without cleft palate. *Eur J Hum Genet* 12(7):521–526, 2004.

222. Stein J, Mulliken JB, Stal S, et al. Nonsyndromic cleft lip with or without cleft palate: Evidence of linkage to BCL3 in 17 multigenerational families. *Am J Hum Genet* 57:257–272, 1995.

223. Wyszynski DF, Maestri N, McIntosh I, et al. Evidence for an association between markers on chromosome 19q and non-syndromic cleft lip with or without cleft palate in two groups of multiplex families. *Hum Genet* 99(1):22–26, 1997.

224. Martinelli M, Scapoli L, Pezzetti F, et al. Suggestive linkage between markers on chromosome 19q13.2 and nonsyndromic orofacial cleft malformation. *Genomics* 51(2):177–181, 1998.

225. Yoshiura KI, Machida J, Daack-Hirsch S, et al. Characterization of a novel gene disrupted by a balanced chromosomal translocation t(2;19)(q11.2;q13.3) in a family with cleft lip and palate*1. *Genomics* 54(2):231–240, 1998.

226. Suzuki K, Hu D, Bustos T, et al. Mutations of PVRL1, encoding a cell-cell adhesion molecule/herpesvirus receptor, in cleft lip/palate-ectodermal dysplasia. *Nat Genet* 25(4):427–430, 2000.

227. Sozen MA, Suzuki K, Tolarova MM, et al. Mutation of PVRL1 is associated with sporadic, non-syndromic cleft lip/palate in northern Venezuela. *Nat Genet* 29(2):141–142, 2001.

228. Scapoli L, Palmieri A, Martinelli M, et al. Study of the PVRL1 gene in Italian nonsyndromic cleft lip patients with or without cleft palate. *Ann Hum Genet* 70(Pt 3):410–413, 2006.

229. Avila JR, Jezewski PA, Vieira AR, et al. PVRL1 variants contribute to non-syndromic cleft lip and palate in multiple populations. *Am J Med Genet A* 140(23):2562–2570, 2006.

230. Warrington A, Vieira AR, Christensen K, et al. Genetic evidence for the role of loci at 19q13 in cleft lip and palate. *J Med Genet* 43(6):e26, 2006.

8

Syndromes of Orofacial Clefting

Marilyn C. Jones, MD • Kenneth L. Jones, MD

This chapter is dedicated to the memory of Robert J. Gorlin, DDS, MS, colleague, friend, and mentor to the authors. Dr. Gorlin was the real master of the syndromes of clefting.

 INTRODUCTION

Evolution of Syndrome Identification

Any textbook presenting a comprehensive approach to the problem of cleft lip and cleft palate will have a chapter devoted to the syndromes of clefting. Why syndromes? Since the early attempts to classify clefts anatomically in the 1940s, investigators have realized that many affected individuals have associated defects that often impacted survival and response to treatment. In the 1960s, the development of chromosome analysis and the simultaneous recognition that environmental agents could adversely impact fetal development spurred an explosion in descriptive syndromology in an attempt to define patterns of malformation with the intent of under-

standing etiology and pathogenesis based upon family history, exposure history, and laboratory evaluation. Associated defects provide a clue as to the etiology and/or pathogenesis of the cleft. Understanding the syndromes of orofacial clefting, therefore, is an essential aspect of clinical management as well as research design. Gorlin[1] has estimated that there are well over 400 distinct syndromes associated with facial clefts. Many of these are quite rare, having been reported in a handful of families or individuals. Organizing a chapter on syndromes thus presents a formidable task.

Knowledge that has been forthcoming from the Human Gene Project has challenged much dogma in genetics, such as the one gene-one disorder hypothesis. It is known, for example, that different mutations in the same gene can produce distinctly different patterns of malformation that may or may not have overlapping phenotypes. A striking example is the group of mutations in COL2A1 that can produce Stickler syndrome (cleft palate, myopia, retinal detachment, and adult onset arthritis), spondyloepiphyseal dysplasia congenita (severe short stature, cleft palate, myopia, and retinal detachment, scoliosis, club feet), and hypochondrogenesis/achondrogenesis type II (a perinatal lethal dwarfing condition with cleft palate). There are other situations in which different genetic mechanisms produce a common, clinically indistinguishable, phenotype. The best example in craniofacial development is Beckwith syndrome, which can be caused by methylation abnormalities at two different genetic loci, uniparental disomy, or point mutations in specific genes, all of which perturb the dosage relationship of imprinted genes on chromosome 11p producing a common phenotype.

From the standpoint of the underlying genetic abnormality, it is tempting to speak of families of genetic conditions such as the collagen II disorders described above. This approach is useful when studying the breadth of clinical ramifications of mutations in a specific gene, but not that helpful for counseling an individual family. Using the collagen II analogy, a child with Stickler syndrome should do well with surgery for the cleft and close ophthalmologic follow up. A child with hypochondrogenesis/achondrogenesis type II would not be expected to survive. Diagnosis of a collagen II disorder without further clarification would not be that helpful to a family.

The purpose of this chapter is to approach syndromes from the standpoint of the clinician at the bedside evaluating an individual patient or family. The primary purpose of a diagnosis is to provide accurate information regarding prognosis and recurrence risk. An accurate diagnosis may dictate a search for occult abnormalities and can outline a strategy for anticipatory guidance and treatment. A diagnosis can also help families understand the options for managing their reproductive risks.

Approach to Diagnosis

In approaching a diagnosis, it is useful first to classify the cleft by pathogenesis (i.e., is the cleft midline, is this a cleft lip with or without cleft palate, is it a V-shaped or U-shaped cleft palate, is the cleft atypical and not following the usual planes of facial closure) and subsequently to address the other major and minor malformations that allow recognition of a syndrome. Syndromes are diagnosed based upon the pattern of major and minor malformations seen in association with the cleft. The most important diagnostic tool, therefore, is a careful physical examination. Helpful references for syndrome identification include *Smith's Recognizable Patterns of Human Malformation,*[2] which has an easy to use index of features to assist with searching, and Gorlin's *Syndromes of the Head and Neck*, which contains the most comprehensive review of disorders of clefting up to the time of its publication in 2001. Searchable databases that are of use include Online Mendelian Inheritance in Man (OMIM),[3] which is available at no charge, and two others, which are available for purchase, the London Dysmorphology Database[4] and POSSUM.[5] Many genetics units have access to one or the other of these diagnostic tools.

Reduced to the most basic level, syndromes are caused by chromosomal abnormalities, single gene disorders, environmental agents, and multifactorial inheritance, involving the interaction of factors in the environment with a susceptible genetic background. In cases in which an underlying diagnosis is suspected but not established, referral to a clinical geneticist is strongly recommended. High-resolution (greater than 550 bands) chromosome analysis is usually warranted. Fluorescent in situ hybridization (FISH) testing is reserved for situations in which a specific clinical condition that can be diagnosed using this technology is suspected. Comparative genomic hybridization (CGH) using targeted microarrays offers a means of screening for a number of well-defined microdeletion/duplication syndromes, chromosomal imbalances, as well as rearrangements involving the telomeres (distal ends) of chromosomes. The yield of CGH in the cleft population remains to be established. With respect to single gene disorders, molecular testing is increasingly available for many conditions. In molecular diagnostics, positive test results will confirm the diagnosis; however, a negative test result typically does not rule out the condition. Before pursuing molecular diagnostic testing in single gene disorders, it is critical to first understand the power of the test to diagnose or exclude the specific condition. The GeneTests web site is very useful for locating laboratories offering clinical testing. It is important to recognize that many single gene disorders can be diagnosed with a high level of certainty based upon delineation of the pattern of malformation. Adjunctive testing such as radiographs and dilated eye evaluations, which may be considered extenders of the physical examination, is often helpful. Environmental agents may be suspected based upon the history of exposure at the critical time in development.

In order to limit the number of references for each syndrome described, the OMIM number(s) will be listed, where available. OMIM contains descriptions of conditions from the first clinical report to the present. In addition, all references relating to localization and identification of the genes responsible are typically referenced. For more recent publications, OMIM provides "hot links" to citations in PubMed. The GeneTests web site[6] contains reviews, called GeneReviews, of many conditions for which molecular testing may be available. GeneReviews are peer-reviewed articles covering diagnosis, strategies for testing, and suggestions for clinical management. If a GeneReview exists for a specific syndrome, such has been noted in the text. Both these web sites are regularly updated. References that may be accessed through either of these two sources will not be duplicated in this text.

Syndromes Associated with Cleft Lip with or without Cleft Palate

The most common type of cleft is cleft lip with or without cleft palate (CL ± P). This anomaly results from failure of fusion of the medial nasal and maxillary processes. Depending upon the age at which the individual is evaluated, the frequency with which associated malformations are encountered in this population ranges from 10 to almost 37%.[7–9] In the fetal and newborn period, the frequency of associated defects is between 26 and 37%.[10,11] In individuals attending a treatment clinic, roughly 10–15% will have associated defects, reflecting the fact that some infants with syndromes and major associated malformations will not survive to present for treatment.

Table 8–1 lists in decreasing order of frequency the most common syndromes associated with CL ± P as seen in the authors' series of 1900 patients presenting for treatment.

Van der Woude syndrome (OMIM #119300, GeneReview) is the most common condition responsible for CL ± P. The associated features are entirely oral, including hypodontia unrelated to the cleft malformation and lower lip pits in roughly 80% of affected individuals (Fig. 8–1). Van der Woude syndrome demonstrates incomplete penetrance. First-degree family members need to be inspected for lip pits prior to genetic counseling. Mutations in interferon inhibiting factor 6 (IRF6) account for the vast majority of cases. Interestingly, different mutations in this gene cause popliteal pterygium syndrome, another syndrome of CL ± P discussed below. Polymorphisms in IRF6 are also associated with nonsyndromic CL ± P and likely contribute to susceptibility in certain populations (Chapters 6 and 7 address this issue more completely).

The CHARGE syndrome (OMIM #214800, GeneReview) is the second most common recognizable pattern of malformation in the CL ± P population. CHARGE is an acronym standing for *c*oloboma, *h*eart defect, *a*tresia choanae, *r*etarded growth and development, *g*enital anomalies and hypogonadism, and *e*ar anomalies and deafness. The disorder was initially felt to represent a nonrandom association of structural defects; however, the recent finding of a common genetic etiology in most patients has supported the concept that this pattern of malformation is a syndrome. In addition to the above abnormalities, facial palsies and esophageal atresia with tracheoesophageal fistula are reported (Fig. 8–2). Hypoplasia of the semicircular canal resulting in vestibular areflexia is a consistent finding. Microdeletion or point mutation in the chromodomain helicase DNA-binding gene (CHD7) causes the CHARGE syndrome. The majority of patients meeting criteria for CHARGE syndrome will have mutations in CHD7. Mutations in semaphoring 3E (SEMA3E) have been identified in two patients. The extent to which mutations in this second locus contribute to the phenotype is not yet clear. Most cases of the CHARGE syndrome occur de novo with a low risk for recurrence for unaffected parents and a 50% risk for the affected individual. Gonadal mosaicism has been documented in one family with sibling recurrence to unaffected parents. The CHARGE syndrome is quite variable with respect to the impact on the individual. Cognitive performance is typically impaired, sometimes severely, although normal intelligence has been reported. Autistic-like behavior has been reported. The combination, when present, of severe sensorineural hearing loss and bilateral macular colobomas presents enormous challenges for habilitation. Multiple cranial nerve palsies may result in feeding difficulties as well as speech problems later on. Postnatal growth failure may reflect growth hormone deficiency.

Down syndrome (OMIM #190685) is the most common pattern of malformation in humans (Fig. 8–3). Although clefts are infrequent findings in children with Down syndrome, the 1:660 incidence of this condition in newborns dictates that Down syndrome is the most common chromosomal anomaly found in treatment populations. In the authors' clinic, Down syndrome accounts for 6% of the syndromic cases of CL ± P. Ninety-four percent of patients have trisomy 21 as a consequence of non-disjunction in the egg (usually) or the sperm. The recurrence risk is 1% for women under 34 years of age and double the age-related risk for women 34 and older.[12] Roughly half of the remaining cases will represent trisomy 21/normal mosaicism, and the rest will result from unbalanced translocations with an increased risk for recurrence for balanced translocation carrier parents. Although the diagnosis of Down syndrome is made on physical examination, the genetic mechanism is established through chromosome analysis. Parental karyotypes are necessary only for individuals with translocations. Down syndrome is associated with mild to moderate mental retardation. Chronic rhinitis is common. Sleep-related upper airway obstruction occurs in about 1/3 of cases. Although dental caries are less common, periodontal disease may be a problem. The American Academy of Pediatrics has published guidelines for the management of children with Down syndrome that are available on the Internet (www.aap.org).[13]

The FAV/OAV spectrum (OMIM #164210) occurs with a frequency of 1:3000 to 1:5000 and has a multitude of names including hemifacial microsomia, facio-auriculo-vertebral malformation spectrum, oculo-auriculo-vertebral spectrum, Goldenhar syndrome, and the first and second branchial arch syndrome. Perturbed and typically asymmetric development of derivatives of the first and second branchial arch constitutes the primary pattern of malformation. In addition to CL/P and CP alone (see below), defects include microtia and/or ear tags and pits, hypoplasia of the malar, maxillary, and mandibular regions, macrostomia, vertebral anomalies (typically cervical), and epibulbar dermoids/lipodermoids. Renal anomalies and cardiac defects also occur (Fig. 8–4). The majority of cases are sporadic events. An empiric 2% recurrence risk for families is commonly cited. The etiology is unknown. Vascular disruption of the structures supplied by the stapedial artery has been implicated in some cases.[14] The disorder has been reported discordantly in one member of a monozygotic twin pair. Maternal diabetes is associated with some cases.[15] The majority of patients have normal intelligence; however, a variety of central nervous system anomalies have been described. Mental retardation is more frequent in the rare case with microphthalmia.

Prenatal exposure to hydantoin, carbamazepine, valproic acid, mysoline, and/or phenobarbital is associated with a pattern of craniofacial features referred to as the "anticonvulsant facies." In addition to oral clefts, which are relatively infrequent, affected individuals have mild ocular hypertelorism, a broad, depressed nasal bridge, short nose, and broad alveolar ridges (Fig. 8–5). In addition, hypoplastic distal phalanges are typical with associated nail hypoplasia and

Table 8–1.

Syndromes Featuring Cleft Lip with or without Cleft Palate Listed in Decreasing Order in which the Diagnosis Occurs in the Author's Clinic Population

Syndrome	Prominent Features	Causation (Gene)
Van der Woude syndrome	Lower lip pits	Autosomal dominant (IRF6)
Charge syndrome	Ocular colobomas, choanal atresia, micropenis, cardiac defect	Autosomal dominant (CDH7)
Down syndrome	Flat face, small ears, cardiac defect, single transverse palm crease	Trisomy 21 (non-disjunction, translocation, mosaic)
FAV/OAV spectrum	Microtia, ear tags, cardiac defect, epibulbar dermoid	Usually sporadic (unknown)
Anticonvulsant embryopathy	Microcephaly, coarse facies, cardiac defect, nail hypoplasia	Exposure to hydantoin, valproic acid, carbamazapine
Amnion rupture sequence*	Ring constrictions, limb amputations, cephaloceles	Sporadic (disruption)
Deletion 22q (VCFS, DiGeorge syndrome)*	Short palpebral fissures, small ears, alar hypoplasia, conotruncal cardiac defect	Deletion 22q11.2
Diabetic embryopathy*	Heart defect, caudal regression, ear tags	Poorly controlled maternal diabetes
Fetal alcohol syndrome*	Microcephaly, short palpebral fissures, smooth philtrum	Alcohol exposure
Trisomy 13 (neonates)	Aplasia cutis congenita, heart defect, omphalocele, polydactyly	Trisomy 13
Trisomy 18 (neonates)	Growth deficiency, petite facies, camptodactyly, short sternum	Trisomy 18
Deletion 4p syndrome**	Hypertelorism, short philtrum, scalp defect, ear pit	Deletion 4p (de novo deletion, inherited translocation)
EEC syndrome**	Ectrodactyly, ectodermal dysplasia	Autosomal dominant (p63, two other loci)
Distal arthrogryposis type 2***	Camptodactyly, dimples	Autosomal dominant
Opitz syndrome***	Hypertelorism, hypospadias, laryngeal cleft	X-linked dominant (MID1) autosomal dominant (22q11.2)
Popliteal pterygium syndrome***	Lip pits, popliteal web, genital anomalies	Autosomal dominant (IRF6)
Roberts syndrome***	Growth deficiency, severe limb reduction defects	Autosomal recessive (unknown)
Waardenburg syndrome***	White forelock, deafness, iris heterochromia	Autosomal dominant (PAX3, MITF, EDNRP, EDN3, SOX 10)
Aarskog syndrome****	Short stature, shawl scrotum, round face	X-linked recessive (FGD1)
Basal cell nevus syndrome (Gorlin syndrome)****	Jaw keratocysts, basal cell carcinomas, bifid ribs	Autosomal dominant (PCTH)
Coffin–Siris syndrome****	Sparse scalp hair, coarse facies, hirsuitism, nail hypoplasia	Mostly sporadic (unknown)

(continued)

Table 8–1.		
(*Continued*)		
Syndrome	**Prominent Features**	**Causation (Gene)**
Fryns syndrome****	Diaphragmatic hernia, coarse face, digital hypoplasia	Autosomal recessive (unknown)
Wildervanck syndrome****	Klippel–Feil anomaly, Duane anomaly, sensorineural deafness	Sporadic, mostly females (unknown)

Note: Symbols following syndrome names denote disorders that occur with equal frequency.

low-arch dermal ridge patterns. A variety of cardiac abnormalities occur. Infants exposed to carbamazepine and valproic acid have an increased have a 1% risk for meningomyelocele. A dose–response curve has not been established, nor has a "safe" dose been found below which there is no increased teratogenic risk. The mechanism through which anticonvulsant drugs produce the phenotype is under investigation. Inherited variation in the activity of a drug-metabolizing enzyme, epoxide hydrolase, has been implicated in some cases.[16]

The amnion rupture sequence (OMIM #217100) is typically associated with clefts that do not follow the normal planes of facial closure. However, some infants will appear to have typical CL ± P. The diagnosis is suspected by the presence of band-related ring constrictions, amputations, or disruptions in other body parts, typically the limbs (Fig. 8–6). Evaluation of the placenta establishes the diagnosis. The cause of amnion rupture is unknown; however, the event is presumed to occur before 12 weeks gestation when separation of amnion and chorion still exists.[17] The extent of malformation depends upon the degree to which the infant becomes entangled in the strands of amnion floating freely in the uterine cavity. Severe fetal entrapment results in cephaloceles, aberrant clefts, thoraco- and abdominoschisis, and limb reduction defects, which are often lethal. The mechanism through which amnion rupture leads to typical CL ± P is unknown.

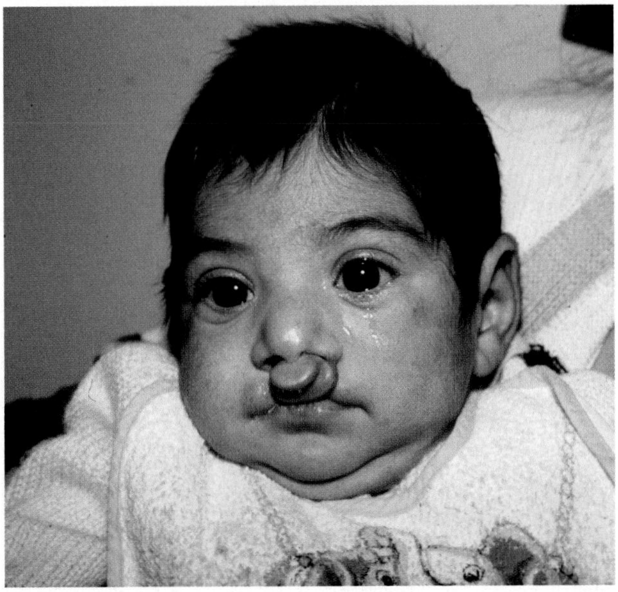

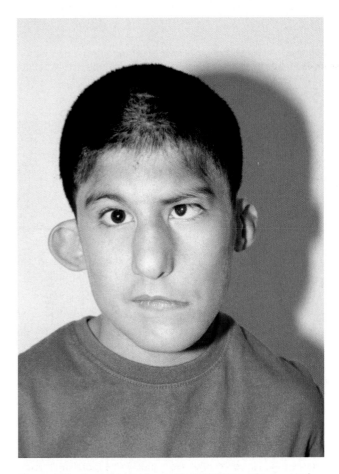

Figure 8–1. Two-month-old with Van der Woude syndrome. In addition to the bilateral cleft lip and palate, she has two lip pits visible as an irregular contour on the lower lip. Individuals with Van der Woude syndrome may present with CL±P, CP alone, or isolated lip pits.

Figure 8–2. Ten-year-old boy with CHARGE syndrome. He has bilateral ear malformations, bilateral retinal colobomas with associated left microphthalmia, a left facial paresis, micropenis and esophageal atresia with a tracheoesophageal fistula. Individuals with CHARGE syndrome may present with CL±P or CP alone.

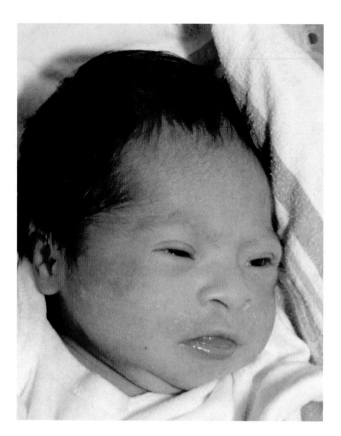

Figure 8–3. Newborn with Down syndrome presenting with a forme fruste of a cleft lip on the right and a complete cleft palate. Individuals with Down syndrome may present with CL±P or CP alone.

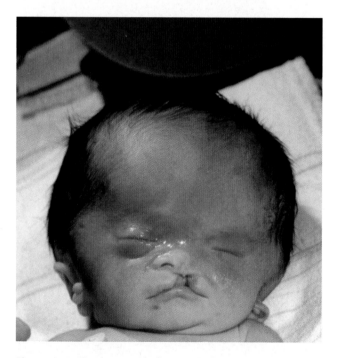

Figure 8–4. Newborn with facio-auriculo-vertebral malformation spectrum. In addition to left microtia, left microphthalmia, a left cleft lip and alveolus, and right preauricular tags, this infant has multiple vertebral malformations and hydrocephalus, an unusual feature for this spectrum of malformations. Individuals with FAV spectrum may present with CL±P or CP alone.

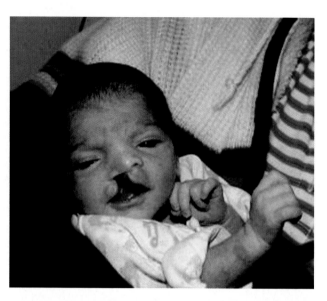

Figure 8–5. One-month-old with the anticonvulsant embryopathy. In addition to the cleft, this infant has mildly coarse facies and 5th nail hypoplasia. She was exposed to Phenobarbital *in utero*. Individuals exposed to teratogenic anticonvulsants may present with CL±P or CP alone.

Although typically associated with cleft palate alone, 22q11.2 deletion syndrome, also known as DiGeorge syndrome, Velocardiofacial syndrome, and Shprintzen syndrome, may also present with CL ± P (OMIM #192430, GeneReview). Affected individuals have typical facies, including short palpebral fissures with a hooded appearance to the eyes, a prominent nose with square nasal root and hypoplastic alae nasi, conotruncal cardiac defects, and long tapered fingers. Because the cleft lip distorts some of the characteristic facial features, the clinical diagnosis may often be

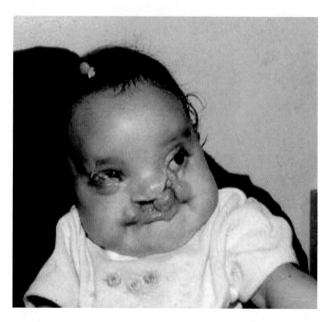

Figure 8–6. Six-month-old baby with multiple band related disruptive defects. In addition to the CL±P, she has ring constrictions on her fingers and eyelid clefts.

missed in the absence of typical cardiac malformations. The phenotype, however, becomes apparent over time. This condition has an autosomal dominant mode of inheritance, with affected individuals having a 50% risk for recurrence. Most cases occur de novo, with only 10–15% of patients having an affected parent. Diagnosis is made using FISH to detect the common microdeletion on chromosome 22q11.2 that is responsible for over 95% of cases. A few patients will have deletions not identified by the commercially available FISH probes. Rarely, point mutations in TBX1, a gene located in the deleted region, account for the phenotype. Hypoplasia of the pharyngeal musculature impacts both feeding and speech, which is typically hypernasal, often despite appropriate surgical management. Although most affected individuals have an intelligence quotient in the borderline to normal range, a variety of learning issues, personality disorders, and problems of socialization impact school performance. Psychiatric disorders occur in about 10% of cases followed longitudinally. Chapter 9 addresses deletion 22q11.2 in detail.

Maternal diabetes in pregnancy is associated with an increased rate of fetal malformations directly related to the degree of glycemic control.[18] As opposed to other environmental agents that produce specific patterns of malformation, poorly controlled maternal diabetes is associated with several recognized phenotypes as well as a list of nonrandomly associated specific malformations.[19,20] Among the phenotypes FAV/OAV spectrum, caudal regression sequence, femoral hypoplasia-unusual facies syndrome, and holoprosencephaly sequence are the best characterized. CL ± P, CP, microtia, cardiac defects, vertebral defects, renal anomalies also occur with increased frequency among infants of diabetics (Fig. 8–7). The maternal hemoglobin A_1C level is an excellent measure of glucose control in the preceding 8 weeks of pregnancy. There is some controversy as to the role of true gestational diabetes in the production of malformation. It is important to recognize that "gestational diabetes" is often type II diabetes that is first recognized in pregnancy. The risk for recurrence of malformation in women with diabetes is related to glycemic control in subsequent pregnancies.

Heavy alcohol exposure in pregnancy produces a characteristic pattern of malformation including pre- and postnatal growth deficiency, microcephaly, short palpebral fissures, a smooth philtrum with thin vermillion of the upper lip, joint contractures, and cardiac defects.[21] In infants with CL ± P, some of the facial features are difficult to assess making the prenatal exposure history and longitudinal assessment of growth, behavior, and performance critical in the diagnosis. Although many affected children test within the normal range for IQ, poor school performance is typical secondary to hyperactivity as well as problems with language, verbal learning, memory, fine-motor speed, and visual-motor integration. Decreased birth size has been documented with as little as two drinks per day. Extensive physical features typically are associated with exposures of 4–6 drinks per day (Fig. 8–8). Since the brain appears to be the most vulnerable organ to the teratogenic effect of alcohol, a "safe" amount of alcohol in pregnancy has not been established.

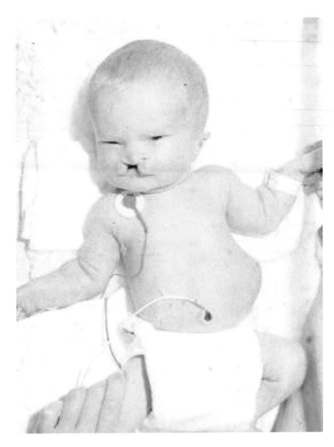

Figure 8–7. Newborn infant with CL±P, hydrocephalus and multiple vertebral and rib defects secondary to poorly controlled maternal diabetes.

Trisomy 13 syndrome is the third most common autosomal trisomy occurring with an incidence of 1:5000 live births. The most characteristic malformations include varying degrees of holoprosencephaly, microphthalmia, scalp defects, cardiac defects, and polydactyly. CL ± P occurs in 60–80% of cases and is midline when associated with holoprosencephaly. Omphalocele and polycystic kidneys are commonly the presenting features prenatally (Fig. 8–9). Trisomy 13 is a common syndromic cause of CL ± P in prenatal diagnosis and in the neonatal nursery. Since the median survival for children with this disorder is 7 days, treatment teams will follow few affected infants. The natural history of survivors has been well documented.[22] Growth deficiency and severe cognitive impairment are typical. Most cases of trisomy 13 are a result of non-disjunction often associated with advanced maternal age. Families are typically counseled that there is a less than 1% recurrence risk.

Trisomy 18 syndrome is the second most common autosomal trisomy. Although more frequent than trisomy 13 syndrome, CL ± P is much less frequent in affected infants. Characteristic features include prenatal growth deficiency, a prominent occiput with hypoplastic supraorbital ridges, a small nose, and small mouth, a short sternum, camptodactyly with nail hypoplasia and a predominance of low-arch dermal ridge patterns, and a short dorsiflexed hallux (Fig. 8–10). The

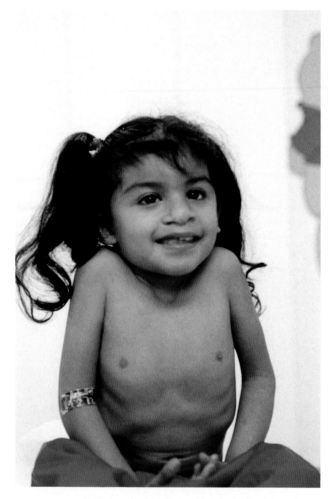

Figure 8–8. Three-year-old girl with profound pre- and postnatal growth deficiency and microcephaly. She has a right CL±P, short palpebral fissures, and 5th finger clinodactyly. Her mother was a chronic alcoholic who continued to drink during the pregnancy.

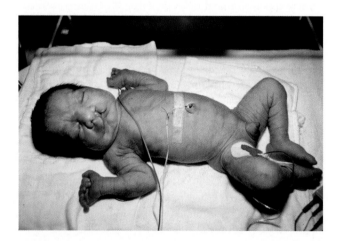

Figure 8–9. Newborn with trisomy 13 syndrome. In addition to the cleft, features that are apparent include the bulbous nose, upsweep to the scalp hair pattern, postaxial polydactyly, and a scrotalized phallus. This baby also had a major cardiac malformation.

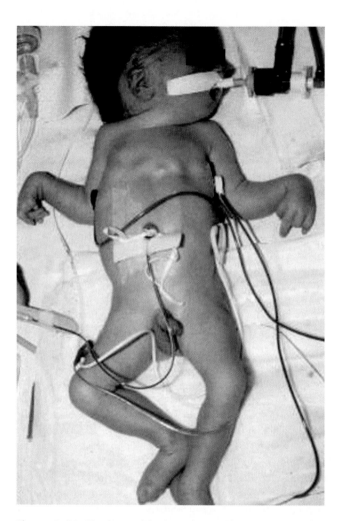

Figure 8–10. Newborn with trisomy 18 syndrome. Features that are apparent include a prominent occiput, posteriorly rotated ears, micrognathia, bilateral redial limb defects, and cocked up great toes. This baby had esophageal atresia with a tracheoesophageal fistula.

median survival for affected infants is 14.5 days. Only 5–10% survive the first year.[23] Severe growth failure and severe mental deficiency are typical. Non-disjunction accounts for the majority of cases of trisomy 18. Advanced maternal age is a risk factor. The empiric risk for recurrence is believed to be less than 1%. Mosaicism may prolong survival in trisomy 18 as well as trisomy 13 syndromes. The natural history for survivors is well documented.[24]

Deletion 4p produces a pattern of malformation characterized by severe prenatal growth deficiency, posterior midline scalp defects, ocular hypertelorism, iris anomalies, arched eye brows that extend onto the nasal bridge, a short upper lip and philtrum, preauricular tags/pits, hypospadias, and cardiac defects. CL ± P is common. Although 87% of cases represent de novo deletions, 13% are the result of translocations in which one of the parents is a balanced translocation carrier. High-resolution cytogenetic studies will detect the majority of cases. Since the phenotype is a consequence of deletion of genes at the extreme end of 4p, FISH studies directed at 4p16.3 should be considered in infants with a characteristic

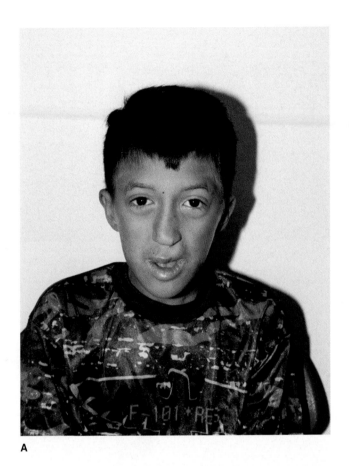

A

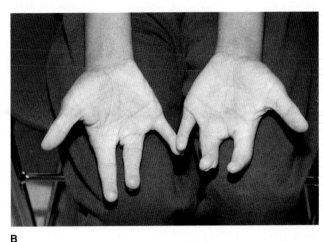

B

Figure 8–11 (a and b). Thirteen-year-old boy with EEC syndrome. His hair is dry and slightly silvery. He had chronic dacrocystitis that was managed with reconstruction of his lacrimal drainage system. His hands show typical split-hand malformations.

phenotype and normal chromosomes. In infancy, seizures and feeding problems are typical. Although mental retardation is usually severe, some children become independent for skills of daily living.[25,26]

The name ectrodactyly-ectodermal dysplasia-clefting (EEC) syndrome (OMIM # 129900, 604292, 602077, GeneReview) well describes the characteristic features of this condition. CL ± P occurs in 68% of cases. Split hand and/or split foot and related anomalies present in 84% of cases. The ectodermal features, which become more evident over time, include light thin scalp hair, mild hyperkeratosis of the skin, partial anodontia, malformed teeth, and lacrimal defects (in 59% of patients; Fig. 8–11). The latter may result in chronic dacryocystitis and corneal injury if not properly managed. Renal abnormalities, some of which require medical or surgical management, occur in 52% of patients. No feature is obligatory. Variable expression among affected family members is documented. EEC syndrome has an autosomal dominant mode of inheritance. Three genetic loci are recognized. Mutations, primarily in the DNA-binding domain in the p63 gene at 3q27, have been identified in some patients with EEC3. Affected individuals have a 50% risk for recurrence. Intelligence is usually normal. Most patients function well with proper management of their specific abnormalities. A variety of polymorphisms in p63 have been identi-

fied as susceptibility factors associated with nonsyndromic CL/P.

The distal arthrogryposis syndromes (OMIM #601680, 114300, 605311) are a group of primarily autosomal dominantly inherited disorders that have recently been characterized as a family of conditions in which mutations in one of the contractile elements of fast-twitch muscle fibers are responsible.[27] The original 1982 paper classifying the distal arthrogryposis syndromes designated type I as typical and type II as atypical based upon the association of other malformations.[28] More recently, these disorders have been reclassified into nine distinct types and two subtypes using family history, physical findings, and genetic linkage data.[29] Clefts are uncommon, with the most distinctive features being the "trisomy 18" appearance of the hand with tightly clenched overlapping fingers but without the nail and dermal ridge hypoplasia seen in trisomy 18 (Fig. 8–12). Positional abnormalities of the feet are extremely common, with contractures at the major joints less frequent. Intelligence is normal. The contractures improve with a combination of physical therapy and orthopedic management.

Opitz syndrome also has a number of synonyms including Opitz–Frias syndrome, Opitz G/BBB syndrome, and hypertelorism–hypospadias syndrome, the latter of which best characterizes the condition (OMIM # 145410, 300000,

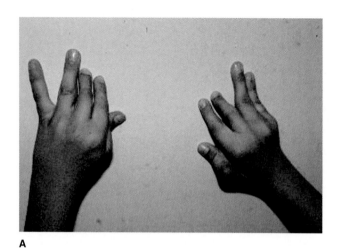

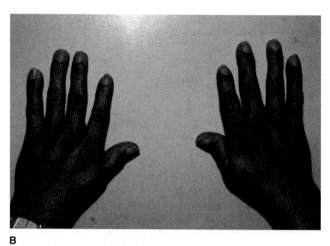

A

B

Figure 8–12 (a and b). Hands of eight-year-old boy (a) and his father (b) demonstrating ulnar drift of the wrist with multiple finger contractures that tend to improve over time.

GeneReview). In addition to CL/P, which occurs frequently, the most distinctive features include a prominent forehead, ocular hypertelorism, a broad nasal bridge with anteverted nares, posteriorly rotated ears, hypospadias, cryptorchidism and a bifid scrotum, and laryngotracheal malformations including laryngotracheal clefts, hypoplastic epiglottis, malformed larynx, and tracheoesophageal fistula (Fig. 8–13). A variety of low-frequency malformations of the central nervous system have been identified. The laryngotracheal malformations are a major source of morbidity and mortality in Optiz syndrome if not identified and managed early. Mild to moderate learning problems occur in roughly two-thirds of patients. Two genetic loci have been identified, an autosomal dominant locus linked to 22q11.2 (the same locus as is deleted in velocardiofacial syndrome) and an X-linked locus at Xp22.3. The gene responsible for the X-linked form of the disorder is MID1. The laryngeal malformations are seen only in the X-linked form of the disorder.

Popliteal pterygium syndrome is characterized by clefts (lip or palate or both) in 90% of cases, salivary lower lip pits in 46%, intraoral fibrous bands in 43%, and popliteal webs in 90% (OMIM # 119500, GeneReview). In extreme form, the latter extend from ischium to the heel. Genital anomalies occur in 51% and include hypoplastic labia or scrotum and cryptorchidism in males. Cutaneous webs between the eyelids occur in 20% of individuals. Intelligence is normal, and most affected individuals function well. The peroneal nerve and popliteal artery run through the fibrous pterygium, complicating attempts at reconstruction. Popliteal pterygium syndrome is inherited as an autosomal dominant condition. Wide variability among family members is typical. Mutations in IRF6 account for this disorder, making it allelic to Van der Woude syndrome, which also features lip pits.

Roberts syndrome (OMIM #268300, GeneReview) is also known as pseudothalidomide syndrome because of the severity of the limb reduction defects in the disorder. In addition to CL/P, craniofacial features include profound prenatal onset growth deficiency, ocular hypertelorism,

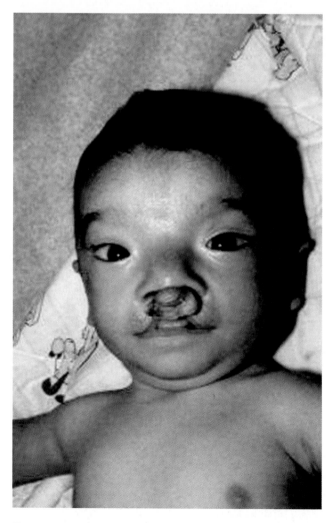

Figure 8–13. Three-month-old boy with Opitz syndrome. In addition to the cleft, he has ocular hypertelorism and hypospadias.

midfacial capillary hemangiomas, shallow orbits, blue sclerae, and sparse silvery blonde hair. Limb defects may include tetra-amelia, tetraphocomelia, humeral, radial, ulnar, femoral, tibial, and/or fibular reduction defects. The upper limbs are usually more severely affected. A variety of intracranial lesions, including encephalocele and hydrocephalus occur with low frequency. Some infants are stillborn or die in the neonatal period; however, survivors, usually diagnosed as having S-C phocomelia, may have only borderline to mild cognitive impairment. The genetic basis for this autosomal recessive syndrome has recently been documented. Mutations in ESCO2 account for both Roberts syndrome and S-C phocomelia. The protein product of this gene is required for the establishment of sister chromatid cohesion during S phase, perhaps accounting for the premature centromere separation on cytogenetic analysis with C-banding that assists clinical diagnosis.

Waardenburg syndrome (OMIM #193500, 193510, 148820, 277580, GeneReview) is usually an autosomal dominant condition characterized by congenital deafness and partial albinism with hypopigmentation of the iris, retina, skin, and hair, typically in the forelock region. In addition to CL/P, which occurs infrequently, affected individuals have a broad, high nasal bridge, a rounded nasal tip, hypoplastic alae nasi, and a medial flare of bushy eyebrows. Four subtypes have been identified. The most common, type I, is characterized by lateral displacement of the medial canthus, giving rise to the appearance of ocular hypertelorism and short palpebral fissures (Fig. 8–14). Deafness is a feature of 25% of WS-I cases. Type II WS lacks the medial canthal changes. Deafness occurs in 50% of WS-II patients. Type III is associated with limb reduction defects and facial changes consistent with WS-I. Type IV shows facial changes consistent with WS-II along with Hirschsprung's disease. WS types I and III are due to mutations in PAX3 located at 2q35. Some cases of WS-II are caused by mutations in MITF. Mutations in EDNRP, its ligand EDN3, and SOX 10 have all produced WS-IV. WS-IV is autosomal recessive when caused by mutations in EDNRP or EDN3. All other forms of WS are inherited in an autosomal dominant manner.

Aarskog syndrome (OMIM #305400) is an X-linked recessive condition featuring short stature. Such stature, which usually mild, but it may present prenatally and be associated with marked failure to thrive. Characteristic physical features include a round face, ptosis and ocular hypertelorism, a small anteverted nose (most apparent in noncleft cases), brachydactyly with an unusual position of the extended fingers, mild interdigital webbing, a prominent umbilicus, and shawl scrotum. CL/P occurs infrequently. Intelligence is usually normal although a variety of attention deficit and learning issues have been reported in some individuals. Aarskog syndrome is due to mutations in FGD1 located at Xp11.21. Carrier females may have minor manifestations in their face and hands.

Gorlin syndrome (OMIM #109400, GeneReview), also known as nevoid basal cell carcinoma syndrome, is an autosomal dominant condition that has a prevalence of 1 in 60,000 individuals. Craniofacial features include macrocephaly, frontal bossing, mild ocular hypertelorism, prominent supra-orbital ridges with heavy eyebrows, and odontogenic keratocysts. Facial clefts including CL/P and CP alone occur in between 4 and 8% of cases. A variety of skeletal changes occur, including short metacarpals, scoliosis, and bifid ribs. Skin changes include dyskeratotic pits on the palms and soles, facial milia, and nevoid basal cell carcinomas over the face, neck, trunk, and arms. A variety of tumors, including medulloblastoma, meningioma, and fibromas of the heart, ovary, peripheral nerves, may also occur. Radiation, as a mode of therapy, should be avoided as this increases the likelihood of malignant transformation of the nevi. Nevoid basal cell carcinomas are rare in young affected children. Mutations in a tumor suppressor gene, PCTH, cause Gorlin syndrome. Polymorphisms in PCTH may represent a rare susceptibility risk factor for nonsyndromic CL/P and CP alone.

Coffin–Siris syndrome (OMIM #135900) features mild pre- and postnatal growth deficiency, coarse facial features with full lips and a broad flat nose, a long philtrum, bushy eyebrows and long eyelashes, and a tendency for hirsuitism with paradoxically relatively sparse scalp hair. Clefts occur infrequently. Hypoplastic to absent 5th finger and toenails are characteristic. Occasionally, absence of the terminal phalanges (typically the 5th) occurs. Other skeletal findings include small patellae, lax joints with dislocation of the radial head, and coxa valga. A long list of internal defects, including Dandy–Walker malformation, diaphragmatic hernia, and cardiac malformation has been documented. Many individuals are significantly delayed. Feeding problems and recurrent infections are typical in early life. The cause of Coffin–Siris syndrome is unknown. Most cases occur sporadically. Sib recurrence with a mildly affected father and sib recurrence to unaffected parents could easily represent mosaicism in a parent.

Fryns syndrome (OMIM # 229850) is a malformation syndrome most often encountered in critically ill neonates since diaphragmatic defects occur in almost 90% of affected individuals. Clefts appear to be common in Fryns syndrome.

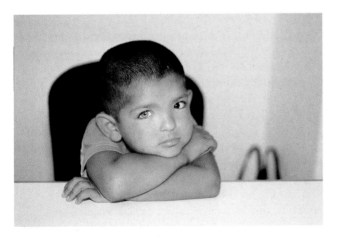

Figure 8–14. Four-year-old boy with type I Waardenburg syndrome. Note iris heterochromia and lateral displacement of the medial canthus.

Facial features are coarse with a broad nasal bridge, short nose, large mouth, and micrognathia. Digital hypoplasia including hypoplastic to absent nails and short terminal phalanges are characteristic. Fifty percent of infants have serious malformations of the central nervous system including Dandy–Walker malformation, arrhinencephaly, and agenesis of the corpus callosum. Abnormalities of the gastrointestinal system including omphalocele, anal anomalies, and duodenal atresia have been reported. Mental retardation is usually significant in the few survivors reported. Fryns syndrome has an autosomal recessive mode of inheritance. The molecular basis for the syndrome is unknown.

Wildervanck syndrome (OMIM #314600), also known as cervico-oculo-acoustic syndrome, is characterized by the Klippel–Feil anomaly with fusion of two or more cervical and sometimes thoracic vertebrae, unilateral or bilateral Duane anomaly, which includes abducens paralysis with retraction of the globe and lid narrowing of adduction of the affected eye, and deafness. The hearing loss may be sensorineural, conductive, or mixed. Malformation of the vestibular labyrinth is common. On examination patients present with short neck, oftentimes severe craniofacial deformation secondary to a structural torticollis and scoliosis, ear tag/pits, and epibulbar dermoids. Clefts are uncommon. Intelligence is usually normal, although a wide variety of central nervous system and spinal cord abnormalities have been reported. The cause of this disorder is unknown. All cases have occurred sporadically. Most have been in females.

Syndromes Associated with Cleft Palate Alone

The second most common type of cleft is cleft palate alone (CP). There are two mechanisms that produce CP. The most common is failure of the palatal shelves to close, producing a V-shaped cleft. Far less commonly, the palate will have a U-shaped cleft. U-shaped clefts are typically part of the Robin sequence, a constellation of anomalies including micrognathia, glossoptosis, and airway obstruction, in which the micrognathia is the initiating event, rather than failure of shelf closure. In contrast to CL ± P, between 40 and 60% of patients with CP will have a syndrome or associated malformations. In the newborn period, the percentage of infants with associated anomalies is close to 50%, with Stoll et al.[11] documenting a 46.7% incidence and Croen et al.[10] a 51.7% figure. Interestingly, the percentage of surviving individuals with syndromes or associated malformations is a bit higher, with an incidence of 55–61% cited in the literature.[7–9] Shprintzen et al.[8] have suggested that 77% of individuals with submucous clefts of the palate will have an associated anomaly. The reason for this paradox has not been fully explored; however, the authors believe that several of the more common syndromes associated with CP have subtle phenotypes not always recognized until an individual has been followed over time.

Prior to palate repair, it is usually possible to determine if the cleft has a V-shaped or a U-shaped appearance. Since the distribution of disorders associated with V-shaped versus U-shaped clefts is somewhat different, it is helpful to start with this distinction when considering syndromes. Table 8–2 lists, in decreasing order of frequency, the most common syndromes associated with CP as seen in the authors' series.

The most common syndrome amongst individuals with both V-shaped and U-shaped CP is Stickler syndrome (OMIM #108300, 604841, 184840, GeneReview). This syndrome accounts for 5% of all patients with CP in the authors' population. Of those patients with Pierre Robin sequence, half appear to have syndromes. Of these, half have Stickler syndrome.[8,30] Stickler syndrome is an autosomal dominant disorder that is due to mutations in the genes that code for either type 2 or type 11 collagen. Three types of Stickler syndrome are distinguished by the ocular phenotype. Those with a vestigial vitreous gel (the majority of patients) link to the gene encoding type 2 collagen (COL2A1). Those with sparse, irregular bundles of fibers in the vitreous link to the alpha 1 chain of type 11 collagen (COL11A1). Individuals with Stickler syndrome but without ophthalmologic manifestations typically have mutations in COL11A2. Characteristic facial features include a flat face with a depressed nasal bridge, short nose, and prominent eyes with or without Pierre Robin sequence (Fig. 8–15). Hypotonia and joint laxity are common. Some infants present with joint deformation, including dislocated hips and clubfeet. Over time, radiographic changes of a mild spondyloepiphyseal dysplasia may become evident, along with physical evidence of scoliosis and enlarged joints. Symptoms may include joint pains. An occasional individual may have a Marfanoid body habitus. Cognitive performance is normal. Affected individuals are at risk for sensorineural hearing loss. Individuals with ocular involvement are at lifetime risk for high myopia, retinal detachment, cataracts, and glaucoma. Since the features of Stickler syndrome may not be obvious in the newborn, it is the authors' practice to refer every infant with CP for a dilated eye evaluation before one year of age whether or not the Robin sequence is present.

The second most common syndrome encountered among individuals with CP is 22q11.2 deletion syndrome (OMIM #192430, GeneReview). Pierre Robin sequence is an unusual presentation in this condition, which is discussed briefly above and covered in detail in Chapter 9.

The FAV/OAV spectrum (OMIM #164210), also discussed above, is the third most commonly encountered disorder in the CP population, occasionally presenting with the Robin sequence.

Kabuki syndrome (OMIM #147920) is fourth on the list of syndromes associated with CP, uncommonly presenting with the Robin sequence. It is characterized by postnatal growth deficiency, hypotonia, and developmental delay. Characteristic craniofacial features including long palpebral fissures with eyelid eversion, arched eyebrows, short nasal septum, protuberant ears, and preauricular pits (Fig. 8–16). The features are often not obvious in neonates. Half of the affected individuals have cardiac defects, including left-sided flow-related lesions, conotruncal malformations, and single ventricle. Joint laxity is very common. Most individuals have persistent fetal finger pads, which may assist in diagnosis. The etiology of Kabuki syndrome is unknown. Most cases occur

Table 8–2.

Syndromes Featuring Cleft Palate Alone Listed in Decreasing Order in which the Diagnosis Occurs in the Author's Clinic Population

Syndrome	Prominent Features	Causation (Gene)
Stickler syndrome	Flat face, myopia, Robin sequence (over half of cases), spondyloepiphyseal dysplasia	Autosomal dominant (COL2A1, COL11A1, COL11A2)
Deletion 22q (VCFS, DiGeorge syndrome)	Short palpebral fissures, small ears, alar hypoplasia, conotruncal cardiac defect	Deletion 22q11.2
FAV/OAV spectrum	Microtia, ear tags, cardiac defect, epibulbar dermoid, Robin sequence (occasional)	Usually sporadic (unknown)
Kabuki syndrome	Large palpebral fissures, fetal finger pads, cardiac defect, Robin sequence (occasional)	Sporadic (unknown)
Down syndrome*	Flat face, small ears, cardiac defect, single transverse palmar creases	Trisomy 21 (non-disjunction, translocation, mosaic)
SED congenita*	Short limb dwarfing, myopia, pulmonary hypoplasia, Robin sequence (over half of cases)	Autosomal dominant
Van der Woude syndrome	Lower lip pits	Autosomal dominant
Anticonvulsant* embryopathy**	Microcephaly, coarse facies, cardiac defect, nail hypoplasia	Exposure to hydantoin, valproic acid, carbamazapine
Fetal alcohol syndrome**	Microcephaly, short palpebral fissures, smooth philtrum	Alcohol exposure
CHARGE syndrome**	Ocular colobomas, choanal atresia, micropenis, cardiac defect	Autosomal dominant
Diastrophic dysplasia**	Short limb dwarfing, hitch-hiker thumb, scoliosis, Robin sequence (common)	Autosomal recessive
Orofacial digital syndrome type 1**	Lobulated tongue, oral frenuli, milia, alopecia	X-linked dominant
Treacher Collins syndrome**	Microtia, zygomatic hypoplasia, micrognathia, Robin sequence (common)	Autosomal dominant
Beckwith syndrome***	Overgrowth, macroglossia, hemihypertrophy, omphalocele, Robin sequence (common)	Multiple mechanisms affecting imprinted loci 11p
Campomelic dysplasia***	Short bowed tibias with dimpling, flat face, sex reversal	Autosomal dominant
de Lange syndrome***	Growth deficiency, hirsuitism, limb defect, cardiac defect, Robin sequence (common)	Autosomal dominant
Distal arthrogryposis type 2***	Camptodactyly, dimples	Autosomal dominant
Mobius sequence***	6th and 7th cranial nerve palsy, clubfoot, other cranial nerve palsy	Sporadic
Nager syndrome***	Radial limb defects, ear malformation, zygomatic hypoplasia, Robin sequence (common)	Autosomal dominant

(continued)

Table 8–2.

(Continued)

Syndrome	Prominent Features	Causation (Gene)
Otopalatodigital syndrome type 1***	Broad nasal root, deafness, broad distal phalanges, Robin sequence (common)	X-linked recessive
Popliteal pterygium syndrome***	Lip pits, popliteal web, genital anomalies	Autosomal dominant
Rapp–Hodgkin ectodermal dysplasia***	Coarse dry hair, anhidrosis, alopecia	Autosomal dominant
Branchio-oto-renal syndrome****	Cup ears, ear pits, branchial arch remnants, Mondini defect	Autosomal dominant
Cleft palate-ankyloglossia****	Ankyloglossia	X-linked recessive
Distichiasis-lymphedema syndrome****	Double row of eyelashes, peripheral edema, cardiac defect	Autosomal dominant
Fragile X syndrome****	Mental retardation, lax joints, large ears, autistic behavior	X-linked (FMR1)
Marshall syndrome****	Flat face, myopia, sensorineural	Autosomal dominant
Diabetic embryopathy maternal diabetes****	Heart defect, caudal regression, diabetes	Poorly controlled maternal diabetes
Multiple pterygium syndrome****	Multiple pterygia, short neck, scoliosis with vertebral defects	Autosomal recessive
Prader–Willi syndrome****	Hypotonia (neonatal), obesity (later)	Deletion SNRPN locus
Retinoic acid embryopathy****	Anotia, conotruncal cardiac defect, brain defect	Isotretinoin exposure
Smith-Lemli-Opitz syndrome****	Ptosis, hypospadias, toe syndactyly	Autosomal recessive
Wildervanck syndrome****	Klippel–Feil anomaly, Duane anomaly, sensorineural deafness (unknown)	Sporadic, mostly females
Williams syndrome****	Mental retardation, friendly personality, supravalvular aortic stenosis	Deletion of elastin locus 7q (by FISH)

Note: Symbols following syndrome names denote disorders that occur with equal frequency. A number of rare lethal short limb dwarfing conditions may present with cleft palate. These diagnoses are not included in this table, which reflect survivors.

sporadically. Rare documentation of parent–child transmission has raised question of autosomal dominant inheritance or microdeletion.

Down syndrome (OMIM #190685) is the most common chromosomal anomaly associated with CP, not usually presenting with the Robin sequence.

Spondyloepiphyseal dysplasia congenital or SED congenita (OMIM #183900) is an autosomal dominant short-limb dwarfing condition. The Robin sequence is very common in this disorder. Features include pre- and severe postnatal growth deficiency with adult stature between 37 and 52 inches. Flat facies, myopia, a small chest, pectus carinatum, and generalized weakness are characteristic (Fig. 8–17). Radiographs demonstrate ovoid vertebral bodies, with lag in ossification of the epiphyses. There is increased mortality in early life secondary to both airway issues and pulmonary hypoplasia. Intelligence is normal. SED congenita is due to mutations in COL2A1, the gene that codes for type 2 collagen. SED congenita and the most common form of Stickler syndrome are therefore allelic. Individuals with SED congenita are at lifetime risk for myopia, vitreoretinal degeneration, and retinal detachment.

Van der Woude syndrome (OMIM #119300, GeneReview) rarely presents with the Robin sequence although cleft palate alone occurs frequently. Airway problems may result if oral synechiae are present.

Prenatal exposure to hydantoin, carbamazepine, valproic acid, mysoline, and/or phenobarbital as well as prenatal

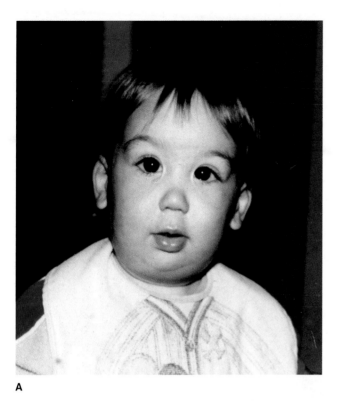

A

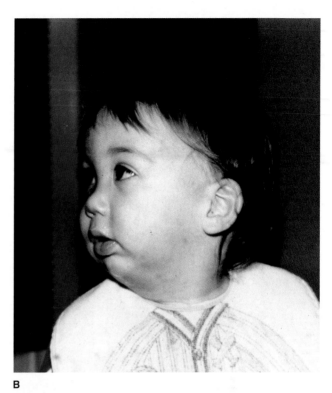

B

Figure 8–15 (a and b). a and b: Eighteen-month-old boy with Stickler syndrome who presented with airway symptoms in infancy. Note his low nasal bridge, mid-face flatness, and micrognathia. He is already significantly myopic.

exposure to alcohol may result in a pattern of malformation associated with CP alone. The Robin sequence is uncommon among this group of disorders.

The CHARGE syndrome (OMIM #214800, GeneReview) may also present with CP alone. Although Pierre Robin sequence is not common, affected infants are often quite ill as a consequence of the associated abnormalities and multiple cranial nerve dysfunctions that may affect feeding. This disorder is discussed above.

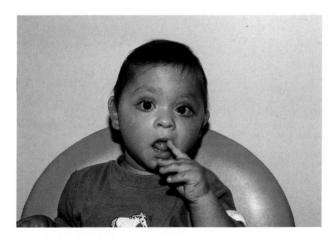

Figure 8–16. Eighteen-month-old boy with Kabuki syndrome. He has arched eyebrows, long palpebral fissures, a short nasal septum, and preauricular pits. He also has prominent fetal pads on the tips of his fingers.

Diastrophic dysplasia (OMIM #222600, GeneReview) is the second most common short-limb dwarfing condition associated with CP, commonly with Pierre Robin sequence. Pre- and postnatal growth deficiency is typical, with final adult height reaching 100–140 cm. Characteristic limb anomalies include a very short first metacarpal with hitchhiker thumb, symphlangism of the proximal interphalangeal joints, and club feet. Severe scoliosis may develop and affected individuals are at risk for spinal cord compression. A characteristic swelling in the ear cartilage develops in 84% of individuals in infancy. Mortality is increased secondary to the airway complications of the Robin sequence, laryngeal stenosis, and pulmonary hypoplasia. Intelligence is normal. Diastrophic dysplasia has an autosomal recessive mode of inheritance. Mutations in the solute carrier family 26 sulfate transporter gene (SLC26A2 or DTDST) account for the condition.

Orofacial digital syndrome type 1 (OMIM #311200) is an X-linked dominant disorder characterized by multiple frenuli between the buccal mucous membrane and the alveolar ridge, a lobulated tongue, mid-line cleft lip in addition to cleft palate, missing and anomalous teeth, hypoplasia of the alar cartilages of the nose, lateral placement of the medial canthus, milia of the face and ears in infancy, sparse dry hair, and a variety of skeletal anomalies including asymmetric shortening of the digits, clinodactyly, and brachydactyly (Fig. 8–18). Mental deficiency, which is usually mild, occurs in 57% of individuals. Multiple structural defects in the central nervous

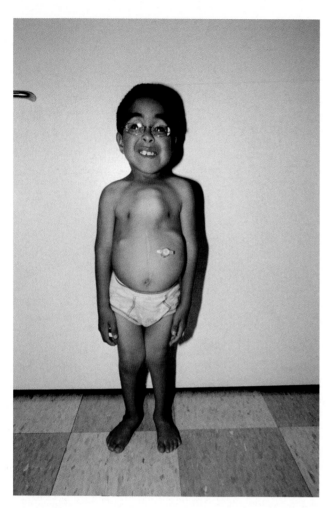

Figure 8–17. Ten-year-old boy with SED congenital. He is very short with a small, flared thorax. He has a flat face, mid-face hypoplasia, and marked myopia.

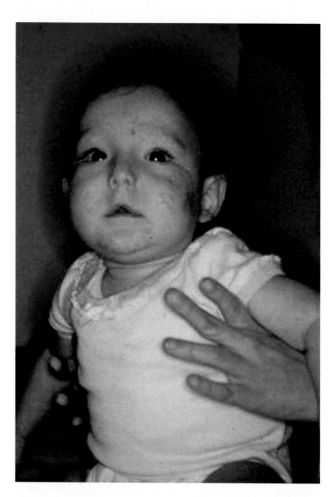

Figure 8–18. Nine-month-old with OFD type 1. Note the hypoplastic alae nasi, the milia, and the midline defects of the lip.

system have been described, including hydrocephalus, porencephaly, absence of the corpus callosum, polymicrogyria, and the Dandy–Walker malformation. Adult type polycystic kidney disease may develop. Mutations in CXORF5 account for the phenotype. Virtually all reported cases are female. The Robin sequence is uncommon.

Treacher Collins syndrome (OMIM #154500, GeneReview) is an autosomal dominant disorder characterized by downslanting palpebral fissures, malar hypoplasia with or without a cleft zygoma, mandibular hypoplasia, lower eyelid colobomas, malformed ears with conductive hearing loss, and occasionally pharyngeal hypoplasia or choanal atresia (Fig. 8–19). Pierre Robin sequence is common in this condition. Affected infants may present with very difficult airway issues. Intelligence and growth are normal. Mutations in the treacle gene (TCOF1) account for Treacher Collins syndrome. The condition is extremely variable. Careful evaluation of parents is necessary before recurrence risk counseling.

Beckwith syndrome (OMIM #130650, GeneReview) is an overgrowth disorder presenting with macroglossia, omphalocele, hemihypertrophy, ear lobe creases, and posterior helical pits. Pierre Robin sequence is common, although some

of the airway issues are the result of macroglossia (Fig. 8–20). Hypoglycemia may be a severe problem in neonates. Affected individuals are usually large for their family. Intelligence is normal, provided the hypoglycemia is managed adequately in the neonatal period. Tumor surveillance is warranted as

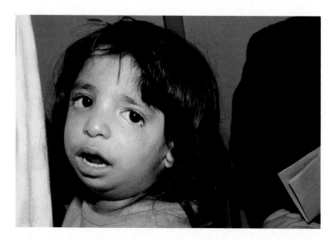

Figure 8–19. Two-year-old with Treacher Collins syndrome. She has downslanting palpebral fissures with colobomas of the lower lids, absent eyelashes on the medial aspect of the lower lids, microtia, micrognathia, and zygomatic defects that are palpable.

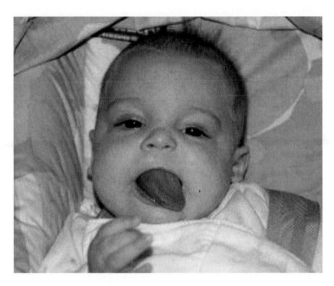

Figure 8–20. Three-month-old with Beckwith syndrome. Her asymmetric macroglossia worsened following delivery. She has infraorbital creases and a glabellar hemangioma.

the risk for developing a malignancy (usually Wilms tumor or hepatoblastoma) is estimated to be 6.5%. Most cases of Beckwith syndrome occur sporadically. The condition is due to a variety of mechanisms that disrupt the balance of genes in either of two imprinted domains on chromosome 11p. Both genetic and epigenetic factors play a role. Roughly 1–2% of cases will have a visible cytogenetic abnormality involving 11p. About 10–20% will have uniparental disomy (where both copies of the genes on 11p are paternally inherited). Fifty percent will have abnormal methylation at KCNQ1OT1 (LIT1). Roughly 5% of cases will have methylation abnormalities at H19. About 5–10% of sporadic cases and 40% of familial cases will have point mutations in CDKN1C. Uniparental disomy and methylation abnormalities at H19 have been associated with an increased risk for Wilms tumor. LIT1 methylation abnormalities are associated with non-Wilms embryonal tumors. However, not enough evidence exists to modify tumor surveillance recommendations based upon the molecular pathogenesis of Beckwith syndrome.

Campomelic dysplasia (OMIM #114290) is another short-limb dwarfing condition that presents with CP, frequently with Pierre Robin sequence. Affected individuals have pre- and postnatal growth deficiency with retarded osseous maturation and macrocephaly. The characteristic finding in the limbs is anterior bowing of the tibiae with skin dimpling over the convex area (Fig. 8–21). Bowed femora, dislocated hips, and clubfeet may also occur. Sex reversal occurs in 75% of chromosomal males (i.e., male chromosomes and apparent female external genitalia). Radiographs document hypoplastic scapulae, absent sternal ossification, and small iliac wings. The vast majority of individuals die in the neonatal period from respiratory insufficiency. Campomelic dysplasia is due to mutations in SOX9. It is inherited in an autosomal dominant fashion. Most cases represent a new gene mutation.

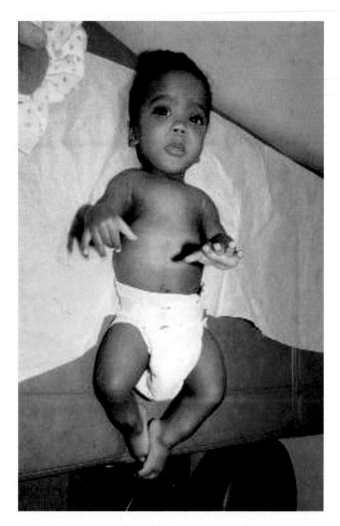

Figure 8–21. Infant with Campomelic dysplasia. She has scoliosis and marginal pulmonary reserves secondary to her small chest cage. Note the anterior bowing and dimpling over the tibias.

The de Lange syndrome (OMIM# 122470, GeneReview) is characterized by profound pre- and postnatal growth deficiency, usually severe mental retardation, hirsuitism, typical facies with synophrys, a short nose and cupid's bow appearance to the mouth, and variable limb reduction defects affecting the ulnar aspect of the limb more severely. Pierre Robin sequence is common. Gastrointestinal problems including gastroesophageal reflux, gut duplications, malrotation and volvulus complicate postnatal management. Mutations in two unrelated genes can produce this phenotype. The de Lange syndrome is usually the result of mutations in NIPBL. This gene functions as an autosomal dominant, with the majority of affected individuals having fresh gene mutations. Mutations in SMC1L1, an X-linked gene, account for a small number of sporadic cases and the rare X-linked cases described in the literature.

The distal arthrogryposes (OMIM #601680, 114300, 605311) are summarized above.

Möbius sequence (OMIM #157500) is usually a sporadically occurring condition characterized by paresis of the 6th and 7th cranial nerves. Micrognathia is common

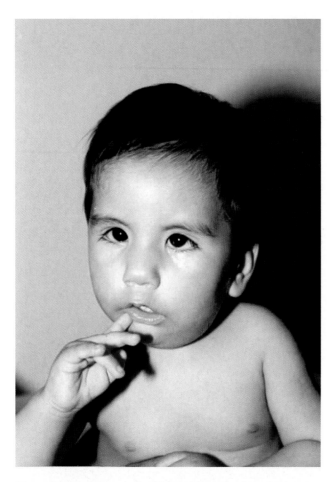

Figure 8–22. Eight-month-old boy bilateral 6th and 7th nerve paresis. He has epicanthal folds and micrognathia.

(Fig. 8–22), as is Pierre Robin sequence. Some patients have more extensive cranial nerve involvement. A variety of central nervous system defects have been documented. Clubfeet occur in roughly 1/3 of cases. Other anomalies include limb reduction defects, the Poland anomaly, and vertebral malformations. Mental retardation occurs in 30% of patients and is usually associated with autism. For the majority of individuals with normal intelligence, gaining social acceptance with an expressionless face is the major challenge. The etiology of Möbius sequence is unknown.

Nager syndrome (OMIM #154400) presents with radial limb reduction defects and mandibulofacial dysostosis, including malar hypoplasia, downslanting palpebral fissures, micrognathia, partial to total absence of eyelashes, micrognathia, and ear malformations which may vary from alterations in placement, tags or pits, to atresia of the external auditory canal with hearing loss. Pierre Robin sequence is common. The limb abnormalities range from hypoplasia of the thumb to a radial club hand with limitation of elbow mobility. Although mental retardation has been observed, intelligence is usually normal. There is an increased incidence of prematurity and a roughly 20% mortality related to airway issues in infancy. The cause of Nager syndrome is unknown. Most cases occur sporadically. The literature documents fa-

milial patterns that support both autosomal dominant and autosomal recessive modes of inheritance.

Otopalatodigital syndrome type 1 (OMIM #311300, GeneReview) is an X-linked recessive disorder due to gain of function mutations in the gene encoding filamin A (FLNA). Features include short stature and mild mental retardation. Craniofacial features include frontal and occipital prominence, ocular hypertelorism, and facial bone hypoplasia which retrudes the midface and results in downslanting palpebral fissures. Pierre Robin sequence is common. Partial anodontia and impacted teeth occur. Skeletal anomalies include pectus excavatum, clinodactyly of multiple digits, and broad distal phalanges. Sensorineural hearing loss progresses over time.

Popliteal pterygium syndrome (OMIM # 119500, GeneReview) is discussed above.

Rapp–Hodgkin ectodermal dysplasia (OMIM#129400) is an autosomal dominant disorder featuring thin, sparse hair, decreased numbers of sweat pores, small nails, hypodontia and conical teeth, and hypospadias. Both CL/P and CP alone may occur in this disorder. The condition is due to mutations in the tumor protein p73-like gene making the disorder allelic to EEC syndrome, with which it shares many features.

Branchio-oto-renal syndrome (OMIM #113650, GeneReview) is an autosomal dominant condition with hearing loss, preauricular pits, branchial fistulas or cysts, stenosis of the auditory canal, lacrimal duct malformation, and renal dysplasia. Abnormalities of the vestibular system and the cochlea (Mondini malformation) are characteristic. Clefts are found infrequently. Intelligence is normal. The hearing loss, which is sensorineural in 25%, conductive in 25%, and mixed in 50%, may be progressive. Mutations in the EYA1 gene are responsible for the phenotype.

Cleft palate-ankyloglossia (OMIM #303400) is an X-linked recessive condition due to mutations in TBX22. Most affected males (~80%) manifest both ankyloglossia and cleft palate. However, 4% have ankyloglossia alone. Of carrier females, 45% have isolated ankyloglossia and 16% have cleft palate. This condition has only oral manifestations. Absent tonsils may be part of the phenotype. Mutations in TBX22 may underlie a significant number of cases of nonsyndromic cleft palate.

Distichiasis-lymphedema syndrome (OMIM #153400) is an autosomal dominant condition due to mutations in the forkhead family transcription factor gene, MFH1 or FOXC2. Distichiasis is an extra row of eyelashes replacing the meibomian glands and occurs in virtually all cases. Cleft palate is a common feature; however, the Robin sequence is infrequent. The lymphedema, which affects primarily the lower extremities, develops between 5 and 20 years of age. Vertebral and cardiac defects are common. Intelligence is normal. Affected individuals may demonstrate short stature.

Fragile X syndrome (OMIM #309550, GeneReview) is an X-linked disorder caused by expansion of a CGG trinucleotide repeat in the promoter of the FMR1 gene. Males and some females with over 200 repeats usually have full manifestations of the syndrome, including mental retardation, autistic behavior, hyperactivity, and macroorchidism in post-pubertal males. Craniofacial features include macrocephaly, large ears, dental crowding, and prognathism in adolescence. Connective tissue abnormalities, including joint laxity and mitral valve prolapse, are common. Cleft palate and submucous cleft palate may be seen in individuals with the full mutation.

Marshall syndrome (OMIM #154780) is an autosomal dominant disorder caused by mutation in the COLL11A1 gene, making the condition allelic to one form of Stickler syndrome. Features include striking nasal hypoplasia, midface deficiency, myopia, and a usually progressive sensorineural or mixed hearing loss. Pierre Robin sequence may occur. Affected individuals need lifetime ophthalmologic follow up.

Maternal diabetes may be associated with CP and is discussed above.

Multiple pterygium syndrome (OMIM #265000) is an autosomal recessive condition caused by mutations in the CHRNG gene encoding the gamma subunit of the acetylcholine receptor. Features include ptosis, micrognathia with limited oral opening, web neck, variable contractures with pterygia across major joints, vertebral abnormalities with scoliosis, and cryptorchidism. CP is infrequent in this condition. Intelligence is normal. The small chest size and kyphoscoliosis are the cause of significant early morbidity and mortality.

Prader–Willi syndrome (OMIM #176270, GeneReview) is characterized by profound hypotonia and feeding issues in infancy and by excessive eating in childhood, resulting in morbid obesity unless caloric restriction is maintained. CP occurs rarely. All individuals have some degree of cognitive impairment, and a characteristic behavior profile has been described. Prader–Willi syndrome is caused by perturbation in dosage of imprinted genes on chromosome 15. Roughly 70% have deletions in the paternally inherited chromosome. The remaining have uniparental (maternal) disomy.

Retinoic acid embryopathy is the result of fetal exposure to isotretinoin (13-*cis*-retinoic acid). A 35% risk for malformation exists in the offspring of women who continue to take this medication beyond the 15th day post-conception. Abnormalities include bilateral microtia or anotia, facial paresis, ocular hypertelorism, mottled teeth, cleft palate, conotruncal cardiac malformations, and a variety of malformations of the central nervous system. Cognitive impairment is common among survivors.[31]

Smith–Lemli–Opitz syndrome (OMIM #270400, GeneReview) is an autosomal recessive disorder caused by an abnormality of cholesterol metabolism secondary to deficiency of the enzyme 7-dehydrocholesterol reductase. Affected individuals have pre- and postnatal growth deficiency, moderate to severe mental deficiency, and a characteristic pattern of malformation including ptosis, a broad nasal tip, anteverted nares, postaxial polydactyly, genital abnormalities typically hypospadias, cardiac malformations, and 2–3 syndactyly of the toes. Cleft palate is common. Many other internal malformations may also occur. Mutations in the gene sterol delta-7-reductase (DHCR7) account for the low enzyme activity and the phenotype.

Wildervanck syndrome (OMIM #314600) may be associated with CP and is discussed above.

Williams syndrome (OMIM #194050, GeneReview) is the result of deletion of a group of genes including the elastin locus on chromosome 7, detectable by FISH analysis. The phenotype includes mild mental retardation, elastin arteriopathy as manifest by supravalvar aortic stenosis, pulmonary stenosis, or hypertension, typical facies with periocular puffiness and full lips, and a characteristic behavior profile, including irritability in infancy followed by the development of an outgoing personality. CP is rare in Williams syndrome. Most cases occur sporadically, although transmission from an affected parent has been documented.

Syndromes Associated with Midline Cleft Lip with or without Cleft Palate

Midline clefts of the lip with or without cleft palate usually reflect a developmental abnormality of the frontonasal process and occur as part of the holoprosencephaly sequence. This condition is encountered primarily in prenatal diagnosis, but it is rarely seen in series of survivors because of the poor overall prognosis. Rarely, midline clefts occur in syndromes associated with accessory frenulae. Table 8–3 list disorders associated with midline clefts.

Holoprosencephaly (OMIM #236100, 157170, 142945, 142946, 605934 GeneReview) results from early loss of

Table 8–3.

Syndromes Featuring Midline Cleft Lip

Syndrome	Prominent Features	Causation
Holoprosencephaly	Cyclopia, hypotelorism, premaxillary agenesis	Chromosomal anomalies, maternal diabetes, single gene disorders
Frontonasal malformation	Hypertelorism, widow's peak, bifid nose	Usually sporadic
OFD syndromes	Oral frenulae, lobulated tongue, digital anomalies	X-linked dominant, autosomal recessive

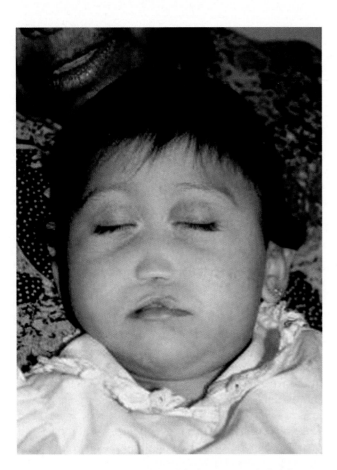

Figure 8–23. Ten-month-old with holoprosencephaly following repair of a midline cleft lip. Note the single nostril, absent columella, and ocular hypotelorism.

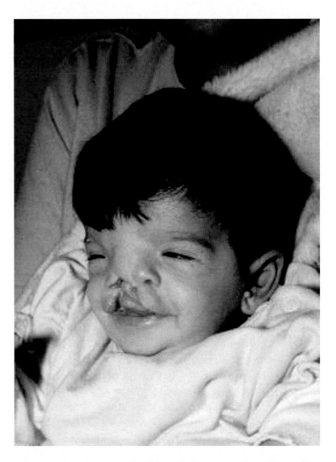

Figure 8–24. Two-month-old with frontonasal malformation. Note the dramatic ocular hypertelorism. Her cranium bifidum is apparent. In addition, she has bilateral preauricular tags.

midline structures in the developing prosencephalon. The phenotype ranges from a single central incisor at the mild end of the spectrum to varying degrees of ocular hypotelorism, with a flap-like nose, an absent columella and midline cleft lip, to cyclopia (Fig. 8–23). Holoprosencephaly is etiologically heterogeneous. Several chromosomal anomaly syndromes include holoprosencephaly as a characteristic feature, including trisomy 13 syndrome, deletion 2p21, duplication 3pter, deletion 7q36, deletion 13q, deletion 18p, and deletion 21q22.3. Holoprosencephaly may occur in single gene disorders such as Smith—Lemli–Opitz syndrome. Mutations in a variety of genes including *Shh*, *ZIC2*, and *tgif* may also produce the phenotype. Holoprosencephaly is also seen in the offspring of women with poorly controlled diabetes in pregnancy. Barr and Cohen[32] have outlined the natural history in survivors with holoprosencephaly.

Frontonasal malformation (OMIM#136760) is usually a sporadically occurring condition of unknown etiology. Features include ocular hypertelorism with lateral displacement of the medial canthus, cranium bifidum occultum, a widow's peak, a notched broad nasal tip to a divided nose, and hypoplasia to absence of the prolabium (Fig. 8–24). Clefts of the lip are uncommon. The majority of affected individuals are of normal intelligence; however, major malformations of the central nervous system are occasionally seen.

Orofacial digital syndrome type 1 (OMIM #311200) is discussed above. There are nine OFD syndromes, any of which may present with midline clefts.

Aberrant Facial Clefts

Aberrant clefts that do not follow the normal planes of facial closure typically have a disruptive pathogenesis, resulting either from amnion rupture or from vascular accidents in utero. The associated anomalies also reflect the disruptive pathogenesis and are typically asymmetrically distributed.

The amnion rupture sequence discussed above under CL ± P is the most common recognizable cause of disruptive facial clefts. Aberrant clefts have been attributed to fetal swallowing of the amniotic strands as well as to attachment of the strands to the developing calvarium. From a treatment standpoint, it is important to recognize that the degree of facial disfigurement from amniotic bands does not always correlate with involvement of the central nervous system. Each affected infant needs careful brain imaging and developmental follow-up, as many are normal with respect to cognitive potential.

The FAV/OAV spectrum (OMIM #164210), which may have a disruptive vascular pathogenesis, is also associated with aberrant facial clefts.

9

22q11.2 Deletion Syndrome

Donna M. McDonald-McGinn, MS, CGC • Elaine H. Zackai, MD

The 22q11.2 deletion has been identified in the vast majority of patients with DiGeorge syndrome,[1-4] velocardiofacial syndrome[5,6] and conotruncal anomaly face syndrome[7,8] and in some patients with the autosomal dominant Opitz G/BBB syndrome[9-11] and Cayler cardiofacial syndrome.[12,13] These syndromes were originally described as individual entities by a number of subspecialists, each concentrating on one particular area of interest. Following the widespread use of fluorescence in situ hybridization (FISH), however, these syndromes became collectively known by their chromosomal etiology: the 22q11.2 deletion.[14]

Historically, the 22q11.2 deletion was identified, cytogenetically, in a small number of patients with DiGeorge syndrome.[1-2] Laboratory advances utilizing FISH with probes (such as N25 or TUPLE) within the commonly deleted "DiGeorge Critical Region" followed,[3,4,15] allowing for the identification of patients with submicroscopic deletions. Since FISH is time consuming, relatively expensive, and limited to just one target sequence within the DGCG, newer techniques such as micro array Comparative Genomic Hybridization, Whole Genome-wide Array, and Multiplex Ligation-Dependent Probe Amplification are also being utilized to identify the deletion[16-18] and will likely replace clinical FISH studies in the near future.

With an estimated prevalence of 1 in 4000 live births, the 22q11.2 deletion is the most common microdeletion syndrome.[19-25] It is present in 1 of 68 children born with congenital heart disease[26]; it is the most common cause of syndromic palatal defects; and it is the second most common cause of developmental delay, accounting for approximately

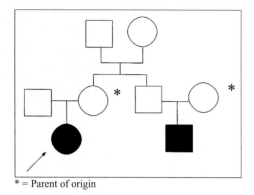

* = Parent of origin

Figure 9–1. This pedigree highlights the frequency of the 22q11.2 deletion as first cousins are affected by chance alone (parent of origin studies revealed the deletion arose in the germ cells of the unrelated mothers—Saitta, 2004).

2.4% of affected individuals.[27] The syndrome is so common, in fact, that affected first cousins have been identified with the 22q11.2 deletion by chance alone[28] (Fig. 9–1). Furthermore, there have been a number of patients found to have both the 22q11.2 deletion and concomitant diagnoses, including familial single gene disorders such as: Marfan syndrome (Stewart D, personal communication, January, 2002); neurofibromatosis (Coleman K, personal communication, May, 2001); familial *FGFR3* mutation[29]; and familial Ehlers-Danlos syndrome, as well as additional sporadic cytogenetic abnormalities including trisomy 8 mosaicism[30] and trisomy 21 (Johnson CJ, personal communication, August, 2007), all of which supports the need to think broadly when evaluating these patients, to examine the parents concurrently for evidence of familial syndromes, and, conversely, to consider deletion studies even in the face of other underlying diagnoses.[30]

The significant clinical features most frequently associated with the 22q11.2 deletion include: immunodeficiency, congenital heart disease, palatal defects (in approximately three-quarters of patients), hypocalcemia, renal anomalies, and dysphagia. Developmental disabilities are present in more than than 90% of affected children.[31–34] Nonetheless, there is wide inter-familial and intra-familial variability, even amongst identical twins, which does not appear to be influenced by the parent of origin in either familial or de novo cases.[30,35,36] In contrast to the early reports on patients with DiGeorge syndrome, the mortality rate for individuals with a 22q11.2 deletion is low (4%), with a median age of death at

4 months, most often due to complications of complex congenital heart disease,[37] reflecting the relatively recent advances in palliative cardiac care and infectious disease management. Thus, there will likely be an increase in the prevalence of the 22q11.2 deletion due to improved reproductive fitness.

The majority of patients (∼90%) have the same large (≥3 Mb) deletion encompassing approximately 30 functional genes, but a subset of patients (∼7%) have a smaller 1.5 Mb "nested deletion" within the "DiGeorge critical region"[38] (Fig. 9–2). Both deletions include a number of well-studied genes including *UFD1L*, *COMT*, and *TBX1*, a member of the T-box family of genes that has been shown to have similar features in haploinsufficient mouse models.[39] Recently, patients with normal 22q11.2 deletion studies using the commercially available FISH probes (N25 or TUPLE) but with overlapping clinical features of the deletion, have been reported with both gain and loss of function mutations in *TBX1*,[40–42] as well as atypical or unique 22q11.2 deletions, some of which include *TBX1* and others of which do not.[35,43–49] With the exception of congenital heart disease and its association with *TBX1*, however, there have thus far been no clear genotype-phenotype correlations in the remainder of the patients, suggesting that the well documented variability is likely due to modifier genes on other chromosomes.[36,49]

From an etiologic perspective, most deletions (93%) occur as a de novo event[34] due to the inherent structure of chromosome 22q11.2—specifically, a number of low copy repeats (blocks of duplicated sequences) which define the breakpoints, flank the deletion structurally, and make this region especially susceptible to rearrangements due to unequal meiotic crossovers and thus aberrant interchromosomal exchanges[28,47,50–52] (Fig. 9–3). It is noteworthy, however, that parents of affected children have been found to have the deletion despite demonstrating minimal clinical findings. In addition, an unaffected adult with somatic mosaicism has also been identified.[37] Thus, parental studies are warranted in all families with an affected child in order to identify mildly affected parents, as well as to rule out low-level mosaicism. Moreover, in counseling families, it is also important to recognize that there are a number of reports of germ line mosaicism[53–56] resulting in a small, yet ill-defined recurrence risk for parents of a child with a de novo deletion. Lastly, like all contiguous gene deletion syndromes, an affected individual has a 50% chance of having an affected child, but due to the variability of the disorder, there is no way to predict the range of manifestations in the offspring. In addition, it is

Cen   **Tel**

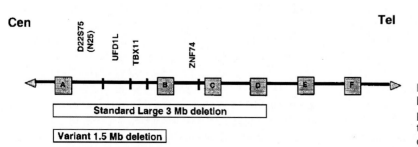

Figure 9–2. The majority of patients (∼90%) have a large (≥3 Mb) deletion encompassing approximately 30 genes, whereas a subset of patients (∼7%) have a smaller (1.5 Mb) "nested" deletion. Both deletions include the *TBX1* gene.

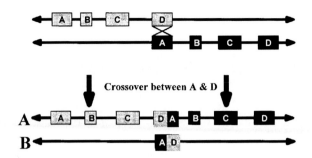

Figure 9–3. Crossing over, due to a number of low copy repeats, results in a duplication on chromosome (**A**) and a deletion on chromosome (**B**). This latter mechanism results in a chromosome 22q11.2 deletion. (*Figure courtesy of Ron O'Connor.*)

notable that the deletion remains unchanged as it passes from parent to child, so there is no evidence of anticipation.

GENETIC COUNSELING AND THE 22Q11.2 DELETION

The topic of genetic counseling can be approached by dividing it into three subtopics[30,37,57]: affected individuals, unaffected parents of an affected child, and the general population:

Genetic counseling for an adult with the 22q11.2 deletion is often quite difficult due, in part, to the wide interfamilial and intra-familial variability of the deletion, as well as to the cognitive limitations of some affected individuals.[38,58] Furthermore, eliciting the risk for medically relevant findings, such as congenital heart disease, is generally complicated by ascertainment bias. To this end, McDonald-McGinn[30] reported findings in 36 affected persons following the diagnosis in a relative. This cohort included 23 parents of affected children and 13 children born before or after the diagnosis of the parent. Four of these children were diagnosed prenatally via amniocentesis. Of this group, 56% had no visceral anomalies, including 65% of affected parents and 39% of children. Remaining findings included congenital heart disease in 19%, overt cleft palate in 11%, hypocalcemic seizures in 6%, a laryngeal web in 3%, and schizophrenia in 3% (Table 9–1). In reviewing the educational background of 20 adults, 70% were high school graduates. However, 30% reported the need for significant learning support while in high school and, despite the high graduation rate and relatively mild phenotype in this adult population, the parents with the 22q11.2 deletion had more difficulty understanding the ramifications of the diagnosis, a poor understanding of their recurrence risk, and greater difficulty in complying with treatment recommendations for themselves, as well as for their affected offspring when compared to their nondeleted counterparts.[59] Nonetheless, many individuals were gainfully employed. In fact, subsequent to this report, the same authors identified one affected adult with a master's degree in family therapy and another with a bachelor's degree in Early Childhood Education.

With respect to prenatal diagnosis for those couples where one partner has the deletion, the options are relatively straightforward (Table 9–2). Knowing that the couple has a

Table 9–1.

Unselected Patients with the 22q11.2 Deletion (*N* = 36) (McDonald-McGinn, 2005)

	Adults (23)	Children (13)
Overt cleft palate	2	2
Congenital heart disease	2	5
Hypocalcemic seizures	2	0
Laryngeal web	1	0
Schizophrenia	1	0
VPI and a vascular ring	0	1
Normal	15 (65%)	5 (39%)

50% recurrence risk and beginning with the least invasive options, the couple may choose noninvasive monitoring, such as a Level II ultrasound, at approximately 16 weeks gestation, followed by serial fetal echocardiography, from approximately 18–22 weeks of gestation. If an abnormality is found, the couple may then proceed to an amniocentesis or percutaneous blood sampling for confirmation of the diagnosis, depending on the timing in the pregnancy. It is important, however, for the couple to understand that level II ultrasonography and fetal echocardiography are screening tools and that they will not definitively exclude the diagnosis of 22q11.2 deletion. Alternatively, a couple may choose a more direct and definitive approach from the outset, that is, chorionic villus sampling (CVS) or amniocentesis at approximately 12 or 16 weeks gestation, respectively. Both amniocentesis and CVS provide diagnostic results early in the pregnancy so that a therapeutic termination can be considered. Alternatives to prenatal testing include donor sperm or oocytes, which reduce the 50% recurrence to that of the general population, as well as preimplantation genetic diagnosis. The latter two procedures involve in vitro fertilization and are therefore quite costly and currently have limited availability, however, they are viable alternatives for those couples who will not consider a termination of pregnancy.

In providing genetic counseling to seemingly unaffected couples who have had one child with the 22q11.2 deletion, parental studies are recommended, as discussed previously, in an effort to ascertain mildly affected individuals and also to rule out low level mosaicism.[30,37,57] Since germ line mosaicism is a true, but ill-defined risk,[53,55,56] the couple may choose to monitor a subsequent pregnancy utilizing either noninvasive techniques, including Level II ultrasonography and fetal echocardiography as outlined above, or couple these studies with a definitive diagnostic test, such as amniocentesis

Table 9–2.

Guidelines for the Prenatal Detection of a 22q11.2 Deletion (McDonald-McGinn, 2005)

	Group 1 Affected Parent	Group II Couples with an Affected Child and Normal Parental Studies	Group III General Population
Risk of having an affected child	50%	Close to zero but with a small and as yet ill-defined chance of germ line mosaicism	~1/4000
Preconception options	Adoption Donor Gametes	—	—
Prenatal diagnostic options	Level II Ultrasound Fetal Echocardiography Amniocentesis* Chorionic Villus Sampling (CVS)* Preimplantation Genetic Diagnosis using in vitro fertilization (IVF)*	Level II Ultrasound Fetal Echocardiography Amniocentesis* CVS*	Level II Ultrasound† Followed by additional studies as needed

Utilizing studies specifically for the 22q11.2 deletion.
†*If structural abnormalities were identified such as a congenital heart defect this could lead to further investigations such as a fetal echocardiogram and possibly followed by an amniocentesis to rule out a 22q11.2 deletion, in addition to another aneuploidy.*

using FISH for the 22q11.2 deletion. The latter is often most justifiable when amniocentesis or chorionic villus sampling is already being considered for another reason, such as advanced maternal age. However, in many instances, parental anxiety is enough to support these studies.

Genetic counseling for the general population is more complicated and should be considered on a case-by-case basis when anatomic abnormalities are found on fetal ultrasonography or when significant findings are identified in a parent following a careful family history. As stated previously, the estimated incidence of the 22q11.2 deletion is 1/4000 at minimum,[20–24] making it the second most frequent chromosome aberration associated with cardiac malformations after Down syndrome.[60] Thus, deletion studies should be considered in any fetus with congenital heart disease, particularly those with conotruncal cardiac anomalies because the 22q11.2 deletion has been identified in 52% of patients with interrupted aortic arch (IAA) Type B, 35% with truncus arteriosus, and 16% with tetralogy of Fallot (TOF).[61,62] Conversely, 76% of patients with the 22q11.2 deletion have congenital heart disease, most often TOF (Table 9–3).[37] This is notable in that amniocentesis is often offered following the prenatal diagnosis of TOF to rule out aneuploidy, such as trisomy 21. However, TOF is found in 20% of patients with a 22q11.2 deletion[37] as compared to just 4% of children with Down syndrome.[63] Thus, 22q11.2 deletion studies are equally justifiable in a fetus with TOF, if not more so.

In addition to congenital heart disease, there are a number of findings in patients with the 22q11.2 deletion that are often identifiable prenatally and that may support intrauterine deletion studies when seen on a Level II ultrasound. These include cleft palate, renal anomalies, polyhydramnios, polydactyly, congenital diaphragmatic hernia (CDH), club feet,

and neural tube defects.[30,37,57] Overt cleft palate is found in 10% of patients with the 22q11.2 deletion, whereas cleft lip and palate is seen in 1%.[31–33,37,64] These figures are significantly greater than those observed in the general population, wherein the incidence of cleft palate is 1/2500 and that of cleft lip and palate is 1/800.[65] However, an unpublished

Table 9–3.

Congenital Heart Disease in Patients with a 22q11.2 Deletion (N = 440) (McDonald-McGinn, 2005)

Tetralogy of fallot	20%
Ventricular septal defect	14%
IAA Type B	13%
Truncus arteriosus	6%
Vascular ring	5.5%
Atrial septal defect/Ventricular septal defect	4%
Atrial septal defect	3.5%
Others*	10%
Normal	24%

Transposition of the great vessels, bicuspid aortic valve, pulmonary valve stenosis, isolated right pulmonary artery atresia, hypoplastic left heart syndrome, aortic root dilatation, AV canal/heterotaxy.

prospective study of 50 children with isolated cleft palate found none to have the 22q11.2 deletion, suggesting that a cleft palate alone does not appear to warrant deletion studies in an otherwise normal child or fetus.[66] Structural renal abnormalities are seen in 31% of patients with the 22q11.2 deletion. Findings which can be seen on prenatal ultrasound include renal agenesis (12%), hydronephrosis (5%), and multicystic/dysplastic kidneys (4%).[67,68] Polyhydramnios has been seen retrospectively in 16% of pregnancies.[37] This incidence is 16 times that of the general population and may be attributable to the presence of fetal palatal anomalies, swallowing difficulties, or esophageal atresia.[69,70] Preaxial and postaxial polydactyly of the hands has been observed in 4% of patients with the deletion, whereas postaxial polydactyly of the feet has been seen in 1%.[71] This is at least 10 times the incidence seen in the general population in both Caucasians and African Americans. Other limb defects that have been reported and that may be identifiable on fetal ultrasonography include radial aplasia,[70] symbrachydactyly,[72] absent/hypoplastic thumb,[73] tibial hemimelia, clubfoot,[74] and a terminal transverse defect of the upper extremity (author's personal experience). CDH is found in 1% of patients with the 22q11.2 deletion,[37] which is 20 times the incidence of CDH in the general population. Like polyhydramnios, CDH is often identifiable prenatally and, as with congenital heart disease, the identification of CDH in a fetus frequently prompts consideration of prenatal cytogenetic studies in order to rule out aneuploidy, particularly tetrasomy 12p.[74] Neural tube defects (NTDs) are occasionally reported in patients with the 22q11.2 deletion,[75] suggesting that they may occur more frequently than in the general population. Thus, prenatal sonographic findings, including overt cleft palate, renal anomalies, polyhydramnios, polydactyly, clubfoot, CDH, and neural tube defects, in combination or in the presence of congenital heart disease, should prompt consideration of intrauterine deletion studies in order to provide appropriate prenatal counseling and clinical management. Furthermore, should such findings lead to prenatal diagnostic testing to rule out any aneuploidy, for example, trisomy 13, 18, 21, etc., the addition of 22q11.2 deletion studies as an adjunct to standard cytogenetics should be considered.

Lastly, it is important to stress the need for a careful family history in the medical setting as children with the 22q11.2 deletion move towards child bearing age and primary care physicians/obstetric practitioners find themselves in a position to identify previously undiagnosed patients. Again, major clues to the diagnosis include congenital heart disease, palatal anomalies including velopharyngeal dysfunction, immune deficiency and a history of chronic infection, hypoparathyroidism, a learning disability or mental retardation, psychiatric illness (most often schizophrenia), and minor facial dysmorphisms, which most often include malar flatness, hooding of the eyelids, hypertelorism, auricular anomalies, a prominent nasal root with a bulbous nasal tip and hypoplastic alae nasae, a nasal dimple or crease, a small mouth, or asymmetric crying facies (Fig. 9–1 to 9–8).[31,33,34,76−80] However, there appears to be a paucity of

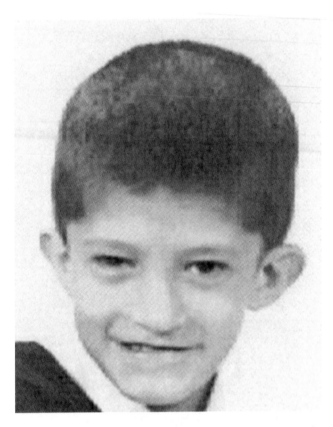

Figure 9–4. This 9-year-old Caucasian male has fairly typical facial features including: A short broad forehead; hooded eyelids with a mild upslant to the palpebral fissures; protuberant ears; some malar flatness; a relatively generous nasal tip with hypoplastic alae nasae; a short philtrum with a thin upper lip; and mild asymmetry of the smile.

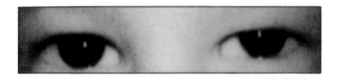
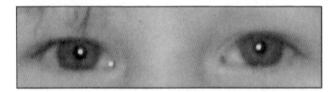
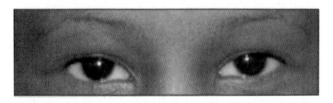

Figure 9–5. These three patients represent the variability in external eye findings including: Significant hooding of the eyelids with no visible eyelashes; mild hooding with +/− telecanthus; no hooding but with a noticeable upslant to the palpebral fissures and mild epicanthus on the left.

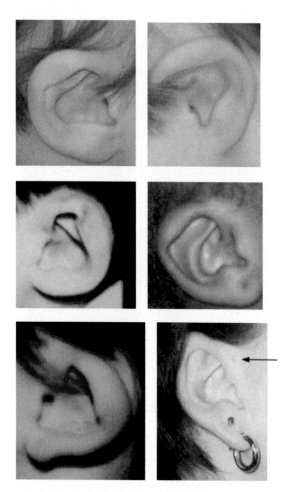

Figure 9–6. Variable auricular anomalies including: Thick over-folded helices; attached lobes; crumpled helices; small ears; cupped and protuberant ears; and preauricular pits. Preauricular tags and microtia have been observed but are not shown here.

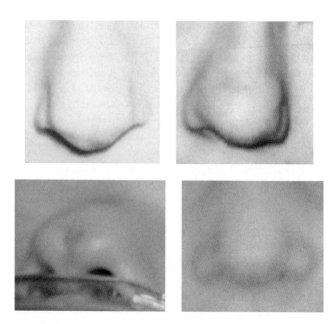

Figure 9–7. Nasal anomalies include a variably bulbous nasal tip with hypoplastic alae nasae and a nasal dimple or crease which at times is punctuated by a strawberry hemangioma.

Immunological

From an immunological perspective, 77% of patients have an immunodeficiency, regardless of their clinical presentation. Of these, 67% have impaired T-cell production, 23% have humoral defects, and 6% have IgA deficiency.[85] Nevertheless, the majority of patients are only mildly immunocompromised and generally do not develop opportunistic or life threatening infections. However, viral infections are often prolonged, and abnormal palatal anatomy and gastroesophageal reflux frequently lead to an increased susceptibility to upper airway bacterial infections and aspiration pneumonia, especially in patients with congenital heart disease.[86] The combination of impaired T-cells and palatal abnormalities is associated with a high frequency of otitis media and sinusitis. Thus, adults and children more than 9 years of age often continue to have infections, including 25–33% with recurrent sinusitis or otitis media and 4–7% with recurrent lower airway infections.[87] Of note, recurrent infections seem to have no correlation with immunologic status, suggesting that these infections have more to do with anatomic and functional airway problems than with defects in the host's defense.[87] In some patients, dysphagia can lead to poor nutrition, further impairing cellular immunity. Despite these issues, very few school-aged children require active management of their immunodeficiency.[86]

In the general population, normal T-cell counts decline rapidly in the first year of life and decline slowly during the next few years. T-cell counts in many patients with the 22q11.2 deletion rise slightly in the first year and then decline more slowly than in children without the deletion.[87] Therefore, the T cell counts in these patients approach normal as they age due to a slight increase in their counts and to the expected decline in normal children.[88] Thus, patients with slight

typical facial features in non-Caucasian individuals (Fig. 9–9) and, therefore, the facies may be less helpful in identifying African American and Asian patients with the 22q11.2 deletion.[81] Thus, one should also be mindful of less common structural anomalies in adults, such as scoliosis, genitourinary anomalies (including hypospadias),[9] craniosynostosis,[33] and laryngeal abnormalities,[9] as well as associated autoimmune disorders (ITP, juvenile rheumatoid arthritis [JRA], psoriasis, vitiligo, Graves disease, autoimmune hemolytic anemia, autoimmune neutropenia)[81–84] and hearing loss, especially in conjunction with a learning disability or psychiatric illness, in order to identify variably affected individuals.[57]

EVALUATION AND MANAGEMENT OF THE PATIENT WITH A 22Q11.2 DELETION

In considering medical management for this diagnosis, each topic must be discussed separately. Here they will be presented in order of frequency:

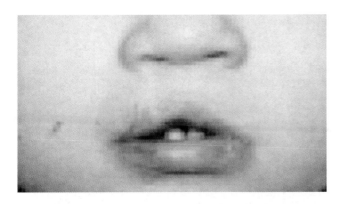

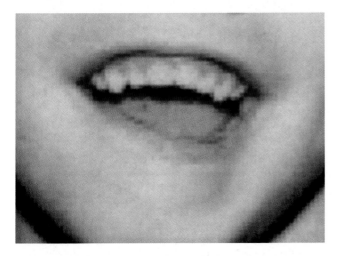

Figure 9–8. Cleft lip is seen in 1% of patients as demonstrated in this child with a repaired unilateral cleft lip, whereas, asymmetric crying facies is more common.

decreases in T-cell numbers have normal defenses against pathogens.[89]

Immunoglobulin levels are usually normal in patients with the 22q11.2 deletion, although subtle immunoglobulin abnormalities may be noted. Hypogammaglobulinemia present in the first year of life usually resolves, and hypergammaglobulinemia may occur after age five.[89] Although the majority of patients have normal antibody function and antibody avidity,[88] some patients have functional antibody defects.[87,90,91] Others, particularly those with recurrent sinopulmonary infections, have frequent immunoglobulin abnormalities, particularly impaired antibody responses to pneumococcal polysaccharide vaccine.[92]

Autoimmune disease in the 22q11.2 deletion is common. However, it does not correlate with severe T-cell dysfunction, and it includes a range of pediatric diseases. Autoimmune cytopenias and JRA appear to be the most common and may occur 20–100 times more frequently than in the general population.[87,92–97] The JRA is often polyarticular and may be difficult to manage.[82,97] Autoimmune thyroid disease and other autoimmune abnormalities have also been described, and it is likely that the T-cell defect acts synergistically with other predisposing factors, such as major histocompatibility complexes, to cause autoimmune disease.[84,87,98] Selective IgA

deficiency may occur in up to 10% of patients with a deletion, and seems to be particularly common in those individuals with autoimmune problems including JRA.[91,97]

From the treatment perspective, live viral vaccines should be withheld in a child with the 22q11.2 deletion and impaired T cell function, an inability to produce functional antibodies, or markedly diminished peripheral blood T cell counts. In the presence of antibody responses to killed vaccines, normal proliferative responses to mitogens and recall antigens, and a CD8 T-cell count of $\geq$250 cells/mm^3 at 1 year of age, live viral vaccines have been administered without sequelae. For patients who have not received varicella vaccine and who are exposed to varicella, varicella-zoster immune globulin or acyclovir prophylaxis is indicated. When the hypogammaglobulinemia is severe or is accompanied by a defect in antibody function, IVIG is warranted. For patients with selective IgA deficiency and recurrent infection, a trial of prophylactic antibiotics can be given.[89]

Cardiovascular

Congenital heart defects are an important feature of the 22q11.2 deletion, as they are present in 74% of affected individuals and are the major cause of mortality ($\geq$90% of all deaths) in patients with this diagnosis.[34,64,99] Further, the 22q11.2 deletion is the second most common syndrome associated with congenital heart disease after Down syndrome.[22] The most frequent anomalies associated with the 22q11.2 deletion are conotruncal defects of the outflow tract of the heart and include TOF (TOF with pulmonary atresia) in 22%, IAA in 15%, conoventricular ventricular septal defect (VSD) in 13%, truncus arteriosus in 7%, and vascular ring in 5% (Fig. 9–10). Less common anomalies include atrial septal defect (ASD), ASD/VSD, isolated aortic arch anomalies such as a right aortic arch, hypoplastic left heart syndrome, pulmonary valve stenosis, double outlet right ventricle, bicuspid aortic valve, heterotaxy, common atrioventricular canal, tricuspid atresia, transposition of the great arteries, coarctation of the aorta, and dilated aortic root.[33,100] Based on this data, deletion studies should be considered in any patient with congenital heart disease, in particular those with conotruncal cardiac anomalies since the 22q11.2 deletion has been identified in 52% of patients with IAA Type B, 35% with truncus arteriosus, and 16% with TOF.[61] Furthermore, it should be noted that the type and severity of congenital heart disease presently varies depending on the age at presentation as neonates and infants most often are more significantly affected whereas older children and adults tend to have less severe findings[100]; however, this too is likely to change as palliative interventions become increasingly successful.

The majority of patients with the 22q11.2 deletion and congenital heart disease requiring surgical interventions do quite well with a very low operative risk and an excellent long-term prognosis.[100] This, of course, is dependent on the preoperative anatomy and any additional confounding factors, such as IUGR, immunodeficiency, laryngotrachealesophageal abnormalities, polymicrogyria, etc., which can also have an

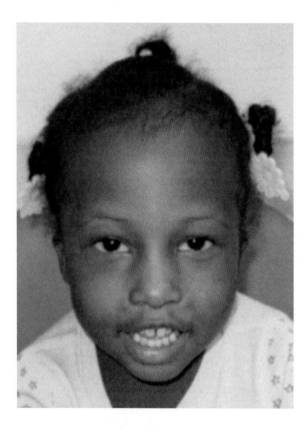

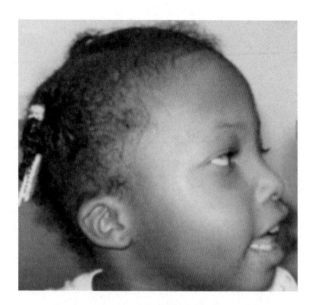

Figure 9–9. This 3-year-old African American female is generally nondysmorphic with mild malar flatness and small ears with thick overfolded helices.

important impact on the postoperative course. With this in mind, patients are often treated with irradiated blood products to avoid the risk of fatal graft-versus-host disease, as well as with prophylactic antibiotics/anti-fungals, depending upon their preoperative immune status (Marino, 2005).

Palata/Velopharyngeal

Palatal anomalies are an important feature of the 22q11.2 deletion, as nearly 70% of individuals with a 22q11.2 deletion have a confirmed palatal abnormality,[33] the most common of which is velopharyngeal incompetence (VPI). It is notable, however, that the reported incidence of palatal anomalies varies widely, ranging from 9% to 98%,[33,58,64,101,102] depending on numerous factors such as the reporting technique, the diligence with which the diagnosis is sought, the age at which the patient is evaluated, and the inherent ascertainment bias within any single center.[103] Thus, the figures presented here are derived from the authors' own experience and are provided as a general guideline for the reader.

VPI may be due to a structural problem, such as a palatal cleft or velopharyngeal disproportion, a functional problem, such as hypotonia of the velopharyngeal musculature, or a combination of both. Frequently, children who are initially diagnosed with a 22q11.2 deletion because of a cardiac defect are subsequently found to have a previously unrecognized but clinically significant VPI.[32] Submucosal clefts and/or a bifid uvula are also fairly prevalent (16%; 5%), whereas, overt cleft palate and cleft lip/cleft lip and palate are less common, accounting for 11% and 2% of palatal anomalies observed

respectively.[33] Conversely, unlike the findings in patients with conotruncal cardiac anomalies, it should be noted that the 22q11.2 deletion does not appear to be responsible for isolated/nonsyndromic cleft palate,[66,104] and therefore screening studies in older patients with overt cleft palate are likely unwarranted.

Overt and classic submucosal clefts are readily diagnosable on physical examination/intraoral inspection, but occult submucosal clefts may require nasendoscopic examination. It is generally agreed that surgical management of palatal anomalies in patients with a 22q11.2 deletion aims to attain normal speech outcome as early as possible, but, in light of the associated delays in emergence of language and concomitant medical problems such as congenital heart disease, there is little consensus regarding the timing or type of procedure, in patients with submucosal cleft palate or VPI. The most commonly performed surgical procedures include a posterior pharyngeal flap and sphincter pharyngoplasty. These are discussed in detail elsewhere in this text. Complications associated with VPI repair include hemorrhage, dehiscence, oronasal fistula formation, pneumonia, and cardiac arrest.[103] Postoperative complications can include nasal airway obstruction and hyponasal speech, which generally resolve once edema subsides. Snoring, obligate mouth breathing, and, rarely, obstructive sleep apnea may occur after surgical management of VPI, especially in those patients with tonsillar hyperplasia. When the tonsils are enlarged, tonsillectomy is generally recommended prior to VPI surgery. Signs of postoperative obstructive sleep apnea include loud snoring, nocturnal arousals, and excessive daytime somnolence.

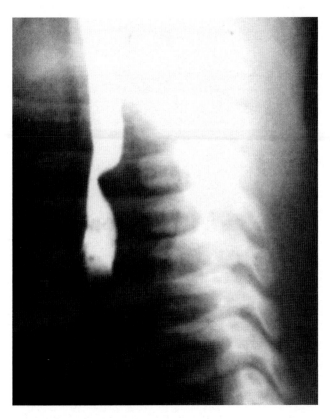

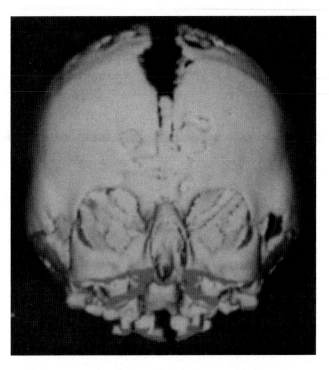

Figure 9–11. This CT scan with 3D reconstruction demonstrates bicoronal craniosynostosis.

Figure 9–10. A vascular ring causing constriction of the esophagus are appreciated here on barium swallow.

Such symptoms should prompt further evaluation and may require a surgical revision of the VPI repair.[103]

It should also be noted that VPI has been observed in patients with the 22q11.2 deletion following adenoidectomy, so the need for this procedure should be weighed against the chance of developing/worsening symptoms of VPI. Furthermore, anomalies of the carotid arteries, specifically medial displacement of the internal carotid arteries at the level of the posterior pharynx, have been described in as many as 25% of patients with the 22q11.2 deletion, placing them at risk for injury at the time of pharyngoplasty.[102] Thus, preoperative imaging studies such as magnetic resonance angiography or computed tomography may be useful in defining the vascular anatomy, thereby allowing for precise surgical planning to minimize the risk of intraoperative vascular injury.[103,105,106]

In light of the high incidence of occult submucosal clefts and VPI in this population and of the fact that early identification of palatal anomalies will allow for appropriate medical intervention and genetic counseling, it is appropriate for all patients with a 22q11.2 deletion to undergo evaluation by a cleft palate team.

Craniofacial

Other craniofacial anomalies that may result in an affected patient presenting initially to the cleft palate/craniofacial team are microtia and craniosynostosis (Fig. 9–11). In fact, both anomalies have led to the diagnosis in individuals followed in this setting when a geneticist was a part of the multidisciplinary team[107] (Digilio, in press). In light of these findings, 22q11.2 deletion studies should be considered in any patient who has features of oculoauricularvertebral spectrum/ Goldenhar syndrome (generally without an epibulbar dermoid), as such patients have numerous overlapping features of the deletion including congenital heart disease, renal anomalies, hemivertebrae/butterfly vertebrae, and microtia/ anotia (Digilio, in press). Furthermore, patients with both unicoronal and bicoronal craniosynostosis are also candidates for deletion studies when all other causes of craniosynostosis have been eliminated, including mutations in FGFR 1, 2 and 3, as well as, mutations and deletions in TWIST.[107]

Well-described craniofacial features of the 22q11.2 deletion which generally do not require intervention but may be clues to the diagnosis include: a variety of auricular abnormalities in addition to microtia/anotia such as thick, overfolded and often "crumpled" helices, protuberant ears, and attached lobes; hooding of the eyelids; hypertelorism; malar flatness; a small mouth; asymmetric crying facies; and micrognathia. It should be noted, however, that some patients have no typical dysmorphic features, especially those of non-Caucasian ancestry.[107] Thus, the diagnosis in non-Caucasians should be considered based on the constellation of medical/ neuropsychological findings rather than on the presence or absence of dysmorphic features.

Endocrine

Congenital or acquired hypocalcemia due to hypoparathyroidism is present in approximately 50% of patients with the

22q11.2 deletion and is typically most serious in the neonatal period.[33] In fact, hypocalcemia is often the presenting symptom in a neonate and frequently leads to the suspicion of the diagnosis of the 22q11.2 deletion. Symptoms may include tremor, tetany, tachypnea, arthymia, irritability, dysphagia, and seizures. Calcium homeostasis generally normalizes with age, although recurrence of hypocalcemia in later childhood or adulthood has been reported during stressors such as illness and/or puberty. Treatment usually includes calcium replacement therapy as well as calcitriol/vitamin D,[108] while being vigilant to avoid causing renal calculi. In some instances, children receiving ongoing care for infantile hypocalcemia may not be diagnosed with the 22q11.2 deletion syndrome until school age. At least one otherwise asymptomatic adult has come to attention following the onset of hypoparathyroidism in the fourth decade (Eagan, a personal communication, April, 2004). With this in mind, periodic monitoring of calcium levels in patients with the 22q11.2 deletion seem warranted and conversely the diagnosis should be considered in patients with hypoparathyroidism.[109]

Another endocrinopathy found occasionally in patients with the 22q11.2 deletion is growth hormone deficiency (GHD) leading to short stature (height less than the 5th percentile), which generally becomes apparent after the first year of life. Additional symptoms, which may or may not be present in such patients, include a delay in pubertal development; a high pitched voice; small hands and feet; a prominent forehead; and underdeveloped male genitalia. Such symptoms should prompt evaluation by a pediatric endocrinologist as these patients respond well to GH therapy.[108]

Gastrointestinal

Approximately 30% of children with the 22q11.2 deletion have significant dysphagia,[69] often requiring nasogastric tube feedings and/or gastrostomy tube placement. Feeding difficulties are independent of cardiac defects as well as palatal anomalies, and it is important to recognize that this aspect of the 22q11.2 deletion is often the most challenging for families, as many feel inadequate when they are unable to feed their offspring. Further evaluation of such children frequently reveals nasopharyngeal reflux (Fig. 9–12), prominence of the cricopharyngeal muscle, abnormal cricopharyngeal closure, and/or diverticulum. The underlying feeding problem in many children appears to be dysmotility in the pharyngoesophageal area, which is derived from the third and fourth pharyngeal pouches, as well as esophageal dysmotility (Fig. 9–13).[69] In addition to dysmotility in the upper gastrointestinal tract, constipation is a chronic feature of the 22q11.2 deletion in the majority of patients (Pasquariello P, personal communication, January, 2006). Other anatomic abnormalities that have been identified include intestinal malrotation, intestinal nonrotation, Hirshprung disease (Mascarenhas M, personal communication, October, 2001), and feeding difficulties secondary to a vascular ring.[33] In light of these findings, children with significant feeding problems will often benefit from an evaluation with a gastroenterolo-

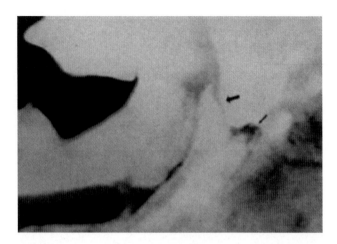

Figure 9–12. Nasopharyngeal reflux is demonstrated here on barium swallow (*Image courtesy of Peggy Eicher, MD*).

gist or feeding specialist, as structural and functional abnormalities generally require imaging studies such as an upper GI with small bowel follow-through, a pH probe, milk scan, swallow study, etc. in order to precisely identify the underlying problem. Chronic feeding issues may be ameliorated once the etiology is identified, since patients' symptoms are generally amenable to therapeutics such as utilizing acid blockades, treating the delayed gastric emptying and/or constipation, facilitating more mature oral motor skills, or performing surgical interventions when necessary.[69]

Renal

Renal abnormalities have been identified in 31% of patients, including single kidney/multicystic/dysplastic kidney (10%), hydronephrosis (5%), vesicoureteral reflux/irregular bladder (6%), and dysfunctional voiding (11%).[67] Additional findings have included small kidneys, renal calculi (often secondary to treatment for hypocalcemia), bladder wall thickening, a horseshoe kidney, a duplicated collecting system, renal tubular acidosis, and enuresis. This high incidence of renal abnormalities is similar to that reported by Devriendt et al.[68] and warrants nephrourological investigation in all patients with a 22q11.2 deletion. In addition, hypospadias (8%), undescended testes (6%)[9,67] and primary amenorrhea due to an absent uterus have also been observed.[110]

Ophthalmic

Eye findings reported in patients with a 22q11.2 deletion include posterior embyotoxin (prominent, anteriorly displaced Schwalbe's line at the corneal limbus or edge) in 49%, tortuous retinal vessels in 34%, hooded eyelids in 20%, strabismus in 18%, ptosis in 4%, amblyopia in 4%, and tilted optic nerves in 1%.[111] In addition, scleracornea, a nonprogressive, noninflammatory condition in which one or both corneas demonstrate some degree of opacification coupled with flattening of the normal corneal curvature, has recently been identified in several patients with the 22q11.2 deletion,[112] whereas

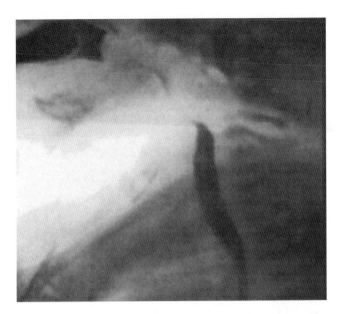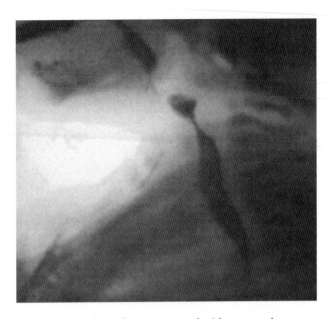

Figure 9–13. Using a barium swallow, esophageal dysmotility is seen on the right as compared with a normal esophageal motility on the left (*Image courtesy of Peggy Eicher, MD*).

Peter's anomaly, a finding with similar embryogenesis, has been seen in one patient to date.[113] As familial cases of scleracornea have been reported previously, including both autosomal dominant and autosomal recessive pedigrees,[114,115] the association with the 22q112 deletion may provide some insight into the etiology of these eye findings. Specifically, the deletion may unmask an autosomal recessive condition, as it has previously with the hematologic disorder Bernard-Soulier syndrome (BSS).[116] Alternatively, the deletion may, in association with other genetic loci previously associated with scleracornea, play multifactorial and interrelated roles in neural crest migration and differentiation.[112] The incidence of astigmatism, myopia, and hyperopia is comparable to that seen in the general population,[111] whereas a small number of patients have cataracts and colobomas (authors' personal experience). Regardless, in light of the high incidence of ocular conditions associated with the 22q11.2 deletion which can potentially affect visual development, it seems prudent that all children with the deletion undergo a comprehensive eye examination upon diagnosis of the condition with follow-up as indicated by the findings in each case.[111]

Otolarynologic

Otolaryngologic abnormalities are an important feature of the 22q11.2 deletion. As mentioned previously, structural auricular anomalies are frequent and include overfolded or squared off helices; cupped, microtic, and protuberant ears; preauricular pits or tags, and narrow external auditory meati. Additionally, many patients have chronic otitis media (88%)[117] and chronic sinusitis due to their underlying immune deficiency and palatal anomalies. Such may result in conductive hearing loss (37%).[33] Sensorineural hearing loss, as well as mixed hearing loss, has also been seen, although the incidence is much lower as compared with conductive

loss.[33,117] A Mondini malformation of the cochlea may also be present and should be considered in any patient with the 22q11.2 deletion, and unexplained meningitis. A prominent nasal root, bulbous nasal tip, hypoplastic alae nasae, and a nasal dimple/bifid nasal tip are also clues to the diagnosis of the deletion.[76] Stridor due to a vascular ring, laryngomalacia, or a laryngeal web can also occur[33] and should be investigated by an otolaryngologist when symptoms are present. Chest MRI or endoscopy may be necessary to define the anatomy.

Musculoskeletal

Occasional significant musculoskeletal anomalies have been observed including preaxial and postaxial polydactyly of the upper extremity in 6% of patients. Lower extremity abnormalities include postaxial polydactyly, clubfoot, overfolded toes, and syndactyly of toes 2 and 3 in 15% (Fig. 9–14).[71] Vertebral anomalies are seen in 19% of patients, including butterfly vertebrae, hemivertebrae, and coronal clefts (Fig. 9–15); rib anomalies, most commonly supernumerary or absent ribs, are seen in 19% of patients, and hypoplastic scapulae are seen in 1.5%.[71] Significant cervical spine abnormalities have been observed in approximately 50% of patients studied, including C2-C3 fusion in 34%, fusion of the posterior elements in 21%, and complete block vertebrae of C2-C3 in 13%.[118] In addition, 56% of persons with cervical spine anomalies have been found to have instability on flexion and extension radiographs, and 33% have increased motion at more than one vertebral level.[118] Of these patients, a small subset (4 of 79), have increased C2-C3 segmental motion with anterior and posterior narrowing of the spinal canal. On further examination with cervical CT scan and/or MRI, two of these four patients underwent surgical stabilization, one of whom required an emergency procedure following onset of symptoms of spinal cord compression (Drummond D,

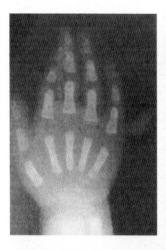
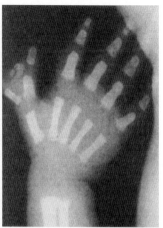

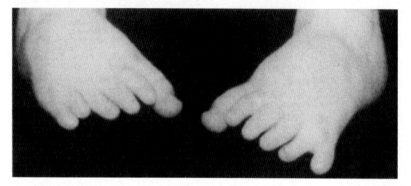

Figure 9–14. Preaxial and postaxial polydactyly of the hands and postaxial polydactyly of the feet are shown here.

personal communication, June, 2004). Thus, 5-view (AP, lateral, flexion, extension, open mouth) cervical spine radiographs are warranted in all patients with the 22q11.2 deletion who are old enough to have full ossification of the cervical spine (usually more than 4 years of age) and who can cooperate for the radiographs (as it is unwise to use force in a potentially unstable cervical spine).

Neurologic

Although the majority of individuals with the 22q11.2 deletion syndrome have a history of hypotonia in infancy and learning disabilities,[119] specific neurologic manifestations are uncommon. Seizures are present in some individuals and are most often associated with hypocalcemia. However, in one study, 7% of 383 patients with the 22q11.2 deletion had unprovoked seizures.[120] Several individuals have asymmetric crying facies, although the etiology of this is unclear.[12,121–123] Rarely, ataxia and atrophy of the cerebellum are observed.[124] Additional CNS abnormalities include multicystic white matter lesions of unknown significance, perisylvian dysplasia,[125] hypoplasia of the pituitary gland,[108] and polymicrogyria.[126] Recent investigations utilizing functional MRI scans revealed significantly-reduced posterior-brain volumes relative to age and sex matched controls with more significant white matter loss in the left occipital and left parietal regions as compared to the frontal lobes.[127–130] Many of these changes in brain structure can be postulated to relate to the specific cognitive deficits

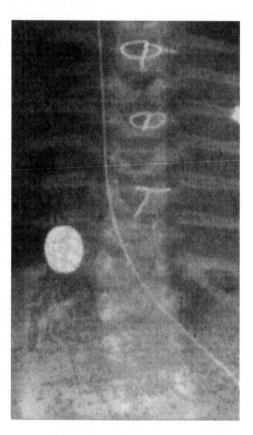

Figure 9–15. Butterfly vertebrae, which have a relatively short differential diagnosis, are seen here.

exhibited in the area of working memory, executive function, visuospatial skill, language and math performance. Overall, the pattern of CNS abnormalities is broad and overlaps with that seen in some cases of Opitz G/BBB syndrome.[131–133] Thus, patients should be referred to neurology when symptoms are present and not necessarily on a prophylactic basis.

Other less common findings observed in individuals with the 22q11.2 deletion include: abnormal lung lobation, imperforate anus, diaphragmatic hernia, umbilical and inguinal hernia, and unexplained leg pain.[9,30,33,37,134] BSS,[116] an autosomal recessive disorder of thrombocytopenia and giant platelets, is caused by a mutation in one of four genes, one of which (*GP1BB*) maps to 22q11.2. BSS is associated with the 22q11.2 deletion in persons whose nondeleted chromosome 22 has a mutation in *GP1BB*. Individuals with both a 22q11.2 deletion and BSS are particularly susceptible to bleeding secondary to any surgical procedures. Lastly, malignancies have been reported in patients with a 22q11.2 deletion, including hepatobastoma, renal cell carcinoma, Wilms tumor, and neuroblastoma.[135–137] Based on these reports, a causal relationship between the 22q11.2 deletion and hepatoblastoma seems, likely, as the population incidence of hepatoblastoma is 1/1,000,000. Neoplasia could conceivably be mediated by the underlying immune deficiency; however, there is too little evidence to invoke a more global causal relationship with the 22q11.2 deletion and cancer.[137]

It is now well established that there is a very wide range of expressions of the "behavioral phenotype" in both children and adults with a 22q11.2 deletion.[34,77,138–141] In general, young children with the 22q11.2 deletion syndrome have delays in motor milestones, with a mean age of walking at 18 months; delays in emergence of language with many who are nonverbal at age 2–3 years; and autism/autistic spectrum disorders in approximately 20%.[142] In a study of 28 toddlers assessed with standardized tests, mental development was average in 21%, mildly delayed in 32%, and significantly delayed in 46%. In motor development, 8% were average, 13% were mildly delayed, and 79% were significantly delayed. In a group of 12 preschoolers assessed using the Weschler Preschool Primary Scale of Intelligence-Revised, the Full Scale IQ was 78 ± 11, the mean Performance IQ was 78 ± 14, and the mean Verbal IQ was 82 ± 15. In total language, 16% were average, 44% were mildly delayed and 40% were significantly delayed.[138] The older individual with 22q11.2 deletion syndrome generally has an atypical neuropsychological profile across multiple domains with the most striking being a significantly higher verbal IQ score than performance IQ score. Moss et al.[119] observed a more than 10-point mean split between the verbal IQ and performance IQ in 66% of 80 school-age children, consistent with a nonverbal learning disability, which is quite rare in the general population.[143] Because the full scale IQ score alone does not accurately represent the abilities of many individuals with the 22q11.2 deletion, verbal and performance IQ scores often need to be considered separately. In addition, affected individuals appear to exhibit relative strengths in the areas of rote verbal learning and memory, reading decoding, and spelling, whereas deficits are found in the areas

of nonverbal processing, visual–spatial skills, complex verbal memory, attention, working memory, visual–spatial memory, and mathematics. This evidence of stronger verbal than visual memory skills and stronger reading than math skills also supports the presence of a nonverbal learning disorder which requires specific cognitive remediation, behavior management, and parental counseling.[119,144–146] It is important to recognize, though, that a "nonverbal learning disability" does not mean that the learning problems of these children only involve nonverbal functions, as a substantial number of these children also have both receptive and expressive language difficulties.[138,141,147] In general, IQ scores in school aged children, using the age-appropriate Weschler IQ test, reveal a mean IQ of between 70 and 76,[77,119] with 18% of patients attaining full scale IQ scores in the average range, 20% in the low-average range, 32% in the borderline range, and 30% in the mentally retarded range.[119]

To date, no direct link between cardiac status and intellectual outcome has been established.[77,148] However, those patients with structural brain malformations such as polymicrogyria are significantly more affected.[126] The mean IQ of individuals with a deletion inherited from a parent is significantly lower than the IQ of individuals with de novo deletions.[77] This finding is not unexpected, as more severe learning disabilities in familial cases can partly be explained by lower educational level and IQ of the affected parent[141] and the unaffected partner of the affected parent has been shown to achieve a lower educational level than the unaffected parents in nonfamilial cases suggesting assortative mating.[77]

Delayed speech and language development is one of the most consistent features in young patients with the 22q11.2 deletion, and like the feeding issues, as such is a source of great frustration for families.[147,149–153] Many affected infants do not babble, and the average age at emergence of language is 2.5 years.[138,145] Thus, sign language is often utilized as an adjunct to verbal communication where needed to avoid frustration and the associated behavioral difficulties.[139,150,153] In looking at total language development, Gerdes et al.[138] reported on a sample of 40 children with the 22q11.2 deletion ages 13–63 months and found 40% to be significantly delayed, 44% mildly delayed, and 16% were in the average range. Although both expressive and receptive language demonstrated a high degree of delay, expressive language was more impaired than receptive. In addition, such delays in expressive language remained significant even after controlling for their cognitive levels. It has also been demonstrated, however, that affected children show remarkable improvement in their speech and language skills by school age,[138,154,155] perhaps as a result of intervention, and over time their verbal skills paradoxically become their strength.[156] Thus, all children with the 22q11.2deletion benefit from speech and language therapy beginning at the time of diagnosis or by 6 months of age, whichever comes earlier.[151]

In addition to their language difficulties, many young children also have significant articulation deficits and speech abnormalities such as a high-pitched voice, hoarseness, compensatory articulation errors, dysarthria, and velopharyngeal incompetence leading to hypernasal speech.[141] Here, too, every child with a 22q11.2 deletion will benefit greatly from early intervention strategies.[139,153]

Psychiatric findings associated with the 22q11.2 deletion include disinhibition and impulsiveness on the one hand and shyness and withdrawal on the other.[144] Anxiety, perseveration, and difficulty with social interactions are also common, along with autism and autistic spectrum disorders.[142,144,157,158] Attention deficits have also been implicated in the behavioral profile of patients[77,138,147,159] and may or may not require behavioral or medical interventions. Additionally, thought problems such as muddled thinking, frequent/easy confusion, ruminations, and repetitive thoughts have been identified.[77,147]

The incidence and type of frank psychiatric disease associated with the 22q11.2 deletion including schizophrenia, bipolar disorder, and depression varies from study to study and has evolved over time.[79,80,160–166] Most recently, a 20–30% prevalence of psychosis, most often schizophrenia, appears to be the most consistent result across differing reports,[158] whereas, "psychosis-like" symptoms have been identified in some adolescents and young adults (age 13–25 years)[165]; however, no precursor symptoms have been identified to date. It should be noted that standard medical treatments appear to be equally effective in this population of patients,[164] and early identification and treatment is essential to minimize future psychiatric morbidity and social isolation or exclusion.[167] Moreover, the behavioral phenotype in patients with a 22q11.2 deletion must be examined further with a specific emphasis on the longitudinal course of symptoms[158] in order to provide more accurate information to patients and their families. Conversely, our understanding of the biological etiology of psychosis and autism in the general population may well benefit greatly from the basic science research involving patients with a 22q11.2 deletion.

DIFFERENTIAL DIAGNOSIS

Each of the anomalies seen in patients with a 22q11.2 deletion can also be found as an isolated anomaly in an otherwise normal individual. Nonetheless, disorders with overlapping features include: Smith-Lemli-Opitz syndrome (when polydactyly and cleft palate are present); Alagille syndrome (when butterfly vertebrae, congenital heart disease, and posterior embryotoxin are present); VATER syndrome (when heart disease, vertebral, renal, and limb anomalies are present); oculoauricularvertebral sequence/Goldenhar syndrome (when ear anomalies, vertebral defects, heart disease, renal anomalies are present); and Kabuki syndrome (when cleft palate, congenital heart disease, and butterfly vertebrae are present). Individuals suspected of having a 22q11.2 deletion but with negative FISH studies may have a chromosome abnormality involving some other chromosomal region, including a cytogenetically visible deletion at 10p13-p14. Alternatively, a smaller deletion which excludes the N25 or TUPLE probes

is possible, as well as a point mutation in *TBX1* (McDonald-McGinn, 2008). Thus, such patients will likely benefit from more sophisticated laboratory studies such as Comparative Genomic Hybridization, whole genome array, Multiplex Ligation-Dependent Probe Amplification, or research studies which will involve sequencing the *TBX1* gene.

Management for patients with a 22q11.2 deletion is age-specific and symptom-specific.[33] Nonetheless, there are some general recommendations. All patients, regardless of their age at presentation, will benefit from the following: a cardiology evaluation, which often includes a chest x-ray, electrocardiogram, and echocardiogram; laboratory studies to assess the presence of hypoparathyroidism and/or an endocrinology examination; a renal ultrasound; and a genetics consultation with parental 22q11.2 deletion studies in order to provide appropriate genetic counseling. Patients more than 4 years of age will benefit from 5-view cervical spine radiographs (AP, lateral, flexion, extension, and open mouth). Most children and some adults will profit from evaluations by a cleft palate team, an immunologist, and child development specialist/psychologist. Patients with specific symptomatology will require a more extensive work-up by other specialties, including: endocrinology, gastroenterology, general surgery, hematology, nephrology, neurology, neurosurgery, oncology, orthopedics, rheumatology, and urology. As is evidenced by this lengthy list of subspecialty evaluations, many patients with a 22q11.2 deletion are quite complex, and they benefit, in particular, from a multi-disciplinary approach, much like that of the cleft palate team model, with one team leader designated to collate the multitude of specialist recommendations and then to provide the family with one unifying message, wherever possible.

References

1. de la Chapelle A, Herva R, Koivisto M, Aula P. A deletion in chromosome 22 can cause DiGeorge syndrome. *Hum Genet* 57:253–256, 1981.
2. Kelley RI, Zackai EH, Emanuel BS, Kistenmacher M, Greenberg F, Punnett HH. The association of the DiGeorge anomalad with partial monosomy of chromosome 22. *J Pediatr* 101:197–200, 1982.
3. Driscoll DA, Budarf ML, Emanuel BS. A genetic etiology for DiGeorge syndrome: Consistent deletions and microdeletions of 22q11. *Am J Hum Genet* 50:924–933, 1992.
4. Scambler PJ, Carey AH, Wyse RK, Roach S, Dumanski JP, Nordenskjold M, Williamson R. Microdeletions within 22q11 associated with sporadic and familial DiGeorge syndrome. *Genomics* 10(1):201–206, 1991.
5. Driscoll DA, Spinner NB, Budarf ML, et al. Deletions and microdeletions of 22q11.2 in Velo-Cardio-Facial syndrome. *Am J Med Genet* 44:261–268,1992.
6. Driscoll DA, Salvin J, Sellinger B, McDonald-McGinn D, Zackai EH, Emanuel BS. Prevalence of 22q11 microdeletions in DGS and VCFS: Implications for genetic counseling and prenatal diagnosis. *J Med Genet* 30:813–817,1993.
7. Burn J, Takao A, Wilson D, et al. Conotruncal anomaly face syndrome is associated with a deletion within chromosome 22. *J Med Genet* 30:822–824, 1993.
8. Matsouka R, Takao A, Kimura M, et al. Confirmation that the conotruncal anomaly face syndrome is associated with a deletion within 22q11.2. *Am J Med Genet* 53:285–289, 1994.

9. McDonald-McGinn DM, Driscoll DA, Bason L, et al. Autosomal dominant "Opitz" GBBB syndrome due to a 22q11.2 deletion. *Am J Med Genet* 59:103–113, 1995.

10. LaCassie Y and Arriaza MI. Letter to the Editor. Opitz GBBB syndrome and the 22q11.2 deletion syndrome. *Am J Med Genet* 62:318, 1996.

11. Fryburg JS, Lin KY, Golden EF. Chromosome 22q11.2 deletion in a boy with Opitz oculo-genito-laryngeal syndrome. *Am J Med Genet* 62:274–275, 1996.

12. Giannotti A, Diglio MC, Marino B, Mingarelli R, Dallapiccola B. Cayler cardiofacial syndrome and del 22q11: Part of the CATCH22 phenotype. *Am J Med Genet* 30:807–812, 1994.

13. Bawle EV, Conard J, Van Dyke DL, Czarnecki P, Driscoll DA. Letter to the Editor. Seven new cases of cayler cardiofacial syndrome with chromosome 22q11.2 deletion, including a familial case. *Am J Med Genet* 79:406–410, 1998.

14. McDonald-McGinn DM, Emanuel BS, Zackai EH. Letter to the Editor. Autosomal dominant "Opitz" GBBB syndrome due to a 22q11.2 deletion. *Am J Med Genet* 64:525–526, 1996.

15. Desmaze C, Scambler P, Prieur M, et al. Routine diagnosis of DiGeorge by fluorescence in situ hybridization. *Hum Genet* 90:663–665, 1993.

16. Kariyazono H, Ohno T, Ihara K, et al. Rapid detection of the 22q11.2 deletion with quantitative real-time PCR. *Mol Cell Probes* 15(2):71–73, 2001.

17. Mantripragada KK, Tapia-Páez I, Blennow E, Nilsson P, Wedell A, Dumanski JP. DNA copy-number analysis of the 22q11 deletion-syndrome region using array-CGH with genomic and PCR-based targets. *Int J Mol Med* 13(2):273–279, 2004.

18. Fernández L, Lapunzina P, Pajares IL, et al. Higher frequency of uncommon 1.5–2 Mb deletions found in familial cases of 22q11.2 deletion syndrome. *Am J Med Genet* 136(1):71–75, 2005.

19. Carey AH, Kelly D, Halford S, et al. Molecular genetic study of the frequency of monosomy 22q11 in DiGeorge syndrome. *Am J Hum Genet* 51(5):964–970, 1992.

20. Wilson DI, Cross IE, Goodship JA, et al. A prospective cytogenetic study of 36 cases of DiGeorge syndrome. *Am J Hum Genet* 51:957–963, 1992.

21. Devriendt K, Fryns JP, Mortier G, van Thienen MN. The annual incidence of DiGeorge/velocardiofacial syndrome. *J Med Genet* 35:789–790, 1998.

22. Goodship J, Cross I, LiLing J, Wren C. A population study of chromosome 22q111998 deletions in infancy. *Arch Dis Child* 79(4):348–351, 1998.

23. Scambler, PJ. The 22q11 deletion syndromes. *Hum Mol Genet* 10(16):2421–2426, 2000.

24. Botto LD, May K, Fernhoff PM, Correa A. A population-based study of the 22q11.2 deletion: Phenotype, incidence, and contribution to major birth defects in the population. *Pediatrics* 112:101–107, 2003.

25. Oskarsdóttir S, Vujic M, Fasth A. Incidence and prevalence of the 22q11 deletion syndrome: A population-based study in Western Sweden. *Arch Dis Child* 89(2):148–151, 2004.

26. Wilson DI, Cross IE, Wren, C. Minimum prevalence of chromosome 22q11 deletions. *Am J Hum Genet Sullp* 55:A169, 1994.

27. Rauch A, Hoyer J, Guth S, et al. Diagnostic yield of various genetic approaches in patients with unexplained developmental delay or mental retardation. *Am J Med Genet A* 140(19):2063–2074, 2006.

28. Saitta SC, Harris SE, McDonald-McGinn DM, et al. Independent de novo 22q11.2 deletions in first cousins with DiGeorge/velocardiofacial syndrome. *Am J Med Genet* 124(A):313–317, 2004.

29. Reardon W, Wilkes D, Rutland P, et al. Craniosynostosis associated with FGFR3 pro 250 arg mutation results in a range of clinical presentations including unisutural craniosynostosis. *J Med Genet* 34:632–636, 1997.

30. McDonald-McGinn DM and Zackai, EH. *Genetic counseling.* In: Murphy KC, Scambler PJ (eds). *Genetic Counseling Velo-Cardio-Facial Syndrome: A Model for Understanding Microdeletion Disorders,* Murphy and Scambler, Cambridge, UK: Cambridge University Press, 200–218, 2005.

31. McDonald-McGinn DM, LaRossa D, Goldmuntz E, et al. The 22q11.2 deletion: Screening, diagnostic workup, and outcome of results. Report on 181 patients. *Genet Test* 1:99–108, 1997.

32. McDonald-McGinn DM, Driscoll DA, Emanuel BS, et al. Detection of a 22q11.2 deletion in cardiac patients suggests a risk for velopharyngeal incompetence. *Pediatrics* 99:1–5, 1997. Also available at http://www.pediatrics.org/cgi/content/full/99/5/e9.

33. McDonald-McGinn DM, Kirschner R, Goldmuntz E, et al. The Philadelphia Story: The 22q11.2 Deletion: Report on 250 Patients. *Genet Couns* 10(1):11–24, 1999.

34. McDonald-McGinn DM, Tonnesen MK, Laufer-Cahana A, et al. Phenotype of the 22q11.2 deletion in individuals identified through an affected relative: Cast a wide FISHing net! *Genet Med* 3:23–29, 2001.

35. Yamagishi H, Ishii C, Maeda J, et al. Phenotypic discordance in monozygotic twins with 22q11.2 deletion. *Am J Med Genet* 78:319–321, 1998.

36. McDonald-McGinn DM, Driscoll DA, Tonnesen M, et al. Parent of origin does not determine phenotype in the 22q11.2 deletion. *Am J Hum Genet* 69:285(A597), 2001.

37. McDonald-McGinn DM, Driscoll DA, Saitta S, et al. Guidelines for prenatal detection of the 22q11.2 deletion. *Am J Hum Genet* 71(4):198 (A173), 2002.

38. Gong W, Emanuel BS, Collins J, et al. A transcription map of the DiGeorge and velo-cardio-facial syndrome minimal critical region on 22q11. *Hum Mol Genet* 58:1377–1381, 1996.

39. Baldini A. Dissecting contiguous gene defects: TBX1. *Curr Opin Genet Dev* 15:279–284, 2005.

40. Yagi H, Furutani Y, Hamad H, et al. Role of TBX1 in human 22q11.2 syndrome. *Lancet* 362:1366–1373, 2003.

41. Zweier C, Sticht H, Aydin-Jaylagul I, Campbell CE, Rauch A. Human TBX1 Missense mutations cause gain of function resulting in the same phenotype as 22q11.2 deletions. *Am J Hum Genet* 80:510–517, 2007.

42. Torres-Juan L, Rosell J, Moria M, et al. Mutations in TBX1 genocopy the 22q11.2 deletion and duplication syndromes: A new susceptibility factor for mental retardation. *Eur J Hum Genet* 15(6):658–663, 2007.

43. Kurahashi H, Nakayama T, Osug Y, et al. Dletion mapping of 22q11 in CATCH22 syndrome: Identification of a second critical region. *Am J Hum Genet* 58:1377–1381, 1996.

44. O'Donnell H, McKeown C, Gould, C, Morrow, B, Scamlbler P. Detection of an atypical 22q11 deletion that has no overlap with the DiGeorge syndrome critical region. *Am J Hum Genet* 60:1544–1548, 1997.

45. Amati F, Conti E, Novelli A, et al. Atypcial deletions suggest five 22q11.2 critical regions related to the DiGeorge/velo-cardio-facial syndrome. *Eur J Hum Genet* 7:903–909, 1999.

46. McQuade L, Christodoulou J, Budarf M, et al. Patient with a 22q11.2 deletion with no overlap of the minimal DiGeorge syndrome critical region (MDGCR). *Am J Med Genet* 86:27–33, 1999.

47. Shaikh TH, Kurahashi H, Saitta SC, et al. Chromosome 22-specific low copy repeats and the 22q11.2 deletion syndrome: Genomic organization and deletion endpoint analysis. *Hum Mol Genet* 9:489–501, 2000.

48. Garcia-Minaur S, Fantes J, Murray RS, et al. A novel atypical 22q11.2 distal deletion in father and son. *J Med Genet* 39:1–5, 2002.

49. McDonald-McGinn DM, Catania C, Saitta S, et al. Atypcial 22q11.2 deletions. *Proc Greenwood Genetic Center* 26:106–107, 2007.

50. Emanuel BS, Budard ML, Shaikh T, Driscoll D. Blocks of duplicated sequence define the endpoints of DGS/VCFS 22q11.2 deletions. *Am J Hum Genet* 63:A11, 1998.

51. Edelman L, Pandita RK, Morrow BE. Low-copy repeats mediate the common 3-Mb deletion in patients with velo-cardio-facial syndrome. *Am J Hum Genet* 64:1076–1086, 1999.

52. Baumer A, Riegel M, Schinzel A. Non-random asynchronous replication at 22q11.2 favours unequal meiotic crossovers leading to the human 22q11.2 deletion. *J Med Genet* 41(6):413–420, 2004.

53. Consevage MW, Seip JR, Belchis DA, Davis AT, Baylen BG, Rogan PK. Association of a mosaic chromosomal 22q11 deletion with hypoplastic left heart syndrome. *Am J Cardiol* 77:1023–1025, 1996.

54. Kasprzak L, Der Kaloustian VM, Elliott AM, Shevell M, Lejtenyi C, Eydoux P. Deletion of 22q11 in two brothers with different phenotype. *Am J Med Genet* 75:288–291, 1998.

55. Hatchwell E, Long F, Wilde J, Crolla J, Temple K. Molecular confirmation of germ line mosaicism for a submicroscopic deletion of chromosome 22q11. *Am J Med Genet* 78:103–106, 1998.

56. Sandrin-Garcia P, Macedo C, Martelli LR. Recurrent 22q11.2 deletion in a sibship suggestive of parental germline mosaicism in velocardiofacial syndrome. *Clin Genet* 61:380–383, 2002.

57. McDonald-McGinn DM, Driscoll DA, Zackai EH. Guidelines for the prenatal detection of the 22q11.2 deletion syndrome *Proc Greenwood Genetic Center* 26:155, 2007.

58. Cohen E, Chow EWC, Weksberg R, Bassett, AS. Phenotype of adults with the 22q deletion syndrome: A review. *Am J Med Genet* 86:359–365, 1999.

59. Tonnesen M, McDonald-McGinn DM, Valverde K, Zackai EH. Affected parents with a 22q11.2 deletion: The need for basic and ongoing educational health, and supportive counseling. *Am J Hum Genet* 69(4):223(A241), 2001.

60. Schinzel A. *Catalogue of Unbalanced Chromosome Aberrations in Man.* Berlin, New York: Walter de Gruyter, Inc., 2001, pp. 846–857.

61. Goldmuntz E, Clark BJ, Mitchell LE, et al. Frequency of 22q11 deletions in patients with conotruncal defects. *J Am Coll Cardiol* 32:492–498, 1998.

62. Marino B, Digilio MC, Toscano A. Anatomic Patterns of conotruncal defects associated with deletion 22q11. *Genet Med* 3(1)45–48, 2001.

63. Freeman SB, Taft LF, Dooley KJ, et al. Population-based study of congenital heart defects in Down syndrome. *Am J Med Genet* 80(3):213–217, 1998.

64. Ryan AK, Goodship JA, Wilson DI, et al. Spectrum of clinical features associated with interstitial chromosome 22q11 deletions: A European collaborative study. *J Med Genet* 34:798–804, 1997.

65. Fraser FC. The genetics of cleft lip and palate: Yet another look. In: Pratt RM, Christiansen RL (eds). *Current Research trends in prenatal craniofacial development.* North Holland, Amsterdam: Elsevier Publishers, 1980.

66. Driscoll D, Randall P, McDonald-McGinn, DM. Are 22q11.2 deletions a major cause of isolated cleft palate? Presented at: 52nd Annual Meeting of the American Cleft Palate-Craniofacial Association; 1995; Tampa, FL.

67. Wu H-Y, Rusnack SL, Bellah RD, et al. Genitourinary malformations in chromosome 22q11.2 deletion. *J Urol* 168:2564–2565, 2002.

68. Devriendt K, Swillen A, Fryns JP, Proesmans W, Gewillig M. Renal and urological tract malformations caused by a 22q11 deletion. *J Med Genet* 33:349, 1996.

69. Eicher PS, McDonald-McGinn DM, Fox CA, Driscoll DA, Emanuel BS, Zackai EH. Dysphagia in children with a 22q11.2 deletion: Unusual pattern found on modified barium swallow. *J Peds* 137(2):158–164, 2000.

70. Diglio MC, Giannotti A, Marino B, Guadagni AM, Orzalesi M, Dallapiccola B. Radial aplasia and chromosome 22q11 deletion. *J Med Genet* 34:942–944, 1997.

71. Ming JE, McDonald-McGinn DM, Megerian TE, et al. Skeletal anomalies in patients with deletions of 22q11. *Am J Med Genet* 72:210–215, 1997.

72. Devriendt K, de Smet L, de Boeck K, Fryns JP. DiGeorge syndrome and unilateral symbrachydactyly. *Genet Couns* 8:345–347, 1997.

73. Cormier-Daire V, Iserin L, Theophile D, et al. Upper limb malformations in DiGeorge syndrome. *Am J Med Geent* 56:39–41, 1995.

74. Bergoffen J, Punnett H, Campbell TJ, Ross AJ III, Ruchelli E, Zackai

EH . Diaphragmatic hernia in tetrasomy 12p mosaicism. *J Pediatr* 122(4):603–606, 1993.

75. Nickel RE, Magenis RE. Neural tube defects and deletions of 22q11. *Am J Med Genet* 66:25–27, 1996.

76. Gripp KW, McDonald-McGinn DM, Driscoll DA, Reed LA, Emanuel BS, Zackai EH. Nasal dimple as part of the 22q11.2 deletion syndrome. *Am J Med Genet* 69:290–292, 1997.

77. Swillen A, Devriendt K, Legius, E. Intelligence and psychological adjustment in velocardiofacial syndrome: A study of 37 children and adolescents with VCFS. *J Med Genet* 34:453–458, 1997.

78. Bassett AS, Hodgkinson K, Chow, EWC. 22q11 deletion syndrome in adults with schizophrenia. *Am J Med Genet* 81;328–337, 1998.

79. Murphy KC, Jones LA, Owen MJ. High rates of schizophrenia in adults with velo-cardio-facial syndrome. *Arch Gen Psychiatry* 56:940–945, 1999.

80. Beauchesne LM, Warnes CA, Connolly HM, et al. Prevalence and clinical manifestations of 22q11.2 microdeletion in adults with slected conotruncal anomalies. *J Am Coll Cardio* 45(4):595–598, 2005.

81. McDonald-McGinn DM, Minugh-Purvis N, Kirschner R, et al. The 22q11.2 deletion in African-American patients: An underdiagnosed population. *Am J Med Genet* 134(3):242–246, 2005.

82. Keenan GF, Sullivan KE, McDonald-McGinn DM, Zackai EH. Letter to the Editor. Arthritis associated with 22q11.2: More common than previously suspected. *Am J Med Genet* 71:488, 1997.

83. Sullivan KE, McDonald-McGinn DM, Driscoll DA, et al. JRA-like polyarthritis in chromosome 22q11.2 deletion syndrome (DiGeorge anomalad/velocardiofacial syndrome/conotruncal anomaly face syndrome). *Arthritis Rheum* 40:430–436, 1997.

84. Kawame H, Adachi M, Tachibana K, et al. Graves' disease in patients with 22q11.2 deletion. *J of Peds* 139(6):892–895, 2001.

85. Sullivan KE. DiGeorge syndrome/chromosome 22q11.2 deletion syndrome. *Curr Allergy Asthma Rep* 1(5):438–444, 2001. Review.

86. Sullivan KE. The clinical, immunological, and molecular spectrum of chromosome 22q11.2 deletion syndrome and DiGeorge syndrome. *Curr Opin Allergy Clin Immunol* 4(6):505–512, 2004.

87. Jawad AF, McDonald-Mcginn DM, Zackai E, Sullivan KE. Immunologic features of chromosome 22q11.2 deletion syndrome (DiGeorge syndrome/velocardiofacial syndrome). *J Pediatr* 139(5):715–723, 2001.

88. Junker AK, Driscoll DA. Humoral immunity in DiGeorge syndrome. *J Pediatr* 127(2):231–237, 1995.

89. Sullivan KE. Immunodeficiency in Velo-cardio-facial syndrome. In: Murphy KC, Scambler PJ (eds). *Velo-Cardio-Facial Syndrome A Model for Understanding Microdeletion Disorders* Cambridge, UK: Cambridge University Press, 2005, pp. 123–134.

90. Schubert MS, Moss RB. Selective polysaccharide antibody deficiency in familial DiGeorge syndrome. *Ann Allergy* 69(3):231–238, 1992.

91. Smith CA, Driscoll DA, Emanuel BS, McDonald-McGinn DM, Zackai EH, Sullivan KE. Increased prevalence of immunoglobulin A deficiency in patients with the chromosome 22q11.2 deletion syndrome (DiGeorge syndrome/velocardiofacial syndrome. *Clin Diagn Lab Immunol* 5(3):415–417, 1998.

92. Gennery AR, Barge D, O'Sullivan JJ, Flood TJ, Abinun M, Cant AJ. Antibody deficiency and autoimmunity in 22q11.2 deletion syndrome. *Arch Dis Child.* 86(6):422–425, 2002.

93. Pinchas-Hamiel O, Mandel M, Engelberg S, Passwell JH. Immune hemolytic anemia, thrombocytopenia and liver disease in a patient with DiGeorge syndrome Isr. *J Med Sci* 30(7):530, 1994.

94. DePiero AD, Lourie EM, Berman BW, Robin NH, Zinn AB, Hostoffer RW. Recurrent immune cytopenias in two patients with DiGeorge/velocardiofacial syndrome. *J Pediatr* 131(3):484–486, 1997.

95. Verloes A, Curry C, Jamar M, et al. Juvenile rheumatoid arthritis and del(22q11) syndrome: A non-random association *J Med Genet* 35(11):943–947, 1998.

96. Duke SG, McGuirt WF Jr, Jewett T, Fasano MB. Velocardiofacial syndrome: Incidence of immune cytopenias. *Arch Otolaryngol Head Neck Surg* 126(9):1141–1145, 2000.

97. Davies K, Stiehm ER, Woo P, Murray KJ. Juvenile idiopathic polyarticular arthritis and IgA deficiency in the 22q11 deletion syndrome. *J Rheumatol* 28(10):2326–2334, 2001.

98. Kawamura T, Nimura I, Hanafusa M, et al. DiGeorge syndrome with Graves' disease: A case report. *Endocr J* 47(1):91–95, 2000.

99. Matsouka R, Kimura M, Scambler, P. Molecular and clinical study of 183 patients with conotruncal anomaly face syndrome. *Hum Genet* 103:70–80, 1998.

100. Marino B, Mileto F, Digilio MC, Carotti A, DiDonato R. Congenital cardiovascular disease and velocardiofacial syndrome. In: Murphy KC, Scambler PJ (eds). *Velo-Cardio-Facial Syndrome A Model for Understanding Microdeletion Disorders*. Cambridge, UK: Cambridge University Press, 2005, pp. 47–82.

101. Finkelstein Y, Zohar Y, Nachmani A. The otolaryngologist and the patient with velocardiofacial syndrome Arch Otolaryngol. *Head and Neck Surg* 119:563–569, 1993.

102. Goldberg R, Motzkin B, Marion R, et al. Velo-cardio-facial syndrome: A review of 120 patients. *Am J Med Genet* 45:313–319, 1993.

103. Kirschner RE. Palatal anomalies and velopharyngeal dysfunction associated with velo-cardio-facial syndrome. In: Murphy KC, Scambler PJ (eds). *Velo-Cardio-Facial Syndrome A Model for Understanding Microdeletion Disorders, Vol 4*. Cambridge, UK: Cambridge University Press, 2005, pp. 83–105.

104. Mingarelli R, Digilio MC, Mari A. The search for hemizygosity at 22q11 in patients with isolated cleft palate. *J Craniofac Genet Dev Biol* 16:118–121, 1996.

105. Mitnick RJ, Bello JA, Golding-Kushner KJ, et al. The use of magnetic resonance angiography prior to pharyngeal flap surgery in patients with velocardiofacial syndrome. *Plast Reconstr Surg* 97:908–919, 1996.

106. Ross DA, Witzel MA, Armstrong DC, Thomson, HG. Is pharyngoplasty a risk in velocardiofacial syndrome? An assessment of medially displaced carotid arteries. *Plast Reconstr Surg* 98:1182–1190, 1996.

107. McDonald-McGinn DM, Gripp KW, Kirschner RE, et al. Craniosynostosis: Another feature of the 22q11.2 deletion syndrome. *Am J Med Genet* 136(4):358–362, 2005.

108. Weinzimer SA, McDonald-McGinn DM, Driscoll DA, Emanuel BS, Zackai EH. Growth hormone deficiency in patients with a 22q11.2 deletion: Expanding the phenotype. *Pediatr* 101:929–932, 1998.

109. Bassett AS, Chow EW, Husted J, et al. Clinical features of 78 adults with 22q11 deletion Syndrome. *Am J Med Genet* 1;138(4):307–313, 2005.

110. Sundaram UT, McDonald-McGinn DM, Huff D, et al. Primary amenorrhea and absent uterus in the 22q11.2 deletion syndrome. *Am J Med Genet A* 143(17):2016–2018, 2007.

111. Forbes BJ, Binenbaum G, Edmond JC, DeLarato N, McDonald-McGinn DM, Zachai EH. Ocular findings in the chromosome 22q11.2 deletion syndrome. *JAAPOS* 11(2):179–182, 2007.

112. Binenbaum G, Forbes B, Zackai EH, McDonald-McGinn DM. Scleracornea associated with the chromosome 22q11.2 deletion syndrome. *Am J Med Genet* 146(7):904–909, 2008.

113. Casteels I, Devriendt K. Unilateral Peters' anomaly in a patient with DiGeorge syndrome. *J Pediatr Ophthalmol Strabismus* 42(5):311–313, 2005.

114. Bloch N. The different types of sclerocornea, their hereditary modes and concomitant congenital malformations. *J Genet Hum* 14(2):133–172, 1965.

115. Tahvanainen E, Forsius H, Damsten M, et al. Linkage disequilibrium mapping of the cornea plana congenita gene CNA2. *Genomics* 30(3):409–414, 1995.

116. Budarf ML, Konkle BA, Ludlow LB, et al. Identification of a patient with Bernard-Soulier syndrome and a deletion in the DiGeorge/Velocardio-facial chromosomal region in 22q11. *Hum Mol Genet* 4:763–766, 1995.

117. Ford LC, Sulprizio SL, Rasgon BM. Otolaryngological manifestations of velocardiofacial syndrome: A retrospective review of 35 patients. *Laryngoscope* 110(3 Pt 1):362–367, 2000.

118. Ricchetti ET, States L, Hosalkar HS, et al. Radiographic study of the upper cervical spine in the 22q11.2 deletion syndrome. *J Bone Joint Surg Am* 6-A(8):1751–1760, 2004.

119. Moss EM, Batshaw ML, Solot CB, et al. Psychoeducational profile of the 22q11.2 microdeletion: A complex pattern. *J Peds* 134:193–198, 1999.

120. Kao A, Mariani J, McDonald-McGinn DM, et al. Increased prevalence of unprovoked seizures in patients with a 22q11.2 deletion. *Am J Med Genet A* 129(1):29–34, 2004.

121. Cayler GG. Cardiofacial syndrome. Congenital heart disease and facial weakness, a hitherto unrecognized association. *Arch Dis Child* 44(233):69–75, 1969.

122. Silengo MC, Bell GL, Biagioli M, et al. Asymmetric crying facies with microcephaly and mental retardation. An autosomal dominant syndrome with variable expressivity. *Clin Genet* (6):481–484, 1986.

123. Sanklecha M, Kher A, Bharucha BA. Asymmetric crying facies: The cardiofacial syndrome. *J Postgrad Med* 38(3):147–148, 1992.

124. Lynch DR, McDonald-McGinn D, Zackai EH, et al. Cerebellar atrophy in a patient with velocardiofacial syndrome. *J Med Genet* 32:561–563, 1995.

125. Bingham P, Zimmerman RA, McDonald-McGinn DM, Driscoll DA, Emanuel BS, Zackai EH. Enlarged Sylvian fissures in infants with interstitial deletion of chromosome 22q11. *Am J Med Genet Neuropsych Genet* 74:538–543, 1997.

126. Robin NH, Taylor CG, McDonald-McGinn DM, et al. Polymicrogyria and deletion 22q11.2 syndrome: Window to the etiology of a common cortical malformation. *Am J Med Genet* 140(22):2416–2425, 2006.

127. Barnea-Goraly N, Menon V, Krasnow B, Ko A, Reiss A, Eliez S. Investigation of white matter structure in velocardiofacial syndrome: A diffusion tensor imaging study. *Am J Psychiatry* 160(10):1863–1869, 2003.

128. Bearden CE, van Erp TG, Monterosso JR, et al. Regional brain abnormalities in 22q11.2 deletion syndrome: Association with cognitive abilities and behavioral symptoms. *Neurocase* 10(3):198–206, 2004.

129. Bish JP, Nguyen V, Ding L, Ferrante S, Simon TJ. Thalamic reductions in children with chromosome 22q11.2 deletion syndrome. *Neuroreport* 15(9):1413–1415, 2004.

130. Kates WR, Burnette CP, Bessette BA, et al. Frontal and caudate alterations in velocardiofacial syndrome (deletion at chromosome 22q11.2). *J Child Neurol* 19(5):337–342, 2004.

131. Cappa M, Borrelli P, Marini R, Neri G. The Opitz syndrome: A new designation for the clinically indistinguishable BBB and G syndromes. *Am J Med Genet* 28(2):303–309, 1987.

132. Guion-Almeida ML, Richieri-Costa A. CNS midline anomalies in the Opitz G/BBB syndrome: Report on 12 Brazilian patients. *Am J Med Genet* 43(6):918–928, 1992.

133. MacDonald MR, Schaefer GB, Olney AH, Tamayo M, Frías JL. Brain magnetic resonance imaging findings in the Opitz G/BBB syndrome: Extension of the spectrum of midline brain anomalies. *Am J Med Genet* 46(6):706–711, 1993.

134. Huff DS, McDonald-McGinn DM, Zackai EH. Autopsy findings in thirteen patients with a 22q11.2 deletion. *Proc Greenwood Genetic Center* 21, 2002.

135. Patrone PM, Chatten J, Weinberg P. Neuroblastoma and DiGeorge anomaly. *Pediatr Pathol* 10(3):425–430, 1990.

136. Scattone A, Caruso G, Marzullo A, et al. Neoplastic disease and deletion 22q11.2: A multicentric study and report of two cases. *Pediatr Pathol Mol Med* 4:323–341, 2003.

137. McDonald-McGinn DM, Reilly A, Wallgren-Pettersson C, et al. Malignancy in chromosome 22q11.2 deletion syndrome (DiGeorge syndrome/velocardiofacial syndrome). *Am J Med Genet A* 140(8):906–909, 2006.

138. Gerdes M, Solot C, Wang PP, et al. Cognitive and behavioral profile of preschool children with chromosome 22q11.2 microdeletion. *Am J Med Genet* 85(2):127–133, 1999.

139. Solot CB, Gerdes M, Kirschner RE, et al. Communication issues in 22q11.2 deletion syndrome: Children at risk. *Genet Med* 3(1):67–71, 2001.

140. DeSmedt B, Swillen A, Ghesquiere P, et al. Pre-academic and early academic achievement in children with velocardiofacial syndrome (del22q11.2) of borderline or normal intelligence. *Genet Coun* 14:15–29, 2003.

141. Campbell LE, Swillen A. The cognitive spectrum in velo-cardio-facial syndrome. In: Murphy KC, Scambler PJ (eds). *Velo-Cardio-Facial Syndrom: A Model for Understanding Microdeletion Disorders.* Cambridge, UK: Cambridge University Press, 2005, pp. 147–165.

142. Fine S, Weissman A, Gerdes M, et al. Autism spectrum disorders and symptoms in children with molecularly confirmed 22q11.2. *J Autism and Developmental Disabilities* 35(4):461–470, 2005.

143. Wang P, Solot C, Gerdes M, et al. Developmental presentation of 22q11.2 deletion. *J Dev Behav Pediatr* 19:342–345, 1998.

144. Swillen A, Devriendt K, Legius E. The behavioral phenotype in velocardiofacial syndrome (VCFS): From infancy to adolescence. *Genet Couns* 10:79–88, 1999.

145. Wang PP, Woodin MF, Kreps-Falk R, Moss EM. Research on behavioral phenotypes: Velocardiofacial syndrome (deletion 22q11.2). *Dev Med Child Neurol* 42(6):422–427, 2000.

146. Bearden CE, Woodin MF, Wang PP, et al. The neurocognitive phenotype of the 22q11.2 deletion syndrome: Selective deficit in visual-spatial memory *J Clin Exp Neuropsychol* 23(4):447–464, 2001.

147. Woodin M, Wang PP, Aleman D, McDonald-McGinn D, Zackai E, Moss E. Neuropsychological profile of children and adolescents with the 22q11.2 microdeletion. *Genet Med* 3(1):34–39, 2001.

148. Gerdes M, Solot C, Wang PP, McDonald-McGinn DM, Zackai EH. Taking advantage of early diagnosis: Preschool children with the 22q11.2 deletion. *Genet Med* 3(1):40–44, 2001.

149. Golding-Kushner KJ, Weller G, Shprintzen RJ. Velo-cardio-facial syndrome: Language and psychological profiles. *J Craniofac Genet Dev Biol* 5(3):259–266, 1985.

150. Scherer NJ, D'Antonio LL, Kalbfleisch JH. Early speech and language development in children with velocardiofacial syndrome. *Am J Med Genet* 15;88(6):714–723, 1999.

151. Solot CB, Knightly C, Handler S, et al. Communication disorders in the 22q11.2 deletion microdeletion syndrome. *J Commun Dis* 33:187–204, 2000.

152. D'Antonio LL, Scherer NJ, Miller LL, Kalbfleisch JH, Bartley JA. Analysis of speech characteristics in children with velocardiofacial syndrome (VCFS) and children with phenotypic overlap without VCFS. *Cleft Palate Craniofac J* 38(5):455–467, 2001.

153. Persson C. Speech and language in patients with an isolated cleft palate and/or 22q11 deletion syndrome. The Sahlgrenska Academy at Goteborg University, Sweden, 2004.

154. Shprintzen RJ. Historical Overview. In: Murphy KC, Scambler PJ (eds). *Velo-Cardio-Facial Syndrome A Model for Understanding Microdeletion Disorders.* Cambridge, UK: Cambridge University Press, 2005, pp. 1–18.

155. Golding-Kushner. Speech and language disorders in velo-cardio-facial syndrome. In: Murphy KC, Scambler PJ (eds). *Velo-Cardio-Facial Syndrome A Model for Understanding Microdeletion Disorders.* Cambridge, UK: Cambridge University Press, 2005, pp. 181–199.

156. Moss E, Wang PP, McDonald-McGinn DM, et al. Characteristic cognitive profile in patients with a 22q11.2 deletion—verbal IQ exceeds nonverbal IQ. *Am J Hum Genet* 57:SS 91, 1995.

157. Niklasson L, Rasmussen P, Oskarsdóttir S, Gillberg C. Neuropsychiatric disorders in the 22q11 deletion syndrome. 1: *Genet Med* 3(1):79–84, 2001.

158. Vorstman JA, Morcus ME, Duijff SN, et al. The 22q11.2 deletion in children: High rate of autistic disorders and early onset of psychotic symptoms. *J Am Acad Child Adolesc Psychiatry* 45(9):1104–1113, 2006.

159. Eliez S, Palacio-Espasa F, Spira A, et al. Young children with Velo-Cardio-Facial syndrome (CATCH-22). Psychological and language phenotypes. *Eur Child Adolesc Psychiatry* 9(2):109–114, 2000.

160. Shprintzen RJ, Goldberg R, Golding-Kushner KJ, Marion R. Late-onset pyschosis in the velo-cardio-facial syndrome. *Am J Med Genet* 42(1):141–142, 1992.

161. Chow EW, Bassett AS, Weksberg R. Velo-cardio-facial syndrome and psychotic disorders: Implications for psychiatric genetics. *Am J Med Genet* 54(2):107–112, 1994.

162. Popolos DF, Faedda GL, Veit S, et al. Bipolar spectrum disorders in patients diagnosed with velo-cardio-facial syndrome: Does a hemizygous deletion of chromosome 22q result in bipolar affective disorder? *Am J Psychiatry* 153:1541–1547, 1996.

163. Yan W, Jacobsen LK, Krasnewich DM, et al. Chromosome 22q11.2 interstitial deletions among childhood-onset schizophrenics and "multidimensionally impaired". *Am J Med Genet* 7;81(1):41–43, 1998.

164. Bassett AS, Chow EWC, AbdeMalik P, et al. The schizophrenia phenotype in 22q11 deletion syndrome. *Am J Psychiatry* 160:1580–1586, 2003.

165. Baker K, Baldeweg T, Sivagnanasundaram S, Scambler P, Skuse D. COMT Val108/158 Met modifies mismatch negativity and cognitive function in 22q11 deletion syndrome. *Biol Psychiatry* 58(1):23–31, 2005.

166. Oskarsdóttir S, Belfrage M, Sandstedt E, Viggedal G, Uvebrant P. Disabilities and cognition in children and adolescents with 22q11 deletion syndrome. *Dev Med Child Neurol* 47(3):177–184, 2005.

167. Stevens AF, Murphy KC. Behavioral and psychiatric disorder in velo-cardio-facial syndrome. In: Murphy KC, Scambler PJ (eds). *Velo-Cardio-Facial Syndrome A Model for Understanding Microdeletion Disorders.* Cambridge, UK: Cambridge University Press, 2005, pp. 135–146.

Nursing and Primary Care

Nursing Care of the Patient with Cleft Lip and Palate

Patricia Chibbaro, RN, MS, CPNP • Joan Barzilai, RN, MS • Mary Breen, RN, MS

THE ROLE OF NURSING IN CLEFT CARE

Introduction

The family of an infant with a cleft has many opportunities to interact with professional nurses. This relationship often begins during a prenatal consultation, at which time the parents meet with the nurse specialist on a cleft lip and palate team. They will encounter nurses in the obstetric office, the birth hospital delivery room, postpartum unit, newborn nursery, and the neonatal intensive care unit (NICU).

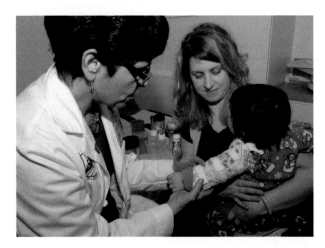

Figure 10–1. Nurse specialist with mother and infant during preoperative teaching session. (*Photo credit: Mary Spano.*)

Once discharged, nurses and nurse practitioners will provide care to the infant and family in the pediatric outpatient clinic or private pediatric office. When surgical procedures are scheduled, nurses in the operating and recovery rooms, as well as on the inpatient pediatric unit, will play important roles in delivering specialized surgical and postoperative care. The nurse specialist on the cleft lip and palate team is available as the consistent resource to the family to help them navigate all phases of their child's treatment. It is common for parents to refer to this nurse as "the glue that helps us to hold everything together" (Fig. 10–1). This chapter provides specific, practical information for all nurses who care for infants and children with clefts and their families.

The Role of the Nurse Specialist on the Cleft Lip and Palate Team

The nurse on the cleft team is often the first contact for the family of a child with a cleft lip and/or palate. By virtue of her specialized nursing education, communication skills, and frequent role as the team coordinator and case manager, a nurse is often the cleft team member with the most comprehensive knowledge of the strengths and needs of families.[1] There is often an immediate emotional connection by the parents, who look to this nurse as the consistent liaison between their child and the entire medical and surgical team. She is the familiar face, the "go to" person who will help them through the often confusing maze that is the hospital and medical system. The nurse on the cleft team will follow the child from birth until the completion of treatment, providing ongoing, comprehensive education, guidance, and emotional support to the patient and the family, as well to all of the nurses and other health care specialists who are involved in the child's care.

In addition, the cleft team nurse is often an advanced practice nurse (clinical nurse specialist and/or pediatric nurse practitioner). The postbaccalaureate curriculum affords her the specific technical knowledge and skills needed to care for the most complicated pediatric patients in both ambulatory and inpatient settings. Advanced education enhances her

Table 10–1.

Role/Responsibilities of Cleft Lip and Palate Nurse Specialist

- Cleft team member
- Cleft team patient care coordinator
- Prenatal nursing counselor
- Consultant to birth hospital
- Feeding instruction—parents, birth hospital nursing staff, caregivers
- Comprehensive case management—patient and family
- Liaison to patient, family, hospital staff and community
- Pre- and postoperative teaching
- Presurgical physical assessment
- Education and support throughout nasoalveolar molding therapy (NAM)
- Postoperative inpatient and outpatient management
- Resource and inservice educator to pediatric nurses and housestaff
- Community outreach and education

ability to provide comprehensive case management, ongoing advocacy, individualized education, and guidance to children with cleft lip and/or palate and their families. She also has additional expertise in the role of staff and outreach educator, resource and consultant/liaison to community providers (Table 10–1).

COMPREHENSIVE NURSING MANAGEMENT

Prenatal Consultation

As a result of the advancements in ultrasound imaging, parents can receive a prenatal cleft diagnosis at as early as 18 weeks gestation.[2] Once a referral to a cleft treatment team has been made, the cleft team nurse specialist may be the initial contact for a couple who may have been informed about their child's diagnosis only a few hours prior to their call. They are often understandably emotional, frequently distraught, and in a state of crisis.

According to Johnson and Sandy,[3] "the wisdom of informing parents of a prenatal cleft diagnosis has been debated in the literature. There are several potential advantages, including planned neonatal care and preparation for feeding, thereby reducing perinatal morbidity." Anecdotal parent reports suggest that prior information gives the family an opportunity to do research about clefts and to identify a treatment team prior to the birth of the baby. Most agree that better preparation results in a more positive delivery and newborn experience. However, many couples relate that the remainder of the pregnancy is more difficult because of the increased worry about the baby, including uncertainty about the severity of the cleft and other potential medical problems.

Table 10–2.

Prenatal Nursing Consultation

- Obtain pregnancy history, delivery plans, and information about family structure and resources
- Clarify information from prenatal meetings with genetics counselor, surgeon and other cleft team members
- Clarify information that parents have read on Internet
- Discuss and support parental feelings about the diagnosis
- Review pre- and postoperative medical and family photographs of cleft-affected infants
- Discuss and demonstrate feeding options and provide samples of bottles and ordering information
- Offer advice on how to explain the diagnosis to family, friends and siblings
- Network to other parents of cleft-affected babies
- Offer nursing guidance in preparation for presurgical nasoalveolar molding therapy (NAM)
- Briefly explain expected hospital and postoperative care following initial cleft lip and palate surgeries
- Refer to the Cleft Palate Foundation—Cleftline, Web site, and feeding video
- Provide team literature and Web site information
- Encourage parents to communicate with birth hospital staff before delivery
- Provide cleft team contact information for family and hospital staff to call after birth of infant

Adapted from Breen ML, Chibbaro PD, Hopper, GM. Nursing care, feeding and nutrition in the first year. In Moller K, Glaze L (eds). Cleft Palate: Interdisciplinary Issues and Treatment. For Clinicians by Clinicians. Austin, TX: Pro-ED, in press.

Protocols for prenatal consultation vary amongst teams. The visit may involve individual meetings with one or several members of the cleft team. Each has specific areas of expertise, but it is common for their information to overlap. The content of the nurse specialist interaction is summarized in Table 10–2. As information is presented, parents may become extremely emotional and confused, often remembering little of what has been said. The nurse can be instrumental in helping parents to deal with their initial reaction to the news of the cleft by providing empathetic reassurance and accurate, nonjudgmental information. An appropriate first response might include: "I can imagine how worried and overwhelmed you must be right now. Let me try to help you to understand what you have been told about the baby's cleft and talk to you about what this all means." Two other important nursing objectives are to attempt to reassure the parents that they did nothing to cause the cleft and particularly to support a parent who may feel guilty and responsible for the infant's cleft.

This visit also provides an ideal opportunity for the nurse to assist the parents to express their concerns about the baby. Sometimes it will be necessary to state what the parents may be thinking but are afraid to say. For example, "Will the baby have other medical problems?", "How will I be able to feed her?", or "Will she be able to have a normal life?" Allowing parents to verbalize their fears can be very helpful for them and will often facilitate their ability to discuss the baby's diagnosis and management more openly with each other, their children, family members, and friends. The nurse should also make the names of the team social worker and psychologist available to the family in order to assist them in adjusting to this new knowledge and to help them deal with the experience.[4,5]

The nurse specialist can provide the phone numbers and email addresses of other families for networking. Team-specific literature, Web site information, and business cards are provided. Parents can be referred to authorized parent support Web sites (e.g., About Face, Cleft Advocate), as well as to the Cleftline (1-800-24-CLEFT) and Web site (www.cleftline.org) of the Cleft Palate Foundation. The prenatal consultation is also a good time to clarify with the parents any information about cleft lip and palate that they may have already obtained from other Internet sources, explaining to them that many sites do not always provide accurate information.

Pre- and postoperative ("before and after") photographs of children with a range of clefts treated at a particular center can be offered by the nurse for review with the parents. To decrease the shock effect that some couples may feel, it may be helpful to show the photos in the opposite order (i.e., start with the "after" photos and then flip back to the "before" photos). This can assist in providing them with a sense of perspective and a realistic idea of what can be accomplished, both surgically and orthodontically.[6] In addition, showing these medical pictures, as well as family photographs of the same infants, can serve to provide the parents with a sense of hope that they can have a healthy, beautiful child, with the potential to lead a normal life, despite some definite challenges.[7]

During the prenatal consultation, the nurse specialist should briefly explain their team's protocol for hospital and postoperative care following the initial cleft lip and palate repairs. Many parents have read Internet accounts of other parents' hospital experiences with their infants and are often quiet overwhelmed. The nurse specialist can help parents to interpret and clarify any misinformation. When the parents complete their prenatal consultation, the nurse (who may also function as the cleft team coordinator) can be the point of contact for them in case they have any further questions or concerns. She is often one of the first people to be contacted following the birth of their baby.

Nursing Care During Labor and Delivery

The birth of an infant is universally recognized as being one of the happiest memories in the life of a couple. In the case of a newborn with a cleft lip and palate, the nursing staff at the birth hospital plays a key role in promoting a positive birth experience. Parents who are aware of the diagnosis prenatally should be encouraged to contact the nursery staff prior to the date of delivery to inform them that their baby will be born with a cleft. They can also enlist the assistance of their obstetrician and pediatrician in preparing the medical team.

If a couple has received a prenatal cleft diagnosis, they may be very anxious during the labor process. As a part of their prenatal consultation, they were likely told that there is a chance of the baby being born with additional medical problems, possibly some type of syndrome. They know that the complete diagnosis, including the exact extent of the cleft lip and palate, can only be determined after their child is delivered and assessed by the medical team. The labor room nurse is in a position to provide tremendous emotional support, to be sensitive to their fears, and to reassure them that the entire staff is prepared to assist them in caring for their baby. This nurse can also be a liaison to the delivery room staff, alerting them in advance to the baby's cleft diagnosis and to other medical problems that may be associated with the cleft.

For parents who have not received a prenatal cleft diagnosis, the birth experience can be much more stressful. There are still many hospitals in which the staff has little or no knowledge about newborn cleft care. Parents can often remember every detail of their child's birth. It is not uncommon for the neonate to be "whisked away" after the delivery, before parents are permitted to see or hold their infant. Anecdotes include observations of nurses and doctors "who gasped or winced" at the sight of the baby and of absolute silence following the delivery. Irrespective of whether or not the cleft is diagnosed prenatally, all parents need tremendous emotional support and empathy during this time. The delivery can often be a very scary, stressful, or sad experience. Nurses in the delivery room can serve as a role model for parents and the entire medical team in terms of the reaction and response to the infant, resulting in a more positive event and a happier memory.

As long as there are no emergent medical concerns, the infant should be treated as a typical newborn, with congratulations expressed to the parents on the birth of their baby. A complete assessment can be postponed until after the parents have seen and held their infant. The parents will interpret silence or whispering in the room as evidence that something is seriously wrong with their baby. If the baby is otherwise healthy, the medical staff explains that the infant has been born with a common, correctable condition. The anatomy of the cleft can then be described in a clear and understandable manner. Parents who did not have prenatal diagnosis or who did not meet with a team prenatally will need to be reassured that there are teams who specialize in caring for infants with clefts. This information may need to be repeated frequently, as parents are often emotionally overwhelmed in the delivery room.

Parents who have never seen a child with a cleft may be afraid to look at or touch their baby. They will be sensitive to the way in which they observe how nurses and other staff react to their baby. The nurse is invaluable as a role model in helping them to connect with their child and should acknowledge the

infant as a baby, not as a "cleft." As parents watch the nurse smiling at their baby, stroking her cheeks, commenting about "her big, beautiful eyes and how she turns to their voice," they are being supported in beginning their bonding process. The nurse can then encourage them to hold, kiss, and speak to their baby. They need to know that is normal to be anxious, sad, and scared and that it is acceptable to cry.[8–10] Parents will appreciate and remember the nurse who sat with them in the delivery room and who supported them in both their grief and their joy.

If the infant does have an unstable airway or other immediate medical problems at the time of delivery, as is sometimes seen in a premature infant, an infant with a cardiac anomaly, or one with Pierre Robin sequence, the parents still need to see their infant and be told about the diagnosis before the baby is transferred to the NICU. It is very traumatic and frightening for parents to have their baby quickly removed from the delivery room, especially if they are not permitted to see their infant. They should be reunited with the baby in the NICU as quickly as possible. Often, because the mother needs more time to rest and recover from the birth, the father will be the first to see the baby. The nursing staff in the NICU must be very sensitive to this situation, providing additional emotional support as needed.

Newborn Nursery/NICU Nursing Care

Unless there is significant prematurity, a cardiac or neurologic abnormality, or airway instability, an infant with a cleft lip and palate need not automatically be placed in an NICU. Some hospitals choose to monitor these babies in the NICU because many of the nurses with expertise in specialized feeding techniques are assigned to this type of unit. If the infant is placed in the NICU solely for feeding support, then it is important for the parents, along with the NICU nurses, to advocate for the baby in order to minimize "overtreating." Babies with clefts, even if they are wide complete unilateral or bilateral clefts, are usually able to tolerate oral feedings. They do not require the placement of intravenous lines. The immediate use of orogastric (OG), nasogastric (NG), or gastrostomy(G) tubes for feeding (prior to attempting oral feeds with cleft palate feeders) are examples of overtreatment. This type of intervention may actually cause the infant to become very orally defensive, making bottle feeding very difficult, even despite the use of proper equipment and feeding techniques (refer to feeding section later in this chapter). Parents should know that it is acceptable for them to question the medical team regarding the rationale for their baby's treatment. If they have already identified with a cleft team, they should share their contact information with the doctors and nurses and ask that they consult with them for advice.

An otherwise healthy infant with a cleft can be transferred directly from the delivery room to the newborn nursery. The nurses caring for the baby can be instructed on feeding methods, either by NICU nurses with cleft feeding experience or by a feeding specialist or cleft palate nurse clinician at the hospital. If this type of support is not available to them onsite, they can contact the Cleft Palate Foundation (www.cleftline.org; 1-800-24-CLEFT). They will be referred to a cleft team specialist who can coach them through this feeding process by phone. In the case of an infant whose parents had prenatal consultation with a cleft team, the nurse can contact the nurse specialist on that team for advice and support. These parents may also already know how to feed their baby and might themselves be able to instruct the newborn nursing staff in the proper techniques.

Postpartum Nursing Care

Even with the benefit of prenatal cleft diagnosis, the postpartum experience can be very isolating for parents, who are likely to be the only couple on the unit with a facially different baby.[11] If sharing a room with another couple, the "perfect" baby is just on the other side of the curtain. For parents who did not know about the cleft diagnosis until their baby was born, this can be a very difficult time. It is common for grandparents or friends to avoid coming to the hospital to visit due to their fear of the unknown and to anxiety about how they will react to the baby's appearance.

The postpartum nurse has many significant roles and responsibilities in working with these families (Table 10–3). It is very important to carefully monitor both the physical and emotional recovery of the mother. Concern over the well-being of the baby often results in her paying little attention to her own needs, particularly those of eating and sleeping. The social worker can be contacted to assess the coping state of both parents and to help to explain the emotions that they might be experiencing. They can be offered assistance regarding how to prepare siblings, in age appropriate terms, for the infant's appearance and how to best explain the diagnosis and treatment to them. Special attention and support should be directed to a cleft-affected parent, who often feels extremely guilty, blaming themselves for "causing the cleft." The baby's birth may also reactivate that parents' unpleasant childhood memories, which can cause distress and possibly lead to depression.

A very important role of nursing is to ensure that the parents have received the basic, yet accurate, medical and nursing information about their baby's cleft during the first 24 hours after delivery. This is especially critical for parents who did not obtain a prenatal cleft diagnosis. Studies have shown[12] that a significant percentage of parents felt that they were not given this information. Parents need to know that there are different treatment options and that the first surgery may not occur until the baby is at least 3 months of age.

Prior to hospital discharge, the nurse must be confident that the parents can feed the infant independently and effectively (see feeding section below). They may need assistance in obtaining the appropriate feeding supplies (bottles, nipples, breast pump). The nurse can facilitate the transition from hospital to home by providing a list of referral numbers for home health care, a lactation specialist, a repeat hearing screening (if the infant failed the newborn screen), an initial pediatric appointment, and contacts on the cleft palate team.

Table 10–3.

Checklist for Use with Parents of Newborn with Cleft Lip and Palate

- Discuss proper cleft lip and palate medical terminology
- Explain that cleft is not their fault and the child is not in pain
- Instruct parents in cleft feeding techniques
- Allow parents to grieve, provide emotional support
- Refer to social worker for assessment of coping, assistance with dealing with reactions of siblings, other family members and the public
- Be sensitive to their feelings of isolation
- Discuss troubleshooting if feeding problems arise at home
- Make contact with cleft team nurse/coordinator if cleft diagnosed prenatally, or if parents have chosen a team
- Consult with onsite cleft team nurse/coordinator, if applicable
- Refer to lactation consultant, if mother desires
- Observe several parent demonstrations of ability to feed (include father if patient not able to exclusively feed at the breast)
- Arrange for baseline hearing test and recommend repeat as outpatient if test failed
- Assist with arrangements for bottles, breast pump, home nursing care
- Instruct parents in routine infant care
- Coordinate referral to cleft palate team for initial postnatal consult (ideally within 2 weeks of hospital discharge)
- Provide written and Web site information from the Cleft Palate Foundation
- Refer to parent support groups (Ameriface, Cleft Advocate, About Face International)
- Recommend pediatric office or cleft team visit at 1 week postdischarge for weight check
- Refer for pediatric primary care visit at 2 weeks postdischarge

Adapted from Young, 2001, Breen ML, Chibbaro PD, Hopper, GM. Nursing care, feeding and nutrition in the first year. In Moller K, Glaze L (eds). Cleft Palate: Interdisciplinary Issues and Treatment. For Clinicians by Clinicians. Austin, TX: Pro-ED, in press.

The baby's birth and discharge weights should be written on the discharge document.

First Contact by Cleft Team Nurse Specialist with Nursery

If the referral of an infant with a cleft is made to a team by the doctors at the birth hospital, the cleft team nurse should call the nursery to begin the assessment and to offer advice and support. The nursery nurses have observed the parents directly and can help to identify family dynamics, structure, and stressors. In addition, several of them have likely been involved in feeding the infant and can provide insight into the infant's feeding behavior and feeding history. Other information from the nursery may indicate that the infant has other associated defects.

The nursery and pediatric staff are often unfamiliar with clefts and feeding techniques, as infants with cleft conditions are rarely seen in most nurseries. In small hospitals, there may be no specialty cleft bottles, or the personnel may be insufficiently experienced in the use of these bottles. This is an important opportunity for the cleft team nurse to educate and support the nursery staff in order to optimize the initial feeding experience for the infant and family and to facilitate an early hospital discharge.

It is frequently reported by parents and nursing staff that infants will often have thick secretions in the first 48 hours of life. The infant may suddenly awaken gagging or dusky and require suctioning. Often, the infant is subsequently moved from the mother's room to the nursery for observation and oxygen administration, causing parental anxiety and fear of similar events after discharge. Another symptom that may present in the first days of life is nasal regurgitation during feeding and after burping. Some infants ignore nasal drainage of formula, and continue to eat. Others will demonstrate distress with head rearing and a facial appearance of anxiety. The baby's distress can often be relieved by sitting the infant forward to allow the formula in the front of the mouth and nose to drain away from the pharynx. The baby will reflexively swallow to clear the fluids that are in the esophagus.[13] Bulb suction of the fluids is sometimes helpful, but parents need careful instruction on positioning, as they often lay the infant back to see what to suction, thereby returning the fluids to the posterior pharynx. It is helpful for the parents and the nursery staff to receive instruction, guidance, and reassurance from the cleft team nurse as the baby learns to manage and resolve these early issues.

The first contact by the cleft team nurse specialist with the parent of the infant is an important one. It may either be in person or over the telephone and can take place while the mother and/or baby are still in the birth hospital or at home following discharge. There are many goals for this first contact. The nurse specialist needs to become acquainted with the parent while exchanging information. It is helpful to converse with the mother or father for a time before any detailed information is provided. After congratulating parents on the baby's birth, they can be asked about the baby's weight, length, the type of cleft, and whether the cleft was diagnosed prenatally. To help the parents to relax a bit more, they can be asked about who the baby looks like and about the color of the baby's eyes and hair. It can be helpful to know whether the mother is married, living with the father, or a single parent and whether there are any other children in the household. Other initial questions may include: Which parent carries health insurance for the family? Have they any babysitting arrangements? Did having a baby with a cleft palate change the arrangements?

Once the parents begin to relax, the topic of feeding can be discussed. The parent should describe the infant's feeding history since birth, including the type of bottle being used, and whether breastfeeding has been attempted. The feeding schedule, including the number of feedings per day, the number of ounces tolerated, and the duration of each feeding are important to review. It is also important to inquire about any of the parents' feeding concerns. A visit is arranged shortly thereafter for an initial face-to-face feeding assessment, so long as the mother's or infant's physical condition does not preclude travel. Other team specialists may also be scheduled to meet with the family at that time.

Regardless of whether or not the infant and family is seen in the first week after hospital discharge, the nurse specialist should make a follow-up phone call to check on the infants' feeding progress and weight gain.

When the infant is first seen by the nurse specialist, the assessment should include the following:

- Cleft type
- Tone and state
- General appearance and associated defects
- Airway
- Family structure, experience, support
- Family response to infant

At the first encounter, the nurse should observe the infant's muscle tone, cleft shape and condition, and parents' response to the infant. For infants with an isolated cleft palate, breathing should be observed for sounds of obstruction, and the neck and chest for substernal, suprasternal, and intercostal retractions. If any of these findings are present, parents should be carefully interviewed for their observations of the infant as well as the behavior seen during feeding, and admission to the hospital for evaluation and monitoring may be needed. A history should be taken for the presence of other birth defects identified in the newborn nursery or since discharge. Family structure and support should be discussed, as well as identification of the primary caretaker. Experience with infant care, breastfeeding, and other children with health or learning problems should be explored.

Primary Pediatric Nursing Care

The infant with a cleft lip and palate should have a weight check at approximately one week after discharge from the nursery. This can be done either by the cleft palate team nurse or by a primary care provider. The first scheduled well-child visit should occur at age 2 weeks. At that point, the baby should have regained birth weight. The goal for weight gain is approximately 5–7 oz/wk. If weight gain is not satisfactory, the pediatric nurse practitioner or pediatrician should consult with the nurse specialist or other feeding specialist on the cleft palate team to discuss strategies to promote more efficient feeding and weight gain.

It is the protocol of most cleft teams to recommend weekly weight checks until adequate weight gain is established. In order to ensure accuracy, the same scale should be used for each weight check. This will not only help to closely monitor the baby's progress with weight gain, but it will also serve to help allay any parental anxiety. Parents should be discouraged from purchasing their own scales, as they might weigh their infant daily, or even multiple times per day, thereby increasing their stress.

If the baby is otherwise healthy, parents can proceed with the routine immunization schedule. It is not necessary to interrupt immunizations prior to surgery, but the administration schedule can be adjusted to prevent an ill-timed postimmunization fever from interfering with the surgical date. The newborn hearing screen (if not performed in the nursery or if failed) should also be scheduled.

FEEDING THE CLEFT–AFFECTED INFANT

Almost as soon as the discovery of the cleft condition occurs, fear and concern about feeding and nurturing the infant may arise. How will my baby eat? Won't food go into the nose and hurt her? Won't she choke when she eats? Will she be able to eat "normal" foods when she is older? Intense emotions surrounding the infant's future will often coalesce into anxiety about feeding.

The mother's ability to give food successfully and the infant's willingness to take food from the mother are central to the development of the early maternal–child relationship.[14] A mother may feel like a failure or may feel rejected by her baby if she is unable to feed the infant, especially if the nurses have been successful, but she has not. Therefore, the sooner the parents learn the skills needed to successfully feed their infant with a cleft, the better. Most parents want to jump right in, but some are tentative and afraid to try to feed their newborn. Within each family, one of the parents often assumes most of the feeding responsibility until the other becomes more comfortable with the technique.

Feeding an infant with a cleft can be relatively straightforward with the proper feeding supplies and instruction, but some infants with clefts will have more complicated feeding problems and will need early and ongoing therapy by a feeding specialist.[15] As with treatment interventions, each cleft team may follow a different feeding protocol.

Feeding Principles and Techniques

The normal feeding process involves an intact, coordinated sequence of sucking, swallowing, and breathing. Suction depends on negative pressure being generated in a sealed oral cavity to draw the fluid from the nipple and into the mouth of the infant. A cleft makes it difficult for an infant to form the seals necessary to create these pressures. A cleft of the lip prevents an anterior seal around the nipple. A cleft palate prevents the formation of a seal in the oral cavity, which is necessary to create negative intraoral suction. Even small clefts of the soft palate and some submucosal clefts (which are often missed) can cause feeding problems.[16]

Infants with clefts are at risk for sucking inefficiency, excessive air intake, frequent nasal regurgitation of milk, excessively long feeding times, and fatigue.[17] These problems can often contribute to inadequate oral intake and poor weight gain. Parents need a professional to provide early, consistent, and ongoing education and guidance to assist them to master and optimize their child's feeding and nutrition. This is one of the most important roles of the cleft team nurse specialist.

When feeding an infant with a cleft, there are some important common principles:

1. Most infants with an isolated cleft lip or cleft of the lip and alveolus can generate normal suction and are able to feed at the breast. The infant with a cleft palate will have an air leak through the cleft that prevents effective suction on a human breast or artificial nipple, and thus, most will not be successful at directly, exclusively breastfeeding (see breastfeeding section for more details).

2. The bottle and feeding system chosen must offer significantly reduced resistance so that milk flows more easily, such as a compressible bottle or nipple, a crosscut in the nipple tip, and/or a one-way flow valve. The flow of milk must be sufficient to keep the infant interested and awake, but slow enough to allow the infant to coordinate breathing between swallows.

3. A free flow of milk allows less air to be swallowed. To avoid adding air to the formula, milk can be mixed and warmed with a minimum of shaking. Powdered formula should be stirred, not shaken.

4. Parents must be able to recognize signs of distress when feeding a young infant with a cleft. These include, but are not limited to:

    a. Pulling the head back and hyperextending the neck away from the bottle and nipple.

    b. A look of alarm, especially paired with a pause in feeding rhythm, or nasal escape of milk.

    c. Coughing or wet inspiration.

    d. Waving, raising, or pushing the hands or arms on the bottle.

    e. Excessive blinking, eye-widening, or frequent pauses in feeding.

5. The length of a feeding should be limited to no more than 30–40 minutes. Longer feedings can cause exhaustion and increased energy expenditure, resulting in less net caloric intake.

6. Infants should return to birth weight by 2 weeks of age, and should be able to gain weight at a rate commensurate with non-cleft affected peers, approximately 0.5–1 oz/day.

7. Parents should be encouraged to investigate their insurance coverage, as some will pay for specialty feeding bottles (under the category of medical supplies), some of which can be costly. A written prescription or letter of medical necessity from the cleft team may improve the chances of successful insurance reimbursement.

Bottle Feeding an Infant with a Cleft Lip and Palate or a Cleft Palate

Step–By–Step Bottle Feeding Instructions

1. Position the infant upright in good alignment, 45 degrees or higher in an attempt to control nasal regurgitation. The head and neck should be in line with the shoulders or slightly flexed toward the chest. Parents need to be reminded not to let the infant's head tip backward into hyperextension. It is helpful to put more volume in the bottle than the infant can consume in order to avoid the need to tip back the head to capture that last half ounce.

2. Tickle the corner of the mouth with the nipple or your finger, alerting the infant that the feeding will begin.

3. Wait for the infant's head to turn toward the nipple and the tongue to drop from the roof of the mouth.

4. Slip the nipple over the center of the tongue and wait for the infant to begin sucking. The baby's lips should begin to close around the nipple. Reposition the nipple so that the tip is in contact with an intact area of the palate. The bottle/nipple should be tipped downward in order to avoid directing the milk up into the vomer or nasal cavity.

5. Observe the suck–swallow pattern to see if the infant breathes every 2–3 swallows. Listen for an audible swallow, followed by a breath.

6. At first, some very young infants will suck and swallow many times and will not be able to stop to breathe. Remove the nipple until the infant catches his or her breath, and then reinsert it. Removing the nipple to decrease the flow is called external pacing. Most infants will develop better organization within a few days, often within a few feedings. Other ways to provide external pacing include tipping the bottle up so that the nipple does not fully fill, pulling the nipple to one side of the mouth to leave room at the edge for a breath, or, if using the Haberman/SpecialNeeds Feeder™, turning the nipple to the no flow setting. Avoid removing the nipple frequently unless the infant is not stopping to take a breath, as this will disrupt the infant's feeding rhythm.

Burping

The infant should be burped, either seated upright on the lap or positioned over the shoulder, after consuming approximately 1 oz. Parents should be instructed to hold the baby upright while tilting the chest and head slightly forward. Often, all that is needed is to straighten the infant's spine, while lifting and supporting the chest and head to elicit a burp.

Feeding Bottles and Nipples

Cross-Cut Nipple on a Hard Bottle[18]

If a specialty feeding bottle is not available in the nursery, the simplest alteration to facilitate the feeding of an infant with a cleft palate is a cross-cut nipple. A sharp, thin blade or scissor is used to cut a small "X" in the tip of an inverted nipple. After every few sucks, the size of the "X" can be increased until the infant is sucking with speed and efficiency. When

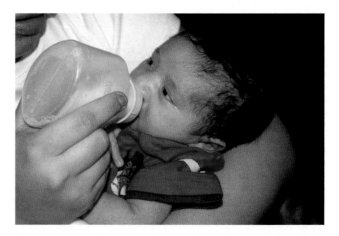

Figure 10–2. Mother feeding infant with Mead Johnson Cleft Feeder. Note the semi-upright positioning. (*Photo credit: Nick Conde Dudding*.)

the nipple cut is too small, the infant becomes easily fatigued and is unable to drink adequately. If the crosscut is too large, the baby is overwhelmed with too much milk and cannot coordinate sucking and breathing. This will often result in nasal regurgitation and/or leakage of milk from the mouth.

To test for correct flow, cut the nipple, attach it to the bottle, invert the bottle, and observe as the milk leaks from the nipple. It will drip quickly and then slow to the proper drip. If the drops are slow, the "X" is too small. If it flows without forming drops, it is too large. If the drops flow rapidly, but with individual drops, it is usually right. The infant's response will tell if the flow is balanced correctly.

A nipple that has been crosscut must be frequently inspected and replaced. Many cleft teams rely exclusively on this type of feeding modification, whereas others never use it, citing concerns about the accuracy of the flow and the possible effect on the integrity of the nipple.

Rapid Flow Nipple on a Commercial Bottle

There are some products on the market that combine a vented bottle with a rapid flow nipple. For some infants with clefts of the lip and palate, this type of bottle/nipple combination is very effective in delivering milk in an efficient manner. Examples of these are the Dr. Brown Natural Flow and the Avent Bottles. Some of the Playtex Bottles (e.g., Ventair) also have a more rapid flow nipple, and the disposable bag can be compressed to assist with the flow.

Enfamil Cleft Palate Feeder (Mead Johnson Nutritionals —800–BABY–123, www.meadjohnson.com)

The Enfamil Cleft Palate Feeder, commonly referred to as the "Mead Johnson Bottle," is distributed by Mead Johnson and is readily available in most newborn nurseries. The 6-oz bottle has soft sides, and can be compressed (Fig. 10–2). The feeder comes packaged with a long, crosscut nipple, although the nipple length and stiffness may be a problem for some infants. Any commercial nipple that has been crosscut can be substituted, and a nipple with a wider base may offer better compression for the infant. Many nurseries combine this bottle with the premature nipple or standard single hole nipple, depending on the needs of the infant. If the opening in the nipple is increased, the amount of compression on the bottle must be carefully tested.

When using this bottle, compression should not begin until after the infant has begun sucking for a few seconds. Compression pressure should then progress from light squeezes to heavier squeezes, with care to observe the infant's face for distress. The testing process will reveal what rate of flow the infant can tolerate. Parents are instructed to compress and release pressure on the bottle every two to three sucks. A stream of bubbles after release indicates adequate compression.

The infant's tongue motion can rub the nipple at the cleft edge, and the feeder will have to hold the nipple firmly in position in the baby's mouth to avoid a friction abrasion along the vomer that can progress to a painful, reddened lesion.

Notes on the Enfamil Feeder:

1. The manufacturer markets this as a disposable bottle. This pertains to how it must be handled in the newborn nursery. Once the baby is at home, however, the bottle can be washed in hot, soapy water and is reusable for up to several weeks. The bottle should not be sterilized, or boiled, or washed in the dishwasher.
2. This is the least expensive of the specialty feeder bottles and can be directly purchased from Mead Johnson Nutritionals, either as individual boxes of 6, or as a case of 72 bottles (12 boxes).

Pigeon Cleft Palate Nipple and Bottle (800–345–6443 or 888–766–8443/www.chmv.respironics.com)

Children's Medical Ventures/Respironics distributes The Cleft Palate Nipple System (commonly known as the Pigeon Bottle), a cleft feeder that is manufactured in Japan. It is composed of an 8-oz bottle, a wide, dual-thickness, vented, Y-cut nipple, and a one-way flow valve (placed in the base of the nipple). The width of the nipple crosses the span of the cleft in many cases, stabilizing the nipple in the mouth. The thick side (the air valve side) of the nipple compresses against the hard palate. The soft, thin side of the nipple is placed above the tongue, to promote optimal compression. When the thin side is compressed, milk is expressed into the infant's mouth. The air vent in the nipple base allows the nipple to refill with milk. The one-way valve prevents backflow of milk from the nipple into the bottle, thus helping to reduce the amount of air ingested during feeding.

This system allows the infant to control the flow of formula. Since the nipple is large, the feeder should observe for signs of infant distress from too rapid a rate of flow. If the infant swallows several times without taking a breath, rears the head back away from the nipple, or coughs, the flow may be too fast, and the nipple should be removed from the mouth (external pacing). Once the infant recovers, the nipple may be reinserted at a shallower angle to slow the flow of milk. Very young newborns will need some time to coordinate the rate of flow and should be watched closely for the first few feedings. Parents should be instructed on the early signs of distress.

Notes on the Pigeon Feeding System:

1. The Pigeon Bottle is sold with two nipples and valves, or a nipple/valve may be purchased separately. The nipple and valve fit on most standard bottles. The valve can sometimes be used successfully in combination with other nipples (e.g., fast-flow silicone nipples on vented bottles).
2. Flow is mostly infant-controlled. This system is not always the best choice for an infant who is unable to feed without assistance.
3. The Pigeon nipple may allow a flow that is too fast for premature infants or infants with poor oral motor or behavioral organization.
4. Prior to using a new nipple, it is necessary to roll the nipple tip between the fingers. The nipple has a tendency to collapse, slowing the flow of milk, which may be relieved by loosening the ring as it screws on the bottle. There is a triangular air vent which must be properly positioned under the infant's nose and which must be dry and patent.
5. The nipples should be washed in mild detergent in order to extend the life of the nipple. They should not be placed in the dishwasher or boiled routinely. The nipple should be replaced after approximately 3 weeks.

Special Needs Feeder/Haberman Feeder

The SpecialNeeds Feeder (Medela Company, www.Medela.com; available for many years as the Haberman Feeder) was designed in the 1980s by Mandy Haberman, the mother of a child with Pierre Robin sequence.[19] It is distributed by Medela, a company that supplies breast pumps.

There are four parts to this feeder that can attach to most bottles. The soft silicone nipple has a reservoir that holds approximately 27 mL of milk and has a slit-valve opening. Three line markings on the reservoir of the nipple indicate the position of the opening relative to the baby's mouth. A white silicone valve is mounted to a polypropylene disk, and these are connected to a feeding bottle (an 80 or 150 mL bottle comes with the nipple) by a polypropylene collar.

To use this feeder, the bottle is filled with breast milk or formula. The assembled nipple/valve/disk/collar is attached to the bottle. To fill the nipple, the bottle is held upright and some air is squeezed out of the nipple. While still squeezing, the bottle is inverted and the nipple released. This is repeated until the nipple/reservoir is completely full.

Flow is controlled according to the direction of the slit in the nipple tip; no flow (smallest line), moderate flow (medium line) at 45 degrees, and high flow (long line) at 90 degrees. The nipple is inserted into the infant's mouth, with the smallest line on the nipple reservoir lined up with the center of the baby's nose; the nipple opening is at the horizontal, or zero flow position. This gives time for the infant to become adjusted and once sucking begins, the nipple can be rotated to increase to a medium or high flow.

Many infants can activate and maintain an adequate flow rate. However, the reservoir may also be squeezed by

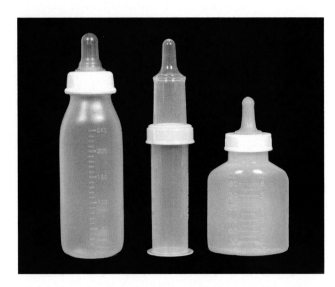

Figure 10–3. Specialty cleft feeding bottles. Left to right: Pigeon nipple and bottle, Special Needs/Haberman Feeder, and Enfamil (Mead Johnson) Cleft Palate Feeder. (*Photo credit: Mary Spano.*)

the feeder to assist the infant in increasing the flow of milk. Assistance with flow may require deep compression of the reservoir. Some feeders compress the nipple with each jaw drop of the infant; others place pressure on the reservoir, releasing compression when the infant pauses.

This is a good feeder for an infant who requires a slower rate of flow or differential flow rates.

Notes on the SpecialNeeds/Haberman Feeder:

1. A "Mini" SpecialNeeds Feeder is also available, providing a smaller size nipple/reservoir for premature infants.
2. This is the most expensive specialty feeder system. Parts of the bottle must be replaced on a regular basis. The high cost may rule this out as a bottle choice for some families, although replacement parts are available to replace worn components at a lower cost.
3. The multiple parts of the nipple can result in improper assembly and problems with successful use of the bottle.
4. The bottle does not have a cover for the nipple and, because of its unusual appearance, often draws attention and questions from strangers.

Commonly used cleft feeding bottles/nipples are shown in Fig. 10–3.

Specialty Feeding Combinations

Sometimes, in order to meet the individual feeding needs of each infant, the following combinations of nipples and bottles have been successfully utilized:

1. A soft (e.g., premature), rapid flow, or wide-based nipple on an Enfamil Feeder.
2. The Pigeon nipple and valve combined with a vented bottle (e.g., Dr. Brown, Ventaire) or the Enfamil Feeder.
3. The Pigeon valve inserted into a slow, moderate, or high flow silicone nipple on a vented bottle.

4. A Playtex Bottle with a wide-based nipple, using bag compression.
5. The SpecialNeeds (Haberman) nipple/valve/disk on any type of commercial bottle.

Note: These combinations are not practices which are recommended by the manufacturers, but anecdotal parent and cleft team reports have noted them to be successful feeding options.

Breast Feeding

The American Academy of Pediatrics[20] and the US Department of Health and Human Services[21] recommend that infants from birth to 6 months be exclusively breastfed. There are many reasons to choose human milk for an infant, particularly in preterm infants, including the immunologic protection provided.[22] Breast milk is well digested and less irritating to the palatal and nasal mucosa of an infant who may experience frequent nasal regurgitation.

Parents should understand that if their baby has an isolated cleft of the lip, they should be able to adequately feed the baby at the breast. Some infants with a cleft lip and alveolus can lose partial suction through the cleft. In this case, the baby may need to be repositioned so that breast tissue fills the cleft. Alternatively, the cleft may need to be covered with a finger.[23] The mother may need to hold her breast in such a way as to have breast tissue pushed into the gap. A feeding position with the infant facing the breast may be needed in order to achieve a good seal (Fig. 10–4).

In rare cases, infants with very small clefts of the soft palate, or with a bifid uvula, can be successful at breastfeeding. However, if there is a cleft of the lip and palate, or if there is an isolated cleft of the hard and/or soft palate, the experience of most cleft palate teams is that it is very unlikely that direct, exclusive breastfeeding will be successful.[24] In breast feeding, suction is required to hold the nipple in place and to allow compression of the lactiferous sinuses by the infant's tongue

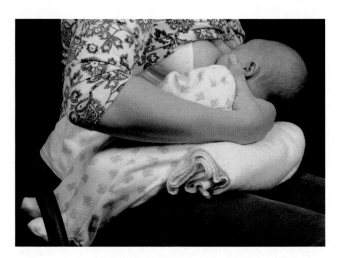

Figure 10–4. Breastfeeding position (modified football hold). (*Photo credit: Mary Spano.*)

against the palatal structures. In most cases, an infant with a cleft in the palate is unable to create adequate intraoral suction and cannot hold the nipple in place. When breast feeding for infants with cleft palate is initiated, the infant often requires frequent feeding, and supplementation with breast milk or formula. The mother must pump to maintain her milk supply. Close monitoring of weight gain is necessary to avoid dehydration and weight loss in a newborn infant with a cleft who is feeding at the breast.

Tips for Breast-Feeding an Infant with a Cleft Palate

For the mother who wants to make a strong effort to directly, exclusively nurse, there are some tips for breastfeeding infants with a cleft palate:

1. A lactation specialist should be sought for in-depth consultation, and ongoing support.
2. The mother must hold her breast in position throughout the feeding or the nipple will become dislodged. It is easier for a baby to latch on the nipple when the mother's nipple anatomy is not flat.
3. Some infants respond to a football hold or straddle-hold position. The infant's mouth is facing mother's nipple, and the infant is sitting more upright. The mother will need to support the baby on or against a pillow so that the mouth is even with mother's nipple.
4. It may be helpful to stimulate letdown with manual expression or with the use of a breast pump before attempting to put the baby to the breast. A helper can drip breast milk down over the breast for the infant to taste during latching-on.
5. The mother should pump after each feeding in order to maintain her milk supply. Ineffective nursing results in reduced stimulation to the breasts and decreased lactation.

The loss of the direct breastfeeding relationship can be devastating for some mothers. However, they want the best opportunity for optimal nutrition for their infant, and the nurse specialist can assist them to achieve this goal. Mothers should be encouraged to put the baby to the breast (if they desire to do so) to support bonding and to assist with the letdown process. A hospital or community lactation specialist can be very helpful in assisting them with the purchase and use of a hospital-grade electric breast pump. They then can be instructed in how to feed expressed breast milk using one of the specialty cleft feeders.

It is common for hospital staff (including lactation specialists), who often have minimal or no experience in feeding cleft-affected infants, to pressure mothers to breastfeed, assuring them that they will eventually be successful. Mothers of infants with clefts often express their feelings of guilt at not delivering "a perfect baby." They need not be burdened with the additional anxiety of not being able to breastfeed. They also need to know that if expressing milk becomes too stressful for them at home, it is perfectly acceptable and not harmful to the baby to supplement with, or to completely switch to, formula.

Expressing Breast Milk

It is important to support the mother who is interested and committed to providing expressed breast milk to her infant. To meet the challenge of pumping breast milk for an actively growing infant, these suggestions can be offered:

1. Use a commercial electric pump. Hand pumping is not efficient enough for the volumes needed and the length of time required.
2. Pump at least five to six times each day, saving the milk for a later feeding. Some mothers try to pump "fresh" milk but may often feel too much stress when pumping while the baby is hungrily crying.
3. To promote the most efficient milk production, massage or warm the breasts before pumping. Actively think about the baby while beginning to pump and try to relax. Have a large glass of liquid nearby.
4. Feed all of the breast milk first before adding formula when there is not enough breast milk for the whole feeding. This will avoid wasting breast milk should the infant not finish the bottle.
5. If the breast milk supply seems inadequate, a consultation with a lactation consultant, obstetrician, or midwife may be helpful.
6. Consult with the baby's pediatrician regarding whether the use of a human milk fortifier is indicated to help supplement the breast milk.

Frequently Asked Questions About Feeding

1. How much should my baby eat?
   In spite of differences between infants, a minimum intake of 2 oz per pound of body weight in 24 hours is suggested. It can take at least several weeks to achieve that goal, depending upon the condition of the child and the level of comfort of the parent.
2. How long should a feeding take?
   Feedings should be limited to no more than 30–40 minutes. Feedings that last an hour or more usually mean an adjustment in the feeding method is needed. Premature infants are very difficult to keep awake and often require shorter, more frequent feedings.
3. How long can I let my baby sleep between feedings?
   Infants in the first weeks of life should not sleep longer than 5 hours between feedings. If the baby is receiving breast milk, more frequent feedings will be needed, as often as every 2 hours. Once adequate fluid volumes and weight gain are achieved, the schedule can be relaxed to a demand-feeding schedule.
4. Does my baby have acid reflux?
   Gastroesophageal reflux is very common in all infants[25] and particularly common with infants with cleft palate

because they often swallow a large amount of air while eating. Parents may become afraid when the infant regurgitates formula from the nose, and they need to be taught to hold the infant forward in order to clear the formula from the nose and mouth. Some infants with reflux will awaken alarmed from sleep long after eating. Parents can be reassured that reflux is very common in young infants and that they have not overfed the infant. They should be taught measures to minimize reflux symptoms, such as to elevate the head of the bed, or to allow the infant to sit up for 30 minutes after eating. The primary care provider can be consulted about the baby's reflux symptoms, and if warranted, a short course of acid-reducing medications may be trialed. If more severe symptoms occur, including pneumonia or poor weight gain, referral to a gastroenterology specialist can be made.

5. Will my baby choke when eating? If so, what should I do?

It is important to differentiate choking from coughing that occurs after nasal regurgitation. It is common for babies with clefts of the palate to leak milk through the nose while being fed. If this happens, the feeding should be stopped and the baby positioned upward and forward. A nasal aspirator (bulb syringe) or, preferably, a soft, damp cloth can be used to clear the milk from the nose and mouth. After a short rest, the feeding can be resumed. Choking or milk entering the lungs (aspiration) is extremely rare. If parents have any concerns about how the baby is managing feedings, they should consult with their pediatrician or cleft team nurse specialist.

6. When should my baby begin to eat solid foods?

At 4–6 months of age as directed by the infant's primary care provider, parents can begin to spoon feed thin solids with the baby in a slightly reclining position. They should begin with small amounts of rice cereal thinned with milk and should not become alarmed if some of the food comes out through the nose. Start with a teaspoon or two, morning and evening, then gradually increase the amount or the thickness of the food. When the consistency of the cereal reaches that of yogurt, parents can begin to add baby jar foods, one food group every 3 days, according to the preference of their pediatrician. A cup may be introduced when the baby is approximately 8–9 months old in order to prepare them for cup feeding after the cleft palate repair. Parents can begin with thickened liquids from an open cup, or they may choose a sippy cup with the no-spill valve removed. Soft table foods may be introduced as recommended by the pediatrician. Parents need not be concerned about food entering the cleft areas. When fluids are given, food in the cleft will loosen and drain. In addition, the baby may automatically "sneeze out" any food that might get stuck in the cleft. Parents can also use very gentle bulb syringe suctioning, if needed, although this is rarely necessary.

NURSING CARE OF THE INFANT WITH PIERRE ROBIN SEQUENCE (PRS)

Pierre Robin Sequence (PRS) is a descriptive diagnosis that includes the triad of micrognathia, glossoptosis, and respiratory obstruction. The condition is often associated with a wide cleft palate and is complicated by a high incidence of feeding difficulties. Neonates with PRS fall in three groups: isolated PRS, PRS associated with a known syndrome, and PRS associated with multiple congenital anomalies.[26]

The birth of an infant with PRS is a stressor for the whole family. The infant may be hospitalized for days to weeks, depending upon the severity of the airway obstruction and feeding issues. The craniofacial nurse specialist can help parents to understand that their infant's airway may require complex management and can support them in coping with the emotional cost of the infant's uncertain immediate future. The parents may need to make difficult decisions about medical treatment, work, insurance, and child care after discharge, and they will need much support during this emotionally vulnerable period.

The first priority in affected infants is the airway. The infant with PRS may be severely compromised from the first moment of life and may need maximum airway support and treatment. The neonate experiencing respiratory obstruction may lift and rotate the entire head from the bed or parent's shoulder in order to create the greatest distance between the posterior pharyngeal wall and the tongue base. There will often be substernal, suprasternal, and intercostal retractions. There may be retraction of the tissues of the neck, and the head may bob when the infant attempts to breathe. The infant's mouth will open and the tongue will not be readily visible. When the infant attempts to inspire, a loud inspiratory gasp may be heard as air is moved past the tongue. The baby may become pale or grey around the mouth and nose as the oxygen saturation drops. Cyanosis expands as the period of obstruction lengthens. Infants should be moved slowly, allowing them a chance to adapt to the new gravitational position of the tongue. The infant with PRS will often be able to relieve the obstruction without assistance, but a gentle push forward at the angle of the mandible, or a finger inserted into the mouth to stimulate a sucking reflex, can be helpful in bringing the tongue forward.

Infants with milder respiratory symptoms are generally stable with prone positioning during sleep, diaper changes, and daily care. This facilitates forward tongue positioning, helping to prevent obstruction and to conserve the infant's energy. Infants with PRS are the published exception to the American Academy of Pediatrics recommendation for supine sleeping to minimize the chance of Sudden Infant Death Syndrome.[27] Oxygen saturation and cardiac function should be monitored to validate clinical observations of respiratory function. Apnea monitors alone are less reliable indicators of respiration because they will pick up respiratory attempts even in the setting of upper airway obstruction and thus often overestimate effective breathing.

Feeding

Feeding management of the infant with PRS will be dependent upon the severity of airway obstruction. While a comprehensive workup is proceeding, a nasogastric (NG) tube may be placed to supply the necessary nutrition until the airway is stable enough for oral feeding attempts. Progression to oral feeding can be made with the NG tube still in place. The presence of orogastric (OG) tubes makes oral feeding a greater challenge, but not impossible. Parents often perceive the feeding tube as a failure, but nurses can demonstrate to them that tubes provide an opportunity to keep the infant well nourished while waiting for oral feeding.

Initially, feedings are accomplished by a nurse or therapist familiar with fragile airways until the infant is stable enough for the entire nursing staff and the parents to be trained. Parents are eager for a feeding trial to begin and often want to observe the feeding process. A running commentary of the infant's behavior during the trial helps the parents to understand what is happening. It must be clear to the family from the outset that the infant's condition and tolerance is the major determinant of the care provided.

In the first 3 months of life, infants with isolated PRS will still be at increased risk for feeding problems requiring tube feedings, even if they do not have airway obstruction severe enough to require surgical management.[28,29] There may be primary oral motor or swallowing abnormalities in addition to the unstable airway and the cleft palate. Infants at the highest risk for more severe and prolonged feeding problems are those with identifiable craniofacial syndromes and multiple anomalies.

Oral Feeding Trial for the Infant with Severe Airway Obstruction

The infant with PRS will expend more energy during the work of breathing than healthy infants of the same age. There are increased energy needs as the tongue is moved into a forward position and accessory chest and neck muscles strain during breathing and feeding. Often, the infant will feed effectively for only a short period of time before exhaustion occurs.

Before beginning a feeding trial, the infant is observed for signs and symptoms of airway obstruction. The anatomy of the cleft and the baby's tongue posture at rest are inspected. To assess tongue position while sucking, a finger is inserted into the baby's mouth. Some infants cannot tolerate a finger or pacifier in the mouth, but sometimes sucking will temporarily relieve an obstruction as the tongue moves forward.

It is challenging to introduce an object into the infant's mouth without pushing the tongue more posterior. The more unstable the infant's airway, the less pacifiers and fingers will be tolerated. Feeding is attempted only with great caution, and with a very low flow rate.

Feeding the infant with Pierre Robin Sequence (Step by Step):

- When the tongue is positioned posteriorly and superiorly, firm tongue massage downward and forward can encourage a flatter posture. This is especially helpful prior to the feeding attempt.[30]
- If the infant tolerates a pacifier and/or finger insertion, the trial begins with a nipple filled with sterile water, then a nipple with a slit, then a crosscut. If the infant responds favorably, then formula or breast milk can be substituted, either before or at the time a specialty cleft palate bottle is tried. If the trial goes well, the above procedure can be accomplished in a few minutes; if not, the trial is terminated and resumed at the next feeding or the next day.
- The infant should be positioned either upright at 90 degrees or side-lying with slight elevation in order to allow gravity to pull the tongue away from the back of the pharynx. The legs and hands should be positioned at midline, with the spine in a gentle curve, and the chin slightly down.
- Gentle downward traction on the mandible may be needed in order to allow the tongue to be seen. The nipple should be inserted with the tip upward over the tongue before the bottle is brought down to a horizontal position.
- Observe the infant's breathing as sucking begins. A finger can be moved to the mandible to monitor sucking and to apply gentle forward traction while feeding. Once the baby is actively sucking and breathing is even and unlabored, a small amount of liquid can be expressed into the baby's mouth. If all continues to go well, more fluids may be expressed with greater volume. A trial with a cleft palate specialty bottle can be tried next.
- The feeder should take care not to abruptly remove the nipple from the infant's mouth, as a sucking motion will continue, and the tongue will be pulled back. If an infant can only tolerate a horizontal side-lying position at the beginning of the feeding, he or she can be slowly elevated to a higher angle while sucking. A more upright position reduces leakage from the dependent side of the mouth and makes the feeding process more efficient.
- If the infant becomes obstructed or experiences oxygen desaturation while feeding, there will be a pause in sucking, and a tense facial expression. To assist the infant, rotate the face down, or reposition the infant on the abdomen. The nipple will still be in place but there will no longer be fluid entering the mouth. If the baby does not then recover, the bottle can be eased from the mouth, and replaced with a finger or a pacifier. Gentle forward traction on the mandible from behind the angle of the jaw can also assist the baby. Lay the infant on the abdomen to recover. The baby may now be exhausted and the feeding will be over. The flow of milk may need to be adjusted, or other bottles and nipples may be trialed. A feeding plan will be chosen for all therapists to follow and changed according to the infant's response.
- The feeding is stopped when the infant tires, sometimes quite suddenly, even without any episode of desaturation. Over time, the infant's behavior will mature and a clearer picture of what intervention is needed will emerge.
- Every attempt should be made to schedule feedings to coincide with the availability of the parents. As the infant becomes more stable, the parents should be coached in feeding

techniques and supervised in providing the feedings. They may become impatient when improvements in feeding are small and slow and may need reassurance and support.

• Continued oral feeding attempts in conjunction with tube feedings to provide adequate nutrition helps the infant organize and maintain feeding skills. Decisions about the feeding plan necessarily include an estimate of time needed to transition to full oral feedings. In some situations, parents will learn the placement and management of NG tubes so they can take their baby home once oral and tube feeding techniques are mastered. For other infants, gastrostomy tubes are placed, and parents manage supplemental feedings using this modality. Parents are understandably anxious about the need to learn tube feeding techniques but are usually willing to do whatever is necessary in order to take their baby home.

• Attempts to orally feed the baby with PRS may provide useful information to the surgical staff while they decide on treatment of the airway. If surgical management is required, feedings are postponed until the infant is recovered, but parents should be cautioned that feeding problems may persist even after surgery and that ongoing feeding therapy may be needed after discharge.[31]

Oral Feeding for the Infant with Moderate Airway Obstruction

Since newborn infants often appear to have small chins, some infants with cleft palate are discharged from the birth hospital before the symptoms of respiratory obstruction, including noisy respirations and mild retractions and feeding difficulty, are identified. Many cleft nursing specialists have reported the experience of hearing the sound of obstruction while speaking on the telephone to a mother holding or feeding her newborn. In that situation, the mother is encouraged to bring the baby in for evaluation by the cleft team as soon as she can travel, and she must be told that the baby may require admission to the hospital for monitoring and assessment.

The baby with moderate obstruction may not have sustained oxygen desaturations, but may only have difficulty with feeding. Such infants should be closely monitored for inadequate weight gain. After the nurse or therapist has reassessed feeding techniques and infant positioning, parents should be instructed to keep a feeding log, and frequent weight measurements should be recommended. Intervention for slow weight gain may include additives or modification of how the formula is reconstituted in order to increase the number of calories per ounce consumed by the infant. Increasing the caloric density of formula may not be effective, as the baby may then simply eat less. In cases of severely compromised weight gain, introduction of tube feeding may need to be considered.

Other factors that impact feeding and weight gain for infants with mild to moderate upper airway obstruction are ear infections, upper respiratory infection, oral thrush, and underlying genetic conditions. Many of the conditions that are associated with PRS include poor weight gain and small

stature as components. If concerns about slow growth persist, referral for a pediatric re-evaluation should be considered.

Despite all efforts by the medical and nursing teams, some infants with PRS may need to be fed (either exclusively or partially) by a gastrostomy. One very positive aspect of this type of feeding is that it will decrease the oral aversion that is very common in infants who have been managed for long periods of time with oral or nasogastric tubes. Other infants may require airway management by tracheostomy, glossopexy, or early mandibular distraction surgery (see Chapters 52 and 63).

Nursing care of the family whose infant is diagnosed with PRS requires empathy, ongoing emotional support, and excellent communication, feeding and teaching skills. The craniofacial nurse specialist plays a central role in educating nursing staff and parents about the signs and symptoms of intermittent respiratory obstruction, as well as in guiding them to safely manage the airway and to successfully feed the infant.

NURSING MANAGEMENT OF THE INFANT AND FAMILY UNDERGOING NASOALVEOLAR MOLDING THERAPY (NAM)

In cleft centers where presurgical nasoalveolar molding therapy, also known as NAM, or PNAM,[32,33] is a component of the treatment plan (see Chapter 46), the nurse specialist is critical to providing ongoing parental education and support. After the NAM therapy is explained to them by the surgeon and orthodontist (either during the prenatal consult or the first postdelivery team visit), it is helpful for the nurse to review and clarify the information with them. The parents can be shown a molding appliance (often referred to as a molding plate, a NAM plate, or simply a "NAM"), as well as photos of other infants with the NAM plate in place and following their surgery. Literature about the treatment, as well as the names of other families who are wiling to share their experience with NAM, can be provided to them. Networking with other parents is optional, but it can be helpful for answering questions that can best be addressed by other parents whose children have undergone this therapy. A tour of the cleft center and dental/orthodontic units can be given during this meeting, with emphasis on introductions being made to all personnel who will be assisting them during the NAM therapy.

This is also a good time for the nurse specialist to discuss and provide guidance to the family regarding some of the logistical issues that they will need to deal with during the NAM process. This includes managing weekly or biweekly appointments, travel, possible associated financial concerns, and additional maternity or family medical leave that may be needed. Parents benefit from reassurance by the nurse specialist, as well as through networking with experienced parents. NAM therapy is a challenging, but very manageable, positive team effort, with parents sharing equal importance with the surgeon and dental/orthodontic team in the baby's care.

The positive "burden of care" aspects of NAM therapy should be discussed with the parents prior to initiating the treatment.

During the initial visit, the nurse can also prepare the family by discussing some possible NAM-related feeding issues. Many parents think that they will be able to successfully breastfeed their infant with the NAM appliance in place, especially if the cleft involves only the lip, nose, and alveolus and if the infant was able to latch on and feed adequately after birth. If the child also has a cleft palate, it is often assumed that the NAM will cover the palatal opening and that the baby can then be successful at breastfeeding. However, the experience at most centers is that the baby will not be able to breastfeed once the NAM appliance has been inserted (ideally by age 2 weeks), as it is often not a comfortable experience for the mother or the infant. Removing the appliance for breastfeeding is discouraged, as such will actually serve to separate the alveolar segments, essentially "undoing" the work that has been accomplished. Many parents report, however, that after the NAM appliance has been inserted and the baby has a few days to adjust to it, feeding does seem to improve. It is likely that feeding would have improved with time, use of the proper bottles, and experience with cleft feeding techniques, as most babies with isolated palatal clefts (who are not fitted with molding appliances or obturators), improve with feeding on their own within the first month of life.[34]

Once the family is ready to proceed with NAM therapy, the next step is for the pediatric dentist/orthodontist/prosthodontist and surgeon to take an impression of the infant's alveolus in order to fabricate the molding appliance. The nurse specialist can describe the procedure to the parents, assuring them that it will take only a few moments to complete and that the baby will be safe and carefully monitored by the dental/orthodontic team. While the impression is taken, the nurse can remain with the parents, using this time to inquire as to how they are adjusting to having a new baby, discussing the status of the baby's feeding, establishing feeding and weight gain parameters, and answering their questions about the NAM treatment process.

Once the appliance is fabricated (this may take several days, depending on whether it is made on-site or sent to an outside laboratory), the family will return to the dental/orthodontic team with the baby for appliance insertion. An effective, non-stressful way of instructing parents in how to properly insert and secure the appliance is to first demonstrate the process on a doll (Fig. 10–5). Once the parents feel comfortable with the technique, the baby's appliance can then be inserted. Parents should be counseled that the baby will need a few days to adjust to the appliance, during which time feeding and sleeping might be affected.

Protocols for the care and management of the molding appliance will differ amongst cleft centers. Clear, written instruction should be given to the parents. In general, the appliance is removed daily for cleaning. Parents can use liquid dish detergent and warm water to clean the appliance. They should not boil the appliance. Parents can be instructed to periodically place their finger in the baby's mouth while the appliance is in place in order to examine it for any sharp edges

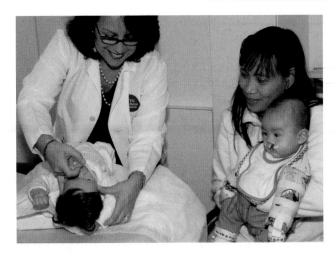

Figure 10–5. Orthodontic team administrator reviewing the proper taping of the NAM appliance. (*Photo credit: Mary Spano.*)

that might irritate the tongue. A penlight and cotton swab can be used to examine the gums for any areas of irritation. The appliance must be removed from the baby's mouth during the examination.

The appliance is generally secured in the mouth through the use of a taping process. Base tapes (e.g., Tegaderm, Duoderm, or Band-Aids) are first placed on the cheeks to help prevent skin irritation from the frequent removal and replacement of the retention tapes that are attached to the appliance. It is important to keep the base tapes dry in order to avoid skin breakdown. The base tapes remain in place for up to 5–7 days and can then be removed by saturating them with warm water, baby oil, or a small amount of liquid adhesive remover. Once the appliance is placed in the mouth, the retention tapes (e.g., Steri-Strips) are connected to orthodontic elastics, which are then attached to the retention buttons on the base of the appliance and stretched over the base tape. Parents can understandably be anxious about the taping process and need detailed instruction and ongoing support. They can be reassured that it can take several weeks to master the process and that they can call someone on the dental/orthodontic team at any time for advice.

During the weekly or biweekly visits for assessment/appliance adjustment, the cleft team nurse will have many opportunities to monitor the baby's progress with feeding, weight gain, and overall growth and development. If the NAM therapy is being managed offsite (e.g., in a dental or orthodontic office/clinic), it is helpful for the nurse specialist to phone the family periodically to offer advice and support. In some cases, a change of nipple or bottle will be indicated. If a pacifier is used, it might need to be modified to accommodate the button. These visits also allow the nurse to observe how the entire family is managing and to provide support as needed, especially as the date of surgery approaches. A preoperative teaching session can be scheduled on the same day as one of the last appliance adjustments. Parents will often need assurance that once the lip and alveolus are repaired, the baby will be able to adjust to feeding without the NAM appliance in place.

The weekly or biweekly visits during NAM treatment provide parents with tremendous support and networking opportunities. Postoperatively, the family will often experience some unexpected anxiety because they will no longer have frequent appointments with the cleft team for NAM adjustments.

NURSING CARE DURING THE SURGICAL PERIOD

The role of the nurse during the surgical period is multifaceted. Initial discussions about the overall process and timeline are included in family education that begins with the prenatal or birth visit. More detailed preoperative preparation occurs closer to the time of surgery. The nurse coordinator may also serve as a resource to staff nurses on the acute care unit for nursing care during the inpatient period. Developing protocols for nursing care, standard orders, and inservice education are often part of the nurse specialist's role, along with discharge teaching and arranging/coordinating team follow-up. The family often views the nurse specialist as the primary resource for postoperative questions when they return home from the hospital. Having a broad focus, from preoperative preparation to discharge teaching and postoperative follow-up, allows the cleft team nurse to provide a seamless transition for the family from the evaluation/preparation phase to the surgical and recovery period. This relationship will be consistent throughout the child's treatment and often until young adulthood.

Cleft Lip Repair

Preoperative Care

The timing of cleft lip repair varies amongst teams but usually occurs by 3–6 months of age. Neonatal cleft lip and palate repair has been reported,[35] but is rare. The use of a presurgical molding appliance (NAM) may delay the primary lip closure in order to take advantage of alveolar and nasal molding changes. Other factors that may contribute to a delayed closure include prematurity and cardiac or other birth defects. In addition, surgery is sometimes postponed due to the presence of a significant respiratory illness, especially during the winter months.

Preoperative preparation for cleft lip repair is aimed at familiarizing the parents with hospital and postoperative routines in order to help prepare them to cope with the experience and to successfully care for their infant. The effectiveness of a preparation program designed to decrease parental anxiety has been documented.[36] Reducing caretaker anxiety often makes the infant's recovery from surgery more successful. In addition, preoperative teaching can help parents to have realistic expectations regarding their infant's appearance after surgery. Most hospitals offer programs giving general information and tours of the outpatient surgical suites, as well as of the inpatient pediatric units. The nurse specialist on the cleft team should supplement general information with information specific to the cleft surgery. Topics to cover include the admissions process, anesthesia instructions, length of the surgical procedure, and postanesthesia care unit routines. Discussions about postoperative routines during hospitalization and after discharge should be included.

Parent participation during hospitalization is important. Separation from the primary caretaker can impact negatively on the recovery of the infant. Parents need to gain confidence in the care they will be providing at home after discharge. They should be encouraged to plan on being present as much as possible throughout the hospital stay, both in the postanesthesia care unit and in the hospital room if an overnight stay is needed. They may need to make arrangements for time off from work, and there may be questions pertaining to day care arrangements for the infant and siblings after surgery. Photographs depicting infants in the immediate postoperative period are helpful adjuncts to verbal information. Networking parents with another family that has undergone the same surgical experience should be included in this preparation process.

Postoperative Care

The goal of cleft lip and palate surgery is to restore normal anatomy and function. Postoperative care routines are aimed at protecting the repair, minimizing pain, and maximizing the physical and psychological comfort of the infant.

Feeding: Depending on the cleft team protocol, changes in usual care practices of feeding may be recommended. Immediate unrestricted feeding without wound complications has been documented,[37] and infants are frequently allowed to return to their preoperative feeding method (bottle/breast). Due to surgeon preference or to infant refusal of a nipple in the initial postoperative period, an alternative method may be required. A 30–60-cc syringe with 1-inch rubber catheter tip or a manufactured soft squeeze bottle with thin tubing (e.g., the Soft-Sipp Bottle) are frequently used postoperatively. Familiarizing parent and infant with this new method before surgery can help make the transition easier. Pacifiers are often not allowed during this recovery period.

Many infants have some degree of postoperative nasal obstruction, resulting from postoperative swelling, the presence of nasal stents, congestion with blood or mucus, or reduced nasal airway area following the closure of the nasal cleft. This can result in problems with coordination of breathing and sucking and can interfere with the postoperative feeding process. An additional impediment may be the absence of an appliance in those infants who underwent presurgical orthodontic (NAM) treatment. Although not necessary for successful feeding, these infants are accustomed to having the appliance in place during feeding and may need time to readjust to feeding without it. It is important for the staff to know that postoperative suctioning of the nose or mouth of an infant after a cleft lip and nose repair should only be done in case of an emergency.

Once it has been assured that the baby has a stable airway, good bowel sounds, and is appropriately awake and alert, oral feeding can be initiated. Clear fluids are offered first, and if the baby tolerates this, the feeding is progressed to full-strength breast milk or formula. Some teams allow a nursing infant to immediately return to the breast. Parenteral IV fluids are continued until the infant is tolerating adequate oral fluids. The IV rate can be decreased to a KVO (keep vein open) rate or capped in order to increase the baby's thirst. If the child refuses to drink, IV access will then still be available, thus avoiding the need for an additional venipuncture. Parents should be instructed as to the amount of fluid that their infant will need to take at home, reassuring them that it is normal and safe for infants to take a few days to resume their presurgical daily volume. The signs and symptoms of dehydration should be explained.

Elbow Restraints: Restraints may be required to keep hands/objects away from the repair site. Parents are taught how to remove and apply these to allow for range of motion exercises and for skin inspection at regular intervals. There is disagreement among cleft teams regarding the value of elbow restraints in protecting the lip repair, and protocols often vary significantly, ranging from not using them at all to requiring that they be worn for up to 3 weeks or longer. The use of restraints does give some parents and surgeons comfort. However, the stress that many parents experience while trying to keep the restraints secured, as well as the frustration and resulting excessive crying they may cause the infant (which itself may serve to put additional stress on suture lines), may outweigh the benefits[38] (Fig. 10–6).

Suture Line Care: Incision care may include cleaning with normal saline on a cotton-tipped applicator or small piece of gauze, as well as the application of an antibiotic ointment. There may be a nasal stent in place, requiring gentle cleansing around the area. Sutures are removed 5–7 days postoperatively, either in the office or as a day surgery procedure with anesthesia. Resorbable sutures may also be used. The use of octyl-2-cyanoacrylate for skin closure is gaining popularity and also avoids the need for suture removal.[39]

Pain Management: Postoperative pain is often difficult to assess in infants after cleft lip repair. The nurse must be aware of verbal and nonverbal cues, such as crying, restlessness, and body movements. It may be difficult to differentiate pain from irritability related to factors such as changes in feeding method, presence of restraints, nasal congestion, and disruption of routines. Pain control measures include holding and comforting by parents, frequent removal of restraints, and administration of non-narcotic or narcotic analgesics every 4–6 hours. Pain medication may be initially given parenterally or rectally, then transitioned to an oral elixir (usually acetaminophen or acetaminophen with codeine) as the infant begins taking fluids by mouth.

Psychological/Emotional Issues: The medical staff must be sensitive to the emotional aspects of surgery that the family may experience. Parents that have anticipated surgery for many months often expect that they will be ecstatic when they see their baby after surgery. Many parents, however, have a difficult time adjusting to their infant's new appearance in the immediate postoperative period. Some will be distressed at first glance in the postanesthesia care unit, even stating

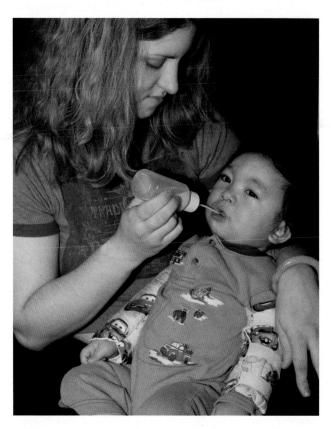

Figure 10–6. Mother and infant following cleft palate repair. Note the Soft-Sipp bottle and elbow splints. (*Photo credit: Mary Spano.*)

that the child "does not look like their baby." These feelings usually pass quickly as parents assimilate the new lip repair and often remark on a resemblance to other family members. Some parents are also very anxious about having to assume immediate responsibility for the baby's postoperative care, especially if the surgery is done on an ambulatory basis.

Discharge: Hospitalization length may vary from that of an outpatient procedure to a 1- or 2-day inpatient stay. Discharge criteria usually include: adequate fluid intake, observable pain control with oral medication, and the absence of significant fever. Before discharge, the nurse should ensure that the parents understand and can demonstrate the child's care at home, including feeding, positioning, suture care, restraints, and medication administration. They may be instructed to continue with administration of acetaminophen every 4–6 hours until approximately the third postoperative day, by which time most infants are comfortable without medication. Antibiotics may be prescribed, according to each individual team's protocol. If prescribed, parents should be alerted to the possibility of the side effects (e.g., rash, diarrhea) and be encouraged to contact the office if these problems are observed.

The nurse instructs the parent to report erythema or drainage at the incision site, a temperature of greater than 101°F, vomiting/diarrhea, decreased oral intake (or refusal to drink), or increasing or unrelieved pain. Parents should be given contact telephone numbers for whom to call with any concerns or questions and to schedule follow-up appointments. They should be assured that it is normal for the infant to require 2 or 3 weeks to return to his/her presurgical routine, particularly if there are postoperative feeding restrictions or if elbow restraints are used.

Cleft Palate Repair

Palate repair is usually performed between 6 and 18 months of age, depending upon factors such as the type of cleft, the surgeon's preference, and the child's weight and overall health. The goal of surgery is to establish normal palatal function before speech development.

Although some parents may have had previous experience with cleft surgery, the difference in age and type of procedure still necessitates thorough preoperative preparation. The length of time for restraints to be worn is center-dependent. Additional topics to cover will include airway concerns and dietary/behavioral changes in an older child.

Airway Management: Postoperative nursing care after palatoplasty is directed toward protecting the repair, monitoring the infant for excessive bleeding, and maintaining the airway. There may be postoperative swelling of the palate and/or tongue as well as thick secretions and drainage. A tongue suture is often in place, taped to the cheek for use in the event of an airway emergency. The appearance of this suture may be frightening to parents, and they should be prepared for such preoperatively by the nurse specialist. Pulling downward on the tongue stitch to reposition the tongue can relieve obstruction. Placing infants in a prone position will facilitate the drainage of secretions. If suctioning is absolutely indicated, a soft catheter must be used, directed away from the operative site.

Feeding: Depending upon the age of the child, transitioning to cup feeding before surgery is helpful. Although some surgeons allow the use of a bottle postoperatively, most children undergoing palate repair are at an age to begin the weaning process. Cups with spouts may or may not be allowed postoperatively. The use of straws and utensils should be avoided. Some centers prescribe a progressive diet, starting with clear liquids and progressing to liquefied foods (e.g., stage 1 or 2 jar foods with added water or blenderized table foods) that can be fed with a spoon held parallel to the lips. Offering water after feeding may help cleanse the mouth and will minimize the child's tendency to attempt to clear the palate with the tongue. Parents need to be given a specific, written feeding protocol so that they can plan accordingly.

Swelling and discomfort during swallowing may delay the initiation of oral feeds. Prompt administration of pain medication so the infant does not associate pain with drinking is important. Careful administration of parenteral narcotics, with appropriate respiratory monitoring, can be safely used until the child is taking fluids and can tolerate oral pain medication. Oral feeds may begin when the child is fully awake and the airway is stable. Offering small amounts of liquids at frequent intervals is helpful. Dietary restrictions are usually in place for 1–3 weeks, with emphasis on the importance of the child being well hydrated during this time.

Restraints/Behavioral Issues: Elbow restraints may be required to keep hands, toys, or other objects out of the mouth. Older infants may be more adept at removing these restraints. Wearing of long-sleeved shirts with the cuff over the restraint or pinning of restraints to the clothes may be helpful suggestions to the parents. The length of time for restraints to be worn is center-dependent.

Owing to their developmental stage, children undergoing palate repair may have more difficulty adapting to limitations on diet and activity. They may be irritable and difficult to console. Parents should be warned of this possibility in order that the behavioral changes may be anticipated and managed with less anxiety.

Discharge: The hospital stay after palate repair is usually 1–2 days, typically a little longer than that required for lip repair. This is often the result of a very willful child refusing to take anything by mouth. Discharge criteria include absence of airway compromise, adequate fluid intake, and effective pain control with oral medication. Discharge instructions should include diet/feeding instructions, use of restraints, and administration of pain medication. Parents should be instructed to report fever over 101°F, bleeding or drainage from palate, inadequate fluid intake, vomiting/diarrhea, and excessive crying or pain unrelieved by medication.

Alveolar Bone Grafting

The timing of bone grafting to repair the alveolar cleft is based on the child's dental development and upon the recommendation of the orthodontist. Secondary alveolar bone grafting is typically performed between 6 and 12 years of age. Although several donor sites are available, bone is usually harvested from the iliac crest.

Preoperative preparation should include the school-aged child as well as the parents. At this age, children are able to understand information relating to surgery, preoperative evaluation, and postoperative changes in routine. They should be encouraged to ask questions about all aspects of the surgery, hospital stay, and any postoperative activity restrictions. This is especially important for children who participate in sports. Networking with another child of the same age who has completed this surgery can be very helpful. Medical play with a child life specialist may allow children to work through fears about surgery and separation. In the rare case of a child who has developed a extreme anxiety regarding medical treatment, referral to a therapist may be indicated.

Postoperative care is aimed at protecting both the graft and donor sites. Both areas need to be observed for bleeding and signs of infection. Intravenous fluids are continued until oral fluids are tolerated. Pain is initially managed with parenteral narcotics in the immediate postoperative period. The overnight use of patient-controlled analgesia (PCA) is very effective in this group of children and may be administered until oral fluids are tolerated. Transition can then be made to oral pain medication, either a liquid preparation or a crushed tablet.

The iliac bone graft site is generally closed with absorbable sutures and may be covered with a waterproof dressing. Discomfort is often greater at the iliac crest harvest site than in the mouth. Surgeons vary in their approach to the use of long-acting local anesthetic agents infiltrated at the harvest site.[40] Pain medication offered 20–30 minutes before ambulation may be helpful. Elevating the head and/or application of ice packs may improve facial swelling, which can be significant, especially in a child who requires bilateral alveolar grafts.

Clear liquids are offered as soon as the child is alert and able to swallow; the diet is progressed to blenderized or soft foods, according to the protocol of the child's cleft team. Daily use of oral liquid supplements can help maximize the child's caloric intake. Utensils and straws should be placed inside the mouth carefully in order to avoid injury to the graft site. A nutritional consult (either preoperatively or prior to hospital discharge) can be very helpful to the family. A written explanation of the diet restrictions, with examples of allowable foods, should be reviewed with the child and parents. These restrictions may need to be followed for up to 8 weeks. Oral hygiene may include mouth rinses with water or a prescription mouthwash. Careful brushing of the upper teeth can begin once the graft site is healed, but the lower teeth and tongue should be brushed immediately after surgery. Depending on the center, a maxillary splint may be inserted for up to 8–12 weeks.

Discharge instructions should include information on diet, medication administration, bathing, oral hygiene, care of the bone graft site, return to school, and activity restrictions. Tub bathing can resume once the suture line at the donor site is completely healed. The child may be slow to ambulate, and climbing stairs may be difficult for a few days. Cleft team-specific activity restrictions (e.g., contact sports, bike-riding, and skateboarding) must be reviewed with the child and family. Children may usually return to school within a few days to 2 weeks after discharge. The school must to be informed of diet and activity restrictions, including non-participation in gym class or recess.

Secondary Palatal Surgery

School-aged children with velopharyngeal dysfunction may be candidates for secondary palatal management. Preoperative evaluation may include a complete speech evaluation, a sleep study, and videoflouroscopy or nasoendoscopy. Tonsillectomy may be indicated and is usually performed at least 6 weeks before secondary palatal surgery. Education and preparation of the child and family for the evaluative procedures is important.

The surgical procedure may be either a sphincter pharyngoplasty or a pharyngeal flap. Postoperative management for both procedures is similar to that after palatoplasty. Potential complications after surgery are bleeding and/or airway obstruction. The nasal airway may be reduced in size and compromised by postoperative swelling. Close monitoring for signs of airway obstruction is necessary.

Feeding restrictions may include elimination of utensils and straws in the mouth. A blenderized diet may be necessary for 2–3 weeks, along with careful oral hygiene practices. A nutritional consult may be helpful to provide creative solutions for the school-aged child's diet preferences.

Pain Management: Oropharyngeal and/or neck pain are common complaints; some children are reluctant to even swallow their saliva. The child may also be irritable due to hunger. The child may also be reluctant to speak immediately after surgery due to discomfort or fear. Adequate pain management is critical to encouraging the school-aged child to drink. Intravenous narcotics are transitioned to oral medication before discharge.

Discharge instructions are similar to those given after the initial palate repair. In addition, information about observing for obstructive sleep apnea should be given to the parents.

Maxillary Advancement

In patients with maxillary hypoplasia, a surgical advancement may be indicated. This is often performed at the end of adolescence, coinciding with the completion of facial growth, and is preceded by extensive orthodontic preparation. Following LeFort I osteotomy, the maxilla is advanced into the desired position and stabilized with internal plates and screws. Another option is to perform a gradual maxillary advancement, a procedure known as maxillary distraction. This involves making a LeFort I osteotomy, placing pins on either side of it, and attaching an internal or external distraction device. After a latency period of 5–7 days, the family is taught how to activate the device. This creates a gap in the bone and stimulates

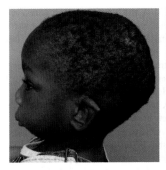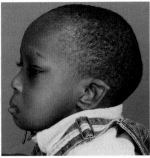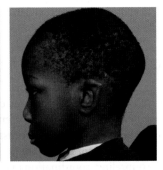

Figure 10–7. Mandibular distraction: pre- and postoperative photos. (*Photo credit: Mary Spano.*)

Pediatric Assessment and Management of Children with Cleft Lip and Palate

Carrie L. Heike, MD, MS, FAAP • Michael Cunningham, MD, PhD, FAAP

INTRODUCTION

A pediatrician caring for a child with an orofacial cleft may be a member of a cleft team or a provider in the community that works closely with a team or individual surgeons.

The multifaceted treatment plan for children with orofacial clefts includes repair of the anomalies (lip, palate, nose), maximization of growth and development, optimization of speech and hearing, intervention to ensure good dental health and functional dental occlusion, and facilitation of optimal psychosocial outcomes. Achievement of these goals requires an interdisciplinary team approach in order to expedite timely assessments, and ensure coordination of care. The pediatrician provides diagnostic evaluations, manages medical problems related to the child's diagnosis, coordinates the specialty care provided by the team, and individualizes care for each child. The pediatrician who works with children with orofacial clefts should be familiar with the medical needs of these children, matching the recommendations of each specialist with the needs and goals of the family. Pediatricians who are members of a cleft team will work with the primary care physician to achieve these goals.

This chapter provides a general overview, addressing aspects of the pediatric evaluation critical to each stage. There are references to other chapters in this text and a short list of additional references for supplementary information on specific topics is provided. The chapter begins with a discussion about prenatal and preadoptive visits, and is subsequently divided according to discrete developmental periods.[1] A comprehensive pediatric evaluation should include all aspects of a general pediatric medical history and physical exam. We have chosen to highlight the aspects of the visit that are particularly important for the management of a child with a cleft lip and/or palate (Table 11–1).

THE PRENATAL VISIT

The prenatal diagnosis of orofacial clefts is becoming more common due to improvements in ultrasonography, and these are further reviewed in chapter 4 on Fetal Diagnosis. A prenatal pediatric consultation offers an excellent opportunity for families to learn about caring for a child with a cleft. Education of the family about what to expect in the first few weeks after delivery can empower the parents and ease their stress in the newborn period.

Prenatal visits with the cleft team are typically scheduled between 20 and 30 weeks gestation and may include consultation with a pediatrician, surgeon, nurse, and a psychosocial professional. A prenatal meeting with members of the team can be reassuring to the parents and familiarize them with the medical team and facility. Parents experience a wide range of emotions during this period, including grief, guilt, and concern over the birth of a child with a visible malformation. The prenatal visit can be used to explore these feelings and connect the parents with additional support services.

Goals

1. Establish a rapport with the family
2. Refer to a cleft lip/palate team
3. Discuss the possibility of a syndrome and genetic counseling (if indicated)
4. Identify risk factors for postnatal complications
5. Discuss feelings and concerns
6. Educate about clefts of the lip and palate
7. Provide feeding instructions and special bottles/nipples
8. Provide contact information and a follow-up plan

Highlights of the Medical History

A thorough pregnancy history includes: parental age, number and outcome of prior pregnancies, access to prenatal care, use of prenatal vitamins or folate, and environmental exposures; further details are reviewed in chapter 5 on Genetic and Prenatal Counseling. This information can be valuable in the assessment of possible postnatal complications. Identification of potential teratogenic exposures should prompt counseling for the current as well as future pregnancies.

Additionally, the pediatrician should determine whether there is a family history of orofacial clefting, other craniofacial conditions, or related syndromes. Family members may have features that are associated with syndromic clefting, such as cardiac malformations, speech impairments, learning delays (22q11.2 deletion syndrome), early myopia (Stickler syndrome), lip pits (van der Woude), or ectodermal dysplasia and these features should be included in the family history. A more in-depth discussion of these issues is addressed in chapter 8 on Syndromes of Orofacial Clefting. The history also should include information concerning family members who have had neonatal respiratory distress or jaw surgery as an adult to identify a family history of micrognathia.

The social history is a critical component of the prenatal evaluation. The history should include an assessment of the family's support system and the parent's reaction to the diagnosis. Variables that may affect the family's feelings include preconceptions regarding etiology, cultural beliefs, and guilt. Anticipation of the reaction of the extended family members and friends can assist parents to develop appropriate responses.

Management

Prenatal imaging is not always precise. As a consequence, the cleft may be more or less severe than initially anticipated. For example, while prenatal ultrasonography often assists in the diagnosis of primary palatal clefting, it frequently misses clefts of the secondary palate; and this is significant as cleft lip and palate is actually twice as common as cleft lip alone. Until technology improves our ability to accurately diagnose clefts of the secondary palate, the prenatal visit should always include a discussion of cleft palate and its management implications. The pediatrician may also recommend a referral for a genetics evaluation to discuss the possibility of additional testing (either during the pregnancy or after delivery depending on the concerns), and evaluate the possibility of a syndromic diagnosis in a child with multiple malformations. A review of this topic is discussed in chapter 5 on Genetic and Prenatal Counseling.

In our experience, professional reassurance to the family is most important at the prenatal visit. The family's opportunity to meet providers with experience caring for children with orofacial clefts, and learn the facts about treatments, can dispel myths and false information while providing the parents with an opportunity to meet their child's providers

Table 11–1.

Key Aspects in the Management of Children with Cleft Lip and/or Palate

Prenatal Visit	Establish a rapport with the family and refer to a cleft lip/palate team Discuss the possibility of a syndrome and genetic counseling Identify risk factors for postnatal complications Discuss feelings and concerns Educate about clefts of the lip and palate Provide feeding instructions and special bottles/nipples Provide contact information and a follow-up plan
Pre-adoption Consultation	Provide information regarding the needs of children with cleft Provide the family with a medical home for their child Assess the possibility of identification of a syndrome Address development
Initial Newborn Visit (Birth–1 month)	Provide feeding instructions and monitor growth Assess respiratory status Evaluate associated anomalies, and recommend genetic referral Begin presurgical orthopedics if indicated Educate the caretakers and provide reassurance Perform a hearing evaluation (OAE or BAER) Outline the short- and long-term plan
Early Infancy (1–4 months)	Monitor feeding and growth Prepare for repair of cleft lip Monitor ear health and hearing Presurgical orthopedics (if indicated)
Transition to Toddlerhood (5–15 months)	Monitor feeding, growth, and development Prepare for palate repair Assess respiratory status Monitor ear health and hearing; consider myringotomy tubes Instruct parents on the importance of good oral hygiene
Speech and Language (16–24 months)	Assess ear health and hearing Assess speech and language development Monitor social, gross and fine motor development, and learning
The Preschool Period (2–5 years)	Evaluate speech and language, manage velopharyngeal insufficiency Assess ear health and hearing Consider lip and/or nose revision before starting school Address psychosocial concerns in the preschool and kindergarten period Optimize developmental services, in and out of school
The Orthodontic Years (6–12 years)	Assess ear health and hearing Assess speech and language, manage velopharyngeal insufficiency Consider orthodontics and determine optimal time for alveolar bone grafting Assess school and psychosocial adjustment, peer acceptance Ensure appropriate educational support in school Assess symptoms of obstructive sleep apnea Begin to redirect the interview to the child
The Teen Years & Transition to Independence (12–21 years)	Accommodate teen's wishes for jaw surgery, rhinoplasty if indicated Optimize orthodontic results Refer for genetic counseling Assess school and psychosocial adjustment Ensure appropriate speech Aid in the transition to adult care

Adapted with permission from Critical Elements of Care: Cleft Lip and Palate, 4th edn. The Center for Children with Special Health Needs, Children's Hospital and Regional Medical Center, Seattle, Washington, 2006.

before their birth. The prenatal visit is also an ideal time to introduce the family to a psychosocial professional. This person can provide additional psychosocial support, help the family access professional and community services, and assist the parents to secure adequate financial resources to care for their child.

An infant with an isolated cleft lip may be able to breastfeed, but those with palatal clefts require special feeding devices, which are reviewed in greater detail in chapter 10 on Nursing Issues for Patients with Cleft Lip and Palate. During the prenatal visit, the provider should demonstrate the use of specialized bottles and/or nipples. Families should also receive specific feeding instructions as well as the necessary supplies. Some mothers may mourn the loss of the chance to breastfeed; and for those mothers who are interested in feeding the infant expressed breast milk, we recommend consultation with a lactation specialist in the perinatal period.

The pediatrician should discuss the possibility of postnatal complications. While most newborns with orofacial clefts do well, some infants may experience difficulty with feeding or respiratory distress. Anticipatory guidance and instructions to monitor for signs of distress may prompt parents to seek timely medical evaluation when indicated. The pediatrician should also mention the possibility that additional malformations could be identified after birth.

Parents have varying methods for processing information. Providing the family with written material on cleft lip and palate, a resource list of educational books and videos, and contact information for the cleft team will allow parents to absorb the information through various modalities. Some families will have facility with web resources prior to the clinic visit. A list of websites with informative and accurate information can minimize misinformation.

The prenatal visit can be exceptionally empowering to the family. After the prenatal visit, they will know more about the management of their unborn infant than most of the providers that will attend the birth. This is a good time to explain to the family that their child will get a great deal of attention after the delivery. The presence of a malformation, even as common as a cleft lip, frequently prompts increased attention from health care providers immediately following birth. Preparing the family for this possibility may reduce their anxiety in the perinatal period. At the end of the visit, the provider should establish a follow-up visit.

Timing of the initial newborn evaluation by the pediatrician varies depending on the comfort level of the family and skill level of the practitioners at the birth hospital. Infants who undergo an early hospital discharge should have a weight check within 48 hours. Ideally, children with orofacial clefts, living in close proximity to the cleft team, should have an initial evaluation in the first one or two weeks of life to establish the health of the newborn and determine candidacy for presurgical orthodontics. The family should be encouraged to contact the cleft team with questions before or after the birth of their child.

PREADOPTION CONSULTATION

Pediatricians associated with cleft lip and palate teams may be asked to consult with families considering the adoption of a child with an orofacial cleft. The majority of these cases represent international adoptions. Much like the prenatal assessment, the clinicians are asked to provide information and recommendations based on limited data. However, adoptive families seeking preadoption counseling are aware that the child has an orofacial cleft, and thus are spared the guilt and sense-of-loss often felt by biologic families. As with the prenatal assessment, the preadoptive evaluation is designed to supply the family with general information about caring for a child with an orofacial cleft and to provide an opportunity to meet members of the cleft lip and palate team.

Goals
1. Provide information regarding the needs for children with clefting
2. Provide the family with a medical home for their child
3. Assess the possibility of identification of a syndrome
4. Address development

Highlights of the Medical History

The primary purpose of the preadoptive visit is to address the family's concerns. Preadoptive families often have some knowledge about clefting and may have major misconceptions. It is helpful to identify the family's source of information, determine their goals for the visit, and inquire about their concerns regarding the potential adoption. The medical histories that are available for preadoptive children vary greatly and most are sparse. Gather as much of the medical history as possible, and remind the family that you will need to confirm these data after the child is adopted. Many medical issues can be "lost in translation" (i.e., a benign heart murmur may be reported as congenital heart disease). Medical information may be exaggerated or underreported depending on the source.

Management

After acquiring information from medical records, photos, and movies, the pediatrician should provide an accurate representation of the ideal management plan for a typical child with orofacial clefting. In addition, they should discuss predictable issues that may arise in international adoptees. For instance, institutional feeding practices vary widely and can include feeding with wide open nipples, bottle propping, and thickening feeds with rice cereal. Hence, some infants may experience feeding difficulties, oral motor delays, and oral aversions beyond those one might observe in a child with an uncomplicated orofacial cleft. These children frequently benefit from guidance from a feeding specialist. Although most internationally adopted children are provided with the standard cleft care, the timing of surgical interventions is often delayed. It is not uncommon for a child who is adopted after 2 years of age to have an unrepaired primary and secondary

Table 11–2.

Contact Information for Pediatricians with Expertise in Adoption Medicine

American Academy of Pediatrics: Pediatricians with a Special Interest in Adoption and Foster Care Medicine: http://www.aap.org/sections/adoption/adopt-states/adoption-map.html.

Orphandoctor. Dr. Aronson and International Pediatric Health Services, PLLC: http://www.orphandoctor.com.

University of Minnesota International Adoption Clinic: http://www.med.umn.edu/peds/iac/

University of Washington Center for Adoption Medicine: http://www.adoptmed.org.

palatal cleft. Delay of the palatal repair is likely to contribute to speech impairments and may contribute to difficulty with communication. Delayed palatal repair can present a surgical challenge with an adverse effect on functional outcomes, but most cases can be managed effectively. It is critical that the family have an opportunity to discuss the details of management with appropriate team members.

One must use caution when discussing the possibility of a syndrome or identifying developmental concerns during a preadoptive consultation. Overt malformations, in addition to the cleft, may be noted on medical or photographic records; however, detailed data is not available for most cases. Growth and developmental delays are often present, but may reflect environmental influences, rather than an underlying genetic condition. For these reasons, diagnosis of a specific syndrome is rarely possible.

If the newly adopted child is medically stable, encourage the family to schedule a team assessment at least two weeks after the adoption is complete. This will give the family an opportunity to get to know their child and develop a set of questions prior to the visit. A medical interpreter should also be scheduled to attend the clinic visit for older adoptive children. Most preadoptive families have also consulted with an international adoption specialist. We have included a list of websites for those families that would like to contact an adoption specialist in their area (Table 11–2).

INITIAL NEWBORN VISIT

The newborn visit is the first pediatric consultation for most families. This encounter serves as an important opportunity to assess the health of the newborn and establish a rapport with the family. Neonates with clefts of the lip and palate require close follow-up with frequent weight checks to monitor feeding and growth. Occasionally, neonates with orofacial clefts will have associated anomalies, such as a micrognathia

or cardiac malformations, requiring early medical or surgical intervention. For example, infants with Robin sequence (micrognathia and glossoptosis with or without a palatal cleft) may appear to breathe comfortably with prone positioning in the first few weeks, but develop significant upper airway obstruction after the first month. Therefore, the pediatrician caring for a newborn with a cleft must perform a through assessment, and anticipate potential complications. Special emphasis should be placed on the evaluation of the child's nutrition and respiratory status, cleft characteristics, and associated physical anomalies.

It is helpful to begin the visit with a brief explanation of how team care functions, with clarification of the roles of the team members that will be involved in the patient's care. It is also beneficial to invite the parents' questions and concerns so that you can address these issues during the visit.

Goals

1. Provide feeding instructions and monitor growth
2. Assess respiratory status
3. Evaluate associated anomalies, and recommend genetic referral (if indicated).
4. Begin presurgical orthopedics if indicated
5. Educate the caretakers and provide reassurance
6. Perform a hearing evaluation (OAE or BAER)
7. Outline the short and long-term plan

Highlights of the Medical History

The prenatal history may provide clues that should prompt further investigation into the possibility of associated physical anomalies; chapter 8 on Syndromes of Orofacial Clefting reviews this topic in much greater detail. As part of the prenatal history, remember to ask about the number of ultrasounds obtained and any other tests that were performed. Answers to these questions may indicate prenatal concerns that might have otherwise been overlooked during the interview. The birth history can also provide valuable information about the general health of the neonate. Questions should include: mode of delivery, complications with delivery, need for resuscitation of the newborn, birth weight, need for additional interventions, and length of hospital stay. The history also includes documentation of the results of tests (including brainstem auditory evoked response (BAER) or otoacoustic emissions (OAE)) that were performed during the birth hospitalization.

The feeding history is an essential part of the evaluation and should include the type of milk (expressed breast milk or formula), and the type of bottle the caregivers are using. Infants with palatal clefts should be using special feeding devices which are reviewed in detail in chapter 10 on Nursing Issues for the Patient with Cleft Lip and Palate. Determining the length of time it takes to feed, time between feedings, and volume taken per feeding can also provide valuable insight into the child's nutritional status. Some infants have clinically significant gastroesophageal reflux; and the provider should inquire about the frequency and volume of regurgitation, as

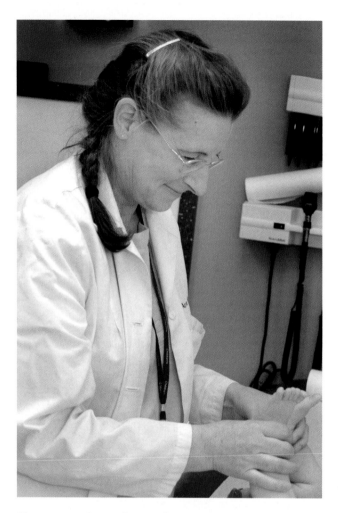

Figure 11–1. A complete newborn exam may be easier to perform if the examiner defers the craniofacial exam until the end.

well as the level of the infant's discomfort with these episodes. Babies who are taking an average of less than 2.5 ounces per pound in each 24-h period, or take more than 30 min to feed, require additional evaluation. The provider should also inquire about the child's respiratory status. It is not uncommon for neonates with orofacial clefts to have "noisy breathing." However, they should not show signs of increased work of breathing. Parental report of respiratory symptoms (e.g., head bobbing, nasal flaring, retractions) warrants further assessment of the child's respiratory status.

Highlights of the Physical Examination

The neonatal exam is often the most comprehensive evaluation, and the pediatrician should be complete and document well. We recommend delaying the evaluation of the cleft until the end of the exam to improve the likelihood of identifying additional malformations (Fig. 11–1). Initiating the exam with the cleft often elicits questions from the family and can distract the examiner from providing a complete examination.

All neonates should have a weight, height, and occipitofrontal head circumference performed as part of each ex-

amination. Infants with orofacial clefts are expected to gain the same amount of weight as infants without clefts, approximately 30 g per day for the first 3 months. Neonates should regain birth weight by 10 days and those who remain less than birth weight by 14 days require additional evaluation. Assessment of body mass index (kilogram per meter squared), subcutaneous fat distribution, activity level, and neurologic status also provides valuable information in assessing overall nutrition status.

The respiratory assessment is particularly important for infants with "isolated" palatal clefts, and includes close observation of the infant's breathing at rest. The presence of subcostal, intercostal, or suprasternal retractions, and/or head bobbing may indicate obstructed breathing. Additional signs of respiratory compromise can include stridor and/or glossoptosis. Positioning the baby on her side or abdomen will frequently relieve distress caused by upper airway obstruction. Assess the infant's jaw size and position, as well as the relative size of the tongue.

An estimated 30% of children with clefts of the lip and palate, and 50% of children with clefts of the secondary palate, have syndromes or associated malformations.[2] For this reason, the pediatrician should examine the neonate for features that are part of the most common syndromes associated with clefting; and these are reviewed in greater depth in chapter 8 on Syndromes of Orofacial Clefting. This includes documentation of dysmorphic facial features, description of ear configuration, presence of ear tags, position and prominence of the eyes, palpebral fissure length, overall facial symmetry, a thorough cardiac exam, and examination of the extremities.[3] Based on the findings from physical exam, additional studies may be indicated.

Finally, the provider should determine whether the cleft is limited to the lip, palate, or involves both the lip and palate. Document whether the cleft is unilateral or bilateral, complete or incomplete, as discussed in chapter 2 on Classification of Orofacial Clefts. It is also essential to identify unusual features of the cleft (e.g., midline location, premaxillary hypoplasia, or agenesis).

Management

Infants demonstrating inadequate weight gain should receive referral to a cleft team nurse or infant-feeding specialist. A pediatric nutritionist can also provide guidelines for caloric requirements and may recommend increasing the caloric density of the breast milk or formula. Although common in children with Robin sequence, infants with isolated cleft lip and palate rarely require supplemental nutrition through a nasogastric tube. In these cases, it is important to address the etiology of the feeding difficulty and to rule out the possibility of descending aspiration. For some infants, difficulty with feeding may be attributable to the infant's inability to coordinate sucking, swallowing, and breathing. Other infants may have anatomic abnormalities of the upper airway, such as Robin sequence or a laryngeal cleft, that make it difficult to protect the airway while feeding. Babies with suspected anatomic abnormalities of the upper airway should also receive consultation with the appropriate subspecialists (e.g., a pediatric otolaryngologist). Although anatomic reasons for poor feeding must be ruled out, inadequate feeding techniques are the most common cause of poor nutritional intake in infants with isolated cleft lip and palate.

Neonates with isolated palatal clefts require close monitoring to ensure that they do not develop breathing difficulty. The ability to feed and adequately gain weight is dependent on the infant's respiratory effort, and inadequate growth may be a result of chronic respiratory distress. For children with Robin sequence, the child's respiratory status can be dynamic in the first several weeks. An infant who appears to breathe comfortably in the first week of life may develop signs of upper airway obstruction by one month of age or later. Newborns with Robin sequence and evidence of respiratory distress require an evaluation for intervention, which may include prone positioning, initiation of nasogastric feedings, placement of a nasopharyngeal tube, a tongue–lip adhesion, mandibular distraction, and/or tracheotomy. Because of the frequency of Robin sequence, an entire chapter is dedicated to its treatment, and the reader is referred to it for further details.

Some cleft lip/palate teams perform presurgical orthopedic interventions in children with clefts of the lip and palate to decrease the size of the cleft and optimize the surgical outcome. These details are reviewed in chapters 45 and 46 on Presurgical Orthopedics and Nasoalveolar Molding. These early interventions require a high degree of cooperation on the part of the caregiver and frequent clinic visits. The pediatrician can help assess the size of the cleft as well as the ability of the family to participate in the molding process, and help determine the neonate's candidacy for preoperative interventions. Those infants who have wide and complete clefts should receive an early consultation with a surgeon and orthodontist.

Finally, all infants should have an initial newborn hearing evaluation with either a brainstem auditory evoked response (BAER) or otoacoustic emissions (OAE).

The frequency of follow-up during this period depends on several factors, including: appropriateness of weight at the initial visit, average daily weight gain, current feeding evaluation, comfort level of parents, level of involvement of the primary care physician, use of presurgical orthodontics, and travel distance from the cleft or craniofacial team. Recommendations for the timing of follow-up visits over the first 3 months should be individualized for each patient.

EARLY INFANCY (1—4 MONTHS)

Clinic visits during early infancy will focus on evaluation of the infant's health, as well as preparation of the family for the patient's cleft lip repair. For babies that are doing well, these visits provide a chance to reinforce the family's current caretaking and answer any questions. Infants demonstrating poor weight gain or other medical issues, require careful assessment and management.

Goals

1. Monitor feeding and growth
2. Prepare for repair of cleft lip
3. Monitor ear health and hearing
4. Presurgical orthopedics (if indicated)

Highlights of the Medical History

The interim history should include a parental assessment of hearing, frequency of otitis media and/or middle ear effusions, and significant illnesses that would preclude the usual timing of lip repair (cheiloplasty). Infants undergoing nasoalveolar molding may be at increased risk for feeding problems and, therefore, a detailed feeding history is important. The provider should also inquire about parental concerns regarding development and upcoming surgery.

Highlights of the Physical Examination

A routine examination of craniofacial features is important at every age, and includes tympanoscopy, evaluation of the jaws, airway, tongue size and position, breathing, and cleft characteristics. A careful pulmonary and cardiac exam is essential in preparation for upcoming general anesthesia for the lip repair. Reduced pulmonary pressures that occur in the first few weeks of life may make a pathologic murmur easier to appreciate at this age. A focused general exam to reevaluate associated anomalies is worthwhile. Assess nutrition status (current weight, weight gain, feeding) and developmental status. The remainder of the exam can be focused on any issues identified in the history.

Management

As with most aspects of pediatric care for a child with orofacial clefting, much of the visit is spent addressing parental concerns. Critical issues include management of poor weight gain and feeding difficulties, significant airway compromise, or illness that may preclude a scheduled surgery. If close communication between the pediatrician and the surgeon occurs during this and future preoperative phases, optimal surgical outcomes will be achieved with a healthy infant.

It is important to remember that not all families are looking forward to lip repair. Although this is a common focus for families in the neonatal period, many families have grown accustomed to their child's appearance and find the cleft to be a part of their infant's personality. It is worth mentioning that this is entirely normal. Families are often uncomfortable asking detailed questions of their surgeons for fear that it will be perceived as challenging the surgeon's recommendations. Thus, the pediatrician can assist the family with their expectations about surgical outcome. The importance of the pediatrician's role as medical "translator" should not be underestimated.

TRANSITION TO TODDLERHOOD (5—15 MONTHS)

Children typically undergo surgical repair of palatal clefts between 9 and 15 months of age. Optimization of the child's health in the pre- and postoperative period is the primary goal of the clinic visits during this phase of care. This is also an active time for growth and development and children with orofacial clefts may have several risk factors that predispose them to developmental delays. These include poor physical growth associated with difficulty feeding, diminished hearing acuity secondary to eustachian tube dysfunction, altered palatal anatomy that may contribute to abnormal speech, associated syndromes, and difficult parent–infant relationships.[4,5] Research has demonstrated that developmental delays and/or learning disabilities may be more common in infants and toddlers with "isolated" orofacial clefting than in the general pediatric population.[4] The pediatrician should screen for developmental delays and provide timely referrals for appropriate developmental services.[6]

Goals

1. Monitor feeding, growth, and development
2. Prepare for palate repair
3. Assess respiratory status
4. Monitor ear health and hearing; consider myringotomy tubes
5. Instruct parents on the importance of good oral hygiene

Highlights of the Medical History

The provider should specifically inquire about the infant's feeding habits, presence of recurrent upper respiratory tract infections, interim diagnoses of otitis media, and history of cough, wheezing, or respiratory distress. Parental report is a critical part of the developmental evaluation. The provider should assess the infant's developmental milestones and ascertain if parents have concerns about their child's hearing, speech and language development, or gross motor skills.

The preoperative visit is an opportunity for the parents to express their concerns about the upcoming surgery. It is also advisable to explore the family's prior surgical experience, for those who have already completed repair of the lip and/or palate.

Highlights of the Physical Examination

This exam includes an assessment of the infant's nutritional status. The presence of caries and health of the gums should be noted when examining the oropharynx. Reexamination of the infant's jaw size, oral airway, as well as relative tongue size and position is essential for those patients with a history of Robin sequence. Assessment of the infant's respiratory status in supine position may reveal subtle signs of upper airway obstruction. In addition, it is important to document the presence of acute otitis media or middle ear effusions. Many standardized and validated screening instruments have been developed to aid in the assessment of early language and communication skills, gross and fine motor milestones, and social and behavioral skills.[6] Most infants are able to complete a formal behavioral audiologic evaluation by 7–9 months of age.

Management

At the preoperative evaluation, the provider should evaluate the overall health of the infant and determine the child's candidacy for palatal repair. Infants that have demonstrated insufficient weight gain, or show other evidence of inadequate nutritional intake, may benefit from nutritional intervention prior to palatoplasty. In addition, the pediatrician should work with the surgeon and speech pathologist to determine the optimal timing of the palatal repair for infants with features of Robin sequence or other causes of respiratory compromise.

The preoperative visit offers the opportunity to answer remaining questions about the upcoming surgery. The parents may be anxious; and the pediatrician, along with other members of the cleft team, can use the visit to prepare the family for the expected postoperative course. Families should be provided with postoperative instructions that include a feeding plan. Rarely, patients without a prior history of respiratory compromise may show signs or symptoms of upper airway obstruction after palatoplasty. Caregivers should be informed about this potential complication and should receive contact phone numbers for timely reassessment if this occurs.

Children with a history of recurrent otitis media or persistent middle ear effusions frequently benefit from tympanostomy tube insertion at the time of palatal repair. Occasionally, infants with recurrent or persistent otitis media, refractory to multiple courses of antimicrobial therapy, may benefit from tube placement prior to the scheduled repair of the palate. For these reasons, we recommend regular evaluations with an otolaryngologist during this period; and, a more detailed review of this topic is discussed in great detail in chapter 50 on Cleft Palate and Middle Ear Disease.

The pediatrician should work with the social worker and psychologist on the cleft team to recommend appropriate referrals for early intervention for children who demonstrate developmental delays.

Finally, the pediatrician can take advantage of visits during this period to emphasize the importance of good oral hygiene and gingival health. The prevalence of poor dental health in children with orofacial clefting is as high (if not higher) as that of the general pediatric population.[7–9] Good oral health is critical to the success of future orthodontic and surgical interventions. The American Academy of Pediatrics Section on Pediatric Dentistry recommends that all infants receive oral health risk assessments beginning at 6 months of age.[10] In addition, parents should be provided with anticipatory guidance for dental care. Caregivers should be instructed to brush the infant's teeth, limit fruit juices to one cup per day during meals only, avoid placing the infant in bed with a bottle containing anything other than water, and provide optimal exposure to systemic fluoride through drinking water or oral supplements.[10] Pediatricians should also facilitate the identification of a dental home for all patients. Further details regarding oral health of children with orofacial clefts are reviewed in detail in the chapter on Pediatric Dentistry.

SPEECH AND LANGUAGE (16—24 MONTHS)

This is a relatively uneventful time for many children with orofacial clefts, and few children require medical and surgical intervention. The primary purpose of the clinic visits during this period is to ensure that the toddler receives a speech and language evaluation and to monitor ear health and hearing. These visits also provide an important opportunity to monitor development.

Goals
1. Assess ear health and hearing
2. Assess speech and language development
3. Monitor social and motor development and learning

Highlights of the Medical History

As with previous visits, the interim history should include a complete review of systems with an emphasis on growth, development, behavior, and recent illnesses. In addition, a good sleep history may uncover subtle symptoms of upper airway obstruction that could be related to the recent palatoplasty and/or physiologic adenoidal hypertrophy. Assessment of the psychological status of the child and family is an essential component of the history.

Highlights of the Physical Examination

Observation of the child during this visit will provide data regarding the child's developmental status and spontaneous speech.[11] Some children are quite cooperative with a structured exam, while others are easier to assess when the provider's attention appears to be focused on the parent. Examination of the tympanic membranes includes evaluation for acute otitis media, middle ear effusions, as well as the presence and patency of tubes. Children should also have a hearing evaluation.

Examination of the oropharynx is indicated, with particular attention to general oral hygiene, evidence of caries, and overall gingival health. This is a good time to reinforce good dental habits and provide instruction for parents who need additional guidance.

Management

Children who demonstrate impairments in speech or language development should receive timely referrals for appropriate speech services. The pediatrician should also review results from the child's hearing evaluation and facilitate consultation with an otolaryngologist for patients with persistent eustachian tube dysfunction. Referral to a pediatric dentist is important for children who do not have a dental home in the community. The pediatrician can also recommend developmental services for children with developmental delays, not already receiving therapy.

Parents that are planning pregnancies in the near future may appreciate the opportunity to discuss their recurrence risks with a genetic counselor. It is also beneficial to readdress the family's psychosocial situation and provide support as indicated.

THE PRESCHOOL PERIOD (2—5 YEARS)

The goal of clinic visits performed during this period is to optimize the child's transition to elementary school. Assessment of speech is often easier at this age and the provider can make recommendations for interventions to maximize the child's ability to communicate. For many children, kindergarten represents the first structured social environment. Preparation of the child and family for cleft-related questions from peers may empower the child and help minimize teasing. Some parents and children may wish to receive secondary cheiloplasty or rhinoplasty prior to entering school.

Goals
1. Evaluate speech and language, manage velopharyngeal insufficiency
2. Assess ear health and hearing
3. Consider lip and/or nose revision before starting school
4. Address psychosocial concerns in the preschool and kindergarten period
5. Optimize developmental services, in and out of school

Highlights of the Medical History

Growth and development, as well as sleep patterns, should be the focus of this history. Children with a history of cleft palate may be at increased risk for obstructive sleep apnea. The provider should ask the parents if the child seems appropriately rested. Questions include the child's bed time, time required to fall asleep, number of hours of sleep, time of wakening, presence of snoring, presence of hyperactivity during the day, and need for daytime naps.

Teachers recommend that children entering kindergarten have the requisite physical, social, and cognitive skills to succeed in the classroom.[12] The parents should be invited to express concerns about the child's development. The pediatrician should assess whether the child can perform simple tasks, such as name colors and letters. Most children will be able to walk, run, and climb stairs, and have the fine motor skills required to use a pen or pencil. The ability to participate in group and individual activities is also critical for success in school. Ask whether the child is able to follow instructions, work with other children, and modify behavior.[12]

Highlights of the Physical Examination

Children are often able to provide a better speech sample during this visit. The perceptual speech evaluation should include a screen for speech intelligibility, ability to express oneself, and the presence of hypernasality. Physical examination focuses on the oropharynx with particular attention to palatal movement, general oral hygiene, tooth eruption, and dental occlusion. Assessment of the middle ears and review of the audiologic evaluations should be included.

Management

Children should undergo annual speech and language evaluations by a speech-language pathologist. Timely referrals for children who could benefit from articulation and/or language therapy are necessary to avoid developing altered and compensatory speech patterns (e.g., glottal stops). Children with evidence of velopharyngeal insufficiency will benefit from additional assessments, including a videofluoroscopic speech study, naso-endoscopy, and/or consultation with a surgeon. The details regarding the assessment and treatment of cleft palate speech can be found in chapters 34–43 within the section on Cleft Palate Speech and Management of Velopharyngeal Dysfunction.

The pediatrician has an important role in identifying areas of developmental delay and providing early referrals for developmental services to optimize the child's transition to school.[12,13]

Families with children that are close to starting kindergarten may benefit from consultation with a psychosocial professional before the school year begins. The psychosocial professional can assist the family with obtaining appropriate support services through the school. In addition, they can provide psychological support and council the patient on helpful ways to respond to questions from peers. The parents' response to the child's transition to school significantly influences the child's success. The pediatrician can use this opportunity to maximize the family's school-readiness and improve the likelihood of a positive experience.

THE ORTHODONTIC YEARS (6—12 YEARS)

This is a relatively quiescent period in the care of a child with cleft lip and palate. Team assessments tend to be less frequent and the focus is on oral health and preparation for alveolar ridge bone grafting. However, it is important to remember that this is a time of great change for children. The transition to middle school can be traumatic. Peers are less likely to simply ask questions about "what" the cleft is and "why" it happened, and more likely to tease and taunt. It is important for the provider to empower the patients by focusing the interview on the child and involving the patient in the decisions about management.

Goals

1. Assess ear health and hearing
2. Assess speech and language, manage velopharyngeal insufficiency
3. Consider orthodontic interventions
4. Determine optimal time for alveolar bone grafting
5. Assess school and psychosocial adjustment, peer acceptance
6. Ensure appropriate educational support in school
7. Assess symptoms of obstructive sleep apnea
8. Begin to redirect the interview to the child

Highlights of the Medical History

Many children with cleft palate will continue to have episodes of otitis media and may still require tympanostomy tubes. This is also an age when the symptoms and severity of obstructive sleep apnea may become more apparent. Ask about snoring, daytime somnolence, decreased school performance, naps, falling asleep in the car, enuresis, and decreased sleep latency period (falling asleep rapidly). The provider will likely need to rely on the parents for much of this history. However, the intake should begin with the patient, and the pediatrician should try to limit discussion with the parents to the health-related details that the patient cannot answer.

Discussion of school performance is an important part of the assessment. Suboptimal school performance may result from inadequately addressed psychosocial issues, health impairment (e.g., obstructive sleep apnea), cognitive problems, and learning disabilities. The pediatrician should also ask about signs of puberty to help determine optimal timing for future orthodontic and/or orthognathic procedures.

Highlights of the Physical Examination

The physical exam should focus on dental hygiene, dental occlusion, and speech quality. Evaluation of ear health and hearing remains an integral part of the assessment. The examination can be used as a tool to open up discussion with the patient. For example, following the oral exam, discuss oral hygiene and any impediments to improved oral health. When examining the lip and alveolus, ask the child about his impression of his appearance and any concerns or desires he may have with regard to additional surgery. At this age it is often helpful to ask "if you could have one thing that was different about your cleft, what would it be?" This simple question may open a dialogue about the child's feelings regarding appearance or speech quality. Children may not want to mention their dissatisfaction with their surgical outcome to their treating surgeon. Speech quality can have also a major psychosocial impact on school-aged children. A sensitive, though direct discussion is the best way to address issues related to appearance and speech.

Management

The major management issues during this period are oral health and readiness for alveolar ridge bone grafting. The pediatrician should work with the child's orthodontist and the surgeon to determine the optimal time to perform this procedure. Providers should also consider prosthetic obturator or surgical management of velopharyngeal insufficiency. Attention to psychosocial development, and school performance is also critical. The pediatrician should facilitate referrals for those children who require additional support services. Involvement of the patient in these discussions is empowering and increases the likelihood of patient participation in the care and satisfaction with treatment.

THE TEEN YEARS AND TRANSITION TO INDEPENDENCE (12—21 YEARS)

Adolescence presents unique challenges for the care of children with cleft lip and palate. It is a time of increased social interactions and greater responsibility. Young adults are often self-conscious and focused on appearance. The presence of a visible facial difference makes adolescence even more challenging.

Visits during the adolescence years provide an opportunity to maximize the surgical results of prior lip, nose, and palate repairs. In addition, the pediatrician can talk with the teen about the possibility of treatments (including addi-

tional orthodontics and/or reconstructive surgery) to maximize dental occlusion. Finally, the provider should address issues that are essential for a seamless transition to independence and adult care.

Goals

1. Accommodate teen's wishes for jaw surgery, rhinoplasty if indicated
2. Optimize orthodontic results
3. Refer for genetic counseling
4. Assess school and psychosocial adjustment
5. Ensure appropriate speech

Highlights of the Medical History

Focus the interaction on the teenager (Fig. 11–2). By asking the patient about their concerns, the provider can learn about the teen's worries and gain insight into their level of self confidence. The teen's self-esteem has as much impact on their self-image as the quality of the reconstructive surgery. Most teens have concerns that fall into one of two categories: *function-* residual concerns about speech, dental, and orthognathic/orthodontic issues, or *form-*perceived need for lip and/or nasal revision or other secondary surgeries. Perhaps the most important aspects of the interaction during the clinic visit are that you direct your conversation to the teen and that you are candid in your discussion about their concerns. The provider needs to remain sensitive to the fact that patients do not want to feel interrogated; however, a direct conversation with the teen about their concerns will help to empower them. At the conclusion of the discussion with the teen, turn to the parents and ask if they have any additional

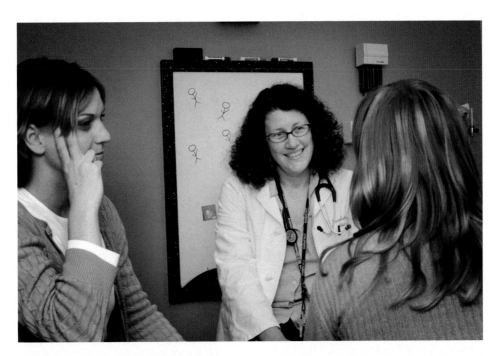

Figure 11–2. The parents and the pediatrician often learn a great deal from a medical interview that is directed to the teenager.

concerns. It is remarkable how often their first comment will be "I had no idea that he was concerned about that." A dialogue often begins between the teen and his parents which can provide insight into the family dynamics and the nature of their concerns. By beginning the dialogue with the teen, the provider can give the patient an appropriate voice in their care.

The review of systems should include a detailed sleep history and address symptoms indicating sleep-disturbed breathing. Inquire about school performance, and elicit concerns on the part of the teen and parents. All adolescents should be screened for risk behaviors (e.g., drug exposure) and mental health status (which should include a screen for depression).

Highlights of the Physical Examination

Repeat the craniofacial exam with particular emphasis on oral hygiene, dental occlusion, and speech quality. Tympanoscopy and a formal hearing assessment should also be performed.

Assess the lip, nose, and palate (including the patency and symmetry of the nares, deviation of the nasal septum, degree of palatal movement, etc.). Document growth parameters and signs of puberty.

Management

The information gathered during the history and exam will dictate the direction of the patient's management. Consultation with a surgeon should be facilitated for teens that express a desire for additional lip or nose revisions. Braces for dental alignment may be an option from some teens. The pediatrician should also monitor jaw growth and work with the orthodontist, surgeon, and teen to determine whether orthognathic surgery would be beneficial for teens with midface retrusion. Teens who are concerned about speech should undergo a formal speech and language evaluation by a speech pathologist. If a psychosocial professional is not already involved in the teen's care, consultation at this time is important to ensure that the teen has appropriate support resources and realistic expectations for surgery. Failure to address the teen's emotional issues and expectations prior to surgery may result in unnecessary surgery and/or dissatisfaction with a technically successful surgical outcome.

Genetics and Heritability

A teen's response to the question: "How likely is it that you will have a child with a cleft?" may vary; and, the response may be, "I know I will have a child with a cleft," "fifty-fifty," or "I don't know." Few teens are considering having children in the near future; however, most are ready and interested to talk about it. The provider should assess the teen's interest in learning about recurrence risks and suggest genetic counseling. Ask the teen if they have ever thought about the possibility that their child will have a cleft. This may start a conversation that is quite interactive. Empowering the teen will improve the patient–provider relationship, provide the pediatrician with a much better idea of the teen's concerns, and increase the likelihood of follow-through. After a general discussion about recurrence risks (which is often much lower than the teen's previous perception), the pediatrician may then recommend a referral to a genetic counselor to discuss the teen's recurrence risks in greater detail, tailored to the patient's family history.

Transition to Adult Care

The teenager's response to transition from the treating team or primary care physician to adult care can vary widely. Some may view this as a statement of completion of numerous stressful surgical interventions, a sense of being "done." Other teens become anxious and fearful that they will not be able to obtain appropriate care. While most cleft and craniofacial teams treat children with orofacial clefts until age 18–21, the nature and coordination of care varies. Most physicians and dentists involved in the care of children with orofacial clefts accept the value of coordinated team care; however, this model may engender dependence. A family who has been required to coordinate cleft care for their child (by making appointments with various providers from different offices on different days) is much more likely to be able to navigate the health care system than a family that has had care coordinated for their child by a large cleft team. This is not to say that we would recommend uncoordinated care; however, the pediatrician on a cleft team must be cognizant of the fact that the team has an obligation to the patient to provide them with the requisite tools to coordinate their own care. Providing your patients with referrals to adult providers as they make this transition can be very helpful.

The details involved in the successful transition to adult care will vary from center to center; however, basic information should be provided to every patient upon their completion of care from the pediatric cleft team (Table 11–3).

Table 11–3.
A List of Documents to Provide to the Teen Transferring Care to Adult Health Care Providers
Principal diagnosis and problem list
Presurgical and surgical treatments
Copies of operative reports
Key clinical reports (genetic counseling, significant illnesses, hospitalizations)
Residual concerns (for plastic or ENT surgery, orthodontics, or orthognathic surgery)

References

1. Critical Elements of Care: Cleft Lip and Palate, 4th edn. The Center for Children with Special Health Needs, Children's Hospital and Regional Medical Center, Seattle, Washington, 2006.
2. Wyszynski DF, Sarkozi A, Czeizel AE. Oral clefts with associated anomalies: Methodological issues. *Cleft Palate Craniofac J* 43:1, 2006.
3. Aase JM. *Diagnostic Dysmorphology*. New York: Plenum Medical Book Company, 1990.
4. Speltz ML, Endriga MC, Hill S, et al. Cognitive and psychomotor development of infants with orofacial clefts. *J Pediatr Psychol* 25:185, 1999.
5. Endriga MC, Kapp-Simon KA. Psychological issues in craniofacial care: State of the art. *Cleft Palate Craniofac J* 36:3, 1999.
6. American Academy of Pediatrics Policy Statement. Identifying infants and young children with developmental disorders in the medical home: An algorithm for developmental surveillance and screening. *Pediatrics* 118:405, 2006.
7. Chapple JR, Nunn JH. The oral health of children with clefts of the lip, palate, or both. *Cleft Palate Craniofac J* 38:525, 2001.
8. Lages EM, Marcos B, Pordeus IA. Oral health of individuals with cleft lip, cleft palate, or both. *Cleft Palate Craniofac J* 41:59, 2004.
9. Kirchberg A, Treide A, Hemprich A. Investigation of caries prevalence in children with cleft lip, alveolus, and palate. *J Craniomaxillofac Surg* 32:216, 2004.
10. Hale KJ. Oral health risk assessment timing and establishment of the dental home. *Pediatrics* 111:1113, 2003.
11. Dixon SD. Two years: Language emerges. In Dixon SD, Stein MT (eds). *Encounters with Children: Pediatric Behavior and Development*, 3rd edn. St. Louis, Mosby, 2000, pp. 301.
12. Nader PR. Five years: Entering school. In Dixon SD, Stein MT (eds). *Encounters with Children: Pediatric Behavior and Development*, 3rd edn. St. Louis: Mosby, 2000, p. 367.
13. Zuckerman B, Halfon N. School readiness: An idea whose time has arrived. *Pediatrics* 111:1435, 2003.

Primary Cleft Lip and Palate Repair

A Short History of Cleft Lip and Cleft Palate

Peter Randall, MD, FACS • Oksana Jackson, MD

ANCIENT HISTORY

Although cleft lip and palate are widespread in the world today, there are few reports from ancient cultures.[1] Some of the oldest representations of cleft lip are found in the 3000-year-old "huacos," or mummy-grave potteries, from Peru (Fig. 12–1).[2] The mysterious female figure shown here has an obvious unilateral cleft lip, but unbelievable symmetry of the nose. The ancient Egyptians wrote about the medical and surgical care of facial trauma (including the use of pressure dressings), but they did not mention clefts or their care.[3] George Dorrance, in the *Operative Story of Cleft Palate*, reports that an Egyptian mummy was discovered with a cleft palate.[3–6] Also, a dental prosthesis made of gold wiring and fixed to the teeth was found in El Gizeh dated approximately 2500 BC, thus representing the first known intraoral prosthesis.[7]

Clefts are scarcely mentioned in the writings from Ancient Greece and Rome. They do not appear in the writings of Hippocrates (460–375 BC) or of A. Cornelius Celsus (25 BC to 50 AD), best known for his medical encyclopedia *De Medicina*. Perhaps the first mention of a cleft in ancient European history is in the writings of the physician Galen (131–206 AD), wherein he refers to clefts of the lip as *colobomatae*.[4] Galen is also credited with first using the word *lagocheilos* or "lip like a hare."[8] According to some reports, prosthetic obturation of palatal clefts was used commonly in the ancient Roman world during the time of Celsus.[7]

Susruta, the great surgeon of ancient India, in his writings from about the 6th century BC, describes a number of

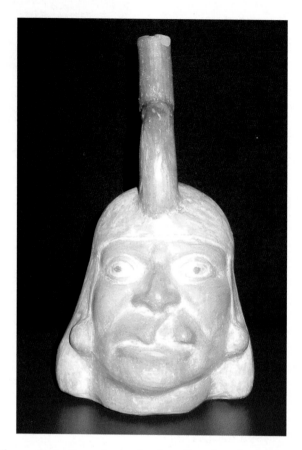

Figure 12–1. Copy of water jug from Lima, Peru thought to be about 3,000 years old, showing a female figure with a cleft lip. This is one of the oldest representations of a cleft lip from the ancient world. Reproduced from H. Landezuri, *History of Plastic Surgery in Peru*, 1992, p. 35–36, with permission from Lippincott, Williams, and Wilkins.

surgical procedures involving the lips and face, but it is unclear whether any of these were for congenital clefts. He describes procedures on the uvula:

... by means of forceps between thumb and finger, drawing the uvula forward, the physician may cut it with a sickle-shaped knife above the top of the tongue.[9]

The written history of ancient China is more illustrative. Translation by Morse and Boo-Chai of ancient Chinese texts reveals many written accounts of cleft lip repairs and cleft lip surgeons:

In the Chin Dynasty (229–317 AD), there was a surgeon who did plastic surgery for harelip. In the Tang Dynasty (618–901 AD) another surgeon, Fang Kan, was designated as "the doctor of lip repair" from which he obtained "considerable repute."[9]

An interesting story, also retold by Boo-Chai, is of a Chinese surgeon who repaired the lip of a poor 18-year-old named Wei Yang-Chi in about 390 AD:

This young man overcame his handicap and became Governor General of six Chinese provinces. This resulted in the perception, which persists in some South Sea Island countries even today, that those with clefts are special and "have been touched by God".[10]

In Turkey, Charaf ed-Din authored the first Turkish surgical manuscript (ca. 1465) and carried on the traditions of the great Arabian surgeon Albucasis (936–1013 AD) of Cordoba, Spain. In his illustrated manuscript, there is an image depicting the cauterization of a lip fissure with a hot iron; this technique was thought by some to be used by Turkish surgeons for clefts of the lip as well (Fig. 12–2). The edges of a cleft lip were touched by a very hot iron, thus creating a third degree burn. After separation of the eschar, the edges were sutured together to repair the cleft. This technique circumvented the need to make an incision and, more importantly, the need to control blood loss.[11,12]

UNILATERAL CLEFT LIP REPAIR

Early European History

Surgical progress was slow in Europe due to frequent postoperative infections, inadequate anesthesia, and inability to control bleeding. The first description of a surgical cleft lip repair did not appear until approximately 950 AD in a book

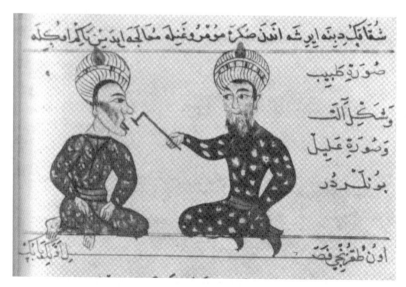

Figure 12–2. Cauterization of a fissure of the lower lip from an illustrated manuscript of the Turkish surgeon Charaf ed-Din written in 1465 A.D.. Reproduced from "Harelip Repair in Colonial America," Blaire O. Rogers in *Plastic and Reconstructive Surgery*, 1964, p. 143, with permission from Lippincott, Williams, and Wilkins.

entitled *The Leech Book of Bald* from pre-Norman Britain.[1] Saxon surgeons at that time were known as "leeches."[13] In this manuscript, it is written:

... fore harelip, pound mastic very small, add white of egg, and mingle as thou dost vermillion, cut with a knife the false edges of the lip, sew with silk, then smear without and within with the salve, ere the silk rot.[14]

Numerous descriptions of cleft lip repairs are found in European literature from the 13 to 17th centuries, all of which fundamentally comprise freshening of the cleft edges and suturing them together with the adjunct of various dressings and salves to promote healing and combat infection. For example, the Flemish surgeon Jehman Yperman (1295–1351) wrote that unilateral and bilateral clefts may be "sutured with needles some distance from the cut margins and wrap around with figure eight." He noted that some surgeons used relaxing incisions externally and laterally in the cheek, but advised against their use because the subsequent facial disfigurement might "compromise the reputation of the surgeon."[14] In France, Ambroise Paré (1510–1590), one of the great surgical figures of the Renaissance, and his student Guillemean used silver needles with tips of steel and thread of waxed linen. Paré, in 1575, popularized the term "bec-de-lieure" or "lip of hare" to describe a cleft lip. He was likely the first surgeon to include an illustration of the repaired lip in his surgical works (Fig. 12–3).[15–18]

Another famous Renaissance surgeon, Gaspar Tagliacozzi (1545–1599) of Bologna, Italy, described his repair in 1597. He used a sharp knife or scissor, and he stressed the importance of full-thickness sutures through the lip. In his writings, Tagliacozzi notes that "the Artist must therefore pass his Needle straight through the Lip from the outside inwards, and on the other side, he must pass the Needle from the inside outwards." He also recommended "some compresses, dipped in Whites of Eggs and Rosewater ... applied both to the inside and the outside of the Wound."[1,19]

In addition to the various ointments and salves used to promote healing, compression bandages frequently were applied during surgery to assist in closure. Fabricius of Aquapendente (1537–1619), a famous anatomist, physiologist, and surgeon who practiced primarily in Padua, Italy, described in 1619 how, in wide clefts, he used an "agglutinative Bandage to bring the edges of the cleft together or to relieve tension on the cleft margins before he started to freshen the edges."[20] In 1686, Johan Philip Hofmann of Heidelberg described a snugly fitting cloth cap with extensions over the cheeks and upper lip. These extensions had hooks around which he would wind thread to pull the edges of the cleft closer together (Fig. 12–4).[21]

Other notable cleft surgeons in early European history were Van Roonhuyse (1622–1672), a surgeon from Amsterdam, who was one of the first to recommend early surgery for cleft lip at the age of 3–4 months,[22] and James Cooke (1614–1688), an English surgeon from Warwick. Cooke advised the following perioperative regimen when operating on such a young child:

"If possible (the infant should be) kept from sleep for ten or twelve hours before the operation, that it may be disposed to sleep presently after. For it have ready a glass of wine or cordial, in case of fainting upon loss of blood. Observe, if there be great deformity, what to do, lest you make it worse than it was."[23]

The Nineteenth Century

Straight line closures of clefts of the lip remained the standard approach for the early part of the 19th century. Two French surgeons, Joseph Malgaigne and Germanicus Mirault, dissatisfied with the inevitable postoperative contracture of the

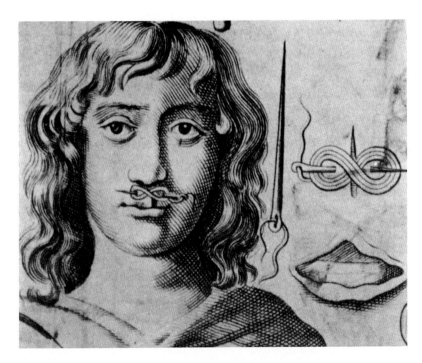

Figure 12–3. Silver needles with sharp steel tips and linen thread were used in a figure of eight fashion in cleft lip repair in 1676. Reproduced from *The Source Book of Plastic Surgery*, ed. Frank McDowell, 1977, p. 194, with permission from Lippincott, Williams, and Wilkins.

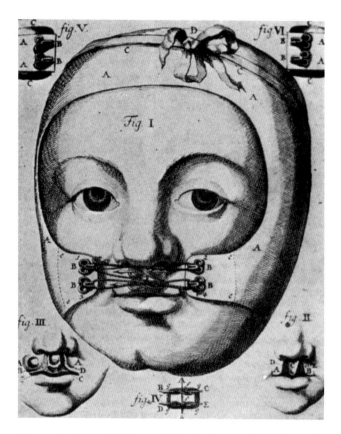

Figure 12–4. In 1686, Johan Philip Hofmann of Heidelberg de-scribed a snugly fitting cloth cap with extensions over the cheeks and upper lip. These extensions had hooks around which he would wind thread to pull the edges of the cleft closer together. Reproduced from *The Source Book of Plastic Surgery*, ed. Frank Mc-Dowell, 1977, p. 193, with permission from Lippincott, Williams, and Wilkins.

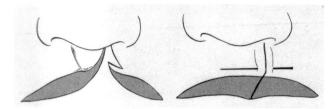

Figure 12–6. Germanicus Mirault's operation made only one horizontal incision on the lateral lip, thus creating a triangular flap of skin and vermillion which was advanced medially. Reproduced from *Cleft Craft*, vol. 1, 1976, p. 102, with permission from D. Ralph Millard.

nique, resecting the turned down medial flap, making only one horizontal incision on the lateral lip and bringing the resulting triangular flap of lateral skin and vermillion across medially (Fig. 12–6).[6] He thus attempted to fill out the vermillion in the line of the incision to avoid the notch or "whistling" deformity. Mirault described many variations of this closure with different flaps from both sides of the cleft; however, he is remembered best for his innovative triangular flap which remained in the cleft surgeon's armamentarium in one form or another for over 100 years.

In the second half of the 19th century, M.H. Collins of Dublin contributed significantly to cleft lip repair by ad-dressing the displaced alar base. He designed a small laterally based flap at the alar base and inserted this into a small in-cision made in the base of the columella. He anchored this flap into the periosteum of the nasal spine. This technique improved alar base symmetry, built a firm nasal floor, and filled out a small "shoulder" in the base of the columella to restore a more normal contour.[6]

In 1879, William Rose proposed curving the incisions away from the center of the cleft to lengthen the closure (Fig. 12–7). In 1912, James Thompson, Professor of Surgery at the University of Texas in Galveston, further refined this tech-nique by paring the cleft edges in the shape of a diamond excision and advocating the use of a compass to mark the an-gled incisions so that they would be precisely matched. This technique of curved incisions became known as the Rose–Thompson repair. Although Rose and Thompson are given

straight line lip repair and resulting "whistling" deformity, were among the first to develop alternative repairs. In 1843, Malgaigne described a two flap operation to lengthen the lip. He turned down flaps of skin from each side of the cleft and made horizontal full thickness cuts on either side of the cleft, which when opened and sutured to each other, lengthening the lip (Fig. 12–5). In 1844, Mirault further refined this tech-

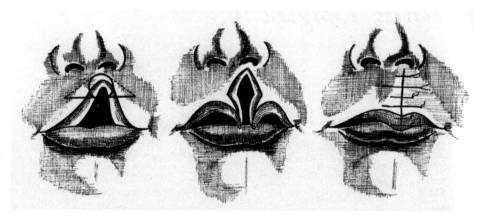

Figure 12–5. The Malgaigne two flap operation designed to lengthen the lip and rebuild the "tubercle." Reproduced from *Cleft Craft*, vol. 1, 1976, p. 102 with permission from D. Ralph Millard.

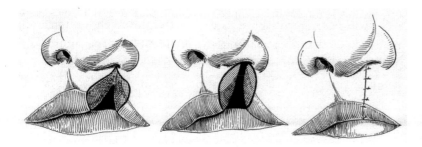

Figure 12–7. The incisions for unilateral cleft lip repair designed by William Rose in 1879, which curved away from the center of the cleft to lengthen the closure. Reproduced from *Cleft Craft*, vol. 1, 1976, p. 90, with permission from D. Ralph Millard.

credit for this design, Von Graefe in 1816 and Husson of Great Britain in 1836 both had previously suggested similar curved incisions in their lip repairs.[6]

The Twentieth Century

Victor Veau of Paris was widely admired in the field of cleft surgery (Fig. 12–8). In 1925, he published a technique for unilateral repair similar to Mirault's final design; however, he quickly abandoned this technique for a more complex variation which sought to lengthen the cleft margins by paring and also to reposition the alar base. He discarded a minimum of tissue and focused on a good muscular approximation with suture, known as his *suture musculaire*. In addition to repositioning the alar base, he also closed the nostril floor and the anterior palatal cleft along with the cleft lip (Fig. 12–9).[6,24] He was criticized by some for the asymmetry of Cupid's bow produced by his repair. Since Veau was such a

prominent surgeon in the field of clefts, however, his design was embraced by many, and he had a significant influence on cleft surgery in Europe.[6]

At the same time, Vilray P. Blair and James Barrett Brown also were experimenting with and perfecting Mirault's original technique in the United States. They were both general surgeons at Washington University in St. Louis, and they dominated the cleft lip surgical scene in the United States in the 1930s and 1940s. Blair is remembered for heading the Head and Neck Team at the Walter Reed Army Hospital in Washington DC during World War I, and, with Dr. Robert Ivy, for forming and instructing teams sent to France to treat the many head and neck injuries resulting from trench warfare. He started the plastic surgery programs at Barnes Hospital

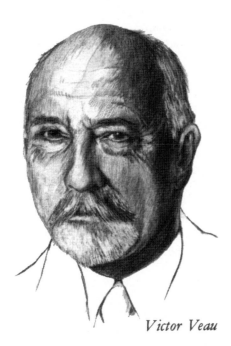

Figure 12–8. Victor Veau of Paris, France was one of the most prominent cleft surgeons of the early 20th century. His contributions to cleft surgery include his *suture musculaire*, or orbicularis muscle approximation during cleft lip repair, and his practice of nasal mucoperiosteal closure of the hard palate in cleft palate surgery. Reproduced from *Cleft Craft*, vol. 1, 1976, p. 94, with permission from D. Ralph Millard.

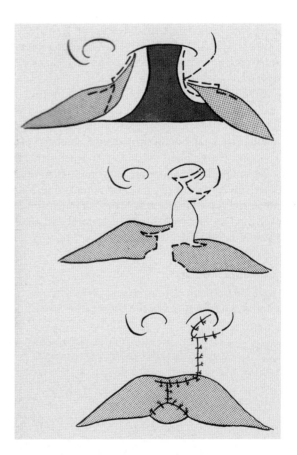

Figure 12–9. Victor Veau's unilateral cleft lip operation designed to lengthen the cleft margins by paring and also reposition the alar base. Reproduced from *Cleft Craft*, vol. 1, 1976, p. 94, with permission from D. Ralph Millard.

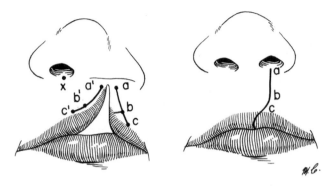

Figure 12–10. The Blair-Brown-Mirault operation, designed by Vilroy Blair and James Barrett Brown in the 1920's and similar to Mirault's original triangular flap design. Reproduced from *Cleft Lip and Palate; Surgical, Dental, and Speech Aspects*, eds. Grabb, Rosenstein, and Bzoch, p. 177, with permission from Little, Brown, and Co.

and the St. Louis Children's Hospital at Washington University. Barrett Brown joined Blair in St. Louis in 1923, and together in 1930, they published *Mirault's Operation for Single Harelip*.[25]

The operation described by Blair and Barrett Brown employed a small triangular flap from the lateral side of the cleft above the vermilion to add length to the incision and fullness to the lower part of the lip (Fig. 12–10). They were also among the first to try to correct the cleft nostril width and flattened nasal tip. Later, Barrett Brown with Frank McDowell, another respected St. Louis surgeon, added measurements related to specific anatomic landmarks so that reliable reproducible results could be obtained and tailored to each child.[26] This Mirault–Blair–Brown–McDowell method became very popular because it achieved good symmetry and excellent nasal correction. It resulted, however, in a high point of the vermilion in the center of the lip and little semblance of a cupid's bow. Moreover, it did not address the maloriented cleft orbicularis muscle.[27] At one point, the Mirault–Blair–Brown–McDowell method was likely the most popular operation for unilateral cleft lip in the United States, although some surgeons, including Professor Kilner of Oxford, still preferred the straight line closure method.[28]

The Quadrilateral Flap

The next milestone in cleft lip repair was to create a cupid's bow, and A.B. Le Mesurier of the Hospital for Sick Children

in Toronto is credited with accomplishing this. He designed a quadrilateral flap from the lateral aspect of the lip which put a curve in the vermilion on the cleft side to mimic the cupid's bow on the noncleft side (Fig. 12–11).[29–31] Le Mesurier admitted his design was not original, but similar to the flap described by the German surgeon Hagedom 50 years before.[29] He presented his operation at the 17th Annual Meeting of the American Society of Plastic and Reconstructive Surgery in West Virginia in November 1948, and he impressed those in the audience, including Barrett Brown and McDowell, with his results.[5] Many surgeons subsequently began using his technique, and some developed their own modifications of it, including Wallace Steffensen, who proposed a triangular wedge excision of the medial lip to facilitate inset of the quadrilateral flap. D. Ralph Millard added an ingenious system of measurements for the technique, and Tom Cronin of Houston advocated using the vertical length of the normal side to calculate the length of the cleft side. One criticism of this technique was that it produced an unnatural scar and another, as stated by Clayton De Haan, was that "measurements made from the cleft side are arbitrary. Even a slight miscalculation in the size of the quadrilateral flap can make the lip too long or too short on the cleft side."[6,32]

The Randall–Tennison Repair

In 1952, Charles Tennison of Houston introduced two concepts: using a stencil to design a triangular flap and using the z-plasty principle to gain vertical length. Tennison used a bent paper clip, sterilized for the operation, to figure out the position of an almost equilateral triangular flap on the lateral lip above the vermilion (Fig. 12–12).[33] He described his technique at the Annual Meeting of the American Society for Plastic and Reconstructive Surgery in Colorado Springs and impressed Kirwin Marcks of Allentown, Pennsylvania. Marcks not only adopted this technique but promoted and popularized it, claiming it was "so much more practical." He emphasized that this triangle should be placed in the most inferior position where he felt the lip was most deficient.[34] The same year that Tennison published his results, A. Duarte Cardoso of San Paulo, Brazil published a technique which similarly sought to preserve the cupid's bow. He noted that the cupid's bow on the cleft side was really not missing but was simply displaced upward and needed to be brought down to the horizontal position.[35] It is not clear whether Tennison

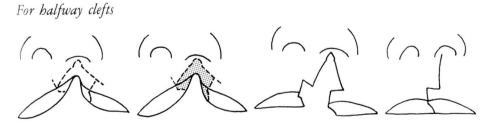

Figure 12–11. Le Mesurier's quadrilateral flap operation put a curve in the vermilion on the cleft side to create a Cupid's bow. Reproduced from *Cleft Craft*, vol. 1, 1976, p. 129, with permission from D. Ralph Millard.

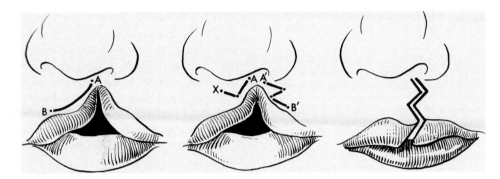

Figure 12–12. The Tennison triangular flap operation created an almost equilateral triangular flap on the lateral lip which was drawn with a stencil for precision. Reproduced from *Cleft Craft*, vol. 1, 1976, p. 139, with permission from D. Ralph Millard.

was aware of Cardoso's contribution, but their ideas complimented one another.

Peter Randall of Philadelphia also adopted Marcks' technique but made some significant alterations. He observed that in incomplete clefts, there was often only a small amount of displacement of the cupid's bow, and he felt that a large triangular flap, as in Tennison's original description, was unnecessary. Working backward from postoperative photographs, he refined the measurements and developed a mathematical system for designing the lip operation. He reduced the size of the triangular flap and significantly simplified the operation (Fig. 12–13).[36–38] This triangular flap approach became known as the Tennison–Randall repair.

The triangular flap operation sustained a long period of popularity with many variations. In 1966, Thomas Cronin from Houston described elevation of the lateral triangular flap 1 mm above the mucocutaneous border in order to facilitate

vermilion alignment. David Davies, Jr. of Cape Town, South Africa advocated two equal flaps of a pure z-plasty to achieve a predetermined height on the cleft side. Another variation popular in Europe was designed by Tord Skoog of Sweden. He used one triangular flap from the lateral side of the cleft just above the skin vermilion border and a second triangle in the top of the lip just beneath the columella (Fig. 12–14). Later, he put this upper flap inside the nostril into the base of the columella, where the scars were hidden.[5,6,38,39]

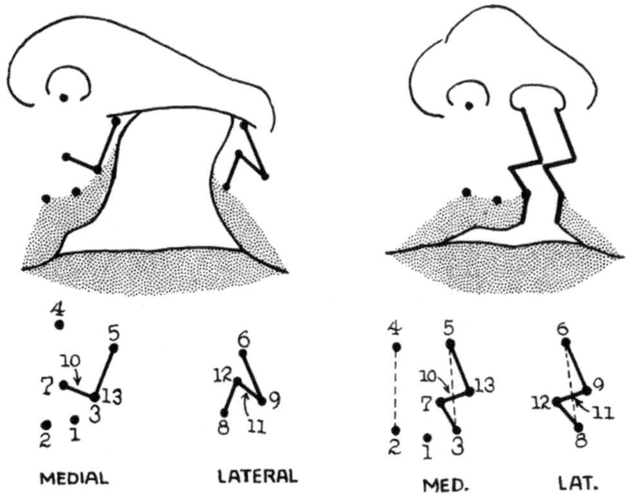

The Rotation–Advancement Technique

The next innovation in unilateral cleft lip repair was the rotation-advancement technique described by D. Ralph Millard. The conception of this novel technique is an interesting story. In 1953, Millard was deployed to Korea as a surgeon with the First Division of the Fleet Marines of the United States Navy. A Korean man who was working for the Americans learned of Millard's interest in cleft surgery and brought him to see his 7-year-old son, who had a wide unrepaired unilateral cleft lip. Dr. Millard performed an excellent Le Mesurier repair, but afterwards pondered its many shortcomings. The division photographer printed out a number of 8 × 10 preoperative photographs of this patient, and Millard worked for hours with these photographs seeking a better solution. One

Figure 12–13. Peter Randall's modifications of Tennison's triangular flap design included a detailed system of measurements which could be applied to clefts of varying severity. Reproduced from "A Triangular Flap Operation for the Primary Repair of Unilateral Clefts of the Lip," Peter Randall, in *Plastic and Reconstructive Surgery*, 1959, p. 486, with permission from Lippincott, Williams, and Wilkins.

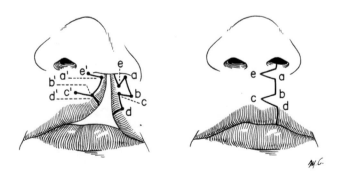

Figure 12–14. Skoog's design for unilateral cleft lip repair, described in 1958, put one triangular flap in the lower third of the lip and another just below the columella. Reproduced from *Cleft Lip and Palate; Surgical, Dental, and Speech Aspects*, eds. Grabb, Rosenstein, and Bzoch, p. 178, with permission from Little, Brown, and Co.

night while working with the prints on a make-shift drawing board, he notes:

I had fallen asleep . . . I opened my eyes . . . the photographs were standing askew. The angle of its position suddenly made me aware that what we had been searching for had been there all the time!"[6]

Thus was born the concept of the rotation-advancement technique: the medial part of the cleft simply had to be detached from its high attachments and rotated down to the proper position, and the lateral lip advanced into the gap created by the rotation. Although the parents of other Korean children with clefts were reluctant to bring their children in for surgery, Millard eventually found his first patient for the technique. He playfully "roped" a 10-year-old boy who did not seem reluctant to "play the game." He was brought to the Quonset Hut Hospital and, without parental knowledge or consent, the first rotation advancement cleft lip repair was performed.[6]

Millard presented the rotation-advancement technique at the First International Congress of Plastic Surgery, held in Stockholm, Sweden, in August 1955. Over the ensuing years, he further refined this technique. In his original description, there were three flaps, labeled A, B, and C: A was the medial rotation flap; B, the lateral advancement flap carrying the flared alar base; and C, the small triangular flap attached to the columella which was originally advanced across the nasal floor (Fig. 12–15). One early concern of many surgeons

was the persistent shortness of the lip on the cleft side which resulted in an unbalanced cupid's bow. Millard felt that this usually was due to inadequate rotation of the medial flap, but it lead to the addition of the back-cut to enable greater downward rotation of the medial lip segment. The function of the C-flap then evolved to fill the defect created by the back-cut, and thus, to lengthen the columella.[6]

The rotation-advancement technique overcame many of the disadvantages of earlier unilateral cleft lip repairs: it preserved the Cupid's bow and the philtral dimple; it improved nasal tip asymmetry; and the scars were aesthetically camouflaged along the philtral columns and within the alar crease. Since his original description, there have been several refinements of Millard's original technique, but the basic principles have remained the same. Several surgeons have advocated the addition of a small triangular or rectangular flap from the lateral element into the lower part of the repair to provide additional length, break up the line of the incision, and preserve the contour of the vermilion.[40,41] Noordhoff suggested that a tiny z-plasty just above the skin-vermillion junction will re-create the slight transverse depression normally seen just above the white roll. He and others also advocated the incorporation of a triangular lateral vermilion flap to augment the deficient vermilion of the medial lip segment.[42,43]

The Mohler Repair

Some have objected that the scar produced by the Millard repair obliquely and unnaturally crosses the philtrum in the upper third of the lip. Lester Mohler of Columbus, Ohio studied the natural philtral shape in children without clefts, and he modified the rotation advancement technique to reposition this scar, creating a "mirror image" of the philtral column on the noncleft side. In 1987, he reported a study of philtral shape in 100 school children without clefts. He classified them into three groups based on whether the philtral columns were divergent or convergent and, in the latter case, whether they converged at or below columellar-lip junction (Fig. 12–16). Whereas Millard's rotation-advancement technique produced a shield-shaped philtrum with the scar and unaffected philtral column converging in the mid-line under the columella, the majority of children in Mohler's study (74%) actually had columns that did not come together in the upper lip. He subsequently altered the design of his repair for such patients in the superior portion of the lip so as to mirror the philtral shape on the noncleft side. In his technique, the rotation incision is drawn in a curvilinear fashion to mimic the shape of the normal philtral column and is extended into the base of the columella. A 90 degree back-cut is made in the columella without crossing the normal philtral column, allowing downward rotation of the medial lip segment. The C-flap is advanced into the defect at the columellar base and used to lengthen the shortened columella on the cleft side (Fig. 12–17).[44] Don LaRossa at the Children's Hospital of Philadelphia has written about a similar approach, using curves in unilateral cleft lip repair.[45] The extended Mohler repair is described by Court Cutting in Chapter 18.

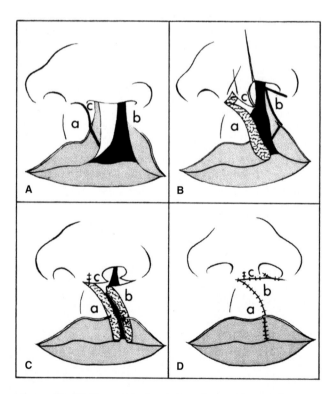

Figure 12–15. The original rotation-advancement design conceived by D. Ralph Millard in Korea and presented at the First International Congress of Plastic Surgery in Stockholm in 1955. Reproduced from *Cleft Lip and Palate; Surgical, Dental, and Speech Aspects*, eds. Grabb, Rosenstein, and Bzoch, p. 195, with permission from Little, Brown, and Co.

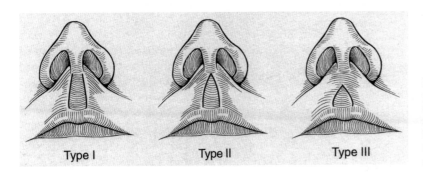

Figure 12–16. Lester Mohler's study of different philtral types in normal school children without clefts showing three primary patterns. Reproduced from "Unilateral Cleft Lip Repair," Lester Mohler, in *Operative Techniques in Plastic Surgery*, eds. Jurkiewicz and Culbertson, Jr, 1995, vol 2, p. 193, with permission from W.B. Saunders Company.

BILATERAL CLEFT LIP REPAIR

James Barrett Brown noted that "the bilateral cleft is more than twice the problem of the unilateral, and the results are less than half as good."[46] Accordingly, bilateral cleft lip repair has progressed slowly. The incisions used have evolved from a straight-line closure on each side to various types of flaps like those used in unilateral clefts. Many surgeons would simply replicate their unilateral repair patterns on each side. Some brought flaps back from the lateral side of the cleft to the midline below the prolabium to lengthen the central lip. In 1891, William Rose pared the central tubercle in a V-shaped manner and curved his incisions in the lateral segments, bringing them together in the midline below the apex of the central segment. Le Mesurier applied his quadrilateral flap design to the bilateral defect, also transposing flaps below the prolabium. Brown, McDowell, and Byars introduced a pair of triangular flaps that were brought together under the prolabium and described several variations to accommodate either a long or short prolabium. Louis Schultz of Chicago contributed significantly to the bilateral repair in the 1940s by emphasizing the importance of muscle approximation from the lateral elements behind the central prolabial segment.[5]

As early as 1790, Pierre Joseph Desault of Paris, advocated surgical closure of both sides at the same time after initial premaxillary compression by a cloth bandage. He pared the cleft edges, approximated the lip segments using the prolabium for the central portion of the lip, and fixed the repair with through-and-through needles and thread in a figure-of-eight fashion. Both Brown and McDowell in St. Louis followed Desault's format; they set the premaxilla back and closed both clefts simultaneously. Other surgeons were in favor of a staged repair of the bilateral cleft deformity. Victor Veau felt that, for complicated bilateral clefts, "closure of the entire defect at one time is too formidable," and he recommended closure of lip and palate in three or more stages, with the lip repaired one side at a time, four weeks apart. Others

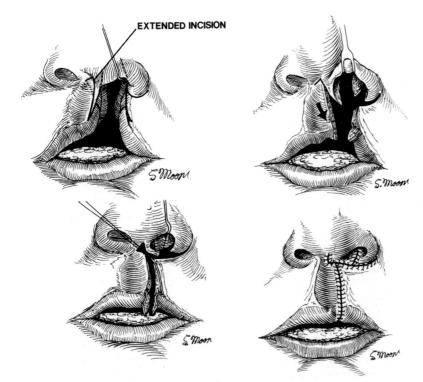

Figure 12–17. Mohler's operation for varying the reconstructed philtral column depending on the configuration of the column on the non-cleft side. Reproduced from "Unilateral Cleft Lip Repair," Lester Mohler, in *Plastic and Reconstructive Surgery*, 1987, p. 513, with permission from Lippincott, Williams, and Wilkins.

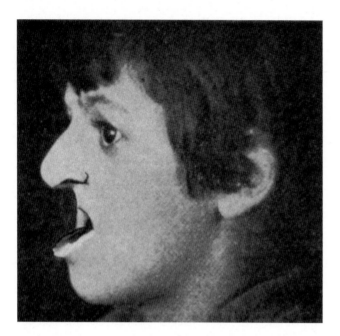

Figure 12–18. A nine year old girl who had the premaxilla removed in infancy with severe maxillary collapse and loss of alveolar tissue presumably by a compression apparatus. Reproduced from *The Operative Story of Cleft Palate*, George M. Dorrance, 1933, p. 412, with permission from W.B. Saunders Company.

who favored staged repair included Kilner and Holdsworth of Britain and Cronin and Bauer of the United States. These surgeons chose to close the wider cleft first in order to pull the deviated premaxilla back to the midline.[5]

The Premaxilla

The protruding premaxilla was one of the first challenges in the history of the bilateral lip repair. In early repairs, it often was excised completely, leading to a loss of incisors, collapse of the lateral maxillary segments, severe restriction of anterior maxillary growth, and a marked anterior cross bite (Fig. 12–18). As early as 1556, Pierre Franco suggested removing the premaxilla completely "with cutting forceps or a small saw, leaving the flesh over them."[47] This suggestion was echoed by Hendrik van Roonhuyse of Amsterdam in 1661, George de al Faye of Paris in 1733, and Guillaume Dupuytren of Paris in 1833.[22,47–49] Pancoast did not excise the premaxilla, but instead forcefully fractured it to a better position.[50] M. Malgaigne in 1844 was one of the first to object "to the removal of two, three, or even four incisors."[51]

Other historic attempts to reposition the protruding premaxilla have included removal of the buccal plate of the alveolus, usually with destruction of the incisor teeth. In 1865, Adolf van Bardeleben of Germany sectioned the vomer subperiosteally through a small incision, allowing "the sectional septal ends to glide past each other without buckling as the premaxilla was repositioned."[52] Section of the septum anterior to the vomerine suture, resection of a segment of bone immediately behind the lingual buccal plate, stapling of the pre-vomerine suture, and a variety of head cups with straps

to place static or elastic pressure on the premaxillary segment have all been tried. More recently, dental appliances have been used to reposition the premaxilla. This has been done with screw attachments for retropositioning the pre-maxilla and for repositioning the lateral maxillary segments or with staged dental plates for passive repositioning. This approach has now reached a high degree of sophistication and has evolved to include additional appliances to reshape the nasal tip cartilages and to lengthen the columella (see Chapter 46).

The lip adhesion procedure was another method developed to reposition the protruding premaxilla. First described by Gustav Simon in 1864, this procedure attached flaps from the lateral lip segments to the prolabium in order to reshape the lip prior to definitive lip repair. In addition to repositioning the premaxilla, the adhesions also acted as tissue expanders of the prolabium, creating more tissue in the central lip segment.[6] Peter Randall was a strong proponent of preliminary lip adhesion and felt it achieved the same results as external elastic pressure or internal dental appliances.[27,53]

The Prolabium

The fate of the prolabium has undergone similar debate. In 1907, the French surgeon Lorenz advanced the prolabium into the columella and closed the lateral lip segments in the midline beneath it. This technique attempted to correct the short columella and flat nasal tip, but it often produced a tight and vertically long lip. Others altered this technique, including Pitanguy in 1967, who divided the entire prolabium creating a "forked flap"; he advanced this into the columella and sutured it to the alar bases, which were advanced medially with the aid of circumalar incisions. Millard later modified this technique. Although he initially described forked flaps created from the bilateral lip scars in a secondary procedure for columellar lengthening, he later banked his forked flaps beneath the nasal sill in the so-called *whisker position* at the time of primary lip repair for later advancement into the columella in a second stage.[5]

There has also been debate as to whether to preserve the prolabial vermilion or to discard it and instead advance vermilion from the lateral segments to the midline below the prolabium. Various techniques have been described to augment the deficient vermillion of the central lip, including advancing denuded lateral vermilion flaps underneath the prolabial vermilion or folding lateral prolabial vermilion under the central segment.[5,6] In 1968, Clayton de Haan of St. Luke's Hospital in New York City described turning down the prolabial vermilion to create an upper labial sulcus and advancing the vermilion from the lateral elements.

Cross Lip Flaps

Another technique developed for augmenting the deficient central lip was the cross lip flap. J.A. Estlander, a Flemish surgeon, was the first to describe this technique, which he used to reconstruct defects of the lower lip caused by typhus. He designed a flap from the upper lip based on the coronary artery

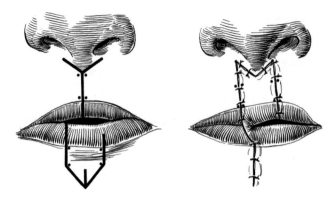

Figure 12–19. Robert Abbé of St. Luke's Hospital in New York was the first surgeon in 1895 to use the Estlander cross-lip flap to augment the central lip for the severe bilateral cleft deformity. Reproduced from *Cleft Craft*, vol. 3, 1980, p. 608, with permission from D. Ralph Millard.

and rotated this flap into the defect on the lower lip; the donor sites were closed by advancing cheek flaps, and the pedicle of the flap became the new commisure.[54,55] Robert Abbé, a surgeon at New York's St. Luke's Hospital, was likely the first to use the cross lip flap for a cleft lip deformity.[5,56,57] His first patient was a 21-year-old man who had had a bilateral cleft lip closed as an infant and who had "extreme flatness and scantiness of the upper lip with an enormous pouting and redundancy of the lower lip." He excised the central upper lip and designed a flap from the mid-lower lip "a little wider than the upper gap" which was hinged into the upper lip defect beneath the columella and divided after 12 days (Fig. 12–19).[56] This soon became a popular solution for the badly scarred tight upper lip. It also gained some popularity in the 1960s and 1970s as a primary solution for the severe bilateral deformity with a short columella and prolabium. Fernando Ortiz-Monastario, among others, advocated shifting the prolabium into the columella and using a primary Abbé flap to fill the lip defect. J.P. Webster, a bibliophile in his own right, researched the technique and found that S.A.C. Stein of Copenhagen had published such a case in 1848 and that Pietro Sabattini of Bologna had also done a similar case in 1837.[58,59]

CLEFT RHINOPLASTY

Prior to Victor Veau in Paris, who had recommended closing the anterior nostril floor and repositioning the alar base, primary cleft rhinoplasty had received little attention.[24] Blair, Brown, and Byars described a more aggressive surgical approach to correct the flattened nasal tip. They completely separated the alar cartilages on the cleft side from the overlying skin, elevated the nasal tip, and maintained this position with through-and-through sutures. Occasionally, they cut the nasal spine with a small chisel and lightly packed the nostril.[25,46] Gustav Aufricht of New York, whose practice primarily included adult rhinoplasties, saw many older patients with clefts whose nasal tips had been badly scarred by injudi-

cious surgery in infancy. These were extremely difficult cases to correct secondarily, and he therefore strongly cautioned cleft surgeons:

> Please don't touch the nose of a patient with a cleft in infancy. Wait at least until late teen age.[60]

Mid-columellar incisions for access to the alar cartilages had been suggested by Blair, and further extension of the incision in the skin over the alar rim was suggested by Figi.[61,62] This approach was later taken even further with excision of a crescent shaped piece of tip skin to elevate the nostril rim, and some, including Berkeley and Royster of Philadelphia, incised the skin of the nasal tip with a columellar extension at the time of the initial surgery.[63,64]

In 1974, Harold McComb of Perth, Australia, described an aggressive cleft nasal tip rhinoplasty with wide separation of the involved nasal cartilages. He used a z-plasty to release the lateral band in the nostril vestibule, and he repositioned the cartilages with through-and-through sutures tied over small cotton bolsters. He stressed the need to re-establish the overlap of the upper edge of the lower lateral cartilage over the lower edge of the upper lateral cartilage.[65] Other authors stressed the need to centralize the deflected septum and nasal spine from the non-cleft side to fully correct the deviation of the nasal tip. Some have scored the septal cartilage on the concave side, and others have used a small chisel to section the nasal spine and reposition it. Conformers and stents within the nostrils also have been used extensively to maintain the shape of the reconstructed alae.

More recently, studies by Matsuo et al. have shown that the alar cartilages can be shaped nonsurgically in the early neonatal period, but that this plasticity disappears by 3 or 4 months of age, the time at which lip repair is most commonly performed. In their experience, cleft lip repair in the first week of life with a retainer placed in the nostril for 3 months results in significantly improved nasal shape and symmetry without additional nasal surgery.[66] Barry Grayson and Court Cutting pursued this principle of early cartilage malleability and developed the technique of presurgical naso-alveolar molding (NAM), which seeks both to reposition the alveolus and to mold the alar cartilages and lengthen the columella to achieve better nasal tip projection and symmetry. This is achieved through a palatal prosthesis with extensions into the nostrils that are adjusted weekly until the desired result is obtained.[67,68]

CLEFT PALATE REPAIR

Early Palatal Surgery

Surgery on the palate was virtually nonexistent in the 16th and 17th centuries in Europe for fear of complications resulting from syphilis, dental decay, scurvy, and tuberculosis. Tertiary lesions from syphilitic infection damaged the buccopharynx and caused severe destruction of the soft palate; the resulting palatal defects were a common problem. Classic descriptions

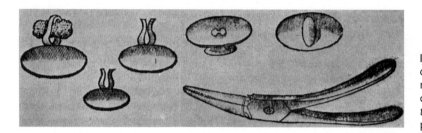

Figure 12–20. Palatal obturators of many different designs were used almost exclusively for the treatment of palatal defects in the 17th and early 18th centuries. Reproduced from *The Source Book of Plastic Surgery*, ed. Frank McDowell, 1977, p. 257, with permission from Lippincott, Williams, and Wilkins.

of this palatal disease can be found nearly half a century before the first description of a congenital palatal cleft by Franco in 1556.[18] During this time, palatal function was also poorly understood. The Frenchman Ambroise Paré, who performed anatomical studies of the palate, emphasized the function of the palate as primarily concerned with eating "hard, acrid, and sharp meats," rather than with producing speech. Paré believed that the uvula, instead, was more essential for speech production and sound quality than the soft palate.[18]

Pierre Franco (1505–1579), the other great Huguenot surgeon and contemporary of Paré, was likely the first to describe the congenital origin of cleft palate which he termed *levre fendu de nativite*. He was also one of the first to recognize the importance of the palate for speech. In 1561, he wrote:

Those who have cleft palate are more difficult to cure: and they always speak through the nose. If the palate is only slightly cleft, and if it is plugged with cotton, the patient will speak more clearly, or perhaps even as well as if there were no cleft.[4,18]

Treatment for palatal defects at this time consisted exclusively of palatal obturation. Obturators of many different designs were created, and most had an extension into the nose for retention. Some held sea sponges on the nasal side which expanded when moistened. Some had mechanical "wings" that could be switched from a vertical to a horizontal position for retention by the use of a key (Fig. 12–20).[7]

One of the first-attempted and reportedly successful repairs was performed by Le Monnier, a dentist from Rouen, France, who operated on a child with a palatal cleft "from the velum to the incisor teeth." As described in 1766 by Robert,

he succeeded in re-uniting the two borders of the cleft, first inserting several points of suture in order to keep them approximated, and afterwards abraded them with the actual cautery. An inflammation supervened, which terminated in suppuration, and was followed by reunion of the two lips of the artificial wound. The child was perfectly cured.[69]

In 1779, Eustache of Beziers, France noted difficulties with swallowing and speech after an operation which involved splitting the palate for extraction of nasal polyps. He proposed to the Academy of Surgery of Paris suturing the defect "after the method of Manne." Four years later, he described his technique for repairing the surgically split velum, and he also suggested that this technique could be applied to congenital clefts of the palate as well. But in 1784, Dubois, another prominent French surgeon, reported to the same Academy and criticized Eustache's procedure for split velum as "impractical."[4]

Nothing more was heard from either Le Monnier or Eustache, and it was not until 37 years later that the first successful surgical palatal repair was reported by von Graefe.[18]

The Nineteenth Century

In 1816, Carl Ferdinand von Graefe, a celebrated German surgeon, known as the "Founder of Modern Plastic Surgery" performed the first surgical closure of a congenital palatal cleft in Berlin (Fig. 12–21).[4] Three years later, Philibert-Joseph Roux of Paris independently completed a similar operation on a Canadian medical student named John Stephenson; he named this operation *staphyloraphie*. John Stephenson was studying medicine at the University of Edinburgh and visited Roux in Paris for his studies. Roux noted Stephenson's poor

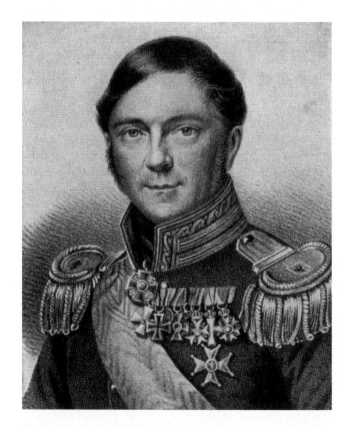

Figure 12–21. Carl Ferdinand von Graefe performed the first surgical closure of a congenital palatal cleft in Berlin in 1816. At age 23, he became Professor of Surgery at the University of Berlin, and at age 26, he became Surgeon General to the Prussian Army. Reproduced from *The Operative Story of Cleft Palate*, George M. Dorrance, 1933, p. 4, with permission from W.B. Saunders Company.

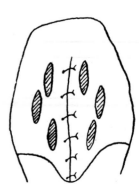

Figure 12–23. Multiple relaxing incisions in the palate were used by Mattauer of Virginia. Reproduced from *The Operative Story of Cleft Palate*, George M. Dorrance, 1933, p. 17, with permission from W.B. Saunders Company.

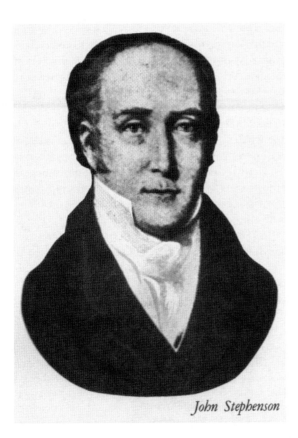

John Stephenson

Figure 12–22. John Stephenson was a Canadian medical student studying under Philbert-Joseph Roux in Paris. He allowed his cleft palate to be repaired by Dr. Roux in 1819, and later described this experience in detail for his graduation thesis from medical school. Reproduced from *Cleft Craft*, vol. 3, 1976, p. 170, with permission from D. Ralph Millard.

speech and volunteered to repair his cleft palate. After recovering from the operation and finding his speech improved, Stephenson described his experiences and his account of the operation itself for his graduation thesis at Edinburg.[70] He later returned to Montreal, where he became a prominent surgeon and Professor at McGill University (Fig. 12–22).[18,71]

Following the work of Von Graefe and Roux, staphylorrhaphy became the accepted treatment for clefts of the velum. This operation was limited initially to simple clefts of the soft palate until Johann Dieffenbach in 1826 introduced his operation for closure of hard palatal clefts, which he called *uranoplasty*. This procedure involved dissecting the mucosa off the hard palate and making relaxing incisions to relieve the tension during closure.[4,72] Subsequently, relaxing incisions gained popularity among surgeons, and they were used in a variety of ways, including multiple small overlapping incisions. Mettauer of Virginia used as many as three to four on each side (Fig. 12–23).[73]

Bernhard von Langenbeck used one long relaxing incision close to the gingiva on each side. In 1859, after noting regeneration of bone after a maxillary resection when he left the periosteum intact, von Langenbeck began to elevate full thickness mucoperiosteal flaps in his hard palate repairs. His technique of raising the periosteum with the mucosa by blunt

elevation from just behind the incisors to the posterior edge of the palatine bones is still in use today and associated with his name.[4,74] Thomas Alcock performed von Langenbeck's operation for the first time in England, and Jonathan Mason Warren studied with Dieffenbach and is credited with bringing the operation to the United States. James Barrett Brown of St. Louis referred to this operation as the "Dieffenbach–Warren Operation," but it is more commonly known as the "von Langenbeck Procedure."[46]

Dieffenbach later suggested cutting through the maxilla laterally and raising bone flaps in continuity with the palatal flaps and closing both in the midline. This was called an *osteal uranoplasty*, later known as "the bone flap technique." He first punched a hole through the bone with a three-cornered awl along the line of his usual relaxing incision, then passed a silver wire through the hole and began twisting. A chisel was used to complete the osteotomies, and the wires twisted again until the bones opposed in the midline. This technique was adopted by many in Europe and in the United States, and was frequently done in two steps, two weeks apart. Proponents of the technique cited fewer fistulae, less reduction in anterior-posterior facial growth, better occlusion, and good speech outcomes.[4]

There subsequently followed numerous designs for specialized instruments and needles, as well as different suturing techniques, suture materials, and bolstering rods. One technique to relieve tension included using strips of cotton or metal which were placed in one lateral relaxing incision, tunneled across on the nasal side of the palate, and brought out through the other relaxing incision; then the two ends were sutured together on the oral side (Fig. 12–24).[4]

Surgical techniques for cleft palate repair become more sophisticated by the mid-19th century, as did the understanding of palatal muscular anatomy and function. The first classic description of the function of palatal muscles was given in 1844 by Sir William Fergusson in a presentation to the Royal Medical and Chirurgical Society of London.[4,75] Philip Gustav Passavant of Frankfort also contributed significantly to the understanding of palatal functions for speech. In 1863, he wrote a monograph on "closure of the palate in speech"

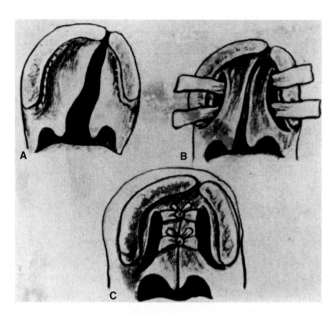

Figure 12–24. One technique used in the early 19th century to relieve tension on the palatal repair included using strips of cotton placed in one lateral relaxing incision, tunneled across the nasal side of the palate, brought out through the other relaxing incision, and then sutured together on the oral side. Reproduced from *The Operative Story of Cleft Palate*, George M. Dorrance, 1933, p. 143, with permission from W.B. Saunders Company.

in which he stressed the movement of the soft palate and noted a "forward swelling (of the posterior pharyngeal wall) at the level of the base of the uvula." This later became known as Passavant's ridge. He felt that it was "essential . . . for normal pronunciation," and further pointed out that "the patient retains a nasal tone, despite the good healing achieved, because the newly formed soft palate is too short to achieve velo-pharyngeal closure." He developed several operations to treat the insufficiency, which included suturing the posterior tonsillar pillars together to form a partial curtain behind the velum and bringing the posterior pharyngeal wall forward by raising a flap and folding in on itself. In 1878, he described another technique in which he transversely incised the palatal mucoperiosteum, posteriorly displaced the entire velum, and sutured the soft palate directly to the posterior pharyngeal wall.[4] This was likely one of the earliest push back procedures. Although his maneuvers did not reliably improve speech, Passavant was one of the first to surgically attempt to improve velopharyngeal dysfunction.[73,76,77]

Compressing the Maxilla

In the early 1800s, it was thought that a cleft of the palate was not an underdevelopment or absence of normal parts but rather a separation of parts of normal size and potential. External pressure was used to diminish the width of the cleft in the maxilla, as it was similarly used to decrease the width of a wide cleft lip and to set back a protruding premaxilla. Extended pressure on the cheeks followed by palatal closure was described by Montin of Paris in 1836. When the borders of the cleft were approximated, they were "denuded with a

red hot iron which was dipped in boiling water." Montin reported that "union resulted in three days," and noted that "this pressure may result in fracturing of the maxillary bones," an incident he considered "of no consequence in the newborn."[78] Numerous devices for mechanical compression were used, some with large clamps and screws that could be gradually tightened, others with circumferential rubber bands placed on the teeth, and others with gruesomely large metal teeth to prevent slippage (Fig. 12–25). Often, wires or silk threads were placed through the maxilla to maintain compression, and most advocates suggested that "the operation should be performed as early as possible after birth, when the bones are in their softest condition."[4,73]

In 1886, Truman W. Brophy, Professor of Oral Surgery at the Chicago College of Dental Surgery, advocated using wire loops placed intraorally for compression. He developed a technique of intraoral wiring in which he passed three loops of silver wire through the maxilla and through holes in lead plates placed in the buccal sulcus (Fig. 12–26).[79,80]

After the wires are twisted, and just before the alveolar processes are brought into contact, a small knife should be passed about one quarter of an inch posterior to the anterior part on either side of the cleft making flaps long enough and thin enough, when sutured to prevent leaving a notch in the bone and to secure a normal bony arch. Horsehair coaptation sutures should be used for fixing the little flaps . . . before the final twist.[4]

This became a popular approach largely because Truman Brophy was a dynamic leader and an influential surgeon. He started the Chicago College of Dental Surgery and then presided over the school as its Dean for 39 years, training many surgeons. In 1921, he founded The American Association of Oral Surgeons and was its president for the first 3 years. This society became the American Association of Plastic Surgeons in 1942.[81] Brophy was much respected for his surgical talents and innovation; in his obituary it is written "if a path to a desired end were not beaten, he never hesitated to break the virgin soil."[82]

Although compression of the maxilla became popular with many surgeons in the United States and in Europe, there were many opponents including Victor Veau of Paris, who criticized this technique in 1931 in his text entitled *Division Palatine*. Another Parisian, Charles Ruppe, also disagreed with this technique and wrote in 1932 that the use of compression "has no anatomic basis."[4,83] Another opponent was Thomas Graber of Chicago who studied facial growth in children with clefts, many of whom likely had been operated on by Dr. Brophy or one of his many trainees. Graber reported in 1949 that there were many severe growth disturbances, and he implicated cleft palate surgery as the cause.[4,84]

The Twentieth Century
The Pushback Procedures

One of the most famous early pushback procedures was the Gillies–Fry operation, described in 1921 by Sir Harold Gilles and Sir Kelsey Fry. They had worked on facial injuries

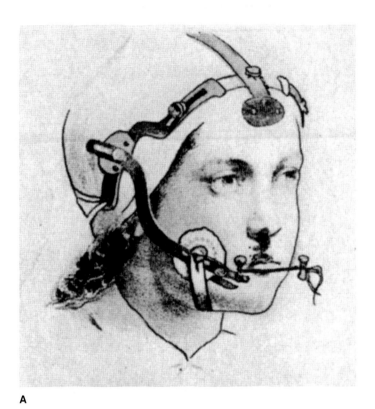

A

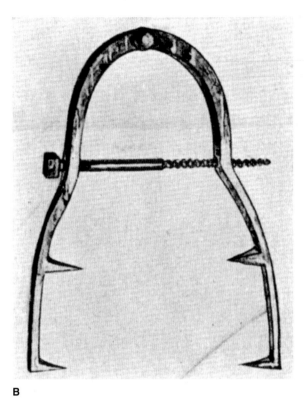

B

Figure 12–25. Compression of the maxilla to narrow the cleft in the hard palate could be applied either externally or internally A) Appliance described by Van Camp placed external pressure on the cheeks. B) Screw activated clamp placed intraorally with teeth to prevent slippage designed by Truman Brophy in 1884. Reproduced from *The Operative Story of Cleft Palate*, George M. Dorrance, 1933, p. 145, 161, with permission from W.B. Saunders Company.

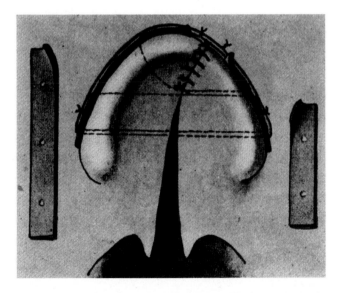

Figure 12–26. Truman Brophy developed his silver wire technique for intraoral compression of the maxilla in 1886. He placed three loops of wire through the maxilla and through holes in lead plates placed in the buccal sulcus and tightened the wires to bring the alveolus together. Reproduced from *The Operative Story of Cleft Palate*, George M. Dorrance, 1933, p. 145, 160, with permission from W.B. Saunders Company.

together in World War I at Aldershot, England, and joined forces again later to collaborate on cleft palate repair. In the procedure they described, Gillies separated the soft palate from the hard palate with a transverse incision at the posterior edge of the hard palate, repaired the soft palate and pushed it back posteriorly until it reached the posterior pharyngeal wall. Fry would fit an immediate prosthesis to cover the hard palatal cleft and to fill the gap between the hard palate and the retro-positioned soft palate. He would augment this from time to time to stretch the newly reconstructed velum (Fig. 12–27).[73] Although he often was successful in improving speech in his patients, Gillies noted that they were "condemned to wear a huge obturator, which necessitated constant dental supervision, irritates the nose, often lodges food and, when the teeth are gone, will not stay in position."[73] He then switched to the laborious external tube pedicle moved into the mouth to fill the defect. These were usually from the arm or neck, introduced either through the mouth or an external incision.[5]

The von Langenbeck operation remained the most commonly performed procedure in the early 1900s until George M. Dorrance introduced his pushback operation. Dorrance was Professor of Maxillofacial Surgery in the School of Dentistry at the University of Pennsylvania in Philadelphia. He recognized the need for additional palatal length to accomplish velopharyngeal closure and achieve normal speech, and in 1925, he presented a new technique to the Philadelphia

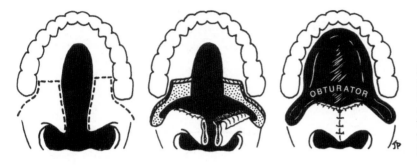

Figure 12–27. In the Gilles-Fry operation, the soft palate was freed from the posterior edge of the hard palate and pushed back as far as possible. The defect and the hard palate cleft were immediately filled with a prosthesis. Reproduced from *Cleft Craft*, vol. 3, 1976, p. 415, with permission from D. Ralph Millard.

Academy of Surgery which became known as "The Pushback Operation" (Fig. 12–28). In his original description, a horseshoe shaped incision was made around the hard palate just inside the alveolar mucosa. The flap was elevated subperiosteally and the posterior neurovascular pedicles were ligated and cut. The hamulus was fractured, the palatal aponeurosis and the nasal mucosal attachment to the bone severed, and the incisions carried around the maxillary tuberosity over the pterygomaxillary fold. The entire palate was thus mobilized and "pushed back"; the anterior hard palate flap was sutured either to drill holes in the posterior edge of the hard palate or to a cuff of nasal mucosa left at this edge. Dorrance subsequently recommended this be done in two stages about

3 months apart to delay the flap.[4,85] Later, Barrett Brown proposed leaving the vascular pedicles intact so that the palate could be set back as an island flap. He recommended stretching the palatine arteries for about 1 cm out of their canals and also dissecting them free from the mucoperiosteum distally to allow such posterior movement.[18]

The Dorrance "Pushback Operation" gained popularity and was performed for primary cleft palate repair, as a secondary procedure for velopharyngeal incompetence, and also for "congenitally short palate."[4] Dorrance initially used an intramuscular aluminum-bronze suture for his repair. He further supported the anterior end of the palatal flap with a heavy piece of silver wire fixed behind the molar teeth around to the incisors. Iodoform gauze was placed under this wire over the denuded hard palate and replaced until granulation tissue covered the bone.[85] He later used a split-thickness skin graft to provide nasal lining for the mucoperiosteal flaps to theoretically reduce palatal shortening from scar contracture. The graft was folded on itself with the raw surface facing outward and placed between the hard palate periosteum and the bare bone. At a second stage, it was divided posteriorly, providing nasal lining on the "pushed-back" flap and also oral lining on the denuded bone. This technique was endorsed by Hamilton Baxter of Montreal who published his version in 1947 in *Plastic and Reconstructive Surgery*; it was used by many surgeons but lost popularity after Barrett Brown complained that it created a foul odor from mucous pooling and epithelial desquamation of the graft.[4,73]

V–Y Palatal Lengthening

Like George Dorrance, Hugo Ganzer, an oral surgeon from Berlin, noted that the von Langenbeck repair resulted in a short palate. In 1920, he proposed lengthening the palate by using a V-Y type of retropositioning, which gained about 1 cm of additional length. He was probably the first of many to utilize the "V-Y principle" in palatal surgery, and subsequently this incision was often referred to as the "V-Y incision of Ganzer" (Fig. 12–29).

Halle and Ernst, also of Berlin, utilized this incision in complete clefts to achieve more posterior displacement of the palate. Their technique also attempted to narrow the pharynx and to make the superior pharyngeal constrictor muscle more effective.[86–88] In their procedure, the lateral relaxing incisions were extended well posteriorly and the dissection

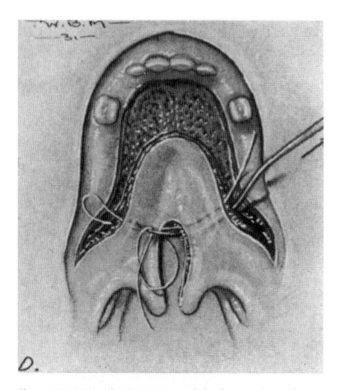

Figure 12–28. In the Dorrance push-back operation, a horseshoe shaped incision was made around the hard palate and flaps were raised sub-periosteally. The entire palate was mobilized and "pushed back;" the anterior hard palate flap was sutured either to drill holes in the posterior edge of the hard palate or to a cuff of nasal mucosa left at this edge. Reproduced from *The Operative Story of Cleft Palate*, George M. Dorrance, 1933, p. 424, with permission from W.B. Saunders Company.

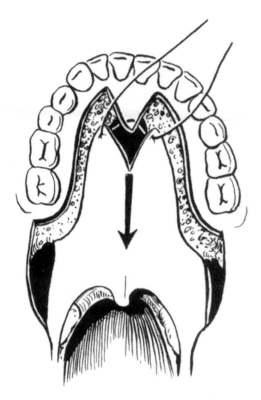

Figure 12–29. The V-Y incision of Ganzer. Reproduced from *Cleft Craft*, vol. 3, 1976, p. 419, with permission from D. Ralph Millard.

was carried into "the space of Ernst," lateral to the superior pharyngeal constrictor muscle. The space was packed with iodoform gauze to move the lateral walls of the pharynx medially. The gauze was changed periodically until the space filled with granulation tissue.[73]

The V-Y incision was also advocated by Victor Veau, one of the great innovators in cleft surgery. As early as 1922, he and Charles Ruppe were using the operation recommended by Ganzer.[83,89] One of Veau's noteworthy contributions to cleft palate surgery was his nasal mucoperiosteal closure of the hard palatal cleft. Veau insisted on careful closure of the nasal mucosa, a step that was often omitted, and in wide clefts, he turned down flaps of vomerine mucosa to achieve this closure. In a first stage, he partially overlapped this nasal closure with mucoperiosteal flaps, and then in a second stage, he used a modified Ganzer V-Y closure without dividing the palatine vessels to lengthen the palate. Although he did not detach the muscles from the posterior edge of the hard palate or reorient their fibers, he felt it was important to bring the "cleft muscles" together in the midline, and he did so with an aluminum bronze wire that encircled the musculature on either side of the cleft.[73,89]

Erich Lexer of Munich loudly denounced Veau's ideas. He preferred to leave the nasal mucosa open to "maintain drainage and to prevent the accumulation of pus between the united muscle layers." He further antagonized Veau by stating that "the French method works only for Frenchmen who speak with the mouth but not for Germans who speak with

the throat."[6] In response, Veau invited Lexer to come to Paris but his invitation was turned down with the response "I shall not cross the Rhine." Later, Madame Veau sent a "Parisian invitation" to Mrs. Lexer and their two daughters. In 1932, all the Lexers did cross the Rhine and were wined and dined in Veau's home state of Burgundy. They were then taken to Paris, where Lexer was shown an "astounding number of clefts" collected for his examination. Mlle. Borel, Veau's speech pathologist, played impressive comparative sound tracings of patients' speech both preoperatively and postoperatively. Lexer was assisted in the performance of a Veau palate operation by Veau himself. The following year, when Veau visited Lexer in Munich, he found that the great German surgeon was using his method.[73]

V-Y lengthening of the palate continued to be very popular. Notable among the proponents was Alexander Limberg of Leningrad, who presented his variation of the technique in 1926 at an International Dental Congress at Convention Hall in Philadelphia before an audience of prominent cleft surgeons including Brophy, Gilmer, Ivy, Blair, and Brown. He criticized ligation of the posterior neurovascular bundle and described an osteotomy of the posterior and medial walls of the foramen with a chisel or bone-cutting forceps so that the vessels could be preserved and further lengthening achieved. He preferred to postpone the final palatal repair until about ten years of age in order to protect the teeth and preserve maxillary growth.[90,91]

Veau's influence spread across the English Channel as well and influenced two British surgeons, William Wardill of Newcastle and T. Pomfret Kilner of London, who independently developed more radical V-Y repositioning procedures than Veau had originally described. In 1937, Wardill described his operation in which he fractured the hamulus, divided the posterior palatine vessels, and transected the mucoperiosteal flaps in their mid-length. He used three flaps for incomplete clefts and four flaps for complete clefts, two based anteriorly and two posteriorly. He also routinely performed a pharyngoplasty (Fig. 12–30).[73] At the same time, Pomfret Kilner was doing a similar lengthening procedure without sacrificing the posterior palatine vessels or routinely performing a pharyngoplasty. Both surgeons favored complete nasal closure following Veau's technique. When socialized medicine came to Britain in 1948, Wardill moved to the Royal Medical College in Baghdad, where he continued to perform cleft surgery.[73]

Wilfred Hynes of Shellfield, England, in 1954 proposed a less severe V-Y closure of the palate in conjunction with a pharyngoplasty. He suggested elevating vertical musculomucosal flaps from the lateral pharyngeal walls which he felt contained the salpingopharyngeus muscle.[92] A transverse incision was made in the posterior pharyngeal wall at about the level of the arch of the atlas, and the flaps were sutured end-to-end within this incision. Later, Hynes proposed overlapping the flaps horizontally and making the flaps fairly wide so that closure of the vertical donor incisions would narrow the pharynx. This became a very popular "pharyngoplasty" in Britain and was often combined with a primary repair

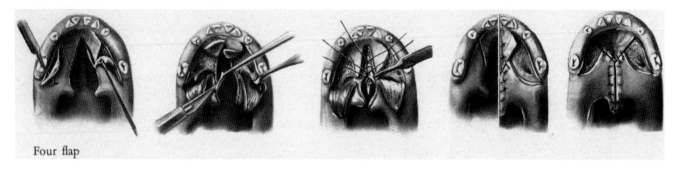

Four flap

Figure 12–30. William Wardill's four-flap operation for complete clefts in which he fractured the hamulus, divided the posterior palatine vessels, and transected the mucoperiosteal flaps in their mid-length. Reproduced from *Cleft Craft*, vol. 3, 1976, p. 426, with permission from D. Ralph Millard.

(Fig. 12–31).[92,93] Jerry Moore of East Grinstead varied this technique by putting these lateral pharyngeal flaps into an incision on the nasal side of the soft palate instead of in the posterior pharyngeal wall.[94]

Intravelar Veloplasty

The next advancement in cleft palate repair was the intravelar veloplasty. In 1967, Otto Kriens of Hamburg, Germany, dissected a stillborn baby with a bilateral cleft and discovered that Veau's "cleft muscle" was the anterior portion of the levator and palatopharyngeal muscles. He performed further anatomic studies to better understand cleft muscular pathology and proposed re-orienting the levator muscles from their abnormal anterior–posterior longitudinal orientation to a more transverse orientation, thus reconstructing the "levator sling." This also reoriented the palatopharyngeus muscle in an operation he called an "intravelar veloplasty." Kriens presented this plan at the first International Cleft Palate Congress in Houston, Texas in 1969.[95,96] An example of Millard's principle of returning "normal to normal," the intravelar veloplasty was an important step forward in improving the function of the reconstructed palate (Fig. 12–32).[6]

Kriens and later David Dickson, a Professor of Anatomy and Speech at the University of Pittsburgh, demonstrated that the abnormal levator muscle inserted along the bony palatal cleft margins. It is appreciably longer than when in the normal

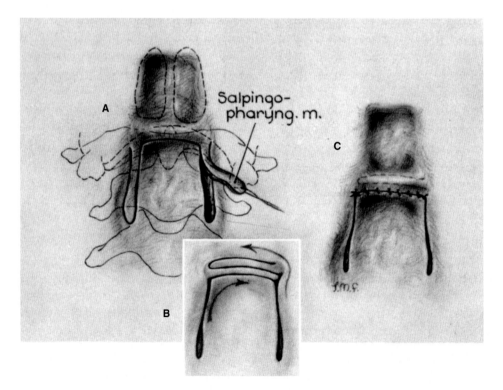

Figure 12–31. The Hynes pharyngoplasty used bilateral musculomucosal flaps from the lateral pharyngeal walls and placed them in an overlapped position within a transverse incision in the posterior pharyngeal wall. Reproduced from *Cleft Lip and Palate; Surgical, Dental, and Speech Aspects*, eds. Grabb, Rosenstein, and Bzoch, p. 195, with permission from Little, Brown, and Co.

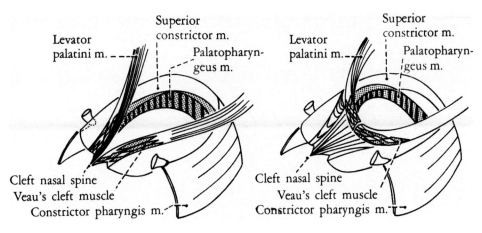

Figure 12–32. Otto Kriens' intravelar veloplasty recreated the "levator sling" by re-orienting the levator muscles from their abnormal anterior-posterior longitudinal orientation in the mid-portion of the soft palate. Reproduced from *Cleft Craft*, vol. 3, 1976, p. 24, with permission from D. Ralph Millard.

transverse position.[73] In his variation of the "intravelar velo-plasty," Peter Randall of Philadelphia dissected the muscles and reoriented them in the transverse position, but instead of suturing them end-to-end as Kriens suggested, he advocated overlapping the two muscle bundles. He believed this would tighten the "levator sling" and thereby improve velopharyngeal competence (Fig. 12–33).[97,98]

Furlow Palatoplasty

In 1978, Dr. Leonard Furlow of Gainesville, Florida, presented a paper at the Annual Meeting of the Southeastern Society of Plastic and Reconstruction Surgeons describing a double opposing z-plasty for cleft palate closure. He presented only four cases, but his technique was novel and ingenious. The time honored z-plasty added length to the soft palate, avoided a straight midline scar in the soft palate which could lead to subsequent palatal shortening, and reoriented the levator muscles to recreate the levator sling. In Furlow's design, one z-plasty was placed in the oral mucosa and another, oriented in the opposite direction, was placed in the nasal mucosa. The levator muscles were completely freed from the posterior hard palate. In each z-plasty the posteriorly based mucosal flap contained the muscle on that side; thus when the z-plasties were completed, the muscles overlapped in the posterior soft palate in a more anatomic position. By leaving the muscles attached to either nasal or oral mucosa on one side, less dissection of the levator was needed, and thus theoretically less scar formation occurred than in an intravelar veloplasty (Fig. 12–34).[99] Klaus Walter and Hans-Henning Meisel of Dusseldorf, also in 1978, reported the same type of double opposing z-plasty for added palatal length, but stated that the incisions were made "without regard for the underlying muscle," which is one of the key considerations in the Furlow cleft palate repair.[100]

Peter Randall was very enthusiastic about Furlow's concepts after hearing his initial presentation, and he brought this operation back to The Children's Hospital of Philadelphia. He and Don LaRossa began performing this procedure routinely with several variations including lateral relaxing

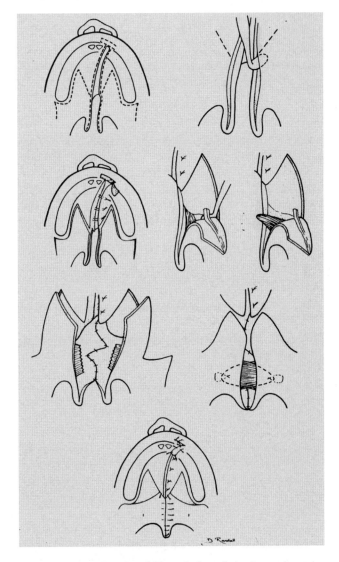

Figure 12–33. Peter Randall's variation of the intravelar veloplasty overlapped the levator muscles in the midline to tighten the levator sling. Reproduced from *Pediatric Plastic Surgery*, ed. Serafin and Georgiade, 1984, p. 293, with permission from Mosby.

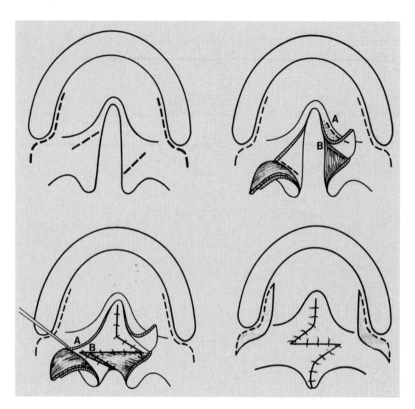

Figure 12–34. Leonard Furlow's double-opposing z-plasty cleft palate repair. A z-plasty is made in the oral mucosa of the soft palate and another in the reverse orientation in the nasal mucosa; each posteriorly based flap contains the levator muscle. Reproduced from *Pediatric Plastic Surgery*, ed. Serafin and Georgiade, 1984, p. 294, with permission from Mosby.

incisions of the von Langenbeck type to achieve a tension-free closure when needed. They reported a series of 106 patients in 1985 with good speech results.[101] The Children's Hospital of Philadelphia has continued to preferentially use this technique and has since accumulated what is likely the largest and longest experience with this technique.[102–104] D. Ralph Millard reported on Furlow's work in *Cleft Craft* in 1980, but it was not until 1986 that Dr. Furlow published his views on the operation.[73,105] Several authors have reported improved speech results when using the Furlow cleft palate repair with a variety of variations.[106–109]

Delayed Hard Palate Closure

In 1944, Herman Schweckendiek of Marburg, Germany, suggested "early" closure of the soft palate and delayed closure of the hard palate. The soft palate closure was done in three layers at about 7–8 months of age. He obturated the hard palatal cleft with a "speech palate," and postponed closure of the hard palate until 12–15 years of age so as not to interfere with bone growth and development.[110] In 1960, his son Wolframm continued his father's plan, and in 1978 he reported on a 25-year experience.[111] He reported "normal maxillary and cranial growth," and normal speech in 57% of cases, minor speech problems in 37%, and velopharyngeal dysfunction requiring pharyngoplasty in only 5%.[111]

Other proponents of delayed hard palate have included Wayne B. Slaughter and Allen Brodie of Chicago. In 1944, they also documented normal facial growth when hard palate repair was delayed.[112] They postulated that interruption of the blood supply by periosteal stripping and fracturing of the bone and postoperative palatal scarring restricted growth.

They further stated that "congenitally deformed parts, unless permanently damaged, grow at normal rates." Samuel Pruzansky later joined this group, and in 1953 he also recommended early closure of the soft palate by 12 months of age with delayed closure of the hard palate.[113] The cleft of the hard palate could be expected to narrow, but if by 2 years it was still too wide for easy closure, a denture was made to obturate the defect.

TEAM CARE

In 1938, Dr. Herbert K. Cooper was practicing orthodontia in Lancaster, Pennsylvania. He realized that children with clefts, in addition to their surgical and dental problems, had other needs, particularly problems with speech, hearing, and even psychological problems. Many of these patients came from poor families, and Dr. Cooper literally took them into his own home so that they could receive better specialty care. He also garnered significant support from the Lancaster Rotary Club to help pay for the costs of this care. Thus began the Lancaster Cleft Palate Clinic and one of the first organized team approaches to the care of children with clefts.

Dr. Robert H. Ivy, a Philadelphia plastic surgeon and dentist, knew Dr. Cooper very well and admired the work he was doing in Lancaster. Dr. Ivy agreed that these patients needed coordinated multi-specialty care to address their many needs. He felt that the care of cleft patients was currently being compromised by the competition amongst surgical specialties which included general surgeons, pediatric surgeons, otolaryngologists, oral surgeons, and plastic surgeons. He also recognized that cleft care was a state health problem, as many families lacked the funds for their child's comprehensive medical care. The surgery itself was seldom a problem because most teaching hospitals at the time provided free care for those unable to pay; however, dental care, speech therapy, and other services were rarely covered. In 1938, Dr. Ivy and Dr. John J. Shaw, the Pennsylvania Secretary of Health, drew up plans to include the care of clefts ("and associated anomalies") in the State of Pennsylvania's Crippled Children's Program. Initially under this plan, cleft cases were assigned only to salaried Board Certified Plastic Surgeons in Philadelphia and Pittsburgh.

By 1949, the State of Pennsylvania acknowledged a greater need for these services. The reported incidence of clefts was 1 in every 776 live births.[114] At this time, the Cleft Palate Program was made into a separate division of the Bureau of Maternal and Child Health, and Dr. Ivy was appointed its Chief. This was the first program of its type in the United States. Dr. Ivy recognized that, through organized clinics, the services of various specialists, including pedodontists, orthodontists, prosthodontists, speech pathologists, otolaryngologists, pediatricians, psychologists or psychiatrists, nurses, and social workers could be coordinated. Soon, there were eight such clinics in the State of Pennsylvania, and they held monthly meetings attended by the team of sub-specialists to review and discuss the cases. Many other groups worldwide followed in adopting the team approach to the care of clefts and craniofacial anomalies. Specialty clinics soon were established elsewhere in the US and Canada, as well as Great Britain, Scandinavia, Germany, France, Switzerland, Mexico, India, Australia, New Zealand, and Japan. The team approach has significantly improved the treatment of patients with clefts by providing truly comprehensive care.

ACKNOWLEDGMENT

This story describing the evolution of the surgical treatment of cleft lip and palate is a tale told previously by many of the masters of cleft surgery and thus borrows richly from their published works. Most prominent among these is the unique three volume work *Cleft Craft*[5,6,73] of D. Ralph Millard, whose rich humor, anecdotes, and detailed descriptions have made it an indispensable asset to any history of cleft care. Other resources include the extensive library of Jerome Webster at the Columbia Presbyterian School of Medicine,[1,13,14] Victor Veau's *Division Palatine*,[83] George M. Dorrance's *The Operative Story of Cleft Palate*,[4] Frank McDowell's *The Source Book*,[18] Robert H. Ivy's *A Link with the Past*,[115] and W.G. Holdsworth's, *Cleft Lip and Palate*.[116]

References

1. Rogers BO. History of cleft palate treatment. In Grabb WC, Rosenstein SW, Bzoch KR (eds). *Cleft Lip and Palate*. Boston, MA: Little Brown and Company, 1971, pp. 142–169.
2. Landazuri H. History of plastic surgery in Peru. In Hinderer U (ed). *X Congress of the International Confederation for Plastic and Reconstructive Surgery; 1992*. Madrid, Spain: Elsevier Science Publishers, 1992, pp. 35–36.
3. Smith G, Dawson WR. Mummification in relation to medicine and pathology. *Egyptian Mummies*. London: George Allen and Unwin Limited, 1924.
4. Dorrance GM. *The Operative Story of Cleft Palate*. Philadelphia: WB Saunders Company, 1933.
5. Millard DR, Jr. *Cleft Craft II*. Boston: Little Brown and Co., 1977.
6. Millard DR, Jr. *Cleft Craft I*. Boston: Little Brown and Co., 1976.
7. Weinberger B. *An Introduction to the History of Dentistry*. St. Louis: Mosby, 1948.
8. Davis AD. Management of the wide unilateral cleft lip with nostril deformity. *Plast Reconstr Surg* 8(3):249–257, 1951.
9. Boo-Chai K. An ancient Chinese text on cleft lip. *Plast Reconstr Surg* 38(2):89–91, 1966.
10. Noordhoff MS. Cleft lip and palate. The Asian connection. In Lee S (ed). *8th International Conference of Cleft Palate and Related Craniofacial Anomalies; 1997*. Singapore, 1997.
11. Rogers BO. Harelip repair in colonial America: A review of 18th century and earlier techniques. In McDowell F (ed). *The Source Book of Plastic Surgery*. Baltimore: The Williams and Wilkins Company, 1977, pp. 180–200.
12. Hnard P, Grmek MD. *Le Premier Manuscript Chirurgical*. Turc Redige par Charaf ed Diu (1465) et Illustre de 140 Miniatures. Paris: Les Eletions, 1960.
13. Rogers BO. Palate surgery prior to von Graefe's pioneering staphylorrhaphy (1819): An historical review of the early causes of surgical indifference in repairing the cleft palate. *Plast Reconstr Surg* 39(1):1–19, 1967.
14. Rogers BO. Harelip repair in Colonial America. A review of 18th century and earlier surgical techniques. *Plast Reconstr Surg* 34:142–162, 1964.
15. Paré A. *Dix livres de chirurgie, avec le magasin des instrumens nécessaires à icelle*. Paris: Impr. Iean le Royer, 1564.
16. Paré A. Les oeuvres de M. Ambroise Paré: Avec les figures & portraits tant de l'anatomie que des instruments de chirurgie, & de plusieurs monstres. Paris: Chez Gabriel Buon, 1575.
17. Johnson T. *The Works of the Famous Chirurgian Ambrose Paré*. London: Richard Cotes and Will Du-gard, 1649.
18. McDowell F (ed). *The Source Book of Plastic Surgery*. Baltimore: The Williams and Wilkins Company, 1977.
19. Gnudi MT, Webster JP. The life and times of Gaspare Tagliacozzi, surgeon of Bologna, 1545–1599. *With a Documented Study of the Scientific and Cultural Life of Bologna in the Sixteenth Century*. New York: H. Reichner, 1950.
20. Aquapendente H. De Chirurgicae In Duas Partes Divisae, 1619.
21. Hofmann JP. De Labis Leporinis: von Hasen-Scharten. Heidelberg: J. Bergmann, 1686.
22. Van Roonhuyse H. *Historischer Heil-Curen in Zwey Theile Verfassete Anmerchungen*. Nurunberg: Michael und Johann Friederich Endtern, 1674.
23. Cooke J. Mellificium chirurgiae: or, The Marrow of Chirurgery. *With the Anatomy of Human Bodies According to the Most Modern Anatomists*, 4th edn. London: Printed for W. Marshall, 1693.
24. Veau V, Recamier J. Bec-de-Lievre: formes cliniques, chirurgie. Paris: Masson et Cie, [n.] 1938.
25. Blair VP, Brown JP. Mirault's operation for single harelip. *Surg Gynecol Obstet* 51:81, 1930.
26. Brown JB, MacDowell F. Simplified design for the repair of single cleft lip. *Surg Gynecol Obstet* 80:12–26, 1945.
27. Randall P, Whitaker LA, LaRossa D. The importance of muscle reconstruction in primary and secondary cleft lip repair. *Plast Reconstr Surg* 54(3):316–323, 1974.
28. Kilner TP. Cleft lip and palate repair technique. *St. Thomas Hosp Rep* 2:127, 1937.
29. Hagedorn W. Operation der hasenchartue mot zickzacknaht. *Zentralbl Chir* 19:281, 1892.

30. Le Mesurier AB. A method for cutting and suturing the lip in the treatment of complete unilateral clefts. *Plast Reconstr Surg* 4:1–12, 1949.

31. Le Mesurier AB. *Hare-Lips and their Treatment*. Baltimore: Williams and Wilkins, 1962.

32. Stark RB. *Cleft palate: A Multidiscipline Approach*. By 19 authors. Edited by Richard B. Stark. New York: Hoeber Medical Division, Harper & Row, 1968.

33. Tennison CW. The repair of the unilateral cleft lip by the stencil method. *Plast Reconstr Surg* 9(2):115–120, 1952.

34. Marcks KM, Trevaskis AE, Dacosta A. Further observation in cleft lip repair. *Plast Reconstr Surg* 12(6):392–402, 1953.

35. Cardoso AD. A new technique for harelips. *Plast Reconstr Surg* 10:92–95, 1952.

36. Brauer RO. A comparison of the Tennison and Le Mesurier lip repairs. *Plast Reconstr Surg* 23(3):249–259, 1959.

37. Randall P. A triangular flap operation for the primary repair of unilateral clefts of the lip. *Plast Reconstr Surg* 23(4):331–347, 1959.

38. Musgrave RH. *General Aspects of Unilateral Cleft Lip Repair*. In Grabb WC, Rosenstein SW, Bzoch KR (eds). Cleft Lip and Palate; Surgical, Dental, and Speech Aspects, 1st edn. Boston: Little, Brown, and Co., 1971, p. xxxiii, 916pp.

39. Skoog TA. Design for the repair of unilateral cleft lips. *Am J Surg* 95(2):223–226, 1958.

40. Onizuka T. A new method for the primary repair of unilateral cleft lip. *Ann Plast Surg* 4(6):516–524, 1980.

41. LaRossa D. *Unilateral Cleft Lip Repair*. Stamford: Appleton and Lange, 1998.

42. Noordhoff MS. Reconstruction of vermilion in unilateral and bilateral cleft lips. *Plast Reconstr Surg* 73(1):52–61, 1984.

43. Noordhoff M, Chen YR, Chen KT. The surgical technique for the complete unilateral cleft lip-nasal deformity. *Oper Tech Plast Reconst Surg* 2:167–181, 1995.

44. Mohler LR. Unilateral cleft lip repair. *Plast Reconstr Surg* 80(4): 511–517, 1987.

45. LaRossa D. Respecting curves in unilateral cleft lip repair. *Oper Tech Plast Recon Surg* 2:182–186, 1995.

46. Brown JB. *Personal Communication*, 1952.

47. Franco P. Traite des hernies, contenant une ample de claration de toutes leurs espe ces, et autres excellentes parties de la chirurgie, assavoir de la pierre, des cataractes des yeux: Lyon, 1561.

48. de la Faye G. Observations on the cleft lip. *Memoires de l'Academie Royale de Chirurgie* 1:603, 1743.

49. Dupuytren G. *Clinical Lectures in Surgery Delivered at Hotel-Dieu in 1832*. Translated by Doane AS. Boston: Carter, Kendec, 1833.

50. Pancoast J. *A Treatise on Operative Surgery*. Philadelphia: Carey and Hart for G. N. Loomis, 1844.

51. Malgaigne JF. Du Bec-de-lieure (new method for the harelip operation). *J Chir* 2:1–6, 1844.

52. Bardeleben A, Vidal A-T. Lehrbuch der Chirurgie und Operationslehre: mit freier Benutzung von Vidal's Traité de pathologie externe et de médicine opératoire, besonders für das Bedürfniss der Studirenden. 4. Ausgabe ed. Berlin: G. Reimer, 1863.

53. Fara M. Anatomy and arteriography of cleft lips in stillborn children. *Plast Reconstr Surg* 42(1):29–36, 1968.

54. Estlander JA. Eine ans der einen lippe substransverluste der anderen Ersitzen. *Arch Klin Chir* 14:622, 1872.

55. Estlander JA. Methode d'autoplastie de la joue on d'une lieure. *Rev Mens Med Chir* 1:344, 1877.

56. Abbe R. A new plastic operation for the relief of deformity due to double harelip. *Med Rec* 53:477, 1898.

57. Stark RB. Robert Abbe: pioneer in plastic surgery. *Bull N Y Acad Med* 31(12):927–950, 1955.

58. Sabattini P. Cenno Storics dell'Orgine e Progresso della Rhinoplastica e Cheiloplastica sequinto della Descrizione de Quests Operazioni Sapra un Solo Individuo. Bologne: Bell'Arte, 1838.

59. Stein S. Hospitals Meddelsen 1:212, 1848.

60. Aufricht G. Recent developments in plastic surgery. *Plast Reconstr Surg* 18:3–25, 1946.

61. Blair VP. Nasal deformities associated with congenital cleft lip. *JAMA* 84:185, 1925.

62. Figi FA. The repair of secondary cleft lip and nasal deformity. *J Int Coll Surg* 17(3):297–305, 1952.

63. Berkeley WT. Correction of the unilateral cleft lip nasal deformity. In Grabb WC, Rosenstein SW, Bzoch KR (eds). *Cleft Lip and Palate; Surgical, Dental, and Speech Aspects*, 1st edn. Boston: Little, Brown, and Co., 1971, pp. 227–242.

64. Royster HP. *Personal Communication*.

65. McComb H. Treatment of the unilateral cleft lip nose. *Plast Reconstr Surg* 55(5):596–601, 1975.

66. Matsuo K, Hirose T, Otagiri T, Norose N. Repair of cleft lip with nonsurgical correction of nasal deformity in the early neonatal period. *Plast Reconstr Surg* 83(1):25–31, 1989.

67. Cutting C, Grayson B, Brecht L, Santiago P, Wood R, Kwon S. Presurgical columellar elongation and primary retrograde nasal reconstruction in one-stage bilateral cleft lip and nose repair. *Plast Reconstr Surg* 101(3):630–639, 1998.

68. Grayson BH, Santiago PE, Brecht LE, Cutting CB. Presurgical nasoalveolar molding in infants with cleft lip and palate. *Cleft Palate Craniofac J* 36(6):486–498, 1999.

69. Robert MJC. Traitâe des principaux objects de mâedecine, avec un sommaire de la plâupart des thâeses soutenues aux âecoles de Paris, depuis 1752 jusqu'en 1764. Paris: Lacombe, 1766.

70. Stephenson J. Dissertatio chirurgica medica inauguralis de velosynthesis, 1820.

71. Martin AE. *Personal Communication*, 1959.

72. Dieffenbach JF. Ueber das Gaumensegel des menschen und der saeugethere. *Litt Ann d ges Heilk* 4:298, 1826.

73. Millard DR, Jr. *Cleft Craft III*. Boston: Little Brown and Co., 1980.

74. Von Langenbeck B. Operation der angeborenen totalem spaltung des harten gaumens nach einer neuer methode. *Deutsche Klin* 8:231, 1861.

75. Fergusson W. The classic reprint. Observations on cleft palate and on staphyloraphy. *Plast Reconstr Surg* 48(4):365–366, 1971.

76. Passavant G. Uber die verschliessung des schludes bien sprechen. *Virchows Arch (apthol. Anat.)* 46:1, 1863.

77. Passavant G. Uber die beseitigter der naeselden sprache bei angebornen spalten des harten und weichen gaumens. *Arch Klin Med* 6:333, 1865.

78. Montin. Bec-de-lievre avec ecartement des os du palais. *Bul gen de therap* 2:231, 1836.

79. Brophy TW. A new operation for cleft palate. *Boston Med and Surg Reporter* 75:576, 1896.

80. Brophy TW. *Cleft Lip and Palate*. Philadephia: Blakiston, 1923.

81. Randall P, McCarthy JG, Wray RC. History of the American association of plastic surgeons, 1921–1996. *Plast Reconstr Surg* 97(6): 1254–1298, 1996.

82. Brophy TW. Obituary. In Archives of Plastic Surgery. Boston: The Countway Library, Harvard University School of Medicine.

83. Veau V. *Division Palatine*. Paris: Masson, 1931.

84. Graber TM. The congenital cleft palate deformity. *J Am Dent Assoc* 48(4):375–395, 1954.

85. Dorrance G. Legthening the soft palate in cleft palate operations. *Ann Surg* 82:208, 1925.

86. Halle H. Gaumensegelplastik, Laryngologische Gellischaft zu Berlin Jan 20, 1922. *Zentralbl Hals Naseu Ohreuheilk* 2:148, 1922–1923.

87. Halle H. Gaumennaht und gaumenplastik. *Zentralbl Hals, Naseu, Ohrenheilk* 12:377, 1925.

88. Ernst F. Zur forage der gaumenplastik etc. *Centralbl f Chir* 52:464, 1925.

89. Veau V. Division palatine, bull et mem. *Soc de chir* 49:838, 1923.

90. Limberg A. Modem chirurgische behandlungsmethodem von spaltbilderlippen, des alveolar fortsatzes und des gaumens, im zusammenhang mit der foederungen der anatomischen,

funktionellen und kosmetischen wiederheustellung. *Nov Kin Mosk* 2:67, 1926.

91. Limberg A. Radikale uranoplastik; osteotomia interlaminaris; resectio marginis foramino palatis plaettchennaht; fissura ossea occulta. *Zhu Souremennoj Chir* 2:809, 1927.

92. Hynes W. Pharyngoplasty by muscle transplantation. *Br J Plast Surg* 3(2):128–135, 1950.

93. Hynes W. Observations on pharyngoplasty. *Br J Plast Surg* 20(3):244–256, 1967.

94. Grabb WC, Rosenstein SW, Bzoch KR. *Cleft Lip and Palate; Surgical, Dental, and Speech Aspects*, 1st edn. Boston: Little, Brown and Co., 1971.

95. Kriens OB. Fundamental anatomic findings for an intravelar veloplasty. *Cleft Palate J* 7:27–36, 1970.

96. Kriens OB. An anatomical approach to veloplasty. *Plast Reconstr Surg* 43(1):29–41, 1969.

97. Randall P. Cleft palate. In Grabb WC, Smith JW (eds). *Plastic Surgery*, 3rd edn. Boston: Little, Brown, 1979, p. 216.

98. Randall P. Clefts of the alveolus and palate. In Serafin D, Georgiade NG (eds). *Pediatric Plastic Surgery*. St. Louis: Mosby; 1976, pp. 290–300.

99. Furlow LT. *Personal Communication*.

100. Walter C, Meisel HH. A new method for the closure of a cleft palate. *J Maxillofac Surg* 6(3):222–226, 1978.

101. Randall P, LaRossa D, Solomon M, Cohen M. Experience with the Furlow double-reversing Z-plasty for cleft palate repair. *Plast Reconstr Surg* 77(4):569–576, 1986.

102. Kirschner RE, Wang P, Jawad AF, et al. Cleft-palate repair by modified Furlow double-opposing Z-plasty: The Children's Hospital of Philadelphia experience. *Plast Reconstr Surg* 104(7):1998–2010, 1999. Discussion 2011–2014.

103. LaRossa D, Jackson OH, Kirschner RE, et al. The Children's Hospital of Philadelphia modification of the Furlow double-opposing z-palatoplasty: Long-term speech and growth results. *Clin Plast Surg* 31(2):243–249, 2004.

104. McWilliams BJ, Randall P, LaRossa D, et al. Speech characteristics associated with the Furlow palatoplasty as compared with other surgical techniques. *Plast Reconstr Surg* 98(4):610–619, 1996. Discussion 620–621.

105. Furlow LT, Jr. Cleft palate repair by double opposing Z-plasty. *Plast Reconstr Surg* 78(6):724–738, 1986.

106. Bardach J, Morris HL, Olin WH. Late results of primary veloplasty: The Marburg project. *Plast Reconstr Surg* 73(2):207–218, 1984.

107. Bardach J, Salyer KE. *Surgical Techniques in Cleft Lip and Palate*, 2nd edn. St. Louis: Mosby-Year Book, 1991.

108. Marsh JL, Grames LM, Holtman B. Intravelar veloplasty: A prospective study. *Cleft Palate J* 26(1):46–50, 1989.

109. Noordhoff MS, Huang CS, Wu J. *Multidisciplinary Management of Cleft Lip and Palate in Taiwan*. Philadelphia: W.B. Saunders, 1990.

110. Schweckendiek W. [Results of formation of a maxilla and speech after primary veloplasty.] *Arch Ohren Nasen Kehlkopfheilkd* 180:541–546, 1962.

111. Schweckendiek W, Doz P. Primary veloplasty: Long-term results without maxillary deformity—a twenty-five year report. *Cleft Palate J* 15(3):268–274, 1978.

112. Slaughter WB, Brodie AG. Facial clefts and their surgical management in view of recent research. *Plast Recon Surg* 4:311–332, 1949.

113. Pruzansky S. Factors determining arch form in cleft of the lip and palate. *Am J Orthod* 41:827–851, 1955.

114. Ivy RH. Experiences in cleft palate surgery. *Ann Surg* 112:775, 1940.

115. Ivy RH. *A Link with the Past*. Baltimore: Williams & Wilkins Co., 1962.

116. Holdsworth WG. *Cleft Lip and Palate*, 3rd edn. London: William Heinemann, 1963.

Anesthesia for Cleft Patients

Franklyn Cladis, MD • Daniela Damian, MD

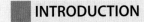

INTRODUCTION

Historically, the repair of the cleft lip and palate was performed with no anesthesia.[1] The early repair of a cleft lip and palate consisted of reapproximating pared tissue edges. These procedures were simple and quick and were performed on older children or adults who could tolerate the pain and inconvenience of the procedure. At most, patients were allowed to gargle with ice water to produce local numbing. It was not until 1847 when John Snow described using ether for a cleft lip repair. Later in 1850, chloroform was reported for the repair of a bilateral lip and palate in a 7 year old.[1]

These anesthetics by today's standards would be considered rather rudimentary and potentially unsafe. The airway was unprotected and compromised secondary to drainage of blood into the posterior pharynx. A refinement in airway management came with the introduction of the nasopharyngeal insufflation technique. A rubber tube was placed down

each nostril, one for inspiration of anesthetics and the other for expiration. Packing could then be applied to the posterior pharynx, which provided a barrier for blood and protected the airway. In 1921, Magill provided the first endotracheal insufflation technique on an infant and later applied this technique for the repair of a cleft palate in 1924.[1] Today, general anesthesia is routinely and safely used for infants and children having cleft lip/palate repairs. Anesthesia management for these patients begins with a thorough preoperative history and physical exam.

PREOPERATIVE CONSIDERATIONS

Children can present for surgical correction of cleft lip and palate from infancy to early adulthood. Typically, surgical repair of the cleft lip is performed at 3–6 months and the repair of the cleft palate at 9–18 months. Pharyngoplasty, when necessary, is usually performed later at 5–15 years of age. Historically, the safe age for cleft lip repair was established at 6–12 weeks in 1964 by an audit of American plastic surgeons[2] and later supported in 1966 by a large retrospective review[3] that showed an increased rate of complications in children with weights less then 10 lbs, hemoglobin less than 10 g/dL, and white cell counts higher than 10 000. There are more recent studies that have highlighted the safety of anesthesia for full and preterm neonates.[4,5] The authors in these studies stress the importance of having a team of surgeons, anesthesiologists, and nursing staff that are experienced and comfortable with the intraoperative and postoperative care of the neonate. The preoperative preparation of the infant for cleft lip and palate surgery begins with a sound understanding of their anatomy, physiology, and associated anomalies.

A hallmark of developmental cardiac physiology is the transition from fetal to neonatal circulation. This transition is characterized by a change from parallel circulation (cardiac output contributes to both pulmonary and systemic perfusion simultaneously allowing mixing of oxygenated and deoxygenated blood) to one that occurs in series (cardiac output contributes to either pulmonary or systemic perfusion with minimal admixture). This change occurs during delivery because pulmonary vascular resistance (PVR) decreases and systemic vascular resistance (SVR) increases allowing for a significant increase in pulmonary blood flow. With a decrease in PVR, pulmonary blood flow and venous return to the left atrium increase. The increase in left atrial pressure and flow closes the foramen ovale. Over the next few months of life, pulmonary vascular resistance decreases even further, and the functional closure of the ductus arteriosus and foramen ovale becomes essentially permanent.[5]

In the newborn period an increase in PVR can lead to a return to fetal circulation with right-to-left shunting across the foramen ovale and ductus arteriosus. Hypoxia and acidosis are important causes of an increase in PVR. Hypoxemia and acidosis can lead to a vicious cycle of increased PVR, increased right-to-left shunting, increased hypoxemia, increased tissue acidosis, and further increase in PVR and shunting.

The neonatal myocardium is immature and continues its development after birth. At delivery and extending into the neonatal period, there are fewer contractile elements and there is less elastin in the newborn's myocardium resulting in a decreased contractile capacity and decreased ventricular compliance, respectively. The consequence is a reduced capacity to adapt to increases in preload or afterload.[6,7] Since the neonatal heart has a limited ability to increase stroke volume,[7] neonates are poorly tolerant of bradycardia; moreover, significant volume loads may more easily cause ventricular overload and failure.

The neonatal/infant lung is less compliant than the adult lung. The immature lung in the pediatric patient is characterized by small and poorly developed alveoli with thickened walls and decreased elastin. Since infants (much like older adults) have less elastin, the closing capacity (the lung volume at which there is airway collapse) occurs at a larger lung volume in the very young and the very old.[8,9] Also the neonatal chest wall is more cartilaginous and compliant than the adult chest wall, making it more likely to collapse. These developmental differences in respiratory physiology make the infant alveoli more prone to closure at end exhalation (closing capacity is larger than functional residual capacity), increasing the infant's risk of developing atelectasis, right-to-left transpulmonary shunting, and hypoxia.

Another significant difference between neonatal and adult respiration is oxygen consumption. Neonatal oxygen consumption is 2–3 times greater than that of the adult (5–8 mL/kg/min vs. 2–3 mL/kg/min).[10] This accounts for the rapid oxygen desaturation during apnea or hypoventilation.

Taking care of the ex-premature infant can pose significant anesthetic concerns. Neonates, especially in the setting of recent prematurity, may have episodes of apnea after exposure to sedation or general anesthesia.[11] The risk of an undetected, untreated apneic event must be balanced with the need for the patient to eventually return home. The younger the postconceptual age (PCA) [PCA = gestational age (weeks) + age of baby (weeks)], the greater the risk for postoperative apneas, and the longer the duration of disordered breathing postoperatively.[12] Fixed risk factors include a history of extreme prematurity (28 weeks vs. 32 weeks) and anemia (hematocrit <30%), regardless of current PCA.[13,14] It is not clear at what post-conceptual age a full-term or ex-premature infant ceases to require postoperative monitoring for these events. In general, a postconceptual age of greater than 45–50 weeks may qualify an otherwise healthy ex-premature infant to return home the day of surgery. Children's hospitals have predetermined ages at which an ex-premature baby having general anesthesia must be admitted overnight for observation. Infants considered at risk for postoperative apnea should be monitored overnight on a bradycardia and apnea monitor.[14]

Acute upper respiratory tract infections increase the incidence of perioperative pulmonary complications, which include laryngospasm, bronchospasm, and oxygen desaturation. Factors that increase the risk of these pulmonary complications include ex-premature status, reactive airway disease, age less than one, airway procedures, endotracheal intubation, and exposure to second-hand smoke. Patients presenting for cleft surgery often exhibit many of these risk factors. Infants with fever, change in behavior from baseline, purulent nasal drainage, and abnormal breath sounds likely have a moderate to severe upper respiratory tract infection and should have their surgery delayed 2–6 weeks.[15]

Many anomalies and syndromes have been associated with facial clefting. In a recent epidemiologic study of nearly 6 million births, almost 30% of cleft lips and palates occur with an associated anomaly or syndrome. Associated congenital malformations involved most organ systems but primarily affected the cardiovascular, musculoskeletal, and central nervous system.[16] Musculoskeletal deformities were the most common and included polydactyly and limb reduction. The majority of central nervous system pathology are categorized as "reduction deformities of the brain." The cardiovascular defects were the third most common associated anomaly and primarily included ventricular and atrial septal defects and tetralogy of fallot. Syndromes that are commonly associated with cleft lip and palate and their anesthetic implications are listed in Table 13–1. The three most common syndromes/sequences are Pierre–Robin sequence, velocardiofacial syndrome (VCFS), and Stickler syndrome.

Other important issues to be considered with these preoperative patients are related to swallowing difficulties, which can lead to malnutrition, anemia, failure to thrive, frequent aspiration and pulmonary infections. Ideally, the nutritional status of the child should be optimized before surgery because of the impact on wound healing and outcome. Significant bleeding from cleft surgery requiring transfusion has been described but this is primarily presented in the older literature.[17] In more recent retrospective evaluations of complications from cleft surgery, bleeding requiring transfusion is a rare event.[4,18,19]

The preoperative evaluation of the cleft patient should include a complete history focusing on significant past medical (obstructive symptoms such as snoring or apnea), surgical, and family history including associated anomalies and syndromes. The exam should identify hidden pathology such as heart murmurs and difficult airways. The airway exam in an infant is challenging. An abnormality in the craniofacial skeleton or mandible may predict difficulty with ventilation or intubation. The infant should be examined en-face and in profile to identify facial anomalies and retrognathia. Associated anomalies may alter the anesthetic management of cleft patients (see Table 13–1). A thorough preoperative evaluation may also include echocardiography and/or brain imaging in infants with suspected cardiac or central nervous system pathology. Infants with associated cardiac malformations may require subacute bacterial endocarditis prophylaxis and meticulous attention to prevent unintentional introduction of intravascular air bubbles.

ANESTHETIC MANAGEMENT

Premedication

Preoperative anxiety is common and can cause adverse effects extending into the postoperative period. Children that display significant preoperative anxiety are more likely to develop postoperative behavioral changes. These changes are characterized by an increase in separation anxiety, eating disturbances, sleeping disturbances, and oppositional defiant behavior. These changes may last for up to two weeks; but, in one study were significantly reduced with the preoperative administration of midazolam.[20] Preoperative anxiety in children is intimately linked to separation anxiety. Separation anxiety usually begins to develop after 10 months of age. Most cleft patients present for surgery when they are less than 1 year old and often do not require premedication for preoperative anxiety. It should be considered in patients over 10 months of age that exhibit preoperative anxiety. Patients with

significant airway obstruction (Treacher Collins, obstructive sleep apnea) should have the dose of midazolam reduced or should not receive it at all.

Induction

Most patients with a cleft lip/palate can be induced with a standard inhalation induction. If an intravenous catheter is in place, an intravenous induction can also be performed. The most important issue related with induction of anesthesia is airway management. Difficulty with mask ventilation and intubation can occur. Infants with craniofacial anomalies in addition to the cleft, or patients with retrognathia, may be difficult to ventilate. Induction for patients with orofacial clefting can be achieved with an inhalational agent such as sevoflurane. Airway management for most of these children is straightforward. Airway obstruction can usually be managed with the insertion of an oropharyngeal airway and continuous positive airway pressure (CPAP).

For the patient with an isolated cleft lip and palate, the incidence of difficult laryngoscopy is common. Several studies have evaluated this, and the reported overall incidence of difficult laryngoscopy (Cormack and Lehane 3 and 4 view) varies from 4 to 7%.[21,22] Factors predicting a more difficult laryngoscopic view include bilateral clefts and retrognathia. Age less than 6 months was not a consistent risk factor. The patients in one study did not receive muscle relaxants, and they all received external laryngeal compression, which may explain some of the differences.[23] Despite this high percentage of poor laryngoscopic view, only 1% of the patients were difficult to intubate, and only one patient had a failed intubation.[21,22]

Cleft patients with associated craniofacial anomalies or retrognathia may be difficult to ventilate or intubate. In these patients, preparations for alternative airway management need to be made. If general anesthesia is induced, the patient should remain spontaneously ventilating until the trachea is secured with an endotracheal tube. Successful intubation through a laryngeal mask with the aide of a fiberoptic scope has been described for pediatric patients with difficult airways.[23] The technique involves placing a fiberoptic scope, previously loaded with an endotracheal tube, through the properly positioned LMA. The scope is then used as a guide to pass the endotracheal tube into the trachea. Another endotracheal tube of equal size can be connected and act as a "pusher," allowing advancement of the first endotracheal tube and facilitating LMA removal. Uncuffed endotracheal tubes are easier to use because the bulb for the cuff is difficult to pass through the lumen of the smaller LMAs (an ETT-LMA sizing chart is provided in Table 13–2). Other intubating devices, including the use of the Shikani Optical Stylet™, have been described.[24] Surgical repair of the cleft palate using a laryngeal mask airway has even been described.[25] Of note, disruption of a previous cleft palate repair, during the placement of an LMA, has also been described: and, this suggests that care should be taken when placing an LMA in a patient with a history of cleft palate repair.[26]

Table 13–1.

Syndromes Associated with Cleft Lip and Palate and Their Anesthetic Implications

Syndrome	Anesthesia Considerations	References
van der Woude syndrome	Associated lip abnormalities	Baum VC, Flaherty JE. *Anesthesia for Genetic, Metabolic and Dysmorphic Syndromes of Childhood.* Philadelphia: Lippincott Williams & Wilkins.
Pierre Robin sequence	Micrognathia, glossoptosis, airway obstruction. May be very difficult to mask ventilate and intubate.	Baum VC, Flaherty JE. *Anesthesia for Genetic, Metabolic and Dysmorphic Syndromes of Childhood.* Philadelphia: Lippincott Williams & Wilkins.
Velocardiofacial syndrome	Microdeletion of chromosome 22, microcephaly, micrognathia, congenital cardiac disease, may have developmental delay, neonatal hypocalcemia, T-cell immune deficiency. May be difficult to intubate, consider preop echo & SBE prophylaxis, blood products need to be irradiated.	Baum VC, Flaherty JE. *Anesthesia for Genetic, Metabolic and Dysmorphic Syndromes of Childhood.* Philadelphia: Lippincott Williams & Wilkins.
Stickler syndrome	Marfanoid appearance. May have Pierre Robin sequence, joint laxity, mitral valve prolapse. May be difficult to intubate if micrognathia present.	Baum VC, Flaherty JE. *Anesthesia for Genetic, Metabolic and Dysmorphic Syndromes of Childhood.* Philadelphia: Lippincott Williams & Wilkins.
DiGeorge syndrome	Same chromosomal abnormality as velocardiofacial syndrome (see above)	Baum VC, Flaherty JE. *Anesthesia for Genetic, Metabolic and Dysmorphic Syndromes of Childhood.* Philadelphia: Lippincott Williams & Wilkins.
Popliteal pterygium syndrome	Eyelid, oral, and popliteal webbing, genital anomalies	Baum VC, Flaherty JE. *Anesthesia for Genetic, Metabolic and Dysmorphic Syndromes of Childhood.* Philadelphia: Lippincott Williams & Wilkins.
Ectrodactyly-ectodermal clefting syndrome	Triad of lobster claw deformity, ectodermal dysplasia, cleft lip/palate. May be prone to hyperthermia.	Mizushima A, Satoyoshi M. Anesthetic problems in a child with ectrodactyly-ectodermal dysplasia and cleft lip/palate: The EEC syndrome. *Anesthesia* 47:137–140, 1992.
Goldenhar syndrome	Hemifacial microsomia, epibulbar dermoids, rib/vertebral/scapular anomalies. May have congenital heart disease. May be very difficult to intubate, consider preop echo & SBE prophylaxis	Baum VC, Flaherty JE. *Anesthesia for Genetic, Metabolic and Dysmorphic Syndromes of Childhood.* Philadelphia: Lippincott Williams & Wilkins.
Treacher–Collins syndrome	Craniofacial clefting, mandibular hypoplasia. May have obstructive sleep apnea, may have congenital heart disease. May be difficult or impossible to intubate, consider preop echo & SBE prophylaxis.	Baum VC, Flaherty JE. *Anesthesia for Genetic, Metabolic and Dysmorphic Syndromes of Childhood.* Philadelphia: Lippincott Williams & Wilkins.
Crouzon syndrome	Craniosynostosis, midface hypoplasia, proptosis, airway obstruction. May be difficult to ventilate and/or intubate.	Baum VC, Flaherty JE. *Anesthesia for Genetic, Metabolic and Dysmorphic Syndromes of Childhood.* Philadelphia: Lippincott Williams & Wilkins.

(continued)

Table 13–1.

(*Continued*)

Syndrome	Anesthesia Considerations	References
Sprintzen syndrome	Same chromosomal abnormality as velocardiofacial syndrome (see above)	Baum VC, Flaherty JE. *Anesthesia for Genetic, Metabolic and Dysmorphic Syndromes of Childhood.* Philadelphia: Lippincott Williams & Wilkins.
Klippel–Feil syndrome	Short webbed neck, micrognathia, may have congenital heart disease. May be difficult to intubate, consider preop echo & SBE prophylaxis.	Baum VC, Flaherty JE. *Anesthesia for Genetic, Metabolic and Dysmorphic Syndromes of Childhood.* Philadelphia: Lippincott Williams & Wilkins.
Trisomy 13	Micrognathia, congenital heart disease, developmental delay, renal anomalies. May be difficult to intubate, consider preop echo & SBE prophylaxis, check preop creatinine.	Baum VC, Flaherty JE. *Anesthesia for Genetic, Metabolic and Dysmorphic Syndromes of Childhood.* Philadelphia: Lippincott Williams & Wilkins.
Trisomy 18	Micrognathia, congenital heart disease, developmental delay, renal anomalies, hypotonia. May be difficult to intubate, consider preop echo & SBE prophylaxis, check preop creatinine.	Baum VC, Flaherty JE. *Anesthesia for Genetic, Metabolic and Dysmorphic Syndromes of Childhood.* Philadelphia: Lippincott Williams & Wilkins.
Trisomy 21	Macroglossia, subglottic stenosis, congenital heart disease, obstructive sleep apnea, pulm HTN, pneumonias, hypothyroidism, atlantoaxial instability. Mask ventilation may be difficult, assess neck for instability, use a smaller than expected endotracheal tube, consider preop echo & SBE prophylaxis.	Baum VC, Flaherty JE. *Anesthesia for Genetic, Metabolic and Dysmorphic Syndromes of Childhood.* Philadelphia: Lippincott Williams & Wilkins.

The oral RAE (Ring, Adaire, Ellwyn) preformed tracheal tube is routinely used for the intubation, as the preformed bend in the tube facilitates the use of the mouth retractor (Fig. 13–1). Extra care should be paid to securing the tube and protecting it from unintentional extubation. Surgical prep can remove the tape from the tube if it is not secured well. An example of an oral RAE secured in place is shown in Fig. 13–2(A)–(G). Owing to the fixed length of the preformed oral RAE tube, there is an increased risk of extubation if an unexpectedly small size is required. An armour reinforced endotracheal tube can also be used to secure the airway in this situation. These endotracheal tubes are reinforced and do not

Table 13–2.

Laryngeal Mask Airway-Endotracheal Tube Compatibility*

LMA size	Endotracheal size
1.5	4.0 uncuffed
2.0	4.5–5.0 uncuffed
2.5	5.5 uncuffed
3.0	6.0 uncuffed
4.0	6.0 cuffed

Hammer G, Anesthesia for pediatric thoracic surgery. Anesth Analg 2001.

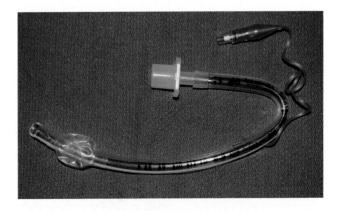

Figure 13–1. Oral RAE tube.

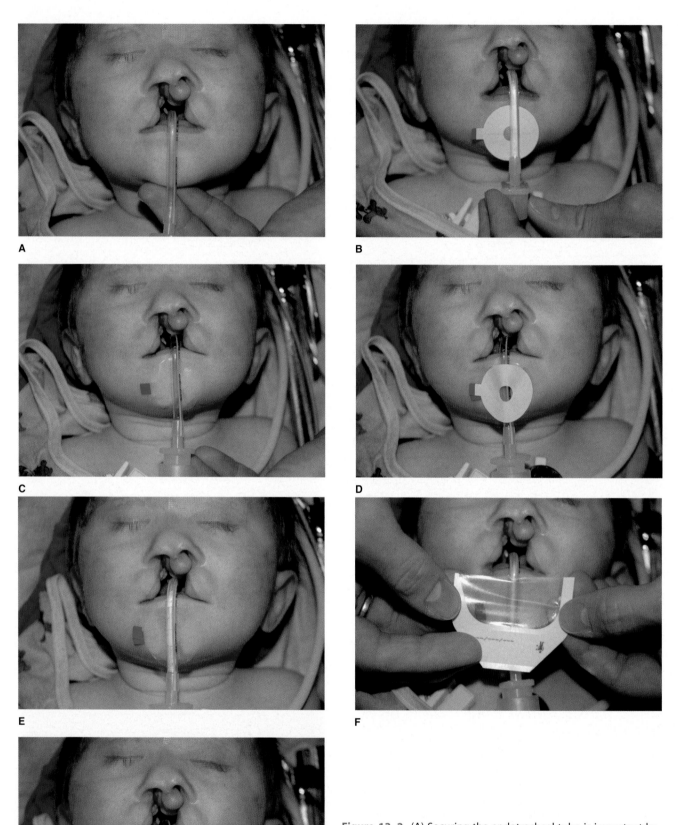

Figure 13–2. (A) Securing the endotracheal tube is important because the surgical preparation will often loosen tape and patient movement can result in dislodgement of the endotracheal tube. (B)–(C) Using the double adhesive tape for precordial stethoscopes provides a solid foundation on which to build. The endotracheal tube can be placed on top of the adhesive. (D)–(E) Another double adhesive tape for precordial stethoscopes can be placed over the endotracheal tube. (F)–(G) Covering the precordial stethoscope adhesives (sandwiching the endotracheal tube) with an occlusive dressing (tegaderm) insures protection from the surgical prep.

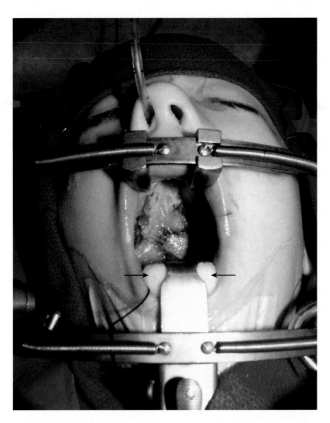

Figure 13–3. Cotton dental rolls are placed on either side of the oral RAE tube (arrows) to prevent compression and/or kinking of the tube at the bend of the metal tongue blade of the mouth retractor.

kink with flexion making them ideal for infants or children who require a smaller than expected endotracheal tube size. Breath sounds should be reevaluated after the mouth gag is in place because of possible compression of the tube or advancement causing single lung ventilation. Of note, an oral RAE tube, when placed into the mouth retractor, may become kinked at the preformed bend as it is compressed between the infant's tongue/teeth and the bend in the metal blade of the mouth retractor. To eliminate this possibility, standard cotton dental rolls can be placed on either side of the oral RAE tube prior to opening the mouth retractor. The dental rolls, which are slightly larger than the RAE tube, serve to block the compression of the tube when the mouth retractor is open, and prevents tube compression (Fig. 13–3).

Maintenance

There is no standard anesthetic technique for the maintenance of anesthesia. Both inhalational anesthetics and total intravenous anesthetics have been described for patients having cleft lip and palate surgery. A balanced anesthetic with any inhalational agent (+/− nitrous oxide), opioid, and muscle relaxant (optional) is effective and safe as long as the autonomic response is blocked, keeping the mean arterial pressure 55–60 mmHg to prevent excessive bleeding. Some studies have attempted to identify a benefit of one technique over

the other. However, there does not appear to be any obvious benefit of one particular technique.

In one study, the use of remifentanil failed to provide any major advantage over sufentanil in infants having cleft palate surgery.[27] Infants receiving remifentanil did use less isoflurane, but time to extubation and postoperative morphine consumption was similar in both groups. The hemodynamic stability provided by remifentanil may be attractive, because it may minimize bleeding. In the study, surgeons described excessive bleeding in three remifentanil patients as compared to six sufentanil patients. This advantage was not seen in another study that compared propofol-remifentanil to sevoflurane-fentanyl in infants presenting for cleft lip and palate repair. In fact, in this study, the propofol-remifentanil group was associated with a higher intraoperative blood pressure. There was no difference in time to extubation or postoperative morphine consumption.[28]

Local infiltration of the palate with epinephrine is performed to prevent excessive bleeding and to facilitate mucosal dissection. It has been demonstrated that inhaled anesthetics sensitize the myocardium and decrease the arrhythmia threshold of epinephrine. Katz, 20 years ago, described ventricular dysrrhythmias when epinephrine was infiltrated during halothane anesthesia.[29] The safe dose of epinephrine is different for adults than for children. Doses as low as 1 μg/kg were found to be arrhythmogenic in adults under halothane anesthesia.[29] In contrast, a study in 1983 found that 10 μg/kg was safe in children under halothane anesthesia.[30] The children in this study ranged from 3 months to 17 years old, were ventilated to maintain an end tidal CO_2 of 40 mm Hg, and did not have congenital heart disease. The other inhaled anesthetics appear to be as safe or safer than halothane. In adults, the arrhythmogenic dose of epinephrine was greater than 5 μg/kg and did not differ between isoflurane, sevoflurane, or desflurane.[31,32]

Positioning and padding is critical during long anesthetics. In particular attention should be paid to protecting the infants chest wall and extremities from the breathing circuit and tight monitoring leads. The patient is often rotated 90–180° and a straight adapter can facilitate the positioning of the circuit.

Emergence

Precautions with the airway management should be taken prior to extubation, especially for those patients with difficult airways. Airway obstruction has been described after palatoplasties.[33] Patients undergoing a palatoplasty that have a history of a difficult airway or have an associated congenital anomaly should have a nasopharyngeal airway placed by the surgeon prior to emergence. This may facilitate ventilation after extubation (Fig. 13–4). For patients with a history of very difficult intubations, a Cook Airway Exchange Catheter (CAEC) can be left in place after extubation until the child is recovered.[34] This is an extreme measure, but can provide a means of oxygenation and reintubation should these become necessary. Throat packs can result in airway obstruction if

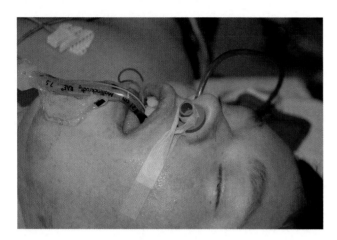

Figure 13–4. A nasopharyngeal airway minimizes the risk of airway obstruction after extubation.

unintentionally left in place and confirmation of their removal must take place prior to extubation.

A particular concern for the anesthesiologist when taking care of the extubated cleft palate patient is tongue edema. Profound tongue, palate, and pharyngeal edema can occur from venous engorgement from the Dingman-Dott mouth retractor. It is prudent for surgeons to regularly release the retractor throughout the procedure to minimize this risk.[35,36] Patients experiencing respiratory distress need to be reintubated and mechanically ventilated (Fig. 13–5). It may take several days for the edema to resolve.[35]

PAIN MANAGEMENT

Systemic Analgesia

Postoperative pain management for cleft lip and palate repair should ideally provide analgesia without respiratory

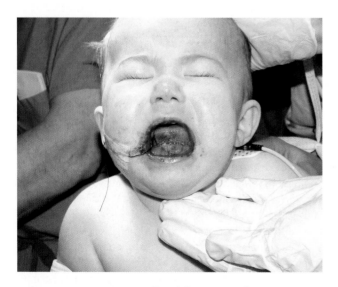

Figure 13–5. Tongue swelling following a cleft palate repair.

depression, nausea, or vomiting. The best solution seems to be the combination of different medications, usually acetaminophen with the occasional addition of an opioid. Acetaminophen when administered rectally is dosed 40 mg/kg followed by 20 mg/kg every 6 hours, 10–15 mg/kg if given orally.[37,38] Acetaminophen may have an opioid sparing effect and some infants require little to no opioids in the postoperative period.[39] One study suggested that there is no opioid sparing effect of prophylactically administered rectal acetaminophen. However, none of the patients in this study received pre or intraoperative opioids, and they were evaluated for only the first 60 minutes of the postoperative period.[40] Nonsteroidal-antiinflammatory agents have been described for analgesia following cleft palate surgery.[41] Although some evidence suggests there may be no increased risk of bleeding, many surgeons and anesthesiologists choose not to routinely use them. Opioids, when administered, should be appropriately dosed to minimize the risk of respiratory compromise in infants. A safe starting dose of morphine for infants is 0.02 mg/kg dosed every 3–4 hours as needed. Infants undergoing cleft surgery who receive postoperative oral or parenteral opioids, should be appropriately monitored (i.e., apnea/bradycardia monitors, EKG, O2 sat, etc.).

Nerve Blockade

The bilateral infraorbital nerve block works very well as an adjunct or as the sole analgesic technique for cleft lip repair.[42] The block can be performed by anesthesiologists or surgeons and provides better analgesia when compared with periincisional infiltration or opioids alone.[43,44] The infraorbital nerve block has been described in all age groups including neonates.[45]

The maxillary division of the trigeminal nerve exits from the infraorbital foramen. The nerve provides the sensory supply to the upper lip, the choana, maxillary sinus, part of the nasal septum, and the tip of the nose. This block can be used to provide analgesia for cleft lip surgery, nasal septal repair, and endoscopic sinus surgery. There are two approaches to the maxillary division of the trigeminal nerve: extraoral (percutaneous) and intraoral. For the extraoral or percutaneous approach, the needle is directed toward the infraorbital foramen externally through the skin. The location of the foramen varies based on age. In children and adults, the foramen is located approximately 5–10 mm below the infraorbital rim in a vertical line from the pupil of the eye (Fig. 13–6A). In neonates the foramen appears to be slightly more inferior at the intersection of a vertical line from the pupil and a horizontal line from the ala of the nose.[45] The correlation between age and the distance of the infraorbital foramen from the midline can be expressed as a mathematical formula [distance from midline to infraorbital foramen in mm = $21.3 + 0.5 \times$ age (in years)].[46] It is suggested that the thumb or a finger of the hand not holding the syringe be placed on the inferior orbital rim as a guide and protector of the eye (Fig. 13–6A).

The intraoral route is accessed through the sub-sulcal area in the buccal mucosa (Fig. 13–6B). The point of insertion

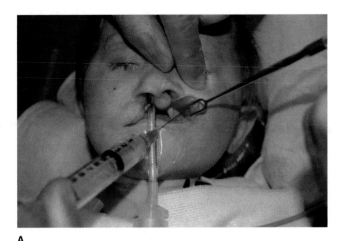

A

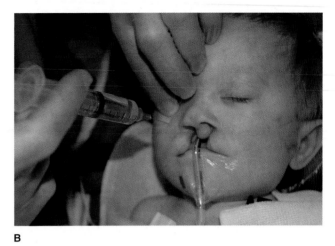

B

Figure 13–6. (A) Left-sided trans-oral infra-orbital nerve block. (B) Right-sided percutaneous infra-orbital nerve block.

is the upper incisor or the second bicuspid on the side to be blocked. A needle is passed through the sub-sulcal route toward the location of the infraorbital foramen. As with the transcutaneous approach, it is suggested that the thumb or a finger of the hand not holding the syringe be placed on the infant's inferior orbital rim and used as a guide and protector of the orbit and eye. Infants scheduled for cleft lip repairs require 0.5–1 mL of local anesthetic solution on each side, for older children and adolescents 1.5–2 mL of local anesthetic solution can be used. Bupivacaine (0.125, 0.25, or 0.5%, with or without epinephrine [5 μg/mL]) or ropivacaine (0.2 or 0.5%) can be used for the block.

The duration of postoperative analgesia depends on the local anesthetic and the concentration being used. For children and adults 0.125% provided analgesia for approximately 4–8 hours.[43] Bupivacaine (0.5%) provides analgesia for 6–24 hours.[42,47] In neonates the block may be shorter at 2–3 hours.[45]

ANESTHESIA IN DEVELOPING COUNTRIES

Medical missions are performed in developing countries for a variety of procedures including cardiac, orthopedic, and genitourinary surgeries. Cleft lip and palate missions are some of the most common and are carried out by multiple organizations around the world. There are several barriers to providing safe effective surgical and anesthesia care in developing countries. Some of these include lack of hospital resources (electricity, lighting), medical resources (anesthesia machines, ventilators, oxygen, surgical equipment, medications), personnel resources (lack of training, temperament), standards of care, language skills, and cultural/social differences.[19,48,49] Despite these barriers, many health care providers volunteer their time and skills to help children with cleft deformities.

There is no standard of care for anesthetizing patients in a developing country. Often the care is tailored to the limited resources that are available. Some of the difficulties described in the literature include limited preoperative evaluations,

number of anesthetizing agents, ventilators, monitoring, and post-anesthesia care units. The preoperative screening process should identify children with obvious cardiovascular and respiratory pathology. Due to the high volume and limited ability to preoperatively prepare these patients, many are not selected for surgery. There are pathologies in developing countries, which may complicate anesthesia care. These include malnutrition, anemia, and parasitic infections to name a few. Unfortunately, many of these patients will not be identified, and it is not clear what impact this has on outcomes. Families may also withhold information for fear of having the surgery cancelled. This may result in increased morbidity and even mortality.[19]

The anesthetic induction, maintenance, and emergence needs to be tailored to the available resources. Patients who present for isolated lip repair, and are old enough, can have the procedure under local anesthesia.[49] Patients that require general anesthesia are induced with either an inhalational or intravenous technique. Halothane is a commonly used inhalational agent because of its cost. The airway is secured with an endotracheal tube in most circumstances; however, endotracheal tubes may be reused. Muscle relaxants in some practices[19] are rarely used because of the lack of mechanical ventilation. In this population, spontaneous ventilation may be safer for the patient and the anesthetist's hands are free. Some groups preferred muscle relaxants because it facilitated rapid recovery in a setting that had no recovery area.[48]

Outcome data for patients having cleft repairs in developing countries is limited. In a recent survey, Fisher identified complications associated with surgical patients from Operation Smile.[19] Most of the surgeries were for cleft lip and palate repair but other common procedures included plastic and orthopedic surgery. The data was collected from voluntary submission of perioperative data sheets. Of the 9422 patients during the time period, data was collected on 6037 patients. Complications in the operating room, which included laryngospasm, bronchospasm, and unintentional extubation, occurred in 5% of these patients. In the recovery area complications such as upper airway obstruction, postextubation croup, bronchospasm, delayed discharge (pain, agitation) occurred in 3.3%. Cardiovascular complications including ventricular ectopy and supraventricular tachycardia occurred in 1.5%. This is likely under reported because not all patients had electrocardiographic monitoring. Significant negative events occurred in 1.8% of the patients and these included return to the operating room for bleeding, intraoperative reintubation, cancellation of surgery after induction, blood transfusion, cardiac arrest, and death. The age of the patient predicted respiratory complications. A significantly larger percentage of children less than 1 year old experienced intraoperative respiratory complications. Death was an uncommon event; however, during the 18-month collection period, there were four deaths among all of the Operation Smile patients. This death rate of 0.4 per 1000[19] is higher than some other reports of pediatric perioperative deaths,[50,51] but it is difficult to compare the different patient populations. Despite this information, countless lives have benefited from medical missions to developing countries, and most of these procedures are accomplished safely. However, it must be recognized that performing surgery and anesthesia in these environments poses unique cultural, patient care, and system-based challenges for the entire surgical team.

References

1. Jones RG. A short history of anaesthesia for hare-lip and cleft palate repair. *Br J Anaesth* 43:796–802, 1971.
2. Lewin ML. Management of cleft lip and palate in the United States and Canada. *Plastic Reconstr Surg* 33:383–394, 1964.
3. Wilhmsen HR, Musgrave RH. Complication of cleft lip surgery. *Cleft J* 3:223–231, 1966.
4. Van Boven MJ, Penderville PE, Veyckemans F, et al. Neonatal cleft lip repair: The anesthetist's point of view. *Cleft Palate Craniofac J* 30:574–577, 1993.
5. Rudolph AM. *Congenital Diseases of the Heart.* Chicago: Year Book Medical Publishers, 1974.
6. Berman W, Musselman J. Myocardial performance in the newborn lamb. *Am J Physiol* 237:H66–H70, 1979.
7. Friedman WF. Intrinsic physiologic properties of the newborn heart. *Prog Cardiovasc Dis* 15:87–111, 1972.
8. Peirce J, Hobcott J. Studies on the collagen and elastin content of the human lung. *J Clin Invest* 39:8, 1960.
9. Mansell A, Bryan C, Levison H. Airway closure in children. *J Applied Physiol* 33:771, 1972.
10. Polgar G, Weng TR. The functional development of the respiratory system: From the period of gestation to adulthood. *Am Rev Respir Dis* 120:625–695, 1979.
11. Welborn LG, Rice LJ, Hannallah RS, et al. Postoperative apnea in former preterm infants: Prospective comparison of spinal and general anesthesia. *Anesthesiology* 72(5):838, 1990.
12. Kurth CD, Spitzer AR, Broennle AM, Downes JJ. Postoperative apnea in preterm infants. *Anesthesiology* 66:483–488, 1987.
13. Welborn LG, Hannallah RS, Luban NLC, et al. Anemia and postoperative apnea in former preterm infants. *Anesthesiology* 74:1003–1006, 1991.
14. Cote CJ, Zaslavsky A, Downes JJ, et al. Postoperative apnea in former preterm infants. *Anesthesiology* 82:809–822, 1995.
15. Tait AR, Malviya S, Voepel-Lewis T, et al. Risk factors for perioperative adverse respiratory events in children with upper respiratory tract infections. *Anesthesiology* 95(2):299, 2001.
16. Calzolari E, Pierini A, Astolfi G, et al. Associated anomalies in multi malformed infants with cleft lip and palate: An epidemiologic study of nearly 6 million births in 23 EUROCAT registries. *Am J Med Genetics part A* 143A:528–537, 2007.
17. Rintala A. Blood loss in cleft palate surgery. *Acta Chir Scand* 129:288–291, 1965.
18. Stephens P, Saunders P, Bingham R. Neonatal cleft repair: A retrospective review of anesthetic complications. *Paediatr Anaesth* 7:33–36, 1997.
19. Fisher QA, Nichols D, Stewart F, et al. Assessing pediatric anesthesia practices for volunteer medical services abroad. *Anesthesiology* 95:1315–1322, 2001.
20. Kain ZN, Mayes LC, Wang SM, et al.. Postoperative behavioral outcomes in children: The effects of sedative premedication. *Anesthesiology* 90(3):758–765, 1999.
21. Gunawardana RH. Difficult laryngoscopy in cleft lip and palate surgery. *Br J Anaesth* 76:757–759, 1996.
22. Xue FS, Zhang GH, Li P, et al. The clinical observation of difficult laryngoscopy and difficult intubation in infants with cleft lip and palate. *Pediatr Anesth* 16:283–289, 2006.
23. Dubreuil M, Ecoffey C. Laryngyeal mask guided tracheal intubation in paediatric anesthesia. *Paediatr Anaesth* 2:334, 1992.
24. Shukry M, Hanson RD, Koveleskie J, et al. Management of the difficult pediatric airway with Shikani Optical Stylet™ *Pediatr Anesth* 15:342–345, 2005.
25. Beveridge ME. Laryngeal mask anesthesia for repair of cleft palate. *Anaesthesia* 44:656–657, 1989.
26. Somerville NS, Fenlon S, Boorman J, Abbot M. Disruption of cleft repair following the use of the laryngeal mask airway. *Anaesthesia* 59:401–403, 2004.
27. Rolla P, Gall O, Dejesus L, et al. Remifentanil for cleft palate surgery in young infants. *Paediatr Anaesth* 13:701–707, 2003.
28. Steinmetz J, Holm-Knusen R, Sorensen MK, et al. Hemodynamic differences between propofol-remifentanil and sevoflurane anesthesia for repair of cleft lip and palate in infants. *Pediatr Anesth* 17:32–37, 2007.
29. Katz RL, Matteo RS, Papper EM. The injection of epinephrine during general anesthesia with halogenated hydrocarbons and cyclopropane in man. *Anesthesiology* 23:597–600, 1962.
30. Karl H, Swedlow DB, Lee KW, Downes J. Epinephrine-halothane interactions in children. *Anesthesiology* 58:142–145, 1983.
31. Moore MA, Weiskopf RB, Eger E, et al. Arrhythmogenic doses of epinephrine are similar during desflurane or isoflurane anesthesia in humans. *Anesthesiology* 79:943–947, 1993.
32. Navarro R, Weiskopf RB, Moore MA, et al. Humans anesthetized with sevoflurane or similar arrhythmic response to epinephrine. *Anesthesiology* 80:545–549, 1994.
33. Anthony AK, Sloan GM. Airway obstruction following palatoplasty: Analysis of 247 consecutive operations. *Cleft Palate Craniofacial J* 39:145–148, 2002.
34. Hammer GB, Funck N, Rosenthal DN, et al. A technique for maintenance of airway access in infants with a difficult airway following tracheal extubation. *Pediatr Anesth* 11:622–625, 2001.
35. Oste CD, Savron F, Pelizzo G, Sarti A. Acute airway obstruction in an infant with Pierre robin syndrome after palatoplasty. *Acta Anaesthesiol Scand* 48:787–789, 2004.
36. Anthony AK, Sloan GM. Airway obstruction following palatoplasty: Analysis of 247 consecutive operations. *Cleft Palate Craniofacial J* 39:145–148, 2002.
37. Birmingham PK, Tobin MJ, Henthom TK, et al. Twenty four hour pharmacokinetics of rectal acetaminophen in children: An old drug with new recommendations. *Anesthesiology* 87(2):244–252, 1997.
38. Birmingham PK, Tobin MJ, Fisher DM, et al. Initial and subsequent dosing of rectal acetaminophen in children: A 24-hour pharmacokinetic study of new dose recommendations. *Anesthesiology* 94(3):385–389, 2001.
39. Stephens P, Saunders P, Bingham R. Neonatal cleft lip repair: A retrospective review of anaesthetic complications. *Pediatr Anaesth* 7:33–36, 1997.

40. Bremerich DH, Neidhart G, Heimann K, et al. Prophylactically administered rectal acetaminophen does not reduce postoperative opioid requirements in infants and small children undergoing elective cleft palate repair. *Anesth Analg* 92:907–912, 2001.

41. Sylaidis P, O'Neill T. Diclofenac analgesia following cleft palate surgery. *Cleft Palate Craniofac J* 35(6):544–545, 1998.

42. Eipe N, Choudhrie A, Pillai AD, et al. Regional anesthesia for cleft lip repair: A preliminary study. *Cleft Palate Craniofacial J* 43(2):138–141, 2006.

43. Pradeep K, Prabhu K, Wig J, et al. Bilateral infraorbital nerve block is superior to peri-incisional infiltration for analgesia after repair of cleft palate. *Scand J Plast Reconstr Hand Surg* 33:83–87, 1999.

44. Rajamani A, Kamat V, Rajavel VP, et al. A comparison of bilateral infraorbital nerve block with intravenous fentanyl for analgesia following cleft lip repair in children. *Pediatr Anesth* 17(2):133–139, 2007.

45. Bosenberg AT, Kible FW. Infraorbital nerve block in neonates for cleft lip repair: Anatomical study and clinical application. *Br J Anaesth* 74:506–508, 1995.

46. Suresh S, Voronov P, Curran J. Infraorbital nerve block in children: A computerized tomographic measurement of the location of the infraorbital foramen. *Pediatr Anesth* 31(3):211–214, 2006.

47. Nicodemus HF, Ferrer MJ, Cristobal VC, de Castro L. Bilateral infraorbital block with 0.5% bupivacaine as postoperative analgesia following cheiloplasty in children. *Scand J Reconstr Surg Hand Surg* 25:253–257, 1991.

48. Ward CM, James I. Surgery of 346 patients with unoperated cleft lip and palate in Sri Lanka. *Cleft Palate J* 27(1):11–17, 1990.

49. Hodges SC, Hodges AM. A protocol for safe anesthesia for cleft lip and palate surgery in developing countries. *Anaesthesia* 55:436–441, 2000.

50. Tiret L, Nivoche Y, Hatton F, et al. Complications related to anesthesia in infants and children. *Br J Anaesth* 61:263–269, 1988.

51. Morray JP, Geiduschek JM, Ramamoorthy C, et al. Anesthesia related cardiac arrest in children: The initial findings of the pediatric perioperative cardiac arrest (POCA) registry. *Anesthesiology* 93: 6–14, 2000.

Anatomy of Cleft Lip and Palate

Martin H.S. Huang, MD • Seng-Teik Lee, MD • Shu-Jin Lee, MD

ANATOMY OF THE LIP

An understanding of the normal anatomy of the upper lip is important in carrying out repairs for unilateral and bilateral cleft lips. In an editorial published in *Plastic and Reconstructive Surgery* in 1967, the late Dr Robert H. Ivy urged more cleft surgeons to be interested in the anatomy of the philtrum of the upper lip so that "eventually a standard procedure will evolve for the correction of the defect".[1] Although notable advances have been made in cleft lip and palate surgery since Ivy made that plea, the knowledge and understanding of normal and abnormal lip anatomy remain limited, and surgery of cleft lip to restore normality to the philtrum remains a challenge.

The upper lip is quite distinct from the lower lip in terms of its embryological development, its anatomy, and its external morphology. Most cleft deformities affect the upper lip, occasionally the commissure of the lips, and very rarely the lower lip. Hence, the attention of most cleft surgeons is directed at the upper lip anatomy, and the surgical aim is at reconstruction of the normal anatomy of the philtrum with its distinctive philtral ridges and midline dimple, as well as the central tubercle of the vermilion and the Cupid's bow (Figs. 14–1A and B).

This section on lip anatomy will cover the following aspects:

- Embryological development of upper lip
- Musculature of upper lip and modiolus
- Blood supply of upper lip
- Anatomy of the philtrum
- Anthropometric measurements of upper lip and nose

EMBRYOLOGY OF UPPER LIP

The comparative anatomical studies by Boyd[2] in 1932 elucidated the roles played by the frontonasal and maxillary processes in the formation of the rhinarium in different mammals and the philtrum in man. His conclusion was that the philtrum is the "median groove in the labial extension of the rhinarium, or the meeting of the two maxillary processes in front of the frontonasal process." He further stated that the appearance of the philtrum in man "is due to a heaping up of the maxillary mesoderm on either side of the middle line." This classical theory of the embryogenesis of the upper lip due to medial migration of the maxillary processes and fusions with the frontonasal or nasomedian process was challenged by Robert Stark[3] in the early 1950s. His detailed studies in 1954 on the volumes of mesoderm present in the cleft area of five rare specimens of embryos with clefts led him to conclude that "normally three masses of mesoderm are present. Each mass grows and joins the mesoderm of the other masses, and a normal upper lip and premaxilla develop. If any of the three masses be absent, a cleft will develop on that side."

The current concept in upper lip embryogenesis is either one of fusion of the maxillary processes to the

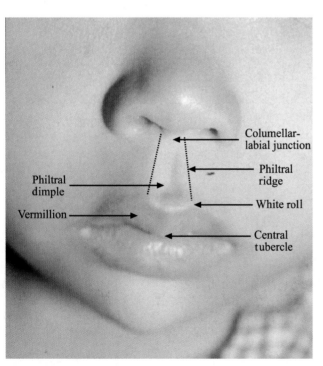

A

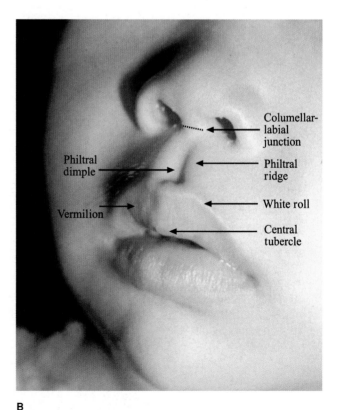

B

Figure 14–1. (A) Normal morphological features of the philtrum of upper lip. (B) Normal appearance of the philtrum-oblique view.

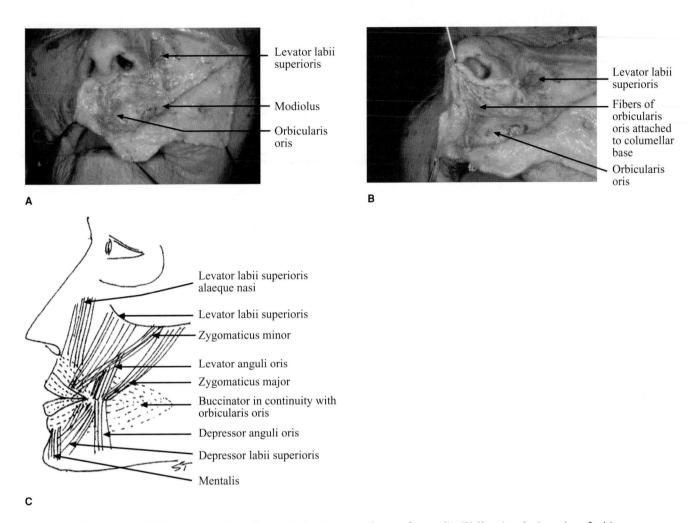

A

B

C

Figure 14–2. (A) Postmortem dissection to display the musculature of upper lip. (B) Showing the insertion of orbicularis oris muscle fibers in the midline. (C) Diagram of the musculature of the upper lip, lower lip and modiolus.

nasomedian or frontonasal process or that an epithelial anlage is present with three mesodermal masses present which grow and fuse. If one mesodermal mass is absent, then the epithelial wall will rupture and result in a unilateral cleft deformity.

MUSCULATURE OF THE UPPER LIP AND MODIOLUS

There is a complex arrangement and a multitude of muscles which form the oral "sphincter" and the modiolus, or angle of the mouth. This not only allows the mouth to open and close, but the intermingling of muscles also allows a variety of movements during speech, mastication, respiration, and facial expression.

Orbicularis Oris Muscle

The orbicularis oris is the main intrinsic muscle encircling the mouth. Other muscles are enmeshed with the orbicularis oris, especially in the region of the modiolus, and they may be considered as extrinsic labial musculature. The orbicularis

oris is only 1 of 14 facial muscles that Nairn[4] has classified into three groups Figs. (Figs. 14–2A to 14–2C). Group I muscles are those that radiate from the modiolus and comprise the orbicularis oris, the buccinator, the levator anguli oris, the depressor anguli oris, and the zygomaticus major. Group II muscles are the retractors of the upper lip that are enmeshed with the orbicularis oris and that comprise the levator labii superioris alaeque nasi, levator labii superioris, and the zygomaticus minor. In their study of the musculature of the upper lip, Latham and Deaton[5] also identified the musculus nasalis, whose fibers arise from the periosteum overlying the incisor teeth, merge with the orbicularis oris, decussate, and insert into the skin at the columellar base. The musculus nasalis rightfully belongs to this group of retractor muscles. Group III muscles are the retractors of the lower lip, comprising the depressor labii inferioris and the mentalis.

Unlike the orbicularis oculi, the orbicularis oris is not a single sheet of circular muscle. The upper lip comprises the superior fibers of the orbicularis oris, which is paired, each half arising from the modiolus of the respective side. The intrinsic fibers of the orbicularis oris insert into the skin, especially in the region of the philtrum of the upper lip, and

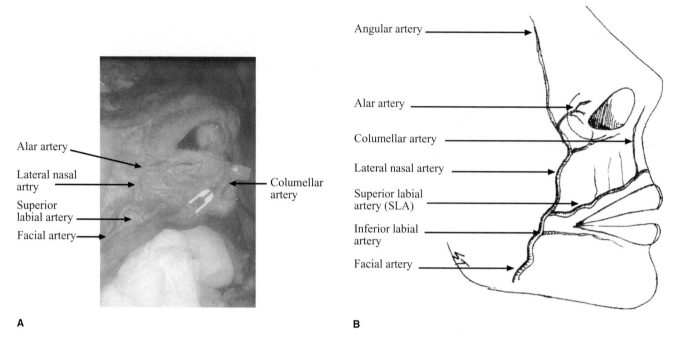

A

B

Figure 14–3. (A) Blood supply to upper lip from branches of facial artery. (B) Branches of facial artery supplying the upper lip (superior labial artery) and lower lip (inferior labial artery).

through the extrinsic muscles enmeshed into its own fibers, the orbicularis oris becomes attached to the maxilla and other parts of the facial skeleton. The inferior fibers of the orbicularis oris run across the lower lip from one modiolus to the other.

Seen in sagittal section, the orbicularis oris has a superficial or marginal part which courses beneath the vermilion of the lip and everts the red lip margin. The main part of the orbicularis oris lies deeper, sandwiched between the skin and the mucosal surface. In the midline, the orbicularis oris demonstrates superficial decussating fibers, which criss-cross in the midline to be attached to the dermis of the overlying skin. Deeper fibers are attached to the region of the anterior nasal spine.

At the modiolus, the orbicularis oris becomes continuous with the fibers of the buccinator muscle, becoming a sheet of muscle across the cheek to the region of the pterygomandibular raphe. When an angular cleft of the lip occurs at the lateral commissure, repair of both the orbicularis oris and the buccinator is necessary in order to reconstitute this continuous sheet and also the modiolus, which is a convergent point not only of the orbicularis oris and buccinator but also of the levator anguli oris, the zygomaticus major muscle, and the depressor anguli oris.

BLOOD SUPPLY OF THE LIP

The main blood supply of the upper and lower lip comes from the facial artery, which gives rise to the superior and inferior labial arteries. The facial artery passes forward in the cheek, lying superficial to the buccinator muscle and deep to

the zygomaticus major muscle. It gives off the superior labial artery and then proceeds upward along the nasolabial groove as the angular artery. Beneath the depressor anguli oris, the inferior labial artery branches and supplies the lower lip.

In his dissection of 20 facial arteries in ten Asian cadavers, Wu[6] found many variations in the course of the facial artery, especially the branches which supply the lip and nose. He found that the superior labial artery, after emerging from beneath the zygomaticus major, plunges into the substance of the orbicularis oris muscle. It may sometimes give rise to the paired columellar arteries, which run in the substance of the orbicularis oris into the columellar base, where they anastomose with the terminal branches of the dorsal nasal artery (Figs. 14–3A and 14–3B).

Niranjan[7] found similar variations of the facial artery in 32% of cases, but in the vast majority (68%) the facial arteries on both sides were symmetrical and terminated as the angular facial arteries. Although there are variations in the arterial blood supply, there is always a rich network of vessels in both the upper and lower lip.

PHILTRUM OF UPPER LIP

The philtrum of the upper lip is one of the key anatomical features that are important in cleft lip repair. It has distinctive morphological features, such as the two lateral philtral ridges and the central midline dimple. With movement of the underlying musculature, the philtral configuration changes, as in the actions of smiling and pursing the lips. Relaxing the orbicularis oris muscle will diminish the philtral features, whereas contraction will exaggerate them. Aging will also gradually

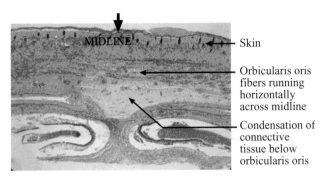

Figure 14–4. Histological section of upper lip in 12 weeks foetus with no philtrum present.

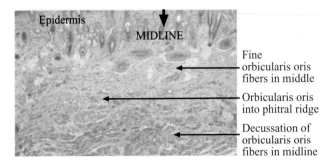

Figure 14–6. Histological section showing insertion of orbicularis oris muscle fibers into dermis of skin after decussating in the midline.

obliterate the philtral ridges and the midline dimple due to the decreased resting tone of the orbicularis oris and other extrinsic musculature of the lip.

In an attempt to explain the features of the philtrum, Latham and Deaton[5] carried out serial sections on six aborted human fetuses in order to show the patterns of origin and insertion of the lip musculature. They used plexiglass tracings to reconstruct and orient the muscles of the upper lip and found that

1. there is considerable insertion of muscle fibers into the skin of the upper lip, lateral to the philtrum;
2. there is a general pattern of muscle fiber decussation in the midline;
3. there are three groups of muscle fibers of the upper lip—the orbicularis oris, the levator labii superioris, and the musculus nasalis.

On the basis of these findings, they concluded that the philtral ridges were formed by the insertion of the orbicularis oris fibers to the skin in this region together with contributions from the musculus nasalis and levator labii superioris. They believed that the philtral groove corresponded to the median decussation of the orbicularis oris, with less bulk due to relative absence of muscle fiber insertion into the skin.

Lee[8] repeated these histological studies of the philtrum using 12 specimens of the upper lip taken from six aborted fetuses at different periods of gestation (12 weeks to 22 weeks), postmortem specimens from children and adults, and 10 operative specimens. In all, over 500 histological sections,

stained with hematoxylin and eosin, Masson's trichrome, and Verhoeff's stains were examined. The findings of this detailed histological study were as follows (Figs. 14–4 to 14–7):

1. The appearance of the philtrum at 20 weeks gestation corresponded with the change in the pattern of the orbicularis oris muscle, especially the decussation of the muscle fibers in the midline and their insertion into the dermis, with oblique as well as vertical muscle fibers.
2. The absence of the philtral configuration in the 12-week fetus. In this instance, there was a midline condensation of connective tissue but the orbicularis oris traversed across the midline in a horizontal bundle without decussation in the midline.

Lee concluded from his histological findings that the philtrum is not embryological in origin. Rather, it makes its appearance after facial development is complete.

The significant histological finding, similar to that of Latham and Deaton's, was the pattern of decussation of the orbicularis oris muscle in the midline, with oblique and vertical muscle fiber extensions into the dermis of the overlying skin. These histological findings were present where the philtrum was present macroscopically.

Lee has postulated a dynamic role of the orbicularis oris in giving form to the upper lip, especially the unique features of the philtrum. He surmised that forcible contraction of the orbicularis oris will accentuate the central philtral

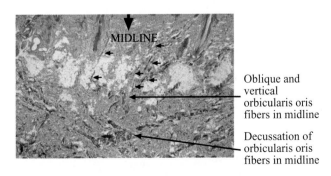

Figure 14–5. Histological section of upper lip in 22 weeks foetus with presence of philtrum.

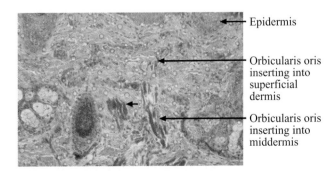

Figure 14–7. Histological section showing the insertion of orbicularis oris muscle fibers into the mid and even superficial dermis of skin.

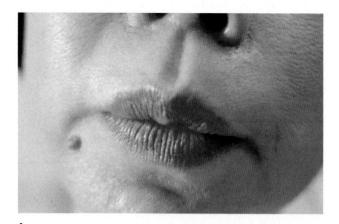

A

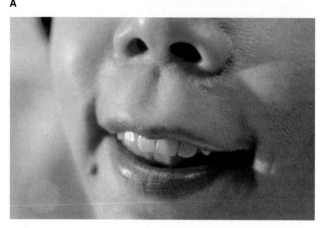

B

Figure 14–8. (A) The morphological features of the philtrum are accentuated by dynamic action of pursing the lips. (B) The appearance of the philtrum change with relaxation of muscle fibers, making the philtral ridges and central dimple less prominent.

depression and the lateral philtral ridges, whilst relaxation of the muscle as in smiling will diminish the philtral configuration (Figs. 14–8A and B). In the normal position of the upper lip, the resting tone and length of the dermal muscle fibers will maintain the features of the philtrum.

ANTHROPOMETRIC MEASUREMENTS OF THE UPPER LIP AND NOSE

A knowledge of the normal philtral dimensions and surface measurements of the upper lip and nose are important for the repair of the cleft deformity. This will allow the correct markings to be placed on the philtrum depending on the age and ethnicity of the patient. It is particularly relevant in complete bilateral cleft lip repair for tailoring the prolabium to the correct size for the creation of the philtrum of the upper lip.

Lee[9] has carried out anthropometric measurements of the lip and nose on a Chinese population in three different age groups (3 months, 4–5 years, and young adults) relevant to the milestones of cleft surgery. Three hundred normal individuals were measured, with 100 in each age group, equally divided between male and female subjects. A reference table of these norms for the three age groups is shown in (Fig. 14–9). Seven parameters were chosen for these anthropometric measurements.

Accurate documentation in cleft lip surgery is important for long-term outcome studies. Anthropometric measurements are simple to carry out once the landmarks have been correctly identified, and they provide an inexpensive and accurate means of long-term documentation of growth of the upper lip and nose.

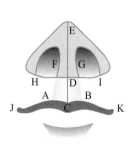
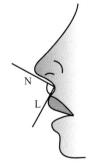

RESULTS

		AB	CD	DE	FG	HI	JK	NL
Group A	M	4.9 mm	7.7 mm	5.7 mm	3.0 mm	12.7 mm	23.0 mm	99.6°
(3 months)	F	4.9 mm	7.2 mm	5.0 mm	2.9 mm	12.8 mm	22.4 mm	103.5°
Group B	M	8.1 mm	12.2 mm	11.0 mm	4.6 mm	18.3 mm	36.3 mm	94.7°
(4–5 years)	F	8.4 mm	11.3 mm	10.9 mm	4.1 mm	17.4 mm	34.7 mm	88.8°
Group C	M	11.6 mm	13.6 mm	15.1 mm	6.2 mm	21.8 mm	50.5 mm	89.6°
(Adult)	F	10.6 mm	12.9 mm	13.7 mm	5.2 mm	20.4 mm	46.1 mm	84.2°

Figure 14–9. Normal lip measurements (seven parameters) in the three different age groups in Chinese population, Singapore. A reference table of anthropometric norms of upper lip relevant to milestones for cleft surgery.

ANATOMY OF THE NORMAL PALATE AND CLEFT PALATE

The palate plays a critical role in velopharyngeal function during speech, swallowing, and respiration. It consists of two parts, the hard and the soft palate. It is important to be acquainted with normal palatal anatomy since cleft palate surgery aims to restore such anatomy or to modify existing anatomy in order to improve velopharyngeal function.

THE HARD PALATE

The hard palate forms the anterior bony part of the palate. It is composed of two lateral palatal shelves that meet each other in the midline and that join anteriorly at the premaxilla, also known as the primary palate. The posterior limit of the premaxilla is marked by the incisive foramen. The posterior border of the palate is notched on each side by the grooves where the posterior palatine nerves and vessels pass between the palatine process and the maxillary wall. The oral mucosa

of the hard palate may be divided into three zones: the thin outermost gingival region, the middle palatine region, which is rough and rasp-like, and the inner zone, which is smooth and thinner.[10] The latter two regions are of importance in cleft palate repair. While the thicker middle region is well vascularized, elevation of its mucoperiosteum is considered to be detrimental to maxillary growth. On the other hand, the inner zone is thinner and heals more slowly. It is also well vascularized, and surgical dissection in this zone is not believed to be detrimental to growth.

THE SOFT PALATE

The soft palate, or velum, is a mobile fibromuscular structure that consists of two parts. Anteriorly, it consists of the palatine aponeurosis, which stretches from the pterygoid processes toward the back of the oral cavity (Fig. 14–10). The aponeurosis is suspended from the skull base by the tensor veli palatini muscle. The posterior part of the soft palate is muscular (Fig. 14–10) and is composed of four paired muscles: levator

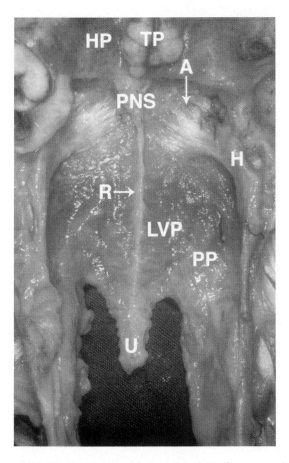

Figure 14–10. Oral surface of the soft palate after removal of mucosa and glandular tissue (HP: hard palate; TP: torus palatinus, present incidentally in this specimen; PNS: posterior nasal spine; A: aponeurosis of tensor veli palatini; H: hamulus; R: (palatine) raphe; LVP: levator veli palatini, which occupies the middle 50% of the velar length; PP: palatopharyngeus; U: uvula).

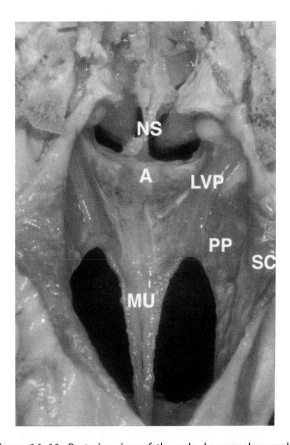

Figure 14–11. Posterior view of the velopharyngeal musculature, with the posterior pharyngeal wall split in the midline (NS: nasal septum; A: aponeurosis of tensor veli palatini; LVP: levator veli palatini, descending from cranial base; PP: palatopharyngeus; SC: superior constrictor, which encircled the velopharyngeal port before division of the posterior pharyngeal wall; MU: musculus uvulae. Note insertion of the palatopharyngeus into the superior constrictor).

veli palatini, palatopharyngeus, palatoglossus, and musculus uvulae. The length of the soft palate, measured from the posterior edge of the hard palate to the base of the free margin of the soft palate excluding the uvula, varies from 30 to 50 mm, with a mean of 40 mm.[11] The three dimensional architecture of the velar muscles has been likened to three loops of muscle that meet in the midline.[12] The superior loop is formed by the levator veli palatini, which forms a sling attached to the base of the skull (Fig. 14–11). The two inferior loops open downward toward the base of the tongue and the pharynx as the anterior and posterior tonsillar pillars. These are formed by the palatoglossus and palatopharyngeus, respectively (Fig. 14–11). The final paired muscle, the musculus uvulae, is intrinsic to the velum (Fig. 14–12). In addition, the superior constrictor (Fig. 14–13) acts in concert with the velar muscles to play a significant role in the valvular action of the velopharyngeal sphincter.[10,13]

The palatine aponeurosis is the fibrous skeleton of the soft palate into which the velar muscles insert directly and indirectly. It is set at a 45-degree angle to the bony vault of the hard palate. It is a quadrangular structure that is fixed on three sides: anteriorly, to the hard palate and laterally, to the tensor veli palatini muscles, the tendons of which terminate in this structure. It occupies the anterior quarter to third of the velar length, measured from the posterior nasal spine to the tip of the uvula (Fig. 14–10).[14,16] The posterior border of the aponeurosis shows a degree of mobility superiorly and inferiorly.[15] The anterior two thirds of the aponeurosis is

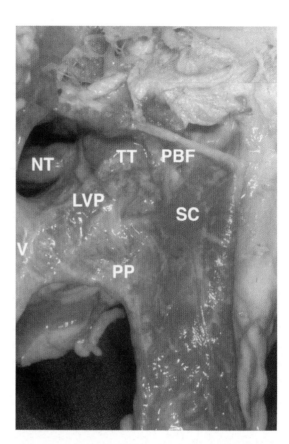

Figure 14–13. Posteromedial view of the right side of the velum and pharyngeal wall. Observe (1) the nasal head of the palatopharyngeus (PP) lying on the nasal surface of the levator veli palatini (LVP) within the velum (V); (2) the superior constrictor (SC), which forms the lateral and posterior pharyngeal walls and whose superior limit consists of a well-defined muscle bundle; and (3) the insertion of fibers of the palatopharyngeus into the superior constrictor in the lateral pharyngeal wall (NT: nasal turbinate; TT: torus tubarius; PBF: pharyngobasilar fascia).

thick, whereas the posterior third is thin. Near the midline, it encloses or fuses with the musculus uvulae (Fig. 14–12), and the levator veli palatini, palatopharyngeus, and palatoglossus are attached to its posterior border (Fig. 14–10). Functionally, the aponeurosis is believed to act as a shock absorber through its lateral continuation as the tensor veli palatini, which regulates the tension of the aponeurosis via its own muscle fiber tension.[10]

THE SUPERIOR VELAR MUSCLES: TENSOR VELI PALATINI AND LEVATOR VELI PALATINI

The superior velar muscles are slinglike structures that suspend the velum from the skull base.

Tensor Veli Palatini

The tensor veli palatini is a flat muscle that arises from the scaphoid fossa of the greater wing of the sphenoid bone between the superior end of the medial pterygoid plate and the spine of the sphenoid, as well as from the adjacent

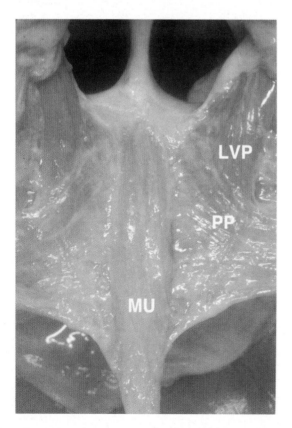

Figure 14–12. Nasal view of soft palate following removal of mucosa and glandular tissue. LVP: levator veli palatini; PP: palatopharyngeus; MU: musculus uvulae.

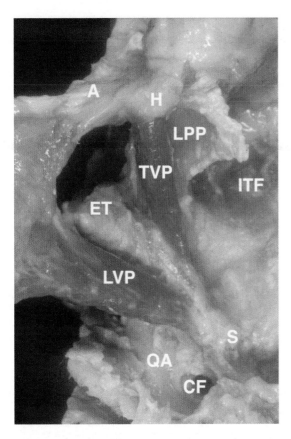

Figure 14–14. Inferior view of the left cranial base at the junction of the sphenoid and petrous temporal bones and of the velum. *Orientation:* Top of picture is anterior, right is lateral, bottom is posterior, left is medial (A: aponeurosis; H: hamulus; LPP: lateral pterygoid plate; ITF: infratemporal fossa; TVP: tensor veli palatini; ET: eustachian tube; LVP: levator veli palatini, reflected medially; QA: quadrate area at apex of petrous temporal bone; CF: carotid foramen; S: spine of sphenoid).

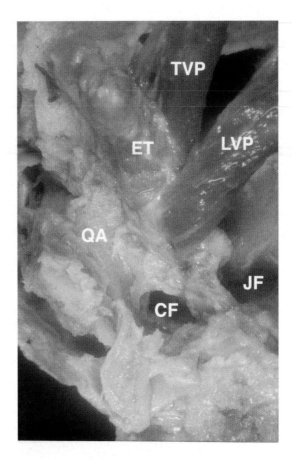

Figure 14–15. Inferior view of the left cranial vase at the junction of the greater wing of the sphenoid and petrous temporal bones. *Orientation:* Same as in Fig. 14–5 (TVP: tensor veli palatini; ET: eustachian tube; LVP: levator veli palatini, reflected laterally; QA: quadrate area at apex of petrous temporal bone; CF: carotid foramen; JF: Jugular foramen). Note that levator veli palatini is attached only to the eustachian tube and not to the quadrate area at apex of petrous temporal bone.

superolateral aspect of the cartilaginous and membranous parts of the eustachian tube along its entire length (Fig. 14–14).[14] Shaped like an inverted triangle, the muscle descends vertically and narrows into a flat tendon as it approaches the hamulus. Some of the fibers are attached to the hamulus, but the majority of the fibers turn a right angle around this structure, fanning out to form the sheet-like palatine aponeurosis (Fig. 14–10).[14,16] The action of the tensor veli palatini on the membranous and cartilaginous portions of the eustachian tube results in tubal dilatation.[14,17] This function is important for the equalization of pressures between the middle ear and the nasopharynx.[18]

In the cleft palate patient, the origin and morphology of the tensor veli palatini is normal,[19] but the muscle is thinner and is inserted abnormally in two ways: commonly as a concentrated, thick bundle into the anterior part of the levator veli palatini, and uncommonly in a dispersed manner into the anterior bundles of the levator muscle.[16]

Levator Veli Palatini

The levator veli palatini is a cylindrical muscle that originates from the inferior aspect of the apical portion of the petrous temporal bone and from the lateral edge of the carotid canal

and cartilaginous eustachian tube (Fig. 14–15).[14,16,20] The levator is oriented in the same direction as the eustachian tube, i.e., the long axes of these structures parallel to one another (Figs. 14–16 and 14–17). It forms a muscular sling that suspends the velum from the cranial base, occupying the space between the superior constrictor and the cranial base (Fig. 14–11).[13] The levator muscle fibers on each side descend anteromedially in a gentle spiral to run parallel and inferior to the eustachian tube (Fig. 14–17). The levator enters the velum by fanning out between the two heads of the palatopharyngeus muscle. Within the velum, the bulk of the muscle fibers run in a transverse direction and occupy the middle half of the velum, measured from the posterior nasal spine to the tip of the uvula (Fig. 14–11).[11,13] The fibers of each side fuse in the midline without significant overlap. Anteriorly, the muscle is attached to the posterior margin of the palatine aponeurosis, with some overlap over its oral surface medially (Fig. 14–10).[13] Anterolateral insertions of the levator have been described, in which fibers from the inferior third of the levator run anterolaterally toward the pterygoid hamulus and lateral part of the palatine aponeurosis. These fibers terminate as fine tendons inserting into the posterior edge of the lateral part of

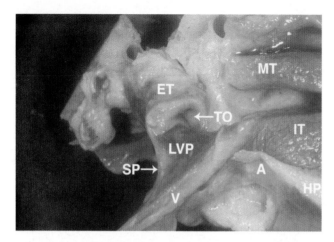

Figure 14–16. Medial view of left lateral wall of nasopharynx (specimen has been split in midsagittal plane). *Orientation:* Top of picture is superior, right is anterior, bottom is inferior, left is posterior (ET: eustachian tube; TO: tubal orifice; MT: middle turbinate; IT: inferior turbinate; HP: hard palate; A: aponeurosis; V: velum; SP: salpingopharyngeus). Note relationship of levator veli palatini to eustachian tube.

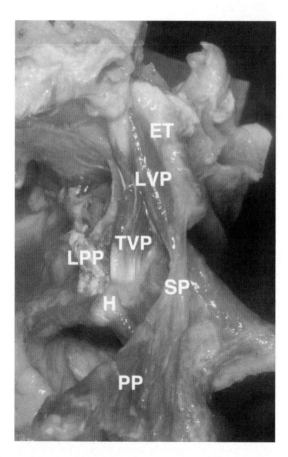

Figure 14–17. Posteromedial view of left eustachian tube (ET), levator veli palatini (LVP), and tensor veli palatini (TVP). *Orientation:* Top of picture is superior, right is anterior, bottom is inferior, left is posterior (SP: salpingopharyngeous; PP: palatopharyngeus). Note relationships of tensor veli palatini and levator veli palatini to eustachian tube.

the aponeurosis in the region of the hamulus.[21] These anterolateral fibers arise from the most lateral part of the muscle's origin from the base of the skull and follow a spiral course inferiorly. Although they do not contribute to the levator sling, their clinical significance lies in the fact that complete release of these tethering anterior attachments of the levator to the aponeurosis in the region of the hamulus during palatoplasty may allow more effective retropositioning of the main part of the levator.[21]

Functionally, the levator's central placement within the velum and its slinglike structure make it well placed to be the primary contributor velopharyngeal closure through the actions of velar elevation and retrodisplacement. The downward, forward, and medial direction of its axis is consistent with the upward, backward, and lateral motion of the velum that occurs in velopharyngeal closure. The distribution of its fibers in the middle half of the velum suggests that it accounts for the "knee" or "genu" observed in velar elevation.[21,22] This positioning allows the muscle to act in concert with the superior constrictor to achieve complete velopharyngeal closure.[10]

Some fibers of the levator veli palatini, together with those of the palatopharyngeus, insert directly into the palatal mucosa about 2 cm posterior to the posterior edge of the hard palate. These mucosal attachments account for the dimpling observed on the oral aspect of the velum during velar elevation.[11] These direct levator insertions not only serve to tether the palatal mucosa to the levator fibers, but may also allow levator contraction to pull the palatal mucosa posteriorly toward the posterior pharyngeal wall during velopharyngeal closure.[11]

The fibers of the levator run in a gentle spiral along the lateral aspect of the nasopharynx, inferior to the eustachian tube. The relationship of the levator veli palatini to the eustachian tube suggests that its action on the tubal cartilage consists of an upward, medial, and posterior displacement of the medial tubal cartilage, mainly along its inferior half and especially in the region of the torus, where there is a greater degree of overhang of the cartilage on the muscle.[14,22–25] This action appears to be the result of an increase in muscle diameter consequent to isotonic contraction, as well as to a superior and posterior displacement of the levator sling. The resulting effect on the eustachian tube is the opening of its lumen. The effect of the levator veli palatini on the membranous part of the tube depends on the resting shape of the tubal lumen. Assuming that this is a vertical or oblique slit, a superior displacement of the membranous part of the tube, caused by a bulging of the contracted levator veli palatini, would tend to change the shape of the lumen from a slitlike opening to a triangle, of which the cross-sectional area would be larger. Thus the effect of the levator veli palatini on the membranous part of the eustachian tube also appears to be a dilatory one.[14]

The significance of medial displacement of the lateral pharyngeal wall during velopharyngeal closure is controversial.[13,26] Movement of the torus is not consistently observed in living subjects. In fact, it is absent in up to 90%

of normal individuals.[27,28] Even in cases where medial movement of the lateral pharyngeal wall occurs, this motion usually occurs at or below the level of the hard palate,[27,28] making it unlikely that it contributes to velopharyngeal closure.[13]

THE INFERIOR VELAR MUSCLES: PALATOPHARYNGEUS AND PALATOGLOSSUS

The inferior velar muscles form two arches that connect the mobile velum above to the mobile pharynx and the tongue below.

Palatopharyngeus

This is a substantial sheet of muscle that originates in the velum, descends inferiorly to form the arch of the posterior tonsillar pillar, and inserts into the lateral pharyngeal wall posteriorly and into the larynx inferiorly (Fig. 14–18).[13] The intravelar portion occupies the middle 50% of the velar length

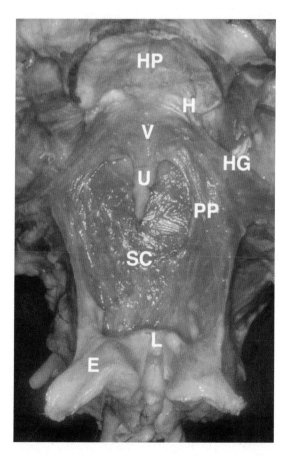

Figure 14–18. Anterior view of the oropharynx, with the tongue split in the midline and reflected laterally out of view (HP: hard palate; H: hamulus; V: velum; U: uvula; HG: hamuloglossus; PP: palatopharyngeus; SC: superior constrictor; L: larynx; E: epiglottis, which has been split in the midline). Observe insertion of fibers of the palatopharyngeus to the superior constrictor posteriorly and to the larynx inferiorly.

(Fig. 14–18). Within the velum, it consists of two heads, which clasp the levator between them.[11,13] The nasal head, lying on the nasal aspect of the levator, is thinner and less developed (Fig. 14–13). The palatal head, lying on the oral surface of the levator, is thicker and more developed (Fig. 14–10). Both heads of the palatopharyngeus are attached to the posterolateral aspect of the aponeurosis anteriorly and to the levator medially. Toward the midline, the muscle fibers thin out and merge in the paramedian zone with those of the levator (Figs. 14–10 and 14–11). In the region where fibers of the levator and palatopharyngeus intermingle, muscle fiber insertions occur into the palatal mucosa at points that correspond to the palatal dimples observed clinically.[29] Lateral to the levator, the two heads of the palatopharyngeus fuse and expand into a broad sheet of muscle. These fibers then run posteroinferiorly and insert over a wide area into the lateral pharyngeal wall, blending imperceptibly with the fibers of the superior constrictor to form part of the longitudinal inner muscular wall of the lower pharynx (Fig. 14–13).[13,20] A minority of muscle fibers insert into the posterior pharyngeal wall. The remainder of the fibers forms a bundle that runs inferiorly through the posterior tonsillar pillar and insert into the pharyngeal raphe and posterior border of the thyroid cartilage in the larynx (Fig. 14–18).[13,20]

The complex and sophisticated anatomy of the palatopharyngeus enables it to fulfill the role of fine-tuning the function of the velopharyngeal sphincter by modulating velar position, size, and shape. Contraction of the palatopharyngeus pulls the velum posteroinferiorly and stretches the velum to allow for velar depression and retrodisplacement, as well as for an increase in the surface area for contact between the surfaces of the velum and pharyngeal walls.[13,30–32] The clasping of the levator by the two heads of the palatopharyngeus serves to interlock the fibers of both muscles during contraction, allowing fine, synergistic control of the antagonistic actions of the inferiorly directed palatopharyngeus and the superiorly directed levator. This micromodulation of velopharyngeal port size, and thereby the control of air emission through the port, may be important for the production of delicate variations in speech sounds. In addition, the insertion of the palatopharyngeus into the superior constrictor muscle in the region of the lower lateral and posterior pharyngeal walls allows the palatopharyngeus to exert a medial pull on the pharyngeal walls.[13] The medial displacement of the lower pharyngeal walls is thought to be important in the production of open vowels.[33–36]

Palatoglossus

The palatoglossus occupies the anterior faucial pillar, connecting the velum and hamulus superiorly with the tongue inferiorly (Fig. 14–18).[15,25,37] Its velar origin is variable.[15,25,37] Its inferior insertion is primarily into the dorsolateral aspect of the posterior tongue.[37]

Functionally, the palatoglossus is capable of velar depression[25,30,35] and glossal elevation.[30,37] Both of these actions may be relevant in the fine modulation of speech sounds during velopharyngeal closure.

SUPERIOR CONSTRICTOR

The superior constrictor is a broad muscle in the shape of a groove that encloses the nasopharynx and upper oropharynx (Fig. 14–11).[10,13] It originates anteriorly from the posterior border of the medial pterygoid plate from the level of the hard palate to the tip of the hamulus. This origin continues on a downward and forward slope along the pterygomandibular ligament. From these anterior attachments the muscle sweeps around the pharynx to form its lateral and posterior walls (Fig. 14–13). The fibers diverge superiorly and inferiorly in the region of the posterior midline to insert into the pharyngeal ligament. In the lateral and posterior pharyngeal walls, there are dense interdigitations between the fibers of the superior constrictor and palatopharyngeus from the level of hard palate downward (Fig. 14–13).[13] The space between the superior margin of the muscle and the cranial base is occupied by the levator veli palatini and the eustachian tube in the lateral nasopharyngeal wall and by the pharyngobasilar fascia in the posterior pharyngeal wall (Fig. 14–13).[13]

The superior constrictor is responsible for the sphincteric closure of the pharynx during the pharyngeal component of velopharyngeal closure. This is important in the functions of swallowing and speech.[25,26] Through its interdigitations with fibers of the palatopharyngeus in the lateral and posterior pharyngeal walls, contraction of the superior constrictor pulls the lateral pharyngeal walls inward, and the simultaneous contraction of bilateral superior constrictor and palatopharyngeus muscles creates a continuous curve of sphincteric action around the pharynx.[13] Additionally, the superior constrictor and palatopharyngeus act together to create the transverse elevation of the posterior pharyngeal wall known as Passavant's ridge.[13]

THE UVULAR MUSCLE: MUSCULUS UVULAE

The musculus uvulae is the only intrinsic velar muscle. It is a paired, longitudinally orientated midline muscle that extends from the posterior nasal spine and dorsal surface of the levator aponeurosis anteriorly to the base of the uvula posteriorly (Figs. 14–12 and 14–19).[11,20,38] The musculus uvulae is the most nasally situated muscle, lying directly above the levator veli palatini muscle (Fig. 14–12 and 14-19).[21,38] The uvula itself is largely devoid of muscle and is composed mainly of glandular and connective tissue (Fig. 14–19). The anterior insertion of the muscle is variable. However, the most common pattern of insertion (observed 90% of the time) is that upon reaching the posterior edge of the aponeurosis, the muscle bundles split into two divergent bundles at a 60–90 degree angle, becoming smaller as they proceed anteriorly.[20,38] These fibers terminate by fusing with the connective tissue of the aponeurosis just short of the hard palate.[38]

Functionally, the musculus uvulae has passive and active roles in velopharyngeal closure. Its passive role is that of a

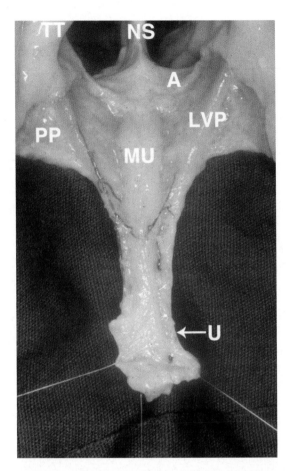

Figure 14–19. Nasal view of velar musculature (NS: nasal septum; TT: torus tubarius; A: aponeurosis; LVP: levator veli palatini; MU: musculus uvulae; PP: palatopharyngeus; U: uvula). Observe absence of muscle in U.

space occupier in the midline of the nasal aspect of the velum, there preventing attenuation of midline bulk caused by lateral traction of the levator during velopharyngeal closure. Augmentation of this passive role occurs during active muscle contraction, which increases midline velar bulk. Contraction of the muscle also results in velar extension toward the posterior pharyngeal wall, which further increases midline contact in velopharyngeal closure.[38] Thus, the musculus uvulae acts synergistically with the levator veli palatini to bulk up, elevate, and extend the velum[24,31,38] during velopharyngeal closure. These actions serve to maximize midline contact between the velum and posterior pharyngeal wall during velopharyngeal closure.

CLINICAL IMPLICATIONS

Fracture of the Hamulus during Palatoplasty

Fracture of the hamulus or division of the tensor tendon near the hamulus during palatoplasty impairs the ability of the tensor to dilate the eustachian tube because of a loss of biomechanical advantage.[13]

Intravelar Veloplasty

Intravelar veloplasty involves repositioning the velar muscles in a transverse orientation during cleft palate repair. This restores the levator sling mechanism, improving velar function, as well as the palatopharyngeus-superior constrictor sphincteric mechanism, which improves pharyngeal wall function. Thus, velopharyngeal function as a whole is enhanced.[13]

Furlow Double Opposing Z-Plasty

This technique involves transverse repositioning of the velar muscles with overlap and simultaneous lengthening and thickening of the velum. When used to repair isolated cleft palate or submucous cleft palate, it obviates the need for hard palatal flaps. However, this technique results in division and malposition of the musculus uvulae.[13]

Pharyngeal Flap

The pharyngeal flap creates a permanent, passive central obturator in the velopharyngeal port in order to reduce velopharyngeal insufficiency. It depends on adequate lateral pharyngeal wall motion to close the lateral gaps during velopharyngeal closure. However, the raising of this myomucosal flap divides the fibers of the superior constrictor and palatopharyngeus, disrupting the sphincteric mechanism that is involved in pharyngeal wall movement.[13]

Sphincter Pharyngoplasty

The sphincter pharyngoplasty reduces the size of the velopharyngeal port along its circumference by augmenting the thickness of the pharyngeal walls. This is achieved by raising superiorly based posterior tonsillar pillar flaps containing the palatopharyngeus muscle and insetting these flaps into the pharyngeal wall at the appropriate level, i.e., the level of velopharyngeal closure. Since the sphincteric mechanism of the pharyngeal walls is preserved, this technique is theoretically more physiologic than the pharyngeal flap.[13]

■ THE NERVE SUPPLY OF THE PALATE

The muscles of the soft palate are innervated by the pharyngeal plexus and the lesser palatine nerve.[20,39–42] Knowledge of palatal innervation is important for the preservation of muscle function, since this innervation is at risk in palatoplasty procedures, especially when radical muscle dissections are performed.[20] The pharyngeal branches of the ninth and tenth nerve branch and intercommunicate as they course between the internal and external carotid arteries to form a pharyngeal plexus with the branches of the sympathetic trunk. This plexus lies on the lateral aspect of the superior constrictor. Branches originating from the plexus pass medially through the superior constrictor into the soft palate musculature. Most anteriorly, the branch to the levator veli palatini penetrates the superior constrictor and enters the levator on its posterior surface to be distributed to the superior part of the muscle.

Posterior to this, branches pass from the pharyngeal plexus toward the superior and middle constrictor, which they innervate, and then continue as small branches into the lateral part of the palatopharyngeus.[20]

The lesser palatine nerve emerges from the lesser palatine foramen to run posteriomedially beneath the palatine aponeurosis and palatopharyngeus to divide into several fine branches. Most of these branches pass into the levator veli palatini near its insertion. Some of the branches pass into the musculus uvulae and into the medial part of the palatopharyngeus. The anterior most branch of the lesser palatine nerve runs beneath the palatine aponeurosis to innervate the palatine glandular tissue and velar mucosa.[20] The fibromucosa is supplied by the anterior and middle palatine nerves.[20]

■ THE BLOOD SUPPLY OF THE PALATE

The blood vessels of the hard and soft palate lie in the plane of glandular tissue located between the mucosa and periosteum (in the hard palate) (Fig. 14–20) and between mucosa and velar muscles (in the soft palate) (Figs. 14–20 and 14–21). Within these tissue planes, they form an extensive anastomotic network. The glandular tissue on the oral side (Fig. 14–20) has a greater density of vessels than that of the nasal aspect[45] (Fig. 14–22).

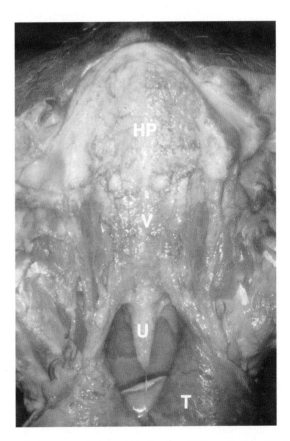

Figure 14–20. Oral view of hard palate (HP) and velum (V) following removal of muscosal and glandular layers (U: uvula; T: tongue). Note richness of blood supply but relative paucity of anastomoses across midline.

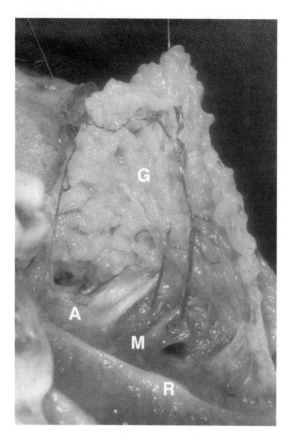

Figure 14–21. Anteromedial view of oral surface of left half of soft palate. Glandular layer (G) has been dissected off muscle layer (M) to show plane of blood vessels (in green). A: aponeurosis; R: midline palatine raphe.

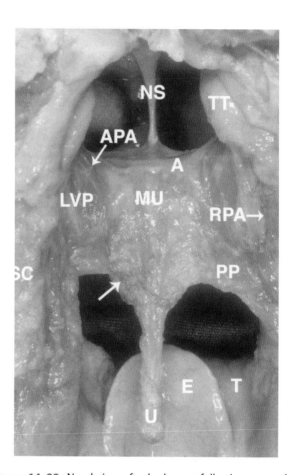

Figure 14–22. Nasal view of velopharynx following removal of mucosal and glandular layers (NS: nasal septum; APA: terminal branch of ascending palatine artery; TT: torus tubarius; A: aponeurosis; LVP: levator veli palatini; MU: musculus uvulae; RPA: recurrent pharyngeal artery; SC: superior constrictor; PP: palatopharyngeus; U: uvula; E: epiglottis; T: tongue). *Arrow* indicates uvular branch of APA to musculus uvulae. Note relatively sparse blood supply, APA supplying LVP, and RPA supplying PP and SC.

The sources of this blood supply are four branches of the external carotid artery. In ascending order, these branches and their territories of supply are as follows:

Ascending Palatine Artery

The ascending palatine artery arises as a branch of the facial artery at the level of the mandibular angle and enters the floor of the mouth. From this area, it ascends toward the palate, and enters the velum at the level of the hamulus, where it lies 1 mm lateral to that structure (Fig. 14–23). It supplies the intravelar part of the levator veli palatini, the palatoglossus, the palatopharyngeus, and the musculus uvulae.[45]

Ascending Pharyngeal Artery

The ascending pharyngeal artery originates from the external carotid artery in the areolar tissue external to the lateral pharyngeal wall at about the level of the uvula. As it ascends vertically toward the skull base, lying in the space of Ernst, numerous perforators branch off to supply the superior constrictor in the lateral and posterior pharyngeal walls (Fig. 14–24).[45]

Recurrent Pharyngeal Artery

The recurrent pharyngeal artery arises from the external carotid artery at the level of the upper third of the stern-

ocleidomastoid muscle. It ascends vertically to the skull base, then turns downward obliquely in recurrent fashion, lying next to the posterolateral aspect of the extravelar part of the levator veli palatini (Fig. 14–25). It supplies that muscle via numerous perforators. It also provides a minor vascular supply to the palatopharyngeus, superior constrictor, and tensor veli palatini.

Maxillary Artery

The maxillary artery branches off from the external carotid artery just below the level of the mastoid and runs horizontally and anteriorly toward the maxilla (Fig. 14–26). It supplies the tensor veli palatini and palatopharyngeus, as well as the hard palate, via its branches, the greater and lesser palatine arteries (Fig. 14–27).[43] The greater palatine artery emerges from the greater palatine foramen of the hard palate and runs parallel to the lateral margin of the hard palate, less than 5 mm from its junction with the alveolus. It supplies the hard palate via medial arcades, which anastomose with branches of the lesser palatine artery (Fig. 14–27). The latter artery exits from the

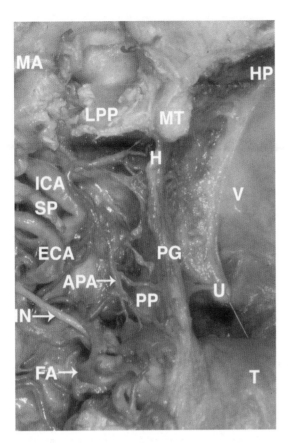

Figure 14–23. Anterolateral view of the right faucial region and palate (FA: facial artery; HN: hypoglossal nerve; APA: ascending palatine artery, retracted away from faucial pillars; ECA: external carotid artery; SP: styloid process; ICA: internal carotid artery; MA: maxillary artery; LPP: lateral pterygoid plate; MT: maxillary tubercle; H: hamulus; PG: palatoglossus; PP: palatopharyngeus; T: tongue; U: uvula; V: velum; HP: hard palate). Observe perforators of ascending palatine artery supplying palatoglossus and palatopharyngeus.

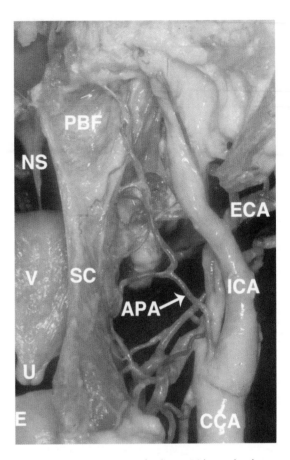

Figure 14–24. Posterior view of right carotid vessels, pharyngeal wall, and soft palate (E: epiglottis; U: uvula; V: velum; NS: nasal septum; PBF: pharyngobasilar fascia; SC: superior constrictor; APA: ascending pharyngeal artery; ECA: external carotid artery; ICA: internal carotid artery; CCA: common carotid artery). Observe horizontal perforators of APA supplying superior constrictor.

lesser palatine foramen of the hard palate, just posterior to the greater palatine foramen, and supplies the aponeurosis (Fig. 14–27). Few anastomoses in the hard palate vasculature cross the midline (Fig. 14–20).[43]

Clinical Implications

The palatoglossus, levator veli palatini, tensor veli palatine, and superior constrictor receive a dual blood supply, and the palatopharyngeus has a multiple blood supply. The midline musculus uvulae receives a bilateral supply from the ascending palatine artery.[43] Because of the multiple sources of blood supply to the velar muscles, their detachment from aberrant insertions and transverse repositioning during palatoplasty is generally safe from a vascular standpoint.[32,43–48]

The generous blood supply of the soft palate also suggests that it is safe to elevate oral and nasal mucosal flaps off the velar muscles during intravelar veloplasty and the Furlow double opposing Z-plasty.[43] However, careful dissection should be performed in the region lateral to the hamulus, along the medial pterygoid plate, and in the space of Ernst in

order to avoid damage to the ascending palatine, ascending pharyngeal, and recurrent pharyngeal arteries, respectively. Based on the vascular supply of the velopharynx, clinical implications for secondary surgery for the correction of velopharyngeal insufficiency are as follows: (1) vertical pharyngeal flaps are random pattern in nature, and (2) the posterior tonsillar pillar flaps of the sphincter pharyngoplasty are axial in nature, supplied by the hamular branch of the ascending palatine artery.[43]

In the hard palate, care should be taken to preserve the greater palatine artery during elevation of mucoperiosteal flaps, as this vessel forms the main vascular supply of these flaps.

PATHOLOGICAL ANATOMY IN CLEFT PALATE

Hard Palate

In complete isolated clefts of the palate, there is a gap between the palatal shelves up to the incisive foramen. The palatal shelves are hypoplastic and steeply angled. The border of the

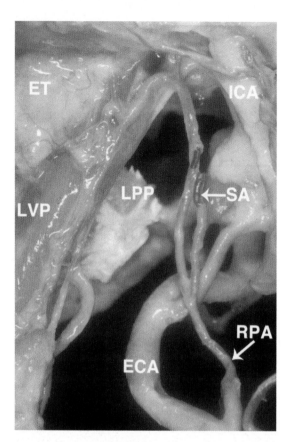

Figure 14–25. Posterior view of extravelar part of right levator veli palatini (LVP) and its blood supply from recurrent pharyngeal artery (RPA) (ET: eustachian tube; LPP: lateral pterygoid plate; ICA: internal carotid artery; SA: sternomastoid artery; ECA: external carotid artery).

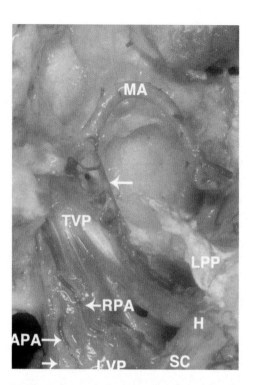

Figure 14–26. Posteroinferior view of right tensor veli palatini (TVP) and its main blood supply (APA: ascending palatine artery; RPA: recurrent pharyngeal artery; MA: maxillary artery; LPP: lateral pterygoid plate; H: hamulus; SC: superior constrictor; LVP: levator veli palatini). *Upper arrow* indicates muscular branch of MA supplying TVP. *Lower arrow* indicates accessory recurrent pharyngeal artery.

bony cleft may be sharply angled or rounded depending on the degree of penetration of the tongue. The distance between the maxillary tuberosities is increased.[49]

MUSCLES AND MUCOSA

The palatine aponeurosis is absent in the midline. Instead, it is present laterally as a small fibrotic bundle. The muscles of the palate are found along the edges of the cleft. The tensor veli palatini aponeurotic insertions are more oblique than usual, with the fibers extending along the cleft edges. The levator veli palatini and palatopharyngeus muscles run parallel to the margins of the cleft and do not join in the midline. The oral mucosa is paler, and the nasal mucosa is redder.[10] The dividing line is visible at the cleft margins. Functionally, cleft palate results in dysfunctions in speech, breathing, hearing, and swallowing. Sucking is also impaired as the oral and nasal cavities communicate with one another.

ACKNOWLEDGEMENTS

The authors wish to thank Dr Roland Chong and also Ms Yong Bee Choon for their kind assistance in the preparation

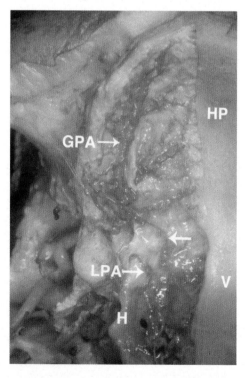

Figure 14–27. Oral view of right hemipalate (GPA: greater palatine artery; HP: hard palate; LPA: lesser palatine artery; V: velum; H: hamulus). Unlabeled arrow indicates accessory LPA arising from GPA.

of the manuscript. The authors would also like to thank the Editor, Annals, Academy of Medicine, Singapore for his kind permission to use some of the published materials in the journal contained in Vol. 12 (2 Suppl):347–51, 1983 and in Vol. 17 (3):328–34, 1988.

References

1. Ivy RH. The philtrum of the upper lip [editorial]. *Plast Reconstr Surg* 40:94–5, 1967.
2. Boyd JD. The classification of the upper lip in mammals. *J Anat* 67:409–16, 1932.
3. Stark RB. The pathogenesis of harelip and cleft palate. *Plast Reconstr Surg* 13:20–39, 1954.
4. Nairn RI. The circumoral musculature: Structure and function. *Br Dent J* 138:49–56, 1975.
5. Latham RA, Deaton TG. The structural basis of the philtrum and the contour of the vermilion border: A study of the musculature of the upper lip. *J Anat* 121:151–60, 1976.
6. Wu WT. The Oriental nose: An anatomical basis for surgery. *Ann Acad Med Singapore* 21:176–89, 1992.
7. Niranjan NS. An anatomical study of the facial artery. *Ann Plast Surg* 21:14–22, 1988.
8. Lee ST. A histological study of the philtrum. *Ann Acad Med Singapore* 17:328–34, 1988.
9. Lee ST. A new approach to bilateral cleft lip repair. *Ann Acad Med Singapore* 12(2 Suppl):347–51, 1983.
10. Malek R. Cleft Lip and Palate: *Lesions, pathophysiology and primary treatment.* New York: Thieme, 2001.
11. Boorman JG, Sommerlad BC. Musculus uvulae and levator palatini: Their anatomical and functional relationship in velopharyngeal closure. *Br J Plast Surg* 38:333–338, 1985.
12. Legent F. Velar tics or pseudo-myoclonus of the palate. *Ann Otolaryngol Chir Cervicofac* 93(7–8):463–470, 1976.
13. Huang MHS, Lee ST, Rajendran K. Anatomic basis of cleft palate and velopharyngeal surgery: Implications from a fresh cadaveric study. *Plast Reconstr Surg* 101(3):613, 1998.
14. Huang MHS, Lee ST, Rajendran K. A fresh cadaveric study of the paratubal muscles: Implications for eustachian tube function in cleft palate. *Plast Reconstr Surg* 100(4):833–842, 1997.
15. Ruding R. Cleft palate: Anatomic and surgical considerations. *Plast Reconstr Surg* 33:132–47, 1964.
16. Fára M. Musculature of the cleft lip and palate. In: Editor. McCarthy JG (ed). *McCarthy Plastic Surgery, Cleft lip & palate and craniofacial anomalies.* Vol 4. Philadelphia: W B Saunders Company. 1990, pp. 2612–2625
17. Maue-Dickson W. Section II. Anatomy and physiology. *Cleft Palate J* 14:270, 1979.
18. Kamerer DB. Electromyographic correlation of tensor tympani and tensor veli palatini muscles in man. 88:651, 1978.
19. Latham RA, Long RE Jr, Latham EA. Cleft palate velopharyngeal musculature in a 5 months old infant: A three dimensional histological reconstruction. *Cleft Palate J* 17(1):1–16, 1980.
20. Shimokawa T, Yi SQ, Tanaka S. Nerve supply to the soft palate muscles with special reference to the distribution of the lesser palatine nerve. *Cleft Palate Craniofac J* 42:495, 2005.
21. Mehendale FV. Surgical anatomy of the levator veli palatini: A previously undescribed tendinous insertion of the anterolateral fibers. *Plast Reconstr Surg* 114(2):307–15, 2004.
22. Dickson DR, Maue Dickson W. Velopharyngeal anatomy. *J Speech Hear Res* 15:372, 1972.
23. Dickson DR. Normal and cleft palate anatomy. *Cleft Palate J* 9:280, 1972.
24. Bosma JF. A correlated study of the anatomy and motor activity of the upper pharynx by cadaver dissection and by cinematic study of patients after maxillofacial surgery. *Ann Otol* 62:51, 1953.
25. Dickson DR. Anatomy of the normal velopharyngeal mechanism. *Clin Plast Surg* 2:235, 1975.
26. Yamawaki Y, Nishimura Y, Suzuki Y. Eustachian tube cartilage and medial movement of lateral pharyngeal wall on phonation. *Plast Reconstr Surg* 104(2):350–356, 1999.
27. Croft CB, Shprintzen RJ, Rakoff SJ. Patterns of velopharyngeal valving in normal and cleft palate subjects: A multi-view videofluoroscopic and nasoendoscopic study. *Laryngoscope* 91:265, 1981.
28. Shprintzen RJ, Croft CB. Abnormalities of the eustachian tube orifice in individuals with cleft palate. *Int J Pediatr Otorhinolaryngol* 3:15, 1981.
29. Boorman JG, Sommerlad BC. Levator palati and palatal dimples: Their anatomy, relationship and clinical significance. *Br J Plast Surg* 38:326, 1985.
30. Last RJ. *Anatomy regional and applied.* 7th edn. London: Churchill Livingstone, 1984
31. Hollinshead WH. Anatomy for surgeons. *The Head and Neck,* Vol 1. New York: Harper & Brothers, 1954.
32. Fara M, Dvorak J. Abnormal anatomy of the muscles of palatopharyngeal closure in cleft palates. *Plast Reconstr Surg* 46:488, 1970.
33. Zazebski JA. Ultrasonic assessment of lateral pharyngeal wall motion at two levels of the vocal tract. *J Speech Hear Res* 18:308, 1975.
34. Iglesias A, Kuehn DP, Morris HL. Simultaneous assessment of pharyngeal wall and velar displacement for selected speech sounds. *J Speech Hear Res* 23:429, 1980.
35. Fritzell B. The velopharyngeal muscles in speech: An Electromyographic and cineradiographic study. *Acta Otolaryngol Suppl* 250:1, 1969.
36. Bell-Berti F. An Electromyographic study of velopharyngeal function in speech. *J Speech Hear Res* 19;2251975.
37. Huang MHS, Lee ST, Rajendran K. A fresh cadaveric study of the palatoglossus muscle: Implications for speech physiology. Submitted for publication.
38. Huang MHS, Lee ST, Rajendran K. Structure of the musculus uvulae: Functional and surgical implications of an anatomic study. *Cleft Palate Craniofac J* 34;466–474, 1997.
39. Broomhead I. The nerve supply to the muscles of the soft palate. *Br J Plast Surg* 4:1, 1951.
40. Nishio J, Matsuya T, Machida J, Miyazaki T. The motor supply of the velopharyngeal muscles. *Cleft Palate J* 13:20–30, 1976.
41. Mitsui T, Shimai K, Yasuda K, Kato S, Kubota K, Inoue Y. *Okajima's anatomy.* New edn. Tokyo: Kyorin Shoin. 1986, pp. 487–500.
42. Leonhaldt H, Tilman B, Tondury G, Ziles K. *Rauber/Kopsch Anatomie des 17 Aud, Bd II.* Leipzig, Germany: Georg Thieme,1948, pp. 61–62.
43. Huang MHS, Lee ST, Rajendran K. Clinical implications of the velopharyngeal blood supply: A fresh cadaveric study. *Plast Reconstr Surg* 102:655–667, 1998.
44. Kriens OB. An anatomical approach to veloplasty. *Plast Reconstr Surg* 43:29, 1969.
45. Furlow LT. Cleft palate repair by double opposing Z-plasty. *Plast Reconstr Surg* 78:724, 1986.
46. Braithwaite F, Maurice DG. The importance of the levator palati muscle in cleft palate closure. *Br J Plast Surg* 21:60, 1968.
47. Edgerton MT, Dellon A. Surgical retrodisplacement of the levator veli palatini muscle. *Plast Reconstr Surg* 47:154, 1971.
48. Brown AS, Cohen MA, Randall P. Levator muscle reconstruction: Does it make a difference? *Plast Reconstr Surg* 72:1, 1983.
49. Brophy M. Bone surgery essential in the treatment of complete cleft palate. *J Am Dent Assoc* 1:23–27, 1923.

Developmental Field Reassignment in Unilateral Cleft Lip: Reconstruction of the Premaxilla

Michael H. Carstens, MD, FACS

I. INTRODUCTION

II. THE PATHOLOGIC ANATOMY OF CLEFT FORMATION

III. RECONSTRUCTION OF THE PMx

IV. PHILOSOPHY OF DFR: THE "4 Ds"

V. SURGICAL TECHNIQUE OF DFR
Preparation and Marking
Dissection Sequence
Closure Sequence

VI. DISCUSSION

INTRODUCTION

In the 21st century, the greatest stimulus for progress in cleft surgery will come from a more accurate model of facial development and how clefts originate. Victor Veau[1] accurately predicted this: "All cleft surgery is merely applied embryology." The revolution in developmental biology has not yet been incorporated into surgical practice. The drawings and terminology used in textbooks today are based on the work of Wilhelm His in the 1870s.[2] Cleft repairs are therefore designed based on the anatomy as it appears in the newborn. Measurements are taken, and the tissues are geometrically manipulated. However, the anatomy of a cleft, as seen at the time of birth, is far different from its original configuration in the embryonic face. From its onset at gastrulation, the clefting event unleashes pathologic processes that predictably alter the original embryonic anatomy over time to produce what we recog-

nize at term as a cleft lip. Left uncorrected, these processes will remain operative throughout facial growth. This explains why geometric cleft repairs relapse over time, requiring revision.

Developmental field reassignment (DFR) is based upon the neuromeric model of craniofacial embryology.[3,4] The goals of DFR surgery are (1) resolution of all pathologic processes of clefting (deficiency, displacement, division, and distortion), (2) dissection along embryonic separation planes (subperiosteal release), (3) preservation of blood supply to the alveolar mucoperiosteum, (4) primary unification of the dental arch, and (5) reassignment of all developmental fields to their correct relationships.

Before describing the surgical technique, certain basic concepts of field theory should be understood. Craniofacial anatomy results from the assembly of specific, identifiable *developmental fields*. Fields are discrete units composed of ectoderm, mesoderm, endoderm, and neural crest. At each

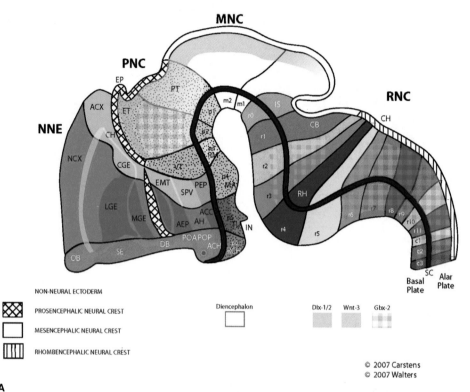

NEUROMERIC CODING OF THE EMBRYO

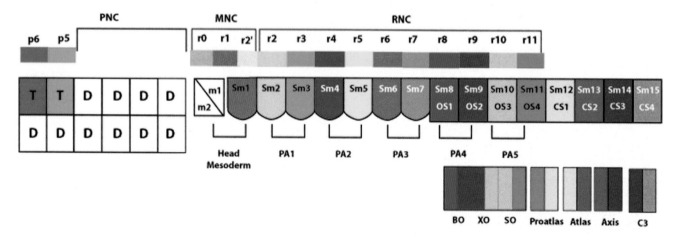

Figure 15–1. Developmental field map of the face. All neuromeres are color coded. Neural crest cells forming ethmoid, presphenoid, vomer, and premaxilla share common embryologic origin from first rhombomere (violet). Maxilla, zygoma, and alisphenoid come from second rhombomere (blue). "Philtral column is interface between p5 philtral dermis and r2 lip dermis." All craniofacial sutures contain neural crest cells. Craniofacial fields are neuroembryologic and follow suture boundaries.

level of the embryo, all germ layers specific to that level can be referenced back to developmental zones of the neuraxis known as *neuromeres*. These are named using the nomenclature of neuroembryology. The master plan of the entire embryo is determined by 6 *prosomeres* (prosencephalon-

forebrain), 2 *mesomeres* (mesencephalon-midbrain), 12 *rhombomeres* (rhomboencephalon-hindbrain), and 31 *myelomeres* (spinal cord)[5–7] (Figs. 15–1 to 15–4).

Applications of neuromeric anatomy provide a potential embryonic "map" of all craniofacial structures with

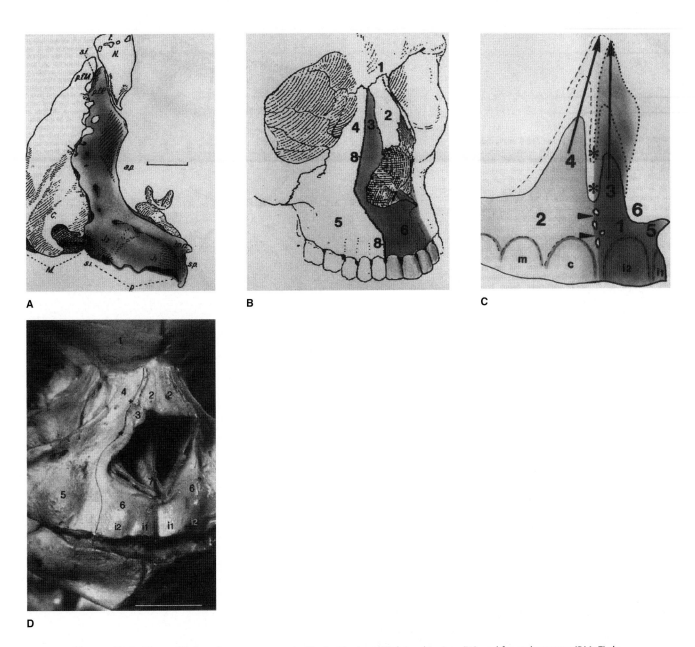

Figure 15–2. Premaxilla has three components. Central incisor (i1), lateral incisor (i2) and frontal process (PMxF) develop in strict spatio-temporal sequence. PMxF grows vertically (3, arrow) to articulate with frontal bone. Clefting affects premaxillary fields *in reverse order*; piriform fossa deficiency is *form fruste* manifestation.

important implications for diagnosis and surgery. Exclusive of the cranial base (basisphenoid and posterior) and parietal bone, the craniofacial skeleton is made exclusively from neural crest. Thus, the cell populations producing the ethmoid, presphenoid, premaxilla (PMx), and vomer (V) all originate in anteroposterior order from the neural folds in genetic register with the first rhombomere (abbreviated r1). The inferior turbinate (IT), palatine bone (P), maxilla (M), alisphenoid (AS) (greater wing), and zygoma (Z) arise from the neural crest of the second rhombomere (r2). The squamous temporal, mandible, malleus, and incus are r3 neural crest bones.

Non-neural crest craniofacial bones (and all muscles) come from paraxial mesoderm (PAM) lying immediately ad-

jacent to the neural tube. PAM is divided into individual units shaped like popcorn balls called *somitomeres* (*Sm*). The first seven somitomeres contain myoblasts for orbit and first three pharyngeal arches: Sm1 (IR, IO, MR), Sm2 (SR, LPS), Sm3 (SO), Sm4 (1st arch), Sm5 (LR), Sm6 (2nd arch), and Sm7 (3rd arch). Beginning with Sm8, all Sm undergo a further transformation into *somites*, each having a dermatome, myotome, and sclerotome. The first four somites (derived from Sm8 to Sm11) produce the cranial base posterior to the sphenoid and the muscles of the tongue and part of the sternocleidomastoid and trapezius. These are called *occipital somites.*

Disturbances at a particular neuromeric level can affect individual or multiple fields to be deficient or absent. Thus,

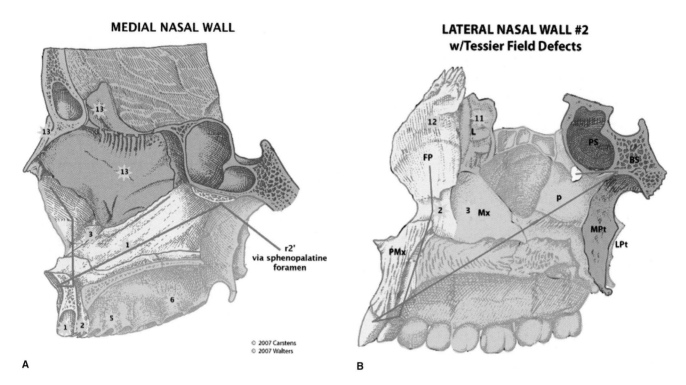

MEDIAL NASAL WALL

A

**LATERAL NASAL WALL #2
w/Tessier Field Defects**

B

© 2007 Carstens
© 2007 Walters

Figure 15–3. Medial and lateral sections of the nasal cavity demonstrate the neuromeric origins of the bone fields. The biosynthetic pathway of the r2' MNC lays down the premaxilla and vomer along the axis of the nasopalatine nerve and the medial branch of the sphenopalatine artery (the absolute terminus of the external carotid). Fields affected by the Tessier clefts are indicated by yellow stars, for example, the #3 cleft is a selective knockout of the inferior turbinate. Because the p5 lacrimal bone is built upon IT the #3 cleft destroys the lacrimal system. The cleft premaxilla is zone #2.

isolated cleft palate (unassociated with cleft lip) represents a deficiency state of the V. This occurs as a spectrum. As the V is progressively deficient or smaller, it lifts away from the plane of the palatal shelves and the resulting cleft extends forward toward the incisive foramen. In mild cases of cleft

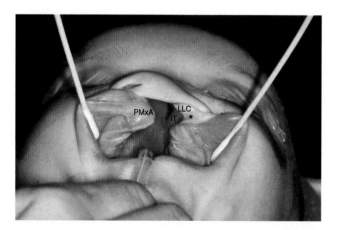

Figure 15–4. Cleft site showing retraction of p5 lateral crus vestibular pulled downward into the premaxillary deficiency site (just in front of the inferior turbinate). LLC is programmed by p5 nasal skin; ULC in programmed by p6 vestibular epithelium. If the LLC is not released and additional tissue provided, the nasal vestibule will be reduced in surface area 30–40% compared to the noncleft side. Standard cleft repairs lead to respiratory dysfunction.

palate associated with *Pierre Robin sequence*, a reduction in the horizontal plate of the r2 P is seen. Soft palate muscles are consequently normal but divided. As the pathology worsens, reduction in the horizontal plate of the r2 Mx creates the well-known "horseshoe" palate cleft. *Submucous cleft palate*, on the other hand, involves pathology in the third pharyngeal arch. Sm7 contains the myoblasts of levator, uvula, palatopharyngeus, and superior constrictor. These can be globally affected. Frequently, persistent VPI follows a seemingly simple palatoplasty, requiring further surgery. *It is our belief that failure to stratify cleft palate by embryologic mechanism may explain much of the confusion currently extent in the speech and surgical literature.*

Finally, *Treacher Collins syndrome* provides an example in which all r2 developmental fields of the midface are affected: the maxillary, palatine, and zygomatic bones are all small. The septum, V, and PMx (being r1 structures) are unaffected. For this reason, the central midface projects normally while the dimensions of the palate, Mx, and Z are constricted.

Developmental fields form in a specific spatiotemporal sequence. Each one builds upon its predecessors. Making a face is much akin to assembling a house with magical pieces of Lego®, each one of which will grow over time. Imagine a Lego house made from 20 pieces (4 on the floor and 5 stories high). All pieces are growing independently. If a cornerstone piece is removed, the 19 remaining pieces undergo a deformation and the house tilts into the deficiency site. *The missing Lego piece in cleft lip is the PMx.* The physiologic basis of DFR is the reconstruction of the premaxillary field.[8,9,10] This chapter presents the reconstructive application of these principles to the surgery of labiomaxillary clefts.

THE PATHOLOGIC ANATOMY OF CLEFT FORMATION

The pathologic anatomy of unilateral and bilateral labiomaxillary clefts stems from a tissue deficiency state localized to the lower lateral piriform fossa. The tissue at fault is the mesenchyme of the ipsilateral PMx. Neural crest stem cells responsible for synthesis of the presphenoid and ethmoid arise from the mesencephalic neural folds and are genetically identified with the r1. Note that the basisphenoid is *not* neural crest in origin; it comes from PAM from somitomere 1 (Sm1). Sm1 lies just outside the neural tube at level r1 and is in register with it. Immediately caudal to this population are neural crest cells immediately above the rostral rhomboencephalon with the r2. *The most rostral zone of r2 (herein referred to as r2′) is the likely source material for the V and PMx.* The more caudal zone of r2 produces IT, P, Mx, AS, and Z.

These cell populations migrate forward into the developing face in a strict temporospatial order. The sphenoid is laid down first, followed by the ethmoid. In like manner, formation of PMx is the prerequisite for the appearance of V. Formation of the PMx and V requires the preexistence of the perpendicular plate of the ethmoid (PPE). The function of the PPE is to provide a cellular scaffold by which r2′ neural crest cells can reach the midline.[10] In holoprosencephaly (HPE), the PPE can be absent. PMx and V cannot develop correctly; a wide bilateral cleft results.[11–13]

The piriform fossa of humans and some high primates is assembled as the fusion of the frontal process of the premaxilla (PMxF) and the frontal process of the maxilla (MxF). In all other vertebrate skulls, PMxF and MxF are readily visible as two distinct entities.[14] Evolution foreshortened the human snout. The two fields became superimposed, *PMxF becoming telescoped internal to MxF.* This lamination is responsible for the strength of the piriform rim. Plating of the piriform "buttress" in fracture repairs takes advantage of this bicortical anatomy.

The developmental field in which the PMx resides consists of an epithelium and a mesenchyme. Formation of the PMx results from interactions between these tissues. The PMx has several anatomic subcomponents, these are assembled in a strict sequence.[15,16] In dental terminology, the central incisor is called "A" and the lateral incisor is called "B." A erupts before B. Therefore, the central incisor field (PMxA) is biologically "older" than the lateral incisor field (PMxB). Neural crest mesenchyme flows forward along the previously established PPE. It first encounters the epithelium corresponding to PmxA and then "spills over" into zone PMxB. The time sequence of dental eruption (central incisor A > lateral incisor B) is a manifestation of the relative biologic "maturity" of the mesenchymal field within which each tooth develops. The

frontal process field (PMxF) is a vertical offshoot of PMxB; this subfield is the biologically "newest" tissue.

Pathology affecting the PMx occurs as a spectrum, based on this original developmental pattern. A deficiency state of the PMx will first occur in the most distal aspect of the frontal process (i.e., at its most cranial extent). As the mesenchymal deficit worsens, frontal process will be reduced in a cranio-caudal gradient. "Scooping out" of the piriform rim results; the nasal lining is pulled down as well. This causes depression of the alar base and a downward lateral displacement of the lateral crus. Biologic signals from PMxF regulate epithelial stability and therefore affect lip formation (vide infra). When the signal strength is minimally disturbed, the lip is normal despite the piriform distortion. Therefore, the *forme fruste* manifestation of premaxillary deficiency is a cleft lip nose deformity, with a perfectly normal lip.[17]

Once the frontal process is eliminated, the deficiency state shows up in the lateral incisor field. Progressive degrees of PMx deficiency in the lateral incisor field cause incremental loss of alveolar bone. Normal alveolar development follows a gradient. It begins at the incisive foramen and progresses forward. Mild deficiency causes notching on the labial surface. As the deficiency worsens, the notch deepens *backward* toward the incisive foramen. A critical lack of alveolar bone mass results in outright failure of lateral incisor development.

BMP-4 signals from this field are directly implicated in the mechanism of fusion between the lateral lip element and the prolabium.[18,19] BMP-4 emanating from PmxB forms a cranio-caudal chemical gradient. The strength of this gradient depends upon the total amount of available BMP-4; this in turn is proportional to the overall mesenchymal mass of PMxB. Reduction in mass of the lateral incisor field results in a diminution of the total BMP-4 signal. Lip fusion follows this same gradient. Mild weakness of the BMP-4 gradient will result in notching of the vermilion. As the situation worsens, the extent of the lip cleft worsens in a cranial direction. The clinical spectrum of the so-called minimal cleft lip deformity faithfully reproduces this biological sequence.[17]

In summation, variations in clefts involving the primary palate and the lip can be understood as interactions between deep plane fields of the PMx, the Mx, and superficial plane field of the lateral lip element. The mesenchyme of the lip has a different embryologic origin. It is genetically identified with the r2. Neural crest cells from r2 provide the dermis and the subcutaneous tissue of the alar base, while PAM from the second somitomere forms the anterior half of the squamous temporal bone and the cranial half of the parotid gland. All derivatives from level r2 can be mapped out within the sensory distribution of V2, the nucleus of which resides within r2.[20–25]

The developmental anatomy of the nose, prolabium, and PMx has been previously described in terms of neuromeric theory by this author.[3,4,8,9] In contrast to the rest of the body, *all dermis and submucosa of the head originates from neural crest cells*, not from a dermatome associated with a somite.[26] Predermal neural crest arises from three distinct zones of the embryo. The dermis of the forehead, nose, and vestibular lining come from the caudal prosencephalon (above prosomeres p4–p1). This prosencephalic neural crest (PNC) migrates forward like a gigantic glacier to occupy the neural folds above prosomeres p6 and p5. The alar half of p6 and p5 creates the telencephalon (cerebrum). The basal halves of p6 and p5 plus all remaining prosomeres (p4–p1) synthesize the diencephalon (epithalamus, thalamus, and hypothalamus). The neural folds above p6 and p5 are "sterile." They contain the pituitary, olfactory, and optic placodes, but no neural crest. When PNC flows forward into this zone, the placodes are activated and dermis is formed. Nasal vestibular lining from the cribriform plate forward to the internal nasal valve comes from p6 PNC. All remaining frontonasal dermis from the internal nasal valve forward to the hairline comes from p5 PNC.

PNC skin shares sensory innervation with the dura of the underlying frontal lobe. V1, the sensory nerve for this common zone, has its nucleus with the r1. The neuroanatomy is analogous for the rest of the face. Rhombomeres r2 and r3 contain neurons supplying all skin and dura innervated by V2 and V3. *This is the embryologic basis for the treatment of migraine headaches with Botox® injected into peripheral trigger points.*

Design of surgical incisions for cleft repair follows this embryology. The boundary between these two fields is sharply demarcated within the naris. The skin of the anterior columella and philtrum is thus a p5 derivative. This skin is supplied by terminal branches of the internal carotid artery, the anterior ethmoid arteries, and innervated by V1.[3] The skin making up the floor of the nose has a different origin. It extends from the base of the columella laterally and makes contact with the alar base. The medial (terminal) branch of the sphenopalatine artery (SPA) innervates this skin. The innervation is from V2 and is shared with the ipsilateral incisors. Continuity between the p5 skin of the lateral columella and the r2′ skin of the nasal floor makes possible the elevation of a skin–cartilage flap containing the medial crura with long skin flaps. Many years ago, Vissarianov described this flap as a means of secondary cleft reconstruction.[27,28]

Based on signals from the underlying PMx, the r2 alar base produces a tongue of tissue that makes contact with the r1 lateral prolabium. This skin bridge sets up the floor of the nose. It also provides a mechanical platform by which mesenchyme from the lateral lip element can make contact with the p5 mesenchyme of the prolabium. Lip closure thus occurs. This process involves mesenchymal "flow" from the lateral lip element toward the prolabium. For this to occur, the epithelium covering the lateral lip element, the r2–r1 skin bridge, and prolabium must undergo a genetically induced breakdown. BMP-4 produced by the premaxillary field causes derepression of *Sonic hedgehog* (*SHH*), a gene localized to these overlying epithelia. The protein product of *SHH* causes epithelial breakdown. Thus, absence or deficiency of an appropriate BMP-4 signal will lead to restricted expression of *SHH*, abnormal persistence of epithelium, and failure of mesenchymal fusion.[29,30]

The volume of the PMx determines whether or not lip closure can occur. First, a small premaxillary field manufactures small amounts of BMP-4. The amount of BMP-4 produced is critical to produce the epithelial breakdown necessary to permit mesenchymal merger. Second, when the PMx is too small, the physical distance between it and Mx will exceed a critical dimension. Epithelial bridge formation between the alar base and the prolabium cannot occur. If this critical distance exists at the level of the incisive foramen, a cleft of the secondary palate will form. This is because the horizontal repositioning of the palatal shelf from the Mx must make contact with the V just posterior to the incisive foramen. The process is just like a zipper. If initial contact is not made, fusion of the palatal shelf to the V cannot take place. Even if initial contact is made, a secondary palatal cleft can still result due to displacement of the V away from the midline. The V can become warped by the inequality of growth forces on either side of the cleft. Thus, the zipper may get started anteriorly but, as the process proceeds posteriorly, when it encounters the deviated V, a palatal cleft will open up.[3]

RECONSTRUCTION OF THE PMx

Cleft surgery that does not reconstruct the missing PMx does not solve the biologic problem. The pediatric face is a set of Lego pieces, all growing over time. If one piece of the set is missing, with subsequent growth the remaining pieces will collapse into the deficiency site. Only when all the Lego pieces are in place can harmonious facial development occur.

The premaxillary developmental field consists of lining (present in its totality) and mesenchyme (missing). Lining can be recreated by (1) subperiosteal dissection of the primary palate (r2′ PMx and r2 Mx); (2) subperichondrial dissection of the p6 septum (sufficient to reduce the septum into the midline; (3) subperiosteal elevation of r2′ V to close the nasal floor (sufficient to reduce the septum into the midline); and (4) subperiosteal rescue of the r2′ nasal floor skin from the lateral prolabium. When these flaps are elevated and sutured, the primary palate becomes a box lined with neural crest stem cells, all of which carry membrane-bound BMP receptors.[30–32]

Mesenchymal replacement can be undertaken using two basic mechanisms. Autogenous bone graft from rib or hip provides mesenchymal cells originating from PAM. Incorporation of the graft into the primary palate occurs by *osteoconduction*. Implantation of recombinant human bone morphogenetic protein-2 (rhBMP-2) in combination with an activated collagen sponge (ACS) results in morphogen-based recruitment of stem cells from the environment into the sponge. Stem cell concentration and differentiation into osteoblasts result in the formation of bone native to the site. This process is known as *osteoinduction*.[33] Extensive preclinical work by Boyne demonstrated the ability of rhBMP-2 to form membranous bone, including reconstitution of surgically created cleft palate defects in primates.[34,35] Studies demonstrating efficacy in maxillary lift combined with absence of donor site morbidity resulted in FDA approval for this indication.[36,37]

The technique of facial bone reconstruction using rhBMP-2/ACS implantation is known as *in situ osteogenesis* (ISO) and has been previously reported by this author and coworkers.[38] Resynthesis of a 12-cm mandibular defect in a 9-year old demonstrated the ability of ISO function effectively outside the range of blood supply associated with a critical-size defect.[39] BMP-2-mediated osteoinduction is accompanied by extensive recruitment of blood vessels from local environment.[40] For this reason, selected bone defects can be resynthesized using ISO alone, without recourse to microsurgical tissue transplantation.

Distraction techniques have been successfully applied to ISO-regenerated bone. In a number #7 lateral cleft with a foreshortened mandibular body and absent ramus, distraction of the recipient periosteal chamber in a posterior and superior direction permitted synthesis of 3.5 cm of mandibular ramus with eventual articulation with the skull base via a pseudoarthrosis.[41] *Distraction-assisted in situ osteogenesis* (DISO) will be an alternative treatment to rib grafts in the reconstruction of the Pruzansky III mandibular defects in craniofacial microsomia. The bone produced will be membranous. The dissection is less problematic. There is avoidance of unpredictable growth of the rib graft outside the natural periosteal environment. Finally, the chest wall donor site is obviated. Histology of ISO-produced membranous bone is indistinguishable from that of the recipient site in both mandible and Mx.

Alveolar clefts are lined with mucoperiosteum containing neural crest stem cells. Blood supply is excellent and the dimensions modest. For this reason, this author and coworkers reported 50 alveolar clefts successfully treated with rhBMP-2.[42] Precise surgical technique of implant placement and of soft tissue closure was emphasized in the current series of 200 cleft sites.[43] Long-term outcome of 43 cleft sites was assessed at 1 year postgrafting with 3D CT. The series was comprised of 23 unilateral clefts (6 primary and 17 secondary) and 12 bilateral clefts (3 primary and 9 secondary). Complete transverse fill (unification of the dental arch) was achieved in all cases. Vertical fill was improved to 75–100% when an inert bulking agent (tricalcium phosphate) was included. For these reasons, primary cleft repair using developmental field reassignment (DFR) technique can ideally be combined with ISO to achieve primary unification of the dental arch without donor site morbidity.

PHILOSOPHY OF DFR: THE "4 Ds"

Faulty embryogenesis of the premaxillary field affects the position and shape of surrounding fields in four distinct ways: (1) *division* of force vectors causes unequal growth, (2) *deficiency*-related collapse of partner fields into the void, (3) displacement of partner fields away from the midline, and (4) *distortion* over time of structures such as the septum.

DFR repair addresses these 4 Ds in reverse order. All distortions should be corrected. The displaced soft tissues of the face should be centralized into the midline. The deficiency site should be restored using neighboring soft tissues and bone graft or ISO and division should be closed via unification of soft tissues.[44]

The execution of DFR surgery is based upon the concepts of Sotereanos.[45] Its guiding principles are five:[6,7] (1) correct all pathologic states in the first operation (as above), (2) respect embryonic developmental planes during dissection, i.e., subperiosteal release of the soft tissue envelope for a tension-free closure, (3) conserve blood supply to the periosteum, safeguarding it for future membranous bone synthesis, (4) align and unite the dental arch into a normal relationship, and (5) reassign all developmental fields into correct relationships with each other.

When properly executed, these principles result in the *restoration of the functional matrix*. When all the bone-forming soft tissue fields are spatially correct, all force vectors exerted upon bone will be correctly aligned. Subsequent growth of the face is directed back toward the normal.[46–48]

A new algorithm: Is lateral nasal wall deficiency relative or absolute?

In keeping with Victor Veau, cleft repair is a constant exploration of nature's experiments. DFR surgery is deliberately designed to address a tissue deficit of the lateral nasal wall and alveolus, the product of a congenitally small premaxillary field. That the lateral crus be entrapped cannot be in doubt. Its release into a normal position occasions a triangular tissue gap that must be filled. Proper airway reconstruction is the name of the game. At the same time, the alveolar cleft (a six-sided box) must be reconstructed. This requires flap coverage for its nasal surface (the "top" of the box). Can these two goals be accomplished with the same tissue?

A skin graft alone (particularly anterior auricular skin and cartilage) will effectively support lateral alar crus advancement. It cannot provide vascular coverage for the alveolar cleft "roof." At first blush, the LLC–NPP flap would seem big enough to accomplish both goals. After 7 years of work with this technique, this author has concluded that paring from the prolabium is not sufficient. *Premaxillary field soft tissues are not just relatively deficient from the lateral nasal wall: an absolute tissue deficit exists.* Use of the premaxillary tissue mismatched to the prolabium is not always sufficient to solve the problem. The new algorithm of DFR surgery now calls for optional composite grafting of the lateral wall, followed by elevation and transposition of the LCC–NPP flap across the nasal surface of the alveolar cleft. The decision to graft is based upon the relative size of the defect versus that of the flap.

SURGICAL TECHNIQUE OF DFR

This operation consists of markings, a five-step dissection sequence, and a five-step closure (Figs. 15–5 to 15–12).

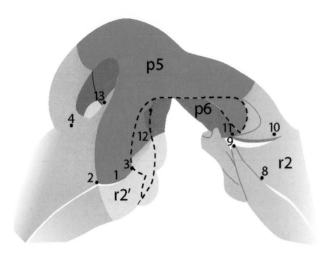

Figure 15–5. Surgical marking and incisions for DFR. Point #3 is 6–10 mm from the normal philtral column. "Lateral NPP-LCC incision can also be directed backward over "shoulder" of premaxilla and into mouth in continuity with vomer flap. Lateral nasal wall incision separates p5 vestibular mucosa (sky blue) from second rhombomere (r2) nasal skin (yellow).

Preparation and Marking

The DFR operation is comprehensive, providing simultaneous correction of the lip, nose, and primary palate. A more extensive dissection is required. The operation takes longer to perform (about 3–4 hours for a unilateral cleft). For this reason, patients come to surgery at 4–6 months of age. Prior to operation, the dental arch is prepared with splinting (a form of infant presurgical orthopedics); this is begun as early as 2 weeks after birth. The emphasis of presurgical splinting is (1) promoting anterior growth of the retro-displaced cleft Mx and (2) maintenance of the space in the alveolar cleft. *If satisfactory maxillary shelf repositioning does not result by age 3 months, a lip adhesion procedure is carried out.* When satisfactory dental arch correction is achieved, DFR repair is performed. This usually occurs 3–4 months after the lip adhesion.

The patient receives antibiotics and corticosteroids for swelling. A central V2 block is performed at the pterygopalatine fossa using 0.25% Marcaine® (bupivacaine hydrochloride). Approximately 3–5 cc per side is sufficient (maximum

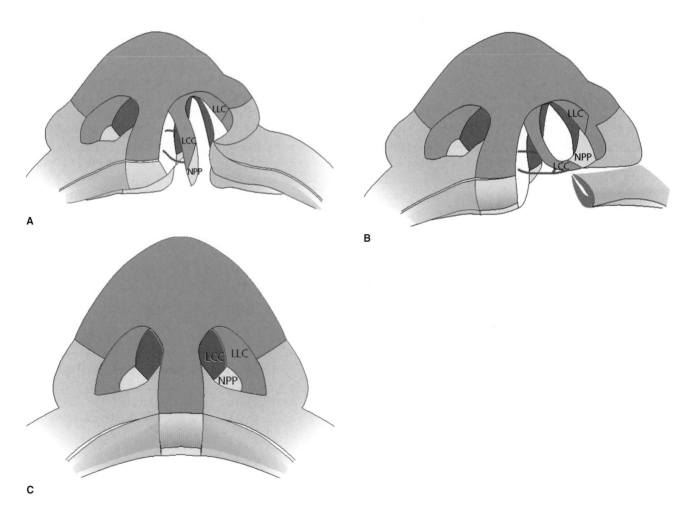

Figure 15–6. Elevation and transposition of NPP–LCC (non-philtral prolabium/lateral columella chondrocutaneous) flap into deficiency site created by release and cephalic rotation of p5 lateral crus. "Composite graft from cymba interposed between NPP and lateral crus reconstructs soft tissue corresponding to premaxillary frontal process."

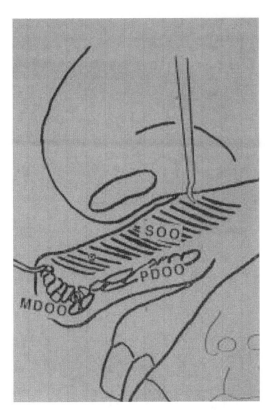

Figure 15–7. Orbicularis oris is structurally and functionally bilaminar. Anatomic dissection by Park demonstrates superficial orbicularis oris (SOO) to attach to the philtral column as a dilator. Deep orbicularis oris (DOO) is separated from SOO by a plane of fat and axial vasculature. DOO is a sphincter. It runs in the plane deep to the p5 mesenchyme of the philtrum and is thus continuous with itself across the midline. All pharyngeal arch muscles follow the same pattern: deep plane muscles appear earlier than superficial, caudal before cranial, and lateral before medial. The very last facial muscle to appear is the oblique head of SOO.

dose for 0.25% bupivacaine being 1 cc/kg). At the end of the case, the central block is reinforced by blocking the infraorbital nerves with bupivacaine, 1–2 cc per side. The child returns to recovery pain-free. The initial block ensures that substance P (a critical mediator in the pain cascade released in response to surgical trauma) will not be produced. In the absence of substance P, the entire postoperative pain response is altered.

The surgical fields of the unilateral cleft are defined as follows: (In neuromeric terms: A = p6 (red) + p5 (turquoise), B = r2′ (pale gold), C is r2 (yellow), and D is r2 + r4 (yellow + orange). The prolabium is divided into two zones. Zone A is the *true philtrum*; it measures the width of the columella. It contains paired anterior ethmoid arteries (the terminal branches of the internal carotid system) and paired terminal branches of V1. Thus, zone A contains two neurovascular developmental fields. Zone B of the prolabium is all tissue lateral to the philtrum: the *non-philtral prolabium* (NPP). The nasopalatine (medial sphenopalatine) artery, the terminal branch from the internal maxillary system, supplies the NPP. Bilateral clefts have two NPP zones.

The cleft-side alar base is zone C. The lateral lip element below the alar groove is zone D. It contains a sphincter layer, the deep orbicularis oris (DOO), and the dilator layer, the superficial orbicularis oris (SOO) muscles. DOO develops in conjunction with the oral mucosa while SOO develops with the skin. A layer of fat conveniently separates these two layers.[49,50]

The true destination of NPP soft tissue is in the nasal floor. NPP represents the soft tissue envelope corresponding to the lateral incisor zone of the PMx. Lateral wall soft tissue corresponds to the PMxF. Nasal floor soft tissue corresponds to the PMxB. The rationale of DFR surgery is to reassign the misplaced fields of the PMx into correct position. When the NPP flap and cymba graft are combined with the reflected mucoperiosteum from the margins of the bony cleft, a surgical "pocket" is created. *This site is subsequently filled with bone graft or a bone-producing cytokine (rhBMP-2) such that missing premaxillary fields are resynthesized.*

Markings are carried out using a modification of the Millard system. (Paired anterior ethmoid neurovascular bundles define the true philtrum; this equals the width of the columella.) First to be marked is point 2, the junction of the normal philtral column with the white roll. The width of the columella at its base is then measured. This distance (usually 6–10 mm) is subsequently marked along the white roll medial to the philtral column as point 3. Distance 2–3 is the *width of the philtrum*; this contains the two anterior ethmoid arteries (approximately 4–6 mm apart). The midpoint of the philtrum (point 1 in the Millard system, or nadir of Cupid's bow) is irrelevant. Point 13, defined by the bulge of the footplate of the medial crus on the noncleft side, marks the "shoulder" of the columella. The corresponding point 12 on the cleft side will be found displaced caudally and internally with respect to point 13. Total *philtral height* 2–13 should equal 3–12. Points 4 and 10 mark the midpoint of the alar bases on noncleft and cleft sides, respectively.

On the lateral side, points 9 and 11 mark the terminus of skin within the nasal cavity. This is located just anterior to the IT. Point 9 is the tip of flap D while point 11 is the tip of the future nostril sill C′, so-called because it is in continuity with the alar base C. The dimensions of C′ can be roughly mapped out by measuring the nostril sill on the noncleft side. This is the distance from the midpoint of the noncleft alar base (point 4) to the ipsilateral footplate point 13. Point 8 marks the natural transition of the white roll. Distance 8–9 should match 3–12.

Dissection Sequence

Step 1. Lateral Dissection: Rescuing the Nostril Sill

The lateral lip is tensed with a single hook and the skin–mucosa margin is incised proceeding upward from 8 to 9, located just below and anterior to the IT. From here the incision swings around laterally to 10, the midpoint of the alar base, (but not beyond it at this point). In this manner, the lateral lip flap D is separated from the alar base C. This step

CLEFT NASAL INCISION SEQUENCE

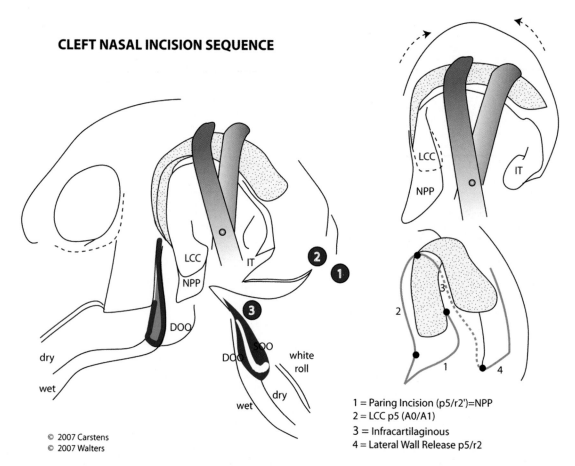

1 = Paring Incision (p5/r2')=NPP
2 = LCC p5 (A0/A1)
3 = Infracartilaginous
4 = Lateral Wall Release p5/r2

© 2007 Carstens
© 2007 Walters

Figure 15–8. Four-step nasal incision sequence achieves advancement of both medial and lateral crura. I have recently modified the infracartilaginous incision, making it discontinuous along the lateral crus to minimize contracture. *Nasal tip is reconstructed by simultaneous elevation of both the medial and lateral crura.* The Delaire sutures are shown. #1 is placed in the levator insertion into the SOO one finger-breadth lateral to the alar base. This centralizes the lip–cheek flap. The noncleft side is done first to the anterior nasal spine (a drill hole is helpful). #2 is placed in the nasalis and is optional (decision made at the end of the case). It adjusts alar base position and nostril sill curvature. #3 suspends the oblique head of SOO from the columellar base. It establishes the "aesthetic drape" of the lip.

separates orbicularis from the nasalis. From point 9, a second, *more internal,* incision defines the triangular flap C'. The base width of C' can be deduced by measuring the dimensions on the noncleft side.

From the lip, a lateral vermilion flap (L) is pared off and dissected down to the alveolar cleft margin. Proper paring of L includes a small strip of lip skin 2–3 mm wide because it is "rolled-in," with an abnormal relationship to the underlying muscle. If the surgeon does not do this, the skin will pucker inward at the final closure. The L flap is the most optional tissue of the entire DFR operation. It is best brought medially and interposed between the nasal vestibular lining and the B flap. It can also be used as a free graft to the lateral nasal wall. *No tissue is sacrificed in DFR.*

With its vermilion stripped off, the lateral lip margin is now entered and the orbicularis is split into its deep (constrictor) and superficial (dilator) components. The DOO is shaped like the letter J and separated from the SOO by a layer of fat. The caudal margin of the two muscles defines the white roll and contains the labial artery.[49]

Step 2. Medial Dissection: the NPP-Lateral Columellar Advancement Flap

The medial margin of the cleft (zone B in our diagram) consists of prolabial tissue lateral to the true philtrum. This is in continuity with lateral columellar skin and the medial crus of the alar cartilage. Conveniently, the blood supply of these two units is a watershed-permitting dissection of a very long flap. The B flap has two parts: (1) a skin/mucosa flap of the NPP and (2) a chondrocutaneous flap containing the lateral columellar skin and medial crus.

$$B = NPP + LCC$$

B has a rich blood supply. The NPP component is irrigated by the nasopalatine artery. The LCC component gets supply from two to three lateral branches of the ipsilateral anterior ethmoid. In addition, vessels in continuity with the lateral nasal system from the facial artery run along the surface of the alar cartilage itself. Once elevated, B is surprisingly long, reaching all the way across the cleft to the lateral nasal rim. Inset of B flap plus composite graft replace the gap created by

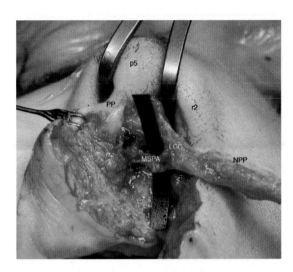

Figure 15–9. NPP–LCC flap has dual blood supply. Behind the surgical tape are (1) lateral branches from the ipsilateral anterior ethmoid artery of the columella and (2) vessels running along the dorsal surface of the lower lateral cartilage that anastomose the nasopalatine artery with the lateral nasal artery. In front of the tape, the nasopalatine (medial sphenopalatine) artery emerges from the septopremaxillary junction. This tissue, otherwise called the B flap, reconstructs the nasal floor (roof of the alveolar cleft) and the lateral nasal wall. This corresponds to the missing premaxillary field.

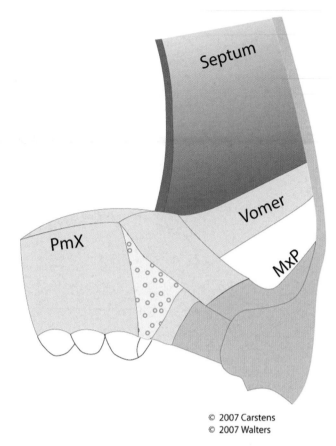

© 2007 Carstens
© 2007 Walters

Figure 15–10. "Alveolar cleft is 6-sided "box." NPP in continuity with mucoperiosteal flap from postero-lateral premaxilla is elevated in direct continuity with vomer flap. Septum is reduced from below. Palatal shelf nasal mucoperiosteum (MxP) is accessed when alar cartilage freed from piriform. Roof (nasal floor) = NPP-Pmx-V flap + MxP flap. Front = M flap + buccal sulcus advancement flap. Sides = alveolar walls. Back and floor = palatal mucoperiosteum elevated at time of alveolar extension palatoplasty. Cleft site "box" filled with osteoinductive rhBMP-2 or osteoconductive graft reconstructs missing premaxillary Lego® piece.

advancement of the p5 lateral vestibular lining (and the lateral crus). This achieves two important surgical goals: (1) cephalic advancement of the medial crus with increased tip projection and (2) soft tissue augmentation of the lateral nasal wall. Inset of B permits release of the tethered lateral vestibular lining. Repositioning the lateral crus now occurs in what would otherwise be a Y–V pattern *without the Y–V closure.* Natural alar cartilage anatomy is accomplished without pinching together an already-deficient lining.

The future cleft-sided philtral column is determined by understanding the embryology of the prolabium. The true philtrum lies between points 2 and 3 and consists of two fields (each supplied by a separate branch of the anterior ethmoid artery). The philtral dermis comes from p5 PNC and is innervated by V1. *The width of the philtrum is roughly equal to that of the columella,* generally measuring 6–10 mm. Because the philtrum develops on top of the r2′ PMx, it receives additional blood supply from the terminal branches of the SPA emerging at the level of the septopremaxillary junction. Thus, *the philtrum has a dual blood supply.* All remaining prolabial skin and mucosa (the NPP) is an r2′ derivative, supplied by the nasopalatine artery and innervated by V2. The prolabium of a bilateral cleft thus consists of four developmental units based on embryology, blood supply, and innervation: two central philtral A fields and two lateral B fields.

The embryology of the columella is as follows: The anterior centrally-located skin comes from p5 and contains the paired anterior ethmoid arteries. On either side of that central swatch, the columellar skin extends backward toward the septum. Just beneath the lateral columellar pillars, lay the medial crura of the lower lateral cartilages (LLC). Because

these pillars serve as the biologic "template" for the cartilage to form, dissection of skin away from the crura is extremely difficult. The LLCs are thus p5 neural crest derivatives. The upper lateral cartilages lie above the p6 vestibular lining and are therefore of p6 neural crest origin.

Correction of the cleft lip nose requires releasing the alar cartilage from two points of entrapment.[51] The deficiency state of the PMx causes a mechanical deformation of perfectly normal p5 skin on both sides of the nasal introitus. In the lateral nasal wall, the r2′ skin overlying the PMxF is reduced or absent. Consequently, p5 skin containing the lateral crus of the alar cartilage is dragged down into this "sinkhole" located just in front of the IT. The lateral crus is therefore flattened. On the medial side, the deficiency of the r2′ PmxB creates a "sinkhole" into which the p5 lateral columellar skin is displaced. This displaces the medial crus of the alar cartilage downward and inward compared with the noncleft side.

The LCC–NPP flap is elevated as follows: Under tension, the NPP skin is elevated in continuity with the lateral

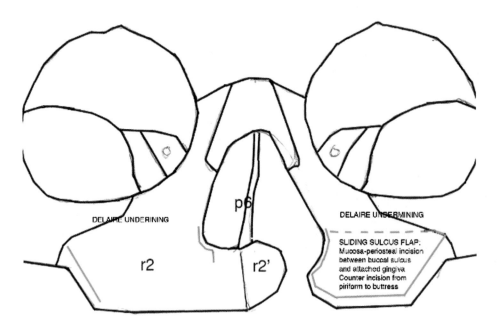

Figure 15–11. Anterior closure of unilateral alveolar cleft using sliding sulcus subperiosteal flaps. On the cleft side two incisions are required. (1) A medial-to-lateral L-shaped *releasing incision* (red line) is placed in the buccal sulcus. It runs from the cleft lateral to the buttress. There, it ascends vertically to the zygomatico–maxillary junction. The subperiosteal flap, elevated widely to the infraorbital foramen, is stiff, being tethered to the orbital rim. (2) A *counter incision* (green line) is made in periosteum alone ***from its undersurface*** begins at the level of the nasal floor and runs transversely from piriform rim to buttress. This releases the lower (alveolar) mucoperiosteal flap. It freely translates two tooth units medially. This closes the anterior wall of the alveolar cleft.

columellar wall. From point 3 the incision is carried postero-laterally over the "shoulder" of premaxilla. Gentle elevation of tissues using a dental amalgam packer avoids the tooth bud. The incision is carried backward into the mouth to elevate an in-continity vomer flap. The septum is reduced from below.

The NPP-LCC + lateral PMx + vomer flap (PMx-V) is very large. When sutured to nasal palatal mucoperiosteum, the floor defect is hermetically sealed.

Scar contracture has not been observed along the columella to date, most likely due to the structural support of the

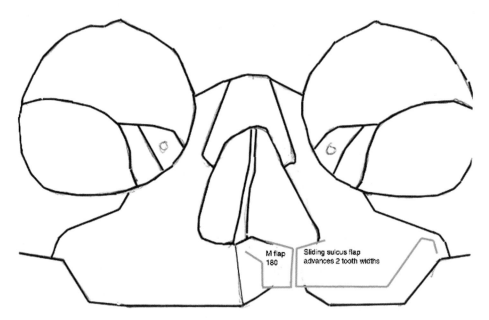

Figure 15–12. Bilateral sliding sulcus flaps. I no longer do gingival releasing incisions except in secondary grafting cases. Furthermore, a one-sided release is sufficient. On the noncleft side, wide subperiosteal mobilization is combined with a full-thickness vertical releasing incision up the buttress. This creates a huge, mobile bipedicle flap. The entire soft tissue complex becomes centralized without tension. *Nota bene*: Surgeons working under extreme condition (very wide clefts in remote areas with no access to orthodontic management) bilateral sliding sulcus flaps are very effective. They will close any size defect.

underlying alar cartilage. The NPP-LCC incision ascends into the nose. At the level of the intermediate crus, it transitions beneath the soft triangle into a standard infracartilagenous incision and is then continued all the way to the piriform margin. It then doubles back as a partial intercartilagenous incision to provide V-Y advancement of the lateral crus. The resulting soft tissue deficit in the lateral nasal wall corresponds to PMxF. A composite graft from the cymba replaces the defect with uncanny accuracy.

The anterior incision of the NPP-LCC flap is not sufficient to advance the medial crus upward. Current use of the combined NPP-LCC-PMx-V flap is very effective, providing simultaneously corrects the medial crus and reduces the septum. In previous publications I described a required second parallel incision to accomplish medial crus elevation. This still has clinical utility in those secondary cases in which one wants to avoid opening the lip. The counter-incison starts in the membranous septum about halfway up. It is then carried downward to the V and then redirected forward to meet the lateral margin of the B flap. Note that the membranous septal incision provides *immediate exposure of the cartilaginous septum.*

The NPP–LCC flap now resembles a long boot, shaped like Italy. The "toe" of the boot extends along the prolabial margin. Beneath the "heel" of the boot lies the footplate of the alar cartilage. This landmark corresponds to point 12. Grasping the heel of B provides instant access to the medial aspect of the medial crus. This is a safe plane permitting dissection of the alar cartilage right into the nasal tip, with the following caveat. The B flap gets blood supply from the nasopalatine artery via —two to three branches emerging at the junction of the PMx and V. Gentle spreading along the medial border of the cartilage will reveal these branches and preserve them. Additional blood supply descends along the skin. Formerly, I would elevate these NPP–LCC flaps completely, never having an issue with ischemia; however, it seems prudent to preserve the nasopalatine branches when possible. In addition, this type of blunt dissection is more than sufficient to advance the nasal tip.

The septum is now dissected out and freed from the maxillary crest until it sits passively in the midline. As growth proceeds, the centralized septum will no longer constitute an abnormal force vector tethering the nasal tip.

Step 3. Nasal Dissection: "Open–Closed" Rhinoplasty

At this juncture, a standard infracartilaginous incision is made. This incision is brought all the way to the piriform rim, following the natural fold between the nasal skin and the vestibular skin. The caudal extent of this incision terminates at the internal border of the triangular nostril sill flap B′. The exposure gained via the lateral columella-infracartilaginous incision allows a complete dissection of the dorsal nasal skin envelope as described by McComb.[52] The success of the McComb dissection is really an embryonic field separation. The deep layer comprises the p6 vestibular epithelium and p6 neural crest upper lateral cartilages, the blood supply to which comes from below via the internal carotid artery (ICA). The

superficial layer is p5 nasal skin and the lower lateral nasal cartilages, the blood supply to which is also of ICA derivation. Interposed between these two layers, like a sandwich, is the superficial musculoaponeurotic system (SMAS) layer of facial muscles derived from the second pharyngeal arch. The myoblasts come from somitomere 6. The nasal muscles are compartmentalized by r4 neural crest fascia (the SMAS). The blood supply to this intermediate second arch layer is from the facial artery, a terminal branch of the external carotid artery (ECA). This mesenchyme provides an additional source of blood supply to the alar cartilages. Careful dissection of the lateral columellar walls from the columella discloses vessels running along the medial surface of the medial crura. These anastomose the lateral nasal vessels with the nasopalatine vessels.

Along the lateral nasal rim, the dissection is carried right down to the piriform margin. The proper plane for separation is achieved by hugging the surface of the cartilage. The overlying r4 SMAS layer and the p5 skin layer are left in anatomic continuity. Very little bleeding is occasioned by this approach. As one reaches the piriform rim, the periosteum is incised and stripped vertically. Subperiosteal elevation of the soft tissues lateral to the piriform rim preserves the facial artery arcade. The nasal skin envelope is then liberated cephalically all the way to the nasal bones.

Despite these maneuvers, the vestibular lining is still tight! The medial crus has been completely released and advanced into the nasal tip but the lateral crus remains splayed out and tethered. Releasing the lateral crus from the vestibular lining has been advocated in the past. This is technically difficult because it violates the embryology (recall that the alar cartilage arises as a neural crest response to a pattern embedded in the vestibular epithelium). The size and shape of the cleft-side alar cartilage has been demonstrated to be normal compared with the noncleft side.[53] Consequently, the p5 vestibular lining "program" must be normal as well. Studies at UNC demonstrate that the overall surface area of the repaired cleft nostril is reduced by 30%.[54] The site of the deficit corresponds to the soft tissues of PMxF. Thus, distortion of the lateral crus is strictly due to deficiency of the PMxF, *the soft tissues of which are located in the prolabium, i.e., the NPP flap!*

Release of the vestibular lining alone leaves behind a soft tissue defect that is roughly equal in size and shape to the missing embryonic tissue, that is, equal to the NPP flap. The release should, therefore, encompass the lateral crus, permitting it to be repositioned medially without tension. To accomplish this, a vertically-oriented Y–V flap is made. The caudal tip of the flap is located just in front of the IT; the base encompasses the lateral crus. When released, the resulting defect will be filled in with NPP.

Exit the turbinate flap!

As the DFR evolved, I employed various solutions to patch the defect created by the vestibular release. One of these solutions made use of an anteriorly-based IT flap as described by Noordhoff.[55,56] Although this tissue worked adequately, I had several reservations about it: (1) The dissection is

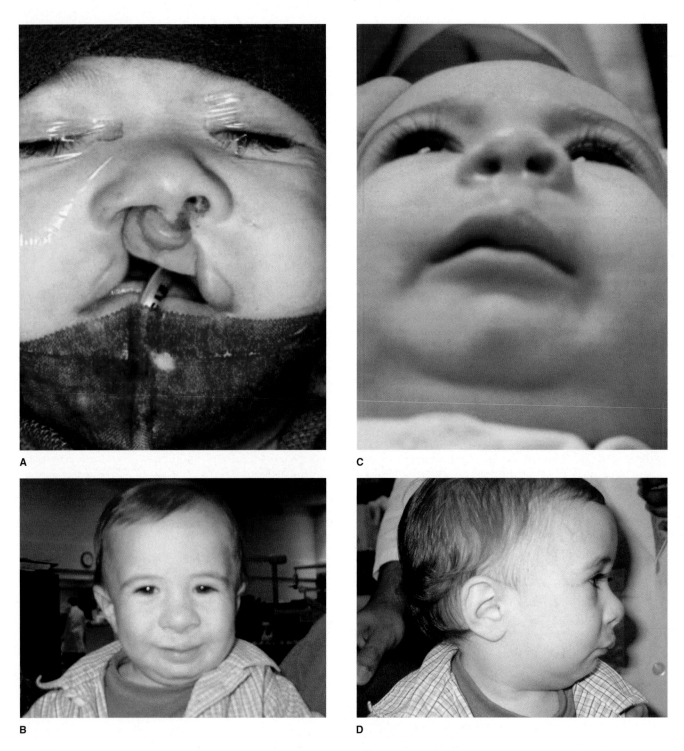

A

B

C

D

Figure 15–13. (Case 1): (a) Preoperative bilateral cleft lip with right unilateral cleft of primary palate and bilateral clefts of secondary palate, (b–e) Soft tissue relationships 1 year after DFR demonstrating stability of nasal tip projection. Comparison of CT scans at 3 months (f–h) and 9 months show bony union of primary palate (i–j). Periapical view of alveolar cleft site (k) shows reconstitution of the periodontal ligament, a neural crest structure. This is not seen with conventional iliac crest graft. Serial 3D skulls (L) taken 9 months apart support the Delaire dissection concept: wide subperiosteal undermining repositions the osteogenic soft tissue fields into a correct, centralized relationship. *Subsequent osteosynthesis of membranous bone now occurs in a correct centric distribution*. Developmental field reassignment promotes normal membranous bone formation *after* the surgical procedure.

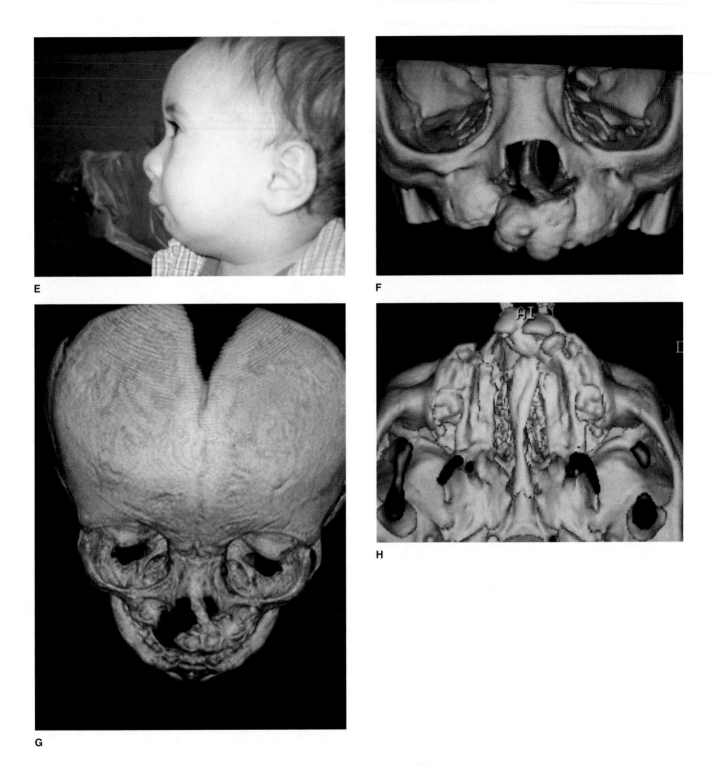

Figure 15–13. (*Continued*)

subtle and difficult to teach; (2) The tissue type is distinct and not native to the nasal rim; (3) Healing of the donor site can be accompanied by crusting and bleeding, and (4) It did not make embryologic sense. Proper dissection and inset of flap NPP, combined with use of a composite FTSG, made the turbinate flap unnecessary. The key to getting the most out of NPP is to include the prolabial vermilion with the skin.

Step 4. Intraoral Dissection: Sliding Sulcus S Flap

The rationale and design of the sliding sulcus mucoperiosteal flap stem directly from pioneering work at the University of Pittsburgh by Sotereanos.[45] This technique involves a gingival release on the cleft side carried out from the alveolar cleft to the buttress.[44] This permits wide subperiosteal dissection over the entire face of the Mx below the infraorbital foramen as described by Delaire.[57,58] A 45° backcut up the buttress is

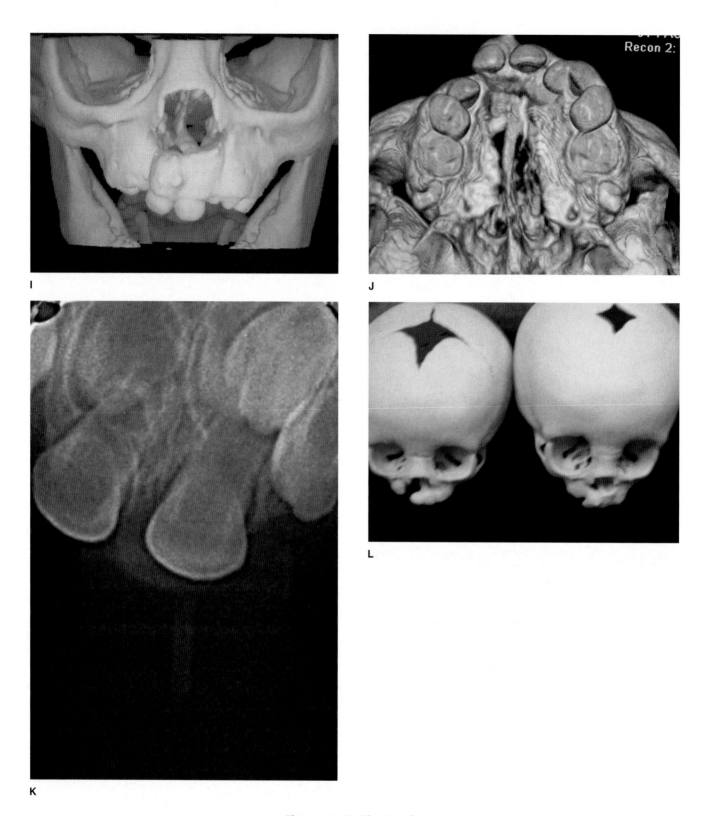

Figure 15–13. (*Continued*).

made. The attached gingival is released. The flap is covered on its undersurface by a sheet of periosteum, rendering it rather stiff. The *Sotereanos maneuver* is a mobilization of the S flap using a counterincision in the periosteal sheet itself parallel to the gum line. The counterincision, located halfway from the gingival margin to the infraorbital foramen, is made by just scoring through periosteum. It extends from the piriform margin straight lateral to the buttress. At this point, it joins up with the previous backcut. These two incisions make a right angle: the periosteal counterincision is transverse across the Mx and the buttress incision is vertical. The combination of these two incisions releases the lower mucoperiosteal S flap from the upper mucoperiosteum attached to the orbit. When the S flap is released, it advances mesially about two tooth units. The S flap advances tooth units; it extends across the alveolar cleft without tension. Like a sliding door, it seals up the anterior aspect of the cleft.

In primary cases I no longer use a gingival releasing incison. A bilateral Delaire-type superiosteal dissection is done. On the cleft side, a buccal sulcus incision is used. On the noncleft side, a piriform access incision (combined with buttress release) generates a bipedicle flap. This permits centralization of the lateralized stem cell-bearing soft tissue envelope. Note, that when cleft lip occurs without an alveolar cleft, bilateral S flaps, elevated *without gingival release,* permit proper tension-free centralization of midface soft tissues.

Step 5. Dissection of the Primary Palate

Release of the lateral crus gives direct access to the piriform rim. Just inside it lies the inferior turbinate. Proceeding beneath it straight backward gives a fast, nearly effortless release of palatal shelf mucoperiosteum. This is sutured to the previously-dissected PMx-V flap using Dingman. I close the nasal floor as far back as the vomer flap permits. Anerior closure of the alveolar cleft is achieved using a combination of two flaps. The large M flap, based on the premaxilla, is rotated 180 degrees. It is sutured to itself and to the mucoperiosteal margin of the S flap.

This technique departs from that used for the cases illustrated. Although these primary palate reconstructions are striking, the geometry of the previous technique was difficult to teach and tedious. Over the past year, DFR has been

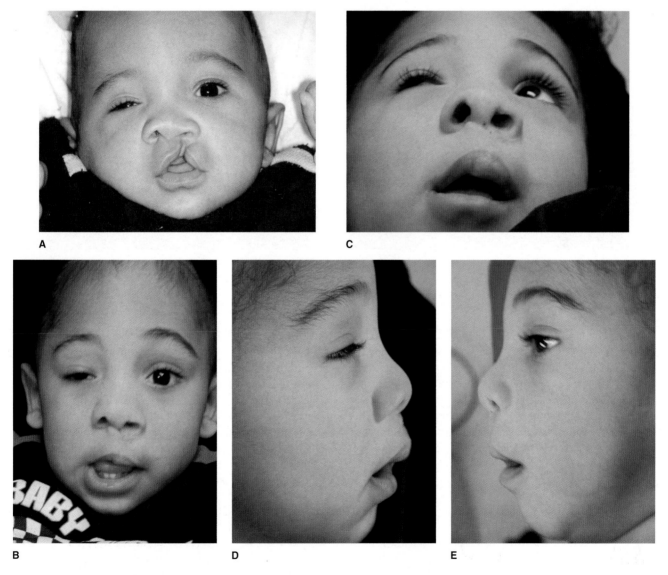

A **B** **C** **D** **E**

Figure 15–14. (Case 2): (a) Preoperative unilateral cleft lip and palate, (b–e) postoperative at 1 year, (f–g) preoperative CT scans, and (h–i) postoperative CT scans of piriform fossa in this challenging cleft demonstrate leveling out of the nasal floor to support the alar base. Consolidation of the alveolar cleft during primary DFR surgery maintains dimensions of the dental arch without collapse even after palatoplasty. Note symmetry of columellar–alar relationships seen in lateral views.

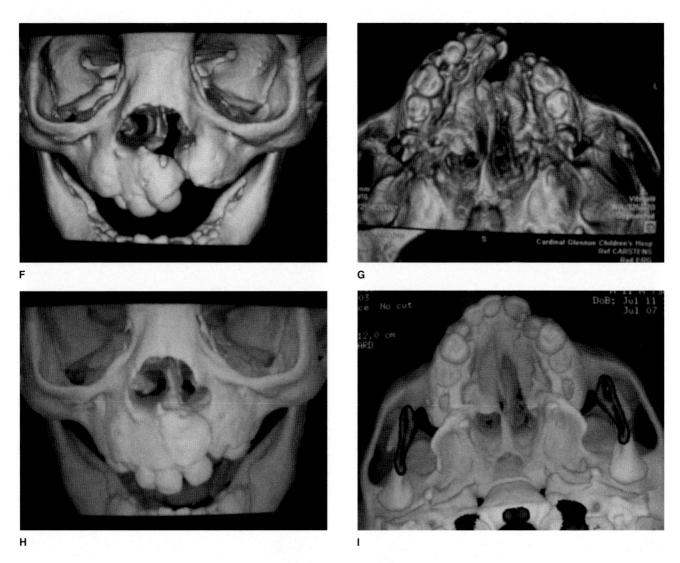

Figure 15–14. (*Continued*).

simplified by 4 factors: the extended M flap, low buccal sulcus release, the LCC-NPP-PMx-V flap, composite graft for the lateral nasal wall, and alveolar extension palatoplasty technique.8 AEP (at 18 months) generates extra-length flaps for secure closure of the cleft "floor." The up-sides of alveolar grafting at palatoplasty are: (1) straightforward design of AEP; and (2) large volume available for grafting. The resulting box is rich in neural crest stem cells. A down-side of this protocol is longer dental arch splinting."

Closure Sequence

Step 1. Elevation of the Nasal Tip

The tip is positioned anatomically using the Cronin nasal retractor (Padgett Instruments). The medial crura are battened together with 5-0 PDS. Suture suspension and modification of the alar cartilage can be readily executed by means of the open–closed approach as per the surgeon's preference. The author approach is predicated on the establishment of normal field relationships. Wide dissection of the nasal soft

tissues combined with release from their "piriform prison" allows all fields to be passively held in position by a nasal stent inserted at the conclusion of the procedure. The author finds the Koken-type silicon stents (Porex Corp., Newman, Georgia) easy-to-use. The stent is placed at the end of the surgery. Closure of the nostril incision starts at the intermediate crus working medially down to the Reinisch flap. One then proceeds laterally to the margin of the lateral nasal wall. This involves placing—two to three sutures over 5 mm. The remainder of the lateral nasal incision will be filled by inset of the B flap. Reconstruction of the (PMxF) adds the missing tissue to the lateral nasal wall (see below). This frequently involves placement of a composite full-thickness graft into the defect. The medial crural complex is then elevated with respect to the septum with 4–0 Vicryl. This also closes the membranous septum counterincision.

Step 2. Soft Tissue Reconstruction of the PMx

The roof of the missing premaxillary field is reconstructed based on meticulous closure of the nasal floor. This is carried out using a mouth gag, starting anteriorly at the incisive fora-men. Because the space is tight using 4-0 Vicryl® on a small P-2 needle is helpful. The medial vomerine and lateral nasal mucoperiosteal flaps are closed all the way posterior to the end of the V flap. This provides correct orientation for inset of the B flap. The *posterior* margin of B is sutured from medial to lateral along the newly-united nostril floor. The tip of B is eventually inset into the donor site of the lateral crural ad-vancement flap. Next, the alar nasal skin flap C is sutured to

the *anterior* margin of B. The surface area of the lateral nasal wall is now restored.

The floor of the missing premaxillary field is recon-structed when the medial and lateral mucoperiosteal flaps harvested from the walls of the alveolar cleft are turned down into the mouth using 4-0 Vicryl. The cleft side sliding sulcus flap S is advanced and secured using 4-0 Vicryl PS-2 around the dental units. Three or four such sutures will suffice. Op-tional suspension of the sulcus to maintain height can be done

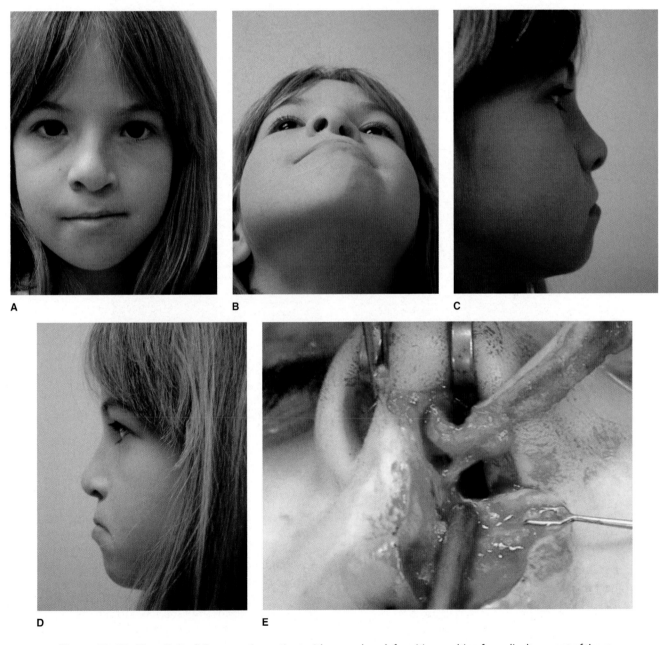

Figure 15–15. (Case 3): (a–d) Preoperative patient with secondary deformities resulting from displacement of tissue from the midline, (e) Vissiarnarov flap harvested from scar simulates non-philtral prolabium and fills lateral piriform defect created by advancement of the lateral crus. Note large pedicle from the external carotid-based nasopalatine artery. These flaps can be harvested in virtually all secondary cleft reconstructions, (f–i) postoperative illustrations demonstrating the corrections made with subperiosteal centralization. Note changes in the non-cleft alar base after DFR. Residual sag in left alar contour will need cartilage batten graft in the future. The straight-line scar in DFR repair simulates philtral column, (j–k) preoperative CT scans, and (l–m) postoperative CT scans.

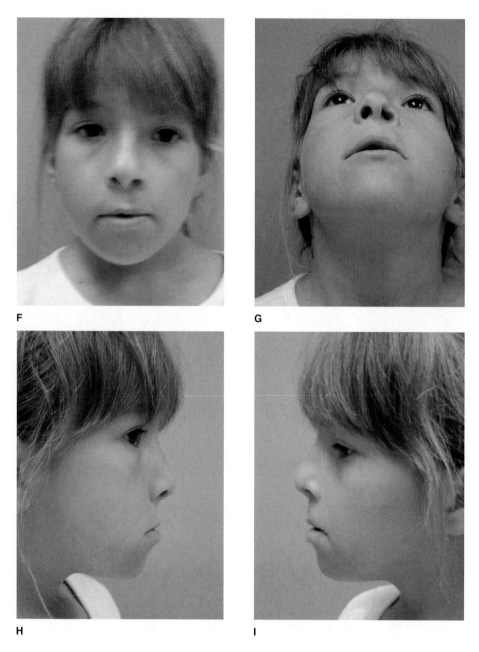

Figure 15–15. (*Continued*)

by passing a 3-0 Vicryl up to the nasal floor and then back down into the sulcus as a mattress suture.

Step 3. Osseous Reconstruction of the (PMx): ISO

The primary palate is reconstructed with Infuse® bone graft (Memphis, Tennessee Sofamor-Danek). The implant is prepared by soaking a Helistat® activated collagen sponge (ACS) (Plainsfield, N.J. Integra Life Sciences) of preselected size with reconstituted rhBMP-2 applied uniformly over the ACS. The minimum time required for protein binding is 15 minutes; however, I usually wait 30 minutes. The Infuse comes in three kit sizes: 4.2 cc, 5.6 cc, and 8.4 cc. These are used as follows: primary unilateral (small), primary bilateral (medium), secondary unilateral (medium), and secondary

bilateral (large). *The volume of the implant should match that of the defect.* "Bulking up" the implantation site is desirable but the ideal agent does not yet exist. In the past, I used tricalcium phosphate but found it persisted. Demineralized bone is a better alternative. The bulking agent can be mixed with diced-up ACS collagen sponge or wrapped within the sponge like a fajita or sushi roll and implanted. I like to place a vertical component into the alveolar walls and a horizontal component below the nasal floor. The pocket created by DFR dissection can be filled with iliac crest graft as well.

Step 4. Closure of the Lip: Delaire Concepts Modified

Many years ago, pioneering work by Delaire demonstrated that wide subperiosteal dissection yield significant aesthetic

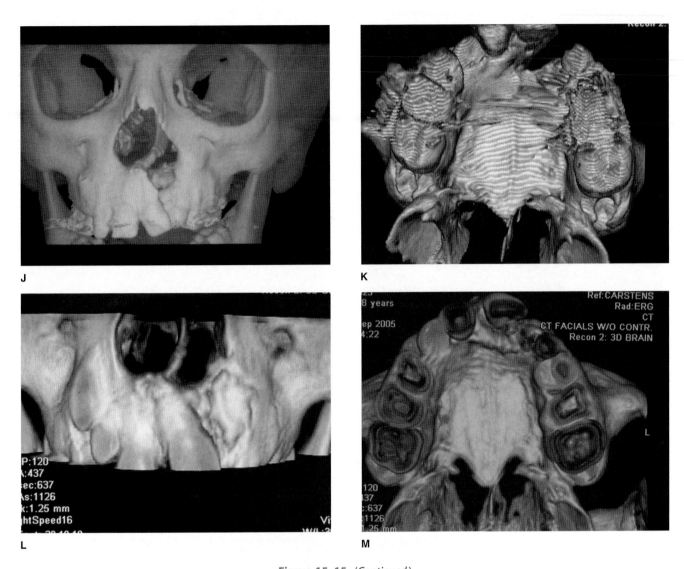

Figure 15–15. (*Continued*).

benefits of tissue draping and, at the same time, did not impair maxillary growth.[57,58] Indeed, when compared with supraperiosteal release, this approach is developmentally correct because it separates the osteogenic functional matrix (the periosteum and overlying soft tissues) from the product (the PMx and Mx).

The suture sequence is as follows:

Delaire 1: Centralization of the bilaterally displaced soft tissues is accomplished with 4-0 nylon sutures placed from below the flap to the paranasalis (levator) insertion into the SOO. This insertion does not involve the alar base. It is generally located one fingerbreadth lateral to the alar base. The noncleft side is sutured first to below the anterior nasal spine. This suture serves as a reference point for a similar suture from the cleft side.

Suspension of the DOO: This suture sets the depth of the sulcus on the cleft side. At the most cephalic margin, the DOO is suspended from the septum with a 4-0 PDS.

Delaire 2: The purpose of this suture is to control the height and curvature of the cleft side nostril. This is accom-

plished by connection of the nasalis to the anterior nasal spine. However, this step is *optional* at this point. If performed, care should be taken to not overtighten this and inadvertently narrow the nostril. When the remaining sutures are placed, a decision can be made if a Delaire 2 is warranted. I usually decide upon a Delaire 2 at the end of the case to accentuate curvature.

Orbicularis closure: Three or four sutures of 4-0 PDS are required for the DOO layer. The SOO layer is closed with 5-0 PDS making sure the loop is at the level of the dermal–epidermal junction.

Delaire 3: The oblique head of SOO sets the aesthetic drape of the lip. The 5-0 PDS is obliquely passed upward from the cephalic edge through the base of the columella and then back down to the SOO as a mattress suture.

Step 5. Final Adjustments: Finessing the Nostril Floor

After closure of the lip, the alar base C is at time compressed medially by the movement of the neighboring D flap (lateral lip element). If so, the alar base must be translocated laterally.

This can be accomplished by excision of a crescent of skin from the lateral lip element. C is then elevated and secured to the lateral lip via a buried 5-0 PDS suture. At times, it is necessary to elevate the ala completely in order to obtain sufficient lateralization. The tip of the nostril sill flap C′ is now sutured just posterior to the columellar shoulder. Continuity between the columellar shoulder and the nostril sill is now reestablished. Perialar suturing with inverted 5-0 PDS sutures restores the alar crease very nicely.

A final caveat concerns the lining of the lateral nasal defect. Experience with this technique shows that prevention of postoperative contraction is paramount. This requires placement of a Porex® silicon conformer sized to the patient. The stent should be sutured in place with 4-0 nylon for 4 weeks. It is important that the B flap not be sutured to the sidewall of C with any tension. If tension exists, I have found it prudent to use a small pinch graft of retroauricular skin (Figs. 15–13 to 15–16).

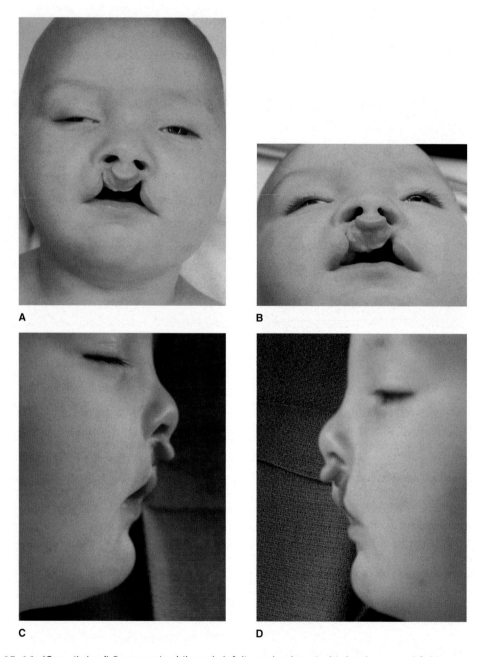

Figure 15–16. (Case 4): (a–d) Preoperative bilateral cleft lip and palate, (e–h) developmental field reassignment of soft tissue fields in bilateral lip/palate cleft repair demonstrates normalization of Cupid's bow. Contrary to current dogma, the philtrum and columella are *not* short in the cleft condition; they are *mismatched*. By recognizing and reconstructing the missing premaxillary field, DFR corrects deficiency-induced field mismatch, (i–j) preoperative CT scans, and (k–l) postoperative CT scans.

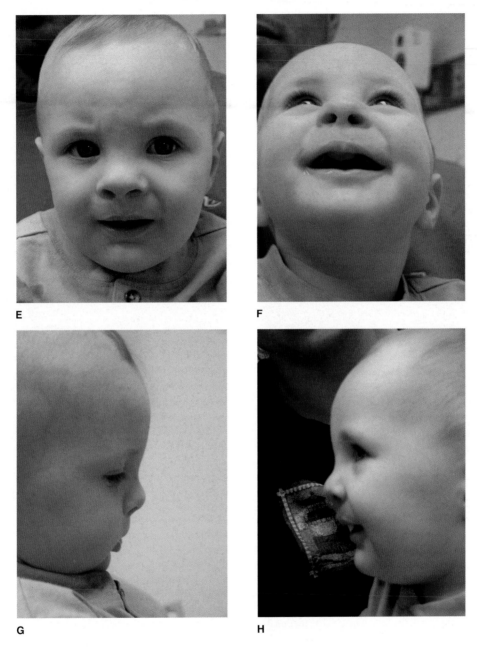

E

F

G

H

Figure 15–16. (*Continued*)

DISCUSSION

Whenever a surgical procedure for a congenital condition in a growing child leads to a predictable pattern of relapse over time, two inescapable conclusions must be drawn: (1) the *biologic rationale of the procedure is incorrect* and (2) the anatomic pattern of relapse *points an accusatory finger at the pathology.* DFR surgery represents a new form of thinking about clefts by identification and rearrangement of specific developmental fields. The primary pathology of cleft lip is hypoplasia or absence of the distal PMx. DFR is designed to reconstruct the missing PMx using osteoinductive technologies for stem cell concentration and differentiation such as rhBMP-2 or by conventional osteoconductive technique (bone grafting).

DFR incisions are made on the basis of vascular supply and embryology, not geometric manipulation. For this reason, the design of DFR presents a series of specific solutions that speak to problems in cleft surgery hitherto inadequately addressed: distortion of the nasal envelope and septum, displacement of soft tissues away from the midline, the entrapped position of the medial crus, and the "hidden" nostril sill. DFR treats mechanisms, not appearance.

The extraoral design of DFR is invariable; it is the same for both unilateral and bilateral clefts. Developmental fields are recognized, separated, and rearranged into correct anatomic relationships. The intraoral design varies with cleft type. If no alveolar cleft is present, subperiosteal release and zygomaticomaxillary buttress backcut are sufficient to achieve

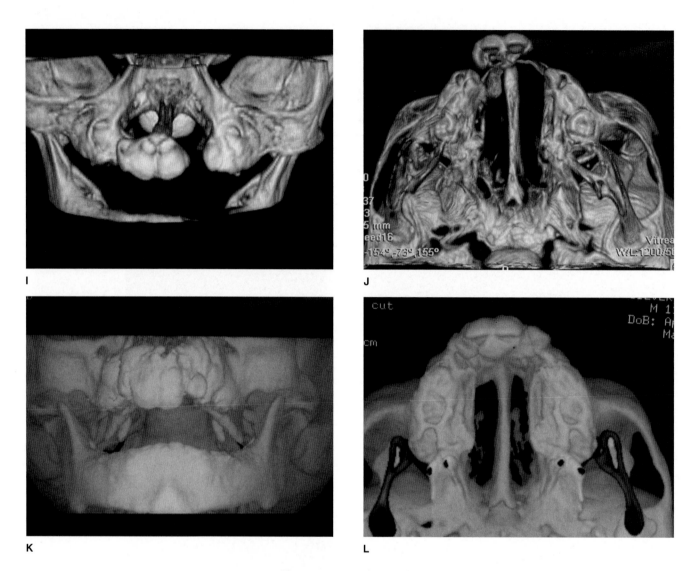

Figure 15–16. (*Continued*).

centralization of the soft tissue envelope. Gingival release is not necessary. If a primary palate cleft exists, a complete sliding sulcus dissection with gingival release will allow for mesial translocation and coverage of the alveolar cleft.

DFR includes a straight-line repair, resulting in an anatomically correct philtral column. The distorted and seemingly foreshortened philtrum in clefts is familiar to all plastic surgeons. For many years, the rotation-advancement technique has been used to reorient the philtrum. So why is philtral rotation not required in DFR? The appearance of the philtrum in clefts stems from the overall malposition of the soft tissue in a falsely lateralized state. Thus, the philtrum and columella appear to be short, but are actually displaced into the nasal tip. DFR achieves derotation of the philtrum and columella by the following: (1) field separation and (2) subperiosteal mobilization. The entire soft tissue complex in a unilateral cleft is laterally displaced "around the corner" of the PMx. When mobilized correctly off the bone, it is brought forward around the curve of the bone and dropped right into place.

The membranous bones of the Mx and PMx are just a product of the soft tissue functional matrix that surrounds them. As the soft tissue grows, new bone is deposited and old bone resorbed according to the mechanical forces placed on the bone. The purpose of subperiosteal centralization in DFR is to change the biologic relationship of the bone product to the functional matrix. Over the time, the former will adapt to the latter in its new, centralized position. Appreciation of the subperiosteal plane as the correct approach to surgically separate the functional matrix from its product (bone) ensures tension-free release and accuracy of muscle repair (individual muscle units can be identified by tugging on them from below). Thirty years of work by Delaire and others confirm the clinical accuracy and safety of this approach.

The concepts and techniques of DFR are applicable to all forms of clefts. Because it separates out osseous pathology from soft tissue pathology, DFR is a true "cut as you go" technique. In secondary cleft surgery, DFR is capable of rescuing previously violated fields and reuniting them into their correct functional relationships. Sliding sulcus flaps function as elastic flaps as defined by Goldstein[59,60] and can readily be brought into the midline. *Abbe flaps are virtually unnecessary,* even in salvage cases involving total loss of the philtrum.

DFR is a practical application of developmental anatomy. It provides a means to analyze membranous bone formation and periosteal physiology. It embodies concepts of facial growth central to orthodontics. It makes use of neuromeric theory to map out and manipulate developmental fields. Proper implementation and study of cleft repair using DFR will provide a forum for dialog along craniofacial surgeons, orthodontists, and developmental biologists.

References

1. Veau V, Recamier J. *Bec-de Lievre: Formes Cliniques-Chirugie.* Paris: Masson et Cie, 1938.
2. His W. Unsere Korperform und das physiologische Problem irhrer Enstehung: Briefe. Leipzig, Germany: *FCW Vogel*, 1874, pp. 204–205.
3. Carstens MH. Development of the facial midline. *J Craniofac Surg* 13:129–187, 2002.
4. Carstens MH. Neural tube programming and craniofacial cleft formation. I. The neuromeric organization of the head and neck. *Eur J Paed Neurol* 8:181–210, 2004.
5. Puelles L, Rubenstein JLR. Development of the central nervous system. In Rossant J, Tam PPL (eds). *Mouse Development: Patterning, Morphogenesis, and Organogenesis.* San Diego: Academic Press, 2002, pp. 37–54.
6. Puelles L, Rubenstein JLR. Forebrain gene expression domains and the evolving prosomeric model. *Trends Neurosci* 26:469–476, 2003.
7. Rubenstein JLR, Puelles L. Development of the nervous system. In Epstein CJ, Erickson RP, Wynshaw-Boris A (eds). *Inborn Errors of Metabolism: The Molecular Basis of Clinical Disorders of Morphogenesis.* Oxford, England: Oxford University Press, 2004, pp. 75–88.
8. Carstens MH. Sequential cleft management with the sliding sulcus technique and alveolar extension palatoplasty. *J Craniofac Surg* 10(6):503–518, 1999.
9. Carstens MH. Function matrix cleft repair: Principles and techniques. *Clin Plast Surg* 31:159–189, 2004.
10. Lemire RJ, Cohen M, Beckwith JB, Kokich VG, Siebert JR. The facial features of holoprosencephaly in anencephalic human specimens. I. Historical review and associated malformations. *Teratology* 23:297–303, 1981.
11. Siebert JR, Kokich VG, Cohen MM, Lemire RJ. The facial features of holoprosencephaly in anencephalic human fetuses. II. Craniofacial anatomy. *Teratology* 23:305–315, 1981.
12. Liem KF, et al. Dorsal differentiation of neural plate cells induced by BMP-mediated signals from epidermal ectoderm. *Cell* 82:969–979, 1995.
13. Liem KF, Bemis WE, Walker WF, Grande L. *Functional Anatomy of the Vertebrates: An Evolutionary Perspective,* 4th edn. Belmont, CA: Thompson, 2006.
14. Carroll RL. *Vertebrate Paleontology and Evolution.* New York: W.H. Freeman, 1988, pp. 360–400.
15. Barteczko K, Jacob M. A re-evaluation of the premaxillary bone in humans. *Anat Embryol (Berlin)* 207:417–437, 2004.
16. Mooney MP, Siegel IP, Kimes KR, Todhunter J. Premaxillary development in normal and cleft lip and palate human fetuses using three dimensional computed tomography. *Cleft Lip Palate J* 28:49–54, 1991.
17. Carstens, MH. The spectrum of minimal clefting: Process-oriented cleft management in the presence of an intact alveolus. *J Craniofac Surg* 11:270–294, 2000.
18. Gong SG, Guo C. *BMP4* gene is expressed at the putative site of fusion in the midfacial region. *Differentiation* 71:228–236, 2003.
19. Ashique AM, Fu K, Richman JM. Endogenous bone morphogenetic proteins regulate outgrowth and epithelial survival during avian lip fusion. *Development* 129:4647–4660, 2002.
20. Lumsden A, Krumflauf R. Patterning the vertebrate neuraxis. *Science* 274:15, 1996.
21. Noden DM. Patterning of avian craniofacial muscles. *Dev Biol* 116: 347–356, 1986.
22. Noden DM. Vertebrate craniofacial development: the relation between ontogenetic process and morphological outcome. *Brain Behav Evol* 38:1990–225, 1991.
23. Noden DM. Origins and patterns of craniofacial mesenchymal tissues. *J Craniofac Genet Dev Biol* 11:192–213, 1991.
24. Noden DM, Trainor PA. Relations and interactions between cranial mesoderm and neural crest populations. *J Anat* 207:575–601, 2005.
25. Helms JA, Cordero D, Tapadia MD. New insights into craniofacial morphogenesis. *Development* 2005;132:851–861, 2005.
26. Carlson BR. *Human Embryology and Developmental Biology,* 3rd edn. Mosby St. Louis, MO, 2004.
27. Vissarionov VA. Analysis of the results of reconstructive plastic surgery of unilateral clefts of the upper lip based on data of the surgical section 1970–1977. In *Pathogenesis, Treatment, and Prophylaxis of Cosmetic Deformities and Deficiencies.* Moscow: Institute of Cosmetology, 1982, pp. 118–121.
28. Vissarionov VA. Correction of the nasal tip deformity following unilateral repair of clefts of the upper lip. *Plast Reconst Surg* 83:341, 1989.
29. Zhang Z, Song Y, Zhao X, Zhang X, Fermin C, ChenY. Rescue of cleft palate in Msx-1 deficient mice by transgenic *Bmp4* reveals a network of BMP and Shh signaling in the regulation of mammalian palatogenesis. *Development* 129:4135–4140, 2002.
30. Gilbert S. *Developmental Biology,* 8th edn. Sunderland, MA: Sinauer, 2006.
31. Wozney J. Overview of bone morphogenetic proteins. *Spine* 27 (165):52–58, 2002.
32. Ebara S, Nakayama K. Mechanisms for the action of bone morphogenetic proteins and regulation of their activity. *Spine* 27(16S):S10–S15, 2002.
33. Valentin-Opran A, Wozney J, Csiima C, Lilly L, Reidel GE. Clinical evaluation of recombinant human bone morphogenetic protein-2. *Clin Orthop Related Res* 395:110–120, 2002.
34. Boyne PJ. Animal studies of application of rhBMP-2 in maxillofacial reconstruction. *Bone* 19(Suppl 1):83S–92S, 1996.
35. Boyne PJ, Nath R, Nakamura A. Human recombinant BMP-2 in osseous reconstruction of simulated cleft palate defects. *Br J Oral Maxillofac Surg* 36:84–30, 1998.
36. Boyne PJ. A feasibility study evaluating rhBMP-2/absorbable collagen sponge for maxillary sinus floor augmentation. *Int J Periodontic Restorative Dent* 17:11–25, 1997.
37. FDA Dental Advisory Board hearing on Infuse® bone graft for maxillary sinus and alveolar extraction socket defects. Gaithersburg, MD, November 9, 2006.
38. Carstens MH, Chin M, Li J. In situ osteogenesis (ISO): Regeneration of 10-cm defect in porcine model using recombinant human bone morphogenetic protein-2 (rhBMP-2) and Helistat ® absorbable collagen sponge. *J Craniofac Surg* 16:1033–1042, 2005.
39. Chao M, Donovan T, Sotelo C, Carstens MH. In situ osteogenesis of hemimandible in a 9-year-old boy: Osteoinduction via stem cell concentration. *J Craniofac Surg* 17:405–412, 2006.
40. Ruberte J, Carretero A, Navarro M, Marcucio RS, Noden DM. Morphogenesis of blood vessels in the head muscles of avian embryos: Spatial, temporal, and VEGF expression analysis. *Dev Dynam* 227:470–483, 2003.
41. Carstens M, Chin M, Ng T, Tom WK. Reconstruction of #7 facial cleft with distraction assisted in situ osteogenesis (DISO): Role of recombinant human bone morphogenetic protein-2 with Helistat activated collagen sponge. *J Craniofac Surg* 16(6):1023–1032, 2005.
42. Chin M, Ng T, Tom WK, Carstens MH. Repair of alveolar clefts with recombinant human bone morphogenetic protein. *J Craniofac Surg* 16(5):778–789, 2005.

43. Chin M, Ng T, Tom WK, Carstens MH. *5th International Conference on Distraction Osteogenesis in Craniofacial Surgery.* Paris, France, June, 2006.

44. Carstens MH. The sliding sulcus procedure: Simultaneous repair of unilateral clefts of the lip and primary palate—a new technique. *J Craniofac Surg* 10:415–434, 1999.

45. Demas P, Sotereanos GC. Closure of alveolar clefts with Cortico-cancellous block grafts and marrow: A retrospective study. *J Oral Maxillofac Surg* 46:682, 1988.

46. Delaire J. The potential role of facial muscles in monitoring maxillary growth and morphogenesis. In Carlson DS, McNamara Jr JA (eds). *Muscle Adaptation and Craniofacial Growth,* Ann Arbor, MI: Center for Human Growth and Development, Craniofacial Growth Monograph No. 8, University of Michigan, 1978, pp. 157–180.

47. Markus AF, Delaire J, Smith WP. Facial balance in cleft lip and palate I. Normal development and cleft palate. *Br J Oral Surg* 30:287–295, 1992.

48. Moss ML, Vilmann H, Das Gupta G, Skalak R. Craniofacial growth in space-time. In Carlson DS, McNamara Jr JA (eds). *Craniofacial Biology.* Ann Arbor, MI: Center for Human Growth and Development, University of Michigan, 1981.

49. Park GC. The importance of accurate orbicularis repair of the orbicularis oris muscle in unilateral cleft lip. *Plast Reconstr Surg* 96:780–788, 1995.

50. Carstens MH. Correction of the bilateral cleft using the sliding sulcus technique. *J Craniofac Surg* 11:136–167, 2000.

51. Carstens MH. Correction of the unilateral cleft lip nasal deformity using the sliding sulcus procedure. *J Craniofac Surg* 10:346–364, 1999.

52. McComb H. Treatment of the unilateral cleft lip nose. *Plast Reconstr Surg* 55:596, 1975.

53. Stenstrom SJ. The nasal deformity in unilateral cleft lip: Some notes on its anatomic bases and secondary treatment. *Plast Reconstr Surg* 28:295–305, 1961.

54. Drake AF, Davis JU, Warren DW. Nasal airway size in cleft and non-cleft children. *Laryngoscope* 103:913–915, 1993.

55. Noordhoff MS, Chen YR, Chen KT, et al. The surgical technique for the complete unilateral cleft lip–nasal deformity. *Op Tech Plast Surg* 2:164–174, 1995.

56. Noordhoff MS. *The Surgical Technique for the Unilateral Cleft Lip-Nasal Deformity.* Taipei, Taiwan: Noordhoff Craniofacial Foundation, 1997.

57. Delaire J, Precious D, Gordeef A. The advantage of wide subperiosteal exposure in primary surgical correction of labial maxillary clefts. *Scand J Plast Recons Surg* 22:147–151, 1989.

58. Precious DA, Delaire J. Surgical considerations in patients with cleft deformities. In Bell WH (ed). *Modern Practice in Orthognathic and Reconstructive Surgery.* Philadelphia, PA: Saunders, 1992, pp. 390–425.

59. Goldstein MH. A tissue expanding vermilion myocutaneous flap for lip repair. *Plast Reconstr Surg* 73:768–770, 1984.

60. Goldstein MH. The elastic flap for lip repair. *Plast Reconstr Surg* 85:446–452, 1990.

Lip Adhesion

Richard E. Kirschner, MD • Joseph E. Losee, MD • Shao Jiang, MD

INTRODUCTION

The complete unilateral and bilateral cleft lip deformities include significant distortion not only of the lip anatomy, but of the nasal anatomy as well.[1] Restoration of skeletal, cartilaginous, and soft tissue relationships prior to definitive lip and nasal repair may offer significant benefits to overall outcome. To this end, numerous methods have been utilized, each with its own advantages and disadvantages, and all with varying degrees of success. Latham popularized the use of an active pin-driven device for presurgical orthopedics.[2] More recently, Grayson et al.[3] have described passive presurgical nasoalveolar molding in infants with cleft lip and palate to assist in achieving improved lip and nasal symmetry after cleft repair. These methods invariably require active parental participation, necessitate frequent travel to the orthodontist's office for appliance fitting and adjustment, and can be costly. To families with economic, geographical, or temporal constraints, presurgical orthopedic management of the complete cleft lip and nasal deformity may represent a very significant burden

of care. For such patients, a staged surgical approach with lip adhesion can be a practical and beneficial alternative.

Lip adhesion was originally described in 1960 as a means to facilitate alveolar approximation in preparation for early primary bone grafting.[4,5] The goal of the procedure was to convert the complete cleft deformity to an incomplete deformity, thereby restoring the normal compressive forces of the intact lip to realign the alveolar arches.[6] In bilateral deformities, the intention was to retract the protruding premaxilla, to expand the soft tissues, and to facilitate the elongation of the severely deficient prolabium.[6] The potential benefit of this procedure to facilitate primary lip and nose repair was clearly evident, and surgeons quickly adopted lip adhesion as a part of their treatment plan for patients with complete unilateral or bilateral cleft lip/nasal deformities. In 1965, Randall published his technique of lip adhesion utilizing broad triangular flaps,[1] and this became the foundation upon which many surgeons added variations and improvements. Walker et al. suggested the potential "physiological molding" of the alveolar segments by a functionally intact lip in 1966. More recently, Mulliken proposed the addition of repositioning of the lower lateral cartilages at the time of the lip adhesion, naming the procedure, "lip-nasal adhesion."[7] He noted the potential advantages of lip adhesion for wide unilateral and bilateral clefts to include not only molding of the alveolar segments, but also improved nasal contour, increased orbicularis oris musculature, and increased vertical height of the lateral and medial lip elements. These benefits were partially validated in his anthropometric study.

Although the advantages of lip adhesion are numerous, the disadvantages are few, namely, the potential anesthetic risks and costs of an additional surgery. Dehiscence rates are reported to be less than 5% in experienced hands.[7,8] When dehiscence occurs, it is usually partial in nature. If a permanent suture is used in the adhesion to approximate the lip element, this often remains intact, and the final result is compromised little, if at all. Since lip adhesion results in unpredictable repositioning of the maxillary segments, passive alveolar molding is required if primary gingivoperiosteoplasty is planned.

In 1983, Osborn et al.[9] reported that only a small percentage of the plastic surgery training programs utilize lip adhesion routinely as a part of their cleft lip treatment plan. Although some have argued that lip adhesion introduces scar into the unrepaired lip, careful design and execution will ensure that such scars remain within tissues that would otherwise be discarded at the time of definitive repair. Bardach and Salyer compared unilateral cleft lip repair with and without lip adhesion and found that children who underwent single-stage repairs had a superior outcome.[10] They partially attributed this to the scarring that occurs after lip adhesion. In the authors' experience, however, scarring has not been a concern; the lip adhesion scar is simply excised at the time of definitive lip repair, and it does not impede the dissection or impact the final aesthetic outcome.

TECHNIQUE

Infants, with wide complete unilateral or bilateral clefts, who are unable to (or whose parents choose not to) participate in a presurgical orthopedic program, are ideal candidates for lip adhesion. The procedure is usually performed under general anesthesia before 2–3 months of age.

Unilateral Lip Adhesion

Initially, the key points for the definitive cleft lip and nose repair are marked on the skin and tattooed with a surgical quill dipped in methylene blue. The key landmarks are delineated so that tissues needed for the repair are not violated during the lip adhesion procedure. Mirror-image rectangular "book flaps" are designed and marked high on the medial and lateral lip elements. The flaps measure 6–8 mm in length and are positioned on the lip just beneath the nostril sill. A short portion of the nostril sill may be included in the flaps, making it a true lip and nose adhesion. On the lateral lip element, a standard buccal sulcus incision is designed, continuing cephalad into the nasal vestibule, and ending just above the inferior turbinate along the pyriform rim. After marking the lip, an epinephrine solution is injected into the planned incisions and nose. Using an ophthalmic knife, the incisions are made on the medial and lateral cleft margins. On the lateral lip element, the upper buccal sulcus incision is made and extended intranasally along the pyriform rim,[7] allowing for complete mobilization and repositioning of the ala. Wide supraperiosteal dissection of the lateral lip element and alar base is critical to achieving tension-free lip adhesion. Through the pyriform rim releasing incision, a subcutaneous dissection of the nasal tip, superficial to the lower lateral cartilage on the cleft side, may be performed. This dissection releases

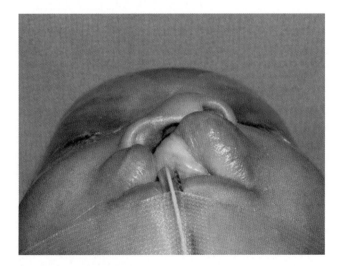

A

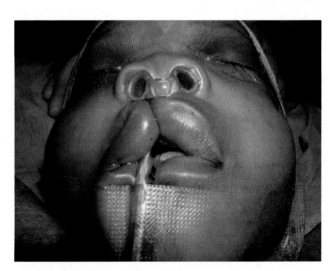

B

Figure 16–1. Infant with a complete unilateral cleft (A) before and (B) immediately after lip adhesion with nasal conformer placement.

the lower lateral cartilage and facilitates its supero-medial repositioning.

After the lip and nose dissection has been performed, a large permanent horizontal mattress suture is used to bring the lip elements together. The suture is passed through the cleft margin incision on the medial lip element, through the substance of the cheek, and exiting through the inner mucosal surface close to the buccal sulcus. A small stab incision is then made on the mucosal surface to allow the needle to be passed back through the cheek substance and to exit the ipsilateral cleft margin incision. Care should be taken to include the orbicularis oris muscle in this loop of suture. This suture is then passed through the lateral cleft margin incision to pass through the lateral lip element in a similar manner. The suture exits the lateral cleft margin incision, and, when tied, brings the cheeks and lip elements in close approximation. The deep mucosal flaps are sutured together, and the orbicularis oris muscle is then approximated using 4-0 Vicryl sutures. The superficial mucosal flaps are then sutured. It should be noted that the horizontal mattress "retention stitch" may produce a small skin dimple on the cheek by the end of the procedure; however, this will disappear with time.[6]

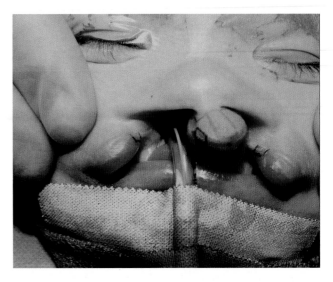

Figure 16–3. Markings for mirror-image "book flaps" for a bilateral lip adhesion in a patient with a bilateral cleft lip.

If complete dissection of the lower lateral cartilage is not adequate to restore convexity of the alar dome, an alar suspension suture, may be used to elevate the alar cartilage, affixing it to the ipsilateral upper lateral cartilage.[7] Silicone nostril retainers, secured across the septum, may also be used to shape the ala and to stretch the shortened columella on the cleft side (Fig. 16–1). The nostril retainers are left in place until definitive repair is undertaken (Fig. 16–2).

Bilateral Lip Adhesion

For patients with bilateral complete cleft lip and nasal deformities, a similar lip adhesion is carried out bilaterally. The procedure is started by tattooing the standard bilateral cleft lip repair markings on the lip. Mucosal "book flaps" are elevated made on the lateral lip elements bilaterally, as well as on both sides of the prolabium (Fig. 16–3). Dissection of the lateral lip elements and the alar cartilages is performed

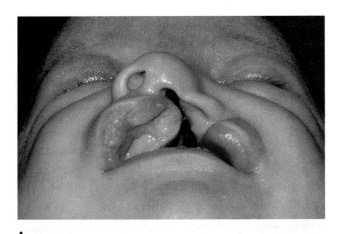

A

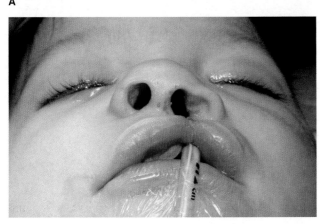

B

Figure 16–2. Infant with a complete unilateral cleft (A) before and (B) 3 months after lip adhesion, just prior to definitive lip repair. The columella has been lengthened on the cleft side, and nasal tip contour has improved.

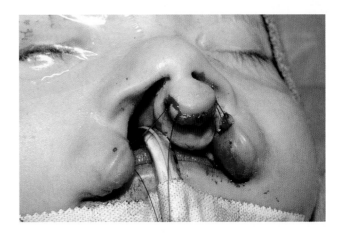

Figure 16–4. Placement of a permanent internal retention suture at the time of bilateral lip adhesion.

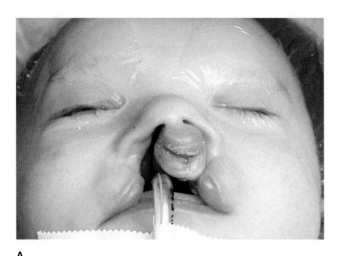

A

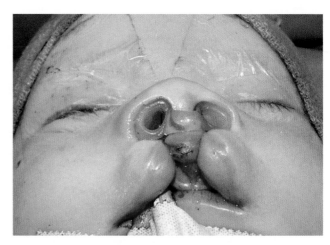

B

Figure 16–5. Infant with a complete bilateral cleft (A) before and (B) immediately after lip adhesion with nasal conformer placement.

in the same fashion as for the unilateral adhesion. Again, a large permanent retention suture is placed through the lateral lip elements, crossing the prolabium, and such is used to approximate the lateral lip elements to the prolabium (Fig. 16–4). The mucosal flaps incisions are then approximated in the same fashion as in the unilateral lip adhesion.

As for unilateral clefts, silicone nasal conformers may be placed at the time of bilateral lip adhesion and should remain in place until the time of definitive lip repair. The conformers help to restore convexity to the lower lateral cartilages and lengthen the columella, while the adhesion retrudes the projecting premaxilla (Fig. 16–5).

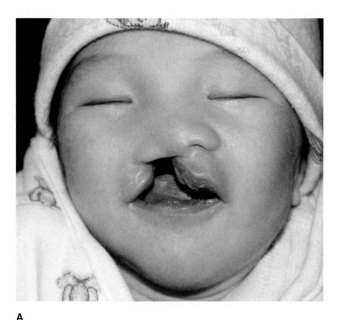

A

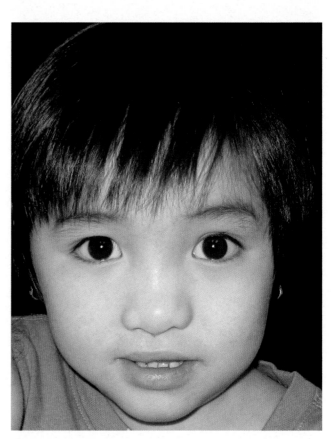

B

Figure 16–6. Infant with a complete unilateral cleft (A) before and (B) after lip adhesion and subsequent definitive lip repair.

POSTOPERATIVE CARE

Postoperatively, the patient is placed on a monitored unit overnight and is usually discharged on postoperative day 1, provided oral intake is adequate. No particular changes in bottle-feeding are recommended. Elbow splints are utilized to prevent inadvertent injury to the lip repair. Topical antibiotic ointment may be used for the first week. Cotton-swab cleansing of the incisions and nostril retainers with half-strength hydrogen peroxide begins on postoperative day 1. Definitive cleft lip and nose repair is then carried out at 4–6 months of age, during which the lip-adhesion scar is excised and the internal retention suture is removed.

CONCLUSION

In treating the infant with a complete cleft of the lip and nose, it is often desirable to narrow the width of the cleft prior to the definitive repair—in essence, converting the complete cleft into an "incomplete" cleft, thereby lessening the preoperative deformity. For those infants with wide unilateral or bilateral clefts who cannot participate in a presurgical orthopedic program, lip adhesion can provide significant benefit. An adhesion not only converts a wide complete cleft to an incomplete one, but it also repositions the abnormally displaced alar cartilage at an early age. The additional use of silicone nostril retainers helps to improve nostril shape and to lengthen the deficient columella. A well-executed cleft lip adhesion will lessen the deformity and prepare the infant for a successful definitive cleft lip and nose repair (Fig. 16–6).

References

1. Randall P. A lip adhesion operation in cleft lip surgery. *Plast Reconstr Surg* 35:371–6, 1965.
2. Millard DR, Jr., Latham R. Improved primary surgical and dental treatment of clefts. *Plast Reconstr Surg.* 86:856–71, 1990.
3. Grayson BH, Santiago PE, Cutting CB. Presurgical nasoalveolar molding in infants with cleft lip and palate. *Cleft Palate Craniofac J* 36:486–98, 1999.
4. Johansson B, Ohlsson A. Die osteoplastik bie spatbehandlung der lippen-kiefer-gaumenspalten. *Arch Klin Chir* 295:876–80, 1960.
5. Nordin KE, Johansson B. Freie knochentransplantation bei defekten im alveolarkamm nach kieferorthopadischer einstellung der maxilla bie lippenkiefer-gaumenspalten. *Fortschr Kiefer Gesichtschir* 1:168–71, 1955.
6. Randall P. Lip adhesion. *Op Tech Plast Reconstr Surg* 2:164–6, 1995.
7. Vander Woude DL, Mulliken JB. Effect of lip adhesion on labial height in two-stage repair of unilateral complete cleft lip. *Plast Reconstr Surg* 100:567–72, 1997.
8. Witt PD, Hardesty RA. Rotation-advancement repair of the unilateral cleft lip: One center's perspective. *Clin Plast Surg* 20:633–45, 1993.
9. Osbuon JM, Kelleher JC. A survey of cleft lip and palate surgery taught in plastic surgery training programs. *Cleft Palate J* 20:166–8, 1983.
10. Bardach J, Salyer KE. *Surgical Technique in Cleft Lip and Palate*, 2nd edn. St. Louis, MO: Mosby, 1987, p. 9.

Microform Cleft Lip

John B. Mulliken, MD

INTRODUCTION

Mother Nature's minor mistakes offer clues to the origins of her major abnormalities. So it is with microform cleft lip. This uncommon anomaly elicits fascination and causes a curious observer to ponder the pathogenesis of a complete cleft lip. Veau called a microform the "first variety" on the "uninterrupted chain" of labial clefting and illustrated variations with drawings traced from photographs.[1] Most moviegoers are familiar with a currently popular actor who has a microform cleft lip.

DEFINITIONS

Microform is a noun to be precise, but it has also gained approval as an adjective. Either designation, microform or microform cleft lip, is now acceptable (Fig. 17–1). Other, less

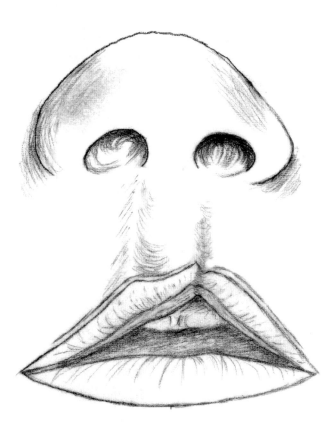

Figure 17–1. Microform cleft lip.

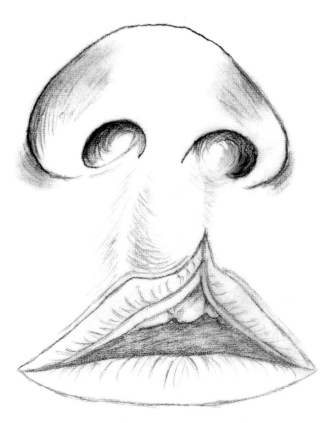

Figure 17–2. Mini-microform cleft lip.

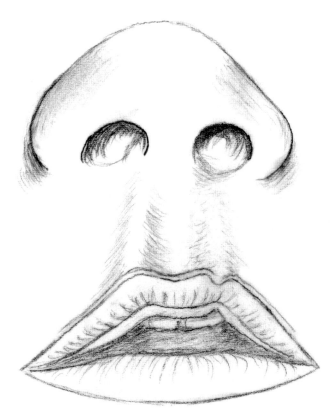

exact, adjectives, used in the past, include "occult," "minor," "minimal," or "congenital healed" cleft lip.[2–4] The old term *forme fruste* (Fr., "defaced," meaning atypical or aborted form) is a sciolism and should be avoided.

The author introduced the term *mini-microform* to describe a more subtle cleft labial anomaly in which there is discontinuity of the vermilion–cutaneous junction, but the split peak of the Cupid's bow is level with the peak on the opposite side.[5] Other features of a mini-microform cleft are slight notching of the mucosal free border, variable nostril deformity, and sometimes a philtral groove that forms on puckering. There usually is no alveolar defect (Fig. 17–2). There are three reported cases of a microform cleft lip in association with an incomplete alveolar cleft and velar cleft or complete unilateral cleft of the secondary palate.[5,6]

The designation *minor* should be reserved for those lesser forms of an incomplete labial cleft. The features that differentiate a minor-form cleft lip from a microform include (1) a vermilion notch that extends 3 mm or more above the level of the Cupid's bow peak point on the normal side; (2) a muscular depression above the cutaneous cleft into the sill; (3) an obvious nasal deformity, i.e., short hemicolumella, dislocated genu, and displaced alar base; and (4) a variable alveolar cleft (Fig. 17–3). Differentiation between minor-form and microform is critical because a modified rotation-advancement type repair, with complete primary nasal correction, is indicated for a minor-form, whereas a less extensive method is possible for repair of a microform.

Figure 17–3. Minor-form cleft lip.

LABIAL ABNORMALITIES

Onizuka listed the following cardinal features of a microform cleft lip: (1) minimal nasal deformity; (2) philtral groove; (3) indented free mucosal margin; and (4) notched vermilion–cutaneous junction, the disruption extending upward less than one fourth of labial height.[7] Other labial abnormalities often present include a slightly narrow medial vermilion and a strip of glabrous skin extending from the Cupid's bow peak, partway up the lip.

MUSCULAR ABNORMALITIES

The orbicularis oris muscular ring is incompletely formed in microform cleft lip; it has been variously described as being either malaligned or fibrotic.[8,9] Stenström and Thilander noted that the *pars alaris* of the nasalis muscle is hypoplastic; this accounts for the laterally displaced alar base.[10] The philtral ridge is usually low; however, sometimes the medial side of the escarpment is overly prominent. A pathognomonic sign is the appearance of a furrow, just lateral to the line of the philtral ridge, as the patient puckers the lips.[9] In my dissections, I have observed that pars marginalis of orbicularis oris is often relatively well formed, whereas pars peripheralis is hypoplastic along the line of the inadequate philtral ridge. Although the white roll is disrupted in a microform, it is well formed in the medial and lateral segments.

There is evidence for a so-called "occult" cleft lip, i.e., one with normal external appearance but with abnormal underlying muscle. In a pilot study, Martin and colleagues used labial ultrasonography and showed a threefold higher prevalence of minor hypoechoic defects of orbicularis oris in first-degree relatives of subjects with cleft lip/palate, as compared with a control group.[11] They suggested that this "subepithelial" orbicular discontinuity is a minor expression of the cleft phenotype. If such an occult cleft lip can be documented, this would be an important finding for estimating recurrence risk, and would increase the power of genetic studies to identify putative genes that cause oral clefting.

NASAL ABNORMALITIES

In a microform, the nasal deformity is often more evident than the labial distortion, although usually less obvious than the nasal distortion in an incomplete cleft lip. The microform nasal tip is slightly flat, the nostril rim is a little drooped, there is nearly normal hemicolumellar length, a minor depression of the sill, and a slightly displaced and underrotated alar base. As a result, the nostril axis is more transverse than on the normal side.

Several investigators have suggested that, in the absence of a microform labial cleft, such minor nostril asymmetry is at the far end of the spectrum of cleft lip. Fukuhara demonstrated unilateral nasopalatal bony abnormalities in a high proportion of apparently normal parents and siblings of children with cleft lip.[12,13] Tolarová found a higher frequency of a depressed nostril in relatives of a child with a labial cleft and suggested this finding was an indicator of a genetic predisposition for this anomaly.[14] Other investigators have shown no differences in the prevalence of nostril asymmetry in relatives of children with cleft lip/palate versus controls.[15,16] Farkas and Cheung concluded that minor nostril distortions, resembling the cleft nasal deformity, are rather common in the general population, present in 1.6% of otherwise healthy individuals.[17]

DENTOALVEOLAR ABNORMALITIES

As microform is the expression of defective development of the primary palate, associated abnormalities of the teeth and alveolus are common. These include bony deficiency around the lateral incisor[12,13], abnormal size/shape and position of the lateral incisor[18], a supernumerary tooth distal to the lateral incisor[3], and impaction of the canine.[19] In one report, fathers of children with cleft lip had a higher prevalence of an impacted upper canine, as compared to a large noncleft control group.[19] Other studies had shown no higher incidence of dental abnormalities in relatives of children with cleft lip/palate.[20,21] Thus, it remains unanswered whether minor nasal asymmetries or dental anomalies represent a carrier state for cleft lip/palate. Nevertheless, for genetic counseling and molecular studies, it is critical to examine for a possible microform in the parents and siblings of the child with overt cleft lip/palate.[22]

CLUES TO PATHOGENESIS OF CLEFT LIP

When observing a complete cleft lip, it is clear that the developmental process was interrupted at an early stage. Whereas in studying a microform cleft lip, it is easier to envision that the process went awry later in nasolabial development. Cosman and Crikelair suggested that microform cleft lip confirms that the defect results from failure of complete mesodermal penetration into an intact ectodermal envelope, rather the older concept of failed fusion of the medial nasal process and maxillary prominence.[2] Furthermore, they posited that the defect begins high in the primary palate, i.e., in the upper lip, nasal floor, and alveolus. An alternative explanation is that the minor abnormalities of muscle, nasal floor and alveolus, seen in a microform, represent a failure to complete the final act of nasolabial development rather than a disruption at an earlier embryonic stage. Another hypothesis, which is doubtful, is that a microform could be the result of an overt cleft lip that "healed" in the late fetal stage.[4]

FREQUENCY

The birth incidence of microform cleft lip is unknown. Too often, this anomaly is either overlooked or given insufficient attention by the neonatologist or the pediatric attending in the nursery. The parents are frequently told not to worry because such a small birth defect is barely noticeable. Sometimes, they are informed that the defect will improve with time, and, if ever necessary, a minor procedure can always be done when the child is older. Thus, the first appointment with a plastic surgeon is often delayed. In my study, the median age at presentation was 11 months (range, 2 weeks to 9 years).[5] Clearly, neonatal specialists and pediatricians need to be educated that an infant with a microform cleft lip should be seen promptly. Referring physicians should know that a scar following an operation in infancy is usually less noticeable than one placed in childhood.

In my series, microform comprised 33/360 (9.2%) of unilateral incomplete cleft lips.[5] About one third of these were mini-microform clefts or 3% of unilateral incomplete cleft lips.

The surgeon who is entirely focused on repair of a unilateral incomplete or complete cleft lip/palate may fail to notice a contralateral microform. In a retrospective review of my unilateral cleft patients, a contralateral microform or mini-microform was present in 4% of incomplete and 2.5% of complete cleft lips. If these contralateral examples were included in demographic studies, the true incidence of bilateral labial clefting would be higher than reported in the literature.

CHRONOLOGY OF SURGICAL REPAIR OF MICROFORM CLEFT LIP

In the literature on microform, it is curious that more attention has been paid to description and pathogenic speculation than to operative repair. Correction of a microform is usually overlooked, or given short schrift, in surgical textbooks and atlases.

In the late nineteenth century, Nélaton used an inverted V-shaped incision, extending just above the cleft, converting the wound to a diamond shape, and followed by vertical closure. The results with this method were considered unsatisfactory by early twentieth century standards. Veau also used a type of straight-line repair, similar to that described earlier by Rose (1891)[23] and Thompson (1912).[24] He pared the edges of the microform, apposed the muscular elements, and completed the closure with careful attention to vermilion–mucosal height.[1] LeMesurier adapted his rectangular flap method for "minor notches," placing the medial joint at the center of the lip.[25] Thomson and Delpero found no differences, based on panel assessment of photographs, between the low triangular flap (Tennison) method and the rotation-advancement (Millard) technique for microform cleft lip.[26]

The Rose–Thompson method for a microform continued to have its advocates. Harding added a small releasing incision at the medial vermilion–cutaneous junction into which he inserted a small, laterally based, triangular flap.[27] Musgrave illustrated an excellent result using straight-line closure,

whereas he followed the rotation-advancement principle in correction of another microform.[28]

Millard noted that, between 1954 and 1977, he repaired only two cleft lips without a cutaneous excision or rotation-advancement: one needed only closure of a vermilion notch and the other presented as a vertical cutaneous groove that was elevated with a dermal graft.[29] Millard also recalled an adult microform cleft lip that he corrected by excising the philtral furrow, "reverse" rotation-advancement of the muscular layers, V–Y roll-down to build up the mucosal deficiency, and advancement of the alar base.

Onizuka devised several techniques to address the particular distortions of a microform cleft lip, rather than follow the conventional methods for complete forms. Many of these techniques for primary repair of microforms derived from methods used for secondary cleft labial deformities.[7] Onizuka visualized the hypoplastic orbicularis oris through Z-plastic incisions in the sill and at the vermilion–cutaneous junction. A superiorly based medial ("central") muscular flap was transposed over the lateral muscular layer, which was "fixed" by through-and-through percutaneous sutures tied over bolsters on each side. In an editorial comment to Onizuka's paper, Millard was adamant that bolster sutures do not give a permanent philtral elevation. Onizuka used a Z-plasty to correct the vermilion–cutaneous notch, and connected it to a second Z-plasty at the free mucosal margin. He also placed a Z-plasty in the nostril sill so that the lateral limb elevated the depressed columellar base. W-plasty was used to correct the minimally slumped alar rim; otherwise, Onizuka undermined, elevated, and secured the lower lateral to the ipsilateral upper lateral cartilage.

For the standard microform, Carstens recommended a short, vertical cutaneous excision, either Z-plasty or tunneled lateral muscle flap to correct the vermilion notch, release of the depressed alar base, and suturing pars alaris to the anterior nasal spine.[30] In cases of mini-microform, Cho avoided a cutaneous scar altogether.[31] Through a sagittal mucosal incision on the posterior side of the lip, he dissects the muscular layers, leaving the most anterior lamella, splits the muscles into two leaves, and interdigitates the orbicular flaps to form the philtral ridge. The anterior leaflet of the lateral muscular flap is sutured to the dermis to emphasize the philtral dimple.

REPAIR OF MINOR-FORM CLEFT LIP

Closure of a minor-form cleft lip follows the rotation-advancement principle with the same, but less extensive, technical maneuvers as for a complete form.[32] The rotation incision is shortened, extending just into the columellar base. The c-flap is taken from the relatively normal medial sill and needs to be only slightly retrogressed to lengthen the hemicolumella. Usually, the alar base does not need to be disjoined from the lateral labial element. To attain mirror–image vertical symmetry, the medial Cupid's bow peak is lowered by advancing a tiny, laterally based, triangular flap of white roll

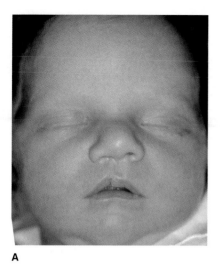
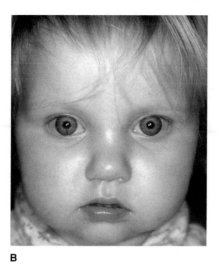
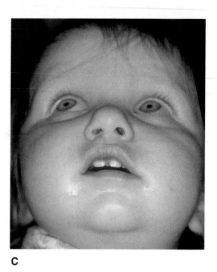

A   B   C

Figure 17–4. (A) Minor-form cleft lip. (B and C) Age 1 year, 7 months following abridged rotation-advancement repair and primary nasal correction.

and cutaneous lip; this is inset into a releasing incision at the medial vermilion–cutaneous junction. The slumped, and usually splayed, lower lateral cartilage is approached through a rim incision and secured to the opposite genu and ipsilateral upper lateral cartilage. The alar base must be placed in a symmetrical position with the normal side and secured to underlying muscle (Fig. 17–4).

REPAIR OF MINI-MICROFORM CLEFT LIP

A mini-microform, the most subtle of labial clefts, may not require an operation. If there is an obvious split in the peak of the Cupid's bow, this can be repaired by a short, vertical lenticular excision, extending just above the vermilion–cutaneous junction. If nasal asymmetry is obvious, this necessitates tightening the alar base, apposition of the uppermost muscle fibers, and sometimes elevation of the lower lateral cartilage. Although the nostrils may appear to be similar following completion of the labial closure, nasal asymmetry often manifests early in the postoperative period. Therefore, never hesitate to undertake semi-open positioning and fixation of the lower lateral cartilage.

REPAIR OF MICRO-FORM CLEFT LIP

Closure of a microform cleft follows the rotation-advancement in principle, but not in technique. The author has devised a method involving a unilimb Z-plasty at the vermilion–cutaneous and vermilion–mucosal junctions; in effect, these are two small rotation-advancements. The repair also includes eversion of the orbicularis oris; augmentation of the philtral ridge with a dermal graft; medial positioning of the alar base, and elevation of the lower lateral cartilage.[5]

Labial Markings

Using Loupe magnification, confirm the presence of normal adnexal structures in the upper portion of the lip, above the glabrous stripe. Mark the vermilion–cutaneous and vermilion–mucosal junctions on both the sides (Fig. 17–5A). Compare the vertical position of the Cupid's bow peak on the normal side (cphi) to the medial and lateral components of the peak on the cleft side. The difference between sn–cphi on the two sides is the distance that the medial side of the microform peak must be lowered to become level with the normal peak point (Fig. 17–5B). To locate this new cphi point, first, draw a horizontal line from the normal side cphi to the cleft side. Measure the distance sn–cphi on the normal side with the Castroveijo caliper, then rotate the caliper to the cleft side, keeping the upper tine on sn point. Mark a point on the medial vermilion–mucosa where the arc of the caliper crosses the horizontal line drawn from normal side cphi: this determines cphi point on the cleft side. An isosceles triangle is formed by the three points, sn, cphi (normal side), and cphi (proposed medial point on cleft side). Draw a laterally based triangular flap on the lateral labial element: the inferior point is the lateral Cupid's bow point and the length of the triangle's base equals the necessary inferior displacement of the medial Cupid's bow point to the proposed cphi point. Next, mark a releasing incision at the medial vermilion–cutaneous junction; its length equals the height of the lateral triangle. Draw a line down from the lateral Cupid's bow point to equal the height of the slightly short medial vermilion and design a laterally based vermilion triangular flap for augmentation of the deficient medial vermilion. The length of the releasing incision at the medial vermilion–mucosal junction equals the height of this lateral isosceles triangle of vermilion (Fig. 17–5B).

With the lip on stretch, the uppermost extent of the abnormal skin can be seen as devoid of fine hair. Draw the shortest possible vertical extension that is necessary to remove

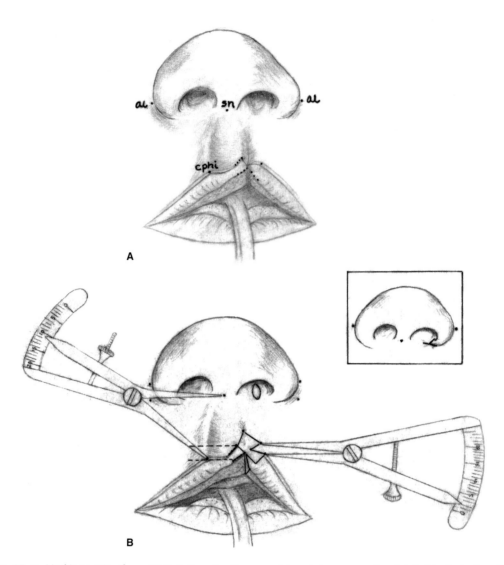

Figure 17–5. Marking a microform: (A) Notation of anthropometric points on normal and cleft side, including dissociated Cupid's bow and vermilion–cutaneous and vermilion–mucosal junctions. (B) Castroviejo caliper used to establish the proposed symmetrical cphi point on cleft side. Cutaneous-white roll, isosceles triangle designed with base equal to difference between sn-cphi on normal versus cleft side (distance medial peak of Cupid's bow must be lowered). Smaller vermilion isosceles triangle drawn with base equal to difference between vermilion height on each side of the cleft. If alar base minimally displaced, use vertical lenticular excision in sill. If alar base more laterally displaced, design Y–V advancement (inset).

this glabrous skin and the "dog ear." Typically, the superior point of excision is one third to one half of labial height.

Nasal Markings

The alar base is usually laterally displaced. If the genu is slightly dislocated, the nostril axis is more transverse as compared to the normal side. The slumped nostril gives the illusion that the alar base is more lateral than its actual position. Measure the sn–al distance on each side (Fig. 17–5A). If the affected alar base is only slightly more lateral (less than 2 mm), then it can be tightened by a vertical lenticular cutaneous excision in the upper sill and plication of the underlying muscle. Alternatively, if the alar base is more than 2 mm laterally

displaced, and particularly if the base is underrotated, draw a Y–V advancement (Fig. 17–5B and insert).

Dissection

After injection of the lip and nose with lidocaine and epinephrine, tattoo the critical points with brilliant green dye, using a 30-gauge needle placed over the end of a cotton-tipped applicator. Also, tattoo the medial vermilion–cutaneous and vermilion–mucosal junctions for several millimeters. Excise the outlined area, skin, vermilion and mucosa, down to orbicularis oris. Begin inferiorly, dissect the orbicular layer from the skin, and continue superiorly as far as possible. This exposure is aided by inferior traction on the muscle with a hook

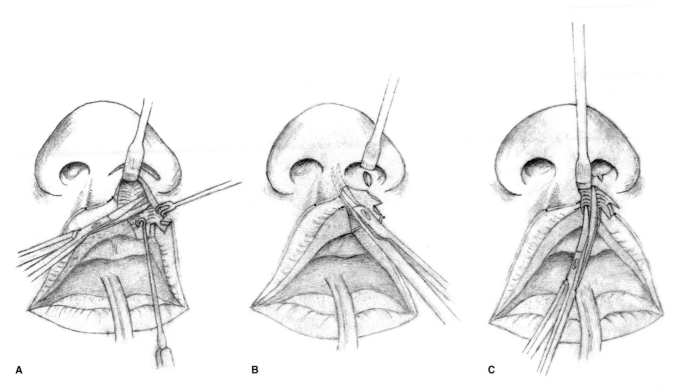

Figure 17–6. Dissecting a microform. (A) Orbicularis muscle separated from dermis through lower Z-plastic excisional wound. (B) Scissors insinuated between middle crura to dissect pocket above lower lateral cartilage. (C) Hypoplastic orbicularis divided along philtral line.

(Fig. 17–6A). The subdermal dissection of the muscular layer is completed through the sill incision (lenticular excisional or Y–V opening). If the lateral philtral furrow persists, carefully score the underside of the reticular dermis that forms the roof of the tunnel. Nasal dissection is next. Insert iris scissors through the sill opening and insinuate upward in the central columella, between the medial and middle crura, into the tip and over the slumped genu (Fig. 17–6B). This dissection permits the lower lateral cartilage to bow and gives a slight upward movement of the medial crus in the hemicolumella.

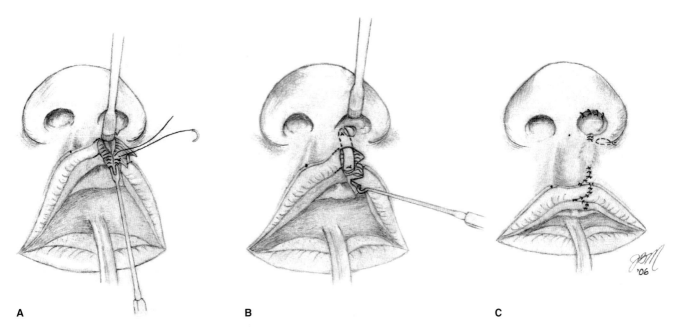

Figure 17–7. Closing a microform. (A) Everting mattress sutures reappose orbicularis oris. (B) Muscular ridge augmented with retroauricular dermal graft. (C) After releasing incisions at the "white" and "red" lines and advancement of cutaneous and vermilion triangular flaps, respectively. Note suture from alar base to muscle; interdomal suture also may be needed.

Complete the dissection by separating the posterior side of orbicularis from submucosa and dividing the muscle from inferior-to-superior, along the philtral line (Fig. 17–6C).

Closure

The orbicular layers are apposed with everting vertical mattress sutures, beginning at pars marginalis. Inferior traction on the suture line helps in the exposure and apposition of pars peripheralis (Fig. 17–7A). The uppermost muscular closure is more easily accomplished through the sill wound. Tighten the splayed pars alaris of nasalis, and, if necessary, secure the lateral muscle to the periosteum of the anterior nasal spine.

Harvest a retroauricular dermal strip for augmentation of the muscular ridge. The graft is tunneled beneath the intact lip and secured at upper pars peripheralis and at pars marginalis beneath the white roll (Fig. 17–7B).

Mirror–image symmetry of the alar bases must be established. If the base on the cleft side is laterally displaced, suture the dermis medially to the orbicular layer. This maneuver advances the base, configures a normal slight depression in the lateral sill, and prevents the base from drifting laterally or elevating with a smile. Verify alar symmetry by comparing sn–al on each side before closing the wound in the sill.

Incise the medial vermilion–cutaneous junction, thus lowering the Cupid's bow point until it is level with the normal side. Advance the lateral cutaneous-white roll flap and secure the junction with dermal and percutaneous sutures. In a similar fashion, incise the medial vermilion–mucosal line and advance the lateral vermilion flap into the defect.

Although nostril symmetry might appear to be satisfactory after labial closure and positioning of the alar base, often this is not sustained in the late postoperative period. To minimize future loss of symmetry, incise the rim and dissect over the slightly slumped lower lateral cartilage; this provides space and allows the genu to rise. An interdomal suture, and possibly an upper–lower intercartilaginous suture, may be necessary to slightly overcorrect the position of the lower lateral cartilage (Fig. 17–7C). An example of double unilimb Z-plastic repair of a microform cleft lip is shown in Fig. 17–8.

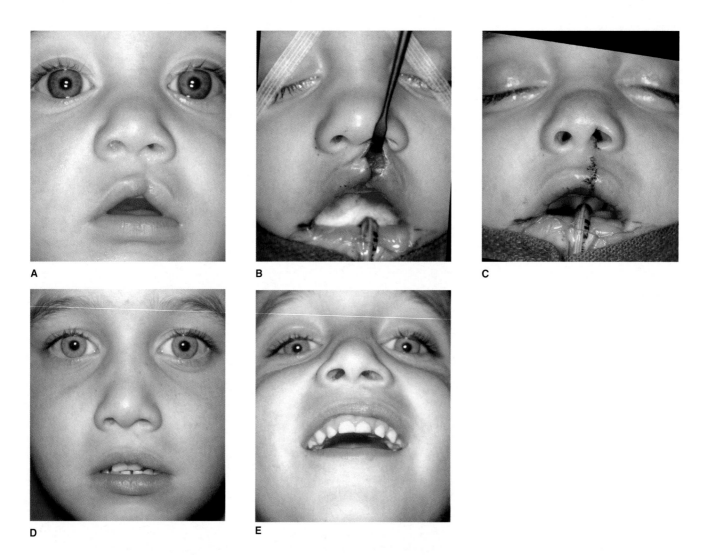

Figure 17–8. (A) Microform cleft lip. (B) Intraoperative photograph showing muscular apposition. (C) After completion of double unilimb Z-plastic repair and tightening alar base. (D and E) Age 4 years, frontal and submental views.

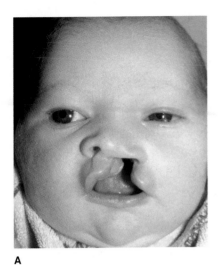
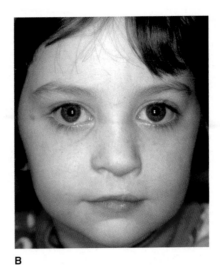
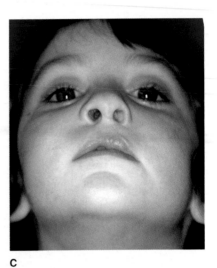

A B C

Figure 17–9. (A) Left unilateral complete cleft lip/palate with right mini-microform. Left labial adhesion at 1 month, followed by rotation-advancement labial repair and primary nasal correction at 5 months, and subsequent palatoplasty. (B and C) At age 4 years; in the future, she will need more procedures to improve symmetry: on the left side, another unilimb Z-plasty at vermilion–cutaneous junction and excision of vestibular web, and, on the right side, lenticular closure of the mini-microform, tightening upper orbicularis oris, advancement of alar base, and dermal graft to median tubercle.

REPAIR OF BILATERAL MICROFORM CLEFT LIP

The unilimb Z-plastic method can be used bilaterally to correct this rare variant, sometimes seen in uncommon disorders, such as branchio-oculo-facial and multiple pterygium syndromes. Special effort is needed to construct sufficient vermilion height at the midline and to augment the median tubercle using any available scraps of de-epithelialized submucosa or dermis. Adjust columellar length to be slightly greater and interalar distance to be slightly less than that of an infant.

REPAIR OF INCOMPLETE/COMPLETE CLEFT LIP AND CONTRALATERAL MINI-MICROFORM

The primary focus is repair of the more severely involved side, a one-stage procedure for an incomplete form and two stages for a complete cleft lip.[32] The question is whether or not to repair the mini-microform at the same time as the major side labial cleft. In my series, one third of repairs were done synchronously, the indication being the split in the Cupid's bow or the notched-free mucosal margin was obvious. The proposed peak of Cupid's bow, both the x and y coordinates, can be accurately placed on the site of the mini-microform. Nevertheless, nothing is lost by waiting at least a year or more to decide whether or not to repair the mini-microform, and sometimes it is best to leave it alone. The goal is symmetrical peaks of the Cupid's bow in the vertical and horizontal axis. The early outcome of staged closure of the

major cleft and postponed correction of the mini-microform is seen in Fig. 17–9. Note there is a slight advantage in this type of asymmetrical bilateral cleft lip because the contralateral mini-microform nasal deformity provides better nostril balance.

Whether as a primary or secondary procedure, a simple lenticular excision at vermilion–cutaneous junction is usually all that is needed to balance the mini-microform and the major side repair. Sometimes, a notch at the free margin needs attention. If necessary, tighten the alar base (for symmetry with the other side) and build up the infra-sill region, either by imbricating the upper orbicular muscle or by inserting a small dermal graft. Usually, the median tubercle is deficient and needs to be augmented later with a dermal graft (Fig. 17–9).

REPAIR OF INCOMPLETE/COMPLETE CLEFT LIP AND CONTRALATERAL MICROFORM

The primary goal is always mirror–image symmetry. A contralateral microform cleft poses potential problems in attaining symmetry with the repaired fully expressed unilateral cleft lip because (1) the median tubercle is deficient; (2) the central vermilion is thin; (3) often the line of the microform defect is slightly laterally displaced resulting in a wide philtrum; and (4) there is no normal Cupid's bow peak on either side for reference. Given these issues, it is usually best to postpone repair of the microform in order to attain symmetry with the healed repair on the greater side labial cleft.

Delayed correction of the contralateral microform permits (1) precise positioning of the Cupid's bow peaks; (2)

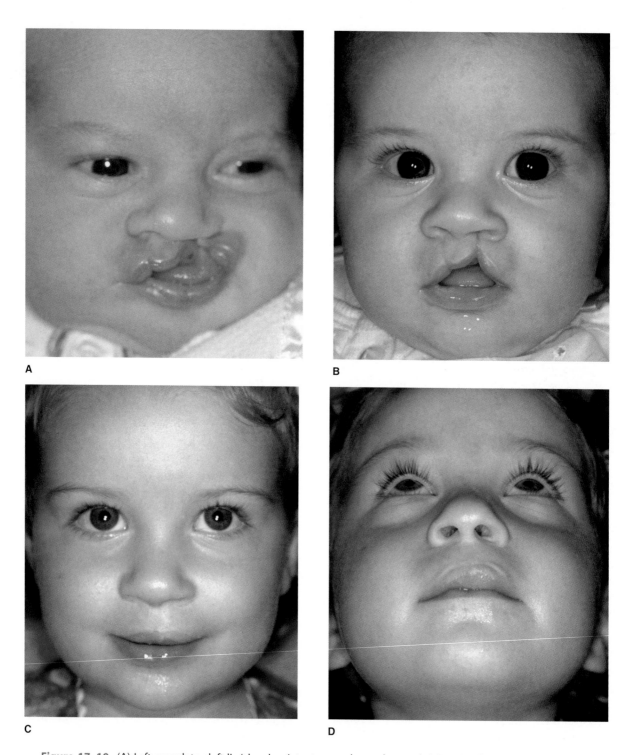

Figure 17–10. (A) Left complete cleft lip/alveolus, intact secondary palate and right microform. (B) Post left labial adhesion and alveolar gingivoperiosteoplasty. (C and D) Age 3 years, following synchronous bilateral nasolabial repair.

adjustment of the alar base position in three dimensions; and (3) observation of labial animation in a cooperative child in order to decide whether or not to repair a muscular furrow.

Simultaneous correction of the microform and major form should be considered in certain instances. While marking the more severely affected side, it is critical to carefully assess the position of the contralateral microform in relation to placement and configuration of the proposed philtral line.

The disrupted Cupid's bow peak on microform side may be displaced laterally such that the lower philtral width (cphi–cphi) is greater than age-matched normal (6–7 mm). Furthermore, the medial peak of the Cupid's bow of the microform may be elevated more than 3 mm above the proposed level on the other side. If either of these findings is present, the microform cleft borders on a minor-form deformity and synchronous bilateral repair is indicated. The old method of bilateral rotation-advancement repairs results in an abnormally bowed philtrum, a nexus of scars at the columellar–labial junction, and unequal height, possible color mismatch, and deficiency of the preserved central vermilion. Given the anatomic disparities between the greater and lesser sides, the best strategy is simultaneous repair, just as for a bilateral cleft lip.[33,34] In this way, it is possible to achieve normal philtral size (narrow) and shape (not bowed), nasal symmetry, and a sufficiently narrow interalar dimension (Fig. 17–10).

CONCLUSIONS

Minor-form, microform, and mini-microform are distinct subcategories of unilateral incomplete cleft lip that constitute the lesser end of the spectrum. They are defined by the severity of the vermilion–cutaneous cleft. Precise anatomic designation of these three types is useful because each is repaired by a different surgical technique: abridged rotation-advancement for a minor-form; vertical lenticular excision for a mini-microform; and double unilimb Z-plasty, muscular closure, and dermal graft for a microform. The nasal deformity is variably expressed in these three forms and should be corrected by the appropriate technique at the time of primary labial repair.

The logic track for repair of an incomplete or complete cleft lip on one side and a contralateral minor-form, mini-microform, or microform is determined by the severity of the deformity on the lesser side. A contralateral minor form constitutes an asymmetrical complete/incomplete bilateral cleft lip. Plan a bilateral repair, possibly with a preliminary labial adhesion on the major side. If there is an obvious contralateral mini-microform, consider synchronous repair, although nothing is lost by postponing the correction. In contrast, defer correction of a typical contralateral microform. However, if the contralateral microform is laterally displaced, follow the recommended method for synchronous bilateral cleft nasolabial repair with emphasis on a narrow philtral flap and overcorrection of the interalar dimension.

References

1. Veau V. Bec-de Lièvre; Formes Cliniques—Chirurgie. *Avec la Collaboration de J. Récamier.* Paris: Masson et Cie, 1938.
2. Cosman B, Crickelair GF. The minimal cleft lip. *Plast Reconstr Surg* 37:334, 1966.
3. Ranta R. Minimal cleft lip: Comparison of associated abnormalities. *Int J Oral Maxillofac Surg* 17:183, 1988.
4. Castilla EE, Martínez-Frías ML. Congenital healed cleft lip. *Am J Med Genet* 58:106, 1995.
5. Mulliken JB. Double unilimb Z-plastic repair of microform cleft lip. *Plast Reconstr Surg* 116:1623, 2005.
6. Thaller SR, Lee TJ. Microform cleft lip associated with complete cleft palate. *Cleft Palate Craniofac J* 32:247, 1995.
7. Onizuka T, Hosaka Y, Aoyama R, et al. Operations for microforms of cleft lip. *Cleft Palate Craniofac J* 28:293, 1991.
8. Lehman JA, Jr., Artz JS. The minimal cleft lip. *Plast Reconstr Surg* 58:306, 1976.
9. Heckler FR, Oesterle LG, Jabaley ME. The minimal cleft lip revisited: Clinical and anatomic correlations. *Cleft Palate J* 16:240, 1979.
10. Stenström SJ, Thilander BL. Cleft lip nasal deformity in the absence of cleft lip. *Plast Reconstr Surg* 35:160, 1965.
11. Martin RA, Hunter V, Neufeld-Kaiser W, et al. Ultrasonographic detection of orbicularis oris defects in first degree relatives of isolated cleft lip patients. *Am J Med Genet* 90:155, 2000.
12. Fukuhara T, Saito S. Genetic consideration on the dysplasia of the nasopalatal segments as a "Forme Fruste" radiologically found in parents of cleft children: A preliminary report. *Jpn J Hum Genet* 7:234, 1962.
13. Fukuhara T. New method and approach to the genetics of cleft lip and cleft palate. *J Dent Res* 44:259, 1965.
14. Tolarová M. Microforms of cleft lip and/or cleft palate. *Acta Chir Plast* 11:96, 1969.
15. Mills LF, Niswander JD, Mazaheri M, Brunelle JA. Minor oral and facial defects in relatives of oral cleft patients. *Angle Orthod* 38:199, 1968.
16. Pashayan H, Fraser FC. Nostril asymmetry not a microform of cleft lip. *Cleft Palate J* 8:185, 1971.
17. Farkas LG, Cheung GCK. Nostril asymmetry: Microform of cleft lip palate? An anthropometrical study of healthy North American Caucasians. *Cleft Palate J* 16:351, 1979.
18. Johnson DB. Some observations on certain developmental dentoalveolar anomalies and dthe stigmata of cleft. *Dent Pract Dent Rec* 17:435, 1967.
19. Takahama Y, Aiyama Y. Maxillary canine impaction as a possible microform of cleft lip and palate. *Eur J Orthodont* 4:275, 1982.
20. Woolf CM, Woolf RM, Broadbent TR. Lateral incisor anomalies: Microforms of cleft lip and palate? *Plast Reconstr Surg* 35:543, 1965.
21. Niswander JD. Laminographic X-ray studies in families with cleft lip and cleft palate. *Arch Oral Biol* 13:1019, 1968.
22. Sigler A, Saavedra-Ontiveros D. Nasal deformity and microform cleft lip in parents of patients with cleft lip. *Cleft Palate Craniofac J* 36:139, 1999.
23. Roe W. *On Harelip and Cleft Palate.* London: HR Lewis, 1891.
24. Thompson JE. An artistic and mathematically accurate method of repairing the defect in cases of harelip. *Surg Gynecol Obstet* 14:498, 1912.
25. LeMesurier AB. *Hare-Lips and Their Treatment.* Baltimore: Williams and Wilkins, 1962, pp. 80–100.
26. Thomson HG, Delpero W. Clinical evaluation of microform cleft lip surgery. *Plast Reconstr Surg* 75:800, 1985.
27. Harding RL. Surgery. In Cooper HK, Harding RL, Krogman WM, et al. (eds). *Cleft Palate and Cleft Lip: A Team Approach to Clinical Management and Rehabilitation of the Patient.* Philadelphia: WB Sauders, 1979, pp. 169–173.
28. Musgrave RH. The unilateral cleft lip. In Converse JM (ed). *Reconstructive Plastic Surgery, Vol 3.* Philadelphia: WB Saunders, 1964, pp. 1371–1373.
29. Millard DR, Jr. *Cleft Craft: The Evolution of Its Surgery, Vol 1.* The Unilateral Deformity. Boston: Little, Brown, 1976, pp. 23–25; 303–304.
30. Carstens MH. The spectrum of minimal clefting: Process-oriented cleft management in the presence of an intact alveolus. *J Craniofac Surg* 11:270, 2000.
31. Cho BC. New technique for correction of the microform cleft lip using vertical interdigitation of the orbicularis muscle through the intraoral incision. *Plast Reconstr Surg* 114:1032, 2004.
32. Mulliken JB, Martinez-Peréz D. The principle of rotation advancement for repair of unilateral complete cleft lip and nasal deformity: Technical variations and analysis of results. *Plast Reconstr Surg* 104:1247, 1999.
33. Mulliken JB. Primary repair of bilateral cleft lip and nasal deformity. *Plast Reconstr Surg* 108:181, 2001.
34. Mulliken JB. Bilateral cleft lip. *Clin Plast Surg* 31:209, 2004.

18

The Extended Mohler Unilateral Cleft Lip Repair

Court Cutting, MD

I. INTRODUCTION

II. HISTORY

III. SURGICAL TECHNIQUE

IV. RESULTS

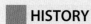 INTRODUCTION

The technique of unilateral lip repair described herein is derived directly from the Millard cleft lip repair that is discussed in the previous chapter. This chapter is not intended to provide a complete description of unilateral cleft lip and nose repair. Rather, its aim is to describe a variation of Millard's unilateral repair that was first described by Mohler in 1987.[1] An expanded version of Mohler's operation has since been adopted by a number of cleft surgeons, the "extended Mohler" unilateral cleft lip repair, which can be applied to all unilateral clefts of the lip.

HISTORY

Prior to the description of the Millard repair in 1957,[2] the dominant method for repair of the unilateral cleft lip was the lower triangular method of Tennison,[3] which was further refined by Randall.[4] The Tennison–Randall method, based on careful measurements of the two sides of the lip, is easy to learn and very reproducible. The triangular repair, however,

suffers from several disadvantages:[5] (1) it tends to flatten the natural Cupid's bow, (2) it places a zig-zag scar in the most visible part of the lip, (3) the triangle breaks up the philtral column, (4) it is strictly a lip repair and adds nothing to primary elongation of the short columella on the cleft side during primary nasal reconstruction, and (5) if the scar heals poorly, the lower triangle cannot be excised in a revision or it will produce too tight a lip.

In 1955, at the International Plastic Surgery Congress in Stockholm, Millard introduced his method for primary unilateral cleft lip repair. His technique employed a back-cut of the medial lip element beneath the columella. Here, the scar is much better hidden. Elongation of the foreshortened medial lip element by a relaxing incision at the top of the lip does not suffer most of the disadvantages of the triangular repair listed above, and thus most major cleft centers have abandoned the lower triangular repair in favor of some variant of the Millard method.

The Millard repair is not without its difficulties. It is a "cut as you go" repair which requires some finesse on the part of the surgeon. There is certainly a significant learning curve associated with the repair. The reader is referred to the

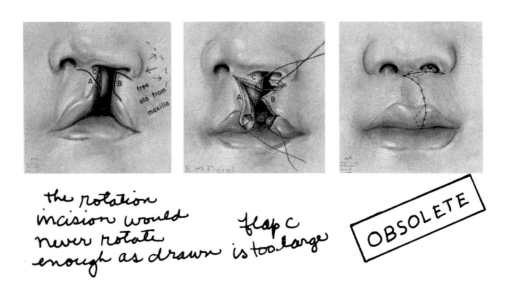

Figure 18–1. One of the earliest drawings of Millard's rotation-advancement unilateral cleft lip repair from *Cleft Craft*. The emphasis at this early stage was on preservation of the natural Cupid's bow. The C flap was used to construct the nasal floor and was not advanced up into the columella. Note also Millard's hand written notation "OBSOLETE" on this design. (*Reproduced with permission from Cleft Craft copyright Little, Brown and Company 1976.*)

previous chapter in this volume for a more complete description of the Millard repair as it is currently practiced.

It is useful to follow the evolution of Millard's repair in his own hands in order to understand how the extended Mohler repair came about. Millard's conceptual development is charted in detail in his magnificent text *Cleft Craft – I. The Unilateral Deformity*.[6] When he first developed the repair while serving in Korea, Millard noted that the Cupid's bow could be preserved through use of a relaxing incision at the top of the lip. This allowed the natural bow, which he found to be nearly normal in shape, to simply rotate downward. The defect created under the base of the nose was filled with an advancement flap from the lateral lip. An illustration of the idea is shown in Fig. 18–1.[6] The focus in this early stage of surgical development was on preservation of the Cupid's bow and not on the nose. Millard's C flap was used to close the floor of the nose at this point in the evolution of his thinking. As can be seen by the handwritten notation under Fig. 18–1, Millard later declared this original design obsolete.

In clefts with a significant vertical shortage of tissue in the medial lip element, Millard gradually began to incorporate a "back-cut" from the cranial-most point of his rotation incision *down* the noncleft philtral column, extended as much as was needed to allow downward rotation of the medial lip element to level the bow. This concept of a "back-cut" became progressively more important to Millard. It is one of the two key elements in Chapter 18 of *Cleft Craft*.[6]

As described in Chapter 18 of *Cleft Craft*, entitled "The Evolution of the Rotation and the Elevation of Flap C," Millard began to radically change his use of the C flap. The top of the rotation flap increasingly took on the appearance of an inverted fish hook, or "button hook,"[6] with the end of the incision cutting down onto, but not through, the noncleft philtral column. This "back-cut" facilitated downward rota-

tion of the medial segment and also began to suggest a new use for the C flap. Now, instead of being used to close the nasal floor, Millard began to use the C flap to advance the skin into the shortened columella on the cleft side. This maneuver was further aided by an incision through the membranous septum on the cleft side.[6] The C flap was rotated into the defect caused by the downward rotation of the medial segment as shown in Fig. 18–2.[6] The C flap had become an integral part of primary nasal reconstruction later championed by McComb,[7] Anderl,[8] Salyer,[9] and a number of others. It should be noted that primary nasal reconstruction in unilateral clefts was described quite well by Vilray Blair in *Surgery, Gynecology and Obstetrics* in 1930.[10] Salyer, McComb, and Anderl were the first to show long-term results of variants of this procedure. They demonstrated that primary nasal reconstruction, if done carefully with preservation of blood supply, was not harmful to nasal growth.[7–10]

Millard's use of the C flap to elongate the foreshortened columella on the cleft side gradually became a permanent fixture in his repair in conjunction with primary nasal reconstruction. Millard credits Holdsworth for incorporating the medial crus on the cleft side in continuity with the C flap for primary nasal correction. This concept is shown in Fig. 18–3. It is interesting to note that, in his book on cleft surgery, Holdsworth credits Vilray Blair for teaching him this maneuver in primary nasal reconstruction.[10,11]

The inverted fish hook design of Millard's complete unilateral cleft lip repair (Fig. 18–4)[6] had the effect of keeping the C flap relatively narrow. Further, as the C flap was brought up to lengthen the columella, the curvilinear design at the lip–columella junction tended to create a dog ear at that site. Millard preserved this inverted fish hook to maintain the basic rotation-advancement principle. The tip of the laterally based flap was advanced to the opposite philtral column, and

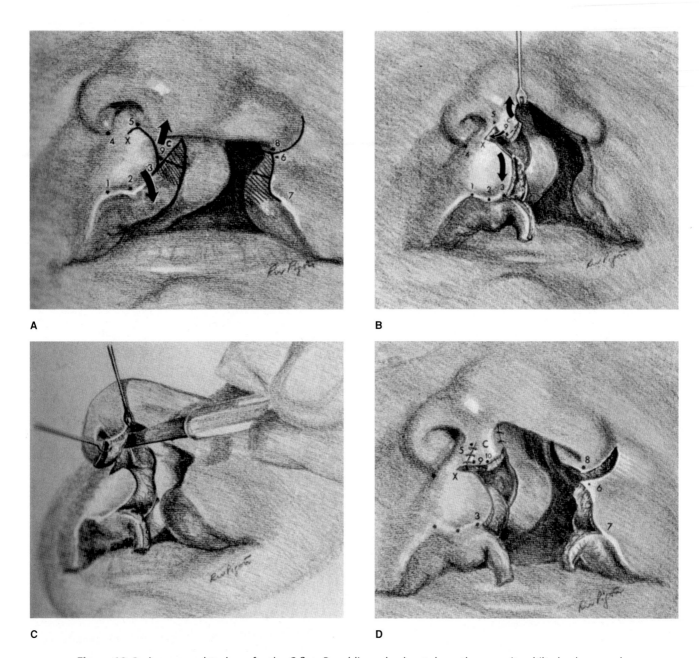

A

B

C

D

Figure 18–2. A more updated use for the C flap. By adding a back-cut down the opposite philtral column and a membranous septum incision, the C flap is used to elongate the short columella on the cleft side. Note that the C flap is no longer used for the nostril floor. It is sutured onto the cranial edge of the back-cut incision to elongate the columella and advance the medial crus up into the nasal tip on the cleft side. (*Reproduced with permission from Cleft Craft copyright Little, Brown and Company 1976.*)

the leading edge of the advancement flap fit smoothly onto the top of the curvilinear rotation incision (Fig. 18–5).[6] The use of the C flap for primary nasal reconstruction was beginning to come into mild conflict with the basic rotation advancement principle. To lengthen the tip of the lateral advancement flap, Millard advocated elongating the flap by using nasal floor skin (see point 9 in Fig. 18–4). Since the C flap was no longer used to create the nasal floor, this often led to nostril stenosis. It is important not to "raid the nasal floor" in an attempt to elongate the lateral lip flap. If the C flap is used to create columella, this nasal floor skin will be important for the creation of a

nostril sill. Further, to get the required advancement of the lateral flap, it was often necessary to make an incision around the alar base (see Fig. 18–2D). The resulting scar, however, is often not a good one. Preservation of the "advancement" part of the rotation-advancement principle also has some negative effects on the nose.

Despite its advantages, several drawbacks of the Millard repair are evident: (1) The philtral column scar ends at the opposite nasal floor. It is certainly possible to create a philtral column using careful suturing of the muscle (Fig. 18–6).[5] It is important not to dissect the skin away from the muscle any

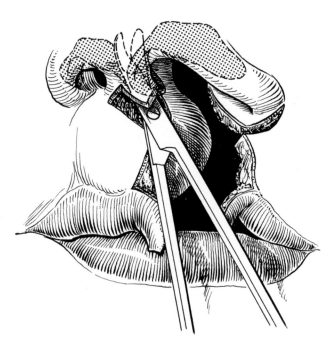

Figure 18–3. Millard's depiction of the use of scissors to separate the medial crura to facilitate advancement of the depressed dome on the cleft side attributed originally to Holdsworth.[11] Primary nasal reconstruction is clearly an integral part of Millard's repair by this stage. (*Reproduced with permission from Cleft Craft copyright Little, Brown and Company 1976.*)

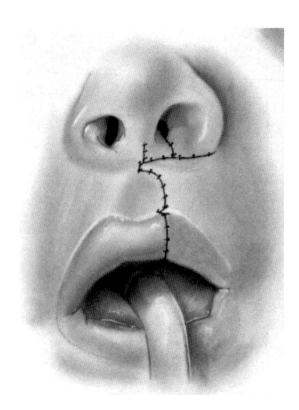

Figure 18–5. The final closure of the Millard repair. Note that the tip of the lateral flap has been advanced to the opposite philtral column. Note also the tiny ''white roll flap'' from the lateral lip which has been inserted into a small back-cut made for it on the white roll of the medial lip element. (*Reproduced with permission from Cleft Craft copyright Little, Brown and Company 1976.*)

further than the depth of the philtral dimple, lest its definition be lost. A major advantage of the Mohler repair is that most of the scar lies at the height of the cleft side philtral column along Langer's lines. This advantage is lost at the height of the classic Millard repair. It is unnatural for the philtral column to end

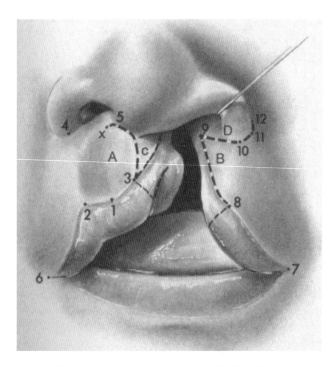

Figure 18–4. The preoperative markings for the Millard cleft lip repair from *Cleft Craft*. Note that point 9 is up in nasal floor skin. This makes it easier for point 9 to reach to the opposite philtral column. The incision around the alar base on the cleft side also facilitates this movement. (*Reproduced with permission from Cleft Craft copyright Little, Brown and Company 1976.*)

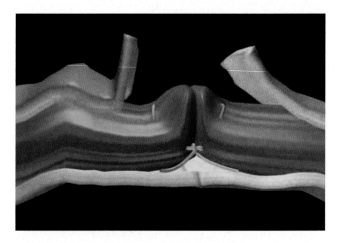

Figure 18–6. The author's method for creating a philtral column in a unilateral cleft lip. The skin must not be undermined beyond the depth of the philtral dimple on the medial side. The muscle is repaired in "praying hands" fashion using a buried absorbable horizontal mattress suture. (*Reproduced with permission from the Smile Train Virtual Surgery Video series, 2001. Animation available from Smile Train at www.smiletrain.org.*)

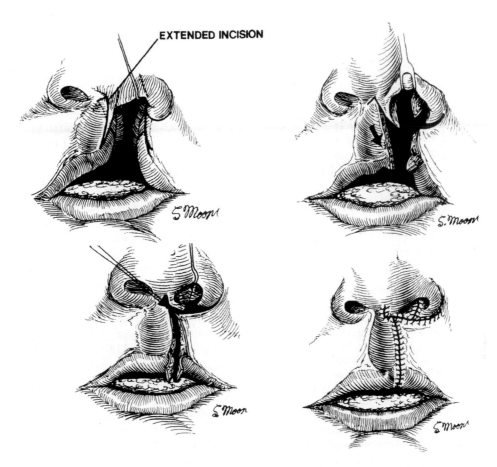

EXTENDED INCISION

Figure 18–7. The diagram of the original Mohler repair. Note that the C flap is narrow and the back-cut extends only to the depth of the philtral dimple. The tip of the C flap is bent such that the tip of it can be used to close the nasal floor. (*Reproduced with permission from Williams and Wilkins copyright 1987.*)

at the opposite nasal floor, and yet this tends to occur with the classic rotation-advancement design. (2) The cranial aspect of the scar along the leading edge of the advancement flap crosses Langer's lines. It is unfortunate that any horizontal scars are required in a lip repair because they cross Langer's relaxed skin tension lines. In the Mohler repair, there is only one horizontal incision crossing Langer's lines. (3) Advancing the lateral flap in the classic rotation-advancement often requires an incision to be made around the alar crease to allow the flap to advance sufficiently. Contrary to popular belief, a scar around the alar crease is often not a good one. Rather, scars in this area often take on a thick, waxy appearance. In the extended Mohler repair, this scar is unnecessary since there is no differential advancement of the lateral skin with respect to the alar base.

Mohler published his modification of the Millard repair in 1987.[1] In his method, the C flap was used to close the entire defect caused by the downward rotation of the medial segment (Fig. 18–7). As can be seen in his original illustration, the back-cut only extended to the middle of the philtral dimple and did not reach to the opposite philtral column, as Millard advocated. In Mohler's design, Millard's lateral advancement flap was not advanced to the opposite philtral column. A straight line closure of the lip was effected instead. Most important was Mohler's placement of a sharply angulated incision *up on the columella* instead of Millard's inverted fish hook incision. This facilitated the closure of the C flap at the columella without a dog ear. In the original Mohler design, the C flap remained quite narrow. This made it impossible to use it to completely fill the entire inter-philtral width. For this reason the back-cut could only extend to the middle of the philtral dimple. In his commentary on Mohler's paper,[12] Millard commented that because the back-cut did not extend to the opposite column, the method would only be useful in incomplete clefts. Note also that Mohler's design retained the incision around the alar base, which is quite unnecessary since the lateral flap is not being advanced. Mohler also retained Millard's point 9 from Fig. 18–4 for reasons that are uncertain. Many plastic surgeons recruit nasal floor skin into the lateral flap in an attempt to lengthen the lateral lip. This does not work effectively, however, because the distance from the lowest point on the alar crease to the height of the bow on the lateral side is not made longer. Mohler paid no price for "raiding the nasal floor" because he used the tip of the C flap to create a nasal floor by folding it laterally, as shown in his diagram.

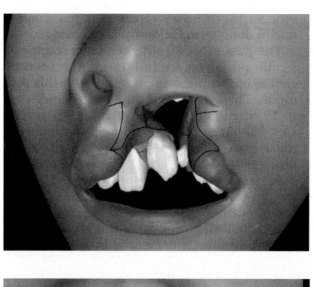
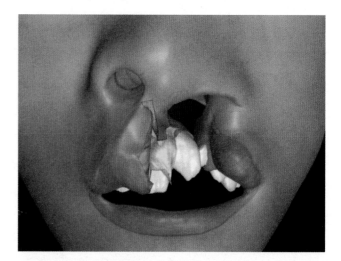
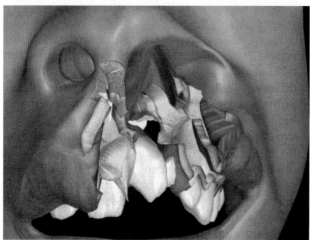
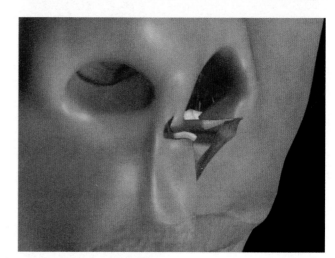
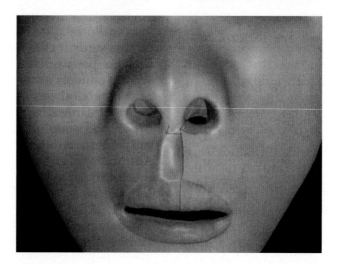

Figure 18–8. The author's "extended Mohler" repair. The critical columellar point at the top of the medial repair is 2 mm up on the columella and is slightly more than half way from the cleft side. A near straight line incision from this point down to the Cupid bow leaves the C flap quite wide. After the C flap is advanced into the short columella, the tip is trimmed off to completely fill the defect created from the downward rotation of the medial segment. The lateral flap is not advanced to the opposite philtral column, but is sewn onto the side of the C flap. It is no longer necessary to include nasal floor skin on the lateral lip flap or use an incision around the alar base. (*Reproduced with permission from Williams and Wilkins copyright 2003.*)

By extending Mohler's design and modifying it slightly, it has now become possible to use it in all complete unilateral clefts.

SURGICAL TECHNIQUE

The extended Mohler repair begins like all others with marking the four cardinal Cupid's bow points (Figs 18–8 and 18–9). The three medial points are marked in the conventional fashion. The height of the Cupid's bow is marked at the white roll on the noncleft side. The depth of the Cupid's bow is then marked on the white roll. In cases where the depth is indistinct, it is possible to make the Cupid's bow a bit narrower to minimize the amount of downward rotation required. The distance between the height of the bow to the depth of the bow on the noncleft side is used to place the height of the bow on the cleft side. This point may be marked slightly shorter than the distance on the noncleft side. It should be remem-

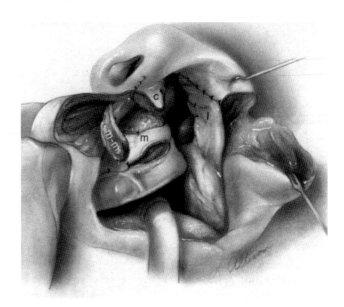

Figure 18–10. Millard's original description of the use of the L flap to close to the defect caused by making an incision along the piriform aperture in continuity with a gingivobuccal sulcus incision and dissection over the face of the maxilla to permit advancement of the alar base. Millard filled the large triangular defect at the piriform aperture to minimize scar contracture at this site. Unfortunately, the blood supply for this flap comes from the alveolus. This creates a mucosa-lined nasolabial fistula. (*Reproduced with permission from Cleft Craft copyright Little, Brown and Company 1976.*)

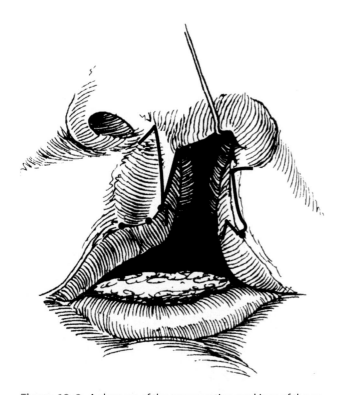

Figure 18–9. A close-up of the preoperative markings of the extended Mohler repair, modified from Mohler's original drawing. The critical point is 2 mm up on the columella and just beyond half way over (approximately 4/7ths) from the cleft side. The back-cut extends onto, but not beyond, the noncleft philtral column as described by Millard. The incision down from the columellar point to just outside the Cupid bow point is nearly a straight line. This leaves the C flap quite wide. This is essential if the C flap is to fill the entire defect caused by the downward rotation of the medial flap. Note also that the Noordhoff vermilion Z-plasty has been added to the design. Note also that the nostril floor has not been used in an attempt to lengthen the lateral lip. Comparison of this drawing with Mohler's original reveals how close in concept they are. The extended Mohler is just a somewhat more aggressive variant of the original.

bered that after the four cardinal points are tattooed with Bonnie Blue dye, the two points on either side of the cleft are suture points, not incision points. These tattooed points must be left on the lip to allow accurate placement of the sutures about the white roll. The scalpel should therefore cut just outside these points, not into them. Careful observation will reveal that the white roll usually disappears within 1–2 mm of the medial Cupid's bow point, fading into a simple skin–mucosa junction with loss of the white roll prominence.

There has been some disagreement amongst authors regarding the position of the Cupid's bow point on the lateral lip element. Noordhoff stresses that the lateral Cupid's bow point is a true anatomic point, found as the point of maximum width of true vermilion between the white roll and the red line separating true vermilion from inner lip mucosa.[13] Although this is a true anatomic point, it is a point on a deficient lateral segment. If this point is used, it will often result in a short lateral lip. The author's lateral lip point is usually marked slightly lateral to this true anatomic point. In order to select the position of the Cupid's bow point on the lateral lip element while preserving adequate lip height, a measurement is made of the distance from the alar crease to the height of the bow on the noncleft side and this distance is duplicated on the cleft side.[5] The lateral Cupid's bow point is marked with no regard to matching the distance from the commissure of mouth to the height of the Cupid's bow as Millard originally described.[6] From an embryological standpoint, the cleft represents a zone of mesodermal deficiency. The volume of tissue

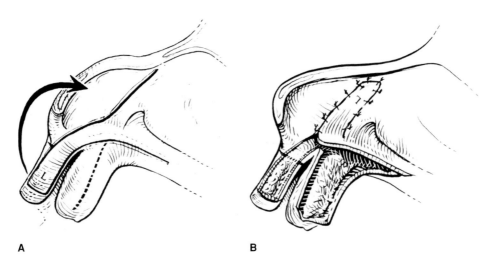

A   **B**

Figure 18–11. The author's modification of Millard's L flap. Note that the vascular supply is from the lateral nasal wall. Turning this flap up to close the piriform aperture defect no longer produces a nasolabial fistula. In fact, the lower edge of this flap is sutured to a septal flap to close the floor of the nose. (*Reproduced with permission from Williams and Wilkins copyright 1993.*)

on the cleft side, therefore, is always less than the volume on the noncleft side. The eye will notice a lip that is vertically short much more than it will notice a slight horizontal deficiency from the Cupid's bow to the commissure. In Millard's original description of his "cut as you go" repair, he states that if the lip appears short at the end of the procedure, the surgeon should just extend the lateral cut along the white roll to increase the vertical height of the lateral lip. Instead, however, this decision can be simply made from the beginning, equalizing the two lateral lip heights at the expense of lip width on the cleft side. It is interesting to note that, in a long-term

quantitative study of the extended Mohler repair, this lateral lip width deficiency tends to normalize with age.[14]

The critical point to mark in the extended Mohler repair is the upper columellar point. This point should be placed 1.5–2 mm up on the columella and 4/7ths of the width of the columella (i.e., slightly more than half way) from the cleft side. Proper marking of this point is crucial to the success of the repair. If this point is marked too close to the cleft side,

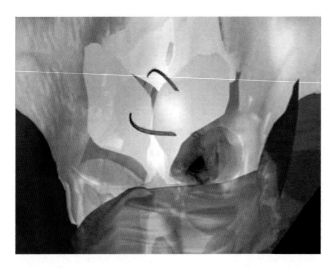

Figure 18–12. The author's method of over-correcting the dome of the lower lateral cartilage on the cleft side without the use of bolsters. An asymmetrically placed polydioxanone suture will stretch slightly in the postoperative period, suggesting the need for some degree of overcorrection. (*Reproduced with permission from the Smile Train Virtual Surgery Video series 2001. Animation available from Smile Train at www.smiletrain.org.*

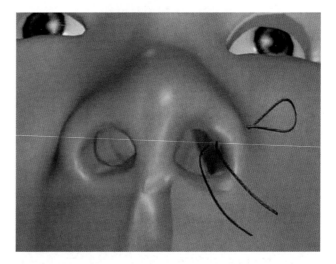

Figure 18–13. The author's method of lateralizing the vestibular web and simultaneously improving the definition of the nasofacial groove. External bolsters are not used. A polydioxanone suture is passed deep to the web then brought out through the nasofacial groove. The suture is passed back through the same hole in the skin and is brought out through the superficial part of the web. Tying the suture down lateralizes the web and deepens the groove without the need for bolsters. Two to three of these sutures are usually used. (*Reproduced with permission from the Smile Train Virtual Surgery Video series 2001. Animation available from Smile Train at www.smiletrain.org.*

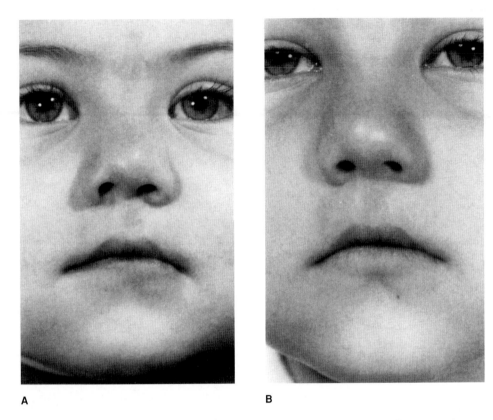

A   B

Figure 18–14. Widening of the initial narrow cleft side of the lip from Cupid's bow height to commissure over time. The picture on the left was taken at 9 months postoperatively. The picture on the right was taken at 68 months postoperatively. (*Reproduced with permission from Williams and Wilkins copyright 2003.*)

the C flap is too narrow to fill the rotation defect. If the point is marked too far over from the cleft side or the point is not high enough on the columella, the C flap will be quite fat, but an adequate inter-philtral width will not be produced at the top of the medial rotation flap.

The incision from this upper columellar point to just lateral to the cleft side Cupid's bow point must be nearly a straight line. The wide curvilinear bowing out of this incision characteristic of the Millard repair must be avoided, or the C flap will be too narrow to fill the rotation defect at the end. A slight bowing out of this incision of less than a millimeter in the middle of the span is permissible. Similarly, great care must be taken to make the incision on the lateral side of the C flap as lateral as possible in order to maximize C flap width. Of course, no vermilion should be included on the lateral edge of the C flap as this would be visible on the front of the lip following closure.

The back-cut point *at*, but not beyond, the noncleft philtral column is the same as that for Millard's repair. It is essential that the point of the back-cut reach the noncleft philtral column, or adequate downward rotation of the medial segment will not be produced. The back-cut can be extended down the opposite column slightly to gain more skin rotation, as described by Millard.[6] As Millard emphasized, the muscle under the skin must also be back-cut to this same point all the way down to the inner lip mucosa in order to allow adequate downward rotation of the medial segment.

After Millard's M flap has been dissected away from the medial lip muscle, it is necessary to back-cut it lateral to the labial frenum approximately two-thirds of the way up the lip toward the gingivobuccal sulcus and to then transect the frenum in order to allow the inner lip mucosa to rotate down as well. The M flap is then rotated into the defect created by this inner mucosal back-cut and is sutured and trimmed as necessary.

The lateral lip element is closed as a straight line repair, adding a small curvilinear element to the bottom of the lateral lip incision. If the lateral lip incision extends directly up the white roll, an undesirable peaking of the Cupid's bow will often result. In the normal lip, the white roll forms a sharp angle with the philtral column of approximately 110 degrees. Cutting directly up along the white roll from the lateral tattoo point creates an angle of 180 degrees which peaks up the Cupid's bow on closure. The lower triangular flap of Noordhoff[13] and Millard's "white roll flap" (see Fig. 18–5)[6] eliminate this tendency to peak the lateral bow. A preferred alternative is to start the incision, nearly perpendicular to the roll, then quickly curve the incision toward the upper skin–mucosa junction point.

Use of Millard's L flap is somewhat different than Millard's original description. In the Millard repair, a gingivobuccal sulcus incision is carried up in continuity with a piriform aperture incision, with dissection over the bone of the lateral maxilla to allow the cleft side alar base to advance up into normal position. This produces a large triangular defect at

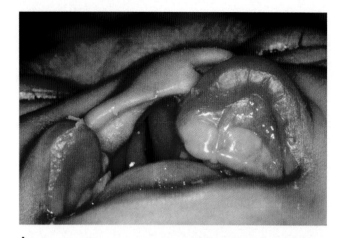

A

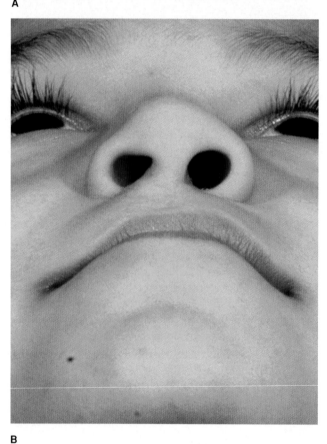

B

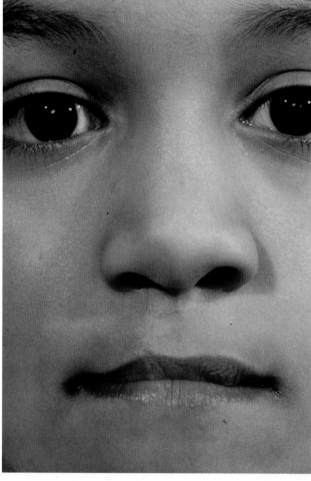

C

Figure 18–15. A,B,C: A patient with a somewhat prominent scar demonstrates the finishing scar pattern after an extended Mohler repair. Note that the lateral flap tip has not been advanced to the opposite philtral column in image C.

the piriform aperture and a large potential fistula between the mouth and nasal passage. Millard originally proposed the use of the strip of mucosa lining the lateral edge of the lip cleft (the L flap) to close this piriform aperture defect. Millard used the alveolar mucosa as the vascular pedicle for this flap (Fig. 18–10),[6] producing a mucosa-lined fistula between mouth and nose. In 1993, the author described an alteration of Millard's design in which the L flap receives its vascular pedicle from the lateral wall of the nose (Fig. 18–11).[5,15] In this way, the L flap can be used to close the triangular defect at the piriform aperture as Millard described and the lower

edge of the flap can be used to attach to a septal flap, thereby closing the nasolabial fistula.

The recent use of nasoalveolar molding (NAM) to mold the nose and alveolar complex prior to surgery (see Chapter 46) permits the surgeon to do a very conservative gingivoperiosteoplasty at the time of lip repair and to produce a more symmetrical nose.[16] Much attention is focused on elongating the short columellar skin and on improving the curvature of the septum and lower lateral cartilages using this method. An underappreciated benefit of NAM is the resultant stretching of the lateral nasal lining

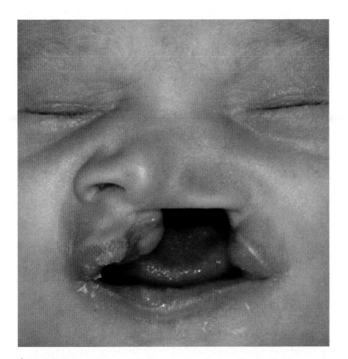

A

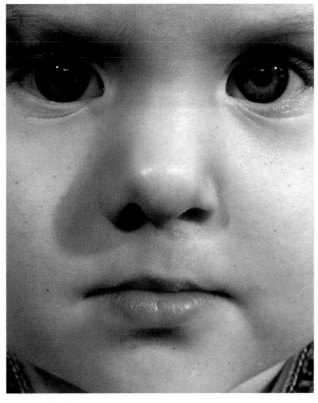

B

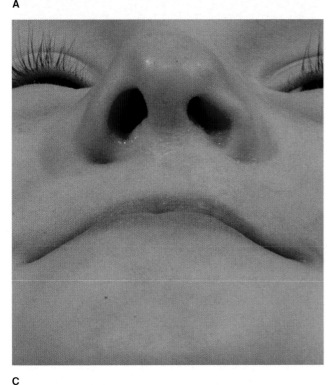

C

Figure 18–16. Two other patients treated using the extended Mohler repair. These patients received a course of preoperative nasoalveolar molding which the author feels significantly improved the quality of the nasal results. Note in the basal view the vertical scar in the columella. This scar heals quite well and is not visible on the frontal view.

and narrowing of the bony gap. This minimizes the need for the L flap and allows for much less dissection over the face of the maxilla, yielding a more reproducible result. NAM also minimizes the need for a membranous septum incision to advance the depressed medial crus on the cleft side.

Primary nasal reconstruction is integral to the extended Mohler repair. The principles of primary nasal reconstruction in unilateral clefts are detailed in the chapter that follows. As Millard and Holdsworth emphasized (see Fig. 18–3), the C

flap is advanced into the short columella on the cleft side in conjunction with advancement of the depressed medial crus of the lower lateral cartilage. This advancement of the chondro-cutaneous C flap is an essential part of the extended Mohler repair. An essential maneuver in primary nasal reconstruction is that of dissecting the skin away from the surface of the lower lateral cartilage on the cleft side all the way down to the inferior edge of the cartilage. There is no soft triangle on the cleft side.[17,18] The cartilage must be advanced anteriorly,

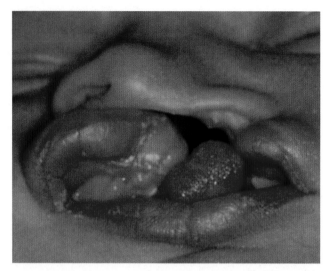

A

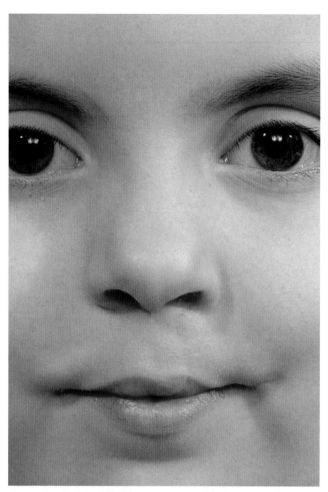

B

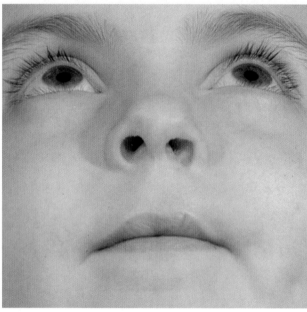

C

Figure 18–17. Two other patients treated using the extended Mohler repair. These patients received a course of preoperative nasoalveolar molding which the author feels significantly improved the quality of the nasal results. Note in the basal view the vertical scar in the columella. This scar heals quite well and is not visible on the frontal view.

but also raised superiorly so that the skin can fold under to become a soft triangle. If the dissection over the cleft side cartilage is incomplete, this is not possible. An internal absorbable polydioxanone (i.e., PDS) suture is used for this purpose, as shown in Fig. 18–12.[5,17] This suture maintains the corrected nasal shape much longer than external bolster sutures. Because the PDS tends to stretch slightly in the postoperative period, it is useful to overcorrect the position of the dome. Similarly, at the lateral vestibular web, a PDS suture is passed deep to the web inside the nose and brought out externally at the nasofacial groove. The suture is then passed back through the same hole in the skin and through a more superficial part of the internal vestibular web (Fig. 18–13). This lateralizes the web and increases the definition of the nasofacial groove, which is usually poorly defined on the cleft side.

Repair of the muscle in the lip proceeds much as in the Millard repair. The muscle pennant under the alar base on the cleft side is sutured just deep to the footplate of the medial crus of the lower lateral cartilage on the noncleft side. The muscle is not sutured to the periosteum in the region of the anterior nasal spine, as is often stated. In the vertical section of the muscle repair, a deep horizontal muscle suture is useful in creating a philtral column (see Fig. 18–6).[5] Care must be taken not to undermine the skin away from the muscle beyond the depth of the vertical philtral dimple. The dimple, like the Cupid's bow, is usually present in the starting form of a unilateral cleft. Overly aggressive muscle dissection can certainly destroy it.

Use of a lateral vermilion advancement flap in unilateral cleft lip repair has been described and popularized by Noordhoff (see Fig. 18–9).[13] Millard described a similar method in

1960,[19] but his attention was focused on alleviation of the vermilion notch and not on the delivery of the much needed vermilion to the medial lip element. Millard preferred moving his vermilion Z-plasty into the back side of the lip. Noordhoff focused on the deficient vermilion at the cleft margin of the medial lip element.[5,13] By inserting a laterally based vermilion flap into the deficiency, true vermilion height is restored and the tendency for a vermilion "whistle" is decreased. It is useful to cut the lateral vermilion flap thick such that muscle is transposed as well. This virtually eliminates the possibility of a vermilion whistle deformity.

Use of the broad C flap to close the entire defect caused by the downward rotation of the medial lip element is the essential maneuver in the extended Mohler lip repair. If the lip has been prepared correctly to this point, the C flap will be broad enough to span the entire width between the philtral columns. It is only necessary to trim off the tip of the flap to fit the defect and suture it into place (see Fig. 18–8). Given that the medial rotation defect has been filled by the C flap, it is no longer necessary to advance the tip of the lateral flap to the opposite philtral column as is done in the classic Millard rotation-advancement repair. In fact, the tip of the lateral flap is trimmed slightly to fit onto the side of the C flap for suturing. This produces two tripoints between the four flaps that come together at this site. The temptation to suture these four flaps together at a single tetrapoint should be resisted. The skin flap at the alar base should be sutured higher on the C flap to properly match the other side.

▌ RESULTS

Long-term results following unilateral cleft lip repair with the extended Mohler technique have recently been reported.[14] Lip height and width were measured, the cleft side compared to the noncleft side in each patient to evaluate symmetry. From a group of 120 patients with complete unilateral clefts, 49 met the study criteria of having photographs taken 13 months or less postoperatively and then a second set at least 2 years postoperatively. The height of the lip from Cupid's bow point to alar base was compared between the cleft and noncleft sides. A similar differential was measured between the Cupid's bow's point and the lateral commissure of the mouth. Lip height was not statistically significantly different between the two sides. As is usually observed in the Millard repair,[6] the lip will initially shorten on the cleft side, maximally at 6–8 weeks postoperatively, but the lip will usually lengthen to normal by 12 months postoperatively.

Lip width from Cupid's bow to commissure was significantly shorter on the cleft side. At ≤13 months, this difference was 8.6% ($p < 0.001$). It is interesting that at 2 years this difference had decreased to 5.8% ($p < 0.001$) (Fig. 18–14). As detailed above, this may be viewed as a necessary consequence of working with a tissue deficiency on the cleft side. It is preferable to have a slightly narrower lip on the cleft side than have a lip which is vertically short.

Several examples of the outcome of successful extended Mohler repairs are shown in Figs. 18–15 to 18–17.

References

1. Mohler L. Unilateral cleft lip repair. *Plast Reconstr Surg* 80:511, 1987.
2. Millard DR. A primary camoflage of the unilateral harelook. Transactions of the 1st International Congress of Plastic Surgery, Stockholm. Baltimore: Williams and Wilkins, 1957, pp 160–166.
3. Tennison CW. The repair of the unilateral cleft lip by the stencil method. *Plast Reconstr Surg* 9:115, 1952.
4. Randall P. A triangular flap operation for the primary repair of unilateral clefts of the lip. *Plast Reconstr Surg* 23:331, 1959.
5. Cutting C, McComb H, Millard DR, Jr., Noordhoff MS. *Disk 1 – Unilateral Cleft. The Smile Train Virtual Surgery Videos.* New York: Smile Train, 2001. Available at www.smiletrain.org.
6. Millard D. *Ralph – Cleft Craft: The Evolution of its Surgery. Volume I – The Unilateral Deformity.* Boston: Little, Brown, and Co, 1976.
7. McComb H. Primary correction of unilateral cleft lip nasal deformity: A 10-year review. *Plast Reconstr Surg* 77:558, 1985.
8. Anderl H. Simultaneous repair of lip and nose in the unilateral cleft (a long term report). In: Jackson I, Sommerland B (eds). *Recent Advances in Plastic Surgery.* London: Churchill Livingstone, 1985, Vol. 3, pp. 1–11.
9. Salyer K. Primary correction of the unilateral cleft lip nose: A 15-year experience. *Plast Reconstr Surg* 77:558, 1986.
10. Blair V, Brown J. Mirault operation for single harelip. *Surg Gynecol Obstet* 51:81, 1930.
11. Holdsworth WG. *Cleft Lip and Palate*, 4th edn. London: Heinemann, 1970.
12. Millard DR, Jr. Discussion: Unilateral cleft lip repair. *Plast Reconstr Surg* 80:517, 1987.
13. Noordhoff MS. *The Surgical Technique for the Unilateral Cleft Lip-Nasal Deformity.* Taipei: Noordhoff Craniofacial Foundation, 1997.
14. Cutting C, Dayan J. Lip height and lip width after extended Mohler unilateral cleft lip repair. *Plast Reconstr Surg* 111:17, 2003.
15. Cutting C, Grayson B. The prolabial unwinding flap method for one stage repair of the bilateral cleft lip, nose, and alveolus. *Plast Reconstr Surg* 91:37, 1993.
16. Maull D, Grayson B, et al. Long-term effects of nasoalveolar molding on three-dimensional nasal shape in unilateral clefts. *Cleft Palate-Craniofac J* 36:391–397, 1999.
17. Cutting C. Cleft lip nasal reconstruction. In Rees T, LaTrenta G (eds). *Aesthetic Plastic Surgery.* Philadelphia: WB Saunders, 1994, pp. 497–532.
18. Cutting C. Secondary cleft lip nasal reconstruction: State of the art. *Cleft Palate-Craniofacial J* 36:538, 2000.
19. Millard DR. Complete unilateral clefts of the lip. *Plast Reconstr Surg* 25:595, 1960.

19

Unilateral Cleft Lip/Nose Repair

Kenneth E. Salyer, MD • Alexandre Marchac, Cheng MS • Michienzi JW • Genecov E.

PROLOGUE TO PRIMARY CLEFT LIP/NOSE AND PALATE SURGERY

The performance of a primary cleft-lip-nose operation presents for the surgeon a major responsibility and challenge, which has a potential magical reward for the infant, family, and surgeon. Achieving an excellent result is the responsibility of the surgeon based on experience, training, and dedication. Achieving perfection in cleft surgery may not always be possible and often just evades even the experienced surgeons. In the hands of the surgeon lies the future of the infant. Society and most cultures are cruel to the facial cripple or those who cannot speak normally. When a surgeon lifts a scalpel to pare or carve a lip or palate, he/she assumes a greater responsibility for restoring the spirit and soul that resides within the child. It is a surgeon's responsibility, through experience and technical skill, to provide the best possible outcome for the child. This can only be achieved by performing a critical number of cases per year in conjunction with multidisciplinary care over time until the child is completely grown. The standard for global cleft care should be nothing less than excellence. We need to create dedicated craniofacial and cleft centers in strategic locations in developing countries globally. Those who perform isolated care or the occasional operation need to examine goals and objectives for themselves and their patients. The goal for all cleft patients needs to be good to excellent facial aesthetics, normal dental occlusion, and normal speech. Long-term outcomes in the literature are sparse. Further studies need to be presented in the literature to document the benefit of multidisciplinary care over time. The timing, sequencing, and treatment modalities, including specific surgical techniques, should be open for discussion as there are differences of opinion. Many approaches are available and must be tailored to the treatment possibilities and team experience. Only one thing counts: patients leading normal lives without social stigmata and being totally accepted in society. The Dallas protocol has been used for over 36 years and is one proven way that works for our team and patients. A large volume of patients throughout the United States has been treated with this protocol at our center. There are many multidisciplinary protocols that provide potential long-term good outcomes. The establishment of dedicated cleft and craniofacial centers globally to treat these children should be the goal of those concerned and responsible for the welfare of our children as well as those in other countries. Optimal protocols for developing countries that are sensitive to regional needs, travel, availability, and many other factors must be developed individually. What has worked for our generally compliant patients in the United States may not work in other unique locations.

INTRODUCTION

The field of cleft surgery has seen major advances over the last 30 years. Normal function and appearance are now a realistic goal and can consistently be achieved.[1] In order to obtain excellent results, a dedicated team approach, following a surgical–orthodontic–speech-oriented protocol, and based on long-term experience treating the patient from infancy through adulthood, is essential. Based on more than three decades of experience, this chapter presents our approach for the care of the primary cleft lip/nose and palate patient emphasizing the importance of interdisciplinary treatment over time.

When treating cleft patients, the most important surgical stage is the primary cleft lip/nose and primary palate repair; however, much more is needed in order to routinely achieve excellence. Without ongoing dedicated multidisciplinary treatment, the outcome of surgery is consistently dismal. Ongoing treatment over time during the period of growth by a multidisciplinary team is necessary in order to achieve excellence. In addition, treatment after the completion of growth is necessary in most cases. Patients with unilateral complete cleft lip and palate are destined for abnormal growth, due to the cleft dysmorphogenesis as well as scarring from surgical correction.

The term unilateral cleft lip is a misnomer. The cleft lip-nose is an integral part of the problem that must be addressed in order to obtain a complete repair and excellent result. There are several key elements, which must be considered in order to obtain the desired result. First, the nasal involvement is almost ubiquitous and therefore must be addressed primarily at the time of lip surgery.[1,2] Second, the treatment should always be multidisciplinary, at a minimum involving a cleft surgeon, orthodontist, and speech pathologist when the palate is involved. Third, the problem confronted is a dynamic one, extending over the child's development. Therefore, treatment protocols spanning the entire period of growth and development, rather than a one-time "home run" solution must be the rule rather than the exception. "Single-stage safari surgery" for clefts can never alone solve the problem of cleft lip/nose and palate deformity. Oro-facial clefting results in deranged skeletal and dental growth and, therefore, a long-term treatment plan is necessary to correct the deformity as the child grows.

Our long-term protocol has evolved gradually over time, and has consistently produced good to excellent results; however, there are other protocols with good results as well. A key tenet in removing cleft stigmata is achieving a full, convex, projecting facial skeleton with minimal soft tissue scarring. This requires ongoing dedicated team care, as well as the thoughtful use and timely execution of proper techniques. Most patients require secondary soft tissue and skeletal surgery.

Early nasal reconstruction is key for enhancing the patient's self esteem from an early age, and this has become the senior author's standard of care in the treatment of patients with unilateral cleft lip/nose and palate. Despite the reluctance of some surgeons to perform early nasal surgery, simultaneous lip/nose reconstruction eliminates the need to correct severe secondary nasal deformities that develop with maturation and growth, producing a thickened skin with more distorted structures and less pliable cartilaginous framework.[3] Early lip-nose repair, followed by early palate closure, provides the foundation for long-term excellent results. Any dedicated cleft surgeon can achieve this goal. It is important to remember that while developing treatment protocols over time, they should be based on ongoing experience, continuous critique, and an accepting attitude to improvements.

Nevertheless, whatever protocol or skin incision technique may be adopted, it is crucial to bare in mind that the surgeon's experience and talent is the single most important factor in determining the final outcome of the cleft lip and nose repair.[4] The type of skin incision for repair of the lip is probably least important. Releasing and repositioning all the displaced nasal and lip elements in all three planes in space is absolutely necessary to achieve excellence. How should we define excellence: normal speech, normal appearance, and normal occlusion. Excellence results from not just repairing the cleft, but by applying and using a protocol over time, that includes techniques which, when growth is complete, result in an attractive face.

HISTORY

The earliest record of hare-lip, found in ancient China with an imaginary explanation for its cause relating to a hare or rabbit, is found in Huainan Zi, a book attributed to Liu An (BC 179–122). It says, "A pregnant woman who saw a hare as a result gave birth to a baby with a 'Que Chun.' "Que" means imperfect, defective, gapped or cleft; and, "Chun" means lip. The use of term "Tu Que" (hare lip), and the first record of cleft lip repair by an unidentified Chinese Physician, are found in the Jin Shu. The operation was carried out between 392 and 395 AD.[5] Yperman (1295–1350), a Flemish surgeon, described the procedure that cut the cleft edges and sutured the margins with needle and twisted waxed thread, reinforcing the closure with hare lip needles secured by a figure-of-8 tie. The popular use of the term harelip was derived from Johnson translation in 1649 of Ambrose Pare writings about bec de lievre (lip of hare) around 1575.[6,7]

The early techniques of cleft lip repair involved a straight-line closure; such as one described by Rose[8] and Thompson.[9] Malgaigne[10] in 1843 introduced the concept of closure of cleft lip by local flaps. The following year, Mirault[11] modified Malgaigne's technique by bringing the lateral flap across the cleft. All subsequent techniques of lip closure are based essentially on this principle. Hagedon[12] in 1884 applied a Z-plasty while popularizing the use of rectangular flap in lip closure. Straight-line closure dominated the field of cleft lip repair in the first half of the 20th century. However, in the 1930s and 1940s, the Blair-Brown[13] and Brown-McDowell[14] repairs, including a triangular flap brought into the lower portion of the lip, were the popular techniques at that time. LeMesurier[15] and Tennison[16] introduced tissue to the lower part of the lip using quadrilateral and triangular flaps respectively. Both techniques shared the advantage of creating a pouting tubercle. Wynn[17] and later Davies[18] introduced variations of triangular flaps into the upper lip, and these techniques became popular in the1950s and early 1960s. Many surgeons today continue to use variations or additions of triangular flaps in their repair.

In 1955 Millard[19] introduced the concept of rotation-advancement technique. This technique preserves both the Cupid's bow and philtral dimple and places the tension of closure under the alar base. This has the advantage of reducing flare as well as promoting better molding of the underlying alveolar process. Millard's method has withstood the test of time and remains the most popular method of closure of the unilateral cleft lip. This rotation-advancement technique was the foundation for the development of the senior author's modification of the lip-nose repair.

In the history of cleft surgery, the management of the cleft lip/nasal deformity, however, has lagged behind in the evolution of the repair. The nasal problem associated with cleft lip was almost totally ignored until recent times.[20] Early illustrations and woodcuts of "harelip repair" in the 18th century often showed rather symmetrical nasal tips with wide clefts of the lips. The existence of the nasal part of cleft lip/nose was largely ignored, as there was little or nothing surgeons could do to correct the deformity at that time. The surgical treatment of cleft nasal deformity only begun after the development of aesthetic rhinoplasty toward the end of 19th century when Jacque Joseph[21] described a new approach for reduction rhinoplasty. Within the next 15–20 years, techniques for correcting the nasal tip deformity began to emerge in different places. Following this, many different approaches and recommendations were made for the management of cleft lip/nose; such as the external tip incision by Gillies and Pomfret Kilner[22] and the "flying gull" tip incision by Erich.[23] Berkeley[24] popularized the open tip approach in the unilateral cleft lip/nose. However, many of the early techniques lacked refinements and ended in a conspicuous and unnatural scar. Today, the technique first developed in 1970 in our center has undergone certain refinements over time, and eliminates extended nasal scarring while allowing internal and external nasal reconstruction.

In the past, procedures to enhance the cleft nasal tip and displaced alar cartilages were described but only enjoyed varying degree of success. Brophy[25] described an external appliance to mold the nasal tip. Humby[26] suggested hinging part of the noncleft side alar cartilage over the top of the cleft side leaving it attached to the medial crura. Byars[27] on the other hand utilized the medial crura on the cleft side after transecting it at the lower end to place over the top of the noncleft side to correct the nasal tip. With these maneuvers attempted by surgeons of varying degrees of expertise, the outcome was an increasing number of patients with noses that were disfigured and heavily scarred. Poor surgical results, with scar tissue distorting growth, subsequently led to surgeons avoiding the nasal tip until the teenage years. Primary repair of the cleft lip/nose had once again fallen into disrepute.[28]

Over the past three decades, with refined techniques, careful surgery, and the avoidance of scars, primary nasal correction at the time of lip repair began to receive increasing attention.[29–31] The senior author developed a primary cleft lip nasal repair incorporating cartilage repositioning in 1970, and this has been improved upon since then. Numerous studies have also disproved the myth that early nose tip surgery negatively affects cartilage growth.[1,30–36] It has also been shown that early nasal surgery sets the stage for more symmetrical growth of the nasal cartilages; and, if a final rhinoplasty is required after completion of nasal growth, the deformity at that time is less severe[2] and more likely to have a better final result.

ANATOMY

Functional reconstruction of a cleft lip should be based upon a good knowledge of the muscular deformity of the lip. The current trend of muscle mobilization and accurate surgical repair of the orbicularis oris muscle in unilateral cleft lip is based upon an understanding of the muscular anatomy in this deformity. Several authors such as Randall,[37] Kernahan,[38] and Nicolau[39] emphasized the importance of the orbicularis oris muscle in lip reconstruction and described their methods of repair. Park[40] believed that the inaccurate and mixed connection between the two different functional muscular components makes the repaired lip distorted and unbalanced. He believed this could get worse during growth, and stressed the importance of accurate repair of the superficial and deep portions of the muscle. We believe that release of the abnormally attached muscles, with realignment and proper approximation with compensation for deficiencies, is necessary. Identification of the specific portions of the cleft muscle is not necessary; however, a full release and reconstruction of the muscle, as a component of the lip and vermilion, is a key to success.

Normal Upper Lip

The presence of two well-defined and functional components of the orbicularis oris muscle is well described.[39–42] They consist of the superficial (pars superficialis) and the deep (pars marginalis) component. The superficial part (pars superficialis) is located under the skin of the lip and is related to other facial muscles of expression (levator labii superioris, alaeque nasi, and zygomaticus minor), and these retract the upper lip as a group. The superficial portion of the muscle consists of an upper and lower bundle. The upper bundle represents the common insertion of the muscles of facial expression, and itself inserts onto the anterior nasal spine, septo-premaxillary[43] ligament, and the nostril sill, passing deep to the alar base. The lower bundle derives its fibers from the depressor anguli oris muscle on each side and decussates in the midline, inserting in the skin, forming the philtral ridges of the contralateral side.

The deep portion of the muscle (pars marginalis), which is responsible for sphincteric action of the mouth, runs under the vermilion from one modiolus to the other.

The two portions of the orbicularis oris muscle thus correspond to the double function of the upper lip. The deep part (pars marginalis), extending from one modiolus to the other, seals the mouth as a constrictor. The superficial part (pars superficialis), on the other hand, mingles with the extrinsic facial muscles to open the mouth as a retractor.

Contraction of the deep part (pars marginalis), when the mouth is pursed, thickens the vermilion and lengthens the upper lip height. Simultaneous relaxation of the superficial portion of the muscle (pars superficialis) produces perioral fine wrinkles and accentuates the philtral columns, while flattening the nasolabial folds. In contrast, when the mouth is opened, the contraction of the superficial part (pars su-

perficialis) leads to flattening of the perioral wrinkles and philtral columns and accentuates the nasolabial fold. As well, the upper lip height shortens. Simultaneous relaxation of the deep part (pars marginalis) decreases the thickness of the vermilion.[40]

Unilateral Cleft Lip

Nicolau[39] and De Mey[42] in their electrical stimulation and histologic study respectively showed that the superficial part of the muscle, which normally inserts on either side of the midline, is misdirected by the cleft. On the cleft side, the lower bundle of the pars superficialis passes from the commissure toward the midline, but changes direction at the level below the displaced alar base to run almost vertically and be abnormally attached to the nostril and the periosteum of the piriform aperture. Contraction of the muscle results in a marked lateral bulge. The upper bundle of the pars superficialis is attached to the lateral aspect of the nasal ala and the nasolabial fold thereby contributing to the nostril deformities. On the contrary, the pars superficialis on the noncleft side appears not to be affected by the cleft. The muscle fibers are scarce and run transversely. A portion of the fibers insert almost perpendicular to the cleft edge and others into the deep dermis. Contraction of this part of muscle recreates philtral ridges and also retracts the free margin of the cleft. Although this part of muscle appears normal and not affected by the cleft, its unopposed lateral and upward pull likely contributes to the anterior septal deformity.

Both authors in their separate studies showed that in both incomplete and complete clefts the pars marginalis, which is located in the vermilion, is minimally displaced. It is simply interrupted by the cleft and ends in the submucosa.

PATHOGENESIS OF CLEFT LIP/NASAL DEFORMITY

Three major factors influence the nasal deformity in both complete and incomplete unilateral clefts: (1) muscle imbalance, (2) skeletal hypoplasia, and (3) asymmetry of the skeletal base.[44]

Muscle imbalance affects nasal symmetry in both complete and incomplete unilateral cleft lip/nose by distorting the position of the ala base and shape of the nostril. With a partial or complete discontinuation of the orbicularis oris muscle in unilateral cleft lip/nose, the extrinsic muscles of facial expression, which are attached to the orbicularis oris muscle on the cleft side, pull the ala base more laterally compared to the noncleft side. The existing muscle imbalance also changes the position of the alar cartilage, as well as the orientation of the nostril from an oblique to a horizontal orientation. Because of the insertion of muscle on the base of septum and columella on the noncleft side, contraction of the muscle pulls the septum and columella toward the noncleft side. Thus, the severity of the cleft nasal deformity depends on the degree of

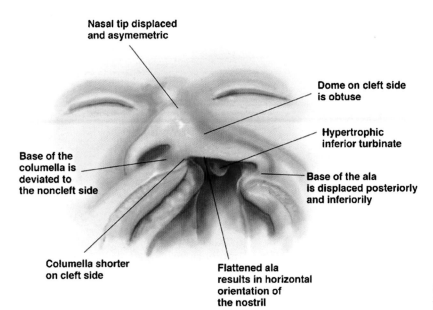

Nasal tip displaced
and asymemetric

Dome on cleft side
is obtuse

Hypertrophic
inferior turbinate

Base of the
columella is
deviated to
the noncleft side

Base of the ala
is displaced posteriorly
and inferiorly

Columella shorter
on cleft side

Flattened ala
results in horizontal
orientation of
the nostril

Figure 19–1. Anatomy of the cleft lip nasal deformity.

separation of the orbicularis oris. Proper repair of the muscle during primary lip repair does not necessarily improve the existing nasal deformity. As the lower lateral cartilage is displaced, lip muscle repair must be combined simultaneously with repositioning of the alar base and lower lateral cartilage.

Skeletal hypoplasia is observed in complete clefts and occasionally in partial clefts, despite the alveolus and palate seeming to be unaffected. Lesser maxillary segment hypoplasia occurs most commonly along its edges, as well as along the ridge of pyriform aperture. This will further accentuate the nasal deformity with the skeletal imbalance and asymmetric alar base.[45]

Malposition of the maxillary segments leads to a nasal deformity that involves all structures of the nose on the cleft side including the septum. Often, the hypoplastic lesser maxillary segment not only leads to malpositioning of the alar base posteriorly and inferiorly, it can also stretch the alar base, resulting in flattening and elongation of the nostril with typical downward deflection of the lateral crus of the alar cartilage. The orientation of the medial to lateral crura of the alar cartilage on the cleft side is also changed. Due to the force of lateral and inferior pull, the medial crus is thus shorter and the lateral crus longer than the noncleft side. The alar cartilage is buckled and deformed. It is rotated downward and drawn into an S-shaped fold. The distortion of the alar cartilage, depending on its severity, can be very difficult to correct during primary lip nose repair. Salyer,[36] Anderl,[30] and McComb[46] have successfully corrected this deformity using their techniques described. As a result of the lateral and inferior pull, as well as from the deformed alar cartilage, the dome on the cleft side is therefore more obtuse and lower than on the noncleft side. The columella is shorter due to the shorter medial crus of the alar cartilage on the cleft side. The columella is also pulled to the noncleft side by the orbicularis oris fibers entering its base.

Septal deformity is common and its severity varies. The caudal septum is usually deviated to the noncleft side. The base of the septum is dislocated from the groove on the maxillary crest and the deviation may lead to nasal obstruction on the cleft side. The degree of obstruction can be presumed by the distortion of the nose.

The following summarizes a list of characteristics typical of a unilateral cleft lip-nose deformity. The degree and severity of the deformities vary and not all of them are present in each patient (Figs. 19–1 to 19–3).

1. The columella is shorter on the cleft side with its foot plate displaced and tethered inferiorly
2. The base of columella is deviated to the noncleft side
3. The medial crus of the alar cartilage is shorter on the cleft side
4. The lateral crus of the alar cartilage is longer and together with the adherent skin are drawn to an S-shaped fold
5. The alar cartilage is displaced in the backward and downward planes

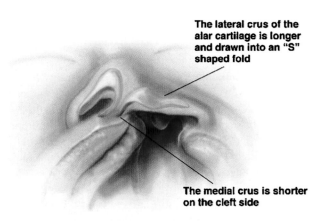

The lateral crus of the
alar cartilage is longer
and drawn into an "S"
shaped fold

The medial crus is shorter
on the cleft side

Figure 19–2. Anatomy of the cleft side alar cartilage.

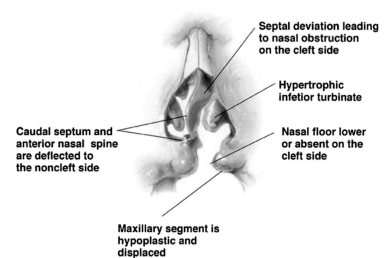

Figure 19–3. Anatomy of the cleft septum, turbinate, and skeleton.

6. The nasal tip is displaced and asymmetric
7. The dome on the cleft side is obtuse
8. The flattened alar results in horizontal orientation of the nostril and it may be smaller or larger than the opposite side
9. The entire nostril is retro-positioned
10. The base of the ala is displaced posterior and inferiorly where it is tethered to the displaced underlying bone
11. The nasal floor is lower or absent on the cleft side
12. The caudal septum and anterior nasal spine are deflected to the noncleft vestibule
13. Septal deviation of varying degrees leading to nasal obstruction on cleft side
14. The lower turbinate on the cleft side is hypertrophic
15. Nasolabial fistula may be present
16. The maxillary segment is hypoplastic and displaced on the cleft side
17. The nasal pyramid is asymmetric.

KEY CONCEPTS IN CLEFT LIP AND NOSE REPAIR

Lip Adhesion

Preliminary lip adhesion in the unilateral complete cleft lip, advocated as early as 1954 by Johanson and Ohlsson,[47] was mainly popularized by Randall[48] in the late '60s. Preliminary lip adhesion decreases the tension of definitive lip closure through its molding effects on the maxillary segments. Seibert[49] discussed the principles of lip adhesion and the possible benefits of the procedure. He recommended minimal soft-tissue undermining of the lateral maxillary segment.[7]

Randall[48] suggested that short, broad triangular flaps be interdigitated and sutured together at the mucosa, muscle, and skin layers. Millard[50] on the other hand, proposed a high adhesion, avoiding scar in the area of the repair, and introducing lateral lip parings into the lateral nasal vestibule. Millard[2] advocated lip adhesion as a substitute for presurgical

orthopedics and incorporated some nasal correction in the adhesion.

It has been our experience that lip adhesion may contribute to unnecessary additional scarring and abnormal tethering of the lip or nasal elements; and in addition, is an unnecessary procedure.[36] Early in our experience, we retrospectively evaluated 50 patients in a blinded fashion, comparing the aesthetic result of those who received lip adhesion to those who did not. We found improved aesthetics in the group that did not undergo lip adhesion, and this brought the author to abandon the use of lip adhesion in our treatment protocol. The senior author has not performed a lip adhesion since our study completed in 1977. Still, many experienced cleft surgeons continue to use preliminary lip adhesion,[51,52] with the purpose of treating the abnormal skeletal base and facilitating the definitive closure of the lip and nose. We believe that lip adhesion may make it easier for the surgeon to close the lip, however, at the potential expense of the overall aesthetic result. Lip adhesion may actually cause fixation or scarring of the alar base and associated adjacent structures in an abnormal position, making it more difficult to obtain a definitive normal contour of the nose.[36] Others have reported benefits to the use of lip taping as a form of "non-surgical" lip adhesion.[53] The current popular use of presurgical orthopedics and nasoalveolar molding has largely eliminated the need for lip adhesion; and, because of this, lip adhesions are being used less by experienced surgical teams.

Timing of the First Stage Repair

The initial repair of the lip/nose and palate is the single most important surgery in the comprehensive care of patients with oro-facial clefts. Every cleft team advocates slightly different timing, ranging from neonatal repairs to reconstructions at 6 months of age or older.

Intrauterine repair of the cleft lip has been contemplated for 25 years, and has been stimulated by the

We also advocate the use of nasal stents postoperatively.[36] They are inserted at the time of primary suture removal 1 week postoperatively. This technique splints the nostril with silicone conformers to limit the effects of scarring and wound contracture, and at the same time, improves the nasal airway. The splints are worn for 3 to 6 months, and we believe they diminish scarring and vestibular stenosis, in primary cases, while improving nasal breathing. The nasal conformer is the Koken stent (Silimed, Porex Surgical, Newnan, Georgia), used in primary and secondary cases. Individually designed postoperative silicone nostril stents may further improve this technique. Preoperative nostril expansion using tissue expansion is another technique in patients with unilateral cleft lip/nose defects, which is time consuming and labor intensive. Nasoalveolar molding (NAM) is advocated by a number of centers for the unilateral cleft lip/nose deformity; however, in our experience, excellent results can consistently be obtained without adding this technique. Many feel that long-term outcome analysis of the efficacy of NAM, in the unilateral cleft lip/nose deformity, is warranted.

PROTOCOL AT OUR CENTER

Passive presurgical orthopedics is begun at 2 weeks of age. Other than the use of the passive device, the abnormal skeletal base is mainly ignored at this stage, and emphasis is placed on the soft tissue repair of the cleft lip/nose complex. The primary cleft lip/nose repair is performed at 3 months of age, as previously discussed. When the palate is involved, two-flap palatoplasty is performed at 8 months of age.[68] Recent long-term outcome data supports normal speech in over 90% of patients treated with this protocol. Approximately, 35% of the senior author's patients benefit from minor secondary correction of the lip and/or nose, generally performed at pre-school age, around 5 years old. Definitive rhinoplasty is performed in most cases at or after completion of growth. This provides definitive normal function and appearance. Palatal expansion is performed at 5.5 years of age, followed by cancellous iliac crest bone grafting when 1/3 to 2/3 of the root of the tooth, destined to erupt in the defect, has developed. Importantly, this is accomplished prior to its eruption into the cleft void. In our experience, bone grafting at this stage provides adequate bone for the orthodontist to achieve orthodontic restoration in 95% of the cases. An open airway promotes normal facial growth; therefore, limited septoplasty and turbinectomy are performed as needed, from the early age of 4 to 5 years, until completion of care. Between 5 and 15 years of age, if maxillary sagittal growth is delayed, secondary to the cleft dysmorphogenesis or scarring, we perform one of two procedures. For those patients with up to 4 mm of midface retrusion at the occlusal plane, a Delaire facemask for protraction is used (Great Lakes Orthodontics, Tonawanda, New York). With retrusion of 12 mm or more, we perform distraction osteogenesis.[36] To achieve optimal facial balance and esthetics, after orthodontic alignment and leveling of the

teeth at skeletal maturity, approximately 40% of patients in our protocol undergo orthognathic surgery. This number has increased as we strive for entirely normal stable occlusion in all patients (Table 19–1).

SURGICAL TECHNIQUE

Overview

The final result in cleft lip and nose surgery is impacted by two major factors. The first, over which we have no control, is the degree of primary dysmorphology. The second is scarring, and this at least partially is dependent upon surgical technique and respect for the tissues. The following description details the latest modifications in our technique for the repair of unilateral cleft lip/nose deformities, and represents our efforts in the quest to achieve consistent symmetry and balance of the nose and lip at the time of the primary repair. The goal is a balanced face that is attractive and reflecting "no" deformity. In our experience, this goal can now be achieved in most cases; however, requires the coordinated surgical-orthodontic treatment from infancy through completion of growth. One of the keys to obtaining the desired final outcome, once growth is complete, is the overcorrection of the skeleton, compensating for the soft tissue deficiency that inevitably exists in the cleft lip and palate patient. In those patients where orthognathic surgery is required, the planning of the surgery is done with the orthodontist and surgeon together, with the patient at rest and in animation. This important treatment planning is performed to plan the positioning of the maxilla, assuring proper balance of the upper and lower lip at the completion of the surgery. The majority of our cleft patients, who come to orthognathic surgery after growth is complete, will have maxillary and mandibular surgery along with malar cheek augmentation using demineralized bone. This has resulted in a projecting facial profile that provides the ideal foundation for an attractive face. When adequate facial and nasal projection has been achieved, then the minimal scar that remains on the lip is less stigmatizing. However, if the same soft tissue facial mask is set on a hypoplastic skeleton, an immediate deformity of the face is apparent. Achieving balance and harmony of the face is important for excellent outcomes in the cleft lip and palate patient.

Lip

There are a large variety of ways to obtain lip closure with excellent results, each one with its own advantages and disadvantages. Many techniques today put an emphasis on exact preoperative skin markings which might commit the surgeon to incisions not always optimal, once full dissection of the muscle and release of the lip and nose from the abnormal skeletal base has been performed. After identification of the peak of the cupids bow on the cleft side of the median segment, a near vertical incision, the length of the noncleft philtral column, is made attempting to mirror

Table 19–1.

Dallas Cleft Algorithm—Infancy to Adulthood

*Integrate team work and timing based on multidisciplinary protocol
*Prenatal evaluation—multiteam approach (surgeon, orthodontist, speech pathologist, prosthodontist, anthropologist, geneticist, pediatric anesthesia, social workerpsychologist, other)

*GOAL ⟶ Bring child's face to normal facial appearance at conversational distance

~Birth

Weeks 1–4 ⟶ Peds evaluation
                  Anthropologist if needed
                  Social worker
          ⟶ Speech pathologist-feeding
          ⟶ Early passive presurgical orthopedics (~2 weeks)
          ⟶ Nasal alveolar molding (see key notes)*
          ⟶ Nonsurgical lip adhesion with tape

~3 months

          ⟶ Lip repair   Single stage or staged repair

          ⟶ Nasal repair ⟨ Broad dissection of the nasal and lip elements off abnormal skeletal base

(Necessary with primary surgery) ⟶ Wide dissection of the nasal cartilage, translocate alar cartilage (goal is contour and tip projection)

*Post surgical nasal splinting or transfixtion bolster sutures (koken stents placed at one week postop when sutures and bolsters are removed)

~8 months

          ⟶ Two flap palatoplasty surgery (always tongue stitch postop)

          ⟶ ENT Evaluation for middle ear disease

                  ⟶ PE tubes

*Speech pathologist and nutritionist to aid in nutritional intake
*No arm restraints for 2–3 weeks
*Soft diet for 3 weeks
*Pulse oximetry and tongue stitch postop for 24 hours
*Remove tongue stitch next day

the noncleft philtral column. A through and through transverse incision, on the lateral lip segment, is performed along the vermilion–cutaneous junction laterally until encountering a normal white roll, thus creating a vermilion flap. Today, with the evolution of our repair, there is little resemblance to the initial Millard procedure.[2,50,69,70] The method is fluid and allows for improvisation and artistry by the surgeon, as well as good access to the nose during the primary repair. The final skin design is determined after the muscle is addressed and alar symmetry obtained.

Muscle

Alignment of the muscle is an important basis for lip reconstruction.[71] Medial and especially lateral preperiosteal dissection releases completely the abnormally positioned muscle from the skeletal base, which is key to accomplishing symmetry of the alar bases. When releasing the muscle within the lip, a small amount of muscle should be left attached to the vermillion to provide an orbicularis marginalis. Dissection of the muscle from the skin of the lip should not be extended for more than 4–5 mm laterally and should avoid crossing the midline of the philtrum medially to avoid effacing the natural philtral lip dimple.

Combined Correction of the Lip and Nose

The peak of the Cupid's bow on the cleft side is marked on the vermillion cutaneous border (the white roll)[72,73] at an equal distance from the midline to that of the noncleft side. In order to facilitate the symmetric design of the philtrum a single arm skin hook may be placed in the middle of the

Table 19–1.

(Continued)

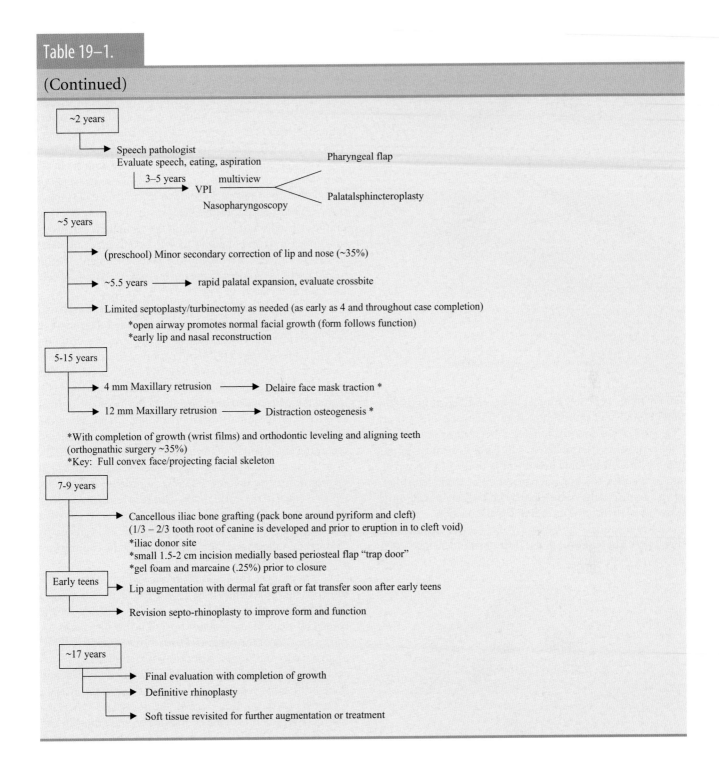

prolabium, retracting the prolabium to the midline and then marking. Another important factor is pre-incision marking of the wet-line (red-line) on the vermillion of each side of the lip; this is critical for a good color match of both sides of the lip, as well as an improved esthetic result as observed by Noordhoff.[73] Also, when performing the transverse incision on the lateral lip, some orbicularis should be left in the new vermilion, creating the orbicularis marginalis and providing a full vermillion.

Surgical Technique for Incomplete Cleft Lip/Nose Repair

The following series of illustrations demonstrates our method for the surgical correction of incomplete and complete cleft lip/nasal deformities, incorporating modifications of the rotation-advancement of the lip and the Salyer cleft nose repair.[31] Surgical repair of the incomplete cleft lip/nose deformity can be as challenging as the complete cleft repair in terms of achieving an excellent result. The surgical sequencing

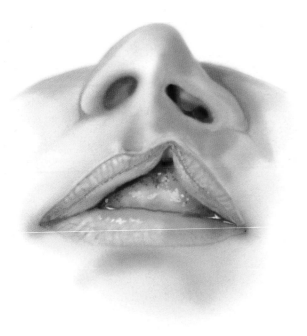

Figure 19–4. Incomplete cleft lip.

and repair are generally similar, however different in certain respects, and are demonstrated in the following illustrations (Fig. 19–4). It is essential to realize that cleft lip, even in its mild expression, is associated with nasal deformity. In patients with cleft lip only, treatment is limited to lip repair, and in the majority of cases, correction of nasal deformity; as, incomplete clefts of the lip may be associated with quite severe nasal deformity, including septal deviation.

Key identifiable points are marked on the lip and nose (Fig. 19–5). The base of each ala is identified and marked using

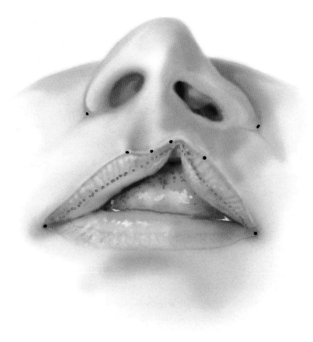

Figure 19–5. Key landmarks identified on the incomplete cleft lip.

methylene blue or appropriate marking pen. The alar base, on the cleft side, is usually elongated and distorted compared to the normal side. The peak of the Cupid's bow is identified and marked on the normal side. The height of the lip, from the alar base to the peak of the cupids bow at rest and without tension on the noncleft side, is measured using a caliper or is just estimated. This is the height to be achieved on the cleft side. This is usually 6–11 mm and averages 7 mm in a 3-month old. The mid-line nadir, or lowest point, of Cupid's bow is identified and marked. An equal distance, from the height of Cupid's bow on the noncleft side to the mid-line of Cupid's bow, is used to identify the peak of the new Cupid's bow on the cleft side, and is marked on the vermilion–cutaneous junction. The exact point may have to be altered a millimeter or two in order to have a lip that is long enough. The lip height needs to be equal to the normal side when completely dissected and placed on tension with a skin hook.

These nuances require surgical judgment, and are based on the particular cleft and the amount of tissue deficiency. The wet-line is marked with dots along its course on the vermilion on both sides of the cleft. Identification of this line provides symmetry and improved color match of the vermilion. The peak of the Cupid's bow and height of the lip on the lateral lip segment is determined by the height of the lip on the normal side, based on the initial measurement. The distance along the vermilion, and down the lateral lip segment, may be altered according to the height of the lip desired. It may be necessary to go along the vermilion cutaneous border, down the lateral lip segment, a few millimeters more in order to create a lip, which is equal to the normal side. This may result in a shorter distance from the new peak of Cupid's bow on the medial cleft side, to the commissure of the lateral lip segment, as compared to the peak of the cupids bow to the commissure on the normal side.

The proposed operation is marked with methylene blue shown as the broken lines (Fig. 19–6). The incision is marked from the peak of the cupids bow on the cleft side on the medial lip element and extends up and below the columella, across the base of the columella toward the opposite normal philtrum edge but stops just short of this landmark. The surgeon should pull the lip down with a single skin hook and hold the lip in its new position while marking. If the incision is carried past the philtral ridge on the normal side, there is a risk that over rotation of the lip may occur, and a long lip created. The lateral lip element is marked along the cleft margin, down to the newly marked peak of the new Cupid's bow (Fig. 19–7). The incision made on the medial lip element attempts to simulate the normal philtrum, creating a normal symmetric shield-shaped Cupid's bow. Again, it is best to mark and cut this incision while pulling the lip element down with a skin hook. The incision can be made with a #15 or #11 standard type blade, or a #65 or #67 beaver blade, which is our preference. The medial incision is cut through and through, including skin and muscle, while along the vestibule of the lip, the mucosa is released and partially separated from the muscle. The medial lip element is dissected and mobilized so that it can be gently pulled down, with a skin hook, to rest at the same

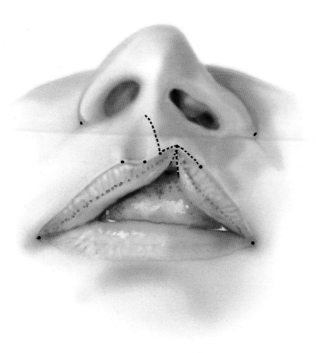

Figure 19–6. Incomplete cleft lip incisions marked with dotted lines.

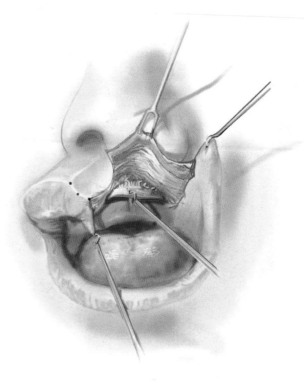

Figure 19–8. Mobilization of the lateral lip element.

level as the normal side, leveling Cupid's bow. The excess vermilion, containing a small amount of muscle, is left attached to the medial lip element at this time. The lateral lip element is likewise incised, leaving an excess vermilion-muscle flap attached to it. These two vermilion-muscle flaps are tailored as the lip is closed, used to produce a full pouting vermilion of the lip. This helps eliminate vermilion notching of the lip at the suture line. The incision of the lateral lip element is car-

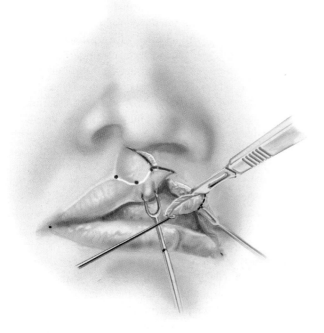

Figure 19–7. Incisions for incomplete cleft lip.

ried along the free border of the lip. The muscle of the lateral lip element, overlying the lesser segment, is completely freed and released above the periosteum so the muscle can be mobilized and sutured creating a normal anatomic muscle with nice pout to the lip (Fig. 19–8). In the incomplete cleft lip, there is usually more muscle available than in the complete cleft lip. Next, the orbicularis oris muscle is pulled with pick-ups, and the dermis undermined 4–5 mm releasing it from the underlying muscle on the lateral lip element. The operation is now carried back to the medial lip element, and the muscle is released from the dermis for a distance of 4–5 mm; however, care is taken to assure that this dissection does not cross or touch the normal philtrum (Fig. 19–9a). With this technique, a natural Cupid's bow, with a central concavity, can be created when the muscle is repaired. The insert Fig. 19–9b demonstrates repair of the orbicularis marginalis from the vermilion-muscle flaps, important in providing fullness to the vermilion.

Using tenotomy scissors, the medial lip element is freed in a pre-periosteal plane, so that the lip and nose can be shifted to the mid-line with muscle suturing. This dissection also facilitates the creation of a symmetric nasal base. Through the skin incision on the medial lip element, the tenotomy scissors are carried between the medial crura, subcutaneously above the cartilage, extending over the nasal tip and dome, freeing the skin of the nasal tip (Fig. 19–10). This is an important step in correcting the cleft lip nasal deformity, and creating a symmetric nasal tip and alar base.

The tenotomy scissors are now used to free the ala laterally by inserting them at the alar base and subcutaneously dissecting the lateral crus of the lower lateral cartilage

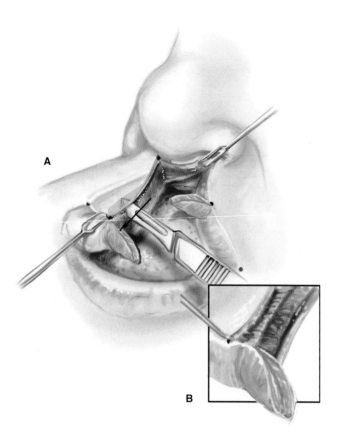

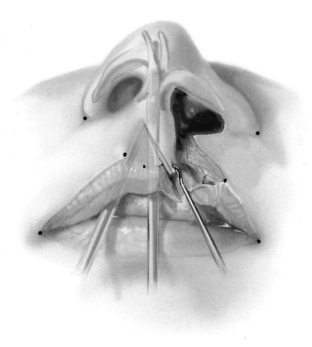

Figure 19–9. (a) Release of the dermis from the underlying muscle. (b) Repair of the orbicularis marginalis.

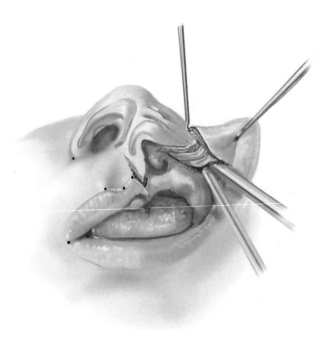

Figure 19–11. Subcutaneous dissection of the lateral ala.

Figure 19–10. Subcutaneous nasal tip dissection.

(Fig. 19–11). The scissors are carried subcutaneously over the alar cartilage, between the cartilage and skin, and connected to the pocket created from the previous medial dissection. This dissection provides for mobility of the ala cartilage, allowing it to be reshaped and contoured, and for the skin to be redraped, allowing the surgeon to create a symmetric nose. In addition, a complete release of the alar base, tethered to the clefted piriform rim, is required for the necessary mobilization and repositioning of the cleft sided ala. One of the keys to achieving a symmetric lip and nose is freeing all of the elements and floating them above the abnormal skeletal base. This allows the elements to be sutured into a symmetric nose and lip, while ignoring the abnormal skeletal base that will likely change and distort the lip-nose repair if tethered to it.

Two straight Keith needles with Prolene are passed through a Dacron pledget, inserted intranasally at a point creating the new ala genu, and brought out through the mucosa, cartilage, and skin in the tip of the nose (Fig. 19–12). The angle and placement of these nasal tip sutures ultimately determine nasal tip symmetry and may require several attempts at placement until symmetry is achieved when the sutures are tied, repositiong the alar cartilages and creating a symmetric nose. This is a key step in achieving nasal symmetry.

While an assistant holds the alar suspension sutures in the proper position, alar base sutures are placed from below (Fig. 19–13). The alar base sutures can be alternatively placed from outside in a transdermal fashion. The orbicularis oris muscle is then repaired so that it fills in the deficiency below the columella in the region of the nostril sill. The muscle is sutured in a rotation advancement fashion, advancing the muscle of the lateral lip element medially and below the columella, superior to the muscle of the medial lip element rotated inferiorly. The initial muscle suture is place deep in

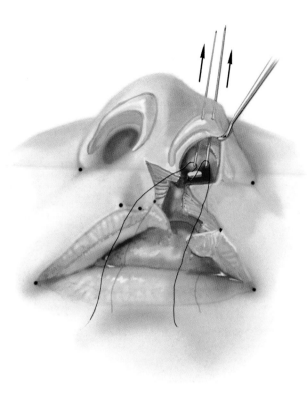

Figure 19–12. Placement of alar cartilage tip sutures.

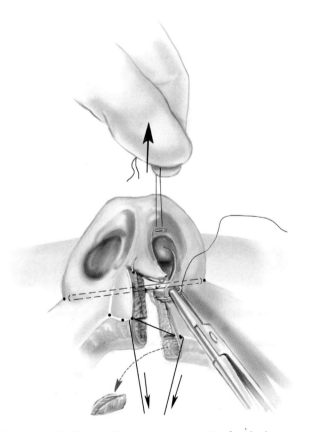

Figure 19–13. Alar cartilage suture suspension for alar base suture placement, noted with dotted lines.

the muscle at the upper angle of the skin incision. Once the suture has been tied, the nose should stay in perfect position; and, if not, the series of steps are repeated until a symmetric nose, with projection of the tip and ala base symmetry, is achieved. The Keith needles are now passed through an additional pledget on the outside of the tip of the nose, tied down, and left in place for 6 days.

Additional pledgets are used to contour the lateral ala; through and through sutures for correction of intranasal webbing, and lateral shaping of the nasal ala are placed (Fig. 19–14). By redraping and adapting the dissected elements of lining, cartilage, and alar base skin, a balanced nose can be created. However, in our experience, the use of pledgets can be more helpful in alar shaping and in gaining symmetry of the nose than using through and through sutures. To be consistently good at reshaping the nose, experience is needed with the placement of these sutures. Alar base cinch sutures, in our experience, have the potential to cause some distortion of the alar contour. The use of these suture techniques to achieve excellent results in nasal reconstruction are highly surgeon dependent but can be taught and learned by experienced surgeons. The main point is that careful surgery with complete dissection of the nose along with proper positioning and suturing can consistently yield improved results using this technique.

The alar base suture, placed from below, helps to gain alar base symmetry (see Figs. 19–13 and 19–14). The muscle sutures in the lip proper are placed to give normal contour and animation of the lip. The way in which the sutures are placed is critical in obtaining a three-dimensional esthetically good result. This technique will be discussed further in the following section on the complete cleft deformity. Another key concept is demonstrated with the insert of Fig. 19–14. Determining and producing an equal height of the new peak of the Cupid's bow is a critical maneuver for a balanced result. In the section that follows addressing the complete cleft lip deformity, techniques to achieve symmetry of Cupid's bow, as well as a proper color match of the vermilion, will be discussed. It is also important to keep enough muscle within the vermilion to provide fullness and eliminating notching.

The muscle is independently sutured to create lip and nose symmetry. The transverse lateral lip incision is brought in to the floor of the nose to create the sill.[74] Once this is achieved, excess skin is trimmed or cut as needed (Fig. 19–15). The proper positioning of the orbicularis oris is the key in gaining symmetry of the lip, rather than putting together premarked "cookie cutter" style skin flaps. A potential problem with this technique is creating a nostril and that is too small on the repaired cleft side. In order to prevent vestibular stenosis, no skin is discarded in the floor of the nose. Because this technique does not utilize a turbinate flap or an L or M flap, it is critical to leave all available skin in the floor of the nose, attempting to prevent a small nostril and possible vestibule stenosis. It is better to error on the side of a larger nostril than to create a smaller nostril. The rotation-advancement procedure as first describe by Millard[2] can produce a small

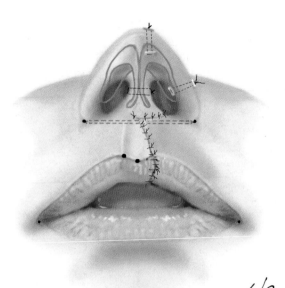

Figure 19–16. Immediate postoperative incomplete cleft lip and nose repair.

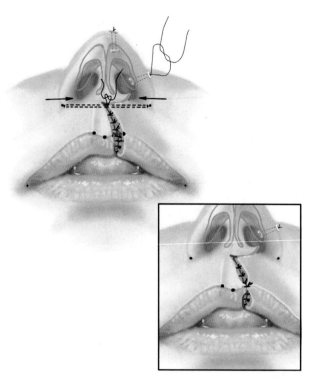

Figure 19–14. Lateral alar percutaneous pledgeted sutures correcting intra-alar webbing and creating lateral alar shape.

nostril; however, with the technique described here, vestibular stenosis, or a small nostril, does not occur very often. As with most things, it is surgeon dependent and can be prevented most of the time. The use of a postoperative silicone stent, placed at the time of suture removal, and used for 6 months, has been found to be very useful in preventing vestibular stenosis, as well as less scarring of the sill and ala rim.

Figure 19–16 demonstrates postoperative symmetry of the alar base with good tip projection and perfect nostril configuration on both sides; however, this rarely can be achieved in the cleft patient. Due to the congenital deformity, there is usually some postoperative asymmetry of the nostril when compared to the normal side, and it is difficult to completely convert a horizontal nostril to a perfectly vertical one. It is possible, however, to consistently achieve alar base symmetry and projection of the nasal tip. This is aided tremendously by the alar base and lip muscle sutures and pledgets, which provide contour and support during early healing. A balanced lip can consistently be achieved with this technique as the surgeon gains experience. The primary repair of the lip-nose complex is strongly recommended and represents the state-of-the-art treatment in primary unilateral cleft lip-nose correction. Additional or secondary surgery on the nose and septum will be necessary; however, the primary cleft lip/nose surgery corrects the major primary deformity. The other important ingredients are experience and dedication to perfection (Figs. 19–17 and 19–18).

Surgical Technique for Unilateral Complete Cleft of the Lip, Alveolus, and Palate

The key points of a unilateral cleft lip and nose repair are marked out on the patient's lip using methyl blue on a sharply pointed wooden stick or an appropriate delicate marking pen, similar to those in the incomplete deformity (Fig. 19–19). The

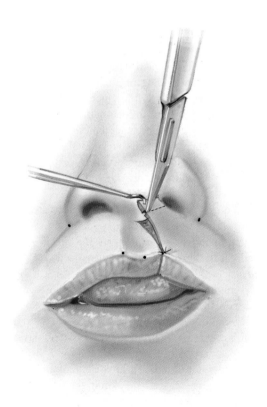

Figure 19–15. Trimming and insetting the lip skin.

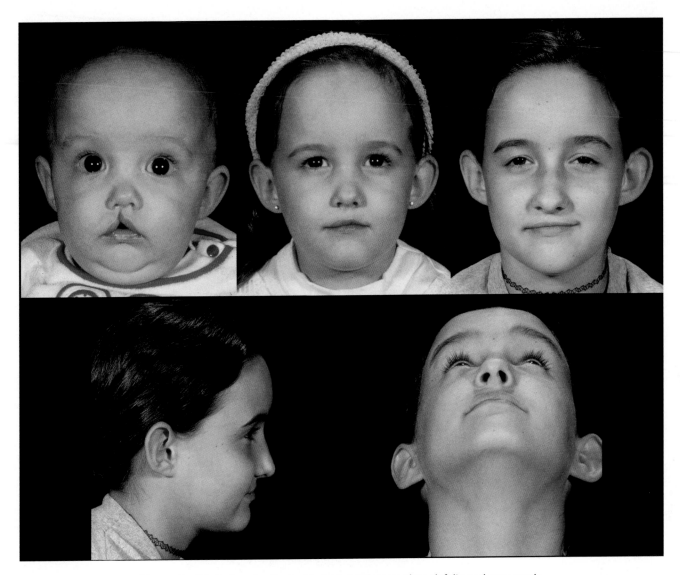

Figure 19–17. Series of patient with right-sided incomplete cleft lip and nose repair.

base of each ala is marked. The peak of the Cupid's bow is first marked on the noncleft side, and then the mid-line of the Cupid's bow is visually identified and marked. At an equal distance from the mid-line to peak of Cupid's bow on the noncleft side, another point is marked, which then becomes peak of the new Cupid's bow. The height of the lip on the noncleft side is measured using a caliper or can be estimated by an experienced surgeon. Laterally, the point corresponding to the new peak of the Cupid's bow is marked on the border of the vermilion–cutaneous junction, along the cleft margin, at a distance equal to the future height of the lip. This measurement should begin superiorly on the lip, however, not in the nose, so that the skin designated for the floor of the nose is not compromised. This is an important step in achieving an adequately reconstructed nose.

The design of the lip repair is the Salyer modification of the rotation advancement procedure, and is noted by the dot-

ted lines (Fig. 19–20). The classical incision around the alar base is not necessary and only adds scar to the final result. The incision on the lateral lip element continues from the vermilion cutaneous border, and enters the nasal cavity and onto the lateral nasal wall above the inferior turbinate. Through this incision, the displaced and abnormally attached soft tissues of the alar base are freed from the underlying abnormal skeletal base. The incision on the medial lip element begins at the newly marked peak of Cupid's bow, and continues up to, but not through, the philtral column on the noncleft side. If the incision is continued past the philtral column on the normal side, it has the potential to create an overly rotated philtrum and abnormally lengthen the cleft side, creating disproportion to the lip. The vermilion and muscle on each side of the lip is cut and maintained until closure of the vermilion. Excess vermilion is tailored to create fullness of the vermilion preventing notching.

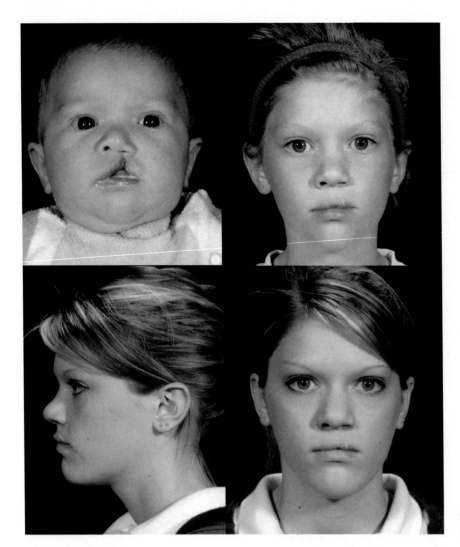

Figure 19–18. Series of patient with left-sided incomplete cleft lip and nose repair.

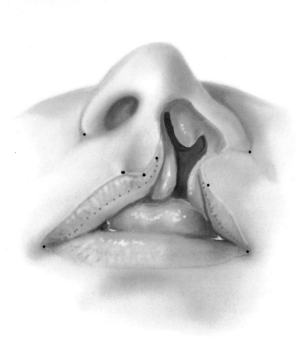

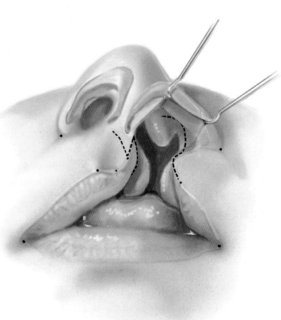

Figure 19–19. Key landmarks identified on the unilateral cleft lip.

Figure 19–20. Complete cleft lip incisions marked with dotted lines.

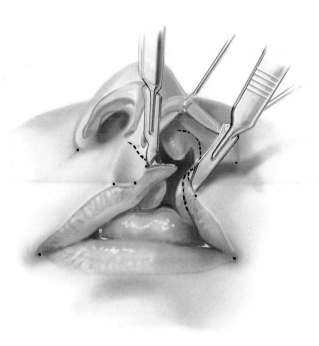

Figure 19–21. Medial and lateral lip element incisions for complete cleft lip.

In Fig. 19–21, the incision on the medial lip element is made with a #15 standard blade but may be performed with a #67 beaver blade or a #11 standard blade as shown on the lateral lip element in the image. This incision should be made perpendicular to the skin and include muscle, creating the C flap, or columellar flap seen retracted by a single skin hook in Fig. 19–26. The incision on the lateral lip segment is carried through and through along the vermilion cutaneous border dissecting a vermilion flap for orbicularis marginalis reconstruction. How the surgeon holds and cuts the lip determines the amount of muscle left in the vermilion. This lateral lip incision extends inferiorly, at least to where an adequate

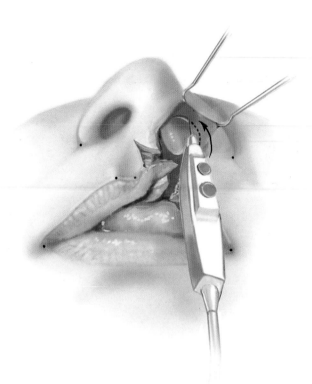

Figure 19–23. Incision carried into the nose on top of the inferior turbinate with the electrocautery.

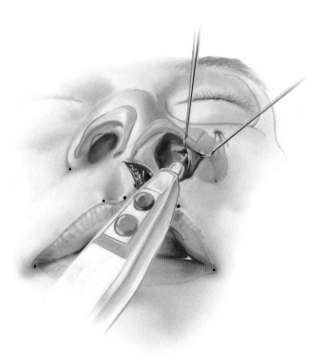

Figure 19–24. Pre-periosteal dissection of the lateral lip element up to the infra-orbital nerve.

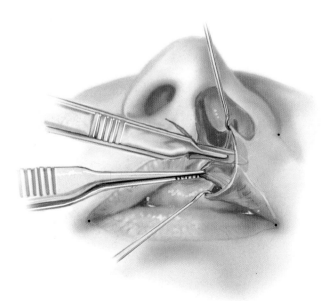

Figure 19–22. Skin of the lateral lip element is undermined.

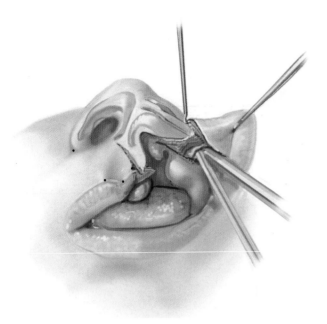

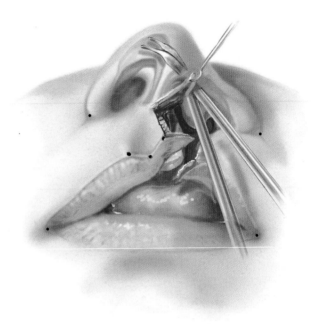

Figure 19–25. Subcutaneous dissection of the lateral crus of the alar cartilage from the alar base incision.

Figure 19–27. Subcutaneous dissection of the noncleft side alar cartilage.

white roll begins, but may be continued down the lateral lip element as lip length is needed.

The freshly cut orbicularis marginalis muscle is pulled with pickups, and the skin of the lateral lip segment is undermined from the underlying muscle for a distance of 4–5 mm from the edge of the incision (Fig. 19–22). The medial lip segment is rotated downward and pulled with a skin hook until its height matches that of the noncleft side. Additional

dissection may be necessary to achieve adequate rotation of the philtrum and lengthening of the lip.

A Colorado needle (Stryker-Leibinger) is used to create the incision through the nasal lining just above the inferior turbinate (Fig. 19–23). This provides a bloodless field for the dissection. Through this intranasal incision, as well as a vestibular buccal sulcus incision beneath the lateral lip element, the Colorado needle is used to dissect above the periosteum to the level of the infraorbital nerve (Fig. 19–24).

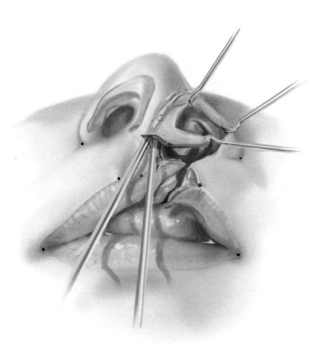

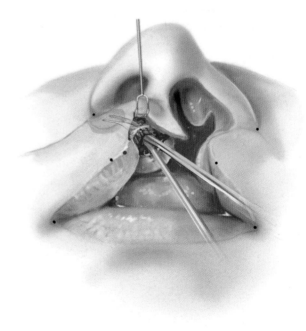

Figure 19–26. Subcutaneous dissection of the nasal tip and alar cartilage from the medial incision.

Figure 19–28. Subcutaneous dissection of the medial lip element lateral to the alar base.

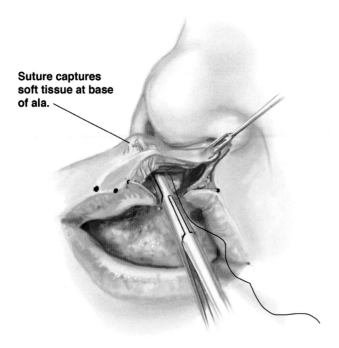

Suture captures soft tissue at base of ala.

Figure 19–29. Placement of alar base suture.

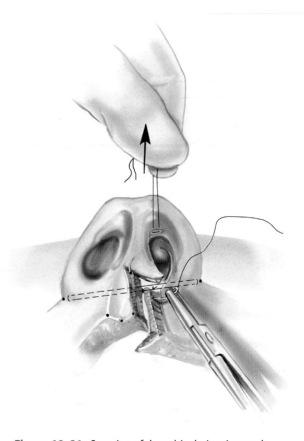

Figure 19–31. Suturing of the orbicularis oris muscle.

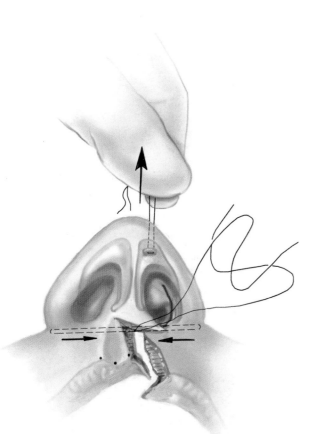

Figure 19–30. Alar base cinch stitch and alar cartilage tip sutures.

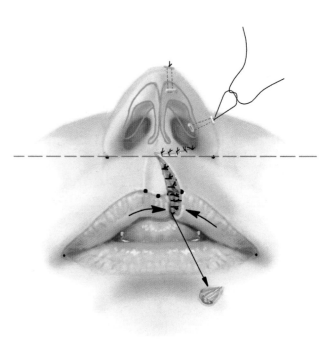

Figure 19–32. Suturing of the muscle and trimming excess vermillion.

This maneuver provides for a bloodless dissection and the appropriate release of the abnormally displaced orbicularis oris muscle in order to provide symmetric closure. Complete pre-periosteal release of the muscles facilitates complete reconstruction of the muscle of the lip.

Scissors are inserted through the incision of the cleft side alar base to dissect the skin from the lateral crus of the lower lateral cartilage (Fig. 19–25). The nasal lining, if distorted, is dissected as well from the lower lateral cartilage as necessary. The nasal lining is left attached, and never dissected at the region of the genu. The scissors are carried over the alar dome and into the subcutaneous pocket to be created from the medial nasal approach over the tip of the nose.

Attention is now turned to the medial lip and nasal tip. Tenotomy scissors are placed through the medial lip incision and used to subcutaneously dissect the nasal dome (Fig. 19–26). The scissors are inserted subcutaneously and between the medial crura, separating the skin of the nasal tip from the alar cartilage, and carried over the nasal dome. The medial lip is freed from the underlying skeleton, in a preperiosteal plane, using scissors. The skin over the noncleft side alar cartilage is likewise freed in order to shift the nose and gain equal projection of the ala cartilages at the tip (Fig. 19–27).

The mucosa is freed from the overlying muscle in the medial lip (Fig. 19–28). Through this approach, the noncleft

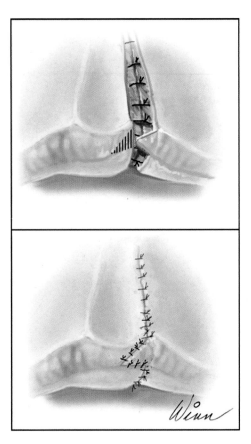

Figure 19–34. Dry vermilion flap of Noordhoff.

side alar base is exposed from below so that it can be sutured to the alar base on the cleft side. This is very important in obtaining alar base symmetry. If alar base symmetry is not achieved, then the suture is placed again until symmetry is obtained. This suture is important in bringing the cleft alar base into the proper position with the normal side.

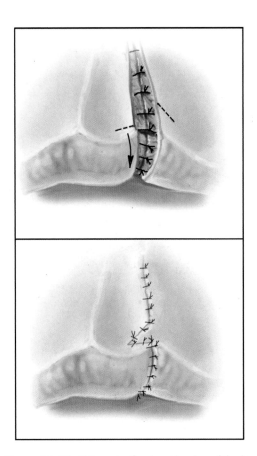

Figure 19–33. Triangular flap lengthening of the lip.

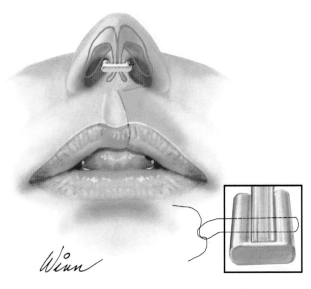

Figure 19–35. Placement of the postoperative silicone nasal stents.

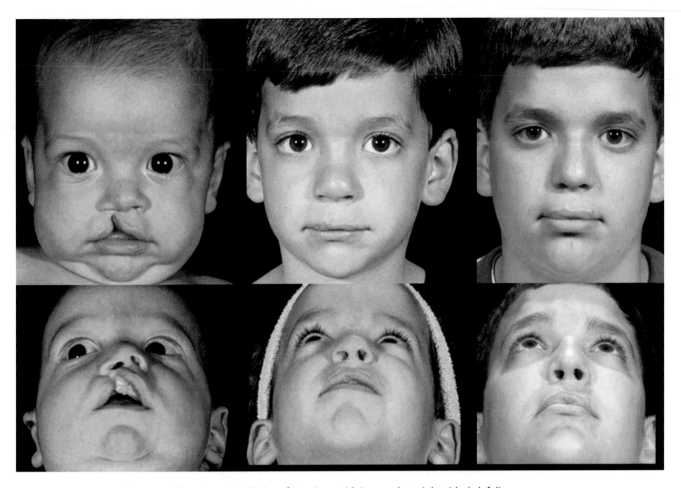

Figure 19–36. Series of a patient with incomplete right-sided cleft lip.

Through the exposure of the medial lip element below the muscle and above the periosteum, a 4-0-monocryl suture is placed in the normal alar base, and then the abnormal alar base is sutured to create alar base symmetry (Fig. 19–29). Symmetry is dependent on how tightly the suture is tied, and after placing the nasal tip sutures as shown in the following illustration (Fig. 19–30). The alar base cinch suture can alternately be placed through a superficial transdermal approach; however, we prefer the technique as described.

A 4-0 Prolene suture threaded on straight Keith needles is placed through a Dacron pledget and brought through the tip of the nose from inside out. While an assistant holds the nasal suture creating nasal tip symmetry, the alar base suture is tied and muscle sutures are placed, creating support for tip symmetry (see Fig. 19–30). The tip of the muscle of the lateral lip element is advanced medially and superior to the muscle of the medical lip element. It is sutured where the skin of the columella and new philtrum join at the corner of the medial skin incision (Fig. 19–31).

At the completion of the muscle repair with 3-0 and 4-0 chromic sutures, the orbicularis oris and marginalis have been positioned to provide symmetry of the lip as well as maintain projection of the nasal tip (see Fig. 19–31). The vermilion excess is trimmed until the proper volume to obtain a full lip remains, preventing notching of the free margin of the lip (Fig. 19–32). An additional suture of nylon over Dacron pledgets is placed through the lateral ala, correcting intra-nasal webbing and providing additional contouring and projection of the nasal tip.

Initiation of skin closure is begun with the nasal sill. The subdermis is closed with interrupted 6-0 PDS (Ethicon, Inc., Somerset, New Jersey). Mucosal closure is performed with a 4-0 chromic and 6-0 nylon is used for the skin closure. To diminish scarring, we utilize lip taping over the scar for 3 to 6 months postoperativelly[75]; and, we educate parents on how to massage the upper lip in hopes of preventing hypertrophic scarring and diminishing postoperative redness and inflammation.[76]

This technique can produce a consistently good result in the hands of experienced surgeons who may make modifications or alterations in each step of the operation as needed. Finally, it is probably better to delay primary nasal surgery if the surgeon and/or technique consistently produce a result with excessive scarring, vestibular stenosis, a small nostril, or any other recurrent deformity.

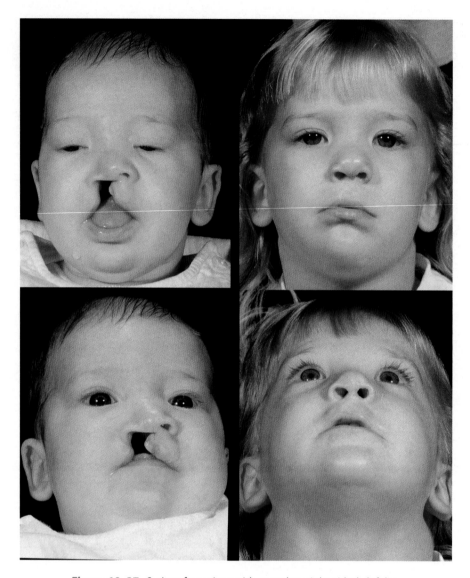

Figure 19–37. Series of a patient with complete right-sided cleft lip.

Triangular Skin Flap for Lengthening the Lip

When the peak of the Cupid's bow on the cleft side is too high (or short), an additional technique that provides lengthening of the lip can be performed (Fig. 19–33). This can be executed at the time of lip closure when the peak of Cupid's bow on the cleft side is not balanced and is short by 1 or 2 mm. The dotted lines in Fig. 19–33 demonstrate the design of the incisions, which create a triangular flap from the lateral lip element to be sutured into the medial lip element. The medial lip incision opens to receive the insertion of the lateral lip triangular flap, and this lengthens the lip on the cleft side. The triangular flap should be designed 3–4 mm above the white roll, and should not to be confused with a white roll flap, which I have found to be inadequate as compared to this technique. We have used this technique on the innumerable occasions finding it to be quite helpful. A variation of this, used by Bardach,[77] is planned at the time of initial marking, and utilizes a larger triangular flap.

Noordhoff's Vermilion Flap Technique

Another useful technique for matching the fullness of the wet and dry vermilion at the time of lip closure is Noordhoff's vermilion flap.[72] This is designed along the wet-line or red-line where the color change in the vermilion occurs between the wet and dry vermilion. Frequently, the vermilion cannot be adequately matched to maintain the width of both the wet and dry vermilion at the level of the peak of Cupid's bow, because the height of the vermilion is inadequate. To correct this mismatch, a triangular flap of dry vermilion is designed from the lateral lip element and sutured into an opening created in the medial vermilion along the wet-line (Fig. 19–34). This eliminates the vermilion color mismatch that occurs in the vermilion border that acts as an obvious visual indicator of an abnormal lip.

Postoperative Care

Six days postoperatively the lip and nose sutures are removed as well as the nasal pledgets. At that time, a silicone Koken

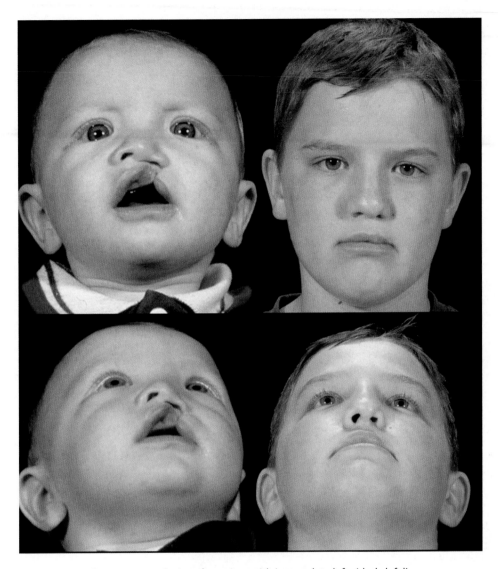

Figure 19–38. Series of a patient with incomplete left-sided cleft lip.

(Silimed) stent is sutured into the nose, carefully suturing it to the cartilaginous septum and not the membranous septum (Fig. 19–35). The silicone stent is maintained for 6 months, and compliant parents can provide proper daily cleaning. We believe this postoperative regimen decreases scarring and maintains the nasal reconstruction (Figs. 19–36 to 19–41).

Primary Lip/Nose with Vomer Flap Closure of the Anterior Palate

When operating without orthodontic support, such as when in a developing country performing mission surgery, primary lip and nose repair with the use of a vomer flap for anterior palate repair is recommended. Figure 19–42 demonstrates a complete cleft of the lip, nose, alveolus, and palate. This procedure is a combination of the primary Salyer-modified lip/nose repair, as described in this chapter, along with an anterior vomer flap at 3 months of age.

When orthodontic support is available, and the Dallas protocol is followed, the lip/nose repair is performed at 3 months of age. At 2 weeks of age, the infant is fitted with a palatal appliance to control the alveolar segments before and after the lip and nose are closed. In the Dallas protocol no attempt is made to close the alveolar segment at the time of the primary repair. This is left open until bone grafting at the age of 7–9 years of age. A palatal appliance cannot be used if this procedure is performed, and that is why it is recommended only when orthodontic support is not available.

This technique involves an anterior vomer flap, which is more easily performed when the lip and nose are open at the time of the primary repair. The proposed incisions are marked out as shown by dotted lines (Fig. 19–43). The lip and nose incision is the same as described above in the Salyer-modified rotation advancement repair. The incision begins medially, turning down a septal flap. This extends through the alveolus of the greater segment and along the junction of mucosa of the

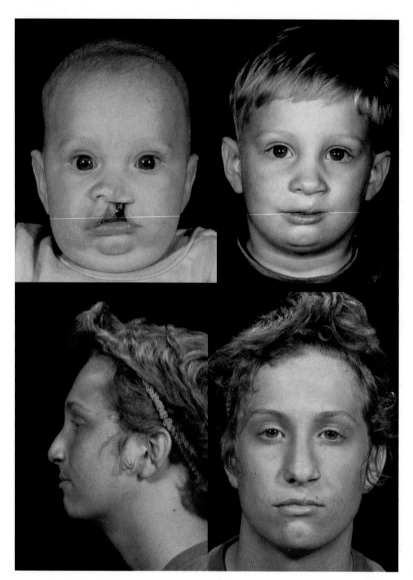

Figure 19–39. Series of a patient with complete left-sided cleft lip.

palate and vomer, to the end of the vomer (Fig. 19–44). The flaps are elevated with a periosteal elevator. The vomer flap is elevated and turned over like the page of the book, sutured beneath the edge of a hard palate mucoperiosteal flap elevated on the opposite side (Fig. 19–45). This technique closes the floor of the nose utilizing the septal flap, which is continuous with the vomer flap. This continuous flap provides closure of the floor of the nose and simultaneously closes the anterior palate and alveolus.

The final closure is shown in Fig. 19–45. Abyholm has used this technique as his primary mode of closure for the last 25 years.[77] This technique has a lot of appeal when resources are limited and has been proven to have good long-term outcomes when carefully executed by experienced surgeons.

COMMON SURGICAL ERRORS AND PITFALLS IN CLEFT SURGERY

Consistently achieving good results in primary cleft lip repair depends upon an in-depth understanding of the cleft lip/nose deformity. Suboptimal outcomes and/or secondary deformities may result from poor operative planning, operative errors, or postoperative scar contraction. Most secondary deformities arise from an inadequate appreciation of how to adequately release, reshape, and reconstruct the lip and nose while minimizing a detrimental scar.

One of the most common mistakes seen in secondary cases arises from the inadequate release of the abnormally attached lower lateral cartilage to the pyriform rim. Utilizing an incision just above the inferior turbinate is the easiest

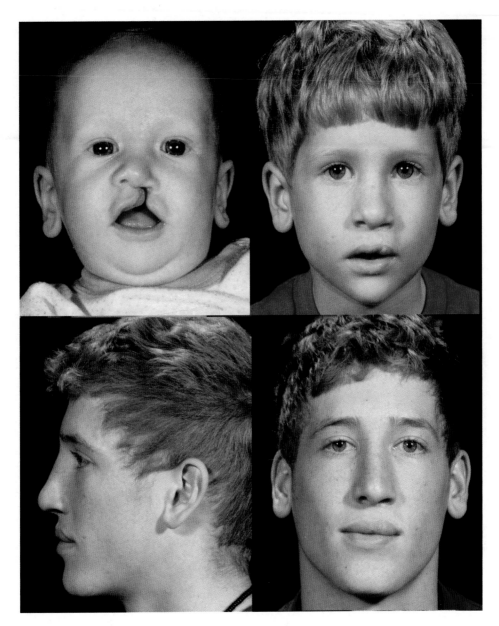

Figure 19–40. Series of a patient with complete left-sided cleft lip.

way to release the displaced alar cartilage from the pyriform rim and advance the alar cartilage to achieve tip projection and nasal symmetry. Another common and related mistake is the inadequate release and mobilization of the nasal lining. This is achieved by a cephalad extension of the incision above the inferior turbinate, allowing for proper mobilization of the alar cartilage and lining.[3] Many authors in my opinion incorrectly believe that the defect in the nasal lining, created by this incision and alar mobilization, should be lined with mucosal flaps from the medial lip paring or turbinate. The author believes that the additional scarring from this mucosal flap closure method may actually tether the alar cartilage instead of enabling mobilization of all the nasal elements. The sentinel concept is sufficient dissection for adequate mobilization of the cartilage.

Another cause of secondary deformities is tension on the primary lip closure. The basic tenet of a tension-free closure applies without exception to the lip repair. A mobile lip, allowing for a tension-free repair, is key in preventing facial growth retardation. If the lip closure is performed under tension, more scarring will result. It is our belief that raising mucoperiosteal flaps for cleft palate repair does not in itself cause significant sagittal growth abnormalities[68]; it does, however, cause alveolar collapse. It is also our belief that any excessive dissection in the space of Ernst will cause severe scarring in the pterygomaxillary region, and this will likely cause growth restriction in an anterior-posterior dimension.

The team approach to comprehensive cleft care is also important in preventing secondary deformities. The use of a interdisciplinary team, particularly integration of the

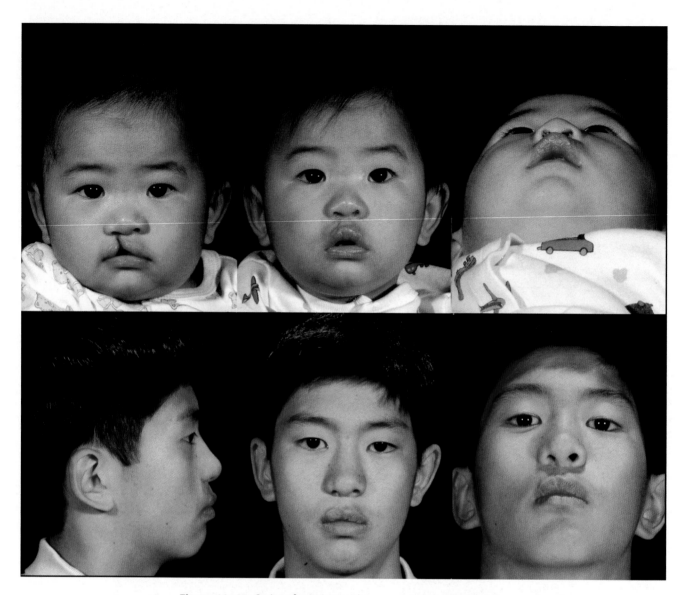

Figure 19–41. Series of a patient with incomplete left-sided cleft lip.

surgical and orthodontic care at critical points in the protocol is key for achieving the best results. Primary surgery without close and continuous orthodontic follow-up and intervention during growth will consistently produce poor results, no matter what surgical technique or protocol is used. Mission surgery, without developing a local team for ongoing surgical-orthodontic-speech treatment is a flawed concept and will not allow for delivery of the best possible result. Interdisciplinary management, with ongoing follow-up care during growth, is vital in all patients who have complete clefts of the lip and palate.[77]

CONCLUSION

Good to excellent results can consistently be achieved in the treatment of primary unilateral cleft lip/nose and palate deformity. The technique for correction of the unilateral cleft

lip and nose presented here, when properly executed and supported by a dedicated team, has resulted in good to excellent results for our Center. Over the years, modifications and improvements have led to improved symmetry, balance, and harmony of the face with less scarring. This technique, when employed by experienced surgeons, will yield consistent, predictable, and reproducible results for all patients with unilateral cleft lip/nose deformities. When treating patients with oro-facial clefts, the goal is normal function and appearance at conversational distance. The achievement of excellent soft tissue and bony restoration, optimized facial growth, and normal appearance and speech depends upon a surgical-orthodontic-speech oriented treatment plan over time. Cleft surgery, performed one time by a surgeon working alone, does not yield a long-term acceptable outcome, despite how good the repair looks postoperatively. In order to obtain excellent results using this primary lip-nose technique, a inter-disciplinary team approach, based on a long-term treatment

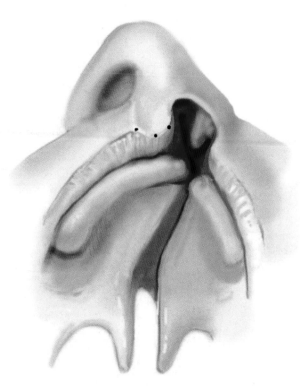

Figure 19–42. Dotted lines marking the primary lip/nose repair combined with vomer flap closure of the anterior palate.

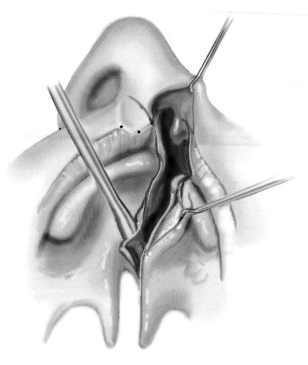

Figure 19–44. Subperiosteal dissection of the vomer flap and opposite hard palate mucoperiosteal flap.

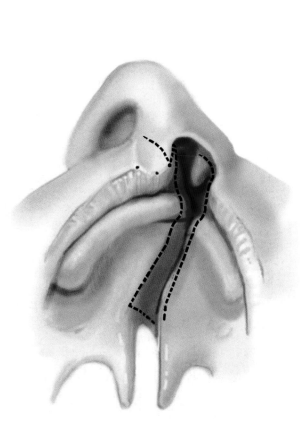

Figure 19–43. Incisions of the vomer flap closure of the anterior palate.

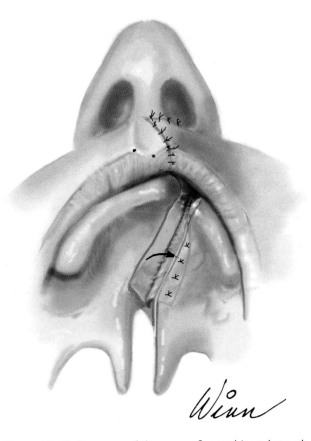

Figure 19–45. Turn-over of the vomer flap and inset beneath the edge of the opposite hard palate mucoperiosteal flap.

protocol, must be carried out until growth is complete. Despite the protocol followed or the technical talent of the surgeon, without ongoing team-oriented treatment after early primary surgery, and overall satisfactory result will not be achieved.

References

1. Salyer KE, Genecov ER, Genecov DG. Unilateral cleft lip-nose repair: a 33-year experience. *J Craniofac Surg* 14(4):549–558, 2003.
2. Millard DR, Jr. Earlier correction of the unilateral cleft lip nose. *Plast Reconstr Surg* 70(1):64–73, 1982.
3. Salyer KE. Early and late treatment of unilateral cleft nasal deformity. *Cleft Palate Craniofac J* 29(6):556–569, 1992.
4. Abyholm F, Salyer KE. *Achieving Excellence in Cleft Lip and Palate: Senior Surgeon's Experience and Protocols.* Oslo, Norway, 2005.
5. Ma KW. Hare-lip surgery in the history of traditional Chinese medicine. *Med Hist* 44:489–512, 2000.
6. Still JM Jr, Georgiade NG. Historical review of management of cleft lip and palate. In Georgiade NG (ed.). Symposium on Management of Cleft Lip and Palate and Associated Deformities. St Louis: CV Mosby, 1974, Chapter 3.
7. Pantaloni M, Byrd HS. Cleft lip I: Primary deformities. *Selected Readings in Plastic Surgery* 9(21):1–43, 2001.
8. Rose W. *Harelip and Cleft Palate.* London: HK Lewis, 1891.
9. Thompson JE. An artistic and mathematically accurate method of repairing the defect in cases of harelip. *Surg Gynecol Obstet* 14:498, 1912.
10. Malgaigne JF. *Manuel de Medecine Operatoire*, 7th edn. Paris: Germer Bailliere, 1861.
11. Mirault G. Deux letters sur l'operation du bec-de-lievre considere dans ses divers etats de simplicite et de complication. *J Chir* (Paris) 2:257, 1844.
12. Hagedorn W. Uber eine modifikation der hasenschartenoperation. *Zentralbl Chir* 11:756, 1884.
13. Blair VP, Brown JB. Mirault operation for single harelip. *Surg Gynaecol Obstet* 51:81, 1930.
14. Brown JB, McDowell F. Simplified design for repair of single cleft lip. *Surg Gynaecol Obstet* 80:12, 1945.
15. LeMesurier AB. Method of cutting and suturing lip in complete unilateral cleft lip. *Plast Reconstr Surg* 4:1, 1949.
16. Tennison CW. The repair of unilateral cleft lip by the stencil method. *Plast Reconstr Surg* 9:115, 1952.
17. Wynn SK. Lateral flap cleft lip surgery technique. *Plast Reconstr Surg* 26:509, 1960.
18. Davies D. The one-stage repair of unilateral cleft lip and palate: A preliminary report. *Plast Reconstr Surg* 38:129, 1966.
19. Millard DR, Jr. A primary camouflage of the unilateral harelook. In Skoog T (ed.). *Transactions of the First International Congress of Plastic Surgery, Stockholm, 1955.* Baltimore: Williams & Wilkins, 1957, pp. 160–166.
20. Randall P. History of cleft lip nasal repair. *Cleft palate Craniofac J* 29(6):527–530, 1992.
21. Joseph J. Operative reduction of the size of a nose (rhinomoisis). *Berl Klin Wochenschr* 40:882, 1898.
22. Gillies HD, Kilner TP. Harelip operation for the correction of secondary deformities. *Lancet* 223:1369, 1932.
23. Erich JB. A technique for correcting a flat nostril in cases of repaired harelip. *Plast Reconstr Surg* 12:322, 1953.
24. Berkeley WT. The cleft-lip nose. *Plast Reconstr Surg* 23:567–575, 1959.
25. Brophy TW. *Cleft Lip and Palate.* Philadelphia: P Blakiston, 1923.
26. Humby G. The nostril in secondary hare-lip. *Lancet* 234:1276, 1938.
27. Byars L. Surgical correction of nasal deformities. *Surg Gynaecol Obstet* 84:65–78, 1947.
28. McIndoe A, Rees TD. Synchronous repair of secondary deformities in cleft lip nose. *Plast Reconstr Surg* 24:150–161, 1959.
29. McComb H. Treatment of the unilateral cleft lip nose. *Plast Reconstr Surg* 55:596–601, 1975.
30. Anderl H. Simultaneous repair of lip and nose in the unilateral cleft (a long term report). In Jackson IT, Sommerlad BC (eds). *Recent Advances in Plastic Surgery*, Vol 3. Edinburgh: Churchill-Livingstone, 1985, p. 1.
31. Salyer KE. Primary correction of the unilateral cleft lip nose: A 15-year experience. *Plast Reconstr Surg* 77:558–566, 1986.
32. McComb H. Primary correction of unilateral cleft lip nasal deformity: A 10-year review. *Plast Reconstr Surg* 75:791, 1985.
33. Sugihara T, Yoshida T, Igawa HH, Homma K. Primary correction of the unilateral cleft lip nose. *Cleft Palate Craniofacial J* 30:231, 1993.
34. McComb H, Coghlan BA. Primary repair of the unilateral cleft lip nose: Completion of a longitudinal study. *Cleft Palate Craniofac J* 33:23, 1996.
35. Byrd HS, Salomon J. Primary correction of the unilateral cleft nasal deformity. *Plast Reconstr Surg* 106(6):1276–1286, 2000.
36. Salyer KE, Genecov ER, Genecov DG. Unilateral cleft lip-nose repair—long-term outcome. *Clin Plast Surg* 31(2):191–208, 2004.
37. Randall P, Whitaker LA, LaRossa D. The importance of muscle reconstruction in primary and secondary cleft lip repair. *Plast Reconstr Surg* 54:316, 1974.
38. Kernahan DA. Muscle repair in unilateral cleft lip, based on findings on electrical stimulation. *Ann Plast Surg* 1:48, 1978.
39. Nicolau PJ. The orbicularis oris muscle: A functional approach to its repair in the cleft lip. *Br J Plast Surg* 36:141, 1983.
40. Park CG, Ha B. The importance of accurate repair of the orbicularis oris muscle in the correction of unilateral cleft lip. *Plast Reconstr Surg* 96:780, 1995.
41. Kernahan DA, Dado DV, Bauer BS. The anatomy of the orbicularis oris muscle in unilateral cleft lip based on a three-dimensional histologic reconstruction. *Plast Reconstr Surg* 73:875, 1984.
42. De Mey A, Van Hoof I, De Roy G, Lejour M. Anatomy of the orbicularis oris muscle in cleft lip. *Br J Plast Surg* 42:710, 1989.
43. Latham RA. The septopremaxillary ligament and maxillary development. *J Anat* 104:584, 1969.
44. Bardach J, Cutting C. Pathogenesis of the cleft lip nasal deformity. In Bardach J, Hughlett LM (eds). *Multidisciplinary Management of Cleft Lip and Palate.* Philadelphia: WB Saunders, 1990.
45. Bardach J, Cutting C. Nasal deformity associated with unilateral clefts. In Bardach J, Hughlett LM (eds). *Multidisciplinary Management of Cleft Lip and Palate.* Philadelphia: WB Saunders, 1990.
46. McComb H. Primary correction of unilateral cleft lip-nose deformity: A 10 year review. *Plast Reconstr Surg* 77:558, 1986.
47. Johanson B, Ohlsson A. Osteoplasty in the late treatment of harelip and cleft palate. *Langenbecks Arch Klin Chir Ver Dtsch Z Chir* 295:876–880, 1960.
48. Randall P. A lip adhesion operation in cleft lip surgery. *Plast Reconstr Surg* 35:371–376, 1965.
49. Seibert RW. Lip adhesion in bilateral cleft lip. *Arch Otolaryngol* 109(7):434–436, 1983.
50. Millard D. *Cleft Craft: The Evolution of its Surgery.* Vols. 1–3. Boston: Little, Brown, and co., 1980.
51. Burt JD, Byrd HS. Cleft lip: unilateral primary deformities. *Plast Reconstr Surg* 105(3):1043–1055, 2000; quiz 1056–1057.
52. Cho B. Unilateral complete cleft lip and palate repair using lip adhesion and passive alveolar molding appliance. *J Craniofac Surg* 12(2):148–156, 2001.
53. Pool R. Tissue mobilization with preoperative lip taping. *Oper Tech Plast Reconstr Surg* 2:155–158, 1995.
54. Hallock GG. In utero cleft lip repair in A/J mice. *Plast Reconstr Surg* 75(6):785–790, 1985.
55. Longaker MT, Stern M, Lorenz P, et al. A model for fetal cleft lip repair in lambs. *Plast Reconstr Surg* 90(5):750–756, 1992.
56. Ortiz-Monasterio F. Personal communication, 1990.
57. Boon L, Manicourt D, Marbaix E, et al. A comparative analysis of healing of surgical cleft lip corrected in utero and neonates. *Plast Reconstr Surg* 89(1):11–17, 1992; discussion 18–20.

58. Kapp-Simon KA. Psychological issues in cleft lip and palate. *Clin Plast Surg* 31(2):347–352, 2004.

59. Delaire J. Theoretical principles and technique of functional closure of the lip and nasal aperture. *J Maxillofac Surg* 6(2):109–116, 1978.

60. Fevre M. Treatment of harelip by the Victor Veau technic completed by a naris plasty. *Presse Med* 73:1761–1762, 1965.

61. Mannucci N, D'Orto O, Bigliolo F, Brusati R. Comparison of the effect of supraperiosteal versus subperiosteal dissection on the growing rabbit maxilla. *Cleft Palate Craniofac J* 39(1):36–39, 2002.

62. Bardach J, Kelly KM, Salyer KE. A comparative study of facial growth following lip and palate repair performed in sequence and simultaneously: An experimental study in beagles. *Plast Reconstr Surg* 91(6):1008–1016, 1993.

63. Shetye PR. Facial growth of adults with unoperated clefts. *Clin Plast Surg* 31(2):361–371, 2004.

64. Berkowitz S, Mejia M, Bystrik A. A comparison of the effects of the Latham-Millard procedure with those of a conservative treatment approach for dental occlusion and facial aesthetics in unilateral and bilateral complete cleft lip and palate: Part I. Dental occlusion. *Plast Reconstr Surg* 113(1):1–18, 2004.

65. Ortiz-Monasterio F, Rebeil AS, Valderrama M, et al. Cephalometric measurements on adult patients with non-operated cleft palates. *Plast Reconstr Surg* 24(1):53–61, 1959.

66. Weinzweig J, Panter KE, Seki J, Pantaloni M, Spangenberger A, Harper JS. The fetal cleft palate: IV. Midfacial growth and bony palatal development following in utero and neonatal repair of the congenital caprine model. *Plast Reconstr Surg* 118(1):81–93, 2006.

67. Talmant JC, Lumineau JP. Therapeutic approach to cleft lip-maxilla-palate: for normal facial growth. A protocol and various technics to restore nasal respiration. *Orthod Fr* 75(4):297–319, 2004.

68. Salyer KE, Sng KW, Sperry EE. Two-flap palatoplasty: 20-year experience and evolution of surgical technique. *Plast Reconstr Surg* 118(1):193–204, 2006.

69. Millard DR, Latham R. Improved primary surgical and dental treatment of clefts. *Plast Reconstr Surg* 86(5):856–871, 1990.

70. Millard DR, Latham R, Huifen X, Spiro S, Morovic C. Cleft lip and palate treated by perisurgical orthopedics, gingivoperiosteoplasty, and lip adhesion (POPLA) compared with previous lip adhesion method: A preliminary study of serial dental casts. *Plast Reconstr Surg* 103(6):1630–1644, 1999.

71. Fara M. The importance of folding down muscle stumps in the operation of unilateral clefts of the lip. *Acta Chir Plast* 13(3):162–169, 1971.

72. Noordhoff MS. Reconstruction of vermilion in unilateral and bilateral cleft lips. *Plast Reconstr Surg* 73(1):52–61, 1984.

73. Noordhoff MS, Chen YR, Chen KT, et al. The surgical technique for the complete unilateral cleft lip-nasal deformity. *Oper Tech Plast Reconstr Surg* 2:167–174, 1995.

74. Noordhoff MS. Personal communication, 1992.

75. Atkinson JA, et al. A randomized, controlled trial to determine the efficacy of paper tape in preventing hypertrophic scar formation in surgical incisions that traverse Langer's skin tension lines. *Plast Reconstr Surg* 116(6):1648–1656, 2005; discussion 1657–1658.

76. Dumas P, Freidel M, Trepsat F. The labial scar of hare lip. Technic and usefulness of early and prolonged postoperative massage. *J Fr Otorhinolaryngol Audiophonol Chir Maxillofac* 26(9):679–681, 1977.

77. Bardach J, Salyer KE. *Surgical Techniques in Cleft Lip and Palate*, 2nd edn. St. Louis, MO: Mosby-Year Book, 1991.

20

Bilateral Cleft Lip and Nose Repair

Philip Kuo-Ting Chen, MD • M. Samuel Noordhoff, MD

INTRODUCTON

The reconstruction of a symmetrically balanced bilateral cleft lip and natural looking nose with adequate columellar length is a difficult challenge. The surgical technique at the

Chang Gung Craniofacial Center has evolved over a period of 30 years. The more common approach was a two stage operation, including a primary lip repair and secondary elongation of the columella.[1–10] An evaluation of 140 complete bilateral clefts, using a staged cheiloplasty with elongation of

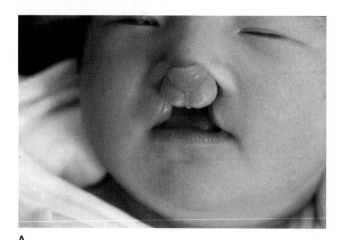

A

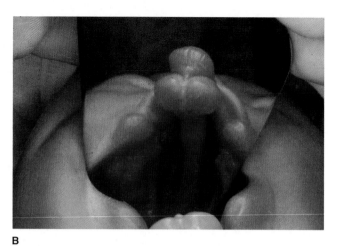

B

Figure 20–1. A newborn with bilateral complete cleft lip and palate.

the columella utilizing four different methods, was reported in 1986.[11] The best results were obtained with the VY open tip approach, which had the disadvantage of leaving a scar on the nasal tip (Figs. 20–1A, B and 20–2 A, B). A one stage cheiloplasty, with primary elongation of the columella by dissecting the prolabium as a pedicled flap on the columellar vessels and rotating the forked flaps superiorly to elongate the columella, was discontinued as being too complicated.[12] More recently, a one staged primary reconstruction of lip and nose, in one procedure, has been advocated and made possible with presurgical nasoalveolar molding (NAM). Trott and Mohan[13] advocated an open rhinoplasty approach with the elevated prolabial flap for approximation of the alar domes. Mulliken[14] reconstructed the nose with intranasal and nasal tip incisions, allowing for the approximation of the splayed lower lateral cartilages (LLC) that results in an accentuation of the columella. Cutting,[15] using presurgical NAM to stretch the columella, advanced the prolabial complex to expose the crus of the LLC, allowing for them to be sutured together for elongation of the columella. Chen and Noordhoff[16] recently

reported the results of a modified Trott approach, and this has led to the present technique of lip and nose repair.

GENERAL PLAN OF MANAGEMENT

Ideally, the initial visit, with a newborn cleft child, is soon as possible after birth. The pediatrician does the initial examination; and basic studies, including dental casts, photographs, and classification of the cleft, are done by the rest of the team. The use of a double-Y numbered classification was initially reported in 1990[17] (Fig. 20–3). This classification provides a numerical means of defining any cleft, and is adaptable for use in computer programs. The family history is obtained and genetic counseling provided. Hands-on counseling regarding feeding is given, and videotapes of the treatment plan are provided. The parents are introduced to parent support groups that explain the course of treatment and help them understand their role in the treatment of their infant. The orthodontist and plastic surgeon carefully

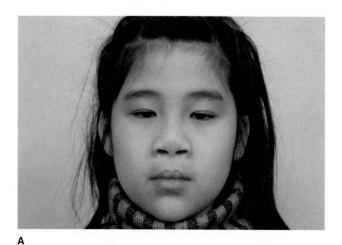

A

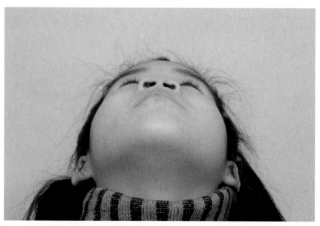

B

Figure 20–2. Patient in Fig. 20–1 at 7 years of age. The lip and nose were repaired with the technique reported in 1986.

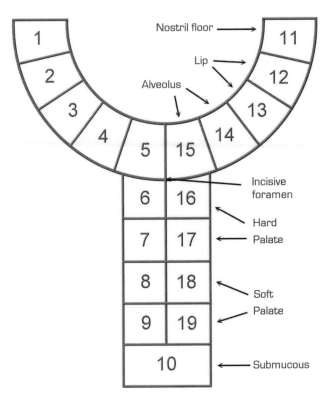

Figure 20–3. A double-Y classification allows for detailed numerical classification of all types of unilateral and bilateral clefts.

examine the infant's cleft, and record details of alveolar segment position and tissue deficiencies. A small premaxilla, deficient vomer, and absence of a frenulum should be noted to rule out median facial dysplasia, as these infants all have severe growth disturbances.[18] Careful recording of tissue deficiencies is helpful in assessing postoperative results. The comprehensive treatment plan is developed and explained to the parents.

Presurgical NAM is started on the first visit. The aim of this molding process is to centralize the premaxilla, narrow alveolar gaps, achieve symmetry of the alar cartilages, and elongate the columella. This process takes 3 to 4 months in order to achieve an optimal outcome, and at this time, the surgery is performed. The timing of the primary lip and nose surgery is also dependent upon the general nutrition and growth of the infant; typically, the infant should be gaining weight, as this is an indication of their general condition. The palate is repaired at approximately 12 months of age, together with insertion of myringotomy tubes when indicated. In our Center, speech assessment is started at 2.5 years of age; and should the patient require speech therapy, it is started at 3.5 years. Velopharyngeal insufficiency (VPI), when diagnosed, is confirmed by nasoendoscopy at 4 years of age, and surgically corrected before the child goes to school. Residual alveolar clefts are closed before eruption of the canine teeth, usually around 9 to 11 years of age. Whenever the patient has psychological problems related to any residual lip or nasal deformity, a revision may be performed; and in our experience, this usually will not be until adolescence.

PRESURGICAL NAM

The key deformities of the bilateral cleft lip include: (1) a protruding/deviated premaxilla with relatively retro-positioned lateral maxillary segments, and (2) shortness of the columellar height with a nasal tip tethered to the prolabium. Approximating the orbicularis muscles from the lateral lip in front of the premaxilla is technically difficult and may result in excess pressure contributing to maxillary retrusion. The nasal shape after a primary lip repair without presurgical orthopedics results in a wide flat nose with inverted nostril axes and a broad nasal tip. The purpose of presurgical NAM is to restore a more normal nasal shape and a balanced skeletal base. The following techniques have all been used in the Chang Gung Craniofacial Center over the past 10 years.

Presurgical Orthopedics

The simplest type of presurgical orthopedics is to apply micropore tape across the lip, with or without traction rubber bands.[19] Having the child sleep on his side, if approved by the pediatrician, also facilitates closure of the cleft.[20] Significant movement of the alveolar segments may be controlled by an acrylic plate. This technique can be utilized in most situations; and is effective in expanding prolabial tissue, and placing the premaxilla in a centralized position[10,11] However, an acrylic plate alone will neither change the nasal morphology nor elongate the columella.

NAM: Grayson's Technique

A passive type of orthopedic appliance is used in coordination with taping of the lip for premaxilla and alveolar molding. Molding the premaxilla into a proper position is initially done, followed by narrowing the alveolar gap. The nasal molding is achieved with a nasal molding device added to the orthopedic appliance. This will lengthen the columella and reshape the alar domes. Tape placed across the upper lip also acts as a lip-adhesion that decreases the width of the nasal base.[21–24]

NAM: Figueroa's Technique

An acrylic plate with a rigid acrylic nasal extension is used to simultaneously achieve satisfactory nasal molding and to reposition the premaxilla backward. Gentle traction of the premaxilla is accomplished with rubber bands connected to the acrylic ball attached to the acrylic plate.[25]

NAM: Liou's Technique[26]

Dental adhesive is used to fix an acrylic dental plate on the maxillary segments. An attached nasal component, made of paired curved stainless steel wires and soft acrylic bulbs on its ends, projects forward and upward bilaterally from the dental plate. The dental plate molds the maxillary segments, and the attached acrylic bulb, positioned beneath the nasal cartilages, molds the nasal cartilages. Micropore tape, placed across the lip, retracts the premaxilla, positions the alar base medially, narrows the alveolar cleft, and helps to give the nose a good configuration. The columella is lengthened by simultaneously pushing the premaxilla backward, as well as, pushing the nasal tip forward. Retraction of the premaxilla and elongation of the columella are done at the same time. The key point is to push the alar domes forward in a sagittal direction for columellar lengthening, instead of a cephalic direction, which results in an up-turned nasal tip. This technique requires follow-up evaluations and adjustments to the device and protocol, every 1 to 2 weeks.

GENERAL SURGICAL PRINCIPLES

Key general surgical principles apply to all cleft surgery,[27] and these include: (1) an understanding of the embryological development and anatomy, (2) an understanding of the nature of the deformity to be corrected, (3) an awareness of the different surgical procedures and their limitations, (4) the use of an atraumatic surgical technique with delicate handling of tissues, sharp dissection and careful hemostasis, (5) limited dissection to avoid surgical trauma to adjacent tissues, (6) knowledge of the healing process, (7) having an alternate plan for complications or unexpected difficulties at the time of surgery, and (8) possessing an understanding and awareness of the problems related to anesthesia as well as pre- and postoperative surgical care.

KEY SURGICAL CONCEPTS

The surgical concepts for bilateral cleft lip and nose repair are as follows: (1) Preserve the presurgical columella length, (2) Keep the prolabial width narrow without compromising blood supply, (3) Advance the prolabial columella complex superiorly to allow for muscle reconstruction in front of the premaxilla, (4) Release of the LLC from its attachment to the upper lateral cartilage (ULC), (5) Reposition the LLC superiorly and reattach it to the ULC, (6) Perform limited dissection on the maxilla above the periosteum, (7) Assure closure of the pyriform area with mucosal flaps that also reconstruct the nostril floor, (8) Reconstruct the prolabial buccal sulcus with prolabial mucosal flaps, (9) Reconstruct the orbicularis muscle and attach it to the anterior nasal spine, (10) Reconstruct a new Cupid's bow with central vermilion and lip tubercle with lateral orbicularis oris marginalis (om) flaps, (11) Balance the height of both lateral lips without incisions around the ala, (12) Maintain the presurgical nasolabial angle, and (13) Accentuate the nasal tip and columellar length with the Tajima procedure.[28]

SURGICAL PROCEDURE

Markings and Measurements

The landmarks of the lip are marked out on the prolabium and lateral segments (Fig. 20–4). The measurements are evaluated

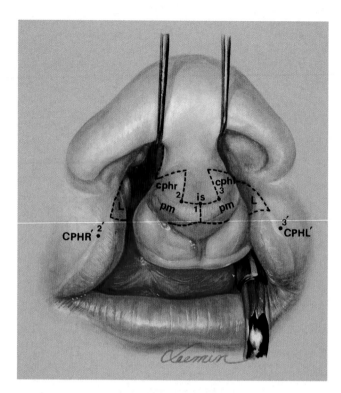

Figure 20–4. Preoperative markings: Point *is-1* is the central point of the Cupid's bow. The lateral points of the Cupid's bow, on the right side (*cphr-2*) and the left side (*cphr-3*) are made to keep the total width of the Cupid's bow at a maximum distance of 4–5 mm. The vertical limbs extend to the base of the columella with the base narrowed to 3–4 mm wide. Points *cphr'2'* and *cphl'3'* are the anatomical points for the base of the philtral column on the lateral lip. These points are approximately 3–4 mm lateral to the converging red-line (the junction of dry vermilion and wet mucosa) and the WSR. This point is usually where the vermilion first becomes it's widest. The prolabial mucosa, *pm*, is used for reconstruction of the nostril floor. The central part of the prolabial mucosa is used for lining the premaxilla. The L flap is elevated from the free edge of the lateral lip and is based on the maxilla.

for symmetry. The width between cphl (left lateral point of cupid's bow) and cphr (right lateral point of cupid's bow) is usually maintained at 4–5 mm. The vertical limbs are straight lines on the prolabium from cphl and cphr, narrowed to a 3–4 mm width at the base of the columella and never extending lateral to the columella. The proposed peak of the Cupid's bow, on the lateral lip, is an anatomical point that is identified and marked.[29] Discrepancies of horizontal and vertical dimensions of the lateral lips should be noticed and recorded for surgical correction as well as the postoperative assessment of results (Fig. 20–4).

Prolabium

A double hook retracts the columella upwards defining the columella lip angle (Fig. 20–4), while a small single hook or a fingertip stabilizes the prolabium for an accurate incision on marked lines. A No. 11 blade is used to make the horizontal and vertical incisions on the prolabium—from point to point. The skin and mucosa (pm), lateral to the vertical

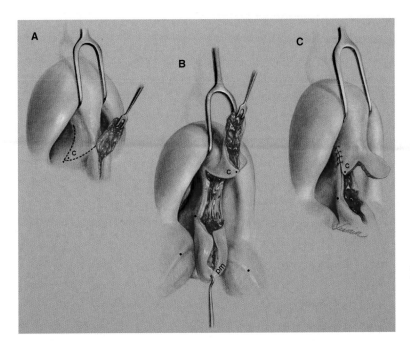

Figure 20–5. Prolabial incisions are extended to point *c* on the premaxilla and continued at the junction of skin and membranous septum to the apex of the upper crus of the LLC (A, B). This prolabial-columellar complex is advanced and sutured in it's elevated position (C). The tip of the *c* flap is inserted posteriorly to maintain the angle of the columella and prolabium (also see Figure 20–9A-B).

incision of the prolabium, is left attached to the premaxilla for reconstruction of the nostril floor (Fig. 20–5A, B). The incision is extended on the premaxilla to point c and continues onto the skin-mucosal junction of the septum behind the columella to the alar domes (Fig. 20–5A-B). This central prolabial-columellar complex is advanced cephalically and sutured into its new-elevated position (Fig. 20–5C). The central part of the prolabial mucosa (pm) is used for lining the lower half of the premaxilla for a buccal alveolar sulcus (Figs. 20–6 and 20–7B). The lateral prolabial mucosa flaps (pm) are used for nasal floor reconstruction (Fig. 20–7B).

Lateral Lip Segments

The incision extends from points cphr' and cphl' along the cleft edge down to the alveolus leaving a 1 mm white skin roll (WSR) for the om flap that is used to reconstruct a new Cupid's bow (Fig. 20–8). An L-mucosal flap is elevated on the cleft edge based on the maxilla. The incision extends along the pyriform rim to the inferior turbinate. The inferior turbinate flap (T) is elevated based on the vestibular skin and the fibrous attachments to the pyriform rim are released (Fig. 20–7). The dissection is extended superiorly to free the fibrous attachments between the LLC and the pyriform rim, as well as the ULC. This allows for elevation and repositioning of the LLC superiorly and reattachment of the LLC to the ULC in an elevated position. The dissection of the orbicularis peripheralis muscle (op) is limited to 2 mm on the mucosal side. The dissection of the op on the skin side is more extensive, extending from cphl' and cphr' to the alar base ipsilaterally. The dissection is then carried beyond the alar base to release the abnormal muscle components that insert into the alar base. This dissection also allows the muscle fibers to be released and gain vertical length to the lateral lip.

Nasal Floor Reconstruction

The T flap my not be necessary in narrow clefts. For moderate to wide clefts it provides a lining in the pyriform area preventing scar contraction. The LLC has been elevated and reattached to the ULC (Fig. 20–7 A). The T flap is rotated 90 degrees attaching it to the vestibular skin and pyriform

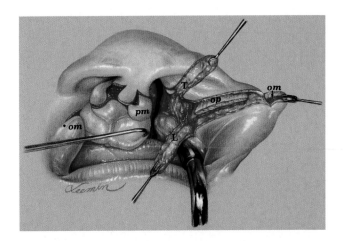

Figure 20–6. The L flap has been elevated from the free border of the lateral lip. The *om* flap is pared from the free border of the lateral lip to create the base of the philtral column. It consists of a 1 mm wide WSR, fibers of the orbicularis oris marginalis muscle, dry vermilion anteriorly, and wet mucosa posteriorly. It is used to reconstruct a new Cupid's bow. The orbicularis oris peripheralis muscle (*op*) is released from the mucosa for a distance of 2 mm and from the skin at the base of the lateral philtral column to the ala. The prolabial mucosal flap (*pm*) is used for nostril floor reconstruction. The T flap is elevated from the inferior turbinate based on the vestibular skin. The fibrous attachments to the pyriform rim at the level of the inferior turbinate and the fibrous attachments between the LLC and ULC are released allowing the LLC to be repositioned superiorly.

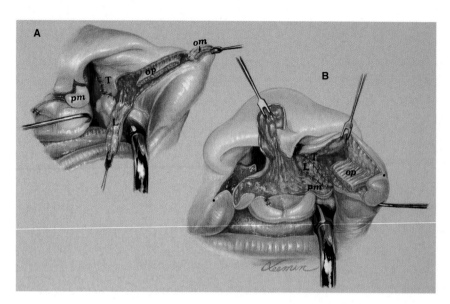

Figure 20–7. The T flap has been rotated into the pyriform area and sutured to the rim of the maxilla and vestibular skin (A). The L flap is advanced and sutured to the apex of the premaxilla and the septum (B). The edge of the T flap is sutured to the L flap. The prolabial flap (*pm*) is sutured laterally to the L flap and maxilla. This creates a complete closure of all operative areas and gives good support for the ala (B).

rim. The L flap is brought across the cleft and sutured to the base of the septal incision to reconstruct the nasal floor (Fig. 20–7B). The inferior margin of the T flap is sutured to the superior margin of the L flap. The pm flap is sutured to the L flap and maxilla providing complete coverage of the nasal floor and pyriform area and support for the ala. Excess tissue of the pm flap is trimmed to avoid redundancy of tissues in the upper sulcus. The vestibulum of the alar base is advanced and sutured to the T and L flap with special emphasis on the width of the nostril. It is very important that the alar base is turned inwards as a flaring open alar is very unattractive.

Muscle Reconstruction

The orbicularis peripheralis muscle and mucosa are approximated in one layer with 4–0 Polyglactin mattress sutures. The upper edge of the muscle is sutured to the caudal edge of the nasal septum (Fig. 20–8).

Cupid's Bow Reconstruction

The skin flap of the prolabium is sutured to the lateral lip with the key suture between points cphl-cphl' and cphr-cphr'. Lateral om flaps are trimmed according to the width of the Cupid's bow leaving a slight excess to form the central tubercle. The skin is closed with 7–0 polyglactin sutures (Figs. 20–9C, and 20–10A).

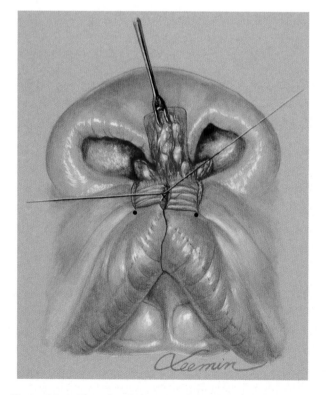

Figure 20–8. The orbicularis oris peripheralis muscle is approximated along with the mucosa posteriorly, and the upper edge of the muscle is attached to the nasal septum.

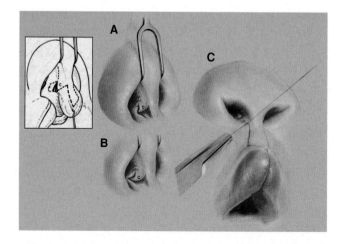

Figure 20–9. The tip of the remaining upper flap is inserted into a back cut on the mucosa at the base of septum and premaxilla, to hold the prolabial-columella junction posteriorly and to accentuate the columella-prolabial angle.

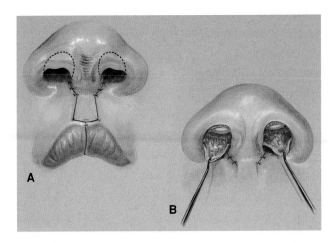

Figure 20–10. Markings are shown for a bilateral Tajima procedure to elongate the columella. This exposes the leading edge of the LLC. Direct visualization of the LLC allows for dissection of the LLC from each side and release of the fibrofatty tissue between and above the LLC.

Restoration of Nasolabial Angle and Nasal Floor

The upper edge of the flap c, is sutured into a back cut on the nasal septum to restore the nasolabial angle and hold it in its proper position (Fig. 20–9A, B). Excess tissue of the nasal floor is trimmed to give a nostril sill and adequate nasal width, around 18–20 mm (Fig. 20–9C).

Nasal Reconstruction

Tajima[28] incisions are made on both alar rims (Fig. 20–10A). The skin is dissected by sharp dissection to expose the leading edge of the LLC (Fig. 20–10B). The LLC's are dissected under direct vision to release all the fibrofatty tissue from between and above the LLC's (Fig. 20–11). The fibrofatty tissue on the nasal tip is brought to the top of the LLC's (Fig. 20–12 insert). The separated LLC's are approximated with 5–0 poly-

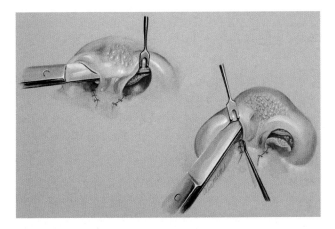

Figure 20–11. The LLC's are identified, and dissection above the LLC releases the fibrofatty tissue from between and above the medial and upper crus of the LLC's. The fibrofatty tissue is displaced above the LLC.

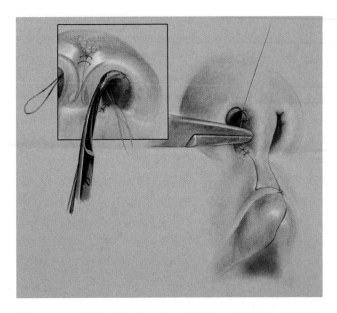

Figure 20–12. The fibrofatty tissue is shown positioned above the LLC's. Mattress sutures of 5–0 Polydioxanone tuck the skin from the Tajima incision behind the columella elongating the columella and supporting the medial crus of the LLC. Any excess skin is excised from the rim of the nostril and the incision closed with 5–0 vicryl sutures.

dioxanone mattress sutures. The approximation of the LLC's with the mattress sutures turns the skin inwards and elongates the columella. The excess tissue at the rim of the nostril is trimmed (Fig. 20–12). The rim incision is closed with 5–0 Polyglactin sutures. Alar transfixion sutures (ATS) (Fig. 20–13) using 5–0 Polydioxanone sutures are placed to accentuate the alar–facial groove, minimize vestibular webbing and support the LLC.[27] The final result (Fig. 20–13) shows the mattress sutures between the LLC, the fat above the LLC's, skin closure, and the reconstruction of a new Cupid's bow.

Postoperative Care

Suture lines are regularly cleaned with normal saline and antibiotic ointment is applied without a dressing to keep blood clots from forming. The sutures are removed in 5–7 days. Micropore tapes, as well as silicone sheets support the lip incisions, for 6 months. A silicone conformer for the nostrils is utilized for 6–9 months. During this period of time, the child continues to grow; however, changing to a larger silicone conformer is not recommended, as it tends to widen the nostrils. Increased height of the conformer is achieved by gradually adding silicone sheets to the domes of the conformer every 1–2 months (Fig. 20–14).

▌ DISCUSSION

Comparison of Molding Techniques

The simplest type of presurgical orthopedics is the use of micropore tape when there is no orthodontist available. It

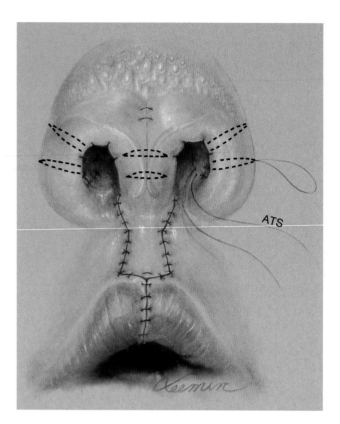

Figure 20–13. The skin incisions are closed with 7–0 absorbable sutures. The *om* flaps have been trimmed and closed with interrupted sutures. There is a clean continuous WSR and paralleling red line, the junction of dry vermillion and wet mucosa. This produces a central tubercle and full central lip with adequate vermillion. Alar Transfixion Sutures (ATS) are placed to accentuate the ala-facial groove, to support the LLC, and to minimize vestibular webbing.

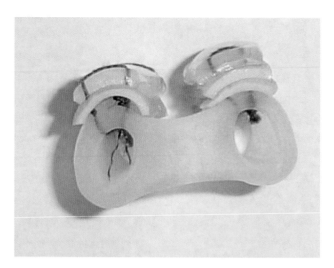

Figure 20–14. A silicone conformer, with silicone sheets added on the dome area, is used for maintenance and further elongation of the columella after the operation. The height of the dome can be adjusted for correction of minor asymmetry.

will expand the tissue on the prolabium and allow for better positioning of the premaxilla but does nothing for nostril molding.[10] A comparison of the three different types of NAM in unilateral clefts showed the Grayson method achieving the best nasal shape, symmetry and skeletal balance.[30] The other techniques of Liou and Figueroa resulted in a larger diameter of the nostril. There was no comparison of the three techniques in bilateral clefts. All methods have been satisfactorily used for bilateral clefts in the Chang Gung Craniofacial Center. Grayson's[22–24] technique produces a closer approximation of the alveolar segments; however, is more time consuming and expensive. Liou's[26] and Figueroa's.[25] methods simultaneously approximate the alveolar segments and elongate the columella. Liou's method achieves a satisfactory approximation of the alveolus, relative retropositioning of the premaxilla, and elongation of the columella. It is cost effective, takes less time, and is easy to accomplish.

Central Segment–Prolabium Width and Length

In the surgical technique without muscle approximation, the central lip tends to become wider and remains vertically short. With muscle approximation, the central lip will have less

widening and more vertical lengthening overt time. Despite beginning with a small prolabium, the lip ultimately will never be short. Noordhoff,[12] attempting primary elongation of columella, interdigitated forked flaps above a prolabial flap based on the columellar vessels. He noted there were always two vessels from the columella supporting the prolabium; however, an extremely narrow central prolabial segment, at the base of the columella, may present a higher risk of compromised blood supply to the prolabium. A width of 3–4 mm, at the base of the columella, and 4–5 mm at points cphr and cphl, will give a proper proportioned central lip segment. Previous reported techniques of central segment reconstruction resulted in an unnaturally wide Cupid's bow,[10,11] and elongation of the prolabium, as described by Cutting, produces an unnaturally long central lip.[31] An initially short prolabium should never be lengthened with lateral flaps, as it will always elongate over time with muscle approximation. A lateral lip that is too long, relative to the vertical length of the prolabium, should always be shortened to match the prolabial length. The Veau technique, as described by Manchester, produces a long lip and unsatisfactory appearance of the Cupid's bow.[32]

Banked Fork Flaps

Millard advocated the use of banked forked flaps to elongate the columella.[2,33] Forked flaps, in our experience, have resulted in unsatisfactory scars on the nostril floor and columella.[11] Pigott,[34] while studying nasal dome to columella measurement ratios in children, noted that the dome/columella ratio was much greater in children compared to adults. In Oriental patients, a nose with a disproportionately long columella and short dome component, often results after using tissue from the nasal floor. Because of the dome/columellar discrepancy, unsightly scars on the nose, and increased scarring of the nostril floor, forked flaps are trimmed and sutured posteriorly to the septum to restore the nasolabial angle. Nakajima has suggested a similar approach to cleft lip nasal reconstruction.[35]

Columella Prolabial Complex

Cutting,[15] Noordhoff,[36] and Chen[16] currently believe that the medial crura and prolabial complex should be elevated superiorly on the septal cartilage to allow for muscle reconstruction. Trott[13] and Mulliken[37] leave the LLC's attached to the septum. Chen,[16] despite reporting the use of an open-tip approach to cleft nasal reconstruction in the past, has abandoned this procedure, adopting the present technique described here.

As the prolabium contains no muscle, the orbicularis must be reconstructed beneath it. If the muscle is to be adequately reconstructed, a space has to be created in front of the premaxilla and behind the prolabium. For this reason, it is our belief that it is necessary to advance the prolabial complex on the septum.

Reconstruction of the Nostril Floor

To prevent postoperative scarring, it is important to have an entirely closed wound. In secondary revisions, it is common to find the mucosa scarred, preventing repositioning of the LLC. Utilizing T and L flaps allows for repositioning the LLCs, reconstruction of the nostril floor, and resurfacing of the pyriform area, thereby preventing scarring. It also permits rotation of the ala inward into a normal position and adequate height of the nostril floor without tension.

Muscle Dissection on the Maxilla

Muscle dissection on the maxilla can be performed above the periosteum or beneath—subperiosteal, and controversy exists over the approach. Advocates of the Functional Matrix closure theory, believe that a subperiosteal dissection is required; however, there is no evidence to support less scarring or better facial growth with this approach.[38,39] With our technique, muscle dissection over the maxilla is supraperiosteal and as minimal as possible for muscle approximation. We believe this results in minimal scarring, and feel it is more important to release the abnormal muscle insertions around the alar base from the ala and maxilla. This maneuver will allow for repositioning the ala and muscle approximation. The angular artery, encountered lateral to the alar base, is a landmark of adequate muscle dissection around the alar base.

Reconstruction of the Orbicularis Oris Peripheralis Muscle

Manchester[32,40] felt that the orbicularis muscle should not be reconstructed as it would cause too much tension and result in growth disturbance. With presurgical molding of the premaxilla, there is less tension on the repair, and may minimize this possibility. In addition, Nagasse[41] showed there was no significant growth disturbance with muscle reconstruction. We believe that muscle reconstruction produces a better functional and aesthetic result; as well, it helps in restoring the alar–facial groove. When reconstructing the orbicularis, it is important to attach the muscle to the nasal spine.

Horizontal Incisions on the Lateral Lip

In both the unilateral[27] and bilateral cheiloplasty, there is seldom any indication for lateral incisions around the ala that result in undesirable scars. Whenever the lateral lip is too long, it can be shortened after muscle reconstruction by advancing the skin into the nostril floor. Excess skin is trimmed in the nostril floor keeping the horizontal incision as short as possible.

Reconstruction of the Cupid's Bow and Lip Tubercle

The native prolabial WSR and vermilion are deficient. Techniques that utilize the WSR and vermilion of the prolabium are unattractive and result with an irregular WSR, a patch of poor vermilion, unnatural scars, and a central deficiency[29] Utilization of the WSR-free border OM flaps, pared from the free edge of the lateral lip with a 1 mm wide WSR, allow for reconstruction of a new Cupid's bow with paralleling WSR/red lines and a full central tubercle[10,11,42]

Restoration of the Nasolabial Angle and Support of the LLC

Wu[43] noted that the nasolabial angle is maintained by a ligament from the subcutaneous tissue to the anterior nasal spine. After raising the columella-prolabium complex, there tends to be a flattening of this angle. The nasolabial angle is restored by advancing the upper edge of the forked flaps posterior to the nasal septum, while a through-and-through suture to the nasal spine might catch the columellar vessels and compromise the blood supply to the prolabium. Wu[43] also noted fibrous attachments from the LLC to the skin that accentuated the alar–facial groove. The use of ATS helps to support the LLC, minimize vestibular webbing, and restore the alar–facial groove.[27]

Open Versus Closed Rhinoplasty

The authors have had experience with the Trott[13] and a modified Trott open tip rhinoplasty.[16] Approximation of the medial crux through an open or closed tip rhinoplasty can be achieved. Technically, a closed rhinoplasty with a bilateral Tajima[28] tip rhinoplasty is easier to do, and there is minimal dissection required to achieve the desired result. Septal incisions, behind the medial crura, have less risk of forming a scar band than those placed in the columella skin, for an open tip rhinoplasty. Adams[44] reviewed the nasal tip support in open versus closed rhinoplasty, and showed the mean loss of tip projection is higher after an open rhinoplasty. This retention of tip projection is another advantage of the closed rhinoplasty with bilateral Tajima[28] incisions.

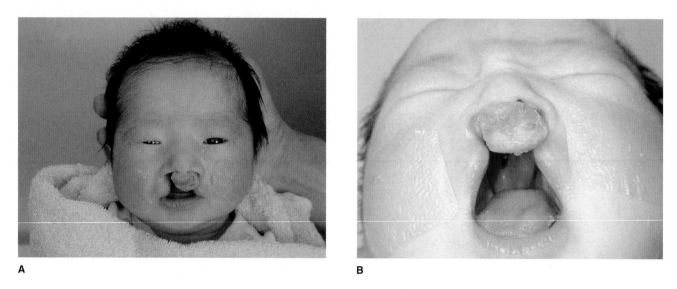

Figure 20–15. A newborn with complete cleft lip, nose, and palate.

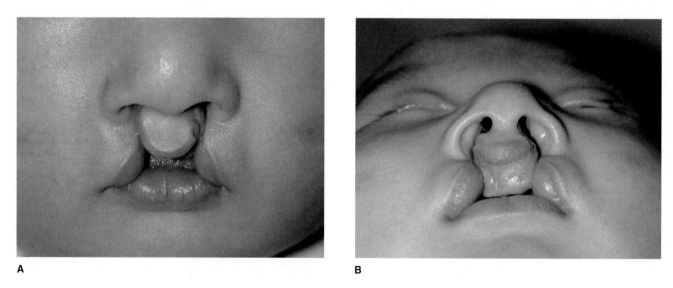

Figure 20–16. The patient in Figure 15, now 3 months of age and after NAM by Grayson's technique and before operation.

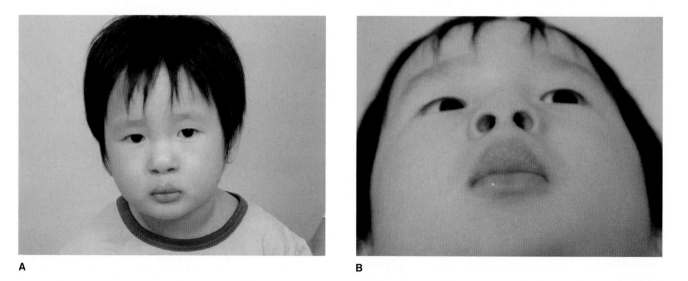

Figure 20–17. The patient in Figure 15 and 16, now 3 years of age, whose lip and nose were repaired with the present technique.

LONG-TERM RESULTS IN NASAL RECONSTRUCTION

In our experience, the long-term results in nasal reconstruction have given the impression of relapse of the nasal shape. However, studies on the long-term results both for unilateral[45] and bilateral clefts, by photometric measurements with 1:1 photos, show that there is a tendency of widening of the nostril width, while the nostril height is maintained postoperatively. This, we believe, gives the impression of relapse. These studies show the importance of over correction of the nostril height and avoiding an excessive nostril width at the time of surgery; however, there is no scientific data suggesting the amount of over correction. Postoperative maintenance of nostril height and columella length can be achieved by gradually adding silicone sheets or soft resin to the nasal conformer postoperatively (Figs. 20–15A, B, 20–16A, B, and 20–17A, B).

The satisfactory long-term result in bilateral cleft surgery is dependent on many factors, including parent/patient cooperation and follow-up. Gradually, our results improve with experience and dedication. The perfect result still eludes the surgeon who continues to strive for perfection in an imperfect world.

References

1. Cronin TD. Lengthening columella by use of skin from nasal floor and alae. *Plast Reconstr Surg* 21:417–426, 1958.
2. Millard DR, Jr. Closure of bilateral cleft lip and elongation of columella by two operations in infancy. *Plast Reconstr Surg* 47:324–31, 1971.
3. McComb H. Primary repair of the bilateral cleft lip nose: A 15-year review and a new treatment plan. *Plast Reconstr Surg* 1990; 86:882–889; discussion 890–893.
4. McComb H. Primary repair of the bilateral cleft lip nose: A 4-year review. *Plast Reconstr Surg* 94:37–47, 1994; discussion 48–50.
5. Millard DRJ, Latham R, Huifen X, Spiro S, Morovic C. Cleft lip and palate treated by presurgical orthopedics, gingivoperiosteoplasty, and lip adhesion (POPLA) compared with previous lip adhesion method: A preliminary study of serial dental casts. *Plast Reconstr Surg* 103:1630–1644, 1999.
6. Mulliken JB. Principles and techniques of bilateral complete cleft lip repair. *Plast Reconstr Surg* 75:477–487, 1985.
7. Tolhurst DE. Primary columella lengthening and lip adhesion. *Br Jr Plast Surg* 38:89, 1985.
8. Salyer KE. Primary Bilateral cleft-lip/nose repair: Salyer's technique. In: Salyer KE, Bardach J, eds. *Atlas of Craniofacial & Cleft Surgery, Vol. I.* Philadelphia: Lippincott-Raven, 1999, pp. 543–567.
9. Hamamoto J. Bilateral cleft lip repairs: The Manchester Method and presurgical orthodontic treatment. *Cong Anom* 24:421–428, 1984.
10. Noordhoff MS. Bilateral cleft lip reconstruction. *Plast Reconstr Surg* 78:45–54, 1986.
11. Noordhoff MS. Bilateral cleft lip and nasal repair. In: Cohen MS, ed. *Masters of Surgery, Vol. 1.* St. Louis MO: Little Brown and Co, 1994, pp. 566–580.
12. Noordhoff M. Primary elongation of the columella in bilateral cleft lip and palate with a prolabial island pedicle flap. The 6th International Congress on Cleft Palate and Related Craniofacial Anomalies, Jerusalem, Israel, 1989.
13. Trott JA, Mohan N. A preliminary report on one stage open tip rhinoplasty at the time of lip repair in bilateral cleft lip and palate: The Alor Setar experience. *Br J Plast Surg* 46:215–222, 1993.
14. Mulliken JB. Correction of the bilateral cleft lip nasal deformity: Evolution of a surgical concept. *Cleft Palate Craniofac J* 29:540–545, 1992.
15. Cutting C, Grayson B, Brecht L, Santiago P, Wood R, Kwon S. Presurgical columellar elongation and primary retrograde nasal reconstruction in one-stage bilateral cleft lip and nose repair. *Plast Reconstr Surg* 101:630–639, 1998.
16. Chen PKT, Noordhoff MS. Treatment of complete bilateral cleft lip-nasal deformity. In: Shenaq SM, Hollier LHJ, Williams JK, eds. *Seminars in Plastic Surgery. Cleft Lip Repair: Trends and Technique, Vol. 19:4.* New York: Stuttgart: Thieme, 2005, pp. 329–341.
17. Noordhoff MS. Mutidisciplinary management of cleft lip and palate in taiwan. In: Bardach J, Morris HL, eds. *Multidisciplinary Management of Cleft Lip and Palate.* Philadelphia: W.B. Saunders Co, 1990, pp. 18–26.
18. Noordhoff MS, Huang CS, Lo LJ. Median facial dysplasia in unilateral and bilateral cleft lip and palate: A subgroup of median cerebrofacial malformations. *Plast Reconstr Surg* 91:996–1005, 1993; discussion 1006–1007.
19. Noordhoff M, Chen PKT, Liou EJW, Lin WY. Recent advances in the treatment of the complete bilateral cleft lip-nasal deformity. In: Habal M, Himel H, Lineaweaver W, Colon G, Parsons R, Woods J, eds. *Key Issues Plast Cosmet Surg, Vol. 17.* Basel, Switzerland: Karger, 2000, pp. 1–21.
20. Huang CS, Cheng HC, Chen YR, Noordhoff MS. Maxillary dental arch affected by different sleep positions in unilateral complete cleft lip and palate infants. *Cleft Palate Craniofac J* 31:179–184, 1994.
21. Grayson BH, Cutting C, Wood R. Preoperative columella lengthening in bilateral cleft lip and palate. *Plast Reconstr Surg* 92:1422–1423, 1993.
22. Grayson BH, Santiago PE, Brecht LE, Cutting CB. Presurgical nasoalveolar molding in infants with cleft lip and palate. *Cleft Palate Craniofac J* 36:486–498, 1999.
23. Grayson BH, Cutting CB. Presurgical nasoalveolar orthopedic molding in primary correction of the nose, lip, and alveolus of infants born with unilateral and bilateral clefts. *Cleft Palate Craniofac J* 38:193–198, 2001.
24. Grayson BH, Maull D. Nasoalveolar molding for infants born with clefts of the lip, alveolus and palate. In: Shenaq SM, Hollier LHJ, Williams JK, eds. *Seminars in Plastic Surgery. Cleft Lip Repair: Trends and Techniques, Vol. 19:4.* New York: Stuttgart: Thieme, 2005, pp. 294–301.
25. Figueroa A. Orthodontics in cleft lip and palate management. In: Mathes SJ, Hentz VF, eds. *Plastic Surgery,* 2nd edn, Vol. 4. Philadelphia: WB Saunders, 2006, pp. 271–310.
26. Liou E, Chen K, Huang C. A modified technique in presurgical columella lengthening in bilateral cleft lip and palate patients. The 4th Asian Pacific cleft lip and palate conference, Fukuoka, Japan, 1999.
27. Noordhoff MS, Chen PKT. Unilateral cheiloplasty. In: Mathes SJ, Hentz VF, eds. *Plastic Surgery,* 2nd edn. Vol. 4. Philadelphia: W.B. Saunders, 2006, pp. 165–215.
28. Tajima S, Maruyama M. Reverse-U incision for secondary repair of cleft lip nose. *Plast Reconstr Surg* 60:256–261, 1977.
29. Noordhoff MS. Reconstruction of vermilion in unilateral and bilateral cleft lips. *Plast Reconstr Surg* 73:52–61, 1984.
30. Lin WY, Grayson BH, Figueroa A, Liou E, Cutting CB. The effect of presurgical molding of the nasal cartilages before lip repair in patients with unilateral cleft lip and palate – an intercenter report. Presented at the 4th Asian Pacific Cleft Lip and Palate Conference, Fukuoka, Japan. Sept 28, 1999 1999.
31. Cutting C, Grayson B. The prolabial unwinding flap method for one-stage repair of bilateral cleft lip, nose, and alveolus. *Plast Reconstr Surg* 91:37–47, 1993.
32. Manchester WM. The repair of the bilateral cleft lip and palate. *Brit J Surg* 52:878–882, 1965.
33. Millard DRJ, Latham RA. Improved primary surgical and dental treatment of clefts. *Plast Reconstr Surg* 86:856, 1990.

34. Pigott RW. Aesthetic considerations related to repair of the bilateral cleft lip nasal deformity. *Br J Plast Surg* 41:593–607, 1988.

35. Nakajima T, Yoshimura Y. Secondary correction of bilateral cleft lip nose deformity. *J Craniomaxillofac Surg* 18:63–67, 1990.

36. Noordhoff MS, Chen PKT, Liou EJW, Lin WY. Recent advances in the treatment of the complete bilateral cleft lip-nasal deformity. In: Habal MB, Himmel HN, Lineweaver WC, eds. *Key Issues Plast Cosmet Surg, Vol. 17.* Basel, Switzerland: Karger, 2001, pp. 51–71.

37. Mulliken JB. Bilateral cleft lip. *Clin Plast Surg* 31:209–220, 2004.

38. Carstens MH. Functional matrix cleft repair: A common strategy for unilateral and bilateral clefts. *J Craniofac Surg* 11:437–469, 2000.

39. Delaire J. Theoretical principles and technique of functional closure of the lip and nasal aperture. *J Maxillofac Surg* 6:109–116, 1978.

40. Manchester WM. The repair of double cleft lip as part of an integrated program. *Plast Reconstr Surg* 45:207–216, 1970.

41. Nagase T, Januszkiewicz JS, Keall HJ, de Geus JJ. The effect of muscle repair on postoperative facial skeletal growth in children with bilateral cleft lip and palate. *Scand J Plast Reconstr Surg Hand Surg* 32:395–405, 1998.

42. Mulliken JB, Pensler JM, Kozakewich HP. The anatomy of Cupid's bow in normal and cleft lip. *Plast Reconstr Surg* 92:395–403, 1993; discussion 404.

43. Wu WTL. The oriental nose: An anatomical basis for surgery. *Ann Acad Med Sing.* 21:176, 1992.

44. Adams WP, Jr., Rohrich RJ, Hollier LH, Minoli J, Thornton LK, Gyimesi I. Anatomic basis and clinical implications for nasal tip support in open versus closed rhinoplasty. *Plast Reconstr Surg* 103:255–261, 1999; discussion 262–264.

45. Liou EJ, Subramanian M, Chen PK, Huang CS. The progressive changes of nasal symmetry and growth after nasoalveolar molding: A three-year follow-up study. *Plast Reconstr Surg* 114:858–864, 2004.

21

Mulliken Repair of Bilateral Cleft Lip and Nasal Deformity

John B. Mulliken, MD

INTRODUCTION

Forty years ago, William Manchester wrote, "No greater problem exists in the whole field of surgery than the successful treatment of a patient suffering from complete, bilateral cleft lip and palate."[1] Although colleagues in other surgical specialities would take umbrage with this statement, Manchester's commitment to these children is clear. He warned that any surgeon who attempts repair of a bilateral cleft lip assumes an "onerous" responsibility because "failure to achieve its objectives" can result in a "lifelong human tragedy" that secondary procedures can only "partially alleviate."

I believe Manchester and all other devoted surgeons before me have struggled to give a semblance of normal appearance to a child born with a double cleft lip. Reader, go no further, unless you have the passion, precision, patience, and perseverance to undertake this operation and accept the obligation for periodic evaluation of your results. In a professional lifetime, you will have the privilege of following only a small number of these patients into adulthood. These children should not suffer because of your technical wanderings and misadventures. The principles to be followed in repair of bilateral cleft lip are established. The techniques have evolved such that the results should be equivalent to those for the unilateral cleft labial counterpart.[2]

Philosophers tell us that those who do not know history are likely to repeat its mistakes. So, before taking a scalpel to an infant with bilateral cleft lip, consider the past and learn from it.

A BRIEF HISTORY OF BILATERAL CLEFT LABIAL REPAIR

The approach to the projecting premaxilla has always been a focus of controversy. From the Renaissance until the early twentieth century, some surgeons summarily excised the intermaxillary bone, either preserving the prolabium as central lip or shifting it upward to form the columella. Our more conservative surgical forbearers struggled with ingenious methods of external compression to force the premaxilla into alignment.[3] These efforts, to reposition the premaxilla, presaged the development of "passive" (removable), and later active (fixed), palatal devices in the middle of the last century.

In 1864, Simon was first to pare the edges of the prolabium and construct bilateral labial adhesions as a way to retrude the premaxilla. This method is probably the source of the dubious eponym "Simonart's bands."[4] Premaxillary surgical "setback" to permit labial closure was advocated by Veau, Brown, and Cronin.[3] Preoperative manipulation of the premaxilla and the concerns about possible deleterious effects on midfacial growth, continue to be controversial.

Techniques for labial repair have evolved to such a level that there is general agreement among most surgeons. At one time, surgeons closed one side first, then the other. The result was loss of symmetry—the one advantage a bilateral cleft lip has over a unilateral cleft lip. There was a misconception that the diminutive prolabium lacked growth potential. Thus, various techniques were used to introduce rectangular or triangular flaps from the lateral labial elements to augment philtral height. These procedures resulted in unsightly geometric scars and a central lip that was tight and too long. Variations on the Veau III or straight-line repair minimized elongation but resulted in an abnormally wide, bowed, or shield-shaped philtrum. For years, there was debate over whether to preserve the prolabial vermilion, either allowing it to grow or augmenting it with lateral vermilion flaps, or excising it and importing lateral vermilion to build

the median tubercle. Closure of the orbicularis muscle was usually not possible over a protruding premaxilla; some surgeons believed that muscular closure would inhibit midfacial growth.

Surgeons seemed puzzled by the obvious nasal distortion in a bilateral cleft lip. They knew that what columella there was did not have the capacity to grow. Surgeons conceded to the complexity of the bilateral nasal deformity and deferred correction. Perhaps, there was a concern that manipulation of the tip cartilages would interfere with growth. Numerous "secondary" procedures were devised, all based on the apparent need to recruit nearby tissue into the columella. There are two basic strategies for columellar elongation. The Cronin technique is rotation of bipedicled straps from the nostril sills.[5] This gives only modest columellar length; often the procedure had to be repeated. The other method, the forked-flap procedure of Millard,[3] once used widely, has fallen out of favor in most centers. Like all secondary procedures, the forked-flap method causes peculiar tertiary distortions. In retrospect, these secondary procedures were incorrectly based on adding soft tissue to build the columella and essentially ignored the dislocated lower lateral cartilages. The primary labial closure accentuates the bilateral nasal deformity by pulling the medial crura inferoposteriorly, further dislocating the domes, and buckling the genua into recurvatum. In short, conventional bilateral labial repair makes the nasal deformity worse.[6] Furthermore, the deformed and malpositioned lower lateral cartilages are difficult to correct secondarily.

LESSONS OF THE BILATERAL CLEFT LIP DEFORMITY

The nasolabial stigmata that remain after bilateral cleft lip repair are all too obvious—even at conversational distance (Fig. 21–1). The child's lip is too long, flat, and lacks the normal protrusion. Upon closer inspection, the philtrum is wide, bowed, and undimpled. The median tubercle is thin and chapped, particularly if the prolabial vermilion-mucosa was retained. The free mucosal margin of the lateral labial elements hangs like swags and there is excessive dental show (the "whistling lip" deformity). The nasal tip is flat and broad, the nostrils have an oblique axis, and the ala nasi are flared (the "cat's knees deformity"). The squatty columella is the centerpiece of these distorted nasolabial features. The snubbed nasal tip and tight upper lip are even more obvious in profile, further accentuated by an everted lower lip and weak chin. This "cleft lip–lower lip deformity" is caused by the child's struggle for bilabial closure over the abnormally positioned premaxilla, i.e., protruded at its base, retroclined inferiorly, and vertically overgrown.[7] As the child puckers, a muscular bulge appears on each side of the lip, and when the child smiles, the alar bases rise abnormally.[8]

The following principles for repair of bilateral cleft lip and correction of the nasal deformity were induced based on

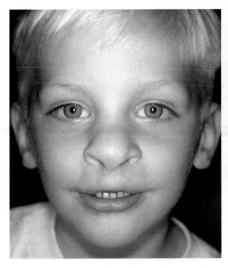 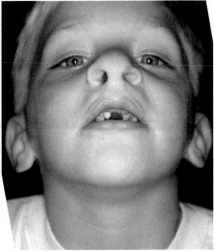 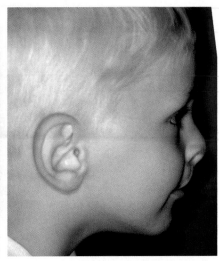

Figure 21–1. Stigmata of repaired bilateral complete cleft lip/palate. Four-year-old boy following labial closure during infancy and columellar lengthening (forked flap) at age 2 years (at a major university center). Nasal width 35 mm (normal 28 mm); columellar length 5.5 mm (normal 6.9 mm); bowed philtrum: peak-to-peak of Cupid's bow 14 mm (normal 8 mm). Also note thin median tubercle.

study of the literature and analysis of the nasolabial distortions that remain using conventional techniques[6]:

1. Preserve symmetry, because even a minor nasolabial difference between the two sides will magnify with growth.
2. Achieve muscular continuity to construct the orbicular ring, eliminate the lateral muscular bulges, and minimize philtral expansion.
3. Design the philtral flap of proper size and shape, because this central labial element will bow and elongate.
4. Construct the median tubercle from the lateral labial elements, because the prolabial vermilion has an abnormal color, lacks a white roll, and does not grow normally.
5. Position the slumped/splayed lower lateral cartilages to form the nasal tip and upper columella.

In the early 1980s, principles 1 through 4 needed definition and interpretation, whereas the principle 5 initiated a fundamental change in approach to the bilateral cleft lip nasal deformity, i.e., primary correction.

SYNCHRONOUS BILATERAL NASOLABIAL REPAIR

Surgical history teaches that complex congenital anomalies, initially corrected in several stages, can be repaired in a single operation by subsequent technical innovation and usually more successfully. This lesson applies to correction of the bilateral cleft lip and nasal deformity.

A few surgeons worked independently toward the goal of primary nasal repair. Intraoperative observation[6] and nasal dissection of a stillborn infant with bilateral cleft lip[9] revealed that the alar domes are splayed and caudally dislocated from their normal position overlying the upper lateral cartilages. Broadbent and Woolf[10] described a single case of primary

medial advancement of the alar domes along with vertical excision of redundant skin in the nasal tip. McComb was in the forefront of primary columellar elongation. He tried elevating a forked flap as the first stage,[11] but was disenchanted with the technique by the time he published his assessment 11 years later.[9] Instead, he proposed a two-staged primary repair, minus the forked flap,[12] and reviewed his early results 4 years later.[13] McComb was clearly on the right track.

Mulliken also struggled to accomplish the goal of primary positioning of the lower lateral cartilages. Initially, he banked the tines of a forked flap, and at a second stage, the tines were retrieved and rotated intranasally to allow the genua and medial crura to ascend. A vertical tip incision was used to elevate the intradomal fat and appose the domes, and the lateral genua were suspended to the upper lateral cartilages through bilateral rim incisions.[6] This approach evolved, such that, by 1987, it became obvious that banked prolabial tines were unnecessary. It also became clear that it was possible to repair a bilateral cleft lip and nasal deformity in a single stage, including construction of the columella.[14,15] The vertical tip incision was abandoned because, with experience, it was possible to position and secure the lower lateral cartilages through bilateral rim incisions by this semi-open approach. Furthermore, caudal extension of the rim incisions permitted the necessary sculpting of the tip and upper columella.[8]

Another way to expose the displaced lower lateral cartilages is to elevate a prolabial–columellar flap, based on the paired columellar arteries. Trott and Mohan dissected the flap on the ventral surface of the cartilages.[16] Cutting and Grayson[17] also employed an open-tip approach, but incised the prolabial–columellar flap along the membranous septum, so that the medial and middle crura are in the flap. The genua were apposed by a transvestibular mattress suture.

Thus, the principle of primary correction of the bilateral cleft nasal deformity has been established, although the techniques continue to evolve. There is no need to secondarily recruit tissue from the lip because "the columella is in the nose."[15] Synchronous nasolabial repair should be the standard procedure. These children no longer need to live with stigmata because a surgeon practiced staged operations.

FOUR-DIMENSIONAL PROBLEMS FOR THREE-DIMENSIONAL MINDS

The surgeon who undertakes repair of a bilateral cleft lip and nasal deformity cannot be compared to the sculptor working in stone. It is not enough to visualize the three-dimensional aspects of size, shape, and proportions of the infantile face. The lip and nose must be constructed in anticipation of the changes that occur with growth. These are not normal growth patterns; instead, they are distortions of normal that befall the child with a repaired bilateral cleft lip.

The nasolabial normal growth patterns in Caucasians from ages 1 to 18 years have been documented by anthropometry.[18] All nasolabial features, with two exceptions, grow rapidly in early childhood, reaching more than two-thirds of adult size by age 5 years. The slow-growing features are columellar length and nasal tip protrusion. This differential rate of growth correlates with the typical stigmata of a repaired bilateral cleft lip and nasal deformity. The fast-growing features become overly long or wide, i.e., nasal length, interalar distance, and all the prolabial dimensions, particularly between the peaks of Cupid's bow. In contrast, the two slow-growing features remain relatively short, i.e., columellar length and nasal protrusion.

The surgeon must make the necessary adjustments in three-dimensional nasolabial features during the repair in expectation of these four-dimensional changes. Features programmed for rapid growth and distortion are crafted on a small scale, whereas, slow-growing features, those that will never reach normal dimensions, should be constructed on a slightly larger than normal size for an infant.[8,19,20] An exception to these guidelines is construction of the median tubercle. Although it is a fast-growing structure in the normal lip, it lags behind in the child with a repaired bilateral cleft lip. Thus, the median tubercle should be made as full as possible, in anticipation of normal show of the secondary dentition.

PREOPERATIVE DENTOFACIAL ORTHOPEDICS

Three- and four-dimensional nasolabial repair cannot be achieved if the premaxilla is procumbent. There are two basic strategies for preoperative premaxillary manipulation: passive and active. A passive appliance is retained by undercuts and dental adhesive; the configuration of the molding plate is altered, by adding or subtracting material, so as to selectively apply pressure on the maxillary elements. A passive appliance maintains, but does not change, the anterior or posterior maxillary width. This can be a problem because sometimes

the lesser maxillary segments have collapsed so there is insufficient space for the premaxilla. Whenever a passive plate is used, an external force is needed to retract the premaxilla. Bilateral labial adhesion was first described in the nineteenth century to apply an external force on the premaxilla; it has been used in conjunction with a passive plate.[21] However, without retracting the premaxilla, labial adhesions are prone to dehisce because there is no muscle in the prolabial element. For years, the conventional way to apply posterior traction on the premaxilla was to fit the infant with a head cap to which an elastic band was attached by hooks and eyes. Steri-Strips® are now used for the same purpose. Cutting and Grayson have described a more sophisticated variation on the passive plate called "nasoalveolar molding."[17,22] Alveolar molding is done first; once the gap is reduced to less than 5 mm, nasal molding begins. The nostrils are pushed upward by prongs on an acrylic extension attached to the palatal plate. To further stretch the columella, a horizontal band of soft denture material is added, across the nasolabial junction, and a vertical tape is placed from prolabium-to-appliance, to give a downward counterforce. At the same time, the premaxilla is gradually retracted by serial application of tape across the outrigger to the cheeks or to the labia. The tapes are changed daily by the parents; the apparatus must be adjusted weekly to modify the alveolar molding plate. In another type of plate, described by Bennun and Figueroa, tape is not used to secure the nasal extension.[23] The acrylic intraoral plate lies loosely in the mouth, and by lingual movement during suction and swallowing, force is transmitted through a flexible spring to a nasal extension fitted with a silicone "bumper."

All external traction techniques tend to focus pressure inferior to the basilar premaxilla causing lingual inclination and bowing of the vomer. Furthermore, it can be difficult to centralize a severely rotated premaxilla using a passive plate and external traction.

The currently used active-type dentofacial orthopedic device is based on the prototypic design by Georgiade and associates,[24] and later refined and popularized by Millard and Latham.[25] A plaster model of the upper jaw is made during early infancy. The custom-made appliance, according to Latham's design, is inserted with the infant under general anesthetic. The acrylic plates are pinned to the maxillary shelves. A looped wire is passed through the neck of the premaxilla, well anterior to the premaxillary–vomerine suture. An elastic chain on each side is connected to the transpremaxillary wire, looped under a pulley in the posterior–superior section of the appliance, and attached to cleats at the anterior edges of the maxillary plate (Fig. 21–2). Each day, the parents turn a ratcheted screw in the middle of the device in order to expand the anterior palatal segments. There is no posterior expansion. The dentist or orthodontist tightens the elastic chains to retract the premaxilla. This requires postinsertion visits at 1, 3, and 5 weeks, then, every 2 weeks until the surgical date. Usually, it takes 6–8 weeks to align the premaxilla between the expanded palatal segments. Latham's fixed appliance is most effective in correcting the premaxilla in the anterior–posterior plane; however, the movement

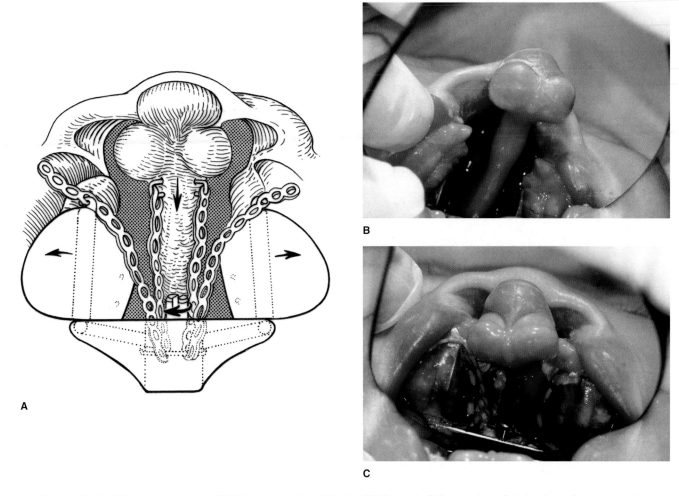

Figure 21–2. (A) Latham appliance. (B) Prior to insertion of device. (C) Six weeks following dentofacial orthopedic manipulation.

is more retroclination than retroposition. The teeth become retroclined, and the vomer may bend slightly. This appliance can also rectify premaxillary rotation, but there is little effect on vertical position.

There is an enduring and pervasive belief that we must never do anything that might interfere with midfacial growth in the habilitation of children born with cleft lip/palate. Thus, there are critics of active premaxillary orthopedics who have shown long-term evidence for minor midfacial retrusion.[26,27] Other longitudinal studies failed to document more serious effects on maxillary growth in children managed with active dentofacial orthopedics, as compared to those who were not.[28,29] Whatever the operative technique, primary repair of bilateral cleft lip/palate causes some inhibition of vertical and forward maxillary growth. The major goals in the repair of bilateral cleft lip/palate are nasolabial appearance and normal speech. These goals should not be forgotten in attempts to minimize restriction of maxillary growth. Midfacial retrusion is predictably corrected by maxillary advancement, with additional aesthetic benefits to nasal, labial, and malar projection.

Whatever might be the effect on facial growth, presurgical dentofacial orthopedics is essential to set the stage for synchronous primary repair of the primary palate. Alignment of the maxillary segments permits design of the philtrum in proper proportions, facilitates nasal correction, and allows closure of the alveolar gaps. Thus, the upper arch is stabilized and oronasal fistulae are eliminated. Furthermore, early retropositioning of the premaxilla minimizes nasolabial distortion as the child grows.

THE OPERATION

Synchronous bilateral cleft labionasal repair should be the first and maybe the only procedure of the day, i.e., there should be no committee meetings, office patients, or other obligations. This is the most important day in the life of your patient since birth.

Markings

While standing at the head of the table, elevate the nostrils with a double-ball retractor and draw the philtral flap using a sharpened toothpick dipped in brilliant green dye. The midpoint at the columellar–labial junction (sn) is noted and dots

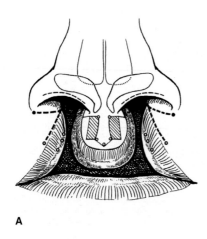

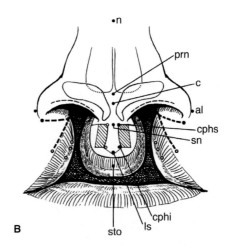

Figure 21–3. (A) Markings for synchronous repair of bilateral cleft lip and nasal deformity. Open circles denote points that are tattooed. (B) Anthropometric points: *nasion* (n); *pronasale* (prn); highest point of *columella nasi* (c); *subnasale* (sn); *ala nasi* (al); *crista philtri superior* (cphs); *crista philtri inferior* (cphi); *labiale superius* (ls); and *stomion* (sto).

are placed 2 mm apart (cphs–cphs) at the base of the flap. The philtral flap is designed to be 6–7 mm in length (sn–ls) and 3.5–4.5 mm from peak-to-peak of Cupid's bow (cphi–cphi). The sides of the philtral flap are drawn slightly biconcave, and on each flank, a tiny rectangular flap is delineated. These flaps will be de-epithelialized and incorporated to simulate philtral ridges. The columellar base flaps are designated up to the prolabial mucosal junction.

The corresponding Cupid's bow peak points on the lateral labial elements are sited such that there will be sufficient white roll for the handle of the bow and ample vermilion for the median tubercle. The alar base flaps are drawn a little inside the junction with the lateral labial element, and the medial edge is extended along the vestibular mucosal–cutaneous junction (Fig. 21–3A).

After completion of the markings, record the anthropometric measurements to document the nasal features: length (sn–al), width (al–al), projection (sn–prn), and columellar length (sn–c) and labial features: philtral flap dimensions (cphs–cphs; cphi–cphi; sn–ls; and sn–sto; and height of the tubercle (ls–sto)[19] (Fig. 21–3B).

The labial elements and nose are infiltrated with xylocaine and epinephrine solution. After a sufficient waiting period, a 30-gauge needle, which is fitted on the end of a cotton-tipped applicator, is used to tattoo the critical anatomic points that must be preserved during the dissection, including the vermilion–mucosal line in the lateral elements. Tattoo punctures made before injection of epinephrine tend to bleed excessively and blur the lines.

Dissection

All the lines are lightly incised; the philtral flanking tabs are de-epithelialized; and the excess prolabial skin is excised. The philtral flap is elevated in the loose areolar plane, extending the dissection up to the anterior nasal spine.

The lateral labial flaps are disjoined from the alar bases and the basilar flaps are freed from the piriform attachments.

The white line vermilion–mucosal flaps are separated from the lower edge of the muscular layer, extending just short of the tattooed lateral Cupid's bow point. With a double hook on the muscle and a protecting ring finger on the infraorbital rim, the lateral labial elements are widely released off the maxilla in the supraperiosteal plane. The orbicular muscular bundles are dissected within the lateral labial elements in the subdermal and submucosal planes (Fig. 21–4A).

Attention is turned to the broad nasal tip and deformed/dislocated lower lateral cartilages. Through bilateral rim incisions, scissor dissection exposes the anterior surface of the slumped and splayed lower lateral cartilages. Fatty tissue is elevated from between the domes (Fig. 21–4B).

Closure

Repair of the lip and nose is integrated, beginning in the lip, then to nose, back to lip, and completed in the nose. The following sequence of steps is suggested as a guide. Minor deviations from this sequence are permissible, but major changes can disrupt and interfere with the construction.

Trim the premaxillary vermilion mucosa and secure the remaining flange to the premaxillary periosteum. This forms the alveolar side of the central gingivolabial sulcus.

The nasal floors are constructed by raising a lateral mucosal flap from below the inferior turbinate and dissecting a medial flap from the premaxillary stem. The alar base flaps are advanced medially and sutured to the constructed nasal floor.

Mirror–image vertical incisions are made through gingival mucosa and periosteum at the ends of the maxillary segments and on each side of the premaxilla. The alveolar repairs (gingivoperiosteoplasties) are completed, first closing the posterior, then the anterior, lamella. Excess premaxillary vermilion-mucosa is excised, and the residual mucosa is sutured high on the premaxilla (Fig. 21–5).

A back-cut is made at the distal end of the sulcal incisions and the lateral labial elements are advanced mesially.

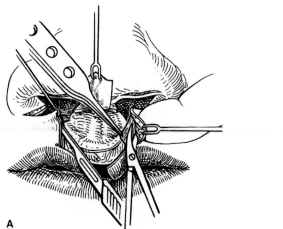
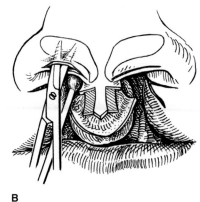

Figure 21–4. (A) Dissection of orbicularis oris muscle in lateral labial elements. (B) Lower lateral cartilages exposed through rim incisions. Cotton-tipped applicator elevates nostril and helps to display tip cartilage.

This advancement of the labial flaps must be accentuated while the buccal sulci are closed; otherwise the muscular layers cannot be apposed. The mucosa of the lateral labial flaps forms the anterior wall of the central sulcus. The orbicular muscles are apposed, inferiorly-to-superiorly; the uppermost suture suspends the pars peripheralis and nasalis to the periosteum of the anterior nasal spine (Fig. 21–6A).

The lateral vermilion–mucosal flaps are trimmed to form the median tubercle. There is a tendency to preserve too much of these flaps, resulting in a central furrow. The closure of the median raphe is completed on the posterior side of the lip (Fig. 21–6B).

Before suturing the philtral flap, return to correction of the nasal deformity. The medial genua are apposed with an interdomal mattress suture of 5-0 PDS (on a half circle cutting needle) (Fig. 21–7A) and the lateral genua are elevated and secured over the corresponding upper lateral cartilage with a mattress suture (Fig. 21–7B). A Q-tip held beneath the genu is helpful during placement and tying these sutures.

The flaps forming the columellar base are cut, leaving 3 mm, on each side. The alar bases are advanced and sutured side-to-end to the c-flaps; the tips are trimmed and closure of the sills is completed. The interalar distance is further narrowed by a "cinch" suture between the alar bases; this suture is tightened until the al–al dimension measures less than 25 mm (Fig. 21–8A). Each alar base is secured by a mattress suture placed through the upper orbicular edge to the underlying maxillary periosteum in order to (1) form the normal cymal configuration of the sill; (2) prevent alar elevation with smiling, i.e., simulate action of the depressor alae nasi; and (3) minimize postoperative widening of the interalar distance (Fig. 21–8B).

Attention returns to the lip. In an effort to simulate a dimple, a suture is placed through the dermis of the philtral flap and into the muscle layer. Next, the dart at the end of the philtral flap is inset into the handle of Cupid's bow. Usually, the leading edges of the lateral labial flaps are not trimmed;

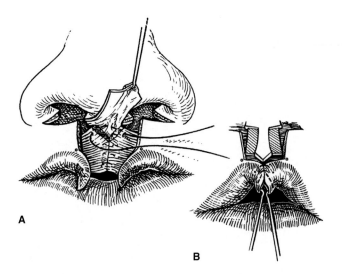

Figure 21–5. Completion of gingivoperiosteoplasty: Redundant premaxillary vermilion mucosa trimmed and remaining mucosa sutured to periosteum to form posterior wall of anterior gingivolabial sulcus.

Figure 21–6. (A) Apposition of orbicularis oris from inferior to superior; uppermost suture placed through periosteum of anterior nasal spine. (B) Lateral white roll vermilion–mucosal flaps trimmed to form median tubercle and Cupid's bow.

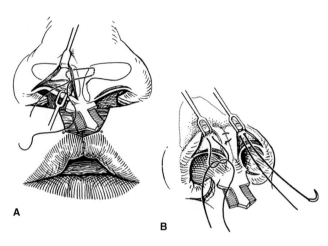

Figure 21–7. Positioning dislocated and splayed lower lateral cartilages: (A) Apposition with interdomal mattress suture. (B) Suspension over ipsilateral upper lateral cartilage with intercartilaginous mattress suture.

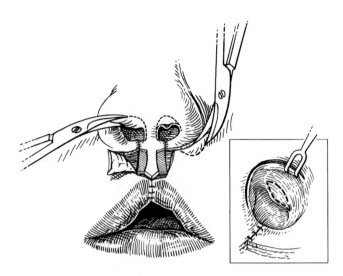

Figure 21–9. Crescentic excision of expanded domal skin and lining extended into upper columella. Cyma-shaped resection of superior margin of lateral labial elements to fit curve of sill. Lenticular excision of lateral vestibular web (Inset).

they are apposed to the philtral flap without tension. The cephalic margin of the lateral labial flaps is trimmed to diminish height and to correspond to the ogee curve of the lower edge of the sills (Fig. 21–9). These flaps are advanced medially as closure proceeds, forming a philtral bulge on each side.

The denouement is sculpting the nasal tip and columella. The excess skin in the soft triangles is obvious after the lower lateral cartilages are secured in anatomic position. The anterior edge of the rim wound is excised as a crescent, extending along each side of the columella (Fig. 21–9). This resection narrows the tip, defines the columella–lobular junction, elongates the upper nostrils, and narrows the columella.

Interdomal apposition accentuates the lateral vestibular web causing the lateral crura to encroach on the vestibule. Lenticular excision on the cutaneous side of the intercarti-

laginous junction obliterates this web and closure supports the lateral crura (Fig. 21–9, inset).

A curved Lactosorb splint, custom-cut from a 1.5-mm-thick panel (W. Lorenz Surgical Inc.), is placed over the newly positioned lower lateral cartilages and the rim wounds are closed[30] (Fig. 21–10A). Nasolabial anthropometry is repeated at the completion of the closure (Fig. 21–10B).

POSTOPERATION

One-quarter inch Xeroform gauze strip is wrapped around a 19-gauge silicone catheter, trimmed, and inserted into each nostril. If necessary, a newly constructed dental appliance is inserted into the palatal cleft (and held with adhesive powder) to maintain maxillary width. A Logan bow is taped to the cheeks for protection; this also serves to hold an iced saline sponge on the repaired lip. The sponge is removed in 24 hours and the infant is discharged on the second postoperative day. The parents are instructed in "suture-line care". Under general anesthesia (mask induction and insufflation), the nostrils are cleaned and the percutaneous nylon sutures are removed 5 days postoperatively. A trimmed one-half inch Steri-Strip (3M Health Care, St. Paul, Minnesota) is applied and changed, as needed, for 6 weeks postoperatively. Thereafter, massage with Pedi-mederma® is encouraged and continued until the scar softens; application of a sunblock solution is emphasized to the parents.

Examples of synchronous repair of bilateral cleft lip, nasal deformity, and alveolar clefts are shown in Figs. 21–11, 21–12, and 21–13. Intraoperative and postoperative anthropometric measurements are compared to values for sex and age-matched normal children.

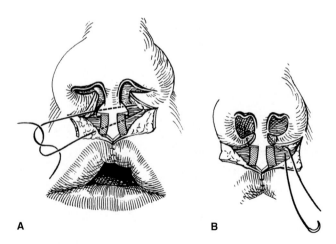

Figure 21–8. (A) Interalar distance narrowed with cinch suture. (B) Alar base flaps trimmed, rotated endonasally and secured (side-to-end) to c-flaps, and sutured to underlying muscle and maxillary periosteum.

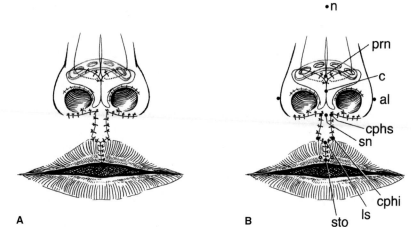

Figure 21–10. (A) Completed repair after insertion of resorbable internal plate. (B) Immediate postoperative nasolabial anthropometry recorded.

MODIFICATIONS IN TECHNIQUES FOR ANATOMICAL VARIANTS

Bilateral Complete Cleft Lip with Intact Secondary Palate

Approximately 10% of infants born with bilateral complete cleft lip and alveolus do not have a defect in the secondary palate. The premaxilla protrudes because of unrestrained growth at the premaxillary–vomerine suture. In such a deformity, a Latham device may be successful in widening the maxillary segments and retruding the premaxilla. Nevertheless, dentofacial orthopedics is not always possible and attempts at external traction are predictably unsuccessful. In some cases, synchronous repair is feasible if the premaxilla is flexible and minimally procumbent. Premaxillary ostectomy and setback is another alternative to permit alveolar closure and nasolabial repair. The mucosal incisions needed for resecting part of the premaxillary neck, retropositioning, and alveolar closure can compromise the premaxillary circulation. Blood supply becomes limited to the preserved septal and vomerine mucosa. If there is a concern during the

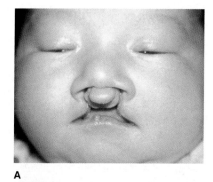

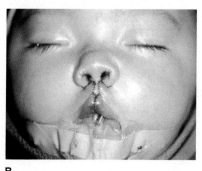

	Pre-	Post-	Normal
	5 mos		4-5 mos
n-sn	22.5	22	NA
al-al	31	23	26.8
sn-prn	7.5	11	7.3
sn-c	1.5	4	4
cphs-cphs	2.0	2.0	NA
cphi-cphi	4	4	NA
sn-ls	6.2	7	9
sn-sto	7	14.5	13
ls-sto	3	7.5	5.6

Normal values expressed as means
NA = not available

Figure 21–11. Chinese girl with bilateral complete cleft lip/palate and Van der Woude syndrome. (A) Prior to synchronous repair and (B) intraoperative appearance, immediately following closure. (C) Anthropometric measures prior to incisions and after repair compared to normal age-matched controls.

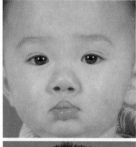
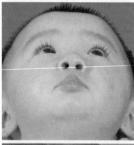
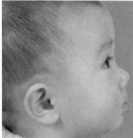

	Patient	Normal
	1 yr	1 yr
n-sn	24.5	NA
al-al	27	27.3
sn-prn	13	8.5
sn-c	4	4.5
cphs-cphs	5.5	NA
cphi-cphi	7.5	NA
sn-ls	8.5	9
sn-sto	16.5	15
ls-sto	8.5	6

Normal values expressed as means
NA = not available

Figure 21–12. Girl in Fig. 21–11 at age 1 year. Note overprojection of nasal tip, columellar length, and alar width in normal range. Compare 1-year anthropometry to intraoperative measures: note rapid growth of philtral height and width. Also, note full median tubercle in anticipation of insufficient growth.

procedure, postpone closing the posterior premaxilla to the anterior edge of the hard palate.

Primary premaxillary positioning performed in infancy is likely to accentuate midfacial retrusion,[31,32] although there are earlier reports to the contrary.[33] Nevertheless, midfacial retrusion is unlikely if the secondary palate is intact.

Symmetrical Bilateral Incomplete Cleft Lip

In this relatively uncommon variant, the secondary palate is usually intact and the alveolar clefts are small. At first glance, repair would seem to be straightforward and it is, if done correctly. The critical decision is whether or not to retain prolabial vermilion-mucosa as the median tubercle or construct it using the lateral labial elements (aforesaid principle 4). As tempting as it might be, the prolabial vermilion-mucosa should almost never be retained as median tubercle unless the clefts are minor and the central white roll is prominent. The design and the technical steps are the same as for a complete bilateral cleft lip, including the adjustments in expectation of nasolabial changes in the fourth dimension. An example of a repaired bilateral symmetrical incomplete cleft lip and nasal deformity is seen in Fig. 21–14, including intraoperative and 5-year postoperative anthropometry.

In a minor form of this variant, positioning the lower lateral cartilages and sculpting the soft triangles may not be indicated, i.e., if tip projection and columellar length are near normal. On the other hand, interalar narrowing is always necessary; this dimension becomes too wide as the child grows.

Asymmetrical (Complete/Incomplete) Bilateral Cleft Lip/Palate

In the asymmetrical variant, the incomplete side presents in a spectrum that ranges from a microform to a nearly complete cleft with a tiny cutaneomucosal band. The guiding principle in planning a strategy is to attain symmetry. A tiny band on the incomplete side often pulls the premaxilla to that side. In this case, it is usually best to divide the band to permit preoperative dentofacial orthopedic centralization of the premaxilla. If there is a microform or mini-microform cleft lip, it is best to postpone its correction and focus on repair of the complete side.[34] In the more common situation of a contralateral incomplete cleft lip, the complete side should be addressed first, i.e., unilateral dentofacial orthopedics followed by lip–nasal adhesion and gingivoperiosteoplasty.[35] This preliminary step levels the surgical field for simultaneous bilateral nasolabial repair.

During the second stage, synchronous bilateral closure, every technical stratagem should be used to achieve mirror–image symmetry. For example, the maneuvers on the complete side should be exaggerated because there is greater distortion than on the incomplete side. At each step in the procedure, it is usually best to execute first on the complete side. It is easier to match the incomplete side to the complete side, rather than vice versa. Exceptions to this sequence become obvious during the procedure. For example, the alar base may be trimmed and secured to the columellar base on the incomplete side, to give a normal nostril width, before the same maneuver on the complete side. Likewise, the lateral labial height (sbal–cphi) can be established initially on the incomplete side. The upper margin of the lateral labial flap is trimmed, advanced medially, and sutured along the sill. The process is repeated on the complete side, and the sill closure is adjusted so that the philtral flap will not be pulled over to that side. Often, the vermilion height is insufficient on complete side; this can be corrected by a vermilion unilimb Z-plastic flap from the incomplete side. Staged correction of a bilateral asymmetrical cleft lip is shown in Fig. 21–15 and the outcome is documented by anthropometry.

Binderoid Bilateral Complete Cleft Lip/Palate

This uncommon variant can disconcert the unwary surgeon. The nasal features include orbital hypotelorism, hypoplastic bony/cartilaginous nasal components, conical columella, and hypoplastic septum with absent anterior nasal spine. The labial features are tiny, floppy premaxilla with hypoplastic prolabium, and thin vermilion in the lateral elements.[36] Usually there is a complete bilateral cleft of the secondary palate, but it can also be intact. The mobile premaxilla often permits

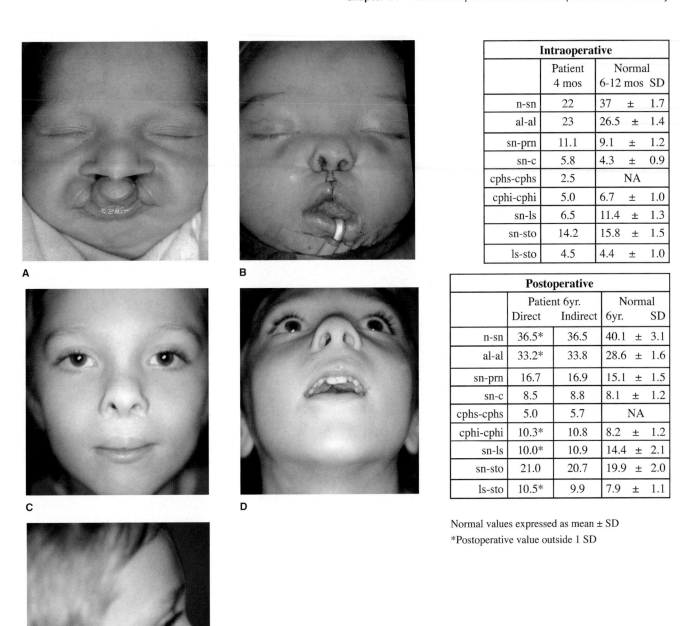

Intraoperative			
	Patient 4 mos	Normal 6-12 mos	SD
n-sn	22	37 ±	1.7
al-al	23	26.5 ±	1.4
sn-prn	11.1	9.1 ±	1.2
sn-c	5.8	4.3 ±	0.9
cphs-cphs	2.5	NA	
cphi-cphi	5.0	6.7 ±	1.0
sn-ls	6.5	11.4 ±	1.3
sn-sto	14.2	15.8 ±	1.5
ls-sto	4.5	4.4 ±	1.0

Postoperative				
	Patient 6yr. Direct	Indirect	Normal 6yr.	SD
n-sn	36.5*	36.5	40.1 ±	3.1
al-al	33.2*	33.8	28.6 ±	1.6
sn-prn	16.7	16.9	15.1 ±	1.5
sn-c	8.5	8.8	8.1 ±	1.2
cphs-cphs	5.0	5.7	NA	
cphi-cphi	10.3*	10.8	8.2 ±	1.2
sn-ls	10.0*	10.9	14.4 ±	2.1
sn-sto	21.0	20.7	19.9 ±	2.0
ls-sto	10.5*	9.9	7.9 ±	1.1

Normal values expressed as mean ± SD

*Postoperative value outside 1 SD

Figure 21–13. Bilateral complete cleft lip/palate. (A) Preoperative. (B) Following synchronous repair: intraoperative nasolabial anthropometry documents undercorrected fast-growing features and overcorrected slow-growing features. (C–E) Appearance at 6 years and postoperative anthropometry (direct and indirect). Note long columella/tip projection and full median tubercle; however, nose and lower philtrum are a little wide. Obtuse columellar–labial angle should diminish with growth.

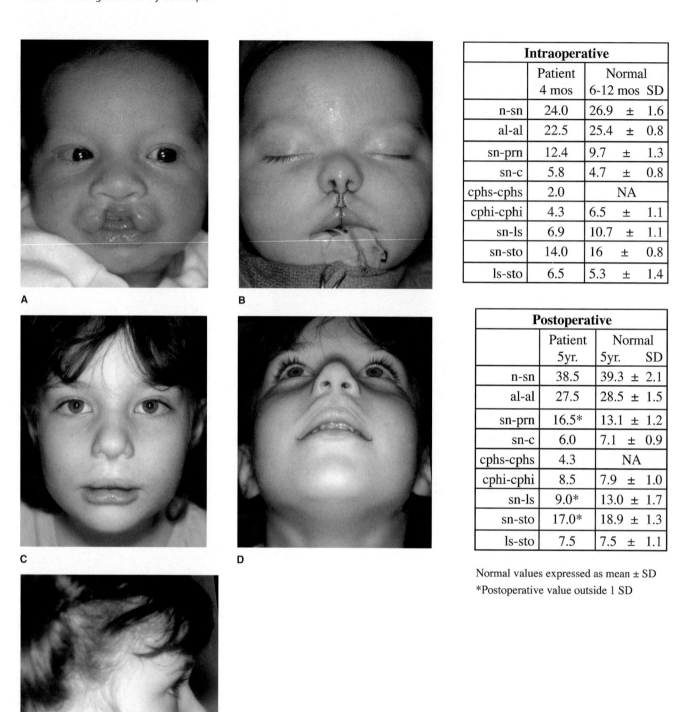

Intraoperative				
	Patient 4 mos	Normal 6-12 mos		SD
n-sn	24.0	26.9	±	1.6
al-al	22.5	25.4	±	0.8
sn-prn	12.4	9.7	±	1.3
sn-c	5.8	4.7	±	0.8
cphs-cphs	2.0	NA		
cphi-cphi	4.3	6.5	±	1.1
sn-ls	6.9	10.7	±	1.1
sn-sto	14.0	16	±	0.8
ls-sto	6.5	5.3	±	1.4

Postoperative				
	Patient 5yr.	Normal 5yr.		SD
n-sn	38.5	39.3	±	2.1
al-al	27.5	28.5	±	1.5
sn-prn	16.5*	13.1	±	1.2
sn-c	6.0	7.1	±	0.9
cphs-cphs	4.3	NA		
cphi-cphi	8.5	7.9	±	1.0
sn-ls	9.0*	13.0	±	1.7
sn-sto	17.0*	18.9	±	1.3
ls-sto	7.5	7.5	±	1.1

Normal values expressed as mean ± SD
*Postoperative value outside 1 SD

Figure 21–14. Symmetrical bilateral incomplete cleft lip. (A) Preoperative. (B) Immediate postoperative. (C–E) Age 5 years.

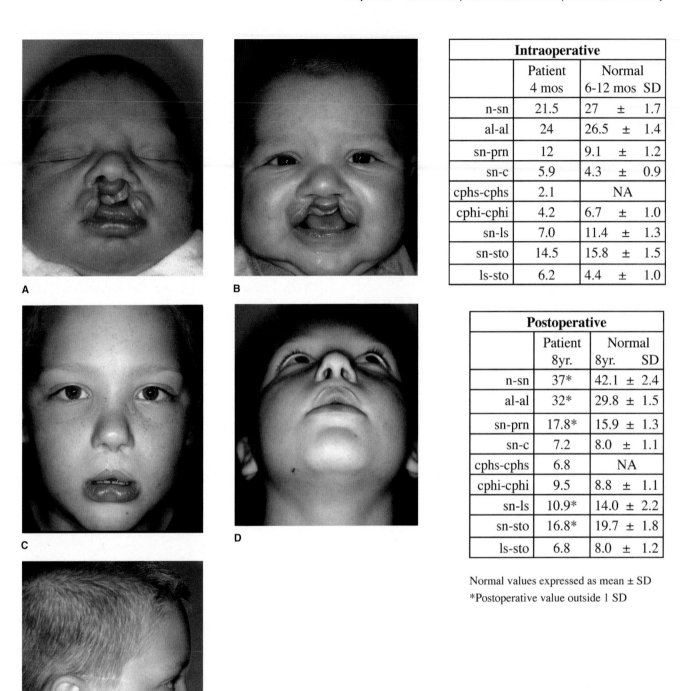

Intraoperative			
	Patient 4 mos	Normal 6-12 mos	SD
n-sn	21.5	27 ±	1.7
al-al	24	26.5 ±	1.4
sn-prn	12	9.1 ±	1.2
sn-c	5.9	4.3 ±	0.9
cphs-cphs	2.1	NA	
cphi-cphi	4.2	6.7 ±	1.0
sn-ls	7.0	11.4 ±	1.3
sn-sto	14.5	15.8 ±	1.5
ls-sto	6.2	4.4 ±	1.0

Postoperative		
	Patient 8yr.	Normal 8yr. SD
n-sn	37*	42.1 ± 2.4
al-al	32*	29.8 ± 1.5
sn-prn	17.8*	15.9 ± 1.3
sn-c	7.2	8.0 ± 1.1
cphs-cphs	6.8	NA
cphi-cphi	9.5	8.8 ± 1.1
sn-ls	10.9*	14.0 ± 2.2
sn-sto	16.8*	19.7 ± 1.8
ls-sto	6.8	8.0 ± 1.2

Normal values expressed as mean ± SD
*Postoperative value outside 1 SD

Figure 21–15. Asymmetrical bilateral (complete/incomplete) cleft lip with intact secondary palate. (A) Preoperative. (B) Following left labial adhesion. (C–E) Age 8 years after second stage (synchronous) nasolabial repair.

synchronous repair of the primary palate without dentofacial orthopedics. This premaxillary segment is difficult to control with a preoperative device and often it is smaller than the interalveolar gap. If necessary, a passive palatal plate can be used to maintain anterior maxillary width following nasolabial closure.

There are some technical nuances that are needed in synchronous repair of the bilateral binderoid variant.[36] Because of nasomaxillary–premaxillary hypoplasia, there is less distortion of labial dimensions with growth. Therefore, the philtral flap should be designed to include the full cutaneous prolabial height and the width need not be excessively narrowed. Primary repair of the hypoplastic nose is difficult. The lower lateral cartilages are small, although they usually can be positioned. The interalar dimension should be narrowed to slightly below age-matched normal because it will widen. The thin columella and its tapered base are augmented with dermal and cartilaginous grafts when the child is older. Likewise the median tubercle must be enlarged with a dermal graft. Correction of the hypoplastic nasomaxillary skeleton is postponed until childhood and adolescence, as in patients with Binder association without cleft lip/palate.

PERIODIC ASSESSMENT

The surgeon's responsibility in caring for the child with bilateral cleft lip does not end after primary repair. There is a tacit understanding that the surgeon will follow the patient throughout childhood and if possible, thereafter. A surgeon also has the obligation to document the changing appearance of the child and to learn from these observations. Periodic assessment is best done with colleagues in an interdisciplinary clinic. In this setting, one also has the opportunity to learn from the work of predecessors and from patients referred from other centers.

Observation alone is probably not sufficient. A surgeon should assess outcome by documenting the number and types of nasolabial revisions. If possible, tabulation of revision rate should include those procedures completed as well as those that will be necessary in the future. Of course, the "true" revision rate cannot be computed until the patients have completed skeletal growth. Nevertheless, neither surgeon nor patient can afford to wait that long. There are three opportunities for nasolabial revision: prior to attending school; during alveolar bone grafting (mixed dentition); following cessation of growth and possible maxillary advancement. These three surgical "windows" are appropriate times to undertake a review of revisions. In so doing, the surgeon can learn from the fourth dimension and modify techniques of primary repair.

Photography

Standardized photography (frontal, lateral, and submental views) is a basic necessity for documentation. Photographs should be taken preoperatively and periodically postopera-

tively, for example, at 2, 5, and 10 years as well as during/after the adolescent growth spurt. Unfortunately, the critical submental photograph is often omitted in the patients' records and in publications. This view should be taken with the head tilted backward so that the nasal tip lies halfway between a line sighted between the medial canthi and medial eyebrows.

Revisions

The conscientious surgeon documents the need for nasolabial revisions, which is obvious early in childhood. The surgeon should keep a mental database of four-dimensional changes so that three-dimensional adjustments can be made in every opportunity to repair a bilateral cleft lip.

Every few years, a more formal assessment can be undertaken. In a study of 50 consecutive nonsyndromic children (median age 5.4 years), the revision rate was 33% for those with bilateral complete cleft lip/palate and 12% for those with bilateral complete cleft lip/alveolus (intact secondary palate).[37] The most frequent revision was resuspension of the anterior gingivolabial sulcus. Once the problem was identified, it is now rarely necessary. Prolapse of the central mucosal is minimized by trimming the extra prolabial vermilion mucosa and securing the remaining mucosal flap and lateral mucosal flaps to the premaxillary periosteum. Two other common problems requiring secondary correction are interalar widening and a thin median tubercle. Technical adjustments are needed at primary repair in anticipation of these shortcomings. None of the children in this analysis required revision for an abnormally wide/long philtrum or for a short columella. Clearly, nasolabial revisions must be reassessed after completion of skeletal growth and likely orthognathic correction.

Panel Rating

There are several studies employing a panel to assess standardized photographs of patients with repaired cleft lip.[38–40] Visual-perceptive analysis, using a rating scale, can be reliable, but this is clumsy, time-consuming, and still subjective.

Direct Anthropometry

Medical anthropometry was pioneered by Farkas; he was first to apply this methodology in children with repaired cleft lip/palate. He has published normal values for Caucasian children from infancy and for a Chinese population older than age 6 years.[41] These measurements can be compared with changes in age- and sex-matched controls during growth. Anthropometry can be used intraoperatively as an aid in primary correction and for documentation of baseline dimensions.[19] Direct anthropometry has its drawbacks. It requires training and experience in using the handheld Vernier caliper. Locating, marking, and measuring the nasolabial landmarks are tedious and demanding, and very difficult in children less than 6 years of age.

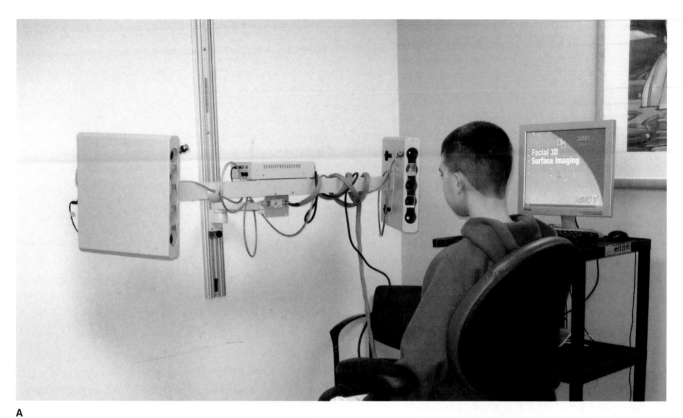

A

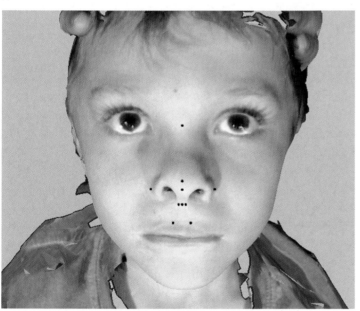

B

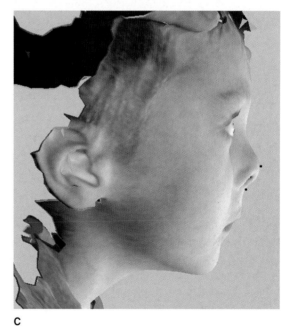

C

Figure 21–16. (A) Three-dimensional photogrammetry with 3dMDface system. (B and C) Anthropometric points placed on frontal and lateral digital images. Direct ("gold standard") and indirect (digital) measurements given in Fig. 21–13.

Indirect Anthropometry

Photogrammetry is one form of indirect anthropometry; however, this two-dimensional format suffers from errors in measurement due to subjective analysis, magnification, parallax, and variation in lighting, head orientation, and subject–camera distance. Two-dimensional photogrammetry is lim-

ited to certain nasolabial dimensions and measurement of proportions and certain angles.[42] Several systems for three-dimensional laser surface imaging eliminate certain measurement errors, especially parallax and magnification, that occur with two-dimensional representations of three-dimensional surfaces.[43,44] While laser surface scanning is reliable and accurate for identification of craniofacial landmarks, the major drawback is the time of image capture (10–20 seconds); this is far too long for a child to hold still. Several new stereophotogrammetric systems are available that obtain images in milliseconds.[45,46] The 3dMDface system[TM] is composed of eight synchronized high-resolution digital cameras arranged in a triangulated configuration (Fig. 21–16A). Software algorithms merge the different overlapping images into one three-dimensional image that can be viewed, manipulated, and analyzed on a computer using the 3dMD software. The standard nasolabial anthropometric points can be easily located on the 3dMD image (Fig. 21–16B-C) and these closely correlate with the direct measurements (Fig. 21–13). The cameras' flash usually highlights the philtral scars, permitting measurement of lower philtral width (cphi–cphi). Locating the points for the upper philtral width (cphs–cphs) is more difficult. This dimension can be accurately determined if ink dots are placed on the subject prior to digital imaging. As in other indirect anthropometric methods, the data are permanently preserved and can be retrieved whenever necessary. The images can be maneuvered for measurements in various views. It is ideal for serial studies and comparative studies among centers. There are some drawbacks: there is a learning curve, analysis is time-consuming, and standardized norms are not yet available. Nevertheless, the validity and reliability of the 3dMDface system has been documented.[47,48] This type of technology should find wide application for quantitative assessment of appearance after cleft lip repair.

CONTROVERSIES AND CONCLUSIONS

Midfacial Growth

Fear of interference with facial growth is an enduring and dominant theme in the habilitation of children born with cleft lip/palate. Some studies have indicted the labial repair, whereas others blame the palatal repair. The debate continues as to whether active preoperative dentofacial orthopedics is potentially more harmful than passive molding methods. It is important to underscore that cephalometric analysis reveals essentially normal facial growth in patients who have reached maturity without the benefit of surgical correction. The sophistic conclusion is that the only way to prevent inhibition of facial development would be to postpone repair of the cleft until growth is completed.

Another viewpoint, sure to raise the hackles of the dental/orthodontic specialists, is to accept some inhibition of facial growth as an unavoidable consequence of surgical intervention. Emphasis should be on protocols and operative techniques that are most likely to give the child the best nasolabial appearance and greatest chance for normal speech, notwithstanding maxillary retrusion.[37] In our unit, the overall frequency of Le Fort I osteotomy is 20%, including all patients with CL/P and CP; however, the frequency of maxillary retrusion correlated with cleft severity: 48% for unilateral complete CL/P and 76% for bilateral complete CL/P.[49] Le Fort

I maxillary advancement and vertical adjustment (often combined with alloplastic onlay of the cheeks) predictably gives a normally convex facial profile. Attempts to compensate the dental inclination at the incisor level will give the young adult a relatively flat facial profile.

Given our current knowledge, midfacial retrusion seems inevitable, particularly in patients with repaired bilateral complete cleft lip/palate. This provides an opportunity for dental specialists to focus on novel ways to distract the upper jaw downward and forward, for example, a buried distractor activated by microchip technology and based on computer-generated preoperative planning. In this way perhaps, the maxilla could be corrected during adolescence, keeping the upper jaw in sagittal harmony with the growing mandible.

Nasoalveolar Molding (NAM)

The New York University protocol for passive preoperative maxillary orthopedics and nasal molding appears to give the diminutive columella a modest stretch.[22] The term passive is a misnomer for NAM, given the amount of exertion necessary and frequent visits required. NAM is complicated, labor-intensive, and slow-paced. NAM also enlarges the nostrils. Taping the NAM appliance can cause irritation of the cheeks; there is also the potential for epidermal erosion, due to pressure, at the columellar–labial junction or the nostril lining. There is also the risk that the molding plate could dislodge and obstruct the airway.[50] In contrast, the Latham device requires only monthly visits and alignment of the maxillary segments is accomplished in 6–8 weeks. Unlike NAM, the Latham device widens the nasal bony–cartilaginous framework (along with the maxillary segments) and does nothing to help the columella. Correction of interalar and interdomal width and construction of the columella must be accomplished by the surgeon.

While NAM is not harmful; it is unnecessary. A columella of slightly greater than age-matched normal length can be constructed in the child with bilateral cleft lip without preoperative NAM. Nasal molding does not obviate the need for anatomic positioning and suture fixation of the lower lateral cartilages. Furthermore, nasal lining need not be stretched because it is already expanded by the pull of the bilateral elements of the cleft lip. The authors of one study noted that NAM was helpful if successful, but if it failed, columellar length was difficult to achieve and maintain.[51] They concluded with a recommendation that a combination of Cutting and Mulliken methods be used, i.e., it is necessary to place an interdomal suture through the anterior side of the lower lateral cartilages in order to narrow the tip and reveal the upper columella. It is easier to position the slumped and splayed lower lateral cartilages after NAM because the anterior maxillary segments are not widened as they are following Latham-type dentofacial orthopedic manipulation.

In the discussion that accompanied the Moravic and Cutting paper,[52] several technical difficulties in the Cutting method of nasolabial repair, unrelated to NAM, were highlighted. The viability of the columellar–philtral unit, raised in a "retrograde" fashion, relies on the paired columellar arteries. This approach limits the possibility of sculpting the nasal tip and columella. Whereas in the Mulliken method, crescentic excision of the excess interdomal skin (in the soft triangle) extended into the columella adds length to the upper columella as well as narrows the nasal tip and columellar waist. Blood supply is also a concern in constructing a narrow base and distal tip of the philtral flap. Tapering the philtral flap appears to be more risky in the Cutting method. The anterior surface of the lower lateral cartilages is not visualized in the Cutting method; the cartilages are apposed with a blindly placed mattress suture. If this suture fails to hold the genua, the nasal tip will remain broad. Finally, the columellar–labial angle tends to be obtuse following the Cutting method. The angle can be reconstructed with a deep suture to the periosteum of the anterior nasal spine, but this too could impair philtral circulation. The columellar–labial angle is also wide following the Mulliken repair; but it has been shown to narrow to normal by early adolescence.[42]

High-volume Surgeons in Centers

The notable studies of poor outcome in cleft care from the United Kingdom led to the recommendation that the National Health Service would only assign newborns with cleft lip/palate to centers staffed by two surgeons, each operating on a minimum of 50 new cases per year.[53] Even such a high-volume surgeon would annually care for about half a dozen new cases of bilateral cleft lip/palate. In contrast, there are over 240 cleft lip/palate centers in the United States; 30% of these units see less than 12 new affected infants per year.[54] Furthermore, in many of these low-volume centers, the newborns are assigned to one of a number of surgeons based on the on-call roster. Given our U.S. health care system, it is difficult for surgeons in small centers to care for a sufficient number of new cases of cleft lip/palate, particularly the bilateral deformity, to gain and maintain expertise.

In the United States, it is well accepted that any newborn with a complicated congenital cardiac anomaly is promptly transferred to a high-volume center of excellence. The mortality rate is unacceptably high in small cardiac units. Unfortunately, this system of triage does not exist for a child born with bilateral cleft lip/palate. Certainly, the child will not die if the initial repair is done by a low-volume surgeon, but there will be an unhappy expression every time the child looks in a mirror. Furthermore, this child will need multiple revisions and despite these attempts, the final outcome may be unsatisfactory in terms of appearance and speech. The ineluctable conclusion is that every child born with bilateral cleft lip/palate should be transferred to a high-volume surgeon who works in a major center.

References

1. Manchester WM. The repair of bilateral cleft lip and palate. *Br J Surg* 52:878, 1965.
2. Mulliken JB. Repair of bilateral complete cleft lip and nasal deformity: State of the art. *Cleft Palate Craniofac J* 37:342, 2000.
3. Millard DR, Jr. *Cleft Craft: The Evolution of Its Surgery, Vol 2.* Boston: Little, Brown, 1977.
4. Gibson T. Pierre-Joseph Celien Simonart (1816–1846) and his intrauterine bands. *Br J Plast Surg* 30:261, 1977.
5. Cronin TD. Lengthening columella by use of skin from nasal floor and alae. *Plast Reconstr Surg* 21:417, 1958.
6. Mulliken JB. Principles and techniques of bilateral complete cleft lip repair. *Plast Reconstr Surg* 75:477, 1985.
7. Pensler JM, Mulliken JB. The cleft lip–lower lip deformity. *Plast Reconstr Surg* 82:602, 1988.
8. Mulliken JB. Primary repair of bilateral cleft lip and nasal deformity. *Plast Reconstr Surg* 108:181, 2001.
9. McComb H. Primary repair of the bilateral cleft lip nose: A 10-year review. *Plast Reconstr Surg* 77:701, 1986.
10. Broadbent TR, Woolf RM. Cleft lip nasal deformity. *Ann Plast Surg* 12:216, 1984.
11. McComb H. Primary repair of the bilateral cleft lip nose. *Br J Plast Surg* 28:262, 1975.
12. McComb H. Primary repair of the bilateral cleft lip nose: A 15-year review and a new treatment plan. *Plast Reconstr Surg* 86:882, 1990.
13. McComb H. Primary repair of the bilateral cleft lip nose: A 4-year review. *Plast Reconstr Surg* 94:37, 1994.
14. Mulliken JB. Correction of the bilateral cleft lip nasal deformity: Evolution of a surgical concept. *Cleft Palate Craniofac J* 29:540, 1992.
15. Mulliken JB. Bilateral complete cleft lip and nasal deformity: An anthropometric analysis of staged to synchronous repair. *Plast Reconstr Surg* 96:9, 1995.
16. Trott JA, Mohan N. A preliminary report on one-stage open tip rhinoplasty at the time of lip repair in bilateral cleft lip and nose repair. *Br J Plast Surg* 46:215, 1993.
17. Cutting CB, Grayson BH, Brecht L, et al. Presurgical columellar elongation and primary retrograde nasal reconstruction in one-stage bilateral cleft lip and nose repair. *Plast Reconstr Surg* 101;630, 1998.
18. Farkas LG, Posnick JC, Hreczko TM, Pron GE. Growth patterns of the nasolabial region: A morphometric study. *Cleft Palate Craniofac J* 29:318, 1992.
19. Mulliken JB, Burvin R, Farkas LG. Repair of bilateral complete cleft lip: Intraoperative nasolabial anthropometry. *Plast Reconstr Surg* 107: 307, 2001.
20. Mulliken JB. Bilateral cleft lip. *Clin Plast Surg* 31:209, 2004.
21. Marsh JL, Martin DS. Bilateral cleft lip: An unorthodox management. *Clin Plast Surg* 20:659, 1993.
22. Grayson BH, Santiago P, Brecht, Cutting CB. Presurgical nasoalveolar molding in patients with cleft lip and palate. *Cleft Palate Craniofac J* 36:486, 1999.
23. Bennun RD, Figueroa AA. Dynamic presurgical nasal remodeling in patients with unilateral and bilateral cleft lip and palate: Modification to the original technique. *Cleft Palate Craniofac J* 43:639, 2006.
24. Georgiade NG, Mason R, Riefkohl R, et al. Preoperative positioning of the protruding premaxilla in the bilateral cleft lip patient. *Plast Reconstr Surg* 83:32, 1989.
25. Millard DR, Jr., Latham RA. Improved primary surgical and dental treatment of clefts. *Plast Reconstr Surg* 86:856, 1990.
26. Henkel KO, Gundlach KKH. Analysis of primary gingivoperiosteoplasty in alveolar cleft repair. Part I: Facial growth. *J Craniomaxillofac Surg* 25:266, 1997.
27. Berkowitz S, Mejia M, Bystrik A. A comparison of the Latham–Millard procedure with those of a conservative treatment approach for dental occlusion and facial aesthetics in unilateral and bilateral complete cleft lip and palate: Part I. Dental occlusion. *Plast Reconstr Surg* 113:1, 2004.
28. Bitter K. Repair of bilateral cleft lip, alveolus and palate. Part 3: Follow-up criteria and late results. *J Craniomaxillofac Surg* 29:49, 2001.
29. Chan K, Hayes C, Shusterman S, et al. The effects of active infant orthopedics on occlusal relationships in unilateral complete cleft lip and palate. *Cleft Palate Craniofac J* 40:511, 2003.

30. Wong GB, Burvin R, Mulliken JB. Resorbable internal splint: An adjunct to primary correction of the unilateral cleft lip–nasal deformity. *Plast Reconstr Surg* 110:385, 2002.

31. Vargervik K. Growth characteristics of the premaxilla and orthodontic treatment principles in bilateral cleft lip and palate. *Cleft Palate J* 20:289, 1983.

32. Friede H and Pruzansky S. Long-term effects of premaxillary setback on facial skeletal profile in complete bilateral cleft lip and palate. *Cleft Palate J* 22:97, 1985.

33. Monroe CW. Recession of the premaxilla in bilateral cleft lip and palate. Follow-up clinic. *Plast Reconstr Surg* 54:482, 1974.

34. Mulliken JB. Unilimb Z-plastic repair of microform cleft lip. *Plast Reconstr Surg* 116:1623, 2005.

35. Mulliken JB, Martinez-Peréz D. The principle of rotation-advancement for repair of unilateral complete cleft lip and nasal deformity: Technical variations and analysis of results. *Plast Reconstr Surg* 104:1247, 1999.

36. Mulliken JB, Burvin R, Padwa BL. Binderoid complete cleft lip/palate. *Plast Reconstr Surg* 111:1000, 2003.

37. Mulliken JB, Wu JK, Padwa BL. Repair of bilateral cleft lip: Review, revisions, and reflections. *J Craniofac Surg* 14:609, 2003.

38. Asher-McDade C, Roberts C, Shaw WC, Gallagher C. Development of a method of rating nasolabial appearance in patients with clefts of the lip and palate. *Cleft Palate Craniofac J* 28:385, 1991.

39. Tobiasen JM, Hiebert JM. Facial impairment scales for clefts. *Plast Reconstr Surg* 93:31, 1994.

40. Lo LJ, Wong FH, Mardina S, Chen YR, Noordhoff MS. Assessment of bilateral cleft lip nose deformity: A comparison of results as judged by cleft surgeons and laypersons. *Plast Reconstr Surg* 110:733, 2002.

41. Farkas LG, (ed). *Anthropometry of the Head and Face*, 2nd edn. New York: Raven Press, 1994.

42. Kohout MP, Monasterio AL, Farkas LG, Mulliken JB. Photogrammetric comparison of two methods for synchronous repair of bilateral cleft lip and nasal deformity. *Plast Reconstr Surg* 102:1339, 1998.

43. Bush K, Antonyshyn O. Three-dimensional facial anthropometry using a laser surface scanner: Validation of the technique. *Plast Reconstr Surg* 98:226, 1996.

44. Yamada T, Mori Y, Minami K, et al. Three-dimensional analysis of facial morphology in normal Japanese children as control data for cleft surgery. *Cleft Palate Craniofac J* 39:517, 2002.

45. Weinberg SM, Scott NM, Neiswanger K, et al. Digital three-dimensional photogrammetry: Evaluation of anthropometric precision and accuracy using a Genex 3D camera system. *Cleft Palate Craniofac J* 41:507, 2004.

46. Krimmel M, Kluba S, Bacher M, et al. Digital surface photogrammetry for anthropometric analysis of the cleft infant face. *Cleft Palate Craniofac J* 43:350, 2006.

47. Weinberg SM, Naidoo S, Govier DP, et al. Anthropometric precision and accuracy of digital three-dimensional photogrammetry: Comparing the Genex and 3dMD imaging systems with one another and with direct anthropometry. *J Craniofac Surg* 17:477, 2006.

48. Wong JY, Oh AK, Ohta E, et al. Validity and reliability of craniofacial anthropometric measurement of 3D digital photogrammetric images. *Cleft Palate Craniofac J* 45:232, 2008.

49. Good PM, Mulliken JB, Padwa BL. Frequency of Le Fort I osteotomy after repaired cleft lip/palate or cleft palate. *Cleft Palate Craniofac J* 44:396, 2004.

50. Grayson BH, Maull D. Nasoalveolar molding for infants born with clefts of the lip, alveolus, and palate. *Clin Plast Surg* 31:149, 2004.

51. Morovic CG, Cutting C. Combining the Cutting and Mulliken methods for primary repair of the bilateral cleft lip nose. *Plast Reconstr Surg* 116:1613, 2005.

52. Mulliken JB. Discussion of combining the Cutting and Mulliken methods for repair of the bilateral cleft lip nose. *Plast Reconstr Surg* 116:1620, 2005.

53. Boorman JG. Treatment of cleft lip and/or palate in the U.K. (Guest Editorial). *Br J Plast Surg* 51:167, 1998.

54. Strauss RP. Cleft palate and craniofacial teams in the United States and Canada: A national survey of team organization and standards of care. *Cleft Palate Craniofac J* 35:473, 1998.

22

Submucous Cleft Palate

Arun K. Gosain, MD • Patrick C. Hettinger, MD

◼ HISTORY AND DEFINITION

Submucous cleft palate was first described by Roux in 1825 during a consultation on a young female with unintelligible speech.[1] On exam, Roux identified a division of the soft palate along with nonunion of the hard palate osseous structures under an intact mucosa.[2,3] Nearly a century later, in 1910, Kelly further described the condition and offered the modern-day name of submucous cleft palate.[4] However, it was not until 1954 that a diagnostic triad was described to identify and diagnose the condition. At that time, Calnan published the three currently recognized stigmata of the overt submucous cleft palate, including (1) a bifid uvula, (2) midline palatal muscle diastasis with an intact mucosa termed "zona pellucida," and (3) a notching defect in the posterior hard palate.[5]

Today, the diagnosis of overt submucous cleft palate remains based on physical exam findings. However, more recently, submucous cleft palate has been shown to exist as a spectrum of disease ranging from overt submucous cleft to lesser defined occult submucous clefts.[6-8] In these occult variants, diagnosis cannot rely on physical exam alone, but rather must employ other means of diagnosis.[6-8] These other means include the use of direct imaging studies and intraoperative exploration. Therefore, submucous cleft palate may be described as a spectrum of disease of the secondary palate that may or may not demonstrate the physical triad laid forth by Calnan. In this chapter, we will discuss submucous cleft palate, its pathogenesis, epidemiology, clinical presentation, diagnosis and evaluation, and modes of therapy.

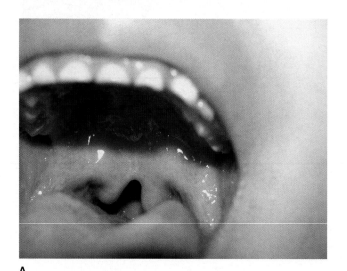

A

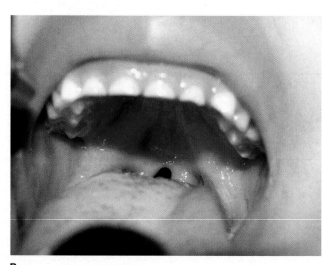

B

Figure 22–1. (A) Classic submucous cleft palate at rest demonstrating a bifid uvula and a "zona pellucida" resulting from diastasis of the levator muscles with the palate joined in the midline only by an overlying thin mucosa. (B) The same patient in phonation demonstrates retraction of the velum with deepening of the zona pellucida due to contraction of the levator muscles, which are abnormally located in the paramedian position and inserted on the posterior margin of the hard palate.

PATHOGENESIS/PATHOLOGY

To fully understand the pathology associated with submucous cleft palate, it is important to have a general concept of the embryology of the primary and secondary palate. The palate is formed in the first trimester of development from the median palatine process (derived from the frontonasal prominence) and the two lateral palatine processes (derived from the maxillary prominences). Initially, each of these structures grows in a vertical orientation surrounding the tongue. However, in the eighth week, there is a change in orientation from vertical to horizontal. This change occurs simultaneously with prognathic growth of the mandible. As a result of this mandibular growth, the tongue is displaced inferiorly, allowing for horizontal growth of the palatal processes without impedance of the tongue. As the palatal shelves continue to grow toward one another, the very medial edge of all three palatal shelves undergoes a process of programmed cell death while the mucosa on the oral and nasal surfaces remains intact. While this is occurring, mesenchymal centers form within each of the shelves. These mesenchymal centers will eventually give rise to the hard palate osseous structures as well as the soft palate musculature. Once the shelves meet, the process of fusion occurs between the lateral palatine processes and the median palatine processes. As this occurs, a downgrowth from the medial nasal prominences, the nasal septum, fuses with the nasal surface of the now-formed palate. The median palatine process subsequently becomes the primary palate, while the lateral palatine processes become the secondary palate.[9] In their study of human fetuses at different stages of development, Cohen et al.[10] demonstrate a definite time line with regard to soft palate mesenchymal maturation and subsequent myogenesis. Furthermore, the osseous structures of

the palate seem to follow a time line that closely parallels myogenesis.

Multiple theories with regard to the pathogenesis of submucous cleft palate have developed since its discovery in the 1800s. However, the failure of mesenchymal proliferation first described by Veau[11] remains the most highly supported in the literature. The reason for this theory is rather intuitive when examining the submucous cleft palate. In all of his initial 18 cases described, Calnan[5] noted a defect of the posterior hard palate with an overlying thin mucosa, midline muscle diastasis, and a bifid muscular uvula (Fig. 22–1). The mucosa, when examined histologically, showed a lack of muscle union across the cleft or poorly developed muscle fibers in a matrix of fibrous tissue. Furthermore, the vomer was typically underdeveloped and attached anteriorly to the bony cleft. As a result of the lack of midline mesenchymal derivatives, Calnan believed that the failure of palate formation resulted from a defect in mesenchymal proliferation. Supporting this theory, Poswillo[12] noted a failure of the maxillary ossification centers to extend to the midline in an induced submucous cleft palate rodent population. More recently, Stal et al.[13] published a histologic study showing similar pathology to that found by Calnan.[5] However, Stal et al.[13] went on to theorize that pathogenesis may involve failure of mesenchymal resorption leading to myocyte fascicular disorganization with haphazard arrangement. To date, the pathogenesis is not completely understood.[13]

As a result of mesenchymal failure, the osseous structures of the posterior hard palate fail to develop. Furthermore, the levator muscles of the soft palate fail to reach the midline for proper insertion. In 1930, Dorrance[14] noted an abnormal insertion of the levator muscles in patients with submucous cleft palate. Normally, the levator muscles insert in the

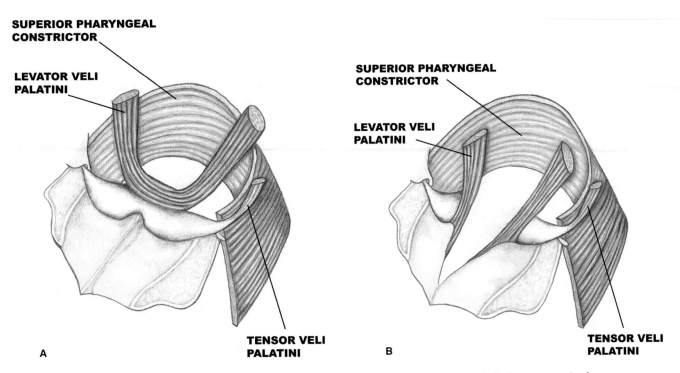

Figure 22–2. (A) Diagrammatic view of the normal velopharyngeal mechanism in which the levator muscles form a sling within the velum. The palatopharyngeal and superior pharyngeal constrictor muscles contribute to the velopharyngeal mechanism, creating a circumferential "valving mechanism," which is open at rest to allow nasal breathing, but is capable of closure during phonation to prevent nasal air escape. (B) Diagrammatic view of the velopharyngeal mechanism in a patient with submucous cleft palate and velopharyngeal inadequacy (VPI). The levator muscles are abnormally located in a paramedian position and inserted on the posterior surface of the hard palate. The posterior nasal spine is absent in the midline of the hard palate. The velopharyngeal mechanism is incapable of achieving complete closure, resulting in nasal air escape during phonation.

palatine aponeurosis at the midline, allowing elevation of the soft palate during contraction. However, in submucous cleft palate, the levator muscles insert too far anteriorly onto the posterior hard palate (Fig. 22–2). The result is a soft palate that is ineffectively raised and actually shortened during levator contraction. This tethering effect of the abnormal insertion is believed to be one of the most important factors in the symptoms associated with submucous cleft palate. These findings were confirmed by Hoopes et al.[15–17] who, using fluoroscopic studies, demonstrated a short palatal length, diminished velar excursion, and a slowed rate of velar ascent in a population of submucous cleft palate patients. The group concluded that the further anterior the insertion, the greater the degree of velopharyngeal inadequacy (VPI).

EPIDEMIOLOGY

The two largest studies examining incidence of submucous cleft palate both screened large populations of school-age children. In the larger of these two studies, Weatherley-White et al.[18] examined 10,836 children and found only 9 (0.08%) to have all 3 stigmata of overt submucous cleft palate.[18] Furthermore, it was found that of these nine children, only one had clinical symptoms of VPI. This relatively high percentage of patients with submucous cleft palate who re-

main asymptomatic has been confirmed by numerous other studies.[4,5,8,19–24] The second large study looked for physical exam findings in 6000 school-age children. However, in this study, Garcia-Velasco et al.[25] required only two physical exam findings, of the three stigmata, to give the diagnosis of submucous cleft palate. In this study, the group found only one child (0.02%) who met their criteria for submucous cleft palate.

While the incidence of overt submucous cleft palate can be evaluated in studies such as those mentioned, the incidence of occult submucous cleft is far more difficult to assess. The reason for this is that within a general population, occult submucous cleft palate is only investigated in patients referred for evaluation of VPI. Furthermore, ethical considerations do not allow for nasoendoscopic studies or intraoperative exploration as a means of screening for submucous cleft palate. However, in using nasal endoscopy to evaluate 25 patients with bifid uvula, Shprintzen et al.[24] found 92% of patients to have landmarks associated with submucous cleft palate. This study suggests that the incidence of occult submucous cleft palate may be considerably higher than what has previously been thought, considering that bifid uvula has been reported in roughly 1–7.5% of the population.[18,22–27] However the true incidence of occult submucous cleft palate remains unknown.

As shown in these and other studies, the incidence of overt submucous cleft palate (0.02–0.08%) is exceedingly rare in the general population; however, when examining populations with VPI, the incidence is markedly increased. In examining 240 patients with VPI, Kaplan[8] found 27% to have diagnoses of submucous cleft palate: 17% of the overt type and 10% of the occult type.[8] In a similar study of 131 patients with VPI, Lewin et al.[7] found 66% of patients demonstrating submucous cleft palates: 44% of the overt type and 22% of the occult type. Therefore, in examining patients with known VPI, there must be a high clinical suspicion for submucous cleft palate.

Although Calnan[5] observed a small proportion of submucous cleft palate patients to have family history of clefts, none of the larger studies have reported a specific familial etiology to submucous cleft palate. While there is no definite familial etiology, submucous cleft palate is commonly associated with other comorbid conditions. In their evaluation of 26 submucous cleft palate patients with evidence of VPI, Kaplan et al.[8] found only 30% to have isolated defects of the palate. Similarly, Weatherly-White et al.[18] found only 35% of 62 submucous cleft palate patients to have the isolated palatal anomaly. Common comorbid conditions include mandibular prognathism/hypognathism, syndactyly, talipes, cleft lip, microtia, neurosensory hearing loss, and mental retardation.[28,29] Furthermore, submucous cleft palate is associated with several syndromes including velocardiofacial, Klippel-Feil, and Treacher Collins syndromes.[18,30]

CLINICAL PRESENTATION

The velopharyngeal valve consists of a complex group of structures that function to separate the oral and nasal cavities for normal speech and deglutition. The soft palate, posterior pharyngeal wall, and lateral pharyngeal walls must all work together for proper closure of this valving mechanism. The muscles primarily responsible for proper velopharyngeal valve closure include the levator veli palatini and superior pharyngeal constrictor, with the palatopharyngeus, salpingopharyngeus, and tensor veli palatini muscles making additional contributions.[31] Valve dysfunction as a result of compromised motion is referred to as velopharyngeal incompetence, while dysfunction due to tissue deficit is referred to as insufficiency. Any combination of these two is more generically termed velopharyngeal inadequacy, which is commonly abbreviated as VPI.[31] However, one must be aware that the "I" in the abbreviation VPI might apply to incompetence, insufficiency, or inadequacy; in addition, many authors are not aware of the different meanings of these terms and often apply the term VPI to apply to any of these conditions. The primary clinical manifestations associated with VPI include nasal escape of air and nasal resonance during nonnasal speech and oronasal reflux of swallowed liquid and solid food.

Depending on the presence of velopharyngeal inadequacy, patients with submucous cleft palate may present at any age or may remain asymptomatic throughout life.[4,5,8,19–24] Those patients presenting in infancy will often have difficulties of prolonged feeding times or nasal regurgitation following feeds. Most commonly, patients will present following the development of speech abnormalities.[32] Primary speech abnormalities arise from inappropriate nasal escape during articulation, producing hypernasal speech. Secondary speech abnormalities arise from articulatory errors learned to compensate for the abnormal nasal escape during speech.[32] When patients present with any of the aforementioned complaints, the diagnosis of submucous cleft palate must be considered. Another presenting symptom is recurrent otitis media and this has also been described in the literature. While the association of cleft palate and otitis media is well established, that of submucous cleft palate and otitis media is less convincing. In children with overt cleft palate, otitis is thought to arise from eustachian tube dysfunction along with a possible impaired tubal dilatory system.[33,34] Children with submucous cleft palate, on the other hand, are thought to have an isolated defect within the levator veli palatini, which is not required for eustachian tube dilatation.[35] Furthermore, while early studies reported increased incidence of otitis media in submucous cleft patients,[19,21,24,36,37] more recent studies have shown an incidence closer to that of the general population.[27,35,38,39]

EVALUATION OF VELOPHARYNGEAL INADEQUACY

Once VPI is suspected, a full workup is indicated as timing of treatment is important in management and outcome. The single most important test performed is a formal perceptual speech evaluation by a trained speech pathologist.[40–42] This evaluation is necessary to establish the diagnosis of velopharyngeal inadequacy. Using articulation measurement, equal-appearing interval scales and global ratings, speech pathologists are able to give subjective assessment of hypernasality.[43–53] Although direct oral examination alone is helpful in identifying features of the overt submucous cleft, it does not allow for assessment of palate length, palate height, pharyngeal wall motion, and velopharyngeal valving.[49] Therefore, direct oral examination provides little information with regard to velopharyngeal inadequacy.

As a result, other means of direct and indirect testing are necessary for adequate assessment. Indirect methods use both qualitative and quantitative measures of velopharyngeal inadequacy, while direct methods allow visualization of the valve mechanism. Indirect methods of evaluation include TONAR (The Oral Nasal Acoustic Ratio),[54–57] air pressure flow measures,[57–61] sound pressure measures,[62] nasal vibratory measurements,[63–65] photodetection,[66–70] and velotrace measuring palatal motion transduction.[71] Electromyography is another indirect method of evaluation, although it has less clinical value.[72,73] Indirect studies allow for objective documentation of velopharyngeal inadequacy and can confirm the perceptual findings of the speech pathologist.

While indirect methods allow for correlation of objective and perceptual findings, they are less beneficial in treatment planning of velopharyngeal inadequacy. Therefore, direct measures of visualization become essential for management. The most common direct techniques in use today include mutiview videofluoroscopy and nasal endoscopy. Direct visualization can identify the closure pattern and contributions of the velum, the lateral and posterior pharyngeal walls, and Passavant's ridge.[31]

One of the two major direct studies in use today is that of multiview videofluoroscopy. This test originated as a plain roentgenogram projected in a lateral view during isolated sound phonation.[74,75] Fluoroscopy has since evolved to allow real-time visualization of the velopharyngeal mechanism in multiple views. By using frontal, lateral, basal, and Towne's projections, the velopharyngeal mechanism can be seen in three dimensions. The basal view is particularly effective for visualization of the lateral pharyngeal walls.[75] Towne's view, on the other hand, is thought to be effective in individuals with large adenoids.[76] Furthermore, it has been shown that by adding Towne's view, sensitivity is significantly increased over lateral view alone.[77] Common findings associated with submucous cleft palate include a shortened soft palate, diminished velar ascent, decreased velar excursion, and palate fatigability.[15–17]

The second major direct study used to evaluate VPI is nasal endoscopy. This study began with the use of a rigid nasendoscope used to view the nasal surface of the velopharyngeal valve.[78,79] Since that time, the use of an end-viewing flexible fiberoptic endoscope has been advocated by numerous studies. During nasal endoscopy, the patient repeats key phrases that stimulate velopharyngeal closure as the scope views the velopharyngeal mechanism. It is important that the investigator views the lateral pharyngeal walls, the posterior pharyngeal wall, and the nasal surface of the velum.[31] Through endoscopy, the velopharyngeal closure pattern can be identified, bearing corrective implications. Furthermore, nasal endoscopy has been shown to be important in the diagnosis of occult submucous cleft palate.[6,7] In such patients, the "seagull sign," demonstrated as a central groove in the nasal surface of the velum, is thought to represent hypoplasia of the musculus uvula.[6,7,80]

More recently, magnetic resonance imaging (MRI) has been employed as a means of direct evaluation of velopharyngeal inadequacy. In a report of two patients with submucous cleft palate, MRI consistently demonstrated interruption of the levator muscle tissue in the midline along with an abnormal anterior insertion. Furthermore, magnetic resonance images demonstrated bilateral encapsulating sheaths interrupting the muscle sling. While MRI is currently not a mainstay in evaluation of velopharyngeal inadequacy, its use may be of importance in the future, as it offers superior soft tissue imaging without ionizing radiation.[81]

MANAGEMENT

One of the long-standing debates in submucous cleft palate literature deals with the most appropriate timing of surgical intervention. In the case of overt cleft palate, it has been well established that speech outcomes are greatly improved when palate repair takes place prior to speech development.[82–84] In overt cleft palate, early surgical intervention is imperative as there is no chance for velopharyngeal competency without treatment. On the other hand, only a small percentage of patients with submucous cleft palate will develop symptoms of velopharyngeal inadequacy.[4,5,8,19–24] Therefore, if surgical intervention were to proceed prior to speech development in this population, a majority of the surgery performed would be unnecessary. More importantly, it would place these patients at unnecessary risk of surgical complications.

Documented VPI that is refractory to speech therapy is the most widely accepted indication for surgical intervention in the treatment of submucous cleft palate. By this indication, 2.5 years would be the earliest acceptable age for surgical intervention, since it is not possible to perform an adequate speech evaluation along with a sufficient trial of speech therapy prior to this age.[32] In 1976, Abyholm evaluated speech outcome in 47 patients with submucous cleft palate operated on before and after age 7 years. Patients underwent either a von Langenbeck palatoplasty or a von Langenbeck repair with a pharyngeal flap. This study found that 84% of patients operated on prior to age 7 years went on to develop normal speech or occasional insignificant hypernasality, while only 64% of those patients operated on after age 7 years achieved an equivalent outcome.[85]

Once the diagnosis of VPI has been established and speech therapy has failed, surgical correction of submucous cleft palate is indicated. As a result of the pathology associated with submucous cleft palate, surgical procedures have been developed to target the specific deficiencies of the secondary palate. Historically, surgical correction has focused on increasing palatal length, improving soft palate motility, reorienting palatal musculature, and recruiting tissue to act as a physical barrier between the oropharynx and nasopharynx. By increasing palatal length or by releasing and reorienting the levator muscles, velar function can be improved. On the other hand, when recruiting tissue to act as a physical barrier, velopharyngeal closure relies on adequate lateral pharyngeal wall motion.

Surgical corrections that have been designed include (1) excision of submucous cleft palate with primary closure, (2) the use of a pharyngeal flap, (3) palatal pushback techniques, (4) intravelar veloplasty, (5) the Furlow Z-plasty, and (6) combined surgical techniques. The following is a brief description of each.

Excision with Primary Closure of Submucous Cleft Palate

Histologic specimens taken from patients with submucous cleft palate demonstrate a failure of muscle fusion at the midline in the region of the cleft. While it would then seem plausible that excision of this region with primary closure may correct the underlying pathology, it has been shown that the palatal musculature does not lie in the correct transverse orientation. Rather, the levator muscles insert abnormally anterior. As a result, primary closure would not recreate the correct palatal anatomy. Therefore, this surgical method is no longer advocated for treatment of VPI in patients with submucous cleft palate. In a report of seven patients undergoing excision of submucous cleft palate with primary closure, Crikelair and colleagues found only one patient to have excellent results 5 months postoperatively.[86]

Pharyngeal Flap

First performed by Schoenborn in 1876, the pharyngeal flap has long been a surgical method for the correction of velopharyngeal inadequacy.[87] In this technique, a myomucosal flap from the posterior pharyngeal wall is raised and insetted into the nasal surface of the soft palate. The pharyngeal flap provides a physical barrier between the oropharynx and nasopharynx. By raising this flap, ports are created on either side of the raised tissue. Velopharyngeal competence is restored as the lateral pharyngeal walls close these ports during speech and deglutition. Therefore, restoration of velopharyngeal competence depends on tailoring flap width to maintain patency of the nasal airway, while relying upon adequate lateral pharyngeal wall motion to achieve velopharyngeal closure. Common side effects of this procedure include obstructive sleep apnea, flap dehiscence, hyponasality, and recurrent velopharyngeal inadequacy. Since its description, this procedure has been one of the most commonly used treatment options for velopharyngeal inadequacy. In 1970, Crikelair et al.[86] reported performing pharyngeal flaps on nine patients in whom velopharyngeal inadequacy was attributed to congenital short palate. Results were judged to be excellent to good in five of the six patients with adequate follow-up and poor in the remaining patient. In a review of 600 palatal pharyngoplasties performed by 1 surgeon, Bronsted et al.[88] reported the results of pharyngeal flap surgery in 104 patients with submucous cleft palate. Eighty-one percent of these patients were reported to have normalization of speech 5 years postoperatively. Similarly, in a series of 76 patients with overt submucous cleft palate, Husein et al.[89] reported significant speech improvement in 80% of patients undergoing a pharyngeal flap procedure.[89] In a series of 50 submucous cleft palate patients undergoing operative repair, Park et al.[90] reported the results of 21 pharyngeal flap procedures. Nineteen of the twenty-one patients achieved "normal" velopharyngeal function. Furthermore, the group reported no complications of obstructive sleep apnea, dehiscence, or consistent hyponasality.[90]

Palatal Pushback

The palatal pushback was first described in 1925 by Dorrance[91] as a modification of the von Langenbeck palatoplasty. In this procedure, bilateral mucoperiosteal flaps were elevated and advanced posteriorly, thereby theoretically increasing the overall length of the palate. Modifications to the procedure have since been made; however, the main principle of palatal lengthening remains. Furthermore, this type of procedure is still in use today for correcting defects of the

secondary palate. In his classic article delineating the physical signs associated with submucous cleft palate, Calnan[5] reported the palatal pushback with excision of the submucous portion of the palate to be the "only treatment for submucous clefts with rhinolalia." Thirteen of the eighteen patients treated in this manner obtained "normal speech"; however, most required is supplemental speech therapy. Similarly, in a series of 13 patients undergoing palatal pushback, Porterfield et al.[92] reported elimination of nasality; however, they also noted that nearly all patients required extensive speech therapy, particularly those in which repairs were done at a later age. In their series of 50 patients with submucous cleft palate, Park et al.[90] reported the results of 18 patients undergoing a palatal pushback procedure. Postoperative velopharyngeal function was judged to be normal in 8 of these 18 patients and good in 3, leaving 7 patients with a result that was less than satisfactory.

Intravelar Veloplasty

Restoration of the levator sling was first popularized in the 1960s following anatomic studies of cleft palate.[93,94] The procedure of intravelar veloplasty was designed to release the levator muscle from its abnormal insertion on the posterior margin of the hard palate and to create apposition of the levator muscles at the midline to restore the levator sling and thereby restore velar function. In 1988, Pensler and Bauer published a report of 15 patients with submucous cleft palate who underwent intravelar veloplasty with palatal pushback. Eight of the fifteen patients underwent repair prior to age 2 years, with six of the eight achieving normal speech. The other seven patients underwent the procedure beyond age 2 years, with only one patient achieving normal speech.[95] However, one must question whether this series represented a selection bias, in that those patients operated on prior to age 2 years were likely repaired before a proper evaluation for VPI could be performed and were selected on an anatomic basis alone. Therefore, many of these patients may never have developed VPI. Those patients repaired after age 2 years, on the other hand, were referred for treatment of VPI associated with submucous cleft palate and therefore may have represented a more complex group of speech disorders than the younger group.

Furlow Z-plasty

In 1978, Furlow[96,97] presented a new technique for repairing palatal clefts using opposing mirror–image Z-plasties elevated from the oral and nasal mucosa, respectively. By transposition of the posteriorly based myomucosal flaps, this Z-plasty reorients the palatal musculature in correct anatomic position, simultaneously increasing palatal length and decreasing pharyngeal width. Since its description, the Furlow Z-plasty has become one of the most widely used procedures for correction of VPI. Furthermore, in recent years, it has been the most highly published of the techniques for correction of VPI related to palatal clefting.

In a well-documented series of 35 patients with submucous cleft palate and VPI, Chen et al.[98] used the selection criteria of sagittal closure pattern—a velopharyngeal gap of <5 mm—and good biofeedback results as indications to perform Furlow Z-plasty. Of 30 patients who underwent the procedure, 29 achieved competent velopharyngeal function and only 1 patient had an unsatisfactory result. In another series of 27 patients with submucous cleft palate, Seagle et al.[99] reported a success rate of 83% when using the Furlow technique.[99] These authors concluded that the Furlow technique was most effective in patients with a velopharyngeal gap of less than 8 mm. Husein et al.[89] reported an overall success rate of 88.9% when using the Furlow technique in nine patients with submucous cleft palate; however, while the group alludes to a short velopharyngeal gap as an indication for Furlow Z-plasty, no objective data on the optimal gap size are provided.[89]

In an attempt to objectively measure postoperative results of the Furlow Z-plasty, D'Antonio et al.[100] used postoperative cephalometric studies to examine the soft palate. These authors found significant increases in both palatal length and palatal thickness in patients who achieved complete velopharyngeal closure following Furlow Z-plasty.

Combined Techniques

These techniques have typically combined two or more of the following: pharyngeal flap, palatal pushback, and intravelar veloplasty. The stated rationale for adding a pharyngeal flap to the palatal pushback is to provide mucosal lining for the defect created by the pushback.[32] In this setting, the palatal pushback, rather than the pharyngeal flap, provides the dynamic component of velopharyngeal competence. After noting poor results with the pushback alone, Hoopes et al.[17] performed a pushback with pharyngeal flap on four patients.[17] Three of the four patients had significant improvement in speech and postoperative cineradiography showed palatal lengthening; however, all patients continued to have some degree of hypernasality. In our opinion, improved speech results have been better documented following the pharyngeal flap alone. Therefore, in patients in whom a pushback and pharyngeal flap are being considered in combination, we would suggest considering performing a pharyngeal flap alone. The pharyngeal flap is a proven technique for correction of VPI in patients with submucous cleft palate and it is difficult to justify its use simply to add lining to another procedure in which results are more marginal than those following pharyngeal flap alone.

In his review of 240 patients with VPI, Kaplan[8] reported 41 of 240 patients to have overt submucous cleft palate based on physical examination and 23 of 240 patients to have occult submucous cleft based on intraoperative exploration. Kaplan performed pharyngeal flap plus pushback, along with intravelar veloplasty on 26 of the patients with overt submucous cleft palate, and on 23 of the patients with occult submucous cleft palate. The average improvement in speech outcome was over three times greater in those patients with overt submucous cleft palate who underwent surgery when compared to those with the occult variety who underwent speech therapy alone. Our opinion is that, although speech outcome improved following this complex regimen of combined procedures, similar or better results may have been achieved with one carefully selected procedure. The rationales for combined procedures cannot be clearly established unless criteria are established by which single procedures are likely to fail. Were the authors able to show that combining procedures in this subgroup of refractory patients results in improvement in speech outcome, then a stronger argument could be made for adapting an initial strategy of combined techniques for the correction of VPI in patients with submucous cleft palate.

CONCLUSION

We feel that the technique for surgical correction of VPI in patients with submucous cleft palate should be chosen based on rational criteria. Given that only a minority of patients with overt submucous cleft palate will develop VPI, surgical correction should not be performed simply because a patient presents with the anatomic stigma of submucous cleft palate. Only after VPI is documented following perceptual speech assessment by a trained speech and language pathologist should surgical intervention be considered. Of note, few, if any, children are able to provide a reliable speech examination prior to age 2½ years, and, it is highly recommended to delay surgical intervention until after this age. We do not feel that the technique for correction of VPI varies between overt and submucous cleft palate; once a proper diagnosis of VPI is established, it is the surgical correction of VPI and not the anatomic features by which submucous cleft palate was defined that is paramount. The technique selected for the correction of VPI must take several factors into account. These factors include velopharyngeal gap size, palate length, lateral pharyngeal wall motion, and velopharyngeal closure pattern. Better documentation of the preoperative factors associated with VPI, and continued follow-up of speech outcomes following surgical correction, will provide more objective data by which future practitioners may choose the best method for surgical correction of this complex problem.

References

1. Roux JP. *Memoires Sur Staphylorrhaphie.* Paris: J.S. Chaude, 1825, p. 84.
2. Dorrance GM. Congenital insufficiency of the palate. *Arch Surg* 21:185, 1930.
3. Roux JP. Congenital fissure of the soft palate. *Lancet* 1:694, 1835.
4. Kelly AB. Congenital insufficiency of the palate. *J Laryngol Otol* 25:281, 1910.
5. Calnan JS. Submucous cleft palate. *Br J Plast Surg* 6:264, 1954.
6. Croft CB, Shprintzen RJ, Daniller A, Lewin ML. The occult submucous cleft palate and the musculus uvulae. *Cleft Palate J* 15:150, 1978.
7. Lewin ML, Croft CB, Shprintzen RJ. Velopharyngeal insufficiency due to hypoplasia of the musculus uvulae and occult submucous cleft palate. *Plast Reconstr Surg* 65:585, 1980.

8. Kaplan EN. The occult submucous cleft palate. *Cleft Palate J* 12:356, 1975.

9. Gosain AK, Nacamuli R. Embryology of the head and neck. In. CH. Thorne, RW. Beasley, J Aston, SP. Bartlett, GC. Gurtner, SL. Spear (Eds). *Grabb and Smith's Plastic Surgery* (Sixth Edition). Philadelphia: Lippincott Williams and Wilkins, 2007, pp. 179–190.

10. Cohen SR, Chen L, Trotman CA, Burdi AR. Soft Palate Myogenesis: A developmental field paradigm. *Cleft Palate Craniofac J* 30:441, 1993.

11. Veau VE. *Division Palatine.* Paris: Masson et Cie, 1931.

12. Poswillo D. The pattogenesis of submucous cleft palate. *Scand J Plast Reconstr Surg* 8:34, 1974.

13. Stal S, Hicks MJ. Classic and occult submucous cleft palates: A histopathologic analysis. *Cleft Palate Craniofac J* 35:351, 1998.

14. Dorrance GM. Congenital insufficiency of the palate. *Arch Surg* 21:185, 1930.

15. Hoopes JE, et al. Cineradiographic definition of the functional anatomy and pathophysiology of the velopharynx. *Cleft Palate J* 7:443, 1970.

16. Hoopes JE, et al. The locus of levator veli palatini muscle function as a measure of velopharyngeal incompetence. *Plast Reconstr Surg* 44:155, 1969.

17. Hoopes JE, et al. Cineradiographic assessment of combined island flap pushback and pharyngeal flap in surgical management of submucous cleft palate. *Brit J Plast Surg* 23:39, 1970.

18. Weatherly-White RCA, et al. Submucous cleft palate. *Plast Reconstr Surg* 49:297, 1972.

19. Beeden AG. The bifid uvula. *J Otolaryngol* 86:813, 1972.

20. McWilliams BJ. Submucous cleft of the palate: How likely are they to be symptomatic? *Cleft Palate Craniofac J* 28:247, 1991.

21. Massengill R, Jr., Pickrell K, Robinson M. Results of pushback operations in treatment of submucous cleft palate. *Plast Reconstr Surg* 51:432, 1973.

22. Porterfield HW, Mohler LR, Sandel A. Submucous cleft palate. *Plast Reconstr Surg* 58:60, 1976.

23. Saad EF. The bifid uvula in ear, nose, and throat practice. *Laryngoscope* 85:734, 1975.

24. Shprintzen RJ, Schwartz RH, Daniller A, Hoch L. Morphologic significance of bifid uvula. *Pediatrics* 75:553, 1985.

25. Garcia-Velasco M, Ysunza A, Hernandez X, Marquez C. Diagnosis and treatment of submucous cleft palate: A review of 108 cases. *Cleft Palate J* 25:171, 1988.

26. Lindemen G, Riis B, Sewerin IB. Prevalence of cleft uvula among 2732 Danes. *Cleft Palate J* 14:226, 1977.

27. Rivron RP. Bifid uvula: Prevalence and association in otitis media with effusion in children admitted for routine otolaryngological operations. *J Laryngol Otol* 103:249, 1989.

28. Minami RT, Kaplan EN, Wu G, Jobe RP. Velopharyngeal incompetence without overt cleft palate. *Plast Reconstr Surg* 55:573, 1975.

29. Fara M, Hrivnakova J, Sedlackova E. Submucous cleft palates. *Acta Chir Plast* 13:221, 1971.

30. Shprintzen RJ, Goldberg RB, Lewin ML, et al. A new syndrome involving cleft palate, cardiac anomalies, typical facies, and learning disabilities: Velocardiofacial syndrome. *Cleft Palate J* 15:56, 1978.

31. Conley SF, Gosain AK, Marks SM, Larson DL. Identification and assessment of velopharyngeal Inadequacy. *Am J Otolaryngol* 18:38, 1997.

32. Gosain AK, Conley SF, Marks S, Larson DL. Submucous cleft palate: Diagnostic methods and outcomes of surgical treatment. *Plast Rerconstr surg* 97:1498, 1996.

33. Doyle WJ, Reilly JS, Jardini L, Rovnack S. Effect of palatoplasty on the function of the eustachian tube in children with cleft palate. *Cleft Palate J* 23:63, 1986.

34. Mastune S, Sando L, Takahashi H. Insertion of the tensor veli palatine muscle and eustachian tube function. *Plast Reconstr Surg* 85:684, 1990.

35. Finklestein Y, Talmi YP, Nachmani A, et al. Levator veli palatini muscle and eustachian tube function. *Plast Reconstr Surg* 85:684, 1990.

36. Saad EF. The underdeveloped palate in ear, nose, and throat practice. *Laryngoscope* 90:1371, 1980.

37. Pensler JM, Bauer BS. Levator repositioning and palatal lengthening for submucous clefts. *Plast Reconstr Surg* 82:765, 1988.

38. Scwartz RH, Hayden GF, Rodriguez WJ, et al. The bifid uvula: Is it a marker for an otitis prone child? *Laryngoscope* 95:1100, 1985.

39. Finkelstein Y, Zohar Y, Nachmani A, et al. The otolaryngologist and the patient with velocardiofacial syndrome. *Arch Otolaryngol Head Neck Surg* 119:563, 1993.

40. Moll KL. Objective measures of nasality. *Cleft Palate J* 1:371, 1964.

41. Phillips BJ. Perceptual evaluation of velopharyngeal competence. *Am Otol Rhinol Laryngol* 89:153, 1980.

42. Phillips BJ. Speech assessment. *Semin Speech Lang* 7:297, 1986.

43. Morris HL, Spriestersbach D, Darley F. An articulation test for assessing competency of velopharyngeal closure. *J Speech Hear Res* 4:48, 1961.

44. Bzoch KR. Measurement and assessment of categorical aspects of cleft palate speech. *Communicative Disorders Related to Cleft Palate.* Boston: Little, Brown, 1979, p. 161.

45. Van Demark DR, Sickard SL. A preschool articulation test to assess velopharyngeal competency: Normative data. *Cleft Palate J* 17:175, 1980.

46. McCabe R, Bradley D. Pre- and post-articulations therapy assessment. *Lang Speech Hear Serv Schools* 4:13, 1973.

47. Fisher HB, Logemann JA. *Fisher-Logemann Test of Articulation Competence.* Boston: Houghton Mifflin, 1971.

48. Boone D. *The Voice and Voice Therapy.* Englewood Cliffs, NJ: Prentice-Hall, 1980, p. 69.

49. McWilliams BJ, Morris HL, Shelton RL. *Cleft Palate Speech.* ST. Louis: Mosby, 1984, p. 286.

50. Wilson DK. Management of voice disorders in children and adolescents. *Semin Speech Lang* 4:245, 1983.

51. Morris HL. Types of velopharyngeal incompetence. *Treating Articulation Disorders.* Baltimore: University Park Press, 1984, pp. 211–222.

52. Subtelny JD, Van Hattum R, Meyers BB. Ratings and measurements of cleft palate speech. *Cleft Palate J* 9:18, 1972.

53. Van Demark DR. Assessment of velopharyngeal competence for children with cleft palate. *Cleft Palate J* 11:310, 1974.

54. Warren DW. The determination of velopharyngeal incompetency by aerodynamic and acoustical techniques. *Clin Plast Surg* 2:299, 1975.

55. Dalston RM, Warren DW. The diagnosis of velopharyngeal inadequacy. *Clin Plast Surg* 12:685, 1985.

56. Hardin MA, Van Demark DR, Morris HL, Payne MM. Correspondence between nasalance scores and listener judgments of hypernasality and hyponasality. *Cleft Palate Craniofac J* 29:346, 1992.

57. Dalston RM, Warren DW, Dalston ET. Use of nasometry as a diagnostic tool for identifying patients with velopharyngeal impairment. *Cleft Palate Craniofac J* 23:184, 1991.

58. Warren DW. PERCI: A method for rating palatal efficiency. *Cleft Palate J* 16:279, 1979.

59. Warren DW, Dalston RM, Trier WC, Holder MB. A pressure-flow technique for quantifying temporal patterns of palatopharyngeal closure. *Cleft Palate J* 22:11, 1985.

60. Morr KE, Warren DW, Dalston RM, Smith LR. Screening of velopharyngeal inadequacy by differential pressure measurements. *Cleft Palate J* 26:42, 1989.

61. D'Antonio LL, Muntz HR, Marsh JL, et al. Practical applications of flexible fiberoptic nasopharyngoscopy for evaluating velopharyngeal function. *Plast Reconstr Surg* 32:611, 1988.

62. Dalston RM, Warren DW Comparison of tonar II, pressure-flow, and listener judgments of hypernasality in the assessment of velopharyngeal function. *Cleft Palate J* 23:108, 1986.

63. Redenbaugh MA, Reich AR. Correspondence between an accelereo-metric nasal/voice amplitude ration and listeners' direct magnitude estimations of hypernasality. *J Speech Hear Res* 28:273, 1985.

64. Reich AR, Redenbaugh MA. Relation between nasal/voice accelerometric values and interval estimates of hypernasality. *Cleft Palate J* 22:237, 1985.

65. Larson PL, Hamlet SL. Coarticulation effects on the nasalization of vowels using nasal/voice amplitude ratio instrumentation. *Cleft Palate J* 24:286, 1987.

66. Dalston RM. Photodetector assessment of velopharyngeal activity. *Cleft Palate J* 19:1, 1982.

67. Dalston RM, Seaver EJ. Nasometric and phototransductive measurements of reaction times among normal adult speakers. *Cleft Palate J* 27:61, 1990.

68. Moon JB, Jones DL. Motor control of velopharyngeal structures during vowel production. *Cleft Palate J* 28:267, 1991.

69. Covello LV, Karnell MP, Seaver EJ. Video-endoscopy and photodetection: Linearity of a new integrated system. *Cleft Palate Craniofac J* 29:168, 1992.

70. Karnell MP, Seaver EJ. Integrated endoscopic/photodetector evaluation of velopharyngeal function. *Cleft Palate Craniofac J* 30:337, 1993.

71. Horiguchi S, Bell-Berti F. The velotrace: A device for monitoring velar position. *Cleft Palate J* 24:104, 1987.

72. Keuhn DP, Folkins JW, Linville RN. An electromyographic study of the musculus uvulae. *Cleft Palate J* 25:348, 1988.

73. Rees TD, Wood-Smith D, Swinyard CA, Converse JM. Electromyographic evaluation of submucous cleft palate: A possible aid to operative planning. *Plast Reconstr Surg* 40:592, 1967.

74. Williams WN, Eisenbach CR. Assessing VP function: The lateral still technique vs. cinefluorography. *Cleft Palate J* 18:45, 1981.

75. Skolnick ML. Videofluoroscopic examination of the velopharyngeal portal during phonation in lateral and base projections—A new technique for studying the mechanics of closure. *Cleft Palate J* 7:803, 1970.

76. Quattromani F, Benton C, Cotton RT. The Towne projection for evaluation of the velopharyngeal sphincter. *Radiology* 125:540, 1977.

77. Stringer DA, Witzel MA. Velopharyngeal insufficiency on videofluoroscopy: Comparison of projections. *Am J Roentgenol* 146:15, 1986.

78. Pigott RW, Benson JF, White FD. Nasendoscopy in the diagnosis of velopharyngeal incompetence. *Plast Reconstr Surg* 43:141, 1969.

79. Pigott RW. The nasendoscopic appearance of normal palatopharyngeal valve. *Plast Reconstr Surg* 43:19, 1969.

80. Pigott RW. The results of nasopharyngoscopic assessment of pharyngoplasty. *Scand J Plast Reconstr Surg* 8:148, 1974.

81. Keuhn DP, Ettema SL, Goldwasser MS, et al. Magnetic resonance imaging in the evaluation of occult submucous cleft palate. *Cleft Palate Craniofac J* 38:421, 2001.

82. McWilliams BJ. The long-term speech results of primary and secondary surgical correction of palatal clefts. *Multidisciplinary Management of Cleft Lip and Palate.* Philadelphia: Saunders, 1990, pp. 815–819.

83. Dorf D, Curtin J. Early cleft palate repair and speech outcome. *Plast Reconstr Surg* 70:74, 1982.

84. Randall P, LaRossa D, Fakhraee S, et al. Cleft palate closure at 3–7 months of age: A preliminary report. *Plast Reconstr Surg* 71:624, 1983.

85. Abyholm FE. Submucous cleft palate. *Scand J Plast Reconstr Surg* 10:209, 1976.

86. Crikelair GF, Striker P, Cosman B. The surgical management treatment of submucous cleft palate. *Plast Reconstr Surg* 45:58, 1970.

87. Schoenborn D. Ueber eine neue methode der staphylorskaphie. *Arch F Klin Chir* 19:528, 1876.

88. Brondsted K, Liisberg WB, Orsted A, et al. Surgical and speech results following palatopharyngoplasty operations in Denmark 1959–1977. *Cleft Palate J* 21:170, 1984.

89. Husein M, Chang E, Cable B, Karnell M, Karnell LH, Canady JW. Outcomes for children with submucous cleft palate and velopharyngeal insufficiency. *J Otolaryngol* 33:222, 2004.

90. Park S, Saso Y, Ito O, Tokioka K, et al. A retrospective study of speech development in patients with submucous cleft palate treated by four operations. *Scan J Plast Reconstr Hand Surg* 34:131, 2000.

91. Dorrance GM. Lengthening the soft palate in cleft palate operations. *Annals Surg* 82:208, 1925.

92. Porterfield HW, Trabue JC. Submucous cleft palate. *Plast Reconstr Surg* 35:45, 1965.

93. Ruding R. Cleft palate: Anatomic and surgical consideration. *Plast Reconstr Surg* 33:132, 1964.

94. Braithwaite F. The importance of the levator muscle in cleft palate closure. *Br J Plast Surg* 21:60, 1968.

95. Pensler JM, Bauer BS. Levator repositioning and palatal lengthening for submucous clefts. *Plast Reconstr Surg* 82:765, 1988.

96. Furlow LT. Cleft palate repair: Preliminary report on lengthening and muscle transportation by Z-Plasty. Presented at the *Annual Meeting of the Southeastern Society of Plastic and Reconstructive Surgeons,* Boca Raton, FL, 1978.

97. Furlow LT. Cleft palate repair by double-opposing Z-plasty. *Plast Reconstr Surg* 78:724, 1986.

98. Chen PK, Wu J, Hung KF, Chen YR, Noordhoff MS. Surgical correction of submucous cleft palate with Furlow palatoplasty. *Plast Reconstr Surg* 97:1136, 1996.

99. Seagle MB, Patti CS, Williams WN, Wood VD. Submucous cleft palate: A 10-year series. *Ann Plast Surg* 42:142, 1999.

100. D'Antonio LL, Eichenberg BJ, Zimmerman GJ, Patel S, et al. Radiographic and aerodynamic measures of velopharyngeal anatomy and function following Furlow Z-plasty. *Plast Reconstr Surg* 106:539, 2000.

23

Double-Opposing Z-Plasty Palate Repair

Leonard T. Furlow, Jr., MD

INTRODUCTION

It has been more than 30 years since the first report of cleft palate repair utilizing the double-opposing Z-plasty,[1] since then the only procedure used by the author for primary palatoplasty. During that time, a number of anatomic clarifications and surgical improvements have become evident: some from thoughts about the operation, some while performing the procedure, and some from assisting, watching,

or listening to other surgeons. This chapter describes the author's concept of the operation after 37 cases in private practice and some 300 cases performed on overseas volunteer surgery trips. This work includes concepts learned over the last decade, not reported in earlier descriptions.[2-9]

While in private practice, the author repaired the palates of 33 consecutive infants by double opposing z-plasty. 12 had unilateral cleft lip and palate, 10 bilateral cleft lip and palate, and 11 cleft palate only. Four older patients underwent double

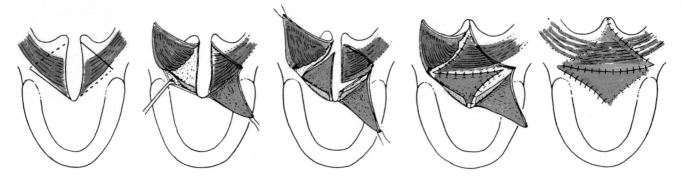

Figure 23–1. The basic design of mirror–image oral and nasal Z-plasties reorients and overlaps the velar muscles into a transverse sling under functional tension. Without taking mucoperiosteum from the hard palate, the geometry of the Z-plasties adds length to the velum and provides both oral- and nasal-side mucosal closure anterior to the muscles. The solid lines indicate the oral mucosal incisions, and dotted lines the nasal mucosal incisions. Red flaps represent musculomucosal flaps and green flaps mucosal flaps only.

opposing z-plasty repair (8). All were followed in the University of Florida Craniofacial Clinic. It became apparent that the double-opposing Z-plasty improved the velopharyngeal competency rate in these patients remarkably, from 48% for my prior von Langenbeck repairs to 91% in the 33 consecutive infants.[8] Most,[10–17] but not all,[18,19] other studies have reported better velopharyngeal competency results with the double-opposing Z-plasty than with comparison procedures.

ANATOMY AND OPERATIVE DESIGN

Soft Palate Anatomic Landmarks

The direction of the lateral limb incisions and resulting angles of the Z-plasties are determined by the patient's 3D

anatomy of the palate (Fig. 23–1). The hamuli, the posterior margin of the hard palate, the base of each uvular half, and the Eustachian orifices are the critical anatomic landmarks.

The Multiple Functions of The Z-Plasties

The velar Z-plasties accomplish more than repair of the cleft, rearrangement of the muscles, and velar lengthening. The Z-plasties' lateral limb incisions *extend to or beyond the hamuli*. They are long enough to expose the underlying anatomy for dissection and repair, which eliminates the need for soft palate lateral relaxing incisions. The lateral limb incisions determine the positioning of the tips of the Z-plasty flaps, and so the orientation and tension of the levator muscles.

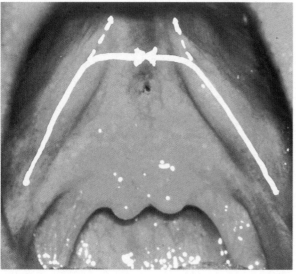

A

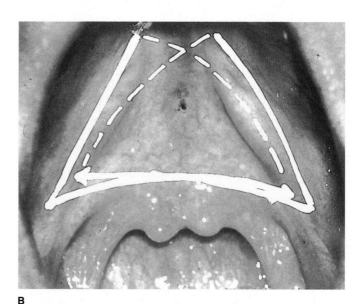

B

Figure 23–2. During phonation, the anteromedial course of the palatal muscles is clear in this patient with a submucous cleft palate. (A) If the palatal muscles are detached from the back of the hard palate but not freed from the aponeurosis, a less effective anterior intravelar veloplasty is constructed (solid lines). (B) When the tensor aponeurosis is divided, the levator muscles are freed to be repositioned horizontally to construct a transverse levator sling (solid arrows). Because the cleft muscles are longer than normal, the levators must be put under functional tension by overlapping.

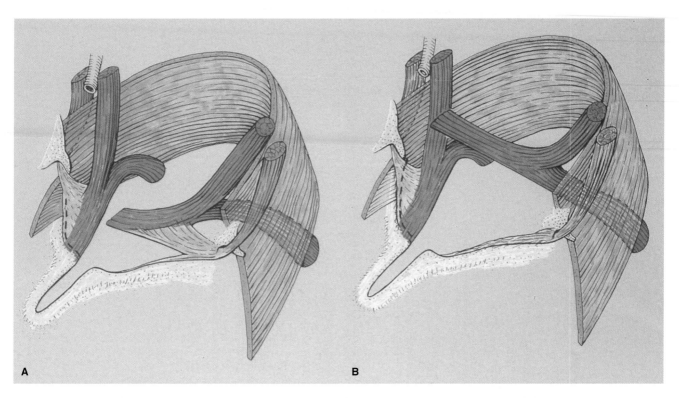

Figure 23–3. (A) When the levator muscles are detached from the posterior edge of the hard palate but the aponeurosis of the tensor is not completely divided (as has been usual in intravelar veloplasty), the levator muscle is tethered, cannot be brought into a transverse position, and a less effective levator sling will be formed in the anterior portion of the velum. (B) By carrying the lateral limb incisions laterally to the point just posterior to the hamulus, the tensor aponeurosis is completely divided and the levator muscles can be swept from the abnormal connections to the superior constrictor, posteriorly into a direct transverse orientation. The hard palate attachments of the aponeurosis are not disturbed, which should protect the tensor muscle function.

Importance of the Palatal Aponeurosis

Freeing the levator palatini muscles, not only from the posterior edge of the hard palate, but also from the attachments to the tensor aponeurosis, is key to completely releasing the levator muscles for construction of an effective intravelar veloplasty (Figs. 23–2A, B and Fig. 23–3).

Posteriorly Based Musculomucosal Flaps

By extending the lateral limb incisions to or beyond the hamuli laterally, the posteriorly based flaps' lateral limb incisions divide the tensor aponeurosis, which frees the flaps to carry the palatal muscles. In our experience, this makes velar lateral relaxing incisions unnecessary, decreases muscle dissection, improves blood supply, and eliminates the need to separately suture the muscles. The author has never found fracture of the hamulus, transection of the tensor tendon, or dissections into the space of Ernst necessary. These maneuvers will not improve the transverse orientation of the levators. The additional scarring from these maneuvers can be avoided, and the superior constrictor is not damaged. Note, that this does not eliminate the need for hard palate lateral relaxing incisions in wide clefts, which the author found in 10–20% of cases on overseas trips were needed for hard palate mucoperiosteal flap closure.

Anteriorly Based Mucosal Flaps

The anteriorly based flaps provide mucosa for complete oral and nasal-side closure anterior to the velar muscles (Fig. 23–4). This eliminates the tendency for the muscles to migrate forward (which has been found to occur very frequently after classical intravelar veloplasty[20]) and prevents

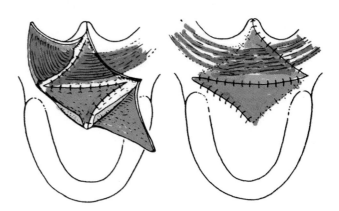

Figure 23–4. The anteriorly based flaps provide mucosa for complete oral- and nasal-side closure anterior to the levator muscle sling reconstruction. This prevents the levator sling from migrating anteriorly, and prevents longitudinal scarring of the velum resulting in shortening of the soft palate. In addition, the Z-plasty design protects the nasal and oral incisions from overlapping.

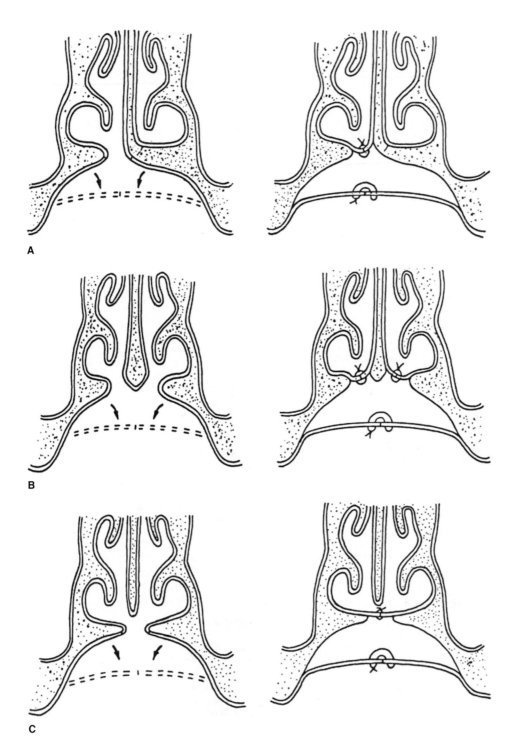

Figure 23–5. Hard palate mucoperiosteal repair without relaxing incisions (A) unilateral cleft palate, (B) bilateral cleft palate, and (C) cleft palate only.

shortening of the velum by wound contraction. Guneren and Uysal[21] have documented an average of 12.5 mm (55%) of permanent lengthening at a mean of 4.5 years postoperatively. This is accomplished without robbing the hard palate of its mucoperiosteum. Because the Z-plasties are mirror images, the oral and nasal incisions do not overlap, which permits the flap bases to protect the lateral limb incisions.

Hard Palate: Midface Growth

Relaxing palatal incisions, along the medial alveolus, result in scars that are one of the factors contributing to maxillary retrusion.[22,23] Although the evidence is weak, mucoperiosteal dissection of the hard palate has also been blamed for maxillary retrusion. However, the amount of hard palate mucoperiosteal elevation is the same with or without relaxing incisions; only hard palate pushback procedures or relaxing

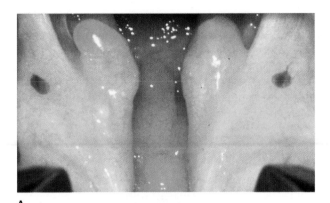

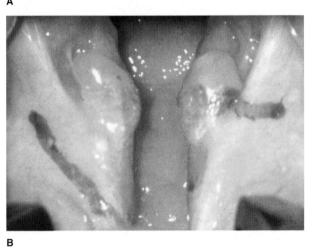

Figure 23–6. The hamulus can be palpated with the fingertip and marked bilaterally (A). The lateral limbs of the Z-plasties are drawn (B). As in the image, the anatomic landmarks may make the flap angles different, approximately 45° on the left and 90° on the right.

incisions produce lateral mucosal scars. Children with cleft lip and palate are also prone to maxillary growth deficits because of their alveolar cleft.

The previously mentioned 33 consecutive patients who underwent double-opposing Z-plasty repair were followed through the University of Florida Craniofacial Clinic. Sixteen of the infants, 8 of the 12 with unilateral cleft lip and palate and 8 of the 10 with bilateral cleft lip and palate, were followed to the age 10.5 to 17.5 years. None of the unilateral clefts, and only one of the bilateral cleft patients, required maxillary advancement for midface hypoplasia.

Hard Palate: Closure

Mucoperiosteal flap repair of the hard palate can be achieved without lateral relaxing incisions by converting the vault of the hard palate to transverse reach. This eliminates the scars around the medial aspect of the palatal alveolus that increase the risk of maxillary growth deficit (Figure 23–5). Repairing the hard palate by converting the vault to a transverse arch utilizes only the midline mucosal incision along the cleft margin. None of the author's 37 private practice cases required lateral relaxing incisions. The residual space space between the vault and the hard palate mucoperiosteal flaps disappeared by the infant's 2-week post-operative appointment, and the vault was reestablished. There were 2 fistulas in these 37 patients (5.4%), both in infants with cleft palate only. The space does not seem to increase the risk of fistulas; perhaps by so widely separating the oral and nasal suture lines, fistulas become less likely.

In order to create the mucosal edges for suturing the hard palate portion of a unilateral cleft plate, a vomer flap must be incised and elevated. Raising the vomer flap is

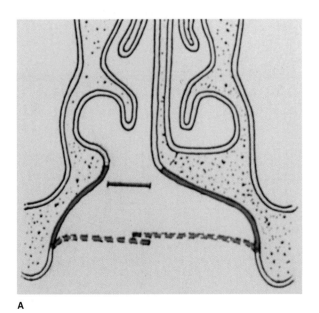

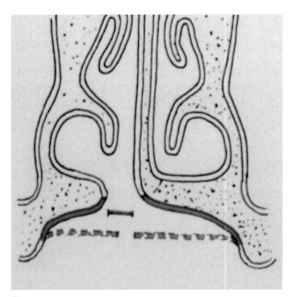

Figure 23–7. Regardless of the width of the cleft one must know if the mucoperiosteal flaps will reach from alveolus to alveolus. (A) Wide cleft, deep vault, mucoperiosteal flaps reach, and (B) narrower cleft, shallow vault, mucoperiosteal flaps do not reach.

necessary to close the nasal side of the hard palate cleft and establish normal anatomy and nasal mucosal continuity. The vomer is large and useful in bilateral cleft repair, but when the cleft is of the palate only, the vomer is small and high.

BEFORE THE INCISION

Soft Palate

Prior to the incision, one should review the design of the velar Z-plasties. The levator muscles are included in each posteriorly based flap, and the nasal Z-plasty is the mirror image of the oral one. Not having these plans firmly in mind invites palatal muscle transection rather than transposition. Although the procedure has routinely been described with the oral posteriorly based musculomucosal flap on the patient's and the surgeon's left, the pattern can of course be reversed.

Prior to injecting the velum with epinephrine, the hamuli are palpated and marked (Fig. 23–6A). The lateral limbs are then drawn (Fig. 23–6B) on the patient's left, from

the hamulus to the cleft's margin at the posterior edge of the hard palate. On the right side, the limb is marked from the base of the uvula, at the junction of the uvula and soft palate, to the hamulus. Because of variations in anatomic landmarks, the flap angles may be different. In Fig. 6B, the left-sided flap is approximately 45°, and the right flap is approximately 90°.

Hard Palate: Planning Ahead for Wide Clefts

It is possible to know *before beginning surgery* whether the hard palate mucoperiosteal flaps will close with medial cleft margin incisions alone. This can be very helpful because if they will not, one can then plan in advance to use another method, such as lateral relaxing incisions and the creation of unipedicled hard palate flaps for hard palate closure.

Regardless of the width of the cleft, we need to know if there is enough mucoperiosteal flap width to reach from alveolus to alveolus (Figs. 23–7A, B).

A simple way to help determine whether the hard palate mucoperiosteal flaps will close without the use of hard palate relaxing incisions is to measure with two Q-tips. With

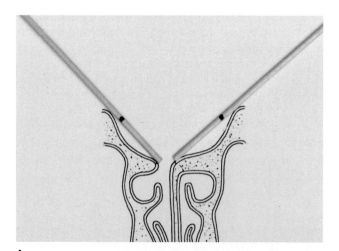

A

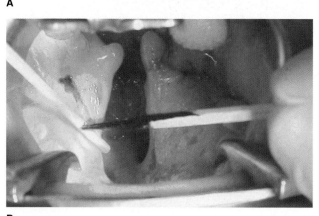

B

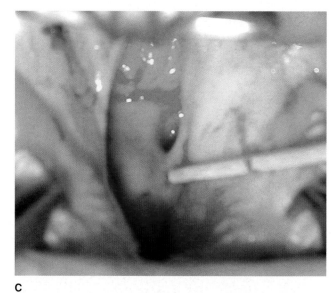

C

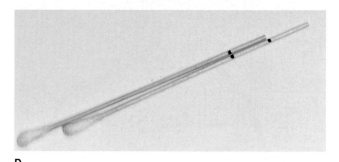

D

Figure 23–8. (A) The distance from the cleft margin along the medial edge of the cleft in the depth of the vault to the base of the alveolus is marked on each side with a Q-tip and methylene blue. (B) Distance measured on the left side. (C) Distance measured on the right side. (D) The distances are added up onto one Q-tip.

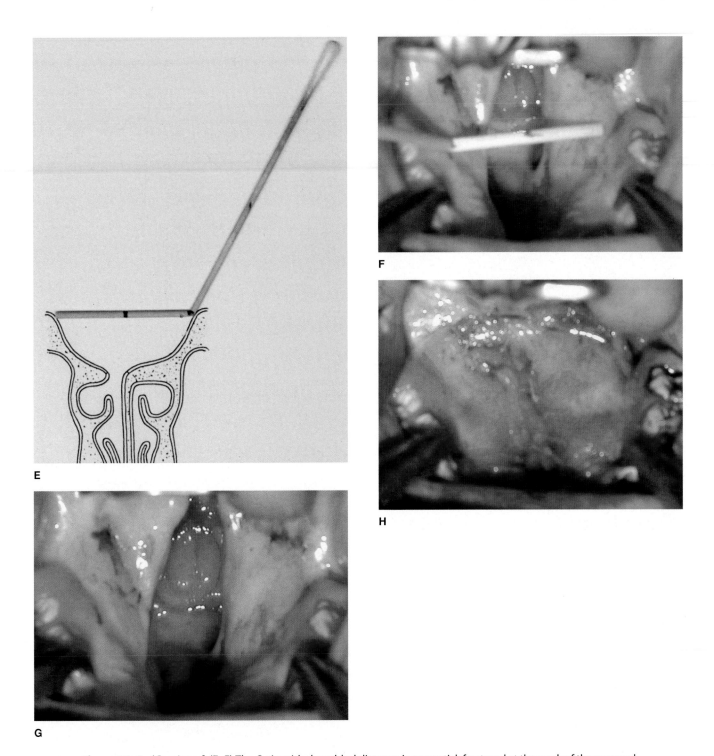

Figure 23–8. (*Continued*) (E–F) The Q-tip with the added distance is greenstick fractured at the mark of the sum and placed at the widest portion of the cleft to see if the flaps will reach. (G–H) Pre- and postoperative view of the cleft.

methylene blue and two Q-tips, on each side measure the depth of the vault at the junction of the hard and soft palates, from the base of the alveolus to the margin of the cleft along the medial edge of the hard palate (Figs. 23–8A, B, and C). The two distances are added up on one Q-tip, (Fig. 23–8D) and that Q-tip is greenstick fractured at the mark indicating the sum of the distances (Figs. 23–8E and F). This distance is used at the widest portion of the cleft, usually the junction

of the hard and soft palates, to assess whether the flaps will come together. Figures 23–8G and H demonstrate the pre- and postoperative palate.

Injection

After marking the position of each hamulus and deciding if the hard palate mucoperiosteal flaps will reach, injection

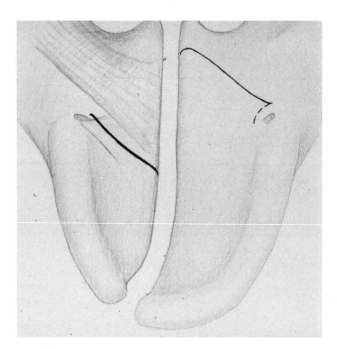

Figure 23–9. The oral lateral limb incisions are shown. On the left side, the incision when carried to the hamulus completely transects the tensor aponeurosis.

with local anesthetic and epinephrine is done, including the incisive foramen. If the uvular halves are injected last and incised immediately after, they are far easier to hold and precisely incise when they are ballooned and tense with local.

OPERATION

Velum

The operation is begun with the velar incisions. This is because blood will flow "downhill" and if hard palate incisions

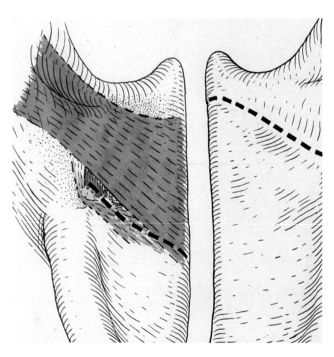

Figure 23–11. The left-sided incision of the posteriorly based musculomucosal flap automatically divides the tensor aponeurosis noted in blue.

are performed first, blood will obstruct the view of the Z-plasty dissections. The oral lateral limb incisions are shown in Fig. 23–9. On the left, note that by extending the incision to the hamulus, the incision completely transects the tensor aponeurosis. The right-sided anteriorly based mucosal flap incision usually requires a backcut around the maxillary tubercle to permit the mucosal flap to move adequately. Once the cleft margin incisions on the velum are made, the tip of the left-sided oral musculomucosal flap is elevated. The levator muscle is cut free from the posterior edge of the hard palate

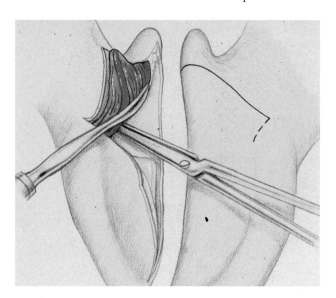

Figure 23–10. The left-sided incision is made and the levator is cut free from the posterior edge of the hard palate and elevated from the underlying nasal mucosa.

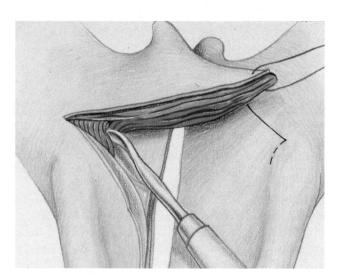

Figure 23–12. The left-sided posteriorly based musculomucosal flap is elevated and pulled across the cleft defect. The elevator pushes the levator muscle in red from the superior constrictor muscle in purple.

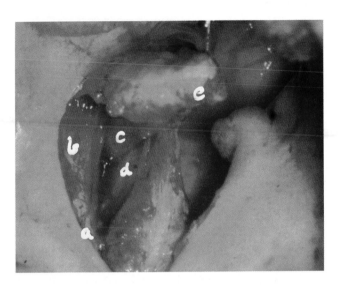

Figure 23–13. The surgical anatomy is marked: (a) Hamulus, (b) Superior constrictor, (c) Levator muscle belly, (d) Nasal mucosa, and (e) Levator muscle ends at the tip of the flap.

and elevated from the underlying nasal mucosa. It is better to leave a few fibers of muscle attached to the nasal mucosa than to perforate it (Fig. 23–10). When the lateral limb incision of the left-sided posteriorly based flap reaches the hamulus, the tensor aponeurosis will have been automatically completely divided. Sharp dissection should stop before the superior constrictor is reached. The entire velar portion of the operation is performed medial to the superior constrictor (Fig. 23–11). The lateral limb incision exposes the superior constrictor. As the flap is pulled across the cleft, the palatal muscles are bluntly pushed posteriorly (not laterally) from the superior constric-

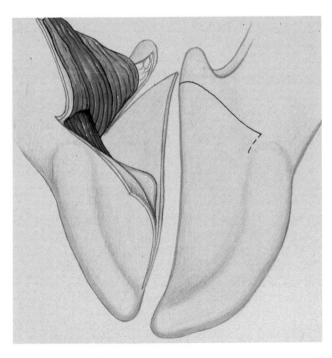

Figure 23–14. With the myomucosal flap retracted, the left-sided anteriorly based nasal mucosal flap is incised.

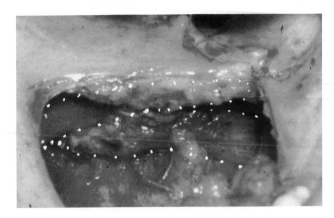

Figure 23–15. Bringing the tip of each posteriorly based musculomucosal flap to the base of the contralateral levator muscle belly and superior constrictor achieves a transverse orientation of the levators and places them on functional tension. Note the levator muscles are outlined in the image.

tor. The levator muscle will become apparent, coming into the flap from the junction between the superior constrictor and the nasal mucosa (Fig. 23–12). Figure 23–13 demonstrates the surgical anatomy. The Eustachian orifice is an important landmark because the levator enters the velum from immediately behind it. A Freer elevator slipped through the cleft and run back and forth laterally will drop into the orifice, identifying its position, and thus the normal position of the levator muscle belly. When dissection of this flap is complete, the flap tip should reach the opposite hamulus and the only structure tethering the flap tip should be the levator muscle.

Lateral Limbs: Levator Orientation and Overlap

With the left-sided posteriorly based myomucosal flap retracted, the anteriorly based nasal mucosal flap is incised. The direction and length of the lateral limb nasal incisions is important as it determines the position of the tip of the

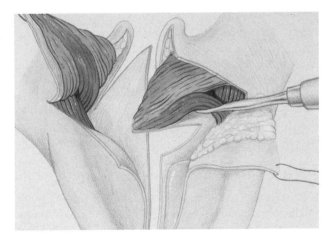

Figure 23–16. The lateral end of the left-sided anteriorly based nasal mucosal flap incision determines the position of the tip of the contralateral posteriorly based nasal musculomucosal flap.

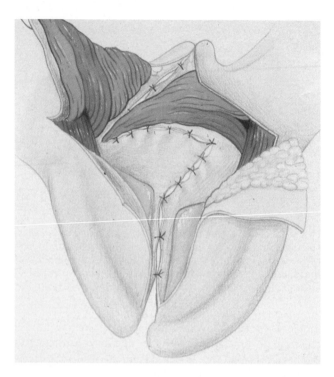

Figure 23–17. To position the levator muscle precisely transversely, the lateral limb of the left-sided anteriorly based nasal mucosal flap must extend to the left-sided superior constrictor and end under the left levator muscle as it enters the velum. Levator muscles noted in red and superior constrictor muscles noted in purple.

right-sided posteriorly based musculomucosal flap, and thus the orientation and tension of the contralateral levator muscle (Fig. 23–14). The primary goal of the Z-plasties is to overlap the levator muscle bellies and place them under "functional tension." Bringing the tip of each posteriorly based musculomucosal flap to the base of the contralateral levator muscle belly achieves a precisely transverse orientation of the levators and puts them on a functional tension. With proper dissection, the tips of the flaps can always be brought to the contralateral superior constrictor, regardless of the cleft width (Fig. 23–15).

When creating the nasal flaps, it is important to appreciate that the anteriorly based left-sided nasal mucosal flap lateral limb incision determines the position of the tip of its contralateral posteriorly based nasal musculomucosal flap bearing the end of the levator muscle (Fig. 23–16). To position the nasal flap levator muscle, the lateral limb incision of the left-sided nasal mucosal flap must extend to the left superior constrictor and end under the left levator muscle as it enters the velum (Fig. 23–17).

Z-Plasty Pitfalls

If a smaller Z-plasty is used, the flap tip will not extend as far, and this has two consequences (Fig. 23–18A). First, the levator muscle will not be brought into the proper functional tension (Fig. 23–18B). Second, because the nasopharynx is tubular and not flat, as the end points of the lateral limb incisions are carried laterally making them longer, the incision moves

posteriorly toward the posterior pharyngeal wall. Therefore, the smaller the Z-plasty, the farther the levator sling will be constructed from the posterior pharyngeal wall, which it must reach for velopharyngeal closure (Fig 23–8C).

If the lateral limb incision of the left-sided anteriorly based nasal mucosal flap is extended too far anteriorly (Fig. 23–19A), the tip of the left-sided posteriorly based nasal musculomucosal flap will be inset in such a way that the levator muscle will not be positioned under the left levator base, the two levator muscles will not overlap, and the levator sling will not be oriented transversely (Fig. 23–19B).

To elevate the right-sided anteriorly based oral mucosal flap, an incision is made along the cleft margin on the right side. The lateral limb incision is made from the base of the uvula to just beyond the hamulus (Fig. 23–20). The plane of elevation is shallow along the cleft margin and posteriorly to avoid cutting the underlying palatopharyngeus and palatoglossus muscles. As the dissection moves anteriorly and the posterior edge of the hard palate is approached, the plane of dissection is deepened beneath the minor salivary glands, taking care not to buttonhole the oral mucosa where it folds over on itself. The flap base is separated from the back edge of the hard palate with an elevator carefully avoiding the greater palatine vessels. This maneuver divides the tensor aponeurosis. If it has been determined that the hard palate mucoperiosteal flaps will reach the midline without the need for lateral hard palate relaxing incisions, the adjacent ipsilateral mucoperiosteal flap is raised, and this gives medial access to the right greater palatine foramen area. The small backcut extension of the lateral limb incision around the maxillary tuberosity can be made as needed to make the flap reach and can be used to access for further dissection around the greater palatine foramen. The flap is then retracted with a suture.

The right-sided posteriorly based nasal musculomucosal flap is elevated by detaching the flap tip and its levator muscle 3 or 4 mm back from the posterior edge of the hard palate, leaving several millimeters of nasal mucosa along the posterior edge of the hard palate for suturing. The lateral limb incision is carried toward the Eustachian orifice and it stops when thinner mucosa is reached. Making this lateral limb incision shorter nearly eliminates the problem of getting the left-sided anteriorly based nasal mucosal flap to reach when transposed, and because it does not position a palatal muscle, there is no functional consequence to making it shorter. The Freer elevator is scooped along the nasal mucosa to lift the levator muscle belly from the mucosa (see Fig. 23–16). As the right-sided posteriorly based nasal musculomucosal flap tip is pulled across the cleft, the elevator is utilized to push the levator muscle posteriorly and away from the superior constrictor into its transverse position. The levator muscle is then freed from the nasal mucosa along the edge of the flap just enough for the flap to be inset under modest tension into the contralateral lateral limb incision (see Fig. 23–17).

4–0 chromic gut suture is used to inset the flaps, taking care not to catch the base of the contralateral levator muscle with the suture. In the small child, three sutures will close the

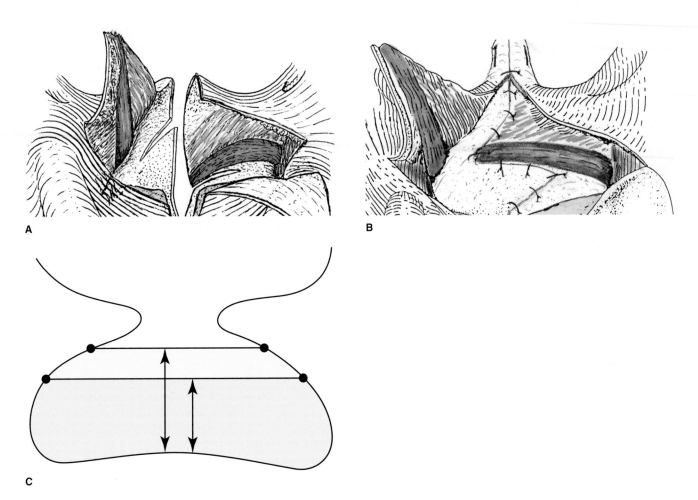

Figure 23–18. (A) If a smaller Z-plasty is created on the left-sided anteriorly based nasal mucosal flap, (B) the levator muscle (demonstrated in red) will be advanced less and so not brought into proper functional tension. (C) As the nasopharynx is tubular and not flat, as the end point of the lateral limb incision is made longer and carried laterally, it also moves posteriorly toward the posterior pharyngeal wall. Therefore, the smaller the Z-plasty, the further the reconstructed levator sling will be from the posterior pharyngeal wall as noted with the longer arrow.

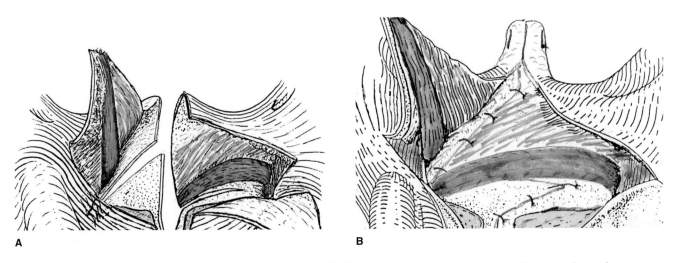

Figure 23–19. (A) If the lateral limb incision of the left-sided anteriorly based nasal mucosal flap extends too far anteriorly, (B) the right levator muscle will not be positioned under the left levator base, the two levator muscles will not overlap, and the levator sling will not be transverse.

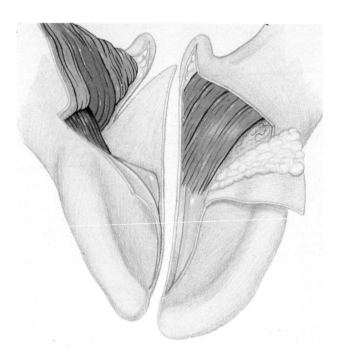

Figure 23–20. To elevate the right-sided anteriorly based oral mucosal flap, the lateral limb incision is made from the base of the uvula to just lateral and beyond the hamulus. The plane of dissection is shallow enough to avoid cutting the underlying muscles, however not so shallow as to buttonhole the oral mucosa.

lateral limb incision to the base of the uvula. The left-sided anteriorly based nasal mucosal flap is freed from the posterior edge of the hard palate shelf, transposed and sutured. It will probably be necessary to lift the levator to find the mucosal edge for suturing the transverse limb. Nasal closure is then continued anteriorly. After the inset of the nasal flaps and reconstruction of the uvula, it is easier to continue with several oral-sided sutures at the junction of the uvula and soft palate at this point rather than while insetting the oral flaps, when access to this area will be more difficult. In Fig. 23–21, the tip of the nasal myomucosal flap has been inset directly beneath the

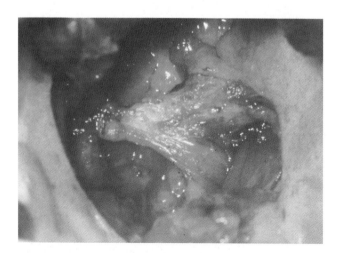

Figure 23–21. The tip of the right-sided posteriorly based nasal musculomucosal flap is inset directly beneath the contralateral levator muscle belly at the contralateral superior constrictor.

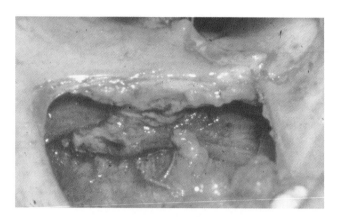

Figure 23–22. The left-sided posteriorly based oral musculomucosal flap is inset by suturing the tip of the flap directly over the base of the right levator muscle, several millimeters posterior to the right hamulus. This completes the reconstruction of the levator sling.

contralateral levator muscle belly at the contralateral superior constrictor.

Oral-side Closure

The left-sided posteriorly based oral musculomucosal flap is inset by suturing the tip of the flap directly over the base of the right-sided levator, several millimeters posterior to the hamulus (Figure 23–22). This completes the precise transverse positioning and overlapping of the two levator muscles. The remainder of the oral-side lateral limb incision is closed to the uvula.

Hard Palate Mucoperiosteal Flap Closure

Elevation of the hard palate mucoperiosteal flaps is done through the cleft margin incision medially. The Blair "hockey stick" elevator is very effective but requires both hands, one near the distal end to stabilize the shaft, and the other to elevate the blade by rotating the handle (Fig. 23–23). Hard palate flap elevation usually needs to extend to the base of the alveolus. To help close the palate anteriorly, the incision

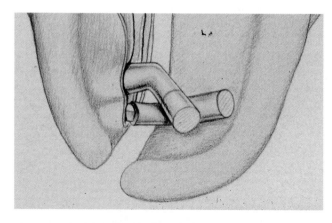

Figure 23–23. The Blair "hockey stick" elevator is used to raise the hard palate mucoperiosteal flaps from the cleft margin incision. Flap elevation proceeds to the base of the alveolus.

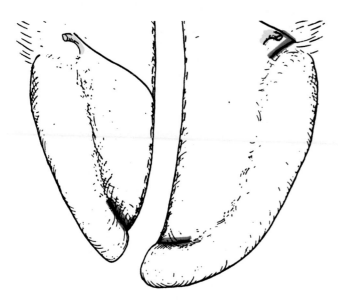

Figure 23–24. To assist in closure of the anterior hard palate, the cleft margin incision is carried along the lingual surface of the alveolus for a short distance. Also, the right-sided oral lateral limb incision is extended around the back of the alveolus. If needed, a lateral relaxing incision is extended anteriorly from this backcut.

along the cleft margin is extended a few millimeters along the lingual aspect of the alveolus (Fig. 23–24).

To facilitate closure of the right-sided anteriorly based oral mucosal flap, extension of the lateral limb incision as a short backcut around the posterior alveolus is performed. This also gives access for dissection of the tough fascial

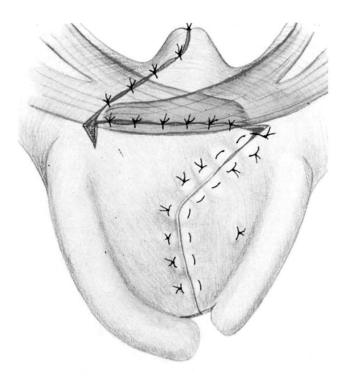

Figure 23–25. After closure is complete, the oral flap bases protect the nasal lateral limb incisions and vice versa. The oral and nasal incisions do not overlap because of the mirror Z-plasties.

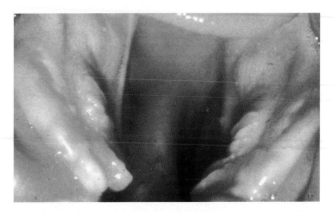

Figure 23–26. Without the use of lateral hard palate relaxing incisions, making the marginal cleft incision may look easy; however, it is often difficult as the cleft margin is hidden and no blade seems properly oriented to make the incision.

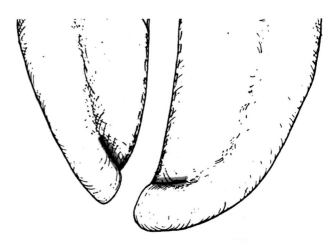

Figure 23–27. Before making the cleft incision, the 0.5 cm incision on the posterior (lingual) aspect of the alveolus is made.

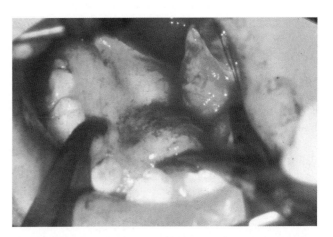

Figure 23–28. Through the 0.5-cm incision along the posterior side of the alveolus, a Freer elevator is used to raise the hard palate flaps. A knife or scissor blade is placed in this incision to incise precisely through he cleft margin.

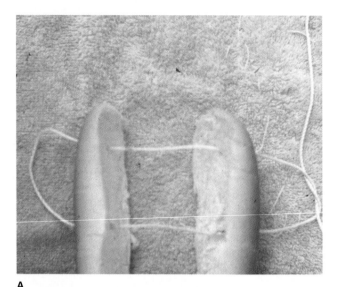

A

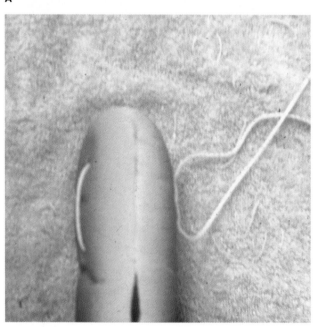

B

Figure 23–29. Dr. Peter Randall's mattress suture method of uvula repair apposes the raw surfaces of the uvular halves. This makes mucosal sutures for the uvula unnecessary.

attachments at the junction of the hard and soft palate. If a lateral relaxing incision is made, there is no mucosal bridge between the flap and the relaxing incision to impair flap mobility (Fig. 23–24).

Oral closure is completed from the tip of the mucosal flap forward. The hard palate mucoperiosteal flaps are apposed with mattress sutures and closed to the back of the alveolus. Always close the hard palate with mattress sutures to avoid fistulas. The mucosal surface of a stiff mucoperiosteal flap margin in the line of closure will prevent healing, and a slit fistula will result. Raw must be a raw. The suggested repair closes the floor of the nose and posterior to the alveolus with lip repair[24] and does not close the alveolar cleft. The author believes that not addressing the alveolar defect with the lip

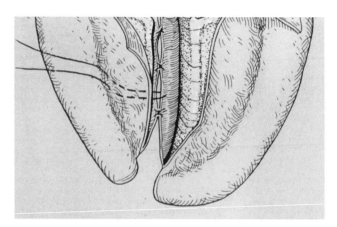

Figure 23–30. When the anterior portion of the hard palate cleft is too narrow for access to suture the nasal layer, a suture is passed through the margin of the hard palate mucosperiosteal flap, through the vomer flap as a mattress stitch, and back out through the hard palate flap. It is tied once the oral hard palate closure is complete.

or palate surgery makes orthodontic arch expansion, prior to alveolar bone grafting, easier and more effective.

After closure is complete, the oral flap bases protect the nasal lateral limb incisions, and vice versa. As the Z-plasties are mirror images, the oral and nasal incisions do not overlap, which decreases the chances of fistula formation postoperatively (Figure 23–25). In addition, the Z-plasty incisions eliminate the longitudinal scar of the velum, reducing the tendency for shortening (Figure 23–25).

HELPFUL HINTS

Hard Palate Flap Elevation

At times it is difficult to make the cleft incision precisely on the cleft argin, which is necessary to preserve maximum

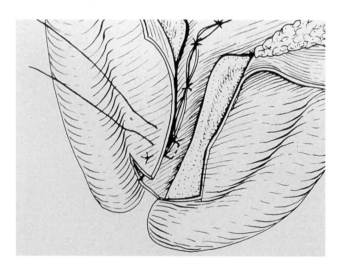

Figure 23–31. When the alveolar gap is wide, extending the vomer flap incision up the midline to the posterior alveolus will add enough reach to the vomer flap allowing it to be tucked beneath the contralateral hard palate mucoperiosteal flap.

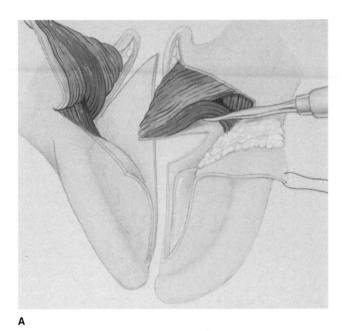

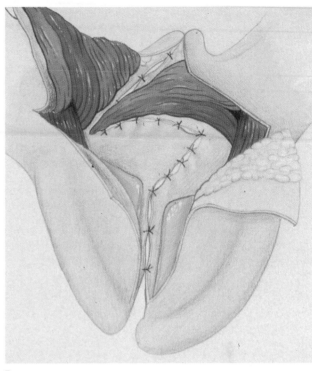

A   **B**

Figure 23–32. Shortening the lateral limb incision of the right-sided posteriorly based nasal musculomucosal flap leaves a smaller area for the left-sided anteriorly based nasal mucosal flap to cover.

mucoperiosteal width for closure. In Fig. 23–26, this may look easy; however, it frequently is not so as the cleft margin is hidden, and no blade seems to be properly oriented to make the incision. Since access for hard palate mucoperiosteal flap elevation is not available through lateral relaxing incisions, a Freer elevator can be placed through the 0.5-cm incision

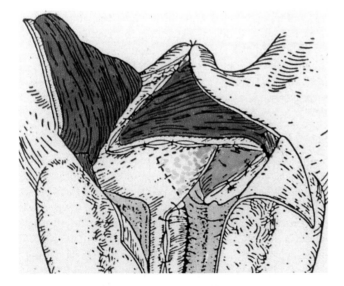

Figure 23–33. If there is still a nasal lining defect at the junction of the hard and soft palates, a posterior vomer flap, noted in yellow, can be turned over to assist in the closure of the nasal lining defect.

along the back side of the alveolus (Fig. 23–27) to elevate the hard palate mucoperiosteal flaps prior to making the cleft margin incision (Fig. 23–28). Elevating the hard palate flaps gives access for a knife or scissor blade to cut accurately along the cleft margin.

Uvular Reconstruction

Dr. Randall's mattress suture method apposes the raw surfaces of the uvular halves, making mucosal sutures for the uvula unnecessary (Fig. 23–29). At the time of nasal lining repair and uvular reconstruction, it is easier to put several sutures on the oral side of the base of the new uvula and junction of the velum, rather than while insetting the oral flaps, when access to this area becomes more difficult.

Hard Palate Closure

It is important to obtain a complete and separate two-layer closure of the hard palate. When the anterior portion of the hard palate cleft is too narrow for access to suture the nasal layer, a suture can be passed through the medial edge of the hard palate mucoperiosteal flap, through the vomer flap, as a mattress suture, and back out through the mucoperiosteal flap (Fig. 23–30). This will pull the vomer flap across the cleft. The suture is tied after the oral layer of the hard palate is completely closed. When the alveolar gap is wide, extending the vomer flap incision up the midline to the posterior edge of the alveolus will add enough reach to the vomer flap to

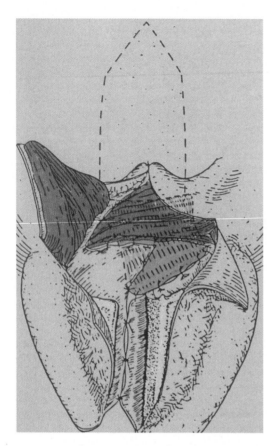

Figure 23–34. A narrow unlined posterior pharyngeal flap, noted in pink, can be brought dorsal to the velar muscle flaps to assist in closure of the nasal lining in larger defects.

tuck it under the contralateral hard palate mucoperiosteal flap (Figure 23–31).

PROBLEM AREAS: WIDE CLEFTS

In the very wide cleft, three areas may present difficulty in obtaining adequate closure. These are (1) inset and closure of the left-sided anteriorly based nasal mucosal flap at the junction of the hard and soft palate, (2) inset and closure of the right-sided anteriorly based oral mucosal flap, and (3) the hard palate mucoperiosteal flaps. The posteriorly based musculomucosal flaps have always reached and not been a problem.

Nasal Mucosal Flap

In wide clefts, there may be difficulty insetting and closing the left-sided anteriorly based nasal mucosal flap. Shortening the lateral limb incision of the right-sided posteriorly based nasal musculomucosal flap will leave a smaller area for the right-sided nasal flap to cover (Figs. 23–32A and B). This has almost eliminated this problem. If the left-sided nasal mucosal flap is still not large enough to close the defect, a posterior vomer flap can be turned over to help close the lateral deficit (Fig. 23–33).

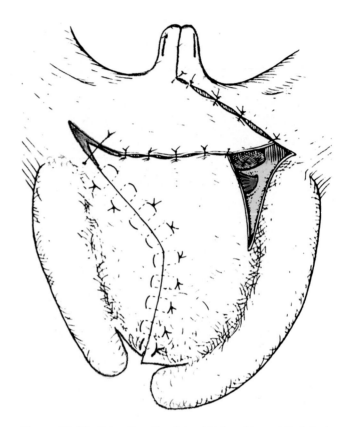

Figure 23–35. Extending the right-sided oral lateral limb incision around the maxillary tuberosity at the posterior end of the alveolus assists with the inset of the right-sided anteriorly based oral mucosal flap.

Rarely, a relatively narrow pharyngeal flap, brought dorsal to the velar muscle flaps, and left unlined, will be necessary to close larger defects (Fig. 23–34).

Oral Mucosal Flap

When the right-sided anteriorly based oral mucosal flap does not fill the defect, extending the right-sided lateral limb incision backcut anteriorly around the posterior alveolus/maxillary tuberosity will usually permit this oral nasal flap to reach (Fig. 23–35). A raw area left laterally will close secondarily just as with lateral relaxing incisions.

Hard Palate Mucoperiosteal Flaps

Think ahead, and at the time of lip repair, if the palatal cleft is wide, consider performing a mucosa-only posterior velar adhesion (Figure 23–36).[23] Oyama et al.[25] found in 13 cases that at 1 year, just before double-opposing Z-plasty, the cleft was significantly narrower than controls at the hard–soft palate junction and at the mid hard palate levels. At the time of palate repair, the mucosal bridge is cut, and the velar double-opposing Z-plasty is performed as usual.

If the preoperative measurements (see Fig. 23–23) indicate that the hard palate mucoperiosteal flaps will not reach, then two unipedicled hard palate flaps can be elevated

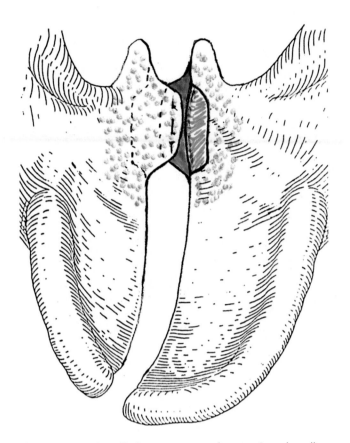

Figure 23–36. A preliminary mucosa-only posterior velar adhesion can be performed at the time of lip repair, which narrows the palatal cleft prior to cleft palate repair.

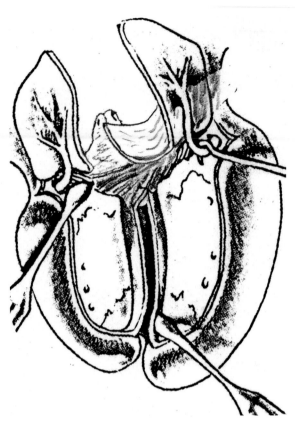

Figure 23–38. Bardach's unipedicled bilateral hard palate mucoperiosteal flap technique.

(Fig. 23–37). Bardach's two-flap approach,[26] once velar and hard palate nasal closure is complete, is a safe way to raise the mucoperiosteal flaps (Fig. 23–38). Raising the hard palate mucoperiosteal flaps, anteriorly to posteriorly, provides excellent visualization of the palatine vessels coming from the greater palatine foramen, which is safer than dissection around the foramen from underneath the flap, where visualization may be difficult (Fig. 23–38). Note that the hard palate lateral relaxing incisions join the lateral ends of the oral velar Z-plasty limbs such that no mucosal bridge is left between the two. Both flaps are attached only by their greater palatine pedicles, and are true island flaps. One must be careful not to let either flap twist on its pedicle; placing one suture holding the flap to the alveolus is prudent.

Alternate Techniques

An alternative technique for large soft tissue deficits at the junction of the hard and soft palates is Bozola's[27] buccinator flap (Fig. 23–39). A posteriorly based axial flap brings tissue into the junction of the hard and soft palates in one stage. Bilateral buccal flaps have also been described by Mann and Fisher.[28] Finally, Seigel's solution, for very wide clefts, is to close the palate in two stages: first, a simple von Langenbeck straight-line repair without an intravelar veloplasty is performed, followed several months later by

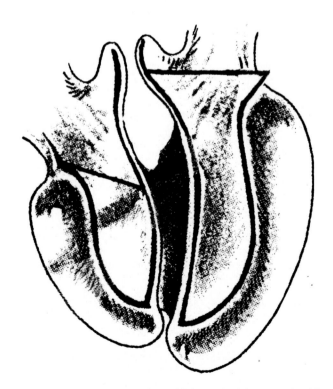

Figure 23–37. Hard palate lateral relaxing incisions creating bilateral unipedicled hard palate mucoperiosteal flaps.

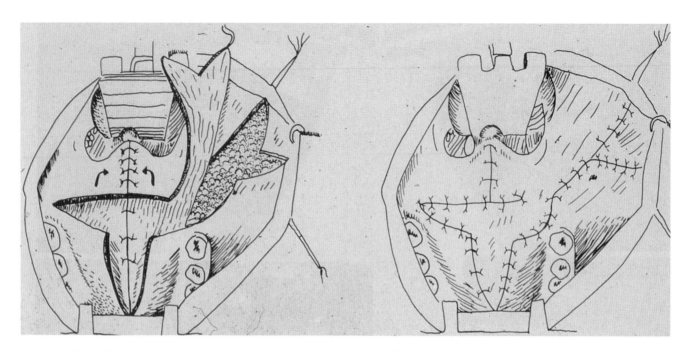

Figure 23–39. Bozola's posteriorly based, axial pattern, buccinator flap that transposes soft tissue into the junction of the hard and soft palates.

double-opposing Z-plasty, made much easier by obliteration of the cleft.

References

1. Furlow LT, Jr. Double opposing z-plasties to repair a cleft palate: A personal account. *Adv Plast Reconstr Surg* 15:203, 1998.
2. Furlow LT, Jr. Cleft palate repair by double opposing z-plasty. *Plast Reconstr Surg* 78:724, 1986.
3. Furlow LT, Jr. Flaps for cleft lip and palate surgery. *Clin Plast Surg* 17:633, 1990.
4. Furlow LT, Jr., Randall P, Brody GS. Cleft Palate Repair by Double Opposing Z-plasty. Plastic Surgery Educational Foundation Teleplast # 9022. May 12, 1990.
5. Furlow LT, Jr. Cleft palate. In Vistnes LM (ed). *Procedures in Plastic and Reconstructive Surgery: How They Do It.* Boston: Little, Brown and Co., 1991, Chapter 19.
6. Furlow LT, Jr. The double opposing z-plasty for palate closure. In Jackson IT, Sommerlad BC, (eds). *Recent Advances in Plastic Surgery,* 4th ed. Edinburgh: Churchill Livingstone, 1992, Chapter 3a.
7. Furlow LT, Jr., Randall P. Double opposing z-plasty in cleft palate repair: Technique, results and analysis. *Perspectives Plast Surg* 7:55, 1993.
8. Furlow LT, Jr. Cleft palate repair by double opposing z-plasty. *Operative Techniques Plast Reconstr Surg* 2:223, 1995.
9. Furlow LT, Jr. Technique of double opposing Z-plasty palate repair. In Salyer K, Bardach J, (eds). *Salyer and Bardach's Atlas of Craniofacial and Cleft Surgery.* New York: Lippincott-Raven, 1999, Chapter 15, pp. 764–767.
10. Spauwen PHM, Goorhuis-Brouwer SM, Schutte HK. Cleft palate repair: Furlow versus von Langenbeck. *J Cranio-Maxillofac Surg* 20:18–20, 1992.
11. Horswell BB, Castiglione CL, Poole AE, Assael LA. The double-reversing Z-plasty in primary palatoplasty: Operative experience and early results. *J Oral Maxillofac Surg* 51:145–150, 1993.
12. Grobbelaar AO, Hudson DA, Fernandes DB, Lentin R. Speech results after repair of the cleft soft palate. *Plast Reconstr Surg* 95:1150, 1995.
13. McWilliams BJ, Randall P, LaRossa D, et al. Speech characteristics associated with the Furlow palatoplasty as compared with other surgical techniques. *Plast Reconstr Surg* 98:610–619, 1996.
14. Gunther E, Wisser JR, Cohen MA, Brown AS. Palatoplasty: Furlow's double reversing Z-plasty versus intravelar veloplasty. *Cleft Palate Craniofac J* 35:546, 1998.
15. Kirschner RE, Wang P, Jawad AF, Duran MB, Cohen M. Cleft-palate repair by modified Furlow double-opposing Z-plasty: The Children's Hospital of Philadelphia Experience. *Plast Reconstr Surg* 104:1998–2010, 1999.
16. Yu CC, Chen PK, Chen YR. Comparison of speech results after Furlow palatoplasty and Von Langenbeck palatoplasty in incomplete clefts of the secondary palate. *Chang Gung Med J* 24:628, 2001.
17. LaRossa D, Jackson OH, Kirschner RE, et al. The Children's Hospital of Philadelphia modification of the Furlow double-opposing z-palatoplasty: Long-term speech and growth results. *Clin Plast Surg* 31:243–249, 2004.
18. Brothers DB, Dalston KW, Peterson HD, Lawrence WT. Comparison of the Furlow double-opposing Z-palatoplasty with the Wardill-Kilner procedure for isolated clefts of the soft palate. *Plast Reconstr Surg* 95:969–977, 1995.
19. Lin KY, Goldberg D, Williams C, Borowitz K, Persing J, Edgerton M. Long-term outcome analysis of two treatment methods for cleft palate: Combined levator retropositioning and pharyngeal flap versus double-opposing Z-plasty. *Cleft Palate Craniofac J* 63:462, 1999.
20. Noorchasm N, Dudas JR, Ford M, et al. Conversion Furlow palatoplasty: Salvage of speech after straight-line palatoplasty and incomplete intravelar veloplasty. *Ann Plast Surg* 56:505, 2006.
21. Guneren E, Uysal OA. The quantitative evaluation of palatal elongation after Furlow palatoplasty. *J Oral Maxillofac Surg* 62:446, 2004.
22. Kremenak CR, Searles JC. Experimental manipulation of midface growth: A synthesis of five years of research at the Iowa Maxillofacial Growth Laboratory. *J Dent Res* 50:1488, 1971.
23. Pigott RW, Albery EH, Hathorn IS, et al. A comparison of three methods of repairing the hard palate. *Cleft Palate Craniofac J* 39:383, 2002.

24. Seagle MB, Furlow LT, Jr. Muscle reconstruction in cleft lip repair. *Plast Reconstr Surg* 113:1537, 2004.

25. Oyama T, Nishimoto S, Ishii N, Hosokawa K. Soft palate mucosal adhesion as preparation for double opposing z-plasty. *Plast Reconstr Surg* 118:469, 2006.

26. Bardach J. Cleft palate repair: Two-flap palatoplasty, research, philosophy technique and results. In Bardach J, Morris HL (eds). *Multidisciplinary Management of Cleft Lip and Palate*, Philadelphia: WB Saunders Co., 1990, Chapter 46.

27. Bozola AR, Lourenco Gasques JA, Carriquiry CE, de Oliviera MC. The buccinator musculo- mucosal flap: Anatomic study and clinical application. *Plast Reconstr Surg* 84:250, 1989.

28. Mann RJ, Fisher DM. Bilateral buccal flaps with double opposing Z-plasty for wider palatal clefts. *Plast Reconstr Surg* 100:1139, 1997.

The Children's Hospital Modification of the Furlow Double-Opposing Z-Palatoplasty

Don LaRossa, MD • Richard E. Kirschner, MD • David W. Low, MD

Attention to muscle repair in cleft surgery evolved in the 1960s and 1970s with contributions from Fara in chieloplasty and Kriens in palatoplasty. It was Veau, however, who originally focused the surgeon's attention on the "cleft muscle." Otto Kriens deserves major credit for introducing and promoting the direct release, reorientation, and repositioning of the cleft palatal muscles in his landmark publications describing the intravelar veloplasty (IVVP).[1-3]

Modifications of the IVVP thereafter became a dominant focus in cleft palate surgery as surgeons attempted to improve speech results through a more thorough restoration of palatal anatomy. In theory, normalization of the muscular anatomy would result in more normal velar function and would thereby reduce the incidence of velopharyngeal incompetence. Most cleft palate surgeons incorporated muscular reconstruction with variations of the IVVP, but the results varied. This variation was thought to be related to variations in technique. In an attempt to evaluate the true value of muscular reconstruction with the IVVP, Marsh conducted a controlled, prospective study. He compared the results of palatoplasty performed with IVVP with those of palatoplasty performed without IVVP. All surgical procedures were performed by two surgeons, each trained as carefully as possible to carry out the operations in a similar fashion. In the end, he could not demonstrate any difference in speech outcome and concluded that the IVVP did not offer any significant advantage.[4]

At the Southeastern Society of Plastic Surgeons meeting in 1978, Leonard Furlow presented his brilliant and novel idea for muscle reconstruction in palatoplasty, referring to the procedure as the *double-opposing Z-palatoplasty*. The result was a major change in how many surgeons treat patients with cleft palate.[5] Furlow described the philosophical and technical aspects of his procedure, which combined a restoration of the velar muscular anatomy with attention to reducing the deleterious effects of scarring of the hard palate on facial growth by limiting the elevation of mucoperiosteal flaps.[6,7] After listening to Furlow's presentation, Peter Randall brought the concept back to The Children's Hospital of Philadelphia (CHOP), where it was quickly embraced by the surgeons there.

Since then, the plastic surgeons at CHOP have used this procedure to treat virtually all patients with cleft palate, regardless of cleft width or type. The operation performed by the surgeons at CHOP, however, is a modification of that described by Furlow. Incorporation of these technical variations in the procedure has been referred to as the "CHOP modification" of the double-opposing Z-palatoplasty.[8]

In an attempt to reduce scarring that might adversely affect maxillary growth, Furlow made a great effort to avoid the use of relaxing incisions in repair of the hard palate. When necessary, he extended the incisions used to create the musculomucosal and mucosal flaps onto the hard palate and undermined just to the extent needed to facilitate a more tension-free closure. CHOP surgeons, however, often found it difficult to obtain a tension-free closure without the more liberal use of relaxing incisions. Other surgeons may also have found it difficult to achieve palatal repair without tension using Furlow's original technique, and some may have experienced a higher incidence of fistula formation, thus discouraging them from using the operation for all but the narrowest clefts.

CHOP surgeons believed that Furlow's approach to repair of the soft palate represented a great advance but did not share his concern regarding the potential for relaxing incisions to significantly impair midfacial growth. With respect to the extent of extraperiosteal dissection, there is seemingly little difference between undermining and lifting the palatal mucoperiosteum out of the palatal arch, as described by Furlow (Fig. 24–1), and using bilateral relaxing incisions of the von Langenbeck type (Fig. 24–2). In contrast, the use of a "pushback" procedure creates an anterior mucosal defect with exposure of a periosteal surface, scarring of which could result in restriction of sagittal maxillary growth. Although some surgeons extend the relaxing incisions anteriorly, as in a two-flap palatoplasty, such practice places the flap at risk for vascular compromise in the event of a vascular accident in the greater palatine vessel leash. Flap necrosis is less likely to occur if tissue bridges are left in the regions connecting the soft and hard palate flaps (Fig. 24–2). Conversely, if one extends the Z-plasty incisions anteriorly, perhaps to the point of creating an

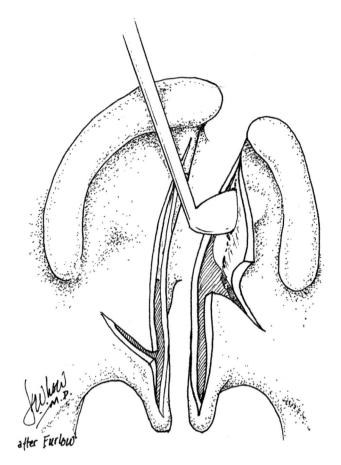

Figure 24–1. From Furlow's illustration of the double-opposing Z-palatoplasty.

island flap as described by Furlow, the risk of mucoperiosteal flap necrosis is increased.

SURGICAL TECHNIQUE: THE CHOP MODIFICATION OF THE FURLOW DOUBLE-OPPOSING Z-PALATOPLASTY

Standard patient positioning and anesthesia, the use of the Dingman or a similar mouth gag for exposure of the surgical field, and local infiltration of palatal soft tissues with epinephrine-containing solutions are used.

The design of the incisions is drawn on the hard and soft palate with methylene blue dye (Fig. 24–3). Most right-handed surgeons will find it easier to dissect the posteriorly based oral musculomucosal flap if it is located on the patient's left side. The Z-plasty incisions are not carried as far laterally as described by Furlow in order to avoid having them intersect with the relaxing incisions, thereby dividing soft tissue bridges that may augment blood flow to the palatal tissues. The angle of the musculomucosal Z-plasty flap is typically 60°, paralleling the direction of the commingled levator and palatopharyngeus muscles and the posterior border of the hard palate.

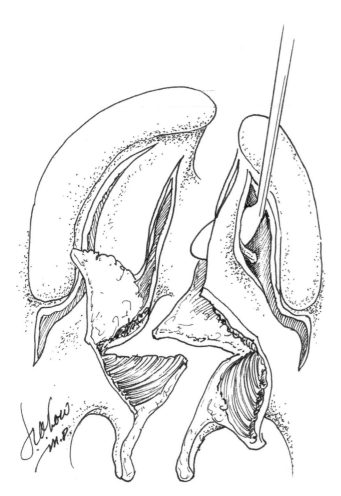

Figure 24–2. The Children's Hospital of Philadelphia (CHOP) modification of the double-opposing Z-palatoplasty.

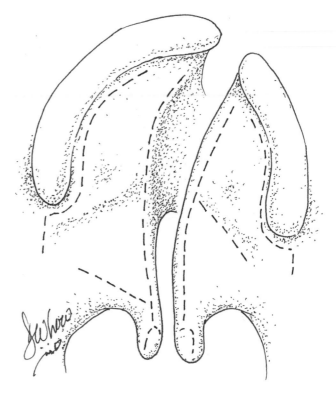

Figure 24–3. Design of incisions for the double-opposing Z-palatoplasty. Note the asymmetrical configuration of the Z-plasty flaps.

The oral mucosal flap on the contralateral side, however, has a variable angle depending upon the length of the soft palate, thus often creating an asymmetrical Z-plasty. The flap is designed with its base just posterior to the hamulus and its tip just anterior to the uvula. In patients with a longer soft palate, the angle approaches 60°. More commonly, however, the angle is more obtuse than that of the musculomucosal flap, approaching 90° when the soft palate is short.

The opposing Z-plasty on the nasal side is similarly designed, with the angle of the posteriorly based flap at approximately 60° and that of the anteriorly based mucosal flap often being more obtuse. The muscular flaps should be placed transversely and as far posteriorly as possible. The actual amount of posterior repositioning of the muscle is determined and limited by its bony origin.

The muscular flaps are dissected laterally and posteriorly until the muscle bundles lie perpendicular to the sagittal plane when they are rotated into the transverse position. Relaxing incisions of the von Langenbeck type, mucoperiosteal undermining of the hard palate, careful dissection into the space of Ernst, infracture of the hamulus, and stretching of the greater palatine neurovascular bundles are used alone or in combination to a degree sufficient to obtain a tension-free closure.

Flaps of vomerine mucoperiosteum are used for closure of the nasal surface in complete clefts of the primary and secondary palate and to close the anterior region in isolated clefts of the secondary palate. Every attempt is made to resurface the nasal side completely, although this is not always possible. Small areas are sometimes left to re-epithelialize. Recently, some cleft surgeons have incorporated the use of acellular dermal grafts to resurface raw areas in the repair in an attempt to reduce the risk of fistula formation.[9,10]

In complete unilateral clefts, particularly in wide clefts wherein the vomer is more slanted toward the noncleft side, the portion of the vomer flap adjacent to the oral mucosa can be fashioned into flap based on the posterior margin of the vomer in order to augment the nasal mucosal flap closure. This works best when the nasal mucosal flap is designed on the noncleft side (Fig. 24–4).

Although many surgeons perform early closure of the anterior palate with a gingivoperiosteoplasty, CHOP surgeons prefer to leave it unrepaired in order to reduce the possible adverse effect of scar in this region on maxillary growth. When a large alveolar gap is present, a medially based buccal mucosal flap can serve to reduce or prevent nasal regurgitation during growth. The alveolar fistula is closed with attached gingival mucosa at the time of alveolar bone grafting prior to eruption of the lateral incisor, if present, at approximately 7 years of age. Even if the lateral incisor is congenitally missing, the bone graft may benefit the central incisor bordering the cleft.

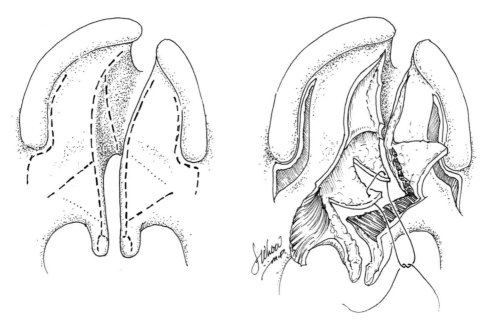

Figure 24–4. Design and inset of a posteriorly based vomer flap to aid in closure of the nasal surface by augmenting the nasal mucosal, soft palate flap. The posteriorly based nasal mucosal flap should be developed on the side opposite the cleft for most efficient use of the combined flaps.

LONG-TERM SPEECH AND GROWTH RESULTS

To date, CHOP surgeons have performed over 900 modified Furlow Z-plasty procedures and have evaluated speech outcomes at 17 and 22 years.[8,11] Separate studies have examined the effects on maxillary growth and occlusion.

Speech Outcome After Palatoplasty Using the CHOP Modification of the Double-Opposing Z-Palatoplasty

A retrospective analysis of the records of 661 patients treated between 1979 and 2001 with a double-opposing Z-palatoplasty by four plastic surgeons at CHOP was undertaken. In initial studies, records of patients treated between 1979 and 1996 were reviewed. Only patients over 5 years of age who had completed a perceptual speech evaluation using the *Pittsburgh Weighted Values for Speech Symptoms Associated with Velopharyngeal Incompetence* instrument were included.[12] Recently, the same group of patients was subjected to analysis at 8 and 10 years following palate repair.

Patients with gross hearing impairment, mental retardation, and syndromic diagnoses were excluded. Also excluded were those individuals who had a primary posterior pharyngeal flap or an oronasal fistula that could potentially affect resonance.

Each patient had at least one standardized perceptual speech evaluation using the Pittsburgh scale by one of two senior speech-language pathologists whose inter-rater reliability had been established.[13] Many patients had longitudinal examinations conducted during their routine evaluations by

the cleft palate team. The latest evaluation was used for the study, provided it was not influenced by other factors such as an upper respiratory infection or allergic rhinitis. Speech outcome was related to age at palatoplasty, and the need for secondary surgery, which in the majority of cases was a PPF, was documented.

Effect of the CHOP Modification of the Double-Opposing Z-Palatoplasty on Maxillary Growth

One of the major differences between the CHOP modification of the double-opposing Z-palatoplasty and that described by Furlow is the use of bilateral relaxing incisions whenever necessary to achieve a tension-free closure. The potential deleterious effects of surgically induced scarring on maxillary growth have been demonstrated in clinical and laboratory studies. For example, Ross et al. demonstrated the negative impact of surgery on facial growth in an extensive review of longitudinal cephalometric radiographs.[14] Bardach et al. confirmed this finding in beagle puppies.[15] Ortiz-Monasterio described more normal midfacial growth in unoperated patients with clefts.[16] Finally, there is an ongoing debate about the possible deleterious effects of primary gingivoperioplasty on maxillary growth.[17,18]

As noted above, the CHOP modification differs from Furlow's operation in its liberal use of relaxing incisions. Since the potential influence of such incisions on maxillary growth remained uncertain, a retrospective analysis of a cohort of 50 consecutively treated patients with left unilateral complete clefts of the lip and palate was undertaken. A cohort of only unilateral complete cleft lip and palate patients was selected in order to maintain as much consistency in cleft morphology as possible. Longitudinal anthropometric evaluation was carried out by a single physical anthropologist with a 5–14 year follow-up. The linear distance from tragion to subnasale was used as the measure of midfacial depth in each patient. Midfacial depth was compared to Farkas' published standards, which served as the controls.

Male and female patients were divided into the following groups: (1) All patients with unilateral complete clefts. (2) Those patients in whom relaxing incisions were used. (3) Those patients in whom relaxing incisions were not used.[19]

Effect of the CHOP Modification of the Double-Opposing Z-Palatoplasty on Dental Occlusion

Because a Z-plasty creates a gain in palatal length at the expense of width, and because relaxing incisions were used liberally in the CHOP modification, the risk of developing anterior and lateral crossbites would theoretically be higher than with a straight-line repair without the use of relaxing incisions. In order to determine the possible negative effects of the CHOP modification on anterior and posterior dental occlusion, dental occlusion was evaluated prospectively in 45 consecutive patients during routine clinic dental evaluations. Patient age, type of cleft, and anterior and posterior occlusion were documented.[20]

Effect of the CHOP Modification of the Double-Opposing Z-Palatoplasty on the Need for Orthognathic Surgery

As an additional determinant of the impact of surgery on facial growth, the need for orthognathic surgery was evaluated. A retrospective analysis of 91 consecutive patients with unilateral and bilateral clefts of the lip and palate under the care of a single orthodontist was undertaken. Patients were analyzed by type of cleft, age, presence or absence of bone grafting, age at bone grafting, and the recommendation or performance of orthognathic surgery.[21]

Results

Speech Outcomes

Between 1979 and 1996, 641 patients with cleft palate were treated, 310 of whom met the inclusion criteria. Three hundred two were excluded because they were under the age of 5 years at the time of their latest speech evaluation or because they had missing or inadequate speech records. Fifteen patients had primary pharyngeal flaps and four had oronasal fistulae felt to be sufficiently large enough to impact resonance. Seven had associated craniofacial malformations, and three had severe hearing loss.

Forty-eight patients (15.5%) had syndromes identified by either their phenotypic findings and/or chromosomal analysis. Two hundred sixty two patients (84.5%) did not have identifiable syndromes other than Van der Woude syndrome. It is likely, however, that some patients had provisionally unique or unidentified syndromes at the time of the analysis.

The distribution of cleft types was typical of a population of this size, with approximately one third presenting with isolated clefts of the secondary palate and two-thirds with complete unilateral and bilateral clefts of the primary and secondary palate. The mean age at palatoplasty was 10.5 months, with a range of 3–66 months.

Children had been followed for a mean of 7 years (85.7 months), and their latest speech evaluation occurred at a mean of 8 years of age (96.1 months), thus allowing sufficient time for developmental errors to resolve.

Speech Results in 262 "Non-Syndromic" Patients

Cleft Type: The distribution of cleft types was similar to that in the general cohort.

Age at Palatoplasty: The majority of patients (72%) underwent palatoplasty before the age of 12 months (mean 10.1 months). Only 5.7% had surgery at or after the age of 18 months.

Nasality: The overall Pittsburgh speech scores indicated absent or mild hypernasality in 92.8% of patients. Nasality was absent in 81.7% and was mild in 11.1%

Nasal Emission: In 85% of patients, nasal emission was absent, inconsistent, or inaudible. Nasoalveolar fistulae remained by intent in the vast majority of patients with complete unilateral and bilateral clefts until the time of alveolar bone grafting. This may account for consistent, but inaudible, nasal escape in 12.6% of patients.

Articulation Errors Related to VPI: Compensatory articulation errors were present in 5.6% of this study population. However, most patients were from urban areas, where good speech therapy was readily available, thus making the weight of this parameter more difficult to assess.

Velopharyngeal Function (Composite Pittsburgh Score): Ninety-four percent of patients had socially functional speech quality, one that would not strike the lay listener as different enough so as to warrant surgical intervention.

Composite scores in the *competent to borderline competent* range were recorded in 74.5% of patients. *Borderline incompetent* scores were noted in 19.9% of patients. These patients were typically monitored, but most did not have speech surgery. Only 5.7% of patients had composite scores indicating a clearly *incompetent* velopharyngeal mechanism.

Incidence of Secondary Surgery

Secondary surgery of the velopharyngeal port was performed in 6.5% of patients. This was a superiorly based posterior pharyngeal flap in 82.4% of patients and a sphincter pharyngoplasty in 17.6%. When patients for whom surgery was

Table 24–1.

Need for Secondary Speech Surgery After Palatoplasty by the CHOP Modification of the Double-Opposing Z-Palatoplasty (N = 262)

	Surgery Performed	Surgery Recommended
Isolated cleft palate	13.2%	15.8%
Unilateral CP	4.5%	5.1%
Bilateral CP	2.3%	4.5%

recommended but not performed were included, the total pharyngoplasty rate would have been 8%.

The Influence of Cleft Type on Speech Outcome

When speech results were compared by cleft type, the poorest outcomes were noted in patients with isolated clefts of the secondary palate. Whereas resonance was normal or mildly hypernasal in 94.2% of patients with unilateral complete clefts and 99.9% of patients with complete bilateral clefts, only 86% patients with isolated clefts of the secondary palate demonstrated a similarly good level of velar function. Audible nasal emission was present in 26.7% of isolated cleft palate patients vs. 6.9% of bilateral and 9.4% of unilateral cleft patients. Similarly, there was an increased need for secondary speech surgery in patients with isolated clefts of the secondary palate (Table 24–1). None of these trends, however, reached statistical significance.

There are some theoretical explanations for these trends. The etiology and development of isolated clefts of the secondary palate is widely held to be distinct from that of clefts of the primary and secondary palate. Hence, there may be skeletal differences that predispose affected patients to velopharyngeal incompetence after palatoplasty. Indeed, Ruotolo et al. have recently demonstrated dramatic differences in velopharyngeal anatomy in individuals with 22q11.21 deletion syndrome. These authors have demonstrated that the cranial base is significantly more obtuse and the volume of the velopharynx is much greater in affected children than in control subjects.[22] Clefts of the secondary palate are far more commonly associated with syndromes,[23] and the differences in speech outcomes between the two groups in this study of non–syndromic patients may indeed have been due to an inability to recognize patients with subtle phenotypic findings or those with provisionally unique syndromes.

The Influence of Age of Palatoplasty on Speech

Until approximately 2 years, the age at which modified Furlow palatoplasty was performed had little effect on speech

outcome. After the age of 2 years, however, speech outcomes were poorer. The data is consistent with previous observations.[24] It is important to note, however, that there may be other factors that influence the outcome in the patients with delayed repair. Important illnesses, airway problems, or unavailability of surgical services (as with adoptees from foreign countries), for example, can all play a role in surgical outcome.

Maxillary Growth Outcomes

Of the 50 patients examined, 36 patients had bilateral relaxing incisions used in their palate closure, 27 males and 9 females; 14 patients did not have relaxing incisions, 8 males and 6 females.

Both male and female patients with repaired clefts had a statistically significant decrease in facial projection when compared to Farkas' norms ($p < 0.001$). However, their growth curves paralleled those of Farkas' norms.

In both male and female patients with repaired clefts, the use of relaxing incisions had no effect on maxillary depth.

Orthodontic Outcomes

Posterior crossbites were not seen on dental evaluation in the study group of 45 consecutive patients. Anterior crossbites were minimal and reflected the severity of the original cleft.[20]

The Need for Orthognathic Surgery

Orthognathic surgery was performed or recommended in 7.1% of 91 unilateral cleft patients and in 14.3% of bilateral cleft patients in the study population.[21] This data may reflect a degree of conservatism in the management of these patients. Indeed, these patients' need for orthognathic surgery is likely to be consistent with reports in the literature from other centers.

SUMMARY AND CONCLUSIONS

Of the 261 non–syndromic patients studied, over 90% had minimal or no hypernasality, almost 86% had inconsistent or no nasal emission, and 95% had no articulation errors related to velar dysfunction. Only 6% of patients had a composite Pittsburgh score indicative of an incompetent velopharyngeal mechanism.

Patients with isolated clefts of the secondary palate did seem to do less well, although their outcomes were not statistically different from those with unilateral and bilateral clefts of the primary and secondary palate. Midfacial growth in patients with repaired unilateral palatal clefts paralleled that of Farkas' standards, but absolute maxillary depth was statistically lower. Relaxing incisions to facilitate a tension-free closure did not adversely impact midfacial depth of male or female patients in the study group. Hence, relaxing incisions of the von Langenbeck type do not seem to affect maxillary growth in patients with unilateral cleft lip and palate treated with the CHOP Modification of the Furlow double-opposing Z-palatoplasty.

Relaxing incisions are felt to have contributed significantly to an acceptably low fistula rate of 6.5%.[25] No major soft palate dehiscences or hard palate flap losses have occurred.

The speech outcomes reported herein represent a significant improvement over historical results at CHOP before introduction of the double-opposing Z-plasty. Similar outcomes with the Furlow repair have been reported by other centers.[26–29]

Despite a better understanding of the various factors that influence outcomes after palate repair, and despite the development of surgical strategies to address these factors, there seems to be a ceiling that can be approached but not exceeded as cleft care providers strive to provide excellent speech and growth outcomes in all patients. There are many variables, both defined and undefined, that can affect palatoplasty outcomes. Disarray of the palatal muscular anatomy is only one of many influences. The quantity, quality, and function of the muscles of the velopharyngeal sphincter can be a critical determinant of speech outcome. Other variables include the severity of the cleft and the angle and position of the cranial base relative to the soft palate. Impediments such as learning disabilities, hearing loss, and variations in soft tissue healing can influence outcomes, even in the face of ideal anatomic factors and skillfully performed surgery.

References

1. Veau V. Discussion on the treatment of cleft palate by operation. *Proc Roy Soc Med* 20(3):156, 1926–1927.
2. Veau V. *Division Palatine*. Paris: Masson, 1931, pp. 16–18, 51–53.
3. Kriens O. An anatomical approach to veloplasty. *Plast Reconstr Surg* 43:29, 1969.
4. Marsh JL, Grames LM, Holtman B. Intravelar veloplasty: A prospective study. *Cleft Palate J* 26:1, 46–50, 1989.
5. Seagle B. Personal communication
6. Furlow LT. Cleft palate repair: Preliminary report on lengthening and muscle transposition z-plasty. Presented at the Annual Meeting of the Southeastern Society of Plastic and Reconstructive Surgeons, Boca Raton, FL, May 16, 1978.
7. Furlow LT. Cleft palate repair by double opposing z-plasty. *Plast Reconst Surg* 78:724–736, 1986.
8. LaRossa D, Hunenko-Jackson O, Kirschner RE, et al. The Children's Hospital of Philadelphia modification of the Furlow double-opposing Z-palatoplasty: Long term speech and growth results. *Clin Plast Surg* 31:2, 243–250, April 2004.
9. Kirschner RE, Cabiling DS, Slemp AE, Siddiqi F, LaRossa D, Losee JE. Repair of oronasal fistulae with acellular dermal matricies. *Plast Reconstr Surg* 118(6):1431–1440, November 2006.
10. Helling ER, Dev VR, Garza J, Barone C, Nelluri P, Wang PT. Low fistula rate in palatal clefts closed with the Furlow technique using decellularized dermis. *Plast Reconstr Surg* 117(7):2361–2365, 2006.
11. Kirschner RE, Wang P, Jawad A, et al. Cleft palate repair by Furlow double opposing Z-palatoplasty: The Children's Hospital of Philadelphia experience. *Plast Reconst Surg* 104:1998–2001, 1999.
12. McWilliams BJ, Morris HL, Shelton RL. In *Cleft Palate Speech*. Philadelphia: Decker, 1984, p. 184.
13. McWilliams BJ, Randall P, LaRossa D, et al. Speech characteristics associated with the Furlow palatoplasty as compared with other surgical techniques. *Plast Reconst Surg* 98:610, 1996.
14. Ross B. Treatment variables affecting facial growth in complete unilateral cleft lip and palate. Part 7: An overview of treatment and facial growth. *Cleft Palate J* 24:1, 71–77, 1987.
15. Bardach J, Klausner EC, Eisbach KJ. The relationship between lip pressure and facial growth after cleft lip repair: An experimental study. *Cleft Palate J* 16:137, 1979.
16. Ortiz-Monasterio F, Rebeil AS, Valderrama M, Cruz R. Cephalometric measurements on adult patients with non-operated clefts. *Plast Reconst Surg* 24:53–61, 1959.
17. Wood RJ, Grayson BH, Cutting CB. Gingivoperiostroplasty and midfacial growth. *Cleft Palate Craniofac J* 34:1, 17–20, 1997.
18. Berkowitz S. A comparison of treatment results in complete bilateral cleft lip and palate using a conservative approach versus Millard-Latham PSOT procedure. *Semin Orthod* (US), 2(3):169–184, 1996.
19. Wang P, Kirschner R, Minugh-Purvis N, Randall P, LaRossa D. Relaxing incisions do not adversely affect the A–P midfacial growth in unilateral cleft lip and palate patients. Presented at the *American Cleft Palate-Craniofacial Association Meeting*, Scottsdale, AZ, 1999.
20. Mayro R, LaRossa D, Randall P, et al. Incidence of posterior dental crossbite post Furlow palatoplasty. Presented at the *American Cleft Palate-Craniofacial Association Meeting*, New Orleans, LA, 1997.
21. Mayro R. Personal communication.
22. Ruotolo R, Arens R, Corbin A, et al. Velopharyngeal anatomy in 22Q11.2 Deletion Syndrome: A three dimensional cephalometric analysis. Presented at the *Annual Meeting of the American Cleft Palate-Craniofacial Meeting*, Asheville, NC, 2003.
23. Jones M, Facial Clefting: Etiology and developmental Pathogenesis. In Advances in Management of Cleft Lip and Palate. *Clin Plast Surg* 20:4, October 1993.
24. Kirschner R, Minugh-Purvis N, Huang K, et al. Very early cleft palate repair: Effects on speech and midfacial Growth. Presented at the *American Cleft Palate-Craniofacial Association Meeting*, Scottsdale, AZ, 1999.
25. Baker S, Kirschner R, Huang K, et al. Incidence and etiology of cleft palate fistulas: Analysis of 429 consecutive Furlow palatoplasties. Presented at the *American Cleft Palate-Craniofacial Meeting*, Atlanta, GA, 2000.
26. Spauwen P, Goorhuis-Brouwer S, Schutte H. Cleft Palate repair: Furlow versus von Langenbeck. *J Craniomaxillofac Surg* 20:18, 1992.
27. Hapcic K, Levine N, Panchal J. Comparing the Furlow palatoplasty to the two-flap repair: a randomized, prospective study. Presented at the *American Cleft Palate-Craniofacial Association Meeting*, Minneapolis, MN, 2001.
28. Havlik R, Ranieri J, Young L, Coleman J. Total release double Opposing Z palatal closure in 180 patients-an evolution of the palatal repair techniques. Presented at the *Annual Meeting of the American Association of Plastic Surgeons*, Baltimore, MD, May 2003.
29. Seagal M, Dutka-Sousa J, Williams W, et al. Presented at the *Annual Meeting of the American Cleft Palate-Craniofacial Association Meeting*, Vancouver, Canada, 2006.

25

Cleft Palate Repair

Brian C. Sommerlad, MB, BS, FRCS Eng, FRCS Ed (Hon), FRCPCH

The aims of cleft palate repair are to improve feeding, to achieve normal speech, and to minimize maxillary growth restriction. The technique of palate repair may also have an impact on middle ear function and hearing. Cleft palate repair is the most important component of cleft surgery not only in that it determines the outcome as far as speech and communication is concerned, but also in that it potentially has the greatest impact on maxillary growth and dental arch relationship.[1]

TIMING

There is considerable support in the literature for the advice that palate repair—at least repair of the soft palate—should be performed before 12 months of age,[2] and there is evidence from a randomized controlled trial[3] that speech outcome is better if the palate is repaired at 6 months rather than 12 months. In the latter study, the children with clefts repaired at 6 months did not develop compensatory articulation, whereas there was an incidence of compensatory articulation in those repaired at 12 months. It seems, therefore, that repair before significant babbling commences provides the best environment for early acquisition of consonants and speech development and also improves feeding. Thus, the author aims to perform cleft palate repair at the age of 6 months. The major argument against early closure is the possible effect of early hard palate surgery on maxillary growth.[4]

There is evidence from countries in which patients often present late with unrepaired cleft palates that palate repair after the age of 8–12 years is unlikely to produce acceptable speech, especially if speech therapy is not available.[5,6] Nevertheless, late closure of the hard palate in such patients may still be indicated for social and psychological reasons. Separating the nasal and oral cavities should be beneficial for eating and swallowing.

PREOPERATIVE AND PEROPERATIVE FACTORS

Above all else, safe cleft palate surgery—particularly in young infants—requires high quality pediatric anaesthesia and postoperative care. Preoperative assessment should ensure that the patient is not anemic and not significantly underweight, although infants with cleft palate do tend to be below the average of weight for age. The airway should also be assessed as palate repair may, at least temporarily, compromise the airway. The general anaesthetic should be administered in such a way that the airway is preserved, allowing the surgeon access to the palate. Intravenous access is secured for fluid and, rarely, blood replacement.

ANATOMICAL CONSIDERATIONS

Although anatomy is covered elsewhere in this book (Chapter 14), certain aspects are of particular relevance to the technique to be described herein:

Hard Palate

The oral mucoperiosteum of the hard palate receives its neurovascular supply from the greater palatine vessels and nerves, which emerge through the greater palatine foramina in the postero–lateral corners of the hard palate. Multiple branches pass both medially toward the cleft margin and laterally toward the alveolus. The latter are divided when lateral releasing incisions are made.

The nasal mucosa of the hard palate is continuous laterally with that of the lateral nasal wall. In a unilateral cleft lip and palate, the nasal layer is formed medially from vomerine mucosa. In a bilateral cleft or an isolated cleft palate involving the hard palate, the vomer is in the midline and not in continuity with the palatal shelves.

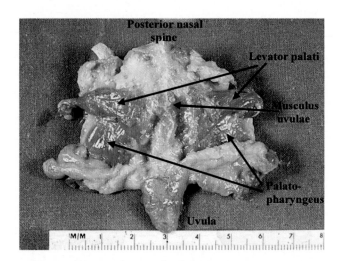

Figure 25–1. Nasal view of a dissected soft palate to illustrate the arrangement of the muscles. *(After Boorman & Sommerlad.[7])*

Soft Palate

In the noncleft palate, the levator veli palatini muscle reaches the midline in the middle 40% of the velum[7,8] (Fig. 25–1). In the cleft palate, the levator passes from its origin at the skull base, downward and medially, to insert into the cleft margin in the anterior half of the velum (but not directly into the back of the hard palate as most texts state). The palatopharyngeus and palatoglossus muscles lie on the oral side of the levator, becoming closely related to the levator in the midline. These muscles fan out from the fauces with some fibers passing forward toward the region of the maxillary tuberosity and pterygoid hamulus and other fibers passing more medially toward the cleft margin (in its anterior two-thirds to three-quarters) and toward the back of the hard palate. The presence of the musculus uvulae muscle in cleft palates is uncertain. The tensor veli palatini muscle passes from the skull base to the pterygoid hamulus to which, in the cleft palate patient, it partially attaches and appears to diverge into two components—a nasal component, which is a triangular tendinous insertion into the lateral part of the posterior border of the hard palate, where it lies adjacent to the nasal mucosa—and a less robust component which passes orally toward the oral mucosa. This component is seen during repair techniques that involve lateral releasing incisions for relief of tension.

The sensory nerve supply of the soft palate is derived predominantly from the lesser palatine nerves, of which there are several branches that pass through lesser palatine foramina in the palatal process of the sphenoid and through the palatal aponeurosis. The motor supply of the levator veli palatini, palatopharyngeus, and palatoglossus muscles is derived from the pharyngeal plexus (cranial nerves IX, X, and XI). The musculus uvulae is said to be supplied by the lesser palatine nerve.[9,10] The tensor veli palatini muscle is supplied by a branch from the trigeminal nerve (V).

The aim of palatal surgery should be to restore anatomy to as close as possible to the normal while minimizing damage to normal anatomical structures.

SURGICAL TECHNIQUE

Principles

The technique used in palate repair depends on the type, extent, and width of the cleft.

Closure of the hard palate should be achieved with minimal dissection. The relative importance of incisions, of mucosal elevation (extraperiosteal or subperiosteal), and of leaving bone exposed at the end of the procedure on maxillary growth impairment is uncertain. Transverse scars across the palate seem to be particularly deleterious.

Soft palate repair involves uniting mucosa and musculature, and the consensus view is that this should also be accompanied by reorientation of the abnormal cleft musculature and "reconstruction of the levator sling."[11] Kriens[12] described his own technique for muscle repair and coined the term "intravelar veloplasty." Cutting,[13] independently of the author, has evolved a technique of radical reconstruction of the palate musculature which differs from the author's technique in some respects.[14] Thus, achieving the aims of velar reconstruction may be accomplished using a number of protocols, some of which are discussed in other chapters of this text.

The management of palatal clefts associated with clefts of the lip depends on the technique used for lip repair and on individual protocols (especially the sequence of repair). Such protocols include:

- Closure of lip and alveolus followed by closure of hard and soft palate (the author's technique until 1993).
- Closure of lip, alveolus and hard palate followed by closure of soft palate (the author's present technique).
- Closure of lip and soft palate followed by closure of hard palate.[15]
- Closure of soft palate followed by closure of the hard palate followed by closure of the lip.[16]
- One-stage closure of lip, palate, and alveolus.

Techniques for Closure of the Palate

Techniques for closure of the palate include:

- von Langenbeck[17,18]
- Veau-Wardill-Kilner pushback[19,20,21,22]
- Two-flap (Bardach[23])
- Furlow double-opposing Z-plasty
- No palatal incisions (Sommerlad[14])

Von Langenbeck Repair (Fig. 25–2)

Early attempts at palate repair involved incision and attempted closure in the midline. Von Langenbeck introduced the concept of lateral releasing incisions to relieve tension in the repair. The technique involves an incision which begins behind the alveolus, passes backward, if required, into the soft palate and forward around the posterior border of the alveolus. The incision then extends anteriorly lateral to the greater palatine neurovascular bundle at the junction of the gingival

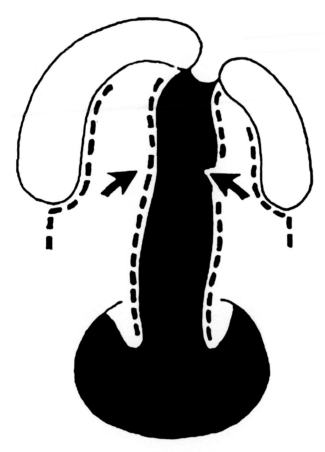

Figure 25–2. Von Langenbeck repair, with lateral releasing incisions.

and oral mucoperiosteal mucosa. The incision is carried down to the bone of the hard palate, and the oral mucoperiosteal flaps are mobilized medially, often with division of the oral component of the tensor palati tendon (described above).

Veau and Wardill-Kilner Pushback Procedures (Fig. 25–3)

These techniques were devised with the belief that V to Y pushback of the oral mucoperiosteum of the hard palate would result in effective palatal lengthening and would therefore improve speech outcome. There is evidence, however, that this did not improve speech outcome,[24] and the greater insult to the hard palate has several potential consequences:

- More transverse collapse
- Potential denervation and devascularization of the alveolus
- Bone exposure
- Probable impairment of antero–posterior maxillary growth
- Difficult fistulae anterior to the pushback flaps (Fig. 25–4)

Unfortunately, this technique has been widely used around the world. The author believes it has accounted for much of the morbidity of palate repair.

Two-Flap Repair (Fig. 25–5)

The two-flap repair is widely used. The technique involves raising two long flaps that extend to the alveolar margin

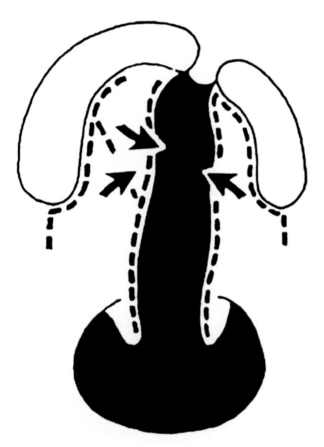

Figure 25–3. Veau-Wardill-Kilner pushback technique.

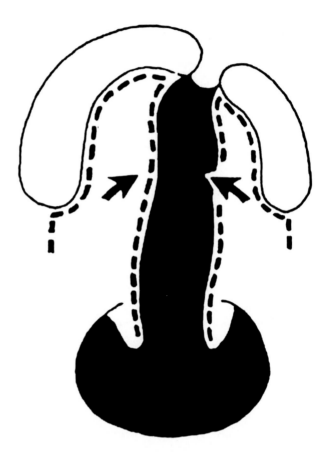

Figure 25–5. Two-flap technique (Bardach).

anteriorly, based posteriorly on the greater palatine neurovascular bundle. Many of the surgeons who use this technique advocate resuturing of the flaps to their original position such that they are not using the flaps to achieve "push-back." Advocates of this technique argue that raising the flaps facilitates

exposure of the soft palate musculature. Further study will be necessary to determine if elevation of these flaps impairs maxillary growth and dental occlusion.

The Furlow Double Opposing Z-plasty

This technique is discussed in Chapters 23 and 24.

AUTHOR'S TECHNIQUE

Instrumentation

The author uses the operating microscope for palate repair.[25] The advantages of the microscope are:

- The operating microscope provides high-quality variable magnification and good lighting, directed at the operating field. It is therefore much more reliable than the alternative of magnifying loupes and headlight. Improvements in visualization have led to refinements of palate repair and palate rerepair.
- By frequently changing the tilt of the binoculars, it is also possible to sit in a relatively comfortable position throughout the entire procedure.
- Magnification can be varied, "zooming up" for more detailed parts of the dissection.
- The assistant obtains an excellent view through the side teaching arm and quickly learns to cut sutures and assist

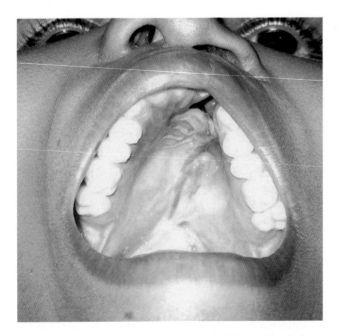

Figure 25–4. A fistula at the anterior end of the pushback flaps.

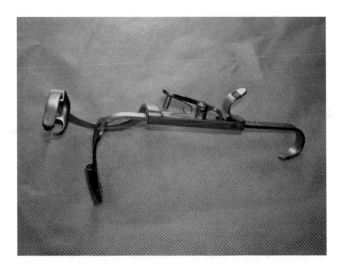

Figure 25–6. Modified gag for cleft palate repair.

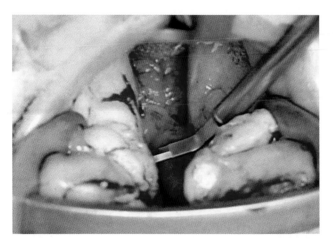

Figure 25–7. The Beaver knife with No. 69 blade, being used here to incise the cleft margin at the time of cleft lip repair.

through this side view. He/she may also view the video monitor. The opportunity to demonstrate the operation to the operating room nurses greatly increases their involvement in the procedure, and it is possible to demonstrate palate surgery adequately to trainees and visitors. Both the assistant and those viewing the video monitor are seeing the same view as the surgeon.

• Still (Figs. 25–10 to 25–18 and 25–20) and video records of the repair can be obtained.

It takes a little time to become used to using the microscope, but the advantages soon become apparent.

If a microscope is not available, the author uses 3.5 × magnifying loupes with attached headlight but believes that this is a compromise and that it makes the soft palate muscular dissection and reconstruction less safe.

A modification of the Dott-Kilner version of the Boyle Davis gag[26] facilitates repair under the operating microscope and helps to avoid compression of the orotracheal tube on the mandible (Fig. 25–6). Other surgeons prefer the Dingman gag, which employs lateral traction of the cheek.

Surgeons vary in their preferences for instruments. A Beaver knife with No. 69 blade is very useful for incisions at the cleft margin and commencement of mobilization of the oral mucoperiosteal flaps (Fig. 25–7).

Technique

Wherever possible, the author closes the palate without lateral releasing incisions. Whether this is possible depends on the type, extent, and width of the cleft.

In isolated clefts of the palate, the need for lateral releasing incisions increases with the extent and width of the cleft, but lateral releasing incisions are required in less than 10% of cases (most often in wide U-shaped clefts, often associated with Pierre Robin sequence). Lateral releasing incisions are likely to be necessary if the width of the cleft at the back of the hard palate is in excess of 10 mm (at the age of repair at 6 months). In very wide U-shaped clefts, if it is determined

early that lateral releasing incisions (Von Langenbeck) will need to be made, and they are made early, with subperiosteal elevation of the oral mucoperiosteum, both laterally and medially.

Closure of the hard palate without lateral releasing incisions depends on:

• The drawbridge effect—converting the sloping palatal mucoperiosteal flaps to become more horizontal
• Unfolding of the flaps, especially if the mucoperiosteum is infolded
• Mobilization of the greater palatine neurovascular pedicles, if necessary
• Division of the oral component of the tensor palati insertion (see above), if necessary

Even in clefts of the soft palate, the incision is extended forward so that the subperiosteal plane at the back of the hard palate can be entered, as this facilitates dissection of the soft palate musculature. The technique of muscle dissection will be described in detail in the following section.

In unilateral clefts of the lip and palate, a single-layer vomerine flap closure of the hard palate is carried out at the time of lip repair at 3 months.[27] This involves an incision at the junction of oral mucoperiosteum and vomerine mucosa on the noncleft side, extending posteriorly down the crest of the vomer and, anteriorly, oral to the groove which exists at the junction of vomer and premaxilla, then forward to become continuous with the lateral incision of the lip repair (Fig. 25–8). By the time the palate is repaired at 6 months, the exposed periosteal surface of the vomerine flap has epithelialised to produce a virtually intact hard palate (Fig. 25–9), although there are frequently small defects that can be probed in the region of the alveolus. At the time of palate repair, a posteriorly-based V-shaped flap can be raised from the neo-epithelialised vomer and turned back to facilitate closure of the anterior nasal layer of the soft palate (Fig. 25–10). An incision is made on the noncleft side, extending down to bony vomer, with care on the cleft side to avoid creating a hole in the nasal layer.

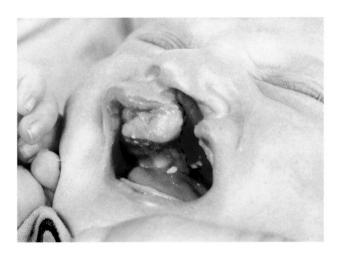

Figure 25–8. Dotted line to demonstrate the incision for the vomerine flap in the patient (aged 3 months) whose palate repair is to be demonstrated in Figs. 25–10 through 25–20.

Unless the cleft is very wide and it is determined at the beginning of the procedure that lateral releasing incisions will be necessary, incisions are made at the junction of oral and nasal mucosa (Fig. 25–11). This junction is usually clearly seen as the nasal mucosa is more pink and telangiectatic and is usually clearly seen on the oral side of the cleft. If the residual cleft extends into the hard palate, the oral flap then needs to be elevated to the edge of the bony palatal cleft. Here a Beaver knife with No. 69 blade is very useful in many cases. With an appropriate dental scaler, the mucoperiosteal flaps are lifted from the hard palate. It is important at this stage to expose the posterior border of the hard palate in a subperiosteal plane.

Most of the remainder of this description is relevant to all cleft types. There are frequently dimples on the oral side of the palate at a point where oral and mucous glands are attached deeply to the posterior border of the hard palate and the white tendinous nasal component of the tensor palati tendon (Fig. 25–12). By extending the incision backward,

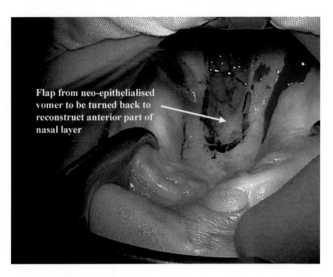

Figure 25–10. Posteriorly-based V-shaped flap raised from neo-epithelialized vomer.

using a combination of dental scaler and knife, the mucous glands are lifted intact from these structures. If the plane is incorrect and the mucous glands are damaged, there is usually more bleeding and mucus and the dissection becomes more difficult.

Depending on the width of the cleft, the oral mucoperiosteal flap is then elevated laterally to expose the greater palatine neurovascular bundle and, if necessary to achieve mobilization, the periosteal sleeve around the greater palatine bundle is incised, a probe passed between the greater palatine bundle and the alveolus, and the neurovascular pedicle elevated out of the foramen. Just behind and lateral to the foramen, a firm structure can be felt, and this is partly composed of the oral component of the tensor palati tendon described above. Lesser palatine neurovascular branches are also present at this point. If necessary to achieve adequate mobilization, the oral component of the tensor is divided with a knife just behind the greater palatine bundle. This degree of

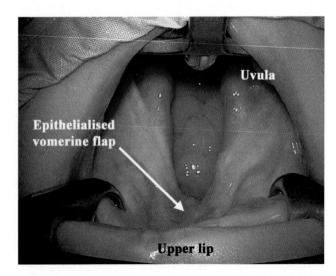

Figure 25–9. The patient shown in Fig. 25–8 at the age of 6 months, showing the epithelialization of the vomerine flap and virtually complete closure of the hard palate.

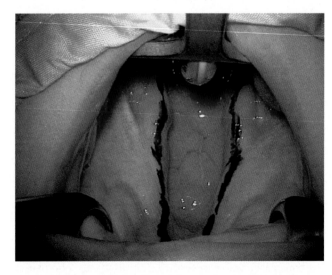

Figure 25–11. Incisions at the junction of oral and nasal mucosa.

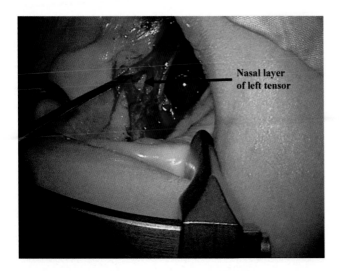

Figure 25–12. Elevation of the oral mucoperiosteum to demonstrate the nasal component of the tensor palati tendon.

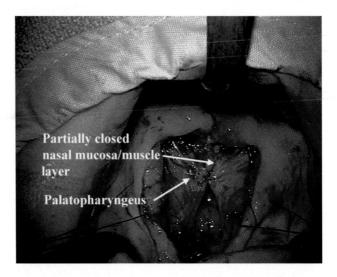

Figure 25–13. Closure of posterior nasal mucosa/muscle layer. The muscle seen is palatopharyngeus.

mobilization is not necessary in narrow clefts and clefts that simply involve the soft palate.

The dissection is continued back into the soft palate, separating the oral mucosa and underlying mucous glands from the underlying musculature, the palatopharyngeus and palatoglossus muscles. This is done by a combination of knife and blunt dissection and extends to the posterior border of the velum and laterally to the pterygoid hamulus.

The nasal mucosa is then mobilized, if necessary, from the nasal surface of the palatal shelves. This is best done after an incision at the edge of the palatal shelves, and then blunt dissection is performed in a subperiosteal plane.

The nasal mucosa, with its attached muscle, is then sutured. Closure of the nasal layer at this stage facilitates the later muscle dissection by placing it under some tension. Sutures (the author uses 5/0 Monocryl) are inserted in the nasal mucosa close to the edge, but then picking up more of the mucous glands (and a little muscle anteriorly). The aim is a suture, which will evert the nasal layer toward the nasal surface. Closure is continued to a point where it is possible without tension (Fig. 25–13). The V-shaped flap is turned back to fill the remainder of the defect (Fig. 25–14).

An incision is then made on each side of the midline, beginning 3–5mm from the midline posteriorly, and closer to the midline anteriorly, just lateral to the previously inserted nasal layer sutures. This knife dissection extends deep to the nasal mucosa, leaving mucous glands medially. The nasal mucosa is recognized because of its almost blue color. Using knife dissection, the plane is then developed between the nasal mucosa and the palatal muscles (Fig. 25–15), extending laterally for 5–10 mm. This allows the nasal surface of the levator veli palatini muscle to be identified as it passes toward the cleft margin in the anterior half of the velum (Fig. 25–16). Laterally, the levator can be seen to pass in a tunnel, surrounded by a thin sheath, toward the skull base, and the dissection between muscle and nasal mucosa can be continued to the posterior border of the velum (Fig. 25–17).

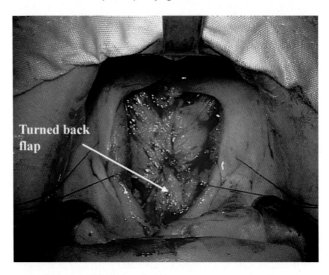

Figure 25–14. Flap of neo-epithelialized vomer turned back to close anterior nasal layer.

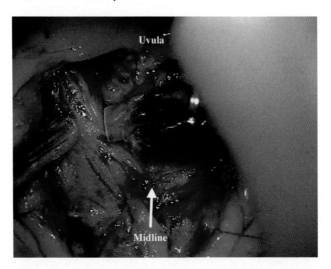

Figure 25–15. Paramedian incision on the left—beginning medial to palatopharyngeus and passing closer to the midline anteriorly.

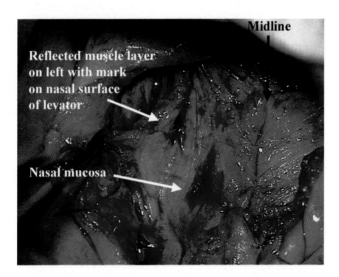

Figure 25–16. Reflected muscle layer after dissection laterally between muscle and nasal mucosa—demonstrating the nasal surface of the levator palati.

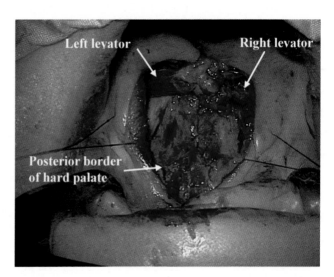

Figure 25–18. The muscle is united with nonabsorbable 4.0 or 5.0 nylon sutures.

With a skin hook in the musculature, the palatopharyngeus medially and the nasal component of the tensor tendon laterally are divided from the back of the hard palate by knife dissection to the bluish colored nasal mucosa. By using the knife to both incise and brush back, retrodisplacement of the musculature is commenced. The knife then turns almost at a right angle in an antero–posterior direction, and most of the tensor veli palatini tendon is divided just medial to the hamulus.

With tension maintained on the muscle, the combined levator veli palatini and palatopharyngeus muscle is further retrodisplaced with a combination of sharp and blunt dissection. When the most posterior fibers of the tensor veli palatini tendon are divided medial to the posterior end of the hamulus, a noticeable freeing is usually achieved. With a dental scaler, the palatopharyngeus fibers can be split to demonstrate the anterior and oral surfaces of the levator veli palatini muscle

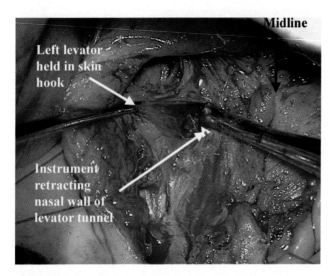

Figure 25–17. Retraction of the nasal wall of the levator tunnel to demonstrate the nasal surface of the levator.

with its thin sheath passing cranially towards the skull base. Frequently, there is a vessel lying anterior to the levator veli palatini muscle, and a small branch passing anteriorly can be divided after coagulation, leaving the major vessel intact as it is retrodisplaced. Dissection continues until the muscle bundle is dissected from the nasal layer and freely mobile. Care is taken to avoid unnecessary damage to the neurovascular structures. A stab incision is made in the nasal mucosa on each side (unless an accidental hole has been created). This helps to avoid a hematoma.

The muscle is united, usually in the posterior half of the velum, with nonabsorbable 4/0 or 5/0 nylon sutures (Fig. 25–18). The anterior of these muscle sutures includes the divided and retrodisplaced tendons of the tensor veli palatini tendon.

Closure of the oral layer commences. The first suture in the oral layer is inserted just in front of the retrodisplaced muscle sling and picks up the nasal mucous glands. A loop mattress suture[28] is used at this point, but with a modification in that the loop is twisted 180 degrees, with the needle inserted through the twisted loop from the side to which it is twisted, thus reducing the likelihood of strangulating small segments of oral mucosa in the loop (Fig. 25–19). One or two further twisted loop mattress sutures are usually inserted anteriorly. The aim of these sutures, uniting oral and nasal layers, is to keep the muscle in a posterior position and to occlude dead space, further reducing the chance of hematoma formation. The author uses a 4/0 monocryl suture on a modified 5/8 curved needle (Ethicon UV-17). Closure of the remainder of the oral layer overlying the muscle and including the uvula and also anteriorly is completed (Fig. 25–20).

In very wide clefts, (usually more than 10mm in width at the back of the hard palate lateral releasing incisions are sometimes necessary (in approximately 10% of cases). These lateral releasing incisions are sometimes made prospectively at the beginning of the procedure if it is thought that they will be necessary, but otherwise they are performed at the

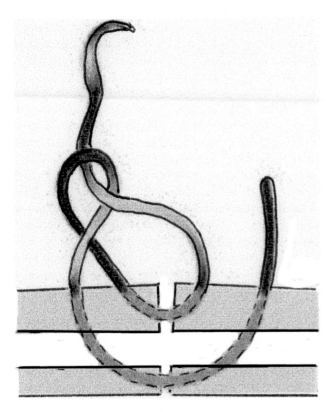

Figure 25–19. Diagram of loop mattress suture used to unite the oral and nasal layers in front of the reconstructed muscle sling.

end of the procedure if closure, particularly at the junction of hard and soft palate, is thought to be too tight. However, the tension in the oral layer is reduced as soon as the gag is released and, if in doubt, it is worth partly releasing the gag and retesting the tension before embarking on late lateral releasing incisions.

In bilateral clefts of the lip and palate a complete vomerine flap is elevated on one side (usually the widest) but only a

limited vomerine flap (posterior to the prevomerine suture) is elevated on the other side, for fear of devascularising the premaxilla and prolabium. Again, at the time of the palate repair a posteriorly-based flap is elevated from the vomer with care not to make a hole in the nasal layer. Lateral releasing incisions are required more frequently in bilateral clefts and closure anteriorly, particularly if the premaxilla is prominent, is less secure.

Submucous Cleft Palate

Repair of submucous cleft palate is covered in Chapter 22. The author uses a similar technique of muscle repair to that described above, leaving the nasal layer intact and leaving, if possible, some mucous glands on the nasal layer in the midline.[29]

Secondary Palatal Surgery

Much of the same operative technique is employed in palate rerepair, which is an alternative to pharyngoplasty.[30]

POSTOPERATIVE CARE

Postoperative care is critical, particularly in the first 24 hours. In vulnerable patients, such as those with Pierre Robin sequence, postoperative oxygen saturation monitoring is mandatory. Some surgeons use a temporary tongue stitch (a loose suture through the tongue which allows the tongue to be pulled forward in the recovery period). The use of a nasopharyngeal airway is a more conventional way of maintaining the airway in a compromised patient in the postoperative period. The airway must be inserted with care, with the distal end at the appropriate level, above the epiglottis but below the posterior border of the tongue. The position should be checked with a lateral X-ray (Fig. 25–21).

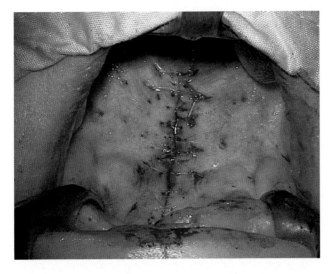

Figure 25–20. Closure without lateral releasing incisions.

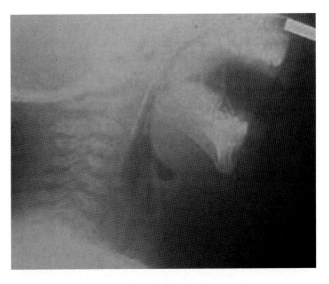

Figure 25–21. Lateral X-ray to check the correct position of the nasopharyngeal airway (prong).

Feeding commences as soon as the baby is awake and often decreases postoperative distress. Most babies with cleft palate are primarily bottle fed, and the same bottle and nipple can be used postoperatively.

Arm splints have traditionally been used on the basis that fingers in the mouth may disrupt the repair and thereby the risk of oronasal fistulae. A randomized controlled trial, however, has demonstrated no benefit,[31] and the use of arm splints has been abandoned by the author.

An earlier study confirmed that blood loss in patients in whom no lateral releasing incisions are made is significantly less than for those requiring such incisions. It is important, moreover, to be aware of "silent blood loss" wherein the baby swallows the blood.

Penicillin V is given as a prophylactic antibiotic against beta haemolytic streptococcus, although this may be unnecessary.

PALATE REPAIR IN SYNDROMIC CLEFTS

Pierre Robin Sequence

In the classical Pierre Robin sequence of micrognathia, glossoptosis, and airway obstruction associated with cleft palate, the clefts are often wide and U-shaped. Lateral releasing incisions are more likely to be necessary. Most infants have largely overcome their early airway and feeding difficulties, but it is to be expected that repair of the palate will, at least temporarily, produce some compromise of the nasal airway. Some surgeons advocate delaying palate repair in infants with Pierre Robin sequence. The author aims to repair at the standard age of 6 months but is prepared to use a nasopharyngeal airway in the early postoperative period (see Fig. 25–21). A preoperative sleep study may be helpful in predicting postoperative airway problems. The operation is occasionally carried out in patients who have continued to require a nasopharyngeal airway from birth, and in rare patients in whom tracheostomy has been necessary.

Treacher Collins Syndrome

Cleft palate in Treacher Collins syndrome may be particularly difficult because of limited mouth opening. The anesthesiologist may have difficulties with intubation, and there is a potential danger of airway compromise postoperatively. Obtaining sufficient exposure to achieve good muscular repair may not be possible, and this may be a situation where a compromise is necessary. It is better not to attempt a muscle repair than to create unnecessary damage.

Apert Syndrome

The cleft palate in Apert syndrome is often atypical. There tends to be a deep groove in the hard palate and, in fact, it is possible to misdiagnose a cleft of the hard palate when in fact the hard palate is intact but grooved and very high. Because children with Apert syndrome have a high incidence of airway obstruction, and because the nasopharynx is crowded, the cleft may not cause significant problems with speech and feeding, and closure may increase airway obstruction. Palatal repair, therefore, should be carried out with care and only after adequate preoperative sleep studies and assessment.

Van der Woude Syndrome

The cleft in Van der Woude and popliteal pterygium syndrome tends to be wide, and the palatal shelves and soft palate are often hypoplastic, making these difficult clefts to repair.

22q11.1 Deletion (Velocardiofacial Syndrome)

22q11.2 deletion syndrome has already been described in Chapter 9. The cleft velar musculature is often hypoplastic and difficult to dissect and suture.

OUTCOME

The outcome of cleft palate repair can be measured in terms of:

1. Speech
2. Maxillary growth
3. Hearing
4. Social and psychological well-being
5. Burden of care

Speech

It is very difficult to compare techniques and protocols. Randomized controlled trials are being undertaken to compare protocols, but because of the requirements for adequate patient numbers in a trial, most are multi-center studies with different operators. Operative techniques are difficult to reproduce. A study comparing "intravelar veloplasty versus none"[32] showed no significant difference in outcomes as far as speech is concerned, but the author has confirmed that the technique of intravelar veloplasty is very different from that described above (personal communication) and that there was considerable variability of technique within the trial.

Most data is therefore provided by reports on series of cases by individual authors, and most use pharyngoplasty rate as the major outcome measure. Pharyngoplasty rates are of little value in comparing outcomes between centers, because they depend on:

• The threshold of the team to recommend pharyngoplasty
• The wishes of patients and parents
• Inclusions and exclusions in the series
• Length and completeness of follow-up

Historical comparisons within one center, using the same criteria for surgery, do have some validity. The author's experience shows an improvement in the rates of secondary surgery for velopharyngeal dysfunction at 10 years associated with a learning curve for the technique of primary repair (Table 25–1).

Table 25–1.	
Some Evidence of the Author's Learning Curve	
Velopharyngeal incompetence (VPI) Surgery (10-y follow-up)	
First 5 y of practice:	10.2%
Second 5 y of practice:	4.9%
Third 5 y of practice:	4.6%

Table 25–2.	
The Increasing Requirement for Secondary Velopharyngeal Surgery with Age	
Secondary Surgery for velopharyngeal incompetence (VPI)	
Up to 5 y:	0.9%
Up to 10 y:	5.9%
Up to 15 y:	8.1%
Up to 20 y:	12.4%

Speech assessment is the primary outcome measure, but it is very difficult to compare between centers as there remain no standardized criteria between centers and across languages. Ideally, speech should be blindly assessed by external speech pathologists. The biggest such study was the Clinical Standards Advisory Group Study in the UK, which was a study of 5–6 year-old and 12–13 year-old patients with complete bony unilateral clefts of lip and palate. This demonstrated that secondary velopharyngeal surgery had been performed or was necessary in 27% and 31% of patients, respectively. The author's results within this study, as one of the five relatively high volume units in the UK, were 0% and 0%, respectively, but numbers in all centers were relatively small.

Many pharyngoplasty rates are given at 5–6 years, but longer follow-up of these patients confirms that a significant number have secondary velopharyngeal surgery up to the age of skeletal maturity (Table 25–2).

Maxillary Growth

There is growing evidence that minimizing surgery of the hard palate decreases the impairment of maxillary growth, although there is also growing evidence from most centers that maxillary growth—particularly in later years—is not as good as in noncleft patients. Maxillary growth is generally measured either by cephalometry or by measures of dental arch relationship such as the GOSLON score.[33] The first major intercenter study was the Eurocleft Study, which demonstrated marked differences in GOSLON scores between six European centers.[34] A consecutive series of the author's patients with similar clefts, where inclusions and exclusions were independently validated, were assessed blindly against the original Eurocleft models and demonstrated outcomes which were at least as good as the best in the study (Fig. 25–22).[35] However, longer term follow-up of these patients, as with most other series, suggests that the growth outcome is poorer at maturity. The large UK Clinical Standards Advisory Group study

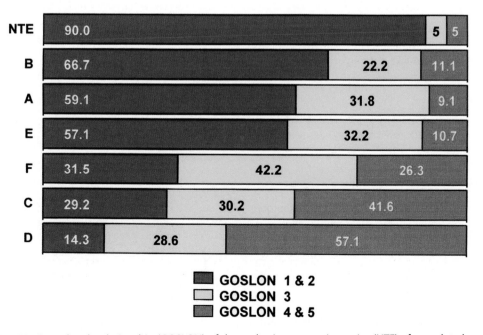

Figure 25–22. Dental arch relationship (GOSLON) of the author's consecutive series (NTE) of complete bony UCLP patients at 9–11 years of age, blindly assessed with the Eurocleft series.

showed that 37% of 5–6-year-olds had 5-year index scores of 4 or 5 and 39% of the 12–13-year-olds had GOSLON scores of 4 or 5, suggesting that at least this number of patients will benefit from future orthognathic surgery.

Growth cannot be assessed until maturity, and very few late outcome studies have been published. Most surgeons only learn about their long-term results toward the end of their careers, and often the number of patients on whom they operated early in their careers is relatively small.

Hearing

It is still unclear to what extent hearing outcome is dependent on the age and type of cleft palate repair. Theoretically, realignment of the palate musculature into a more normal configuration may improve Eustachian tube function. Some authorities have been concerned that tensor tenotomy may impair the tensor veli palatini in its Eustachian tube function. However, the early evidence from the author's series suggests that this is concern is not borne out.[36]

Once again, good intercenter comparisons are not available. Both the number of interventions (such as the insertion of ventilating tubes) and the long-term outcome need to be assessed.

Social and Psychological Well-being

The ultimate aim of cleft surgery is a patient who is happy and well adjusted. It has been shown in our own center and elsewhere that the patients' psychological well-being and satisfaction with results are not directly related to objective assessments of outcome. Because palate repair is so critical for communication and appearance, it is, however, a significant factor in this ultimate measure of final outcome.

Burden of Care

Both the outcome and the burden borne by the patient and his/her parents in order to achieve this outcome need consideration. The burden of care includes:

• Number of operations
• Number of hospital visits
• Amount of speech therapy
• Speech during childhood
• Appearance during childhood
• Teasing during childhood

An acceptable long-term result achieved by many operations may be at the expense of a patient who has suffered psychological scars in the process.

CONCLUSION

Cleft palate repair is the key to cleft surgery in that it is fundamental not only to communication but also to maxillary growth and appearance. The search continues for a proto-

col and a technique of palate repair that produces minimal impairment of maxillary growth while maximizing palatal function to optimize speech.

References

1. Mars M, Houston WJB. A preliminary study of facial growth and morphology in unoperated male unilateral cleft lip and palate subjects over 13 years of age. *Cleft Palate J* 27:7–10, 1990.
2. Dorf D, Curtin JW. Early cleft palate repair and speech outcome. *Plast Reconstr Surg* 70:75, 1982.
3. Ysunza A, Pamplona MC, Mendoza M, et al. Speech outcome and maxillary growth in patients with unilateral complete cleft lip/palate operated on 6 versus 12 months of age. *Plast Reconstr Surg* 102: 675–679, 1998.
4. Friede H, Enemark H. Long-term evidence for favorable midfacial growth after delayed hard palate repair in UCLP patients. *Cleft Palate Craniofac J* 38:323–329, 2001.
5. Ortiz-Monasterio F, Serrano A, Barrera G, et al. A study of untreated adult cleft palate patients. *Plast Reconstr Surg* 38:36, 1966.
6. Sell D, Grunwell P. Speech studies and the unoperated cleft palate subject. *Eur J Disord Commun* 29(2):151–164, 1994. Review.
7. Boorman JG, Sommerlad BC. Levator palati and palatal dimples—their anatomy, relationship and clinical significance" 1985 *Br J Plast Surg* 38, 326–332.
8. Huang MHS, Lee ST, Rajendran K. Anatomic basis of cleft palate and velopharyngeal surgery: Implications from a fresh cadaveric study. *Plast Reconstr Surg* 101:613, 1998.
9. Broomhead IW. The nerve supply of the muscles of the soft palate. *Br J Plast Surg* 4:1, 1951.
10. Broomhead IW. The nerve supply of the soft palate. *Br J Plast Surg* 10:81, 1951.
11. Braithwaite F. Cleft palate repair. In Gibson T, (ed). *Modern Trends in Plastic Surgery.* London: Butterworths, 1964.
12. Kriens OB. Fundamental anatomic findings for an intravelar veloplasty. *Cleft Palate J.* 7:27, 1970.
13. Cutting CB, Rosenbaum J, Rovati L. The technique of muscle repair in the cleft soft palate. *Operative Tech Plast Reconstr Surg* 2:215, 1995.
14. Sommerlad BC. A technique for palate repair *Plast Reconstr Surg* 112:1542–1548, 2003.
15. Lilja J, Mars M, Elander A, et al. Analysis of dental arch relationships in Swedish unilateral cleft lip and palate subjects: 20-year longitudinal consecutive series treated with delayed hard palate closure *Cleft Palate Craniofac J* 43:5, 606–611, 2006.
16. Malek R, Martinez H, Mousset M-R, Trichet C. Muldisciplinary management of cleft lip and palate in Paris, France. In: Bardach J, Morris HL, eds. *Multidisciplinary Management of Cleft lip and Palate.* Philadelphia: WB Saunders, 1990.
17. Langenbeck B von. Weitere Erfahrungen im Gebiete der Uranoplastic mittels Ablusung des mucosperriostealen Gaumenüberzuges. *Arch Klin Chir* 5:170, 1861.
18. Langenbeck, B von. Die Uranoplastik mittles Ablosung des microsperiostalen Gaumenüberzuges. *Arch Klin Chir* 2:205, 1862.
19. Veau V, Ruppie C. Anatomie chirurgicale de la division palatine. *J Chir (Paris).* 20:1, 1992.
20. Veau V. *Division Palatine* Paris: Masson & Cie, 1931.
21. Wardill WEM. Technique of operation for cleft lip and palate. *Br J Surg* 25:97, 1937.
22. Kilner TP. Cleft lip and palate repair technique. In: Maingot R, (ed). *Postgraduate Surgery. Vol 3.* London: Medical Publishers, 1937.
23. Bardach J, Salyer KE. Cleft palate repair. In: Bardach J, Salyer KE, (eds). *Surgical Techniques in Cleft Lip and Palate.* St Louis, MO: Mosby. 1991, pp. 224–273.
24. Witzel MA, Clarke JA, Lindsay WK, et al. Comparison of results of pushback or von Langenbeck repair of isolated cleft of the hard and soft palate. *Plast Reconstr Surg* 64:347, 1979.

25. Sommerlad BC. The use of the operating microscope in cleft palate repair and pharyngoplasty. *Plast Reconstr Surgery* 112:1540–1541, 2003.

26. Sommerlad BC, Mehendale FV. A modified gag for cleft palate repair. *Br J of Plast Surg* 53:63–64, 2000.

27. Pichler H. Zur operation der doppelten lippen-gaumenspalten. *Dtsch Z Cir* 195:104, 1926.

28. Gault DT, Brain A, Sommerlad BC, Ferguson DJP. The Loop Mattress Suture *Br. J Surg* 74:820–821, 1987.

29. Sommerlad BC, Fenn C, Harland K, Sell D, et al. Submucous cleft palate—a system of grading and a review of a consecutive series of 40 submucous cleft palate repairs *Cleft Palate Craniofac J* 41:114–123, 2004.

30. Sommerlad BC, Mehendale FV, Birch MJ, et al. Palate re-repair revisited. *Cleft Palate-Craniofac J* 39(3):295–307, 2002.

31. Jigjinni V, Kangesu T, Sommerlad BC. Do babies require arm splints after cleft palate repair? *Br J Plast Surg* 46:681–685, 1993.

32. Marsh JL, Grames LM, Holtman B. Intravelar veloplasty; a prospective study. *Cleft Palate J* 26:46–50, 1989.

33. Mars M, Plint DA, Houston WJB, et al. The GOSLON Yardstick: A new system of assessing dental arch relationships in children with unilateral clefts of the lip and palate. *Cleft Palate J* 24:314–322, 1987.

34. Mars M, Asher-McDade C, Brattstrom V, et al. A six-center international study of treatment outcome in patients with clefts of the lip and palate: Part 3. Dental arch relationships. *Cleft Palate J* 29:405, 1992.

35. Chate R, DiBiase D, Ball J, et al. A comparison of the dental occlusions from a United Kingdom sample of complete unilateral cleft lip and palate patients with those from the Eurocleft Study. *Transactions of the 8th International Congress on Cleft Palate and Related Craniofacial Anomalies*, Singapore, 1997.

36. Andrews PJ, Chorbachi R, Sirimanna T, et al. Evaluation of hearing thresholds in 3-month-old children with cleft palate: The basis for a selective policy for ventilation tube insertion at time of palate repair. *Clin Otolaryngol* 29(1):10–17, 2004.

26

Two-Stage Palate Repair

Hans Friede, DDS

INTRODUCTION

In the early history of cleft palate repair, it took a confident surgeon, Dr. Harold Gillies (later Sir. Harold due to his surgical accomplishments) to suggest that the surgery of a wide palatal cleft should be done in stages.[1] His recommendation was to start with soft palate repair (SPR) to be followed by a much delayed, maybe indefinitely deferred, hard palate repair (HPR). Dr. Gillies admitted his limited experience in cleft palate repair, but he expressed a strong opinion that, particularly in severe cases, *none* of the surgical methods used at that time would lead to a satisfactory result. He felt that most patients would never develop good speech, perfect mastication/occlusion, normal nasal breathing, or proper facial esthetics. Since then, many opinions about the two-stage method have been expressed. Presently, the advocates for the two-stage cleft palate repair generally stress the positive influence on maxillary growth. The adversaries, on the other hand, mainly emphasize the danger of poor speech development, and some maintain that the claimed facial growth advantages might not occur.

MAXILLARY GROWTH AND SPEECH DEVELOPMENT BASICS

Maxillary Growth

Before describing variations in surgical timing and methods for different two-stage protocols, some relevant principles of normal maxillary growth will be briefly considered. It should be noted that, commonly, and so also in this chapter, the maxilla is used as a synonym for the upper jaw, which actually consist of two maxillary and two palatine bones.

During bone growth, certain zones of the maxilla are active (Fig. 26–1). Both sutures, and the periosteal lining, are functioning to achieve the change in size and shape that occurs during maxillary development.[2–4] The midpalatal suture contributes to growth in width, while the transverse palatine suture is important for growth in length of the maxilla. The sutural growth activities are supplemented by periosteal bone apposition, particularly in the sagittal dimension, with bone deposited at the posterior palate and at the tuberosities, making space for the molar teeth. In the vertical dimension, the major increase in maxillary height occurs by bone apposition along the alveolar process, and in connection with the eruption of teeth. In addition, the whole palatal vault is relocated downwards by bone deposition on the oral side of the palate, and bone resorption on the surface facing the nasal cavity. There is also some vertical growth in most sutures bordering the maxilla, however, because of its proximity to the surgical field at cleft palate repair, only the maxillary-vomerine suture will be mentioned here. This suture allows the entire maxilla to be displaced inferiorly, and in the early years, also in an anterior direction.[5,6]

It has been proposed that the composition of the mucosa covering different parts of the palate should be considered at cleft palate surgery.[7] The mucosa inside the dental arch can be separated into three distinctive zones (Fig. 26–2). In the middle portion of the palate, there is thin mucosa covering the palatal shelves. Further laterally, much thicker mucosa is overlaying the maxillary body. Finally, close to the dental arch, a gradually thinning gingival mucosa covers the alveolar process and surrounds the necks of the teeth. Scars occurring in the thin midline mucosa, or in the lateral most zone, adjacent to the teeth, are much less harmful to normal maxillary growth, than scar tissue in the area between these zones[8]. Scars in this middle region seem to distort dentoalveolar growth in particular (Fig. 26–2).

Speech Development

At around 4–5 months of age, typical development of prespeech starts with combinations of vowels and consonant-like sounds, which develop into canonical babbling at around six months.[9] Canonical babbling, in typically developed infants, consists of rapid transitions between vowels and predominantly anteriorly produced consonants (dental/alveolar and labial placement). A prerequisite for making these sounds is the baby's proficiency to achieve velopharyngeal closure. This is in contrast to infants with unoperated cleft palates

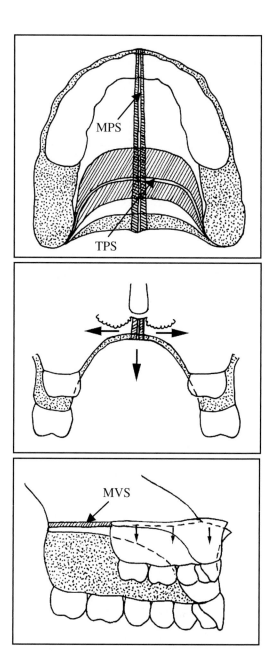

Figure 26–1. Schematic drawing of maxillary bone growth in three dimensions. Hatched lines indicate sutural growth while punctate areas designate appositional growth. Note the pronounced bone deposition at the posterior maxilla and particularly at the alveolar process. MPS = Midpalatal suture; TPS = Transverse palatine suture; MVS = Maxillary-vomerine suture.

who, at sound production, lack the ability to separate the oral cavity from the nasal cavity. Such children will instead develop a predominance of posteriorly articulated consonant sounds. These seem to more often be glottally placed if the whole palate is unoperated; whereas, an oral, but posterior, velar placement is more common in babies after early velar closure.[10,11] It is debated whether the preponderance of posterior sounds at babbling, in children with clefts, carries over to misarticulations in speech. It seems likely, though, in development from babbling/prespeech to normal early speech, the

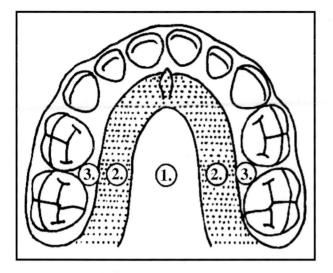

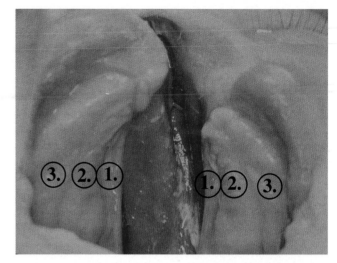

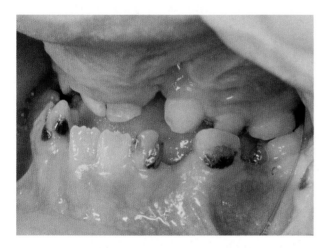

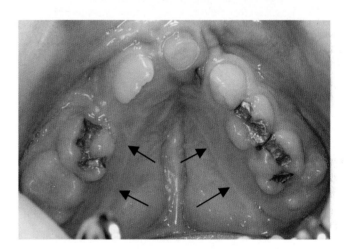

Figure 26–2. Three zones of palatal mucosa which cover: the palatal shelves (=1); the maxillary body (=2); and the alveolar process (=3). Scar tissue (arrows) in the mucosa covering the maxillary body (=2), created at cleft palate surgery, contributed to growth restriction of the upper jaw including its dental arch. The three photographs are from the same patient. *(The schematic figure is redrawn after Markus AF, Smith WP, Delaire J. Primary closure of cleft palate: A functional approach. Br J Oral Maxillofac Surg 31:71, 1993.)*

manner of articulation of certain anterior consonants (plosives) necessitates a competent velopharyngeal mechanism. In addition, an intact palate, allowing the build-up of necessary intraoral pressure is required (Fig. 26–3A). If any of these features are missing in a patient with a palatal cleft, there is risk for the development of compensatory articulations of the anterior pressure consonants. With velopharyngeal incompetence (VPI), these sounds (plosives and fricatives), normally produced in the dento-alveolar area, will be compensatorily articulated in the pharyngeal and/or glottal tract (Fig. 26–3B). On the other hand, some patients with velopharyngeal competence (VPC), but with a residual cleft or fistula in the palate, will retract their articulation of plosives. They will move those normally articulated in front of the palatal opening or fistula, to a place behind the opening in the palate (retracted oral articulation) (Fig. 26–3C).[12] Other patients, though, will keep the place of their articulation anterior to the palatal defect, and plosives will be produced with deviances such as weakness

or nasal leakage. It is not clear which patients will retract their articulation and which will not.

VARIATIONS IN SURGICAL TIMING AND METHODS

The controversies over the benefits of the two-stage palate repair method are caused by the many variations of surgical protocol, regarding both the particular techniques used and their timing. In the literature, the recommended age for SPR has varied from 3-24 months, and similar data for HPR has ranged from 6 months to more than 16 years. These age recommendations are, as a rule, reflections of the personal experience of the individual surgeon, and without any scientific evaluation of their relevance. Specific age concerns regarding early SPR can be related both to intraoperative technical difficulties and other matters, such as breathing problems and

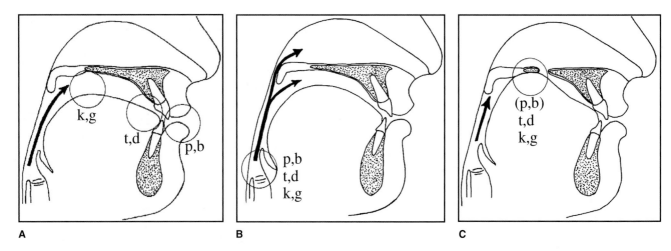

Figure 26–3. Illustration of place of articulation of plosive consonants. (A) Normal articulation with placements for the different sounds indicated with circles. (B) Compensatory glottal articulation due to VPI. (C) Retracted oral articulation of t and d sounds and sometimes also of p and b sounds. These speech deficits are caused by a residual cleft or fistula of the hard palate. (*Redrawn after Lohmander-Agerskov A. Speech outcome after cleft palate surgery with the Göteborg regimen including delayed hard palate closure. Scand J Plast Surg Hand Surg 32:63, 1998.*)

bleeding during the postoperative period. For HPR, the variation in timing has been caused by similar personal opinions, often reflecting the preferences of the most influential members of the cleft team, whether to promote speech development or maxillary growth and facial esthetics. Unfortunately, when evaluating outcomes of the repair, the timing of the palatal procedures has seldom been viewed in relation to the surgical details of the methods used. By concentrating mainly on the timing factor to describe the two-stage protocol, much confusion about the results of the method has been created.

During the evolution of surgical methods for SPR (Fig. 26–4), some specific points have proven very important for a good result. Though Gillies and Fry,[1] in their introductory two-stage technique, separated part of velum from the hard palate to improve subsequent velopharyngeal closure, this surgical component was not included in the concept a few decades later, when some surgeons published renewed interest in the method.[13,14] However, soon it became obvious that separation of the velar mucosa and muscles, from the posterior hard palate, was necessary to obtain a long soft palate after repair.[15] The velar muscles were dissected from their abnormal attachment to the posterior palatine bones. After muscle reorientation, from a sagittal to transverse direction, the repaired velum is brought closer to the pharyngeal wall, enhancing the possibilities for adequate velopharyngeal function.

When the covering oral mucosa was to be separated at the border region between soft and hard palate, surgeons differed in their interpretations of where to make the ideal dissection (Fig. 26–4). Some raised the flaps at the border area,[16] while others dissected the palatal mucosa[15] or most often the whole mucoperiosteum[17] further anteriorly. By extending the flaps forward, particularly medially, the size of the residual; hard palatal cleft became smaller.[18] From the point of view of interim speech development before HPR, this was

a desirable goal. However, the downside was increased risk for maxillary growth impairment, particularly when bone, in growth sensitive palatal areas such as the transverse palatine suture, was left denuded (Fig. 26–5). Thus, the surgeon had to strike a reasonable compromise between the two goals to obtain the best overall outcome for the patient.

To obtain a stable repair of the velum, the nasal mucosa must be sutured in the midline, and particularly at the anterior margin of the soft palate, this might cause tension, and furthermore, shortening of the repaired velum. Therefore, to facilitate the midline closure, the medial parts of the nasal mucosa have to be separated from the posterior palatal shelves. Some surgeons have included a vomer flap in the repair of the anterior nasal mucosa layer of the velum.[15,18,19] This flap is raised from the posterior vomer and then rotated 180° to fit between the two anterior edges of the nasal mucosa (Figs. 26–4B, E, and F). By anchoring the anterior part of the sutured velum to the lower nasal septum, the soft palate is elevated to the level of the palatal shelves, which further helps reduce the size of the residual cleft in the hard palate.

At the HPR, different methods have been devised, in part related to the size of the residual cleft, but also to the age of the patient, and the surgeon's personal preference. In patients with minor residual clefts of the hard palate, some surgeons have reported successful two-layer closures without extensive mucoperiosteal undermining or lateral relaxing incisions on the oral side. Others have advocated small, uni- or bilateral mucoperiosteal flaps from the palate for the oral repair, after closure of the nasal mucosa[15] (Fig. 26–6). The mucoperiosteal flaps were shifted medially to cover the residual cleft, and only a relatively small area of palatal bone, near the cleft, was left denuded for secondary healing. Another method for closure of the residual cleft has included the use of a turn-over vomer flap with its raw surface facing orally.[20] By utilizing a single-layered flap, no new bone will form that

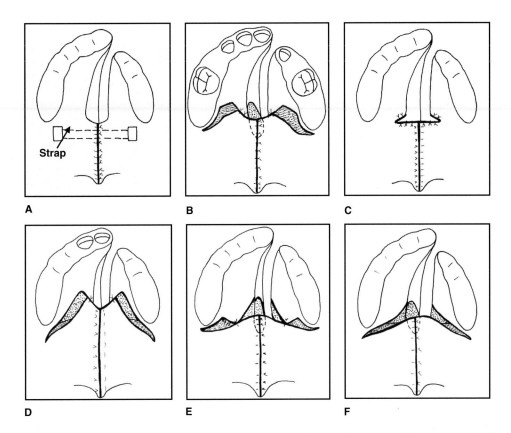

Figure 26–4. (A–F) Schematic illustration of six different methods for SPR Subperiosteal dissections are indicated as punctate areas while supraperiosteal/mucosal dissections are shown with zigzag lines. (*Redrawn from the literature of: (A) Schweckendiek W. Primary veloplasty: Long-term results without maxillary deformity. A twenty-five year report. Cleft Palate J 15:268, 1978; (B) Perko MA. Two-stage closure of cleft palate. J Maxillofac Surg 7:76, 1979; (C) Tanino R, Akamatsu T, Osada M. The influence of different types of hard palate closure in two-stage palatoplasty upon palatal growth: Dental cast analysis. Keio J Med 46:27, 1997; (D) Chait L, Gavron G, Graham C, et al .Modifying the two-stage cleft palate surgical correction. Cleft Palate Craniofac J 39:226, 2002; (E) Lilja J, Friede H, Johanson B, et al. Changing philosophy of surgery of the cleft lip and palate in Göteborg, Sweden. In Berkowitz S (ed.). Cleft Lip and Palate; Perspectives in Management, Vol. II. San Diego, Singular Publishing Group, 1996, p. 15; (F) Malek R, Martinez H, Mousset MR, et al. Multidisciplinary management of cleft lip and palate in Paris, France. In Bardach J, Morris HL (eds). Multidisciplinary Management of Cleft Lip and Palate. Philadelphia, Saunders, 1990, p. 1.*)

might secondarily block growth occurring at the maxillary-vomerine suture. However, the method carries an increased risk for postoperative fistula development. As a way to reduce the risk of postoperative fistula, it has been suggested to add a periosteal graft from the tibia,[19] or a full thickness skin graft as the oral layer.[16] It has not been reported whether the use of periosteum, together with the vomer flap, would adversely affect maxillary growth. When attempting to close wider residual clefts of the hard palate, some surgeons have employed more extensive mucoperiosteal flaps, dissected according to Veau, von Langenbeck or Wardill.[16] These methods generally result in greater areas of palatal scar tissue, and increase the risk for maxillary growth restriction in length at the transverse palatine suture. As well, this potential growth restriction might also cause distortion of dentoalveolar growth.[3]

In the early development of the two-stage palatal repair, the HPR was delayed until most of the maxillary growth had occurred, and therefore, the choice of surgical method was less important from growth point of view. In protocols were the HPR was performed together with alveolar bone grafting,

during mixed dentition, the soft tissue surgery, especially in the anterior palate, was crucial for survival of the graft. In this variant of the two-stage method, the entire palatal mucoperiosteum within the dental arch was raised to facilitate repair of the nasal mucosa.[18] After the palatal flaps were joined in the midline, they were redraped on the maxilla, leaving no or only minimal areas of uncovered palatal bone close to the teeth.

OUTCOME ANALYSES

Historical Background

In the evaluation of treatment protocols for cleft lip and palate, outcomes in different areas of habilitation have to be considered together, because, the total outcome will determine how the protocol is rated. Therefore, in this section, the effects of surgery on maxillary growth and speech development will be discussed together.

A, B, C: Case UCLP

D, E, F: Case Incompl.BCLP

G, H, I: Case BCLP

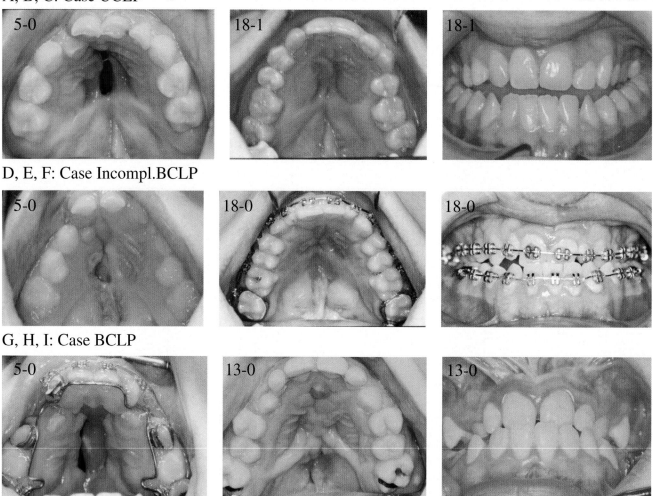

Figure 26–5. (A–I) Intraoral photographs demonstrating unsatisfactory SPR in three patients with different diagnoses: (A–C) UCLP, (D–F) incomplete bilateral cleft lip and palate, and (G–I) bilateral cleft lip and palate. The palatal scars after the velar surgery indicate that dissections were extended too far forward not only medially but also laterally. Sagittal maxillary growth in particular was impeded as seen in the views of occlusion in the right column. Ages are given in years and months.

When the two-stage palatal surgery with delayed HPR was reintroduced in the 1950s, improvement of maxillary growth was stressed. Not only occlusion was thought to improve, but also the residual cleft in the hard palate was expected to narrow considerably during the development after SPR. However, speech results were only described in general terms, and there were insufficient speech outcomes to make comparisons between the protocols. Therefore, it was not until the 1980s that increasing emphasis was placed on the importance of the patient's speech development.

The concern over speech outcomes resulted in several surgeons publishing objections against the two-stage method.[20–22] The criticism had certain specifics. First, after SPR, the residual cleft in the hard palate narrowed, but did not develop functional closure as often as expected. A substantial number of palatal obturators were therefore needed. Secondly, when the repaired velum was functioning at speech,

frequently it was too short to obtain solid contact with the pharyngeal wall, resulting in VPI. A potential explanation maybe, these early surgeons performed insufficient dissections to separate the anterior velum from the posterior hard palate. Neither did they include any posterior vomer flap in the repair of the nasal layer of the anterior soft palate. With such closure, the sutured velum was pulled forward at surgery, causing later VPI, which necessitated pharyngeal flaps in many patients. Thirdly, residual clefts in the hard palate, both narrow and wide, were not as simple to close as expected. In a narrow residual cleft, it was said to be technically difficult to reach and repair the nasal layer. A wide cleft was, in some ways, easier to repair. However, scar tissue in the anterior velum from the primary surgery increased the risk for postoperative fistulae, especially if simple closure was attempted. A forth argument against the two-stage palatal repair protocol was that the occlusion did not improve as much as was hoped for.

Case 1

Case 2

Case 3

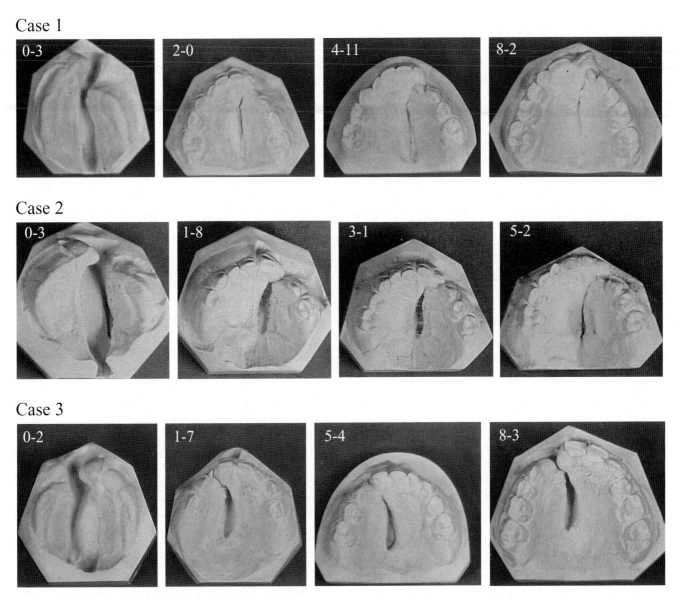

Figure 26–8. Composite of maxillary casts from three UCLP patients. The ages when the casts were obtained are given in years and months. Note the different patterns of narrowing of the residual cleft of the hard palate.

HPR, almost all children demonstrated VPC. Less than 10% of the patients needed velopharyngeal flap surgery, and none used glottal compensatory articulations during preschool age. Interestingly, the incidence of hypernasality was rather high among the children at ages 3 and 5 years, but was markedly reduced at age 7, which actually was before HPR. Presumably, this was caused by the gradual reduction in size of the remaining cleft of the hard palate during the time period. The major speech disadvantage, found in the Göteborg patients, was the development of retracted oral articulations of the anterior pressure consonants, due to the residual cleft of the hard palate. Even if regarded as serious, these compensatory speech sounds are considered less detrimental for intelligibility than glottal or pharyngeal substitutions. Like hypernasality, the incidence of the retracted oral articulations decreased with age, from occurrence in every second patient

at age 3 years, to about every third at ages 5 and 7. Follow-up, at 1–2 years after HPR, showed the existence of the orally retracted speech substitutions in only about every tenth patient, and at age 16, these speech compensations had generally disappeared.

The size and effect of a residual cleft of the hard palate has been the subject of several studies by the Göteborg team. Follow-up of UCLP study casts indicated variation in development of the residual hard palate cleft after SPR (Fig. 26–8). Most often the greatest reduction in width of the hard palatal cleft occurred during the first year after SPR.[38] Then, generally the cleft width was stable for the majority of children. However, in a few patients, narrowing continued, while in a few others, the remaining cleft actually increased in width. In about one-fifth of the patients, the residual cleft narrowed to such an extent that it became functionally closed before

HPR. Another investigation compared speech development of these patients to those who showed an open residual cleft before HPR, and the most important difference was in the prevalence of retracted oral articulations.[39] Children who ended up with functionally closed residual clefts displayed speech *without* retracted oral articulations. As the functional hard palate closure predominantly occurred during the 18–36 months age interval, it was decided, in 1996, to perform HPR in all children with cleft lip and palate (CLP) at age 3 years. Unfortunately, this change in timing of HPR, from age 8–9 years down to age 3, did not result in the expected speech improvement.[40] Presumably, the articulation errors might have been developed and established long before age 3 years, possibly already during the babbling stage. Luckily, however, these patients with earlier HPR did not show any different maxillary growth than the children with later repair, at least as studied up to 10 years of age.[41]

As a final comment regarding the Göteborg experience with the two-stage protocol, it should be pointed out that unfortunately, no external assessor has made a comprehensive evaluation of the results from this center similar to what was done in Marburg and Zürich. However, examiners from other Scandinavian teams have been used in some of the published studies from the Göteborg center.

Three Center Summary

The long-term outcome for patients with UCLP from the three selected centers can be *summarized* as follows. Both excellent growth and more or less normal speech can be accomplished. All three centers have published reports revealing very satisfactory maxillofacial development of their patients, actually much better than demonstrated by proponents of more "conventional" protocols. The weak point, of the two-stage protocol, is speech development before HPR. The technique for SPR, advocated by Schweckendiek, and his preference to wait until puberty before HPR, cannot be considered acceptable today. The SPR method used in Zürich and Göteborg is very similar, and gives a predictably long and mobile soft palate. Despite the difference in timing of SPR (18 months in Zürich and 6–8 months in Göteborg), and use of early maxillary orthopedics to support development (birth to 18 months versus presently none), the long-term outcome is by and large similar. Velopharyngeal function has improved to such an extent that the severe speech errors such as glottal stops have essentially been eliminated. Furthermore, pharyngeal flaps are more rare than after "conventional" protocols. The remaining problem is how to avoid development of retracted oral articulations by closing the residual cleft as early as possible. Timing and method for HPR have to be considered together. An early HPR, possibly at 12–18 months of age is desirable; however, the surgeon has to be very careful to use a method that does not violate sensitive palatal growth zones. The narrower the residual cleft, the easier it can be closed by means of flaps raised close to the midline. A turnover vomer flap, possibly extending slightly into the palatal mucosa of the non-cleft side, seems logical to use for such

surgery. However, there is the reported risk for postoperative fistula development. Whether this can be avoided by utilizing more experienced surgeons or by making a two-layer closure (e.g., adding a layer of periosteum or skin graft to cover the vomer flap) has not been sufficiently studied in a large group of patients. Neither do we know if a double layer repair using periosteum would affect the descent of the maxilla during growth. If the remaining cleft is very wide, it seems appropriate to postpone closure at least up to the age of full deciduous dentition. Then flaps of the whole palatal mucoperiosteum, within the dental arch, might be dissected and used, similar to when HPR is performed together with the alveolar bone grafting procedure. Hopefully, the Scandcleft project for UCLP patients, a multicenter randomized clinical trial performed by Scandinavian teams,[42] will provide improved scientific guidance on how to achieve both favorable speech development, and satisfactory maxillary/facial growth, with a two-stage protocol for palatal repair.

OUTCOME RELATED TO OTHER PATIENT FACTORS

Racial Background

A few studies have reported data after using the two-stage palatal closure in cleft patients not being of Caucasian origin. Noordhoff et al.,[43] from a cleft center in Taiwan, reported dissatisfaction with a two-stage surgical protocol, following the protocol of Perko[15] from the successful Zürich cleft center. The reason for discontinuation of the protocol in Taiwan, after use in over 400 patients, was poor speech development. The patients with delayed HPR showed high incidence of articulation deficits, particularly in the form of substitutions. The size of the residual cleft was measured and used in analyses, but no actual size figures were reported. However, some of the data were split into subgroups of patients with a "fistula size" of more than or less than 50 mm^2. These figures make one suspect that the residual clefts of the Taiwan patients were much larger than found in Göteborg, where a median value of about 12 mm^2 was reported for a group of 5-year-old UCLP children.[44] The reason for the wide residual cleft might be both racial difference, and variation in the execution of the SPR method. In the Perko reference[15] referred to for the Taiwan study, nothing is mentioned about inclusion of a posterior vomer flap at velar closure. In Göteborg experience, this is a crucial step to reduce the size of the residual cleft of hard palate. A preliminary roentgencephalometric study of midfacial growth in 7-year-old Taiwanese UCLP patients have also been published.[45] At that stage, the intermaxillary relation and skeletal profile was more favorable after treatment with delayed closure of the hard palate, than after early repair. However, the difference was only statistically significant for the males. No long-term study of maxillary growth after the two-stage protocol seems to have been reported from this Taiwanese center.

The theory that Asians, with brachycephalic head shapes and wider faces, as well as dental arches, also would have wider residual clefts, was supported by a Japanese study.[46] Similar hard palate cleft sizes were reported, as mentioned in the Taiwanese investigation above. In only 5% of the UCLP patients the remaining hard palate cleft narrowed to functional closure, which is a much lower figure than reported for Caucasians, around 20% in Göteborg.[38] The two-stage protocol reported in the Japanese study was similar to that used in Zürich, and the growth results were similarly excellent, at least as studied in 10–13 years old UCLP subjects.[47,48] Regarding speech development, VPC was satisfactory in 90% of the patients at age 8 years, two years after HPR.[49] Normal articulation was achieved in about three-fourth of the patients at age 8, but intensive speech therapy was necessary in two-thirds of them to get such a result.

The two-stage protocol has also been used and studied in South American subjects. Kontos et al.,[50] reported on Brazilian patients with UCLP after SPR performed by a surgeon from Göteborg. The technique used was the same as in Göteborg, and the maxillary growth results were compared to those from the Swedish center. It was found that the deciduous occlusion was similarly satisfactory in both groups. However, the average maxilla was wider in the Brazilian children than in the Swedish sample, and so was the residual cleft of the hard palate. How this difference in size of the remaining hard palate cleft carried over regarding speech development in the two samples has not been studied.

Another Brazilian cleft center, in Bauru, compared facial development in deciduous/ early mixed dentition in children with UCLP treated either with a two-stage protocol or with complete palatal repair.[51] No growth advantage was found after delaying HPR to age 1.5 years. Nothing has been reported about the size of the residual hard palate cleft or how speech developed in the two groups.

To summarize the influence of racial background, it seems that the two-stage protocol can be successfully used in different racial populations. However, in many patients the residual cleft appears to narrow less than found in Caucasian patients. To enhance speech development, this might necessitate earlier HPR in spite of the risks of growth restrictions due to repair of the wide residual cleft. An alternative would be to delay HPR, allowing for more palatal growth before surgery, and give most patients extensive speech therapy postoperatively.[49]

TWO–STAGE PALATE REPAIR IN OTHER CLEFT TYPES

Bilateral Cleft Lip and Palate

Most studies regarding the two-stage protocol have dealt with UCLP clefts. Likely reasons for such a preference may include the greater incidence of UCLP than Bilateral Cleft Lip and Palate (BCLP), and possibly the fact that UCLP patients are at greater risk for unfavorable growth than patients with cleft palate only. A few teams though have reported their expe-

rience with two-stage palatal repair in BCLP. Of course, the surgical details differ somewhat from what is applied in UCLP. However, also in the bilateral cleft type, the vomer mucosa can be used to attach the repaired velum to the nasal septum for better reduction in size of the residual cleft in the hard palate as reported by the Zürich cleft team.[26] In that study, speech data for 10-year-old children with BCLP was reported. No patient required pharyngeal flap surgery, and velopharyngeal function was judged competent or marginal in more than 90% of the subjects. After HPR, about half of the patients received speech therapy, supposedly aiming to eliminate compensatory articulations. About 90% of the children met normal standards for speech at the start of school around 7 years. With respect to facial growth, a study from the Zürich center addressing the skeletal profile in 15–20-year-old patients with BCLP,[52] reports that none of the 17 consecutively studied subjects needed any maxillary osteotomy. In fact, the facial convexity was very close to non-cleft control values. Good growth outcome after treatment of BCLP, with the Zürich protocol, has also been reported from the previously mentioned Japanese center.[53]

Patients with BCLP have been followed up to adolescence and adulthood by the Göteborg team. A rather small group ($n = 16$), treated according to the two-stage protocol, was evaluated for maxillary growth, and compared to a similar group of patients having undergone more traditional palatal surgery.[54] As with the UCLP patients, the two-stage BCLP patients demonstrated superior maxillary growth and occlusion. Due to the great variation between patients, and the relatively small numbers of subjects studied, statistical significance could only be obtained for children in the early stages of treatment. As with the growth evaluations, speech outcome after the two-stage protocol in Göteborg patients with BCLP has been studied less than in subjects with UCLP. Glottal and retracted oral articulations, as well as reduced intelligibility, were slightly more common in BCLP than in UCLP. However, in general the speech results showed clear resemblance between the two cleft types.[12]

Isolated Cleft Palate

Treatment results in subjects with isolated Cleft Palate (CP), involving both the hard and soft palate, and repaired according to the two-stage protocol, have been reported in a few publications. It should be remembered that in this cleft type, the remaining cleft in the hard palate does not spontaneously narrow as well as in UCLP.[38] Therefore, HPR is usually performed prior to, or at, complete eruption of the deciduous dentition. Before commenting on speech outcomes in CP patients treated with the two-stage protocol, it should be remembered that this cleft group generally has worse speech outcomes than patients with CLP. One reason might be that any cohort of CP patients is likely to include cases of syndromic children, and those with additional malformations in addition to the CP. In a doctoral thesis from Uppsala, Sweden, speech outcomes for CP patients treated with the two-stage protocol were investigated.[55] An early group of patients with CP

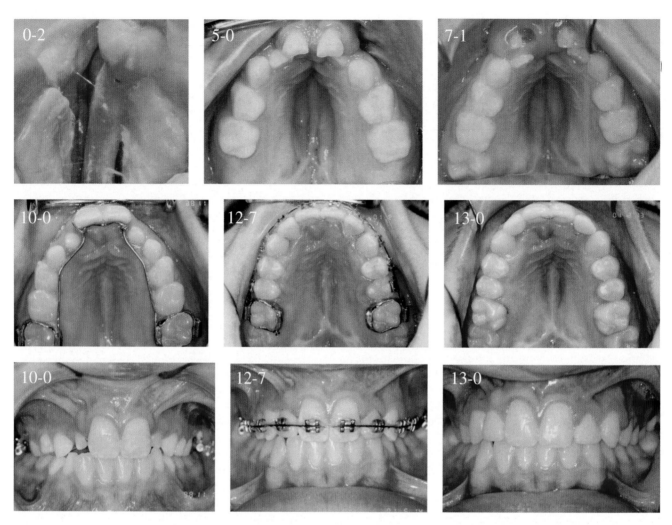

Figure 26–9. Composite of intraoral views of a patient born with BCLP and treated according to the two-stage protocol in Göteborg, Sweden. The photographs were obtained at various ages (shown in years and months). Scars from surgery only in the posterior palate and therefore, maxillary development was very good resulting in normal occlusion at puberty.

had been treated with a one stage pushback repair at around 1.5–2 years of age. Speech data for these children was mostly retrieved from hospital charts. A later cohort of CP patients, treated with the two-stage protocol, had better speech samples. However, the ages for the two surgical procedures were gradually changed; for SPR from 18 to 6 months of age, and for HPR from 6 to 2 years. It was reported that the one-stage repair group generally demonstrated better speech results at about 6–7 years of age. This was true except for "articulation faults," where no difference was found between the two surgical methods. However, these findings have to be carefully interpreted, particularly due to the shortcomings in data collection, and variation in age at the time of surgical repair in the two-stage group. Maxillary growth data, obtained at around age 8 years, demonstrated no major difference between the groups, except for some measurements of dental arch width. In the two-stage group, the transverse distance at the level of the second deciduous molar was significantly greater than after the one-stage pushback surgery.

At our cleft center in Göteborg, a one-stage protocol for patients with CP was advocated until the late 1980s, when the two-stage palatal repair protocol was introduced. With the two-stage protocol, the timing and method for SPR remained the same as with the one-stage pushback surgery (6–8 months).[56] Closure of the hard palate, was carried out at approximately 4 years of age, and performed with different methods according to size of the residual cleft. For residual hard palate clefts that were small, local mucoperiosteal flaps, raised close to the midline, were employed. In wider clefts, and particularly in complete clefts of the secondary palate, the mucoperiosteal flaps were dissected laterally reaching the dental arch. After both methods of HPR in CP, only relatively minor portions of palatal bone was left denuded following surgery. In addition, as these areas were reepithelialized from the edges of the thin palatal mucosa in areas 1 or 3 (Fig. 26–2), formation of growth impeding scar tissue was minimal. This was in great contrast to what occurred after the earlier pushback closure, where much scar tissue developed after

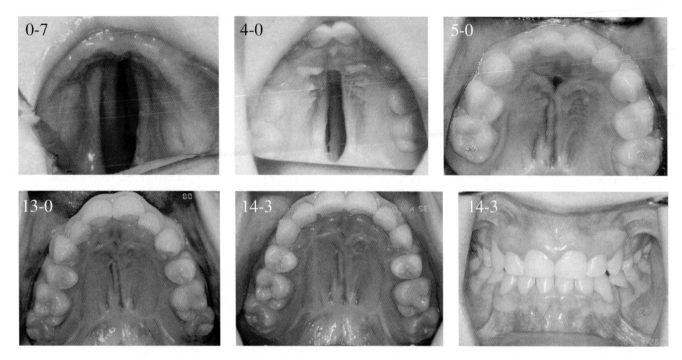

Figure 26–10. Composite of intraoral photographs of a patient with complete cleft of the secondary palate treated according to the two-stage method as employed in Göteborg, Sweden. The soft palate was repaired at age 7 months and the hard palate at 4 years. Note the satisfactory growth of the maxillary dental arch. Only minor scar tissue had developed in the palatal mucosa covering the maxillary body. Ages are given in years and months.

denudation of palatal bone in area 2. Here the reepithelialization of the denuded bone occurred from the edges of the thick part of the palatal mucosa. As might be expected, maxillary growth after the one-stage pushback surgery became more restricted across the dental arch than after the two-stage repair.[57] This is in agreement with what was reported from Uppsala.[55] In contrast, however, speech in the Göteborg children definitely improved after introduction of the two-stage protocol.[56] At age 5 years, only about 14% of these patients had moderate to severe VPI. These speech results were much better than those obtained after the pushback surgery, where approximately 40% of the children had VPI before any treatment with pharyngeal flaps. Secondary speech surgery was necessary in 23% of one-stage patients, in contrast to 7% after palatal closure in two stages. None of the patients treated according to the new-staged regime developed any compensatory articulations.

To *summarize* treatment for cleft types other than UCLP, the two-stage protocol seems to result in favorable outcomes also in patients with BCLP and CP. Improved midfacial growth appears especially important for the bilateral clefts, because, both better occlusion (Fig. 26–9) and more normal facial profiles can be achieved in the majority of cases. In the CP only patients, the occlusal improvement after palatal repair in two stages, mostly relates to development of wider dental arches in the deciduous molar/premolar region (Fig. 26–10). With respect to speech development, BCLP patients appear to have near similar satisfactory outcomes, as subjects with UCLP. A high prevalence of VPC can be expected, with minimal need for secondary palatopharyngeal flap surgery.

In a patient born with CP alone, and no other malformations or syndromes, there is also a great chance for speech development with adequate velopharyngeal function and no compensatory articulations.

GENERAL SUMMARY: SUGGESTIONS FOR SURGICAL TIMING AND METHODS

The purpose of this chapter is to map controversies regarding the two-stage palatal surgery protocol, and attempt to understand why reported outcomes have varied. Such knowledge would be helpful when trying to suggest a variant of the protocol, where speech, as well as maxillofacial growth, can develop normally in the same patient.

Great variations in timing, as well as surgical methods, for the two surgical stages have been reported, and this may explain why outcomes after some two-stage protocols have been more successful than others. The following suggestions for palatal repair can be employed in many cleft types, and also be used for patients of all races.

In a small child born with a complete CLP, many teams around the world advocate palatal surgery in two stages of short duration, instead of one long operation. Frequently, the HPR is done first together with the lip closure. However, the sequence of starting with SPR affords the advantage of substantially narrowing the remaining cleft of the hard palate. This reduction in hard palate defect severity following initial SPR is analogous to lip adhesion, and is more beneficial for subsequent maxillary growth than if HPR was performed as a first stage.[7] Furthermore, initial velar closure will result in a long soft palate, if its muscles are dissected from the posterior palatal shelves and reoriented to a transverse course. In addition, the inclusion of a posterior vomer flap to help repair the anterior nasal layer of the velum is another important step in the creation of a long soft palate. It is also valuable to use a pushback procedure at the closure of the oral layer with only minor denudation of palatal bone. The favorable reconstruction of the soft palate will result in early VPC, reducing the risk for the development of compensatory glottal/pharyngeal articulation of pressure consonants. To avoid development of other compensatory speech patterns (e.g., retracted oral articulations) the residual cleft in the hard palate must narrow as much as possible. To increase this likelihood, use of the posterior vomer flap is important, especially in wide clefts, as it anchors the anterior velum to the lower septum. To maximize speech outcomes, repair of the residual hard palatal cleft is performed as early as possible; however, with techniques that introduce the least amount of postoperative growth restriction and are most favorable for maxillary growth. The smaller the cleft, the easier it is to accomplish this goal by use of narrow mucoperioseal flaps, raised from the vomer or from the palatal area close to the cleft. However, for wider clefts, there are methods for HPR that do not leave large areas of denuded bone in growth sensitive areas.

The following timing and methods for two-stage palatal surgery is suggested for closure of an average case of UCLP:

1. At age 4–5 months of age, SPR (possibly together with lip adhesion or final lip closure) with the inclusion of a posterior vomer flap.
2. At age 1–1.5 years of age, HPR with the use of a vomer flap or narrow mucoperiosteal flaps raised from the hard palate close to the cleft. In wide clefts, the repair might be postponed until around 3 years of age. Flaps of the entire palatal mucosa may then be dissected, connected in the midline, and redraped on the palate with none or only minor areas of bone left denuded.

These suggestions are based on our extensive experience and retrospective outcome studies published in the literature. In addition, we await future data and outcomes of the prospective clinical Scandcleft trial.[42]

References

1. Gillies HD, Fry WK. A new principle in the surgical treatment of "congenital cleft-palate," and its mechanical counterpart. *Br Med J* 1:335, 1921.
2. Björk A, Skieller V. Growth of the maxilla in three dimensions as revealed radiographically by the implant method. *Br J Orthod* 4:53, 1977.
3. Ross RB, Johnston MC. *Cleft Lip and Palate.* New York: Krieger, 1978.
4. Enlow DH, Hans MG. *Essentials of Facial Growth.* Philadelphia: Saunders, 1996.
5. Friede H. The vomero-premaxillary suture- a neglected growth site in mid-facial development of unilateral cleft lip and palate patients. *Cleft Palate J* 15:398, 1978.
6. Delaire J, Precious D. Avoidance of the use of vomerine mucosa in primary surgical management of velopalatine clefts. *Oral Surg Oral Med Oral Pathol* 60:589, 1985.

7. Markus AF, Smith WP, Delaire J. Primary closure of cleft palate: A functional approach. *Br J Oral Maxillofac Surg* 31:71, 1993.
8. Ishikawa H, Nakamura S, Misaki K, et al. Scar tissue distribution on palates and its relation to maxillary dental arch form. *Cleft Palate Craniofac J* 35:313, 1998.
9. Oller DK. The emergence of the sounds of speech in infancy. In Yeni-Komshian G, Kavanaugh J, Ferguson CA (eds). *Child Phonology. Vol 1.* New York, Academic Press, 1980, p. 96.
10. Lohmander-Agerskov A, Söderpalm E, Friede H, et al. A comparison of babbling and speech at pre-speech level, 3, and 5 years of age in children with cleft lip and palate treated with delayed hard palate closure. *Folia Phoniatr Logop* 50:320, 1998.
11. Willadsen E, Albrechtsen H. Phonethic description of babbling in Danish toddlers born with and without unilateral cleft lip and palate. *Cleft Palate Craniofacial J* 43:189, 2006.
12. Lohmander-Agerskov A. Speech outcome after cleft palate surgery with the Göteborg regimen including delayed hard palate closure. *Scand J Plast Surg Hand Surg* 32:63, 1998.
13. Schweckendiek H. Zur zweiphasigen Gaumenspaltenoperation bei primärem Velumversluss. *Fortschr Kiefer Gesichtschir* 1:73, 1955.
14. Schweckendiek W. Primary veloplasty: Long-term results without maxillary deformity. A twenty-five year report. *Cleft Palate J* 15:268, 1978.
15. Perko MA. Two-stage closure of cleft palate. *J Maxillofac Surg* 7:76, 1979.
16. Tanino R, Akamatsu T, Osada M. The influence of different types of hard palate closure in two-stage palatoplasty upon palatal growth: Dental cast analysis. *Keio J Med* 46:27, 1997.
17. Chait L, Gavron G, Graham C, et al. Modifying the two-stage cleft palate surgical correction. *Cleft Palate Craniofac J* 39:226, 2002.
18. Lilja J, Friede H, Johanson B. Changing philosophy of surgery of the cleft lip and palate in Göteborg, Sweden. In Berkowitz S (ed). *Cleft Lip and Palate; Perspectives in Management, Vol. II.* San Diego, Singular Publishing Group, 1996, p. 155.
19. Malek R, Martinez H, Mousset MR, et al. Multidisciplinary management of cleft lip and palate in Paris, France. In Bardach J, Morris HL (eds). *Multidisciplinary Management of Cleft Lip and Palate.* Philadelphia, Saunders, 1990, p. 1.
20. Cosman B, Falk AS. Delayed hard palate repair and speech deficiencies: A cautionary report. *Cleft Palate J* 17:27, 1980.
21. Jackson IT, McLennan G, Scheker LR. Primary veloplasty or primary palatoplasty: Some preliminary findings. *Plast Reconst Surg* 72:153, 1983.
22. Robertson NRE, Jolleys A. A further look at the effects of delaying repair of the hard palate. In Huddart AG, Ferguson MJW (eds). *Cleft Lip and Palate. Long-term results and Future Prospects. Proceedings of the First International Meeting of Craniofacial Society of Great Britain, Vol. 2.* Manchester University Press, England, 1990, p. 176.
23. Bardach J, Morris HL, Olin WH. Late results of primary veloplasty: The Marburg project. *Plast Reconstr Surg* 73:207, 1984.
24. Ross RB. Treatment variables affecting growth in unilateral cleft lip and palate. Part 5: Timing of palate repair. *Cleft Palate J* 24:54, 1987.
25. Hotz M, Gnoinski W. Comprehensive care of cleft lip and palate children at Zürich University: A preliminary report. *Am J Orthod* 70:481, 1976.
26. Hotz M, Gnoinski W, Perko M, et al. The Zürich approach 1964–1984. In Hotz M, Gnoinski W, Perko M, et al. (eds). *Early Treatment of Cleft Lip and Palate.* Toronto, Huber, 1986, p. 42.
27. Gnoinski WM. Infant orthopedics and later orthodontic monitoring for unilateral cleft lip and palate patients in Zurich. In Bardach J, Morris HL (eds). *Multidisciplinary Management of Cleft Lip and Palate.* Philadelphia, Saunders, 1990, p. 578.
28. Gnoinski W. Orofacial development up to age 15 in complete unilateral cleft lip and palate cases treated according to the Zürich concept. In Pfeifer G (ed). *Craniofacial Abnormalities and Clefts of the Lip, Alveolus and Palate (4th Hamburg International Symposium).* Stuttgart, Thieme, 1991, p. 270.

29. Gnoinski WM, Haubensak RR. Facial patterns and long-term growth in patients with complete unilateral cleft lip and palate. In Lee ST (ed). *Transactions 8th International Congress on Cleft Palate and Related Craniofacial Anomalies.* Singapore, Academy of Medicine, 1997, p. 764.

30. Hotz MM, Gnoinski WM, Nussbaumer H, et al. Early maxillary orthopedics in CLP cases: Guidelines for surgery. *Cleft Palate J* 15:405, 1978.

31. Van Demark DR, Gnoinski W, Hotz MM, et al. Speech results of the Zürich approach in the treatment of unilateral cleft lip and palate. *Plast Reconstr Surg* 83:605, 1989.

32. Lohmander A, Lillvik M, Friede H. The impact of early infant jaw-orthopaedics on early speech production in toddlers with unilateral cleft lip and palate. *Clin Linguist Phon* 18:259, 2004.

33. Friede H, Möller M, Lilja J, et al. Facial morphology and occlusion at the stage of early mixed dentition in cleft lip and palate patients treated with delayed closure of the hard palate. *Scand J Plast Reconstr Surg* 21:65, 1987.

34. Friede H, Enemark H. Long-term evidence for favorable midfacial growth after delayed hard palate repair in UCLP patients. *Cleft Palate Craniofac J* 38:323, 2001.

35. Lilja J, Mars M, Elander A, et al. Analysis of dental arch relationships in Swedish unilateral cleft lip and palate subjects: 20-year longitudinal consecutive series treated with delayed hard palate closure. *Cleft Palate Craniofac J* 43:606–611, 2006.

36. Lohmander-Agerskov A, Willadsen E. A comparison of long-term speech results following the delayed hard palate closure concept and a conventional two-stage vomer flap/push back procedure in UCLP patients. Presented at the *Sixth European Craniofacial Congress,* Manchester, England, Abstract, 1999.

37. Lohmander-Agerskov A. *Speech in Children with Cleft Lip and Palate Treated with Delayed Closure of the Hard Palate.* Doctoral Thesis. University of Göteborg, Sweden, 1996.

38. Owman-Moll P, Katsaros C, Friede H. Development of the residual cleft in the hard palate after velar repair in a 2-stage palatal repair regimen. *J Orofac Orthop* 59:286, 1998.

39. Lohmander-Agerskov A, Friede H, Lilja J, et al. Delayed closure of the hard palate: A comparison of speech in children with open and functionally closed residual clefts. *Scand J Plast Reconstr Surg Hand Surg* 30:121, 1996.

40. Lohmander A, Friede H, Elander A, et al. Speech development in patients with unilateral cleft lip and palate treated with different delays in closure of the hard palate after early velar repair: A longitudinal perspective. *Scand J Plast Reconstr Surg Hand Surg* 40:267, 2006.

41. Friede H, Lohmander A, Hagberg C, et al. Maxillary dental arch and occlusion in patients with unilateral cleft lip and palate treated with different delays in closure of the hard palate after early velar repair. *Scand J Plast Reconstr Surg Hand Surg* 40:261, 2006.

42. Rautio J, Semb G, Lohmander A. International randomized control trial of primary surgery. Presented at the *9th International Congress on Cleft Palate and Craniofacial Anomalies,* Göteborg, Sweden, Abstract 758, 2001.

43. Noordhoff MS, Kuo J, Wang F, et al. Development of articulation before delayed hard-palate closure in children with cleft palate: A cross-sectional study. *Plast Reconstr Surg* 80:518, 1987.

44. Lohmander A, Persson C, Owman-Moll P. Unrepaired clefts in the hard palate: Speech deficits at the ages of 5 and 7 years and their relationship to size of the cleft. *Scand J Plast Reconstr Surg Hand Surg* 36:332, 2002.

45. Wang F, Cheng WS, Huang CS, et al. Roentgencephalometric study of complete unilateral cleft lip and palate patients treated with delayed closure of the hard palate a preliminary report. *Ann Acad Med Singapore* 17:394, 1988.

46. Ono K, Ohashi Y, Takagi R, et al. Spontaneous narrowing of residual hard palate cleft after velar closure in two-stage palatoplasty. *J Jpn Cleft Palate Assoc* 21:126, 1996.

47. Ishii K, Arai T, Saito I, et al. Effects of Hotz' plate-based two-stage palatoplasty in unilateral cleft lip and palate. *Orthod Waves* 59:402, 2000.

48. Ono K, Iida A, Imai N, et al. Effects of two-stage palatoplasty combined with Hotz's plate on maxillary growth in unilateral cleft lip and palate. *J Jpn Cleft Palate Assoc* 25:36, 2000.

49. Isono S. Speech results and speech development after two-stage palatoplasty combined with Hotz's plate in cleft lip and palate children. *Niigata Dent J* 28:15, 1998.

50. Kontos K, Friede H, Cintras H, et al. Maxillary development and dental occlusion in patients with unilateral cleft lip and palate after combined velar closure and lip-nose repair at different ages. *Scand J Plast Reconstr Surg Hand Surg* 35:377, 2001.

51. Siva Filho OG, Calvano F, Alcoforado Assuncao AG, et al. Craniofacial morphology in children with complete unilateral cleft lip and palate: A comparison of two surgical protocols. *Angle Orthod* 71:274, 2001.

52. Perko M, Gnoinski W. Skeletal facial profile in 15–20 year old patients with complete BCLP. Presented at *7th International Congress on Cleft Palate and Related Craniofacial Anomalies,* Broadbeach, Australia, Abstract 194, 1993.

53. Silvera QAE, Isii K, Arai T, et al. Long-term results of the two-stage palatoplasty/Hotz' plate approach for complete bilateral cleft lip, alveolus and palate patients. *J Craniomaxillofac Surg* 31:215, 2003.

54. Melissaratou A, Friede H. Dental arches and occlusion in bilateral cleft lip and palate patients after two different routines for palatal surgery. *J Orofac Orthop* 63:300, 2002.

55. Jacobsson OP. Repair of Isolated Cleft Palate. Doctoral Thesis, University of Uppsala, Sweden, 1990.

56. Lilja J, Elander A, Lohmander A, et al. Isolated cleft palate and submucous cleft palate. *Oral Maxillofac Surg Clin North Amer* 12:455, 2000.

57. Friede H, Enocson L, Möller M, et al. Maxillary dental arch and occlusion in repaired clefts of the secondary palate: Influence of surgical closure with minimal denudation of bone. *Scand J Plast Reconstr Surg Hand Surg* 34:213; 2000.

27

Rare Craniofacial Clefts

Fernando O. Monasterio, MD • Jesse A. Taylor, MD

OBJECTIVE

The main objective of this chapter is to define the etiology, classification, and treatment of rare craniofacial clefts. Our series of 490 patients with rare craniofacial clefts is presented, as well as the treatment philosophy and treatment protocol have evolved over 40 years of following these challenging patients.

ETIOLOGY

Craniofacial clefts, other than clefts of the lip and palate, are relatively rare malformations. These fissures may follow the lines of union of the processes responsible for the development of the face early in embryonic life, and thus may be considered primary clefts. Secondary clefts that interrupt the continuity of facial anatomic structures along axes not related to embryonic development develop after the facial processes have already fused. Their pathogenesis is not well understood but is likely the result of a complex, interrelated series of events such as incorrect genetic translation, cell deposition, cell differentiation, cell proliferation, and tissue remodeling. The type and severity of the clefts is also related to the stage of the development when the disruption occurred.[1]

Owing to the rarity of these malformations, it is difficult to establish an epidemiologic profile for facial clefts. Most reports in the literature are based on relatively small number of patients or meta-analyses from various regions. One example is the analysis published by Kawamoto[2] concluding that the incidence of facial clefts varies from 1.43 to 4.84 for 10,000 live births. This is a wide range, and it is difficult to determine its validity.

In our center, we have examined 490 patients with craniofacial clefts among a population of 23,000 clefts of lip and palate from 1968 to 2005, giving us a ratio of 21 per 10,000 patients. This ratio cannot be considered the true relationship between cleft lip and palate and major craniofacial clefts because these patients have been referred to a specialized center, so the numbers do not coincide with the true incidence. We suspect this skewed view may also be present in reports in the literature.

CLASSIFICATION

Attempts to classify craniofacial clefts have a long history in the literature based mainly on clinical and anatomic judgment. Some classification schemes have focused on morphogenesis in an effort to explain the mechanism involved in the formation of clefts. Others, like the Tessier system, focus on surgical anatomy. The term dysmorphia was proposed to cover all clefts or disruptions of development describing the clinical aspect and disregarding morphogenesis. The majority of these systems are inadequate because they rely on soft tissue landmarks. The term dysplasia, or abnormal development, covers all pathogenic and clinical aspects of craniofacial malformations and has been proposed by Van der Meulen et al. with a classification based on morphogenesis.[3] Although these comprehensive classifications explain most craniofacial malformations, it goes beyond the scope of this chapter limited only to facial clefts.

We prefer to use the classification proposed by Tessier[4] based on surgical anatomy and integrating external findings with the underlying skeletal malformation. This classification does not pretend to explain the morphogenesis of facial clefts, but it provides a topographic description that has been widely accepted. It proposes a simplified numeral system from 0 to 14 for all clefts depending on their relationship to the 0 line,

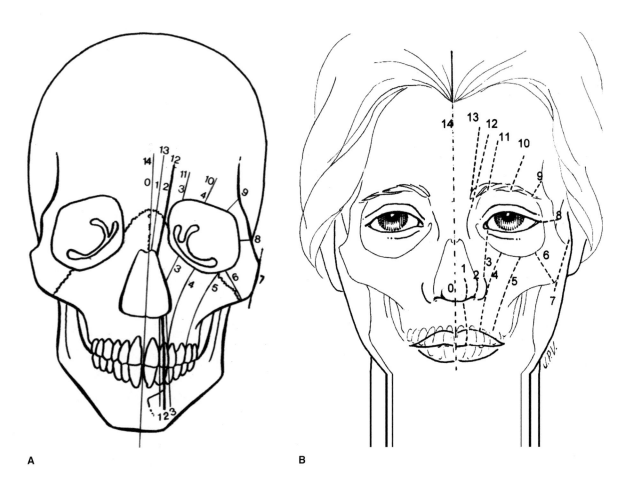

Figure 27–1. (A) Tessier classification of major craniofacial clefts, skeleton. (B) Tessier classification of major craniofacial clefts, soft tissue.

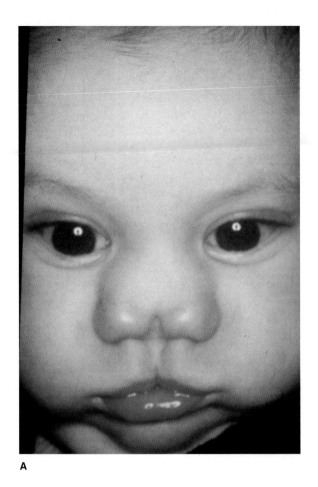

A

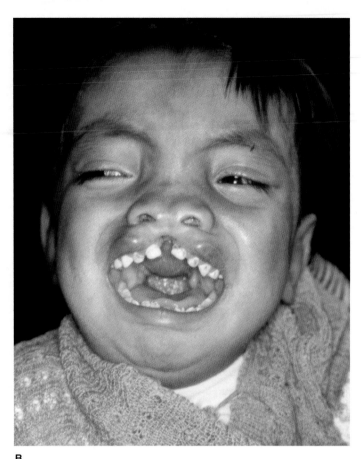

B

Figure 27–2. (A) Tessier cleft number 0 affecting the lip and nose. (B) Tessier cleft number 0–14 with pharyngeal encephalocele extending to the floor of the anterior cranial fossa.

which is a vertical cleft of the midline of the face (Fig. 27–1). The palpebral fissures separate facial from cranial clefts. Some of the cranial clefts follow the same axis as those of the cheek and lip.

Number 0 and 14

Cleft number 0 and 14 are located at the midline of the face that may present a bifid frontal bone with a central encephalocele extending caudally with a bifid nose and a central cleft of the upper lip (Fig. 27–2A). They are accompanied by hypertelorism, and may extend along the cranial base with herniation of the cranial contents (pharyngeal encephalocele), which displaces the orbits laterally (Fig. 27–2B).

Number 1

Cleft number 1 is a paramedian cleft crossing through the olfactory groove of the cribiform plate and extending between the nasal bone and the nasal process of the maxilla. Caudally, it may affect the dome of the alar cartilage and corresponds to the common unilateral cleft of the lip. Patients often present with telecanthus, a vertical furrowing of the nasal ala, and cleft palate (Fig. 27–3A).

Number 2

Cleft number 2 is slightly more lateral, traversing the nasal dome at the lateral crura of the alar cartilage. Cranially, it cuts through the lateral mass of the ethmoid. The lachrymal apparatus is absent and hemiatrophy or aplasia of the heminose is common. It corresponds superiorly to cleft number 12 (Fig. 27–3B).

Number 3

Cleft number 3 is a paranasal cleft crossing through the medial canthus or medial third of the lower lid; the frontal process of the maxilla may be absent. Caudally, it proceeds around the alar base, cutting through the lip and the alveolar ridge exiting the midface lateral to the lateral incisor (Fig. 27–4A).

Number 4

Cleft number 4 cuts through the lower lid lateral to the punctum and medial to the infraorbital nerve. It extends through the orbital floor and the maxilla to the upper lip between the philtrum and the buccal commissure. There is usually

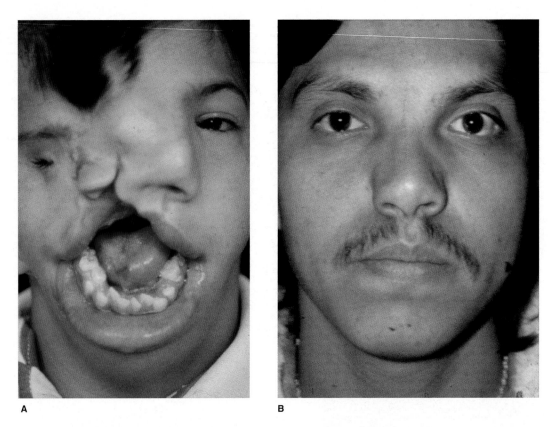

A   B

Figure 27–3. (A) Right Tessier cleft number 1 severely affecting the skeleton and soft tissues of the midface. (B) Right Tessier cleft number 2 affecting alar cartilages and the frontal process of the maxilla.

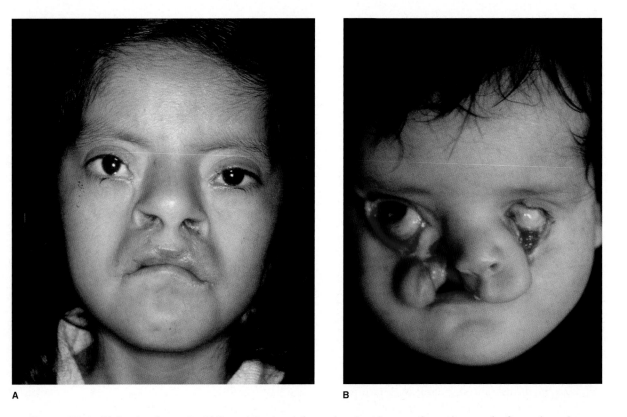

A   B

Figure 27–4. (A) Previously repaired bilateral Tessier cleft number 3 with a scar from closure of a fissure lateral to the nasal ala extending to the medial canthus. (B) Bilateral Tessier cleft number 4 with variable penetration. Fissures extend from lateral lip segment to the medial third of the lower eyelid. Upper eyelid coloboma reveals the presence of a soft tissue Tessier cleft number 10.

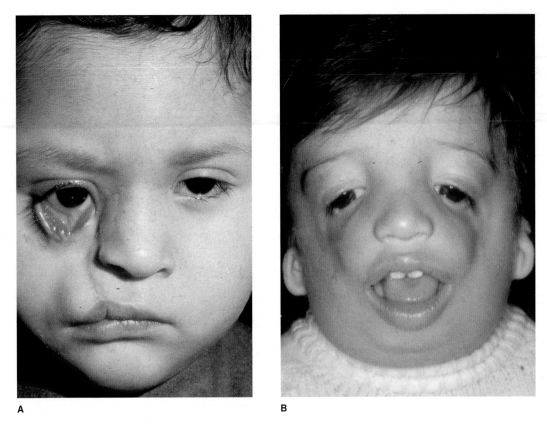

Figure 27–5. (A) Tessier cleft number with a lower lid coloboma and previous lip repair. (B) Tessier skeletal cleft numbers 6, 7, and 8 corresponding to the Treacher Collins syndrome.

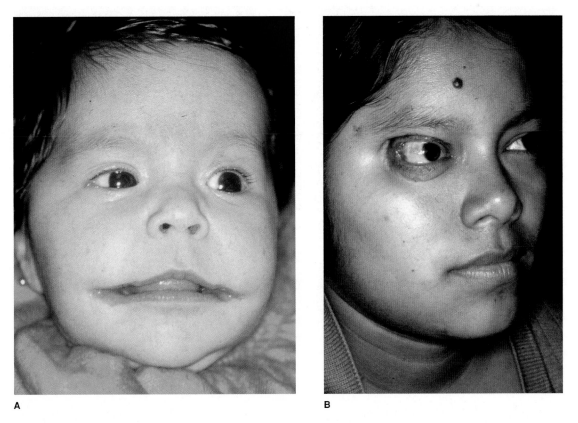

Figure 27–6. (A) Bilateral Tessier cleft number 7 of the soft tissue as denoted by bilateral microstomia. (B) Bilateral Tessier cleft number 8 affecting the lateral canthi.

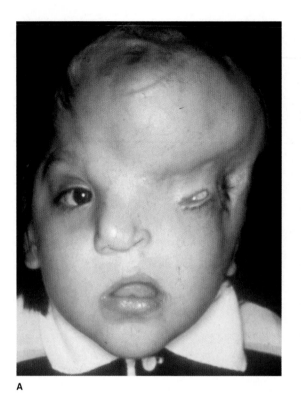
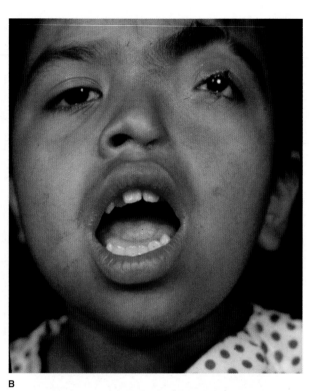

A   **B**

Figure 27–7. (A) Tessier cleft number 9 extending from the superolateral orbit onto the frontal bone with an associated frontal encephalocele. (B) Left Tessier cleft number 10 extending from the orbital roof lateral to the supraorbital nerve, through the eyebrow, and onto the frontal bone. Upper eyelid coloboma is also present, as is left heminasal hypoplasia perhaps representing a mild cleft number 3.

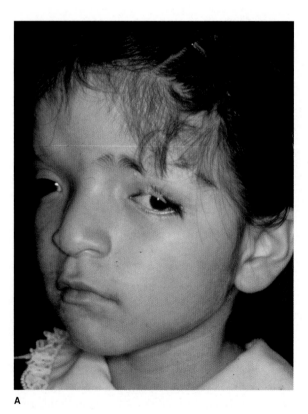
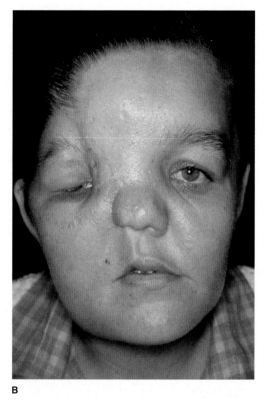

A   **B**

Figure 27–8. (A) Left Tessier cleft number 11 extending from the orbital roof medial to the supraorbital nerve onto the forehead with associated upper eyelid coloboma. (B) Right Tessier cleft number 12 extending from the nasofrontal process onto the forehead with associated upper eyelid coloboma, aplasia of the medial brow, and a mild cleft number 2.

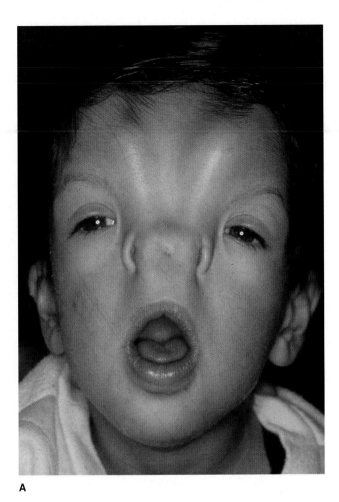

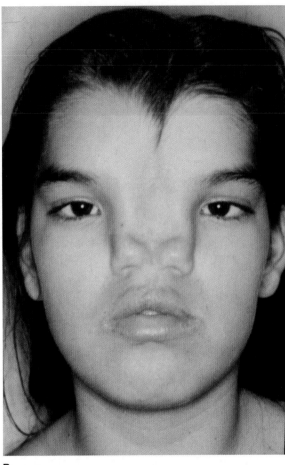

A   **B**

Figure 27–9. (A) Bilateral Tessier cleft number 13 with hypertelorism and a small encephalocele. There is also a cleft number 1 on the right side. (B) Tessier cleft number 14 with grade III hypertelorism. Associated cleft number 0 is also present.

marked shortening of the midface on the affected side, marked dystopia of the affected globe, and a coloboma of the lower lid (Fig. 27–4B).

Number 5

Cleft number 5 divides the lower eyelid at the junction of the middle and the lateral third extending caudally through the orbital rim and the maxilla lateral to the infraorbital nerve to the alveolar ridge behind the canine. On the cheek, it may appear as a ridge extending to the buccal commissure or as fully blown cleft cutting through the soft tissues (Fig. 27–5A).

Numbers 6, 7, and 8

The next three clefts numbers 6, 7, and 8 correspond to the Treacher Collins syndrome that mainly affects the skeleton (Fig. 27–5B). In these three clefts, there is a deficiency or an absence of temporal, zygomatic, frontal, and maxillary bones, which may occur in multiple combinations. Cleft number 6 manifests as a soft tissue cleft extending from the oral com-

missure to the lateral lower eyelid. Skeletally, cleft number 6 affects the zygomaticomaxillary suture, entering the orbital floor at its lateral third. Cleft number 7, which is also found in hemifacial microsomia, may be associated with hypoplasia of the mandibular ramus, the condyle, and the coronoid process. It manifests as a soft tissue cleft extending horizontally from the buccal commissure to involve the ear with corresponding macrostomia. (Fig. 27–6A). The cleft number 8, or frontozygomatic cleft, extends from the lateral canthus to the temporal region presenting as a coloboma of the lateral eyelid (Fig. 27–6B). Occasionally, clefting of the frontozygomatic suture is present.

Number 9

Cleft number 9 extends from the lateral third of the upper eyelid through the superolateral angle of the orbit to the forehead. The bony deficiency may result in abnormal lateral positioning of the globe. Often the frontal branch of the facial nerve is affected. This rare cleft corresponds to cleft number 5 in the face (Fig. 27–7A).

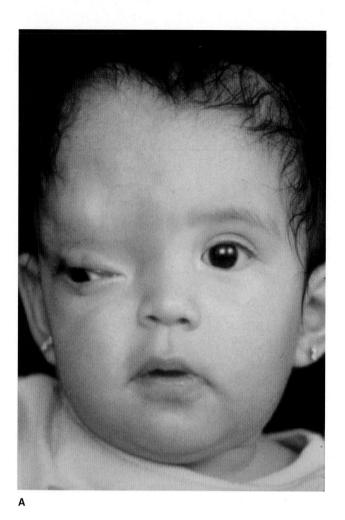

A

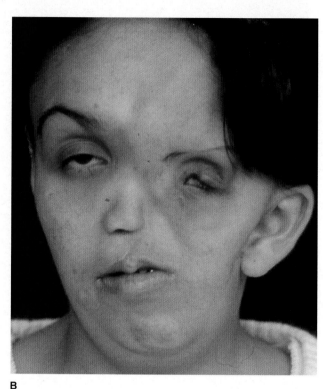

B

Figure 27–10. Craniofacial clefts associated with anterior plagiocephaly.

Number 10

Cleft number 10 cuts through the supraorbital rim and orbital roof lateral to the supraorbital nerve, ascending through the frontal bone. There is a central coloboma of the upper eyelid and the eyebrow is divided. Coloboma of the iris may be present. This cleft is the cranial continuity of cleft number 4 (Fig. 27–7B).

Numbers 11, 12, and 13

Cleft number 11 follows the same axis as cleft number 3 over the medial third of the upper lid and it, more often than not, occurs in concert with cleft number 3 (Fig. 27–8A). Cleft number 12 is located medial to the medial canthus of the upper eyelid, extending through the ethmoid (Fig. 27–8B). As with cleft number 11, it occurs most frequently in concert with cleft number 2. Cleft number 13 is the cranial extension of cleft number 1. It is located between the nasal bone and the frontal process of the maxilla (Fig. 27–9A). It is often bilateral resulting in severe hypertelorism. The cleft number 14, as previously discussed, extends cranially in the midline, often causing hypertelorism and furrowing of the midline forehead (Fig. 27–9B).

Most clefts of the soft tissues also present with bony cleft; the reverse is not true. Facial clefts are often bilateral with different degrees of severity on each side. They are frequently multiple, with two or three different types in the same patient. As observed by Tessier, facial clefts never pass through foramina that may be converted into grooves by hypoplasia at the lateral edges. The correlation of facial clefts with their cranial counterparts is sometimes difficult, and the frequent presentation of multiple clefts further complicates this task. Due to the radial pattern of craniofacial clefting, all except for cleft numbers 0 and 14 cross aesthetic units of the face, which further complicates their surgical correction.[5]

OUR SERIES

We have operated on 490 patients with major craniofacial clefts in our unit from 1965 to 2005.[6–8] One of the main objectives of this chapter is to present the evolution of our treatment plan and our present protocol, which is based on long-term observations. We are including in this series patients with Treacher Collins syndrome. We have excluded a group of 339 patients with hemifacial microsomia treated during

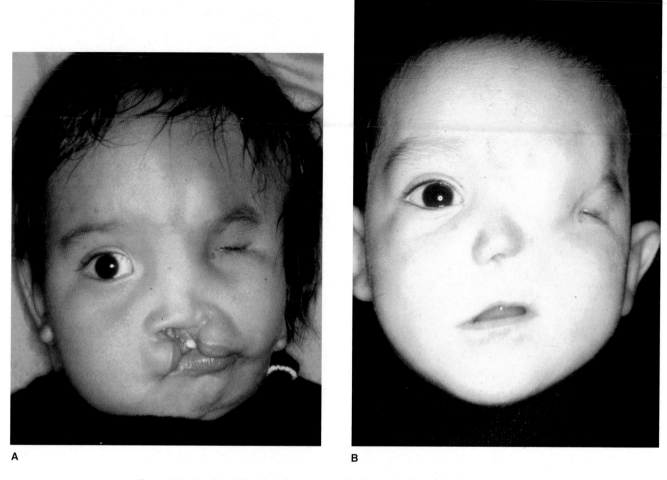

A

B

Figure 27–11. Craniofacial clefts associated with anophthalmia and microorbitism.

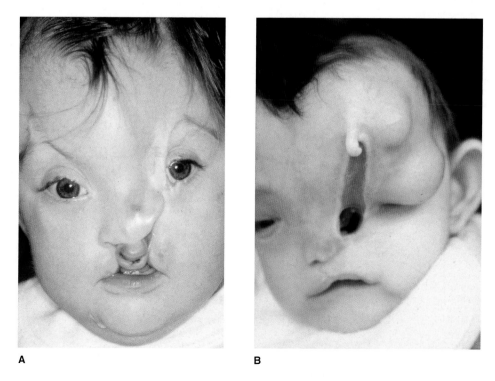

A

B

Figure 27–12. Craniofacial clefts associated with amniotic bands.

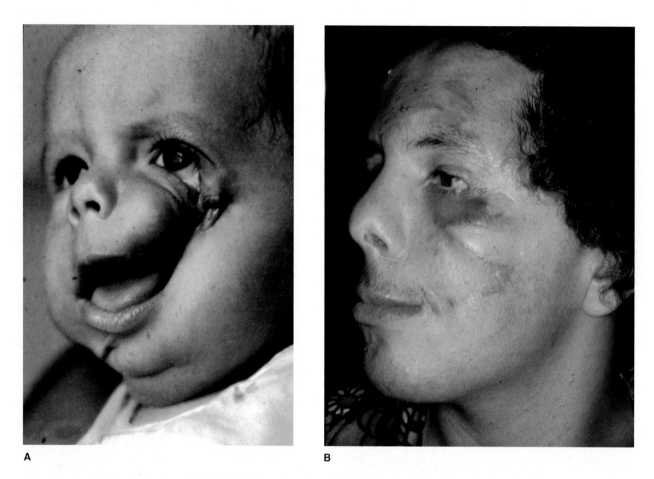

Figure 27–13. (A) Profound left-sided cleft number 6 repaired in infancy. (B) Note the patchwork effect of Z-plasty and local flap reconstruction in the 35-year follow-up.

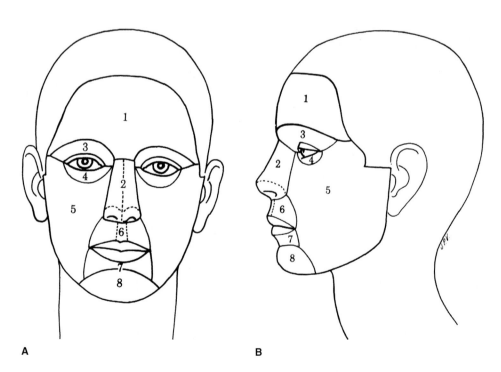

Figure 27–14. (A) Aesthetic units of the face, frontal view. (B) Aesthetic units of the face, lateral view.

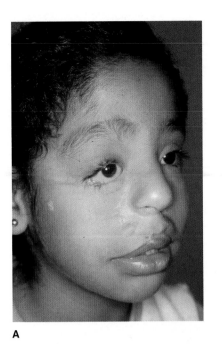
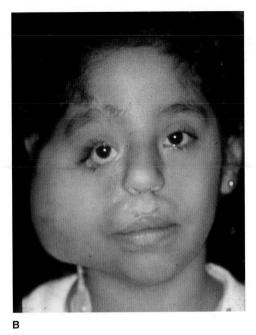
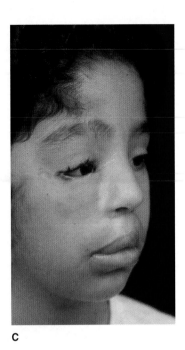

A   **B**   **C**

Figure 27–15. (A) Closure of cleft number 4 with Z-plasty and local flaps with scars traversing the cheek aesthetic unit. (B) Tissue expansion of cheek to allow for aesthetic unit reconstruction. (C) Same patient 5 years after aesthetic unit reconstruction of the cheek.

the same period. Although patients with hemifacial microsomia may correspond to a Tessier cleft number 7, their surgical treatment follows an entirely different philosophy that must be discussed separately.

Of our series of 490 patients, 54% were male and 46% female, which corresponds to a ratio of 1:8, but which is not statistically significant. Three hundred and nineteen (65%) patients presented with multiple clefts and 171 (34%)patients with a single fissure. In 159 (32%) patients, the malformation was unilateral, the rest (68%) were bilateral. In absolute terms, the most common cleft was cleft number 0 (17%) followed by cleft number 7 (15%) and cleft number 14 (12%). Considering only single clefts, the most frequent were, in descending order, cleft number 7 (34%), cleft number 0 (23%), cleft number 3 (12%), cleft number 2 (8%), cleft number 4 (7%), cleft number 8 (4%), cleft number 1 (3%), cleft numbers 5 and 10 together (2%), cleft numbers 6, 13, and 14 (1%), and cleft number 12 (0.6%) (Table 27–1).

Regarding patients with multiple clefts, the most common combination was 0–14 (36%), followed by 1–13 (22%), and combinations of 6–7–8 represented by the Treacher Collins syndrome (13%). Less frequent were combinations of 2–12 (10%), 3–11 (3.%), 0–13 (1%), and 3–12 (0.3%) (Table 27–2). From clinical observation and radiological studies, we found that in 71% of the patients both the soft tissues and the skeleton were affected. In 23% only the soft tissues were affected, and in 6% only the skeleton.

Bony clefts of the nasal skeleton were present in 72% of cases, clefts of the orbit in 61%, clefts of the maxilla in 43%, and clefts of the frontal bone in 42%. Craniosynostosis, mainly coronal, was found in 11.3% of the patients and was usually associated with multiple clefting (Fig. 27–10). Anophthalmia was present in 5.1% of patients with orbitopalpebral clefts of which 3.7% were unilateral and 1.4% bilateral (Fig. 27–11). Microphthalmia was present in 4.5%, 3.9% of them affecting both eyes. Palpebral clefts were present in 19.5% of the patients; 13.4% had coloboma of the lower lid and 6.1% of the upper lid. Complete arhinia was observed in 10 patients and hemiarhinia in 5. Orbital hypertelorism was the most frequent skeletal deformation, found in 38% of our patients, mainly in the 2–12, 1–13, and 0–14 clefts. Eighteen patients had craniofacial clefts associated with amniotic bands (Fig. 27–12).

Frontal encephalocele was observed in six patients with 10, 12, 13, and 14 clefts, and pharyngeal encephalocele corresponding to a cleft of the floor of the anterior cerebral fossa was found in three patients with 0–14 clefts, representing complete central craniofacial dysraphia (Fig. 27–2B).

TREATMENT

Historical Perspective

Because of the unlimited number of combinations of the craniofacial clefts and the variations of soft tissue and skeleton affected in each particular case, it is almost impossible to propose standard techniques for their correction. Many ingenious operations have been described over the last two centuries for the correction of individual clefts. These techniques are often based on the observation and treatment of small numbers of patients followed for short periods of time. Very little information is available on the long-term results

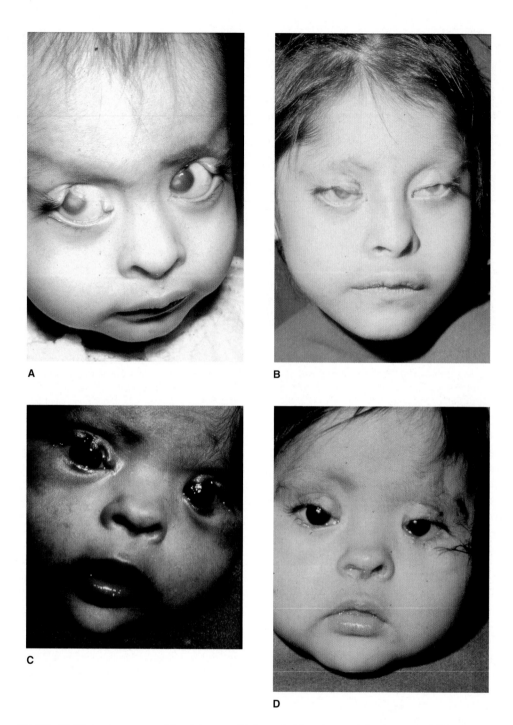

Figure 27–16. (A) Bilateral upper eyelid coloboma with loss of vision due to delay in repair. (B) Postoperative aesthetic result with bilateral upper lid–switch flaps. (C) Preoperative view of sister to patient in Fig. 27–17A with bilateral upper lid coloboma. (D) Postoperative view of patient after immediate repair with lid–switch flaps. Vision is intact due to immediate treatment.

of these techniques regarding the location of surgical scars, quality of skin cover, growth of facial and cranial structures, and restoration of craniofacial contours.[2,9–12]

Generally, most techniques have been focused on the closure of soft tissue clefts by direct approximation or by the rotation of flaps from the edges of the cleft. For major or more complex defects, the rotation or advancement of regional flaps has been employed, sometimes in combination

with skin grafts. Skeletal defects have been corrected by the use of bone grafts and osteotomies or a combination of the two, simultaneous with soft tissue correction. In some major craniofacial clefts, it has been considered desirable to reconstruct the skeleton before the soft tissue; in others, skeletal correction followed soft tissue correction.

The interposition of flaps from different regions of the face produced a patchwork effect because of the differences

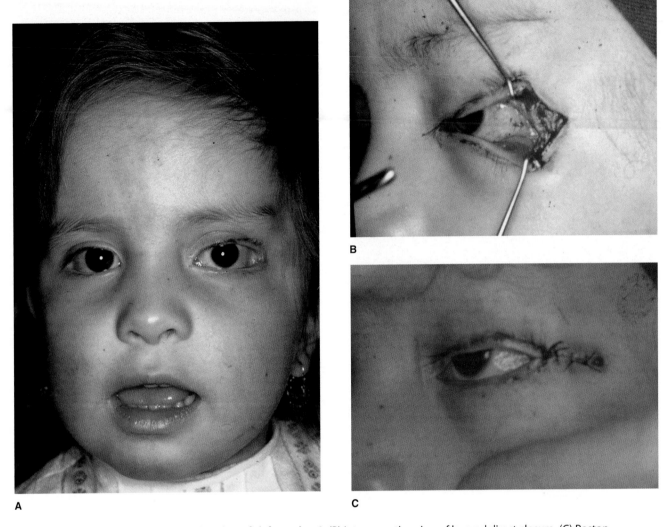

Figure 27–17. (A) Preoperative view of cleft number 8. (B) Intraoperative view of layered direct closure. (C) Postoperative view of direct closure of cleft number 8.

in color, texture, and thickness of the skin. Z-plasties have often been used to elongate the resulting scars, increasing the patchy effect, and resulting in scars crossing the face in many directions and in conspicuous locations (Fig. 27–13).[5]

The concept of aesthetic units in facial reconstruction was first proposed by Aufricht[13] in 1943 showing that better surgical results could be obtained when complete units were replaced even when some normal skin had to be resected (Fig. 27–14). This concept has evolved over the years, establishing well-defined units and subunits. Since these units are limited by facial prominences and depressions that reflect light in different directions, the scars located exactly at the boundaries between two units are less visible. In contrast, a scar is more evident when it traverses a subunit.

A classic example is the long-term result after the correction of a number 5 cleft extending from the junction of the lateral and middle thirds of the lower eyelid through the cheek to the lateral third of the upper lip. This cleft is always associated with an ectropion of the lower lid. The closure of

the cleft by multiple Z-plasties to correct the ectropion and to achieve elongation was the standard technique for many years, and the resulting scar crisscrossing the cheek was considered acceptable. Fig. 27–15 demonstrates the reconstruction of a 15-year-old female whose cleft number 4 was repaired first with local flaps and Z-plasties, and later with tissue expansion and subsequent aesthetic unit reconstruction. It illustrates the importance of hiding scars at the boundaries of aesthetic units.[14]

Current Treatment Philosophy and Protocol

In following these patients over more than four decades, it has become clear that incorrectly placed scars do not improve with time, differences of skin color and texture are permanent, and facial asymmetry due to bony and soft tissue irregularities distracts from an aesthetically pleasing appearance. Based on this experience, we have developed a treatment protocol with the following objectives:

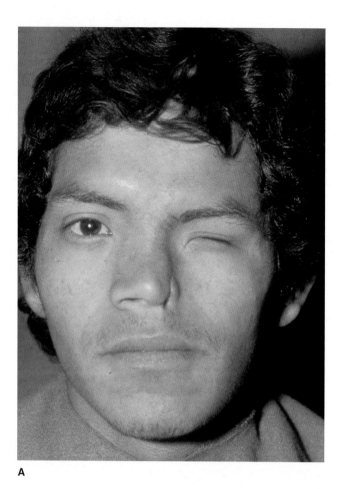

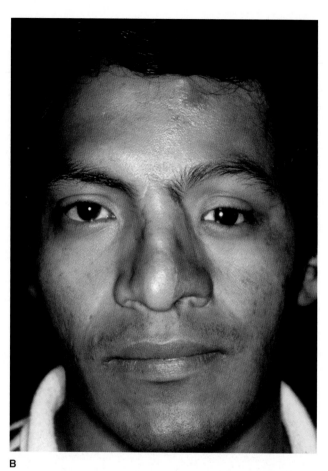

A **B**

Figure 27–18. (A) Adult male with left-sided Tessier number 2 cleft number and heminasal aplasia. (B) Postoperative view after reconstruction with forehead flap for reconstruction of the heminose and ocular prosthesis.

- Restoration of the craniofacial skeleton
- Reconstruction with skin and soft tissue of like color and texture
- Generous use of tissue expanders
- Aesthetic subunit reconstruction
- Scar location at limits of aesthetic subunits
- Symmetric repositioning of key facial landmarks

Urgent Treatment Considerations

Rarely do patients with craniofacial clefts require urgent or emergent therapy. Most are able to maintain an adequate airway, though severe cases of Treacher Collins syndrome are known to require prolonged airway management. In these patients, urgent mandibular distraction osteogenesis has been shown to improve airway mechanics and avoid the need for tracheostomy.

Another urgent matter is globe exposure due to coloboma of the upper eyelid. Coloboma of the lower eyelid rarely results in blindness due to Bell's phenomenon, while that of the upper eyelid frequently leads to blindness if not treated directly. Short-term solutions include an ocular moistening chamber. Definitive treatment consists of direct

closure, local flap closure of the coloboma, or one of a number of lid–switch operations (Fig. 27–16).

Soft Tissue Reconstruction

Every effort is made at reconstruction with skin and soft tissue of like color and texture. This can be accomplished most readily through direct approximation and local flap rotation or advancement. We use tissue expanders frequently to achieve aesthetic subunit reconstruction with scars located at the limits of aesthetic subunits.[14,15]

Direct Approximation

When involvement of the soft tissues is minimal, as in many median and paramedian clefts, direct closure is the optimal treatment even with severe skeletal malformations. This scenario is common in cleft number 0 affecting the upper lip and nose in which a vertical midline scar produces very acceptable results. Through these incisions, it is easy to medialize the alar domes, the nasal bones, and even the medial orbital walls.[6,8]

Direct approximation is also indicated in minor coloboma of the upper eyelid and closure of cleft number

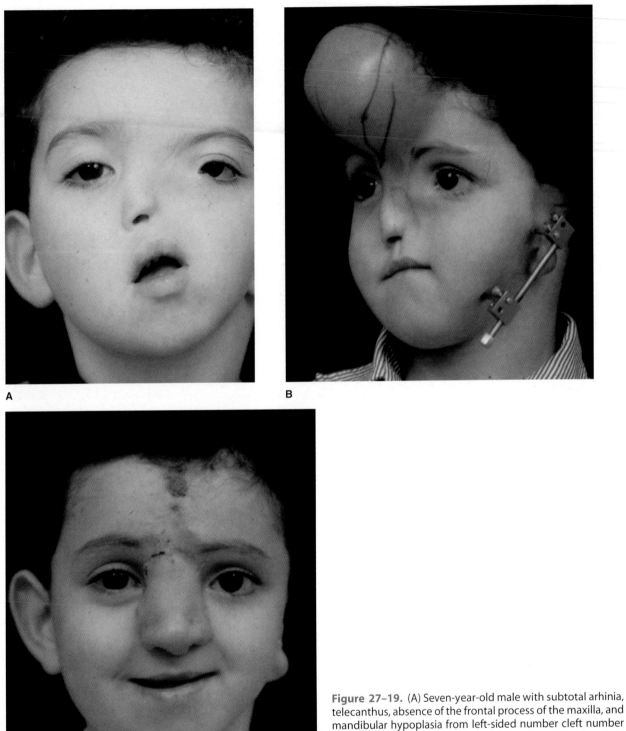

Figure 27–19. (A) Seven-year-old male with subtotal arhinia, telecanthus, absence of the frontal process of the maxilla, and mandibular hypoplasia from left-sided number cleft number 2 and hemifacial microsomia. (B) Expansion of the forehead flap simultaneous with mandibular distraction osteogenesis. (C) Early postoperative result after complete nasal reconstruction with the expanded paramedian forehead flap and costochondral grafts.

8, which cut across the lateral canthal ligament. Layered closure of the conjunctiva, orbicularis muscle, and skin results in excellent form and function (Fig. 27–17).

Finally, direct approximation can function as a temporary measure in cases of severe clefting in which formal recon-

struction is not possible. This includes patients with severe nasomaxillary dysplasia and severe cerebral malformation in which survival is doubtful. If the patient survives, the direct closure can be replaced by more formal flap reconstruction that might consist of a lid–switch flap, a microvascular bone

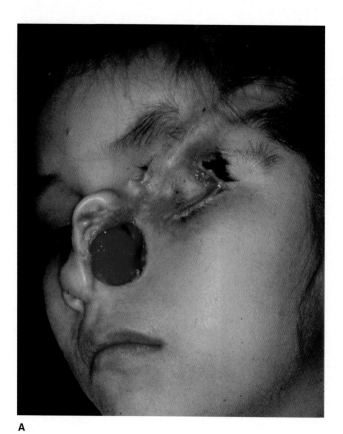

A

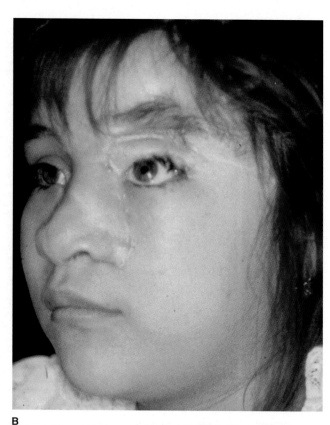

B

Figure 27–20. (A) Cleft numbers 2–12 from amniotic bands with heminasal aplasia, left-sided blindness due to exposure, and telecanthus. (B) Nose reconstructed with an expanded paramedian forehead flap. Medial and cephalic advancement of cheek tissues, canthal repositioning, and upper lid reconstruction leaving scars at the limits of aesthetic units. Symmetric repositioning of key facial landmarks such as the canthi, alae, and nasal base greatly improve the aesthetic result.

flap to the premaxillary region, and a forehead flap for nasal reconstruction.

Local Flap Reconstruction

Local flap reconstruction, with or without tissue expansion, plays an important role in the closure of paramedian, naso-oro-ocular, and lateral clefts. Multiple local flaps exist to close coloboma of the eyelids, examples of which are the Hemi-Tripier flap[16] and the Mustarde[17] lid–switch flap (Figs. 27–16B and D).

Our workhorse for nasal reconstruction is the expanded paramedian forehead flap. We have found tissue expansion to be the critical advancement to allow the forehead flap to reconstruct the entire nose in children while allowing for donor site closure. We have not experienced the problems others have with this technique, and it has provided reliable cutaneous coverage for our bone grafts and costal cartilage grafts for years.[8,18] Perhaps the use of stronger structural support in the form of costal cartilage, in place of ear cartilage, is what has led to this success. Fig. 27–18 demonstrates the paramedian forehead flap's ability to reconstruct the heminose. Fig. 27–19 demonstrates its ability to reconstruct the entire nose.

Local Flap Advancement

The area in which tissue expanders have aided our reconstructions the most has been in the preexpansion of cheek advancement flaps. Tissue expansion allows us to excise scars from the middle of the cheek all the way to the medial canthus, and cover the entire cheek with neck and lower facial skin that has been expanded. Perhaps no other advancement has led to such dramatic improvements in our aesthetic results, as it routinely allows us to perform aesthetic unit reconstruction (Fig. 27–20).

Tissue expansion has also aided in nasal reconstruction with an advancement flap from the forehead in cases when the paramedian forehead flap is not available. This is particularly helpful in dramatic cases of multiple clefts involving large portions of the midface in which a cheek flap will close the cheek defect and a forehead flap can provide nasal cutaneous coverage.

Skeletal Reconstruction

Even normal overlying soft tissues cannot hide a deficient or defective skeleton, and thus it is imperative to restore the craniofacial skeleton in major facial clefts. In cases with

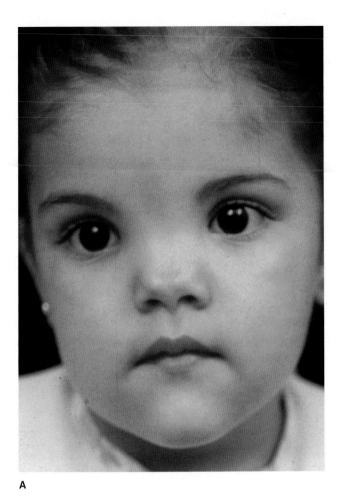

A

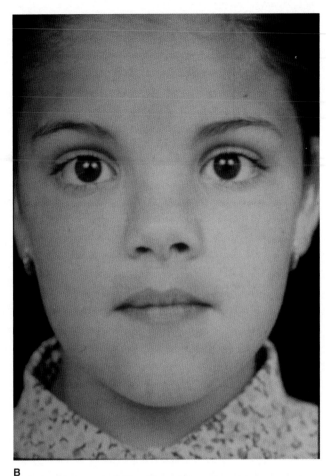

B

Figure 27–21. (A) Cleft numbers 0–14 with mild hypertelorism. (B) Eight years after medialization of medial orbital walls via a coronal approach.

minor bony defects, bone grafts may suffice. As defects become larger and more complex, osteotomies are required, either in combination with rigid fixation or with distraction osteogenesis. The main regions of prominence in the skeleton are the position and shape of the orbits, the nose, and the chin. Also dependent on the skeleton are key prominences and depressions of the face. Key prominences include the supraorbital ridge, the malar eminences, the nose, the zygomatic arch, the mandibular angles, and the chin. Key depressions in the face include the temporal region, the inferior orbits, the central hollow of the cheeks, and the submandibular region.[19]

Orbital Repositioning

Orbital hypertelorism occurs with some frequency and to varying degrees in facial clefting. Treatment of orbital hypertelorism ranges from medialization of the medial orbital walls in minor cases to complete orbital repositioning and hemifacial rotation. All of these operations can be performed through coronal and vestibular incisions, avoiding the addition of scars to the soft tissues of the face.

Medialization of the medial orbital walls is indicated in patients with minor orbital hypertelorism (intercanthal

distance less than 40 mm) without an increased distance between the lateral orbital rims. This procedure is performed extracranially through a coronal incision. The osteotomies extend from the medial orbital rims to the supraorbital and infraorbital nerves. After repositioning the osteotomized segments, care is taken in performing a transnasal canthopexy (Fig. 27–21).[20]

Formal orbital repositioning in the form of "box" osteotomies is indicated in adult patients with moderate to severe orbital hypertelorism (intercanthal distance greater than 40 mm). Children are not candidates for these procedures because they cause retardation of midfacial growth, resulting in hypoplasia. Coronal and vestibular incisions are used to access the bony orbits. The bony orbit is dissected from its periosteum and circumferential osteotomies are performed in order to medialize the orbit. Medialization can be performed symmetrically or asymmetrically.[21] Intracranial box osteotomies are shown in Fig. 27–22. Importantly, all intraorbital osteotomies must be carried out at least 1 cm posterior to the lachrymal crest so as to avoid injury to the lachrymal apparatus. Equally important is fastidious resuspension of the midface soft tissues so as to avoid soft tissue ptosis, which can prematurely age the face. Though care is taken to perform a

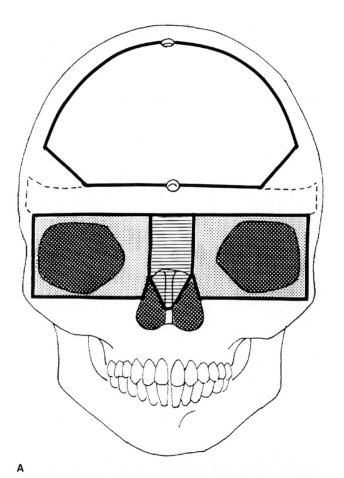

A

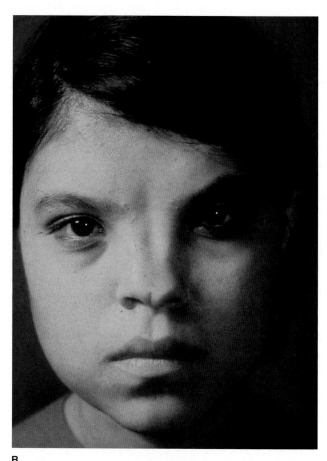

B

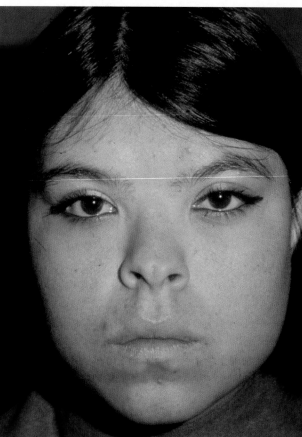

C

Figure 27–22. (A) Schematic of intracranial orbital repositioning. (B) Preoperative view of a 20-year-old female with a 0–14 cleft and moderate hyptertelorism. (C) Postoperative result after intracranial orbital repositioning.

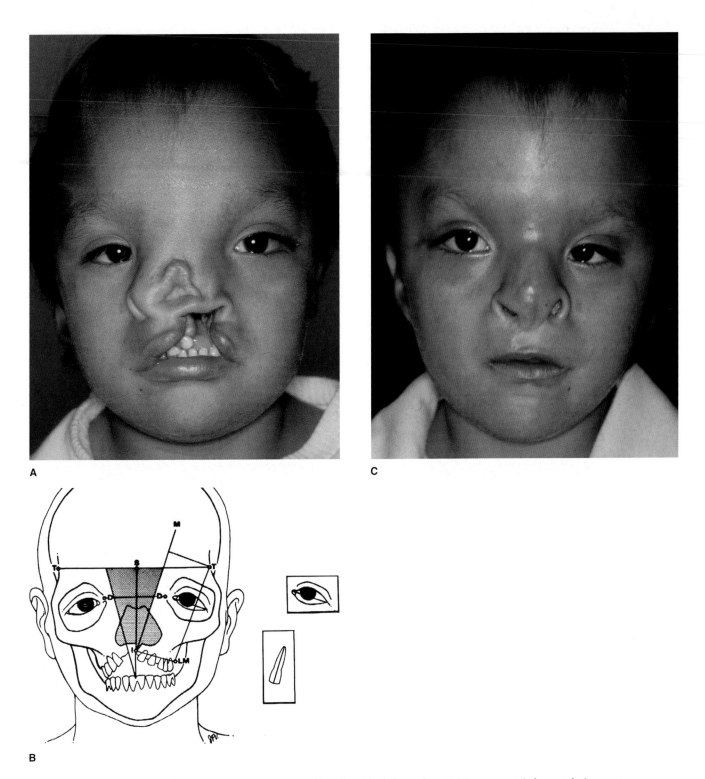

Figure 27–23. (A) Preoperative view of 8-year-old male with cleft numbers 1–13, asymmetric hypertelorism, anterior open bite, shortened midface, cleft of the lip and palate, and nasal malformation with *cutis gyrate* (B) Schematic demonstrating the geometric planning of an asymmetric hemifacial rotation to approximate the orbits, close the open bite, and lengthen the midface (C) Postoperative view of patient after asymmetric hemifacial rotation, nasal correction, and closure of the clefts of the lip and palate.

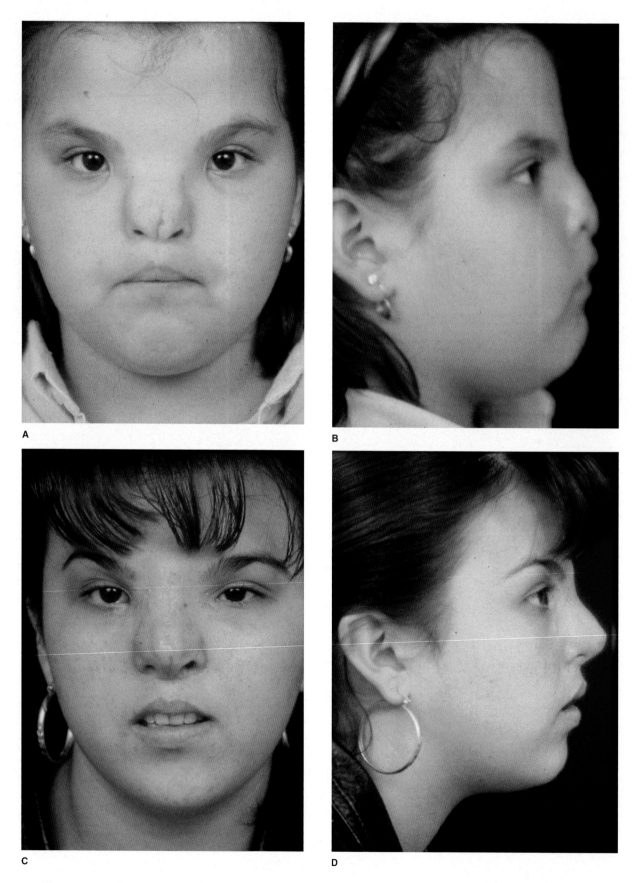

Figure 27–24. (A) Preoperative frontal view of 14-year-old female with a 0–14 cleft, moderate hypertelorism, and anterior open bite (B) Preoperative lateral view of same patient (C) Five-year postoperative result after symmetric hemifacial rotation and costochondral grafting of the nasal dorsum (D) Postoperative lateral view. Note the increased length of the midface and the increased projection of the nasal dorsum.

sturdy medial canthopexy, increased intercanthal distance is the most common reason for reoperation in these patients.

Hemifacial rotation[22] is indicated in children and adults with moderate to severe orbital hypertelorism, an anterior open bite, and a shortened midface. It, too, can be performed intracranially or extracranially, symmetrically or asymmetrically. Planning a hemifacial rotation requires attention to maxillary cant as well as interorbital distance.[23] Proper planning and clinical photos of symmetric and asymmetric hemifacial rotation are shown in Figs. 27–23 and 27–24. As with orbital box osteotomies, the most common reason for reoperation is increased intercanthal distance, and thus every attempt is made to avoid this late complication.[24]

Symmetric Repositioning of Key Facial Landmarks

Facial asymmetries are routinely detected by the casual observer, and facial asymmetries in these patients are a source of anguish for them and their relatives. It is paramount to restore facial symmetry, and one of the most important steps to doing so is the repositioning of key facial landmarks. Repositioning of the bony skeleton brings the orbits, nasal pyramid, and chin into alignment. The soft tissues overlying those structures, including the medial and lateral canthi, nasal alae, nasal base, and buccal commissures must also be placed in a symmetric position either by flap rotation or suture techniques.

CONCLUSIONS

The etiologic basis for major facial clefts is varied, with both genetics and environmental factors playing a role. Major facial clefts have been classified based on a multitude of factors, and the most widely used classification scheme is Tessier's that numbers clefts from 0 to 14 based on their anatomic location.

Treatment of these conditions has evolved over the past century to provide improved aesthetic and functional results. Current tenets of treatment include the following:

- Restoration of the craniofacial skeleton
- Reconstruction with skin and soft tissue of like color and texture
- Generous use of tissue expanders
- Aesthetic subunit reconstruction
- Scar location at limits of aesthetic subunits
- Symmetric repositioning of key facial landmarks

References

1. Niemeyer MF, Van der Meulen J. The genetics of craniofacial malformations. In Stricker M, Van der Meulen J, Rápale B, Mazzola R (eds). *Craniofacial Malformations*. London: Churchill Livingstone, 1990.
2. Kawamoto HK. The kaleidoscopic world of rare craniofacial clefts: Order out of chaos. *Clin Plast Surg* 3:529, 1976.
3. Van der Meulen J, Mazzola R, Vermeij-Keers C, Stricker M, Raphael B. A morphogenetic classification of craniofacial malformations. *Plast Reconstr Surg* 71:560, 1983.
4. Tessier P. Anatomical classification of facial, craniofacial, and laterofacial clefts. *J Maxillofac Surg* 4:69, 1976.
5. Tessier P. Fentes orbito-faciales verticals et obliques (colobomas), copletes en frustes. *Ann Chir Plast* 14:301, 1969.
6. Ortiz-Monasterio F, Olmedo A. Reconstruction of major nasal defects. *Clin Plast Surg* 8:3, 1981.
7. Ortiz-Monasterio F, Fuente del Campo F, Dimopulos A. Nasal clefts. *Clin Plast Surg* 18:5, 1987.
8. Ortiz-Monasterio F, Fuente del Campo A, Longato F, Saint Martin R. Schisi Facciali rare. *Rev. Italiana de chir.* Plast. 2:3, 1989.
9. Fogh-Anderson B. Rare clefts of the face. *Acta Chir Scand.* 129:275, 1965.
10. Pitanguy I, Franco T. Nonoperated facial tissues in adults. *Plast Reconstr Surg* 39:569, 1967.
11. Boo Chai K. The transverse facial cleft: Its repair. *Br J Plast Surg* 22:119, 1969.
12. Moore MH. Rare craniofacial clefts. *J Craniofac Surg* 7:408, 1996.
13. Aufricht G. Evaluation of pedicle flap versus skin graft, reconstruction of surface defects and scar contractures of the chin, cheeks, and neck. *Surgery* 15:1, 1944.
14. Ortiz-Monasterio F. The concept of aesthetic units for the correction of craniofacial clefts. In David D (ed). *Craniofacial Surgery* 11. Bologna: Medimond, 2005.
15. Argenta LC, Vander Kolk CA. Tissue expansion in craniofacial surgery. *Clin Plast Surg* 14:143, 1987.
16. Tripier L. Musculocutantous flap in the form of a bridge, applied to the reconstruction of the eyelids. *Compt rend adac sc (Paris)* 109:620, 1889.
17. Mustarde JC. *Repair and Reconstruction in the Orbital Region*. Edinborough: Chruchill Livingstone, 1966.
18. Ortiz-Monasterio F, Molina F. Nasal reconstruction in hypertelorism. The problem of blood supply. In Lauritzen CK (ed). *Craniofacial Surgery*. Italy: Monduzzi Editori, 2001.
19. Ortiz-Monasterio F. Analysis estetica de la cara. In Ortiz Monasterio F, Molina F (eds). *Cirugía Estetica Del Esqueleto Facial*. Buenos Aires: Panamericana, 2005, Chapter 3.
20. Ortiz-Monasterio F, Molina F. Orbital hypertelorism. *Clin Plast Surg* 21:4, 1994.
21. Tessier P. The definitive treatment of orbital hypertelorism by craniofacial or extracranial osteotomies. *Scand J Plast Reconstr Surg* 6:135, 1972.
22. Van der Meulen JC. Medial faciotomy. *Br J Plast Surg* 32:339, 1979.
23. Ortiz-Monasterio F, Medina O, Musolas A. Geometrical planning for the correction of hypertelorism. *Plast Reconstr Surg* 86:650, 1990.
24. Ortiz-Monasterio F. Orbital hypertelorism. In Goldwin RM, Cohen MN (eds). *The Unfavorable Result in Plastic Surgery: Avoidance and Treatment*. Hagerstown: Lippincott Williams and Wilkins, 2001.

28

Transverse Facial Clefts of Macrostomia

Peter J. Taub, MD, FACS, FAAP • Lisa Vecchione, DMD, MDS • Joseph E. Losee, MD, FACS, FAAP

◼ INTRODUCTION

Distinct from typical clefts of the lip and/or palate, transverse facial clefts of macrostomia are relatively rare anomalies. Such transverse lateral clefts, involving the oral commissure, constitute less than 1% of all facial clefts. They are commonly associated with anomalies affecting structures derived from the first and second branchial arches, and may affect either one or both sides of the face. The embryologic process resulting in a transverse cleft is postulated to be a failure in obliteration of the normal grooves that exist between the fetal maxillary and mandibular prominences, a process which normally occurs in the fourth and fifth weeks of gestation.[1,2]

Transverse facial clefts are most recognizable by the larger than normal width of the mouth or macrostomia, and the deficiency of soft tissue (and possibly bone) just lateral to the oral commissure (Fig. 28–1). The normal oral commissure is not a simple union of upper and lower lip elements, but rather a continuous, circumoral band of vermilion mucosa.[3,4]

Beneath the mucosa are interdigitating fibers of the orbicularis oris muscle, which parallel the upper and lower lip elements. Accurate reconstruction of the oral commissure needs to recreate this anatomic configuration, which is important for both feeding and speaking.[5]

In the transverse cleft, the normal anatomy is lost as the bands of muscle continue to remain parallel to the margins of the cleft, and fail to interdigitate with one another as they course laterally (Fig. 28–2). The upper lip band often interdigitates with the superiorly based zygomaticus muscle and the lower band limb interdigitates with the inferiorly based risorius muscle. As a result, there is a reduced distance between the commissure and the tragus of the ear on the affected side of the face. At rest there is no closure of the commissure, and with whistling and speaking, the lips fail to completely purse. The dehiscence of the commissure and lack of lip competence results in drooling and the inability to control secretions. In addition, the unrepaired deformity creates an unusual smile with facial animation.

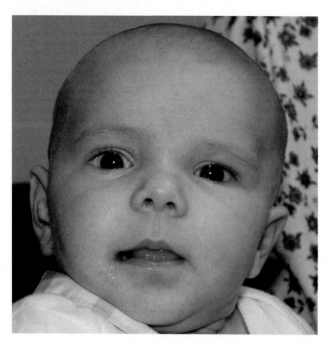

Figure 28–1. Right-sided transverse facial cleft of macrostomia.

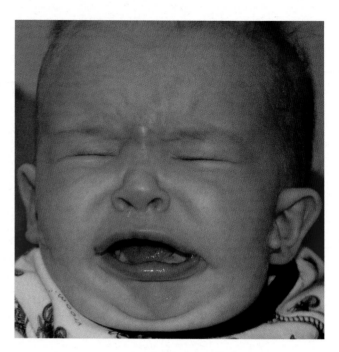

Figure 28–3. Bilateral transverse facial clefts.

The transverse cleft and resulting macrostomia may present as an isolated finding, but may be found with associated anomalies of the ears, parotid gland and duct, facial nerve branches, and other first and second branchial arch structures. In addition, macrostomia may be associated with numerous syndromes, including Noonan, Treacher Collins, Goldenhar, and William. In such cases, it is important to identify congenital anomalies related to other organ systems early. Infrequently, macrostomia can occur bilaterally, with clefting at each commissure (Fig. 28–3).

SURGICAL RECONSTRUCTION

For the transverse facial cleft, the principles of repair include accurate placement of the commissure to restore symmetry to the lower third of the face, recreation of the orbicularis oris muscle as a sphincter around the mouth, minimizing external scarring, and avoidance of secondary contracture that serves to displace a correctly positioned commissure (Fig. 28–4).

Numerous techniques for reconstructing macrostomia have been proposed in the literature to achieve acceptable results. The more established procedures utilize flaps of skin and/or mucosa that place the suture line over the bulk of either the upper or lower lip, in efforts to avoid a scar at the corner of the mouth. Borrowing from the principles of Estlander for lip reconstruction, May advocated rotation of a full-thickness, vermilion-lined flap, including muscle, from the lower lip to the upper as a means of reconstructing the commissure.[6] Longacre et al. proposed a lateral Z-plasty of the cheek incision to more closely reconstruct the normal creases of skin.[7] Torkut applied the double-reversing Z-plasty, similar to that used for cleft palate repair, to address the transverse facial cleft.[8] One lip margin contributed an external flap of skin and an internal composite flap of orbicularis muscle and oral mucosa. The other lip contributed an external flap of skin and muscle and an internal flap solely of mucosa. More recently, Fukada and Takeda described the advancement of the entire corner of the mouth as a composite flap from its existing location to a more anatomic one.[9] The intervening medial segments of vermilion were excised together with a triangle of oral mucosa and the resulting ends were reapproximated with the commissure in a more medial position. Eguchi et al. designed a vermilion

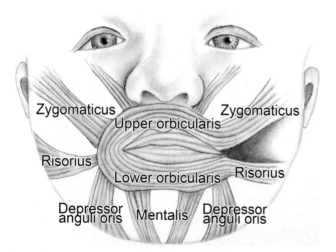

Figure 28–2. Illustration of the abnormal anatomy of left-sided macrostomia.

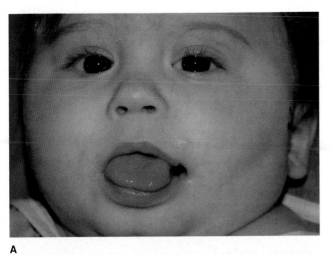

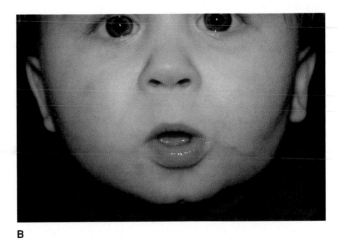

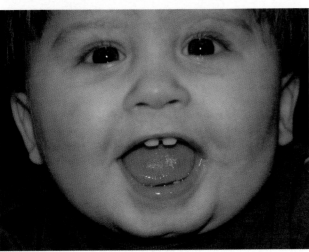

Figure 28–4. (A) Left-sided macrostomia preoperative photo. (B) Repair left-sided macrostomia in repose. (C) Repaired left-sided macrostomia with animation.

square flap method that straddled the mucocutaneous border and crossed the commissure to place the suture line away from the corner of the mouth.[10] They specifically raised their vermilion flap off the lower lip because the resultant scar would rest on the upper lip. They believed lower lip scars become more conspicuous over time as a result of continuous tension with opening the mouth, which is not similarly seen in the upper lip. A W-plasty was used to reapproximate the lateral cheek skin.

AUTHOR'S PREFERRED OPERATIVE TECHNIQUE

The technique of repair, as proposed by Kaplan,[11] is what the authors have adopted as their primary choice of reconstruction. Similar to more conventional cleft lip repairs, surgery is perhaps best performed around 3 months of age when the anesthetic risk to the infant begins to diminish. Earlier closure may improve any unlikely feeding difficulty resulting from the

macrostomia, but should have no appreciable effect on speech and language development. As stated above, associated congenital anomalies should be identified and addressed prior to surgery.

Preoperative Marking

There are several ways to determine the proper position of the new commissure. First, the face should be inspected in static, forward repose. The normal commissure should fall along a straight line dropped from the medial limbus of the iris. Next, the cleft side should be carefully inspected for a distinct change in the color, contour, and quality of the vermilion edge. This change in vermilion quality should also correspond to the normal commissure position. Third, the distance from the unaffected contralateral commissure to the height of the ipsilateral Cupid's bow can be accurately measured. This distance may be transferred to the affected side, and the new position for the reconstructed commissure marked. Finally, data from established normative tables may be used to gauge an

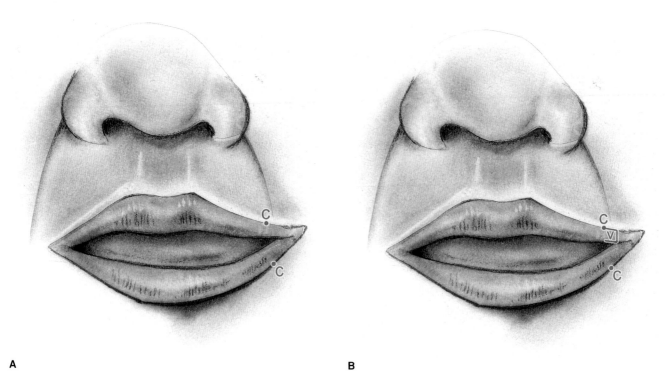

A

B

Figure 28–5. (A) Preoperative marking of c points. (B) Preoperative marking of c points and v flap.

appropriate distance.[12,13] The distance from commissure to high point of Cupid's Bow in a 3-year-old infant ranges from 16 to 20 mm depending on race. Utilizing these techniques, the commissure points (c point) on the upper and lower lateral lip elements are marked and tattooed (Fig. 28–5A). Additional ink marks can be made *just* medial to the points of the commissure junction, facilitating identification of the placement of sutures.

A vermilion commissure flap (v flap), whose base is medially pedicled at the upper lip commissure point (c point), and whose length is approximately 3–4 mm, is marked out

(Fig. 28–5B). The v flap is ultimately transposed to the lower lip, so that the suture line is not placed within the new commissure. In addition, it is designed to have the v flap created from "pale" cleft vermilion to line the newly reconstructed commissure. As a modification, a V-shaped notch may be designed on the distal aspect of the v flap to break up the straight-line scar at the site of closure (Fig. 28–6). Following this, buccal mucosal turnover flaps (b flaps) are then designed on the upper and lower lips to be pedicled on the internal mucosa (Fig. 28–7). The b flaps reconstruct the intraoral lining of the cleft reconstruction. Of note, the lower lip b flap extends medially, beyond the lower lip c point—a distance equal to the upper lip v flap—approximately 3–4 mm. It is important to include the white roll and vermilion–cutaneous junction

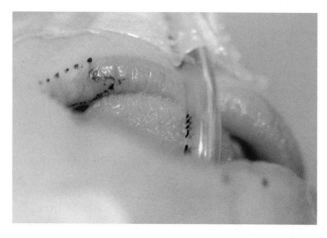

Figure 28–6. An above view of the left lower lip demonstrating an alternative technique incorporating a "dart" of vermilion tissue designed to break up the scar.

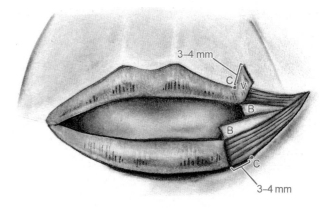

Figure 28–7. Preoperative markings of c points, v flap measuring 3–4 mm, and b flaps.

with the b flaps, so that vermilion or white roll is not included in the skin closure of the cheek skin, lateral to the newly reconstructed commissure. The area is then infiltrated with a solution of lidocaine and epinephrine to provide adequate hemostasis and analgesia.

Surgical Procedure

The procedure is begun by elevating the v flap off of the upper lip musculature, and basing it medially at the upper lip c point (Figs. 28–7 and 28–8A, B). This is performed with a #15 blade, a #67 Beaver blade, or ophthalmic knife. Next, the

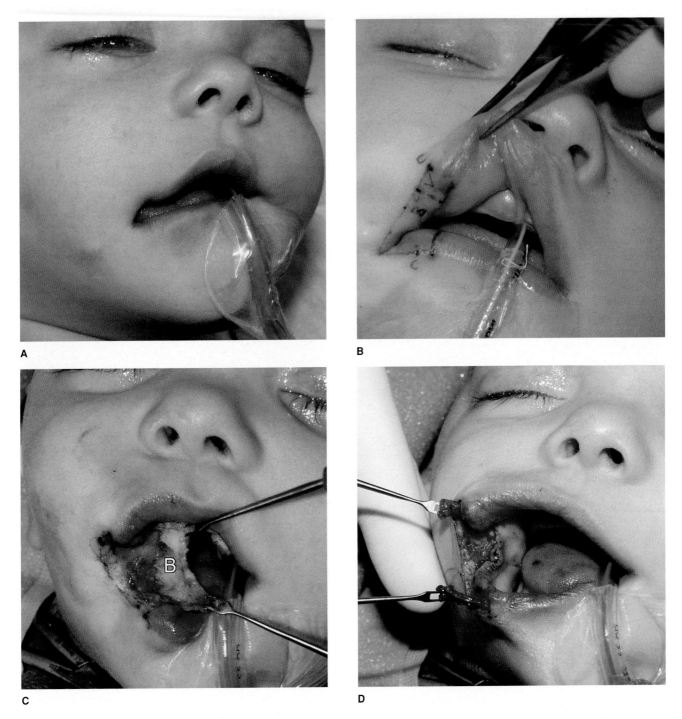

Figure 28–8. (A) Preoperative photo of right lateral facial cleft. (B) Preoperative markings including the c points, v flap, and b flaps. (C) Skin hooks retracting the b flaps. (D) Skin hooks holding the upper and lower orbicularis oris muscles. (E) Skin hooks overlapping the upper and lower orbicularis oris muscles. (F) Z-plasty cutaneous closure orienting the central vertical limb along the nasolabial crease. (G) 1-year follow-up following right lateral cleft repair. (H) Three-year follow-up following right lateral cleft repair.

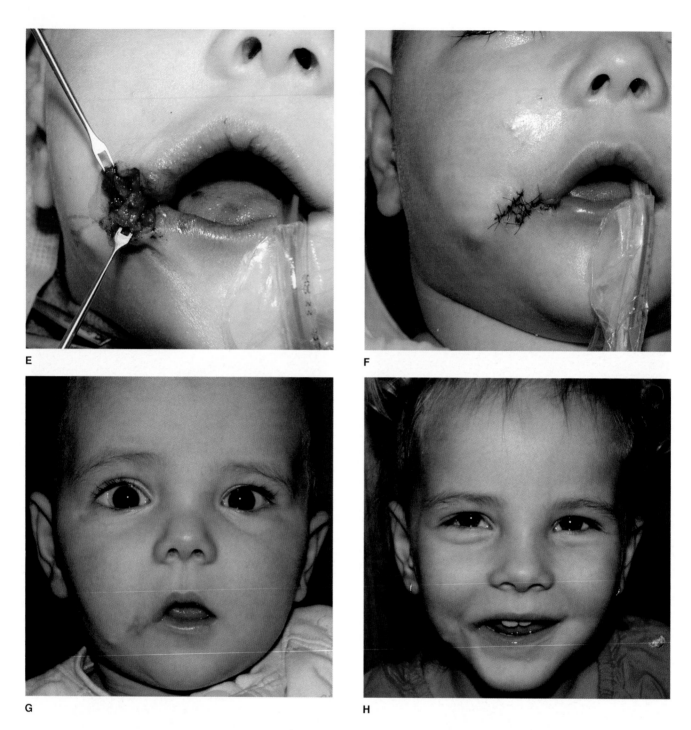

Figure 28–8. (*Continued*).

b flaps are elevated off of the upper and lower lip musculature and pedicled on the intraoral mucosa (Figs. 28–7 and 28–8C). Again, when raising the b flaps, it is important to include the red–white roll of the lateral lip elements and include them in the b flaps, so that at final skin closure, no white roll is included in the cutaneous repair.

The aberrant orbicularis oris muscle is then dissected free from the surrounding tissues farther laterally than simply the end of the cleft margin (Fig. 28–9). The upper and

lower muscles are dissected, and the muscle ends are transected approximately 5 mm beyond the c points (Figs. 28–10 and 28–8D). The muscle flaps are then transposed medially, and overlapped with the upper lip muscle on top of the lower muscle, to recreate the sphincter mechanism (Figs. 28–8E). The upper muscle limb is placed anterior to the inferior muscle limb since the upper lip tends to lie slightly anterior to the lower lip when recumbent. To facilitate a durable and accurate muscle reconstruction, a cutaneous commissure suture

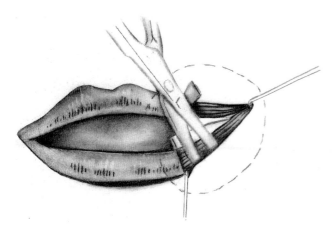

Figure 28–9. The aberrant orbicularis oris muscle is then dissected free of surrounding tissues farther laterally than simply the end of the cleft margin.

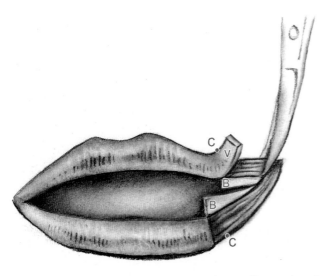

Figure 28–10. The upper and lower muscles are dissected, and the muscle ends are elevated and transected approximately 5 mm beyond the c points.

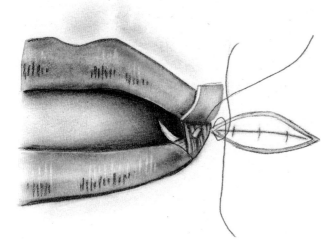

Figure 28–11. A cutaneous suture is placed at the new commissure and temporally cinched, but not tied, facilitating the alignment of the orbicularis oris muscles.

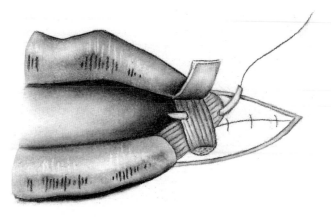

Figure 28–12. The muscle limbs are sewn with long-lasting absorbable sutures in a horizontal mattress fashion.

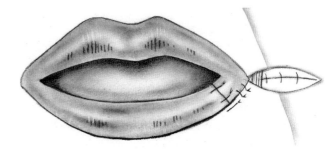

Figure 28–13. The v flap is transposed and inset in the lower lip.

is placed through the upper and lower lip c points and temporally cinched, but not tied (Figs. 28–11 and 28–8E). This allows for the accurate gauging of muscle overlap and tension required for muscle reconstruction. The muscle limbs are then sewn with long-lasting absorbable sutures in a horizontal mattress fashion (Fig. 28–12).

The b flaps are sewn together to reconstitute the intraoral buccal mucosa. As a modification, a Z-plasty of the intraoral mucosa may be included to minimize lateral scar retraction. If there was a lateral subcutaneous grove or crease,

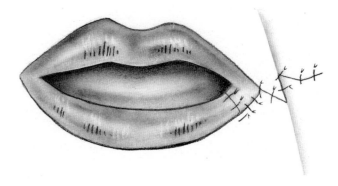

Figure 28–14. A cutaneous Z-plasty is designed to reorient the lateral cheek skin incision into the nasolabial crease. The central limb of the Z-plasty should lie in the oblique direction of the nasolabial crease.

it can be partially obliterated by the advancement and suturing of adjacent tissue to add bulk to the region.

The v flap is then transposed and inset in the lower lip (Fig. 28–13). The corner commissure sutures are tied, and the skin of the lateral cheek is trimmed and modified to facilitate a straight-line closure. It is rare today for the authors to place percutaneous epithelial sutures, but rather rely upon a meticulously repaired dermal layer, and this has resulted in superior final scar results.

At this time, a cutaneous Z-plasty, if utilized, is designed to reorient the lateral cheek skin incision into the nasolabial crease (Fig. 28–14). The central limb of the Z-plasty should lie in the oblique direction of the nasolabial crease (Fig. 28–8F, G, and H). Some authors believe that a Z-plasty should be

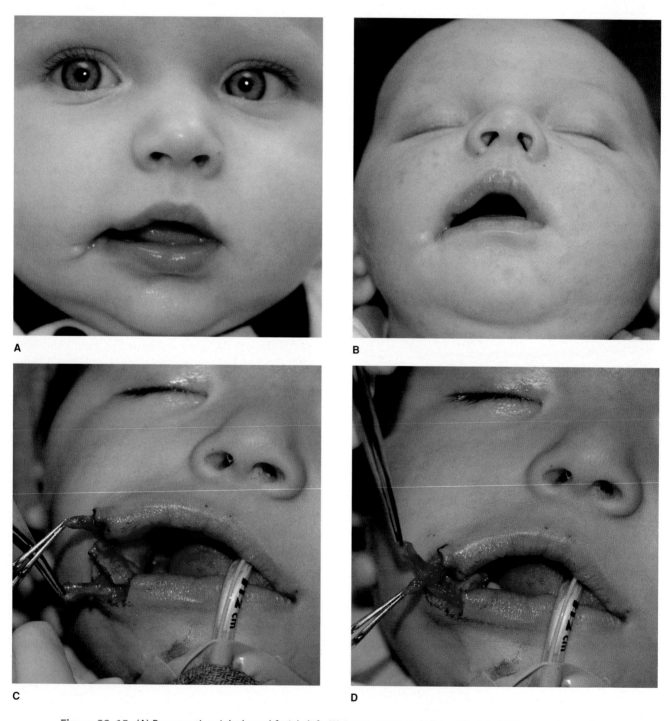

Figure 28–15. (A) Preoperative right lateral facial cleft. (B) Preoperative right lateral facial cleft in worm's eye view. (C) Forceps holding upper and lower orbicularis oris muscles. (D) Forceps overlapping the orbicularis oris muscles. (E) Follow-up at time of suture removal. (F) Early 1-year follow-up repair right lateral facial cleft. (G) Early 1-year follow-up repair right lateral facial cleft, worm's eye view.

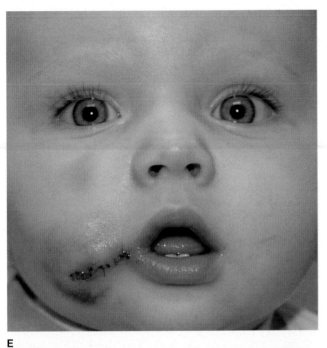

E

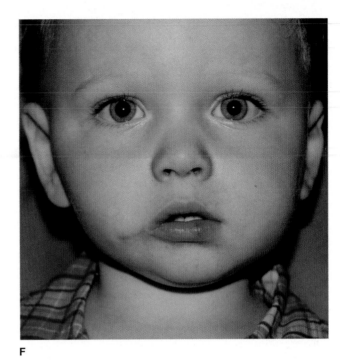

F

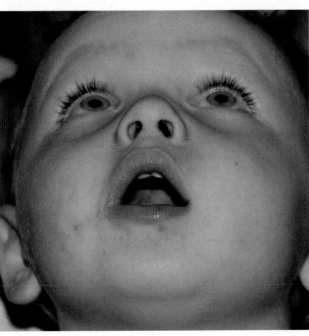

G

Figure 28–15. (*Continued*).

avoided on the cheek if possible since the scar on the cheek will always be conspicuous, and instead, suggest a "lazy" W-plasty closure.[14] Furthermore, a formal Z-plasty may be better designed after some time has elapsed and a more distinct nasolabial fold is present.

In the rare instance of a lateral facial cleft occurring with a classic paramidline cleft of the lip and nose, some authors have suggested repair of the typical cleft prior to correction of the macrostomia.[10] This is felt to reestablish balance of the upper and lower lips, which is an important initial step, that may then be followed by transverse cleft repair in a reasonable amount of time.

POSTOPERATIVE CARE

Following surgery, the patient is placed in a monitored unit at least overnight and given intravenous and parenteral pain medication as needed. Oral feeds, as pre-operatively administered, are provided when the infant is awake enough to tolerate. Instructions to place the nipple on the contralateral side of the mouth and away from the surgical site are provided. A routine pre-operative dose of a first-generation cephalosporin is given; however, routine postoperative antibiotics are not utilized. Wound care consists of preventing crusting and scabbing by carefully cleansing the wound with half-strength peroxide on a cotton-tip applicator, followed by a light layer of topical antibiotic ointment. If skin sutures were placed during the procedure, these are removed in the office 4 or 5 days later. The child is brought to the office in the morning for suture removal, having had the routine and feeding withheld; and, when given a bottle and preoccupied with feeding, suture removal can be performed with little difficulty. After complete cutaneous healing, approximately 1–2 weeks following surgery, scar massage can begin. The child then receives routine follow-up through the cleft-craniofacial center as any child with an orofacial cleft. Note example of patient example with a right-sided lateral facial cleft with 1-year follow-up at the cleft-craniofacial center (Fig. 28–15).

COMPLICATIONS

The most worrisome early complication following repair of the transverse facial cleft is dehiscence at the surgical site. Numerous case series report their results with the repair of transverse facial clefts, and uniformly describe good results; however, the number of cases is comparatively low. The disheartening early complication of hypertrophic scaring is difficult to prevent and treat. Early aggressive scar management with massage, silicone gel sheeting, and/or local steroids may be offered. Later, lateral displacement of the commissure may occur with healing at the surgical site due to linear scar contracture.[15,16,17] Should this lateral commissure displacement occur, a scar revision may be performed, and the addition of a Z-plasty may be performed if not done at the primary surgery.

References

1. Stark RB, Saunders DE. The first branchial arch syndrome. *Plast Reconstr Surg* 29:229, 1962.
2. Powell WJ, Jenkins HP. Transverse facial clefts. *Plast Reconstr Surg* 42:454, 1968.
3. Onizuka T. Treatment of the deformities of the mouth corner. *Jap J Plast Reconstr Surg* 8:132, 1965.
4. Anderson R, Kurtay M. Reconstruction of the corner of the mouth. *Plast Reconstr Surg* 4:463, 1971.
5. Habal MB, Scheuerle J. Lateral facial clefts: Closure with W-plasty and implications of speech and language development. *Ann Plast Surg* 11:182, 1983.
6. May H. Transverse facial clefts and their repair. *Plast Reconstr Surg* 29:240, 1962.
7. Longacre JJ, deStefano GA, Holmstrand KE. The surgical management of first and second branchial arch syndromes. *Plast Reconstr Surg* 31:507, 1963.
8. Torkut A, Coskunfirat OK. Double reversing Z-plasty for correction of transverse facial cleft. *Plast Reconstr Surg* 99(3):885, 1997.
9. Fukada O, Takeda H. Advancement of oral commissure in correcting mild macrostomia. *Ann Plast Surg* 14:205, 1985.
10. Eguchi T, Asato H, Takushima A, Takato T, Harii K. Surgical repair for congenital macrostomia: Vermilion square flap method. *Ann Plast Surg* 47:6, 2001.
11. Kaplan, EN. Commissuroplasty and myoplasty for macrostomia. *Ann Plast Surg* 7(2):136–144, 1981.
12. Boo-Chai K. The transverse facial cleft: Its repair. *Br J Plast Surg* 29:119, 1962.
13. Cervenka J, Gorlin R, Anderson V. The syndrome of pits of the lower lip and cleft lip and/or palate: Genetic considerations. *Am J Hum Genet* 19:416, 1967.
14. Fukada O, Takeda H. Advancement of oral commissure in correcting mild macrostomia. *Ann Plast Surg* 14:205, 1985.
15. Boo-Kai K. The transverse facial cleft: Its repair. *Br J Plast Surg* 29:119, 1962.
16. Nagia I, Weinstein I. Surgical repair of horizontal facial cleft: Report of a case. *J Oral Surg* 21:251, 1963.
17. Aketa J, Kuga Y, Yamada N, et al. A method for the repair of transverse facial clefts. *Cleft Palate J* 17:235, 1980.

Secondary Cleft Lip and Palate Repair

29

Complications of Cleft Lip and Palate Surgery

John F. Reinisch, MD, FACS • Wai-Yee Ii, MB ChB • Mark Urata, MD, DDS

INTRODUCTION

Cleft lip with or without cleft palate is one of the most common congenital malformations in humans, with an incidence of up to 1 in 500 live births.[1-3] The goal of surgical treatment is the restoration of function and appearance. The procedures to repair cleft lip and palate have many variations.[4] This chapter will discuss the common complications that may arise following lip and palate repair. With a better understanding of these complications, the majority can be avoided. Complications can be considered in terms of timing, i.e. early and late, as well as those specifically related to cleft lip and cleft palate repair, respectively.

CLEFT LIP REPAIR

Preoperative work up for cleft lip repair varies by institution and country. Unless there are specific clinical indications (anemia, clotting disorder), the authors do not routinely obtain preoperative blood work. Length of hospitalization postoperatively also varies significantly.[5-7] For over two decades, unilateral and bilateral cleft lip repair at our facility have been successfully performed as an outpatient procedure. In a recent study of complications of 155 cleft lip patients, there were no significant difference in outcome reported between inpatient and outpatient cleft lip repairs.[8]

EARLY COMPLICATIONS

In cleft lip repair, a number of early complications may arise during the first 2 weeks following surgery. These complications include: bleeding, wound infection, wound dehiscence, nasal airway obstruction, and flap necrosis.

Bleeding

Following cleft lip repair, significant bleeding is unusual.[6,9] We have not had to perform blood transfusion in children following cleft lip surgery. Early postoperative bleeding is readily observed and easily controlled with direct pressure.[6] In our study of 157 cleft lip repairs, we found one patient who presented 2 days postsurgery with epistaxis and bleeding in the mouth.[8] This patient was evaluated in the emergency room and sent home without any further intervention. It is likely that this bleeding resulted from the relatively blind dissection of the nasal cartilages, which is done if the cleft lip is associated with marked cleft nasal distortion.

Wound Infection

Postoperative infection in cleft lip is unusual. *Reinisch and Sloan* reported an incidence of 2.3% in 132 cases of cleft lip repair.[10] All cases resolved with oral antibiotics, without any wound separation or unsatisfactory scarring. We give a single dose of intravenous prophylactic antibiotics at the time of anesthesia induction, followed by 5 days of oral suspension postoperatively. All patients are seen within a week of surgery and advised to call us if there is any significant redness or swelling. In patients with cardiac defects, we follow the prophylactic antibiotics policy as recommended by the American Heart Association. Localized infection from a buried suture is occasionally seen and should be treated with suture removal, since prolonged inflammation can lead to hypertrophic scarring.

Wound Dehiscence

Wound dehiscence is a rare complication in unilateral cleft lip repair. Because of greater tension secondary to a protruding premaxilla, the incidence is higher in patients having had bilateral cleft lip repair.[10] For unilateral and bilateral cleft lip repair there is an overall reported incidence ranging from 1% to 7.4%.[11-14] In our experience, the majority of patients with wound dehiscence following cleft lip repair are older, more mobile infants, with a higher risk of causing direct trauma

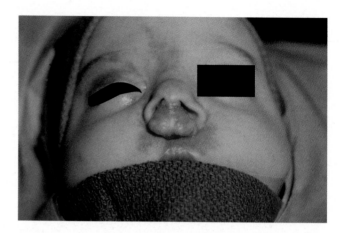

Figure 29–1. Protrusion of the premaxilla at the junction of the lip and nose. The intact repair is seen posterior to the premaxilla. The redness of the lip is a vascular birthmark.

to the early repair. Despite this, we still advocate outpatient surgery in these children, feeling that keeping such patients in hospital overnight or longer would not prevent this from occurring. We advise parents of older infants of the increased risk of traumatic wound separation. In children with a prominent premaxillary segment, we have seen dehiscence of the upper lip with protrusion of the premaxilla at the junction of the lip and nose (Fig. 29–1). While the lip repair remained intact, inferior migration resulted in the repair coming to lie posterior to the protruding premaxilla. Placing a suture to anchor the repaired upper lip to the nasal spine can reduce this tendency for inferior migration. The increasing use of preoperative nasoalveolar molding should minimize the likelihood of lip separation by reducing lip tension prior to repair.

Nasal Airway Obstruction

Following cleft lip surgery, nasal airway obstruction can occur from nostril narrowing, postoperative edema, or clotted blood in the vestibule. This can cause breathing difficulties in young infants who are obligate nasal breathers. With negative inspiratory pressure, breathing difficulties may occur because the floppy lower lip has a tendency to seal against the upper lip. One can minimize this problem by hyperextension of the neck or stiffening the lower lip by applying layers of adhesive tape. During the first few days after surgery, cleansing the nose of dried blood is helpful and can improve feeding.

Flap Necrosis

For unilateral cleft lip, we use a modified rotation-advancement repair and have not seen necrosis of this flap. For bilateral cleft lip, we advocate simultaneous repair of both sides in one-stage to achieve optimum symmetry. In order to mimic the natural philtrum, we design our prolabial flap to be narrower at the superior base. We also tend to make the flap narrow, as the philtrum has a tendency to widen. Caution must be taken to avoid over-thinning the flap or inadvertent injury to the superior pedicle. When flap necrosis does occur, we recommend the use of topical antibiotics until the necrotic area has declared itself. Skin loss is usually minor and the lip generally heals without the need for further intervention. Delayed healing increases the risk of hypertrophic scarring. Only in cases of significant skin loss, would we replace the missing tissue with a full-thickness skin graft from the posterior auricular region or an Abbé flap.

LATE COMPLICATIONS

The late complications of cleft lip repair are seen after the immediate postoperative period (i.e., 2 weeks postsurgery) and are generally esthetic in nature. They tend to be iatrogenic, resulting from avoidable errors of planning or execution. Since patients wear these complications so prominently, a surgeon should learn to avoid or minimize their occurrence. Although subsequent revision surgery can be performed, the result is rarely comparable to a well-performed initial procedure. These late complications include deformities of the lip, muscle, and nose.

Lip Deformities

The upper lip is an important landmark of the face and the maintenance of symmetry is critical for a successful cleft lip repair. Lip deformities can be divided into vertical height discrepancies, tissue mismatch, muscle deformities, and external scars.

Vertical Height Discrepancy

In order to achieve a natural appearing lip, the vertical height of the vermilion–cutaneous junction must be aligned, and the peak of Cupid's bow on the cleft side placed level with the corresponding peak of the normal side. During the first few months postsurgery, scar contracture and lip shortening can occur and may be worrisome to parents. If the height of the repaired side of the lip was adequate at the time of surgery, it usually resumes the on-table result, as the scar tissue matures and softens. Occasionally, lip scar contraction can be extreme and permanently ruin the appearance of the lip (Fig. 29–2). Excision of the scar and revision of the lip is necessary in these unusual cases. Relatively normal scar healing can occur following revision of these cases; however, we routinely use immediate postoperative radiation in these cases.

The lower border of the upper lip vermilion should be even, without notching, thinning, or excess fullness. Since the red vermilion sits anterior to the white teeth, this contrast makes any vermilion asymmetry very noticeable. Many surgeons, in an effort to preserve as much tissue as possible, tend to mark the vermilion more centrally, where the vermilion is thinner. If this is done, approximating these thinner segments of vermilion will result in vermilion notching (Fig. 29–3). To avoid this, we recommend marking the vermilion slightly more lateral, where it is thicker. Approximation of these segments will then result in a more uniform vermilion appearance. It is helpful to mark and align the junction between the dry vermilion and the wet mucosa of the lip. The vertical height of the dry vermilion is frequently deficient on the medial segment. A flap of dry vermilion from the lateral segment can be used to augment the vertical height of the central lip and improve symmetry.[15] If notching does occur and is identified at the time of the lip repair, it can be remedied either by incising the flaps more laterally and re-approximating the lip, or by performing a vermilion Z-plasty.

In bilateral cleft lip repair, central vermilion thinness is seen frequently in procedures where the vermilion of the prolabium is preserved in the central lip. Even when the prolabial vermilion is replaced by vermilion from each lateral

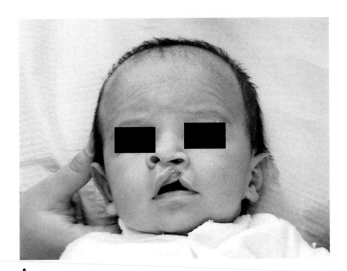

A

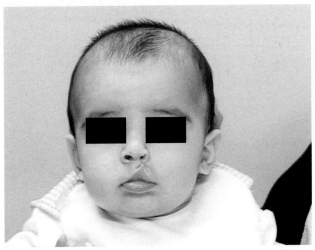

B

Figure 29–2. Left unilateral cleft lip with excessive scar contracture, unrelated to postoperative infection or tissue loss. (A) Preoperative and (B) postoperative showing scar contracture.

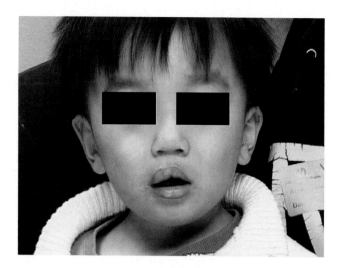

Figure 29–3. Vermillion notching.

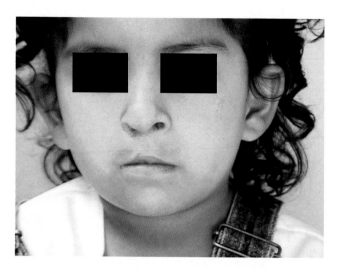

Figure 29–5. Misalignment of the white roll.

lip segment, there is a tendency to get some central vermilion thinning, the so-called "whistle deformity"[16] (Fig. 29–4). When the lateral lip segments are used, more vermilion will be available for central tubercle reconstruction. It is important to compensate for thinning of the central vermilion by creating an excessively full tubercle at the end of the procedure, with the knowledge that the tubercle will thin during the first week or two after surgery. Leaving apparent excess central tissue is usually difficult for plastic surgeons, who tend to seek a perfect result when the patient leaves the operating room. In comparison with vermilion deficiency, excess vermilion is rarely a problem and can be easily corrected if necessary.

Tissue Mismatch

Mismatch occurs when tissues with different characteristics are approximated. These tend to be iatrogenic, occurring as

a result of poor planning or execution by the surgeon. Mismatch of the white roll is a common and noticeable complication of cleft lip repair (Fig. 29–5). The chance of this occurring can be minimized by tattooing the superior and inferior margins of the white roll, prior to infiltration with local anesthetic. The use of marks above and below the white roll, on each lip segment, allows accurate alignment of this visually important structure. This "four-mark" method has also been useful in the occasional instances in which one tattoo mark is difficult to see or has been inadvertently excised.

Poor alignment can also occur when approximating the wet and dry portions of the vermilion. This can manifest itself either by contrast in color or in peeling and scaling of the vermilion. Color mismatch can occur when the central lip is composed of prolabial vermilion, which occasionally is of a different color than the lateral segment vermilion (see Fig. 29–4). This can be overcome by discarding the prolabial

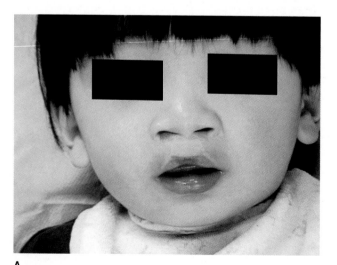

A

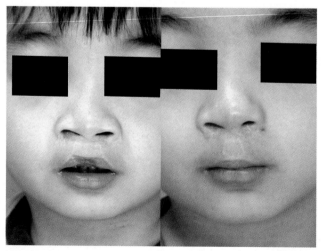

B

Figure 29–4. (A) Whistle deformity showing the different color of the prolabial vermilion retained in this cleft lip repair. (B) Same patient, preoperatively and following postoperative correction, with narrowing of the philtrum and use of the lateral segment vermillion flaps to replace the original prolabial vermilion.

vermilion, and moving the vermilion from the lateral segments beneath the cutaneous part of the philtrum and suturing it in the midline. Peeling and scaling of the lip is observed when the wet portions of the vermilion are exposed and allowed to dry. This mismatch can be avoided by recognizing the distinct characteristics of these regions within the vermilion, aligning them accordingly, and preventing exposure of the wet vermilion.

Muscle Deformity

During cleft lip repair, the main emphasis has been on the skin incision and reconstruction. Recently, the importance of an accurate and sturdy repair of the orbicularis oris muscle has come to light.[17,18] It is now known that an inadequate muscle repair will cause the upper lips to undergo abnormal shape change, particularly during animation, with the appearance of lateral bulging. This problem, seen more frequently in bilateral cleft lip repairs, can be prevented by adequate muscle dissection and careful suturing with permanent material, such as nylon. In addition, a good muscle repair will minimize tension on the skin closure, as discussed below.

External Scars

The lips are generally sites of good wound healing and scar formation. The majority of complications relating to scars from cleft lip repair are due to the thickness and location of the scar.

Fortunately, the vermilion tends to heal with minimal adverse scar formation, and hypertrophic scarring is a rare event. However, scarring of the skin above the vermilion is not uncommon and can detract from a good repair. Feeling that dermal trauma can increase the risk of adverse scarring, we avoid external sutures by using individual subcuticular sutures. This has the added advantage of not having to remove fine sutures from a young and often uncooperative patient. Furthermore, we can minimize the number of buried dermal sutures, through a good muscle closure. Tensionless skin approximation can be achieved by first resecting 3–4 mm from the medial edges of the orbicularis oris. Approximation of the shortened muscle will then bring the skin together, minimizing the need for dermal sutures.

The location of a lip repair scar should be designed to mirror the normal philtral column. A common error is to place the medial lip marking exactly where the philtral column should be, without considering the pull of the lateral segment once the repair is completed. In this scenario, the scar ends up being too lateral to mimic the philtral column (Fig. 29–6). To avoid this, the authors compensate by placing the lip incision slightly more medially, anticipating that the lateral segment will pull the lip scar into a more natural position once healed.

Nasal Deformity

The cleft lip nasal deformity is worthy of a chapter in itself and will not be discussed in great detail here. While the nasal

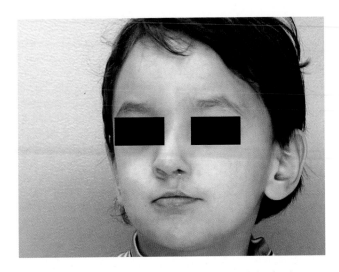

Figure 29–6. Lip scar asymmetric to normal philtral column.

deformity is determined by the initial severity of the cleft lip, the cleft lip repair can improve or even worsen the nasal appearance. How much of the nasal deformity is tackled during the initial cleft lip repair varies by the surgeon's preference and experience. Recent studies suggest that the conventional fear of radical nasal correction resulting in growth retardation in the younger patient appear unfounded.[19–21] While there is little data to support a superior outcome between initial or delayed nasal reconstruction, advocates for the former justify early correction based upon the psychosocial benefits to the patient and their families.[21] However, aggressive nostril dissection can lead to nostril stenosis.

Nostril Stenosis

Distortion of the nasal tip cartilages accompanies the cleft lip deformity. Most surgeons attempt some degree of nasal tip correction at the time of cleft lip repair and will have occasionally experienced nostril stenosis as a complication (Fig. 29–7). This is a very difficult problem to manage successfully.

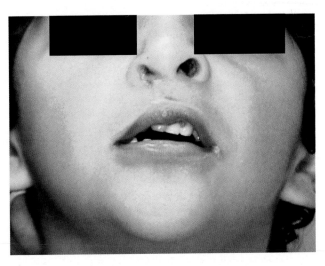

Figure 29–7. Right nostril stenosis.

Nostril stents are frequently used after nasal tip reconstruction. However, the length of time required to prevent nostril contraction (several months) is generally longer than the stents that can be maintained in place. The risk of stenosis is proportionate to the degree to which the vestibular lining is disturbed. Surgeons who have experienced significant nostril stenosis generally have tempered their initial enthusiasm for aggressive dissection of the vestibular lining. Correction of nostril stenosis has been attempted using local flaps and grafts, with varying degrees of success.[22–25]

CLEFT PALATE REPAIR

Cleft palate closure can be performed at the same time as cleft lip repair, but is generally done as a separate procedure, months after the cleft lip repair. Unlike repair of the cleft lip, palatoplasty is never carried out as an outpatient procedure because of the potential for significant early complications.

Early Complications

The early complications following cleft palate repair occur during the first week after surgery. The principle complications are bleeding, airway obstruction, and poor feeding. A less common early complication can be traumatic disruption. A child with a feeding tube and a tracheostomy would be an ideal patient for a palatoplasty since feeding and airway obstruction would not be problematic.

Bleeding

Bleeding usually occurs immediately following repair. It rarely occurs as a delayed event without preceding trauma. Prior to extubation, careful inspection of the palate and suctioning of the stomach needs to be carried out. If oozing is seen at this point, gentle palatal pressure can be applied to control the bleeding. Once the patient is extubated and in the recovery room, slow palatal bleeding can go undetected until hematemesis occurs. Therefore, it is important to place the patient in a prone position while in the recovery room, to more quickly identify postoperative bleeding. Rarely, bleeding requires a return to the operating room for control under anesthesia.

Airway Obstruction

Airway obstruction is the most important early complication following palatoplasty. Postoperative edema is the principle cause of airway obstruction. This is more likely to occur in children who have an anatomic tendency for airway obstruction, such as those with Pierre-Robin sequence. In a study of 247 patients, using the Furlow repair, 14 (5.7%) patients were reported to have perioperative or postoperative airway compromise.[26] Half of these patients with airway obstruction following cleft palate repair had Pierre-Robin sequence. All cases occurred during the first 48 hours of surgery, with

8 (57%) occurring in the operating room upon extubation. Mild to moderate postoperative airways obstruction can be improved with the temporary placement of a nasopharyngeal tube, which can be removed once the patient is more alert.

Severe tongue swelling from the use of a mouth gag during surgery can cause airway obstruction and require reintubation. Postoperatively, some surgeons place a tongue suture to allow traction in the event of significant tongue swelling. Others will routinely admit children to the intensive care unit for postoperative monitoring. The authors have found that tongue swelling can be virtually eliminated by simply releasing the gag every 30–40 minutes during surgery for a 5 minutes period, thus limiting the length of time the tongue is continuously compressed. The majority of cases of postoperative airways obstruction is temporary and resolves as postoperative swelling subsides.

Poor Feeding

Following palatoplasty, poor feeding is expected. All our cleft palate patients receive fluids, antibiotics, and analgesia intravenously. While the infiltration of long-acting local anesthetic to the surgery site at the end of the operation minimizes discomfort, we have not found that it significantly improves oral intake in these patients. Our practice is to encourage oral intake as soon as possible, using the same nipple and bottle as the patient and their parents used preoperatively. Many surgeons discharge patients only after oral intake in the hospital is sufficient, resulting in a 2–4 day stay after palatoplasty. Often, intravenous fluids have to be reduced in order to encourage oral intake. For the last decade, we have discharged patients on the morning following palate repair, provided there are no signs of bleeding or airways obstruction, placing less emphasis on oral intake. These infants begin feeding later that same afternoon at home. Although their oral intake is still reduced at this point, hydration is not usually a problem because they have received overnight intravenous fluids. Oral feeding continues to improve thereafter and we have not had to readmit any patients for rehydration using this protocol.

Wound Dehiscence

Wound dehiscence can occur following palatoplasty. Although it can be caused by excessive tension due to inadequate dissection, dehiscence is usually a result of direct trauma. Parents are cautioned against placing anything in the mouth that can cause injury to the healing palate. We have not seen wound dehiscence resulting from the use of a feeding nipple. Long objects such as pens, pencils, and straws should be kept away from the child to minimize the risk of injury during the first month after surgery. A low-grade fever following cleft palate repair will frequently bring the patient to their pediatrician or emergency room. Parents should be warned against allowing medical personnel to use a tongue depressor during examination, which could disrupt a recently repaired palate. If wound dehiscence occurs, we would allow the tissues to heal before attempting a secondary palatoplasty.

LATE COMPLICATIONS

The late complications of cleft palate repair are seen after the first postoperative week. They include: oro-nasal fistula, velo-pharyngeal incompetence, tooth bud injury, and maxillary growth disturbance. Velo-pharyngeal incompetence is a large topic and beyond the scope of this chapter.

Oro-nasal Fistula

Fistulae vary in severity and clinical presentation. They can be very large, resulting from dehiscence or tissue loss, or so small that they are only detectable years later, following palatal expansion in preparation for bone grafting. Fistula formation may result in fluid and food regurgitation into the nasal cavity, as well as speech difficulties secondary to nasal air escape. The severity of the symptoms is directly related to the size of the fistula. The ability to accurately detect the presence of a fistula varies since small ones are often asymptomatic. This may account for the reported incidence of fistula formation following palatoplasty ranging from 0 to 63%.[27] The main factors believed to influence this incidence include the experience of the surgeon,[27,28] the severity of the initial cleft, and the repair procedure employed.[29] In a recent study, the highest fistula rate was seen with pushback repairs, followed by von Langenbeck and then Furlow palatoplasty.[29] The same study reported that close to 90% of fistulas are found in the area of the hard palate closure, and half are found immediately posterior to the alveolus.

It is far better to perform a sound initial repair than to revise a fistula once formed, as subsequent closure of a palatal fistula has a high recurrence rate. Following initial fistula repair, Cohen et al. reported a recurrence rate of 37%, while Muzaffar et al. reported a rate of 33%.[29,30]

Tooth Bud Injury

Elevation of the mucoperiosteum can cause inadvertent injury to the tooth buds of the primary teeth. Although primary teeth are not permanent, this injury should be avoided as the primary teeth act as space maintainers and guide the future eruption of the permanent teeth.

Damage to developing teeth is most likely to occur at the time of gingivoperiostealplasty or palatoplasty. If gingivoperiostealplasty is performed at 3 months of age, the typical time of cleft lip repair, care must be taken to avoid damage to the developing deciduous central and lateral incisors. The central and lateral incisors will complete their crown development at approximately 2.5 months, but will remain unerupted until 10–11 months of age.[31] There is usually little to no bone over the unerupted crown, and inadvertent dissection into the surrounding follicle may disturb the early root formation. Dissection with periosteal elevators from a superior to inferior direction will reduce the potential of injury to the tooth bud.

Similarly, when performing a palatoplasty between 10 and 14 months of age, the maxillary central and lateral incisors are usually erupted in the mouth. The primary first molars will erupt around 16 months of age and lie directly under the gingiva, protected only by their follicle, with no overlying bone.[32] Incisions and dissection over the alveolar ridge can place the tooth follicles at risk. To avoid this, we prefer to make our palatal incisions just medial or lingual to the crest of the alveolus, theoretically preserving the periodontal ligaments of the teeth. We initiate our dissection posterior to the erupted central and lateral incisors, as this is a dentally "safe" zone. By elevating the central palate first, followed by a sweeping motion with our elevators laterally and caudally, we avoid entering the follicles of the unerupted molars.

If a tooth or follicle is inadvertently avulsed, it should be placed back into its bony socket, with the original orientation, as soon as possible. Local gingival flaps or sutures through the neighboring bone are then used to secure the avulsed structure. Eventually, referral to a pediatric dentist is recommended in order to monitor teeth eruption.

Maxillary Growth Disturbance

Maxillary growth disturbance as a result of surgical repair of cleft lip and palate has been a subject of debate for some time. It is thought by many that this is a consequence of tissue fibrosis, which is directly related to lip repair and/or stripping of the mucoperiosteum during palate repair. Ortiz-Monasterio et al. studied untreated adults with complete cleft lip/palate and found that maxillary growth was normal, but they did not have a control group and the cohort consisted of only 14 patients.[33] Using surgically created cleft lip and palate in beagles, Bardach accumulated a wealth of data. His important conclusions include: Repair of cleft lip and palate results in increased lip pressure,[34] maxillary growth inhibition was related to the degree of mucoperiosteum stripping,[35] and that the sequence of cleft lip and palate repair was related to the degree of maxillary growth inhibition. The latter study showed that repairing the lip first, followed by the palate, resulted in the least inhibition, compared to either palate repair first or simultaneous lip and palate repair.[35]

Kapacu et al. compared adults with unilateral cleft lip and palate who had lip repair only with those who had undergone lip and palate repair during childhood.[36] They concluded that both groups had significant maxillary retrusion compared with the noncleft controls, but there was no difference between lip repair alone or lip and palate repair. This suggests that maxillary retrusion, resulting from cleft lip repair alone, is not compounded by palate repair. However, since palate repair is not routinely carried out without lip repair, there are no available studies with a group having undergone isolated palate repair for comparison. Another possible explanation is that perhaps both lip repair and palate repair contribute equally to maxillary retrusion, but one procedure alone may result in maximal maxillary growth disturbance, thus masking the effects of any additional factors.

Overall, it can be concluded that abnormalities in craniofacial development seen in children and adults with operated clefts result from intrinsic and iatrogenic factors. It must be remembered that in animals with surgically created clefts one is ignoring the intrinsic patient factors: i.e. any innate abnormal craniofacial growth pattern that may occur in children with cleft lip and palate. However, findings from these studies suggest that to minimize maxillary growth disturbance, it would be prudent to repair the lip first, followed by the palate: and, be mindful to minimize stripping of the mucoperiosteum as much as possible.

When it does occur, maxillary growth disturbance is generally seen late, but in severe cases can present in the first several years after surgery. It can adversely affect appearance, mastication, and speech. In most cases, orthodontic manipulation and orthognathic surgery can be used successfully to compensate for the resultant growth deficiency.

CONCLUSION

In conclusion, the spectrum of complications related to cleft lip and palate surgery is fairly well defined and has been experienced by all cleft surgeons. With increased clinical experience, the frequency and severity of these complications can be minimized. Generally, the initial repair is most likely to yield success and is worthy of careful planning to achieve the optimum result.

References

1. Chung CS, Myrianthopoulos NC. Racial and prenatal factors in major congenital malformations. *Am J Hum Genet* 20:44, 1968.
2. Fraser FC. The genetics of cleft lip and cleft palate. *Am J Hum Genet* 22:336–352, 1970.
3. Neel JV. A study of major congenital defects in Japanese infants. *Am J Hum Genet* 10:398, 1958.
4. Sadove AM, van Aalst JA, Culp JA. Cleft palate repair: Art and issues. *Clin Plast Surg* 31:231–241, 2004.
5. Lees VC, Pigott RW. Early postoperative complications in primary cleft lip and palate surgery – how soon may we discharge patients from hospital? *Br J Plast Surg* 45:232–234, 1992.
6. Demay A, Vadoud-Seyedi J, Demol F, Govaerts M. Early postoperative complications in primary cleft lip and palate surgery. *Eur J Plast Surg* 20:77–79, 1997.
7. Eaton AC, Marsh JL, Pilgram TK. Does reduced hospital stay affect morbidity and mortality rates following cleft lip and palate repair in infancy? *Plast Reconstr Surg* 94:911–915;discussion 16–18, 1994.
8. Rosen H, Barrios LM, Reinisch JF, Macgill K, Meara JG. Outpatient cleft lip repair. *Plast Reconstr Surg* 112:381–387;discussion 88–89, 2003.
9. Dingman RO, Ricker L, Lob V. Blood loss in infant cleft lip and palate surgery. *Plast Reconstr Surg* 4:333, 1949.
10. Reinisch JF, Sloan GM. Complications of cleft lip repair. In Bardach JaM H (ed). *Multidisciplinary Management of Cleft Lip and Palate*. Philadelphia: Saunders, 1990, pp. 247–252.
11. Schettler D. Intra- and postoperative complications in surgical repair of clefts in infancy. *J Maxillofac Surg* 1:40–44, 1973.
12. Weatherley-White RC, Kuehn DP, Mirrett P, Gilman JI, Weatherley-White CC. Early repair and breast-feeding for infants with cleft lip. *Plast Reconstr Surg* 79:879–887, 1987.

13. Wilhelmsen HR, Musgrave RH. Complications of cleft lip surgery. *Cleft Palate J* 3:223–231, 1966.
14. Bromley GS, Rothaus KO, Goulian D, Jr. Cleft lip: Morbidity and mortality in early repair. *Ann Plast Surg* 10:214–217, 1983.
15. Fisher DM. Unilateral cleft lip repair: An anatomical subunit approximation technique. *Plast Reconstr Surg* 116:61–71, 2005.
16. Holmstrom H. The Abbe island flap for the correction of whistle deformity. *Br J Plast Surg* 40:176–180, 1987.
17. Park CG, Ha B. The importance of accurate repair of the orbicularis oris muscle in the correction of unilateral cleft lip. *Plast Reconstr Surg* 96:780–788, 1995.
18. Schendel SA. Unilateral cleft lip repair – state of the art. *Cleft Palate Craniofac J* 37:335–341, 2000.
19. Mulliken JB. Repair of bilateral complete cleft lip and nasal deformity – state of the art. *Cleft Palate Craniofac J* 37:342–347, 2000.
20. Thomas C, Mishra P. Open tip rhinoplasty along with the repair of cleft lip in cleft lip and palate cases. *Br J Plast Surg* 53:1–6, 2000.
21. Nakajima T, Ogata H, Sakuma H. Long-term outcome of simultaneous repair of bilateral cleft lip and nose (a 15 year experience). *Br J Plast Surg* 56:205–217, 2003.
22. Blandini D, Tremolada C, Beretta M, Mascetti M. Iatrogenic nostril stenosis: Aesthetic correction using a vestibular labial mucosa flap. *Plast Reconstr Surg* 95:569–571, 1995.
23. Aydogdu E, Akan M, Gideroglu K, Akoz T. Alar transposition flap for stenosis of the nostril. *Scand J Plast Reconstr Surg Hand Surg* 40:311–314, 2006.
24. Constantian MB. An alar base flap to correct nostril and vestibular stenosis and alar base malposition in rhinoplasty. *Plast Reconstr Surg* 101:1666–1674, 1998.
25. al-Qattan MM, Robertson GA. Acquired nostril stenosis. *Ann Plast Surg* 27:382–386, 1991.
26. Antony AK, Sloan GM. Airway obstruction following palatoplasty: Analysis of 247 consecutive operations. *Cleft Palate Craniofac J* 39:145–148, 2002.
27. Emory RE, Jr., Clay RP, Bite U, Jackson IT. Fistula formation and repair after palatal closure: An institutional perspective. *Plast Reconstr Surg* 99:1535–1538, 1997.
28. Shaw WC, Dahl E, Asher-McDade C, et al. A six-center international study of treatment outcome in patients with clefts of the lip and palate: Part 5. General discussion and conclusions. *Cleft Palate Craniofac J* 29:413–418, 1992.
29. Cohen SR, Kalinowski J, LaRossa D, Randall P. Cleft palate fistulas: A multivariate statistical analysis of prevalence, etiology, and surgical management. *Plast Reconstr Surg* 87:1041–1047, 1991.
30. Muzaffar AR, Byrd HS, Rohrich RJ, et al. Incidence of cleft palate fistula: An institutional experience with two-stage palatal repair. *Plast Reconstr Surg* 108:1515–1518, 2001.
31. Ten Cate AR. *Oral Histology: Development, Structure and Function*, 5th edn. St Louis, Mosby, 1998.
32. Harris EF. Tooth eruption. In *Craniofacial Growth and Development*. 2002. Wheeler's Dental Anatomy, Physiology, and Occlusion. 8th edn., Eds Ash and Nelson, Philadelphia: W.B. Saunders, 2003, p. 53.
33. Ortiz-Monasterio F, Serrano A, Barrera G, Rodriguez-Hoffman H, Vinageras E. A study of untreated adult cleft palate patients. *Plast Reconstr Surg* 38:36–41, 1966.
34. Bardach J, Mooney MP. The relationship between lip pressure following lip repair and craniofacial growth: An experimental study in beagles. *Plast Reconstr Surg* 73:544–555, 1984.
35. Bardach J, Kelly KM, Salyer KE. Relationship between the sequence of lip and palate repair and maxillary growth: An experimental study in beagles. *Plast Reconstr Surg* 93:269–278, 1994.
36. Kapucu MR, Gursu KG, Enacar A, Aras S. The effect of cleft lip repair on maxillary morphology in patients with unilateral complete cleft lip and palate. *Plast Reconstr Surg* 97:1371–1375;discussion 76–78, 1996.

30

Correction of Secondary Unilateral Cleft Lip and Nose Deformity

H. Steve Byrd, MD • Kusai A. El-Musa, MD • Arjang Yazdani, MD

INTRODUCTION

Major advances have been made in cleft care in the past 50 years. Deformity can consistently be transformed early in life to minimal or residual variations from normal, so that predictable outcomes for patients with unilateral cleft lip and cleft nasal deformity can be achieved. Normal appearance and function is a realistic treatment goal.

Despite careful planning and constant effort by the surgeon to achieve the best possible result in the primary operation of a cleft, secondary cleft deformities are frequent events, occurring 35–75% of the time,[1,2] and even higher in the cleft nose deformity. They are referred to, by multiple authors, as the "rule rather than exception."[3,4] Secondary deformities are both intrinsic to the anomaly and iatrogenic as well.[3] The causes include lack of surgeon experience, deficiencies of tissues, individual scar formation, and the effects of facial growth. The best treatment for secondary deformities of the cleft lip and nose is prevention at the initial operation, when every effort should be made to achieve a balanced correction of the lip and nose.[3]

SECONDARY UNILATERAL CHEILOPLASTY

Introduction

Knowledge of normal lip and nasal anatomy is essential for an understanding of the distortion caused by a facial cleft. The most important element of a cleft repair is realignment of the muscles. Accurate release and realignment of the muscles comprising the lip and nose are key features in the correction of both the primary and secondary cleft lip and nasal deformity. The ideal lip repair results in symmetrically shaped nostrils, nasal sills and alar bases, a well-defined philtral dimple and columns, and a natural appearing cupid's bow with a pout to the vermilion tubercle. In addition, it results in a functional muscle repair that with animation mimics a normal lip. While ideally the lip scars approximate natural landmarks, ultimately the eye first focuses on symmetry and then normal contours of the lip at rest and in animation. The fullness and shape of the free border of the upper lip is a key to these contours.[5,6]

Analysis of Secondary Cleft Lip Deformities

When we analyze the secondary cleft lip deformity, we have to consider multiple aspects in these patients: the degree of asymmetry, the type of primary cleft repair,[7–15] the presence of underlying skeletal deformity, and the degree of soft tissue deficiency contributing to the deformity. Although anthropometric knowledge may be used consciously or unconsciously during planning and evaluation of treatment by plastic surgeons, Vegter and Hage[16] could find no evidence that patients have an anthropometric interest in their appearance. When asking for correction of the lip, for example, the patient may not want the shortness or flatness to be corrected but, rather, may want to correct an irregular vermilion border or scar. Even though we may not be content with residual stigmata in our patients, it is the patient who decides whether and which further corrections are indicated. Careful recording of the patient's history and objectives will prevent misjudgments and mistreatment by the surgeon.[16]

Before embarking on secondary surgery for the cleft deformity, the surgeon must accurately diagnose all problems associated with the lip. The examiner must note the lip scar, the status of the orbicularis muscle, the orientation of the vermilion and white roll, the Cupid's bow, and the mucosa. Skeletal imbalance from maxillary hypoplasia contributes significantly to the secondary problems commonly seen after initial lip repair.[17]

Once the deformity has been accurately diagnosed, one must make every effort to determine the underlying cause. Although hypoplasia and distortion occur as a result of the malformation, and set the stage for many of the commonly seen secondary deformities, poor preoperative design of the primary operation contributes as well. For example, a short lip may be caused by something as simple as a tight contracted scar. On the other hand, underrotation of the initial lip repair may be the source of the problem, as may be failure to anatomically reunite the underlying orbicularis. The design of the secondary surgery should be focused to correct the specific problem. The solution must take into account the soft tissue, muscle, and the underlying skeleton. Addressing all short lips with the same operation is not sufficient.

Numerous classification schemes have been devised to simplify the evaluation of secondary cleft lip and nasal deformities.[18] However, they tend to be very cumbersome and do very little to facilitate the diagnosis and its underlying cause.[19,20]

Determining the age to surgically intervene is an important component of a successful outcome. The timing of the surgical intervention should be predicated on the severity of the deformity, the psychosocial and functional effect of the deformity on the child, the stage of facial growth, and the expected effects of such growth on the repair.[21] The need for further surgeries at the completion of growth and the timing of other cleft-related surgical procedures (i.e., cleft palate repair, pharyngeal flap, alveolar cleft repair with bone graft, maxillary LeFort I advancement, and rhinoplasty) may also contribute to timing of revisional surgery. The most common age for revisional soft-tissue surgery, in our practice, is in the preschool period from 5 to 6 years of age. The goal is to achieve a socially acceptable appearance by the second grade (7–8 years of age), when peer interactions change from awareness and curiosity to harmful teasing and ostracism. Another common period for surgical correction is during early adolescence. Post-pubescent development may enhance the deformity through asymmetric growth threatening the child's self esteem at this vulnerable age.

Deformities of the Vermilion Border, White Roll, and Cupid's Bow

The vermilion border, the distinct convex white roll, and the precise relationship between these two structures are absolutely critical in lip repair. The vermilion border at the level of the cleft repair may be malaligned or appear peaked because of a short vertical dimension to the lip (Fig. 30–1A). Mild deformities of the vermilion are commonly seen early, within the first 6 months after the rotation advancement repair.[22] This is attributable to a degree of scar contracture, which usually resolves with time. We think it is beneficial to encourage the parents to participate in active massage and taping of the scar to facilitate scar resolution and softening of the repair. In general, we defer decision toward revisional surgery on these children until the preschool age.

In cases in which there is a vermilion mismatch or widened white roll scar, we perform a diamond or keel-shape excision of the scar, which involves the cutaneous and vermilion element above and below the white roll (Fig. 30–1B). We avoid cutaneous undermining so that the deep stitch in the deep dermal and muscular area can be used to help avoid further widening and separation. It is also possible to design a small Z-plasty along the affected column; however, it places additional scars on the lip that do not fall along anatomic landmarks.

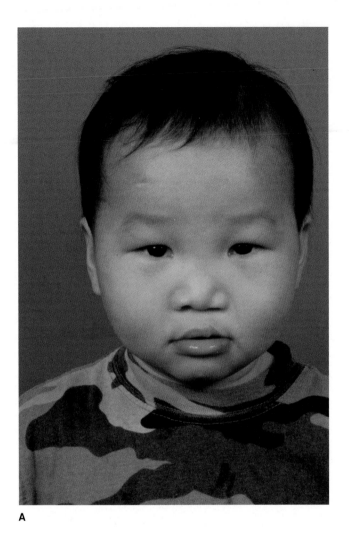

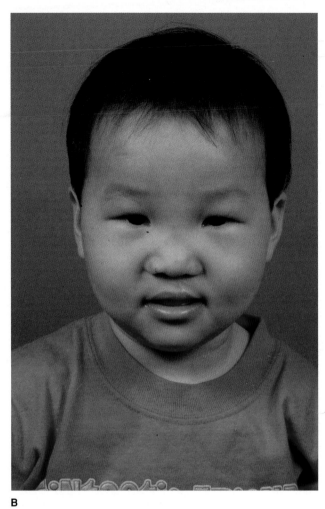

A

B

Figure 30–1. (A) Malalignment of the vermilion border is visible at short distances. (B) A diamond-shaped excision of the mismatched vermilion will align the vermilion border and slightly lengthen the lip.

Reconstruction of the Cupid's bow and the white roll is crucial in preserving the aesthetic nature of the lip; even slight alterations or misalignments of these areas are overtly noticeable. The white roll is a structure that cannot be duplicated surgically. We no longer advocate Millard's white roll triangular flap as part of the primary repair, as it may introduce cutaneous and dry vermilion scarring above and below the inset that is noticeable and difficult to correct. However, in secondary cases of white roll separation but with good cutaneous lip scars, it can be used to not only reconstruct the white roll, but additionally gain some lip length.

Deficient Vermilion

Vermilion notching is a common secondary deformity of the vermilion in patients with cleft lip. The free border of the lip is a composite structure consisting of the orbicularis oris and the overlying tissues, namely subcutaneous fat, vermilion, and mucosa. A deficiency of all or one of these structures is responsible for the vermilion notch.[5]

Careful analysis of the deformity may reveal malalignment of the profundus muscle, vermilion, or labial mucosa, as well as fullness or hypoplasia of the medial or lateral segment. Malalignment without significant tissue deficit can be corrected by readjustment of available local tissue. This may involve a complete revision of the lip with mobilization and realignment of the superficialis and profundus components of the muscle. Realignment of the vermilion redline can be achieved by advancing the lateral segment excess into a medial segment redline incision or back cut.

Fullness in the lateral segment can be treated with a horizontal linear excision on the inner aspect of the lip along the maxillary labial sulcus (Fig. 30–2).

Hypoplasia or tissue deficiency can be noted in either the medial or lateral segment. Vermilion augmentation can be performed using microfat grafting.[23] Fat harvested from the periumbilical area may be centrifuged and injected along the area of deficiency[24] (Fig. 30–3). However, do not combine fat grafting with scar revision. Perform the fat grafting first, and then come back and do scar revision. A V-Y mucosal advancement, from the inner lip, can address lining deficiency. Care must be taken when advancing wet mucosa, however, to align the redline of the upper and lower lip.

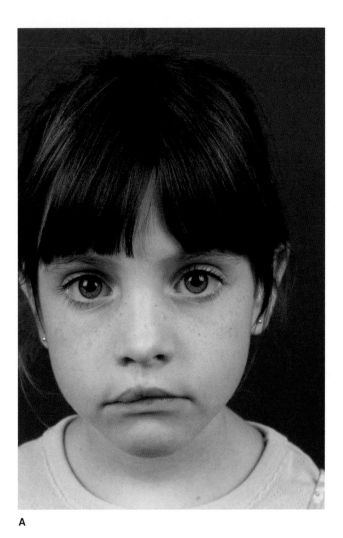
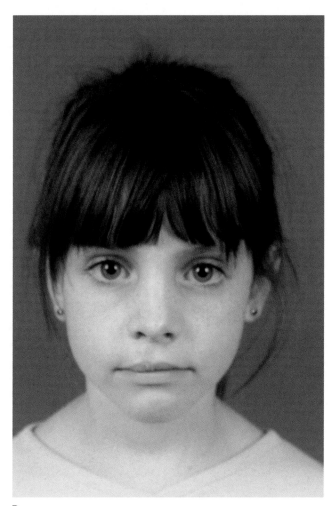

A

B

Figure 30–2. (A) A child with fullness of the lateral segment vermilion. (B) Lateral fullness reduced with a horizontal linear excision of vermilion.

Vermilion redistribution can be performed using a transverse twist flap.[25] This involves the transposition of a transversely oriented flap of mucosa, elevated on a connective tissue and muscle pedicle. The flap is rotated 180° from the contralateral side of the lip (or from both sides for a deficient vermilion tubercle), to help fill the defect. The flap is asymmetrical, thus enabling the transposition of more tissue into the primary defect than is lost from the donor site.

When severe notching is associated with scarring, the reconstruction requires unscarred tissue. Even in the unilateral deformity, we think the Abbé flap is the best choice to correct the problem. It should be used when lip disproportion exists in conjunction with normal occlusion and central lip deficiency (Fig. 30–4).

Short Lip

A lip is considered short when the philtral column on the cleft side is shorter than the contralateral noncleft philtrum. This may be confirmed by measuring the distance from the cupids bow peak points to the alar base on the respective sides. As mentioned previously, it is common to see shortening in the rotation/advancement repair the first 6 months after surgery. The cause may be active underlying scar contracture that improves over time (6–8 months), as the scar matures and softens. More severe cases are usually caused by inadequate rotation of the lip at the time of the primary operation, and are most often seen with an improperly designed rotation advancement repair. Furthermore, unrepaired or dehisced orbicularis muscle may contribute to a short lip. This can be diagnosed preoperatively by the presence of a muscle bulge when asking the patient to purse their lips. In addition, a hypoplastic, vertically short, lateral lip orbicularis muscle segment may be the most common cause of short lip. This condition can be prevented, if recognized during the primary surgery, and treated with muscle scoring along the direction of the muscle fibers, aiming to expand the muscle vertically.

In cases where there is clear underrotation, and a vertically short lip is present, the repair should be taken down and repeat rotation and advancement performed. Lip length should be controlled with precise muscle alignment. The muscle repair should fully rotate and visually level the Cupid's

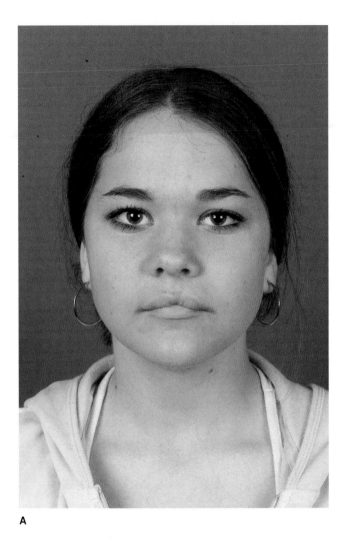

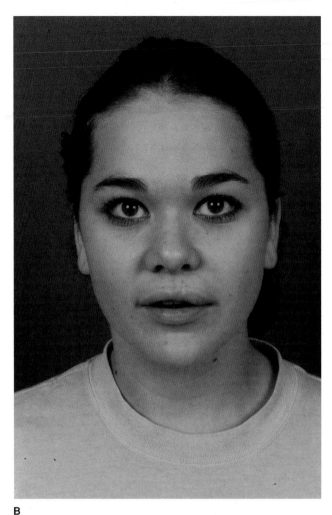

A   B

Figure 30–3. (A) Medial segment vermilion deficiency. (B) Microfat grafting to deficient tubercle.

bow peaks. These cases often originate from a short lateral lip segment where the muscle itself is bunched and short. Liberating and "un-bunching" the lateral lip muscle, and suturing it so as to maximally rotate the medial segment, is key (Fig. 30–5). The Rose–Thompson excision is seldom indicated, as it unnecessarily sacrifices philtral tissue.

As for the triangular flap repair, further advancement of the lateral segment triangular flap, or a diamond or keel-shaped excision, may lengthen the lip up to 2 mm. If more than 2 mm lengthening is required, the repair should be taken down with redesigning of the triangular flap repair, paying special attention to lip muscle repair. It is advisable to avoid converting a triangular flap repair into a rotation advancement flap repair, since such conversion will sacrifice excessive normal lip tissues.

Long Lip

A postoperative long lip is frequently seen with the Tennison repair.[26] Very rarely does the rotation advancement lip repair produce a long lip, and mostly it is due to overrotation of the lip medial segment. In correcting a long lip secondary

to a rotation advancement repair, complete takedown with muscle realignment is frequently indicated.

In treating the long lip secondary to a triangular flap repair, a lip excision from the alar base on the cleft side will give adequate elevation of the lip. This can be combined with permanent suspension suture to the ipsilateral maxilla to maintain elevation during the healing phase. Furthermore, width reduction of the lateral segment triangular flap, by partial excision of the lower portion of the triangular flap along its lower limb, can shorten the lip in mild cases. In severe cases, the entire repair should be taken down and repair redesigned using the same triangular Tennison repair.

Tight Upper Lip

Although a tight lip may be seen in unilateral clefts, it is more common in bilateral cases. In unilateral cases, it often results from the repair of a wide cleft with associated maxillary hypoplasia. Significant tissue deficiency, or excessive tissue excision, at the primary repair can also result in a tight lip. When a tight lip is present, the maxillary skeleton should be addressed first. Correction may involve orthodontics, as well

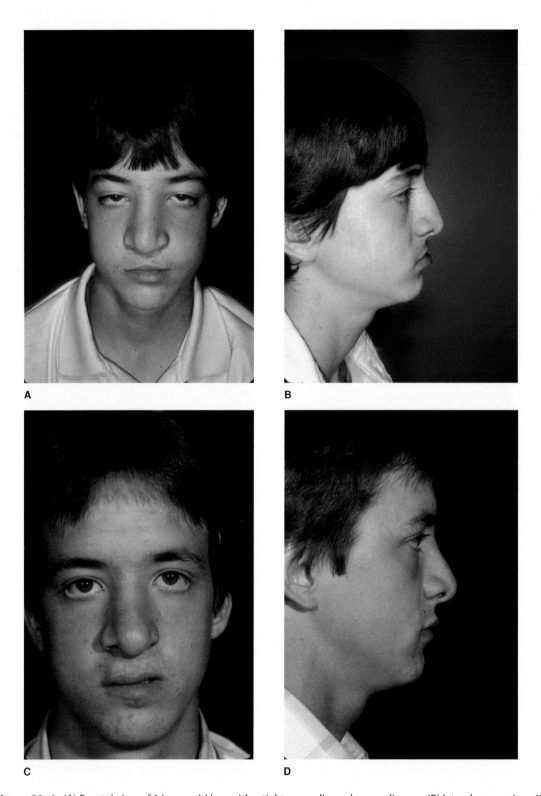

Figure 30–4. (A) Frontal view of 14-year-old boy with a tight upper lip and a poor lip scar; (B) lateral preop view; (C) postop frontal view after Abbe flap; (D) postop lateral view.

as LeFort I advancement. If the lip is still tight and deficient, the cleft nasal deformity is addressed using a rib columella strut, to advance the lip and columella up and out. Persisting deficiencies may be corrected by microfat augmentation to the upper lip vermilion, and combined with lower lip reduction.

The lower lip reduction is done with a horizontal ellipse, whose central axis is the redline between the wet and dry mucosa, and includes a wedge of vermilion muscle. In more severe cases, a cross-lip Abbé flap may be the only remaining option (see Fig. 30–4).

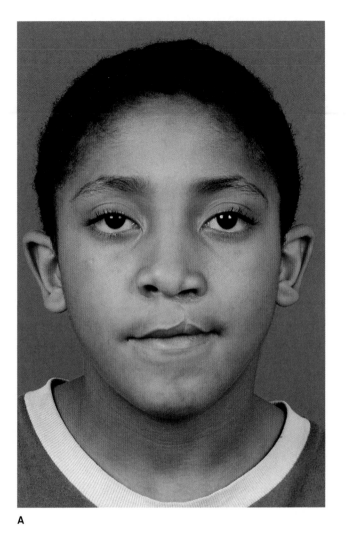

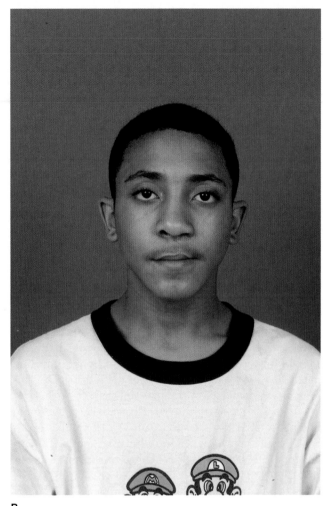

A

B

Figure 30–5. (A) Frontal view of a 10-year-old boy with a short lip and a lateral bulge. (B) The repair was redone and the lateral segment orbicularis was re-elevated and "unbunched" to restore adequate lip height.

Scar Deformity

The best possible scar in the repair of the unilateral lip is at the primary repair. Unsatisfactory scars deserve special evaluation. If the cutaneous scar is universally poor, but lip alignment is good, caution should be used in any revision, as this most likely indicates an underlying tendency to scar poorly. Exceptions to this are those cases in which there is a history of infection or traumatic dehiscence that would account for the initial poor scar. If the poor scarring is in association with lip imbalance or malalignment, then revision is indicated. If portions of the cutaneous scar have healed well, and other areas are hypertrophic, limited revision, eliminating tension, may be warranted.

Animation Deformity (Unrepaired or Dehisced Orbicularis Oris Muscle)

Interruption of the orbicularis muscle, or its components, can lead to a wide range of deformities that can be static or dynamic. These include a short lip, lip notching, a widened depressed scar, or an animation-induced muscular bulge. Regardless of the nature of the deformity created by the muscle, the correction requires a total revision of the repair paying special attention to dissect, release, redirect, and repair the superficial and deep heads of the orbicularis oris muscle. When a muscle bulge is part of the deformity, wide undermining of the skin, with scoring to "un-bunch" the muscle, is indicated. Despite these efforts, muscle bulges frequently persist after correction.

SECONDARY REPAIR OF THE UNILATERAL CLEFT LIP NASAL DEFORMITY

Introduction

With improved outcomes in the management of cleft defects, the repair of the nasal deformity has become more important to families and patients, whose ultimate goal is to restore the face to its full functional and aesthetic capacity. The cleft lip nasal deformity offers a unique challenge to the reconstructive surgeon. Despite the current trend toward nasal reconstruction at the time of primary lip repair, the prevalence of the historic dogma against primary cleft nasal correction results in two classes of patients with secondary cleft nasal deformities: those with primary repair and those with no primary correction.

In general, patients who have had primary nasal correction are less severely deformed, and can be approached with more normal rhinoplasty techniques. Early repair has a major role in balancing the muscle forces on the nose, and will decrease the degree of lasting nasal deformity, if proper release of the tethering forces is achieved. As a result, the algorithm for secondary cleft rhinoplasty varies widely between groups with and without primary nasal correction.

Cleft Nose Anatomy

Controversy persists as to whether the cleft nasal deformity is secondary to tissue malposition, or if it is associated with tissue deficiencies. McComb[27,28] has shown, from his dissections of stillborn fetuses with clefts, that anatomic distortion and malposition is the primary factor in the deformity. This opinion was reinforced by Huffman and Lierie,[28–30] who proposed that the cleft deformity was due to tissue malposition, and not to a relative size discrepancy.[31] Despite these published results, our experience in the dissection of stillborn children with clefts, as well as in open rhinoplasty, suggests that hypoplasia of the lower lateral cartilage complex may be found in association with malposition.[32]

Malposition is felt to be secondary to an imbalance of muscle forces across the cleft. This would explain the deviation of the septum away from the cleft, as well as the lateralization of the cleft dome and lateral crus.[33] Equally significant is the abnormal fixation of the lateral crus to the periosteum of the pyriform through a continuation of cartilaginous and fibrous structures.

Hence, we feel that the primary cleft nasal deformity is characterized by some or all of the following components: malposition of the lower lateral cartilage, hypoplasia of the lower lateral cartilage, interruption of the muscle ring across the nasal sill, fixation of the accessory chain of the lateral crus through fibrous connections to the pyriform, soft tissue deficiency to the nasal floor, septal deviation, and abnormal muscle insertions at the alar base to the cheek and lip.

Secondary Cleft Lip Nasal Deformities

All the features of the unrepaired primary deformity may characterize the secondary cleft nasal deformity, plus the added distortion induced by growth.[34–36] Lesser degrees of the primary deformity are seen, depending on what was done at the time of lip repair. The surgical steps at primary repair that most influence the outcome of the nasal deformity are (1) adequate release of the lateral crus from its attachments to the pyriform and reattachment to the cheek muscles, (2)

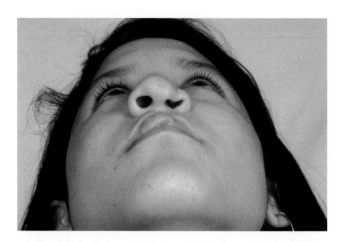

Figure 30–6. The unrepaired alar cartilage is weak and contributes to a collapse of the ala.

reconstruction of the muscle ring across the sill and floor, and (3) reposition of the caudally rotated lateral crus and dome.

The Cleft Ala and Tip

The major defect of primarily unrepaired or inadequately repaired cleft lip nasal deformity concerns the position of the ala.[37–39] The ala lies caudal and lateral to the contralateral side, and is tethered by a pathologic attachment of the accessory chain to the pyriform aperture.[36] The ala rests on an underdeveloped maxilla, which partly accounts for alar base lowering and horizontal nostril seating. The ala may be underdeveloped, hypoplastic, and weak, exhibiting a convoluted shape (Fig. 30–6). This contributes further to dome lowering on the cleft side. The clefted orbicularis muscle ring across the nasal sill places unequal muscular pull on the cleft and noncleft sides, and adds to the nasal asymmetry and deformity. Malfunction of the cleft ala external valve may be due to the position of the cleft alar base, imbalanced muscular pull, or abnormal attachment of the cheek muscles to the lateral crus. Because of the abnormal ala, the columella is foreshortened and lies obliquely, with its base directed away from the cleft side.

The Septum

The septum may be displaced from the vomerine groove, and the cartilaginous portion may be buckled, both of which contribute to nasal tip deviation and narrowing or obstruction of the nasal airway. The caudal septum is displaced away from the cleft, and dorsal septal curvature is present. Clinically significant posterior bony airway obstruction involving the vomer and ethmoid is frequently present.

The Skeletal Framework

The nasal bones are frequently widened both at the dorsum and at the frontal process of the maxilla. The dorsum may be low, normal, or overprojecting. Deviation may affect the bony as well as the cartilaginous segments. Generally,

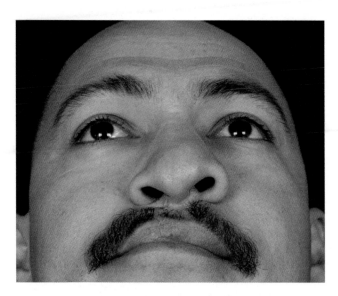

Figure 30–7. Midvault curvature can be seen with concavity on the cleft side and convexity on the noncleft side.

mid-vault curvature is present, with collapse on the concave side, and fullness on the convex side (Fig. 30–7).

Obstruction of the Airway

Besides the narrowing expected from the deviated septum and bony obstruction, nasal rhinometry has demonstrated statistically significant findings of smaller airways in patients with cleft deformity, when compared to patients without cleft deformity. Furthermore, external valve malfunction may add to the airway problem.

Timing of Secondary Surgical Procedure

We plan the secondary cleft lip nose repair after the age of 14 in females, and after the age of 16 in males. The goal is to allow the completion of the postpubertal growth spurt in the anterior septum and in the bony dorsum. We do not favor repetitive rhinoplasty procedures throughout the course of childhood, as we believe the final long-term result is greatly compromised. Occasionally, a failed primary repair will result in such a severe nasal stigmata, that nasal tip plasty is performed. Such occurrences are almost always in association with severe hypoplasia of the lower lateral cartilage complex, require ear cartilage augmentation, and are generally repaired before the second grade.

Analysis of Cleft Nasal Deformities

The key points of our analysis that influence the algorithm of repair are:

1. Was primary cleft nasal repair done:
   a. Was the lateral crus released from the pyriform?
   b. Is the nasal lining deficient?
   c. Was muscle reconstruction across the nasal sill accomplished?
   d. Is the external valve patent and functional?
   e. Was malposition of the lateral crus and dome corrected?
2. Is tip projection adequate?
3. Is the cleft lateral crus deformed by a persisting alar crease or buckle?
4. Is the alar base recessed and tethered to the pyriform?
5. Is the pyriform and maxilla hypoplastic?
6. Is projection of the bony dorsum deficient, normal, or overprojecting?

Surgical Algorithm

Despite multiple technical procedures described, no one protocol has proven to be completely satisfactory in the repair of all cleft lip nasal deformities.[40] Still, controversy remains as to the optimum corrective approach, the best techniques for exposure and repair, and most significantly, the timing of the correction. In the following section, we will present our personal surgical algorithm, based on the residual nasal deformity.

First, in those children who have had successful primary correction of the nasal deformity, surgical treatment ranges from the management of airway obstruction and the correction of minor contour deformities, to fairly traditional rhinoplasty procedures to balance the tip and dorsum. Unfortunately, a few of these patients have enough residual deformity to place them into the category of unrepaired cleft noses. Hypoplasia of the septum, the maxilla, and the lower lateral cartilage complex, are frequently found in association with these patients, and may be more responsible for the poor outcome than inadequacy of the primary repair per se. Clefts with central facial dysplasia (~5%) are unique to this group and have practically no septal development and support.

In patients with no nasal repair, or failed primary repair, the presence of dorsal deficiency or inadequate tip projection, in association with a deformed ala, are the driving forces toward rib graft reconstruction. The great majority of these patients are approached with an open rhinoplasty, employing a transcolumella step incision connected with an infracartilaginous incision for soft tissue degloving.[41–44] A dorsal approach to the septum is carried out detaching the upper lateral cartilages submucoperichondrially from the septum. The submucoperichondrial dissection is connected with subperiosteal tunnels developed over the vomer and ethmoid. These tunnels are initiated anteriorly off the spine and maxilla, as opposed to posteriorly. A wide vomerine–septal–ethmoid resection is carried out under direct vision leaving an 8–10 mm dorsal and caudal L-strut. The base of the caudal septum is mobilized and repositioned to the aesthetic midline with suture anchorage. If the dorsum is overprojecting, the septum and bony dorsum are reduced, and lateral percutaneous J-osteotomies made. The excess of the upper lateral cartilages are turned in as alar spreader flaps, and nasal bone in-fracture carried out. A traditional spreader graft is frequently added to the concave side of the septal curvature. If the dorsal projection is normal, medial oblique osteotomies, with lateral percutaneous osteotomies, are carried out to narrow the bony width. A spreader graft is used on the concave side, and clocking sutures between the upper lateral cartilage and septum are adjusted to bring the septum to midline. If the dorsum is deficient or the nose is short, reconstruction of the dorsum with rib graft is employed.

The algorithm now turns to the tip and the deformed ala. If tip projection is inadequate, the lateral crus collapsed by a persisting crease, or if the columella labial angle is acute and recessed, then tip support is provided by a columella strut taken from the cartilage of the tenth rib. The choice of rib cartilage for the columella strut in these instances is threefold: (1) To provide enough strength and bulk to the premaxilla in the area of the nasal spine, (2) to adequately support the soft tissues, the base of the columella and tip, and lift the base of the lip to achieve a more obtuse columella–

lip angle, (This creates an aesthetic fullness in the area, and restores the youthful curve to the central lip.) and (3) to allow all of the harvested septal cartilage to be used in tip and alar reconstruction, and provide enough tip support to resist the soft tissue shortage in the columella and lateral nasal sidewall.

The convexity of this rib graft is placed cephalad and secured to the caudal septum. This leaves the concavity caudal allowing the medial crus to be joined in front of the graft thereby avoiding excess widening of the columella. The length of this graft is generally in the range of 32 mm.

A number 0.028 threaded K-wire is placed in the midline of the maxilla in the base of the anterior nasal spine extending approximately 3 mm into the maxillary bone. The rib graft is impaled over the threaded K-wire. A hole is created in the base of the columellar strut with a 19-gauge needle to receive the exposed K-wire, which extends into the graft approximately 5 mm.

The algorithm expands at this point depending on the characteristics of the alar base and lateral crus. If the accessory

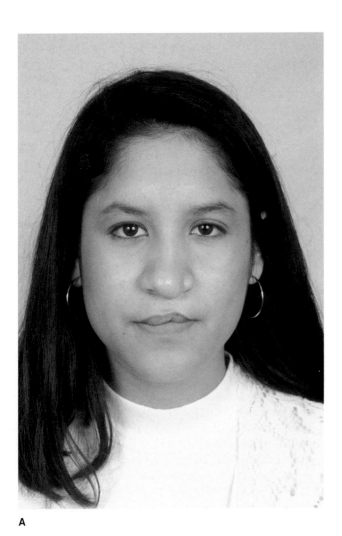 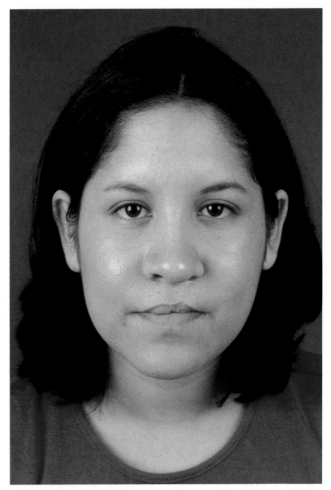

A   **B**

Figure 30–8. A 17-year-old female with inadequate primary nasal correction. Her secondary rhinoplasty consisted of dorsal hump reduction and osteotomies, right spreader graft, columellar strut graft, and release of lower lateral cartilage with alar strut and contour graft. (A and B) Pre- and postoperative frontal view. (C and D) Pre- and postoperative lateral view. (E and F) Pre- and postoperative worm's eye view.

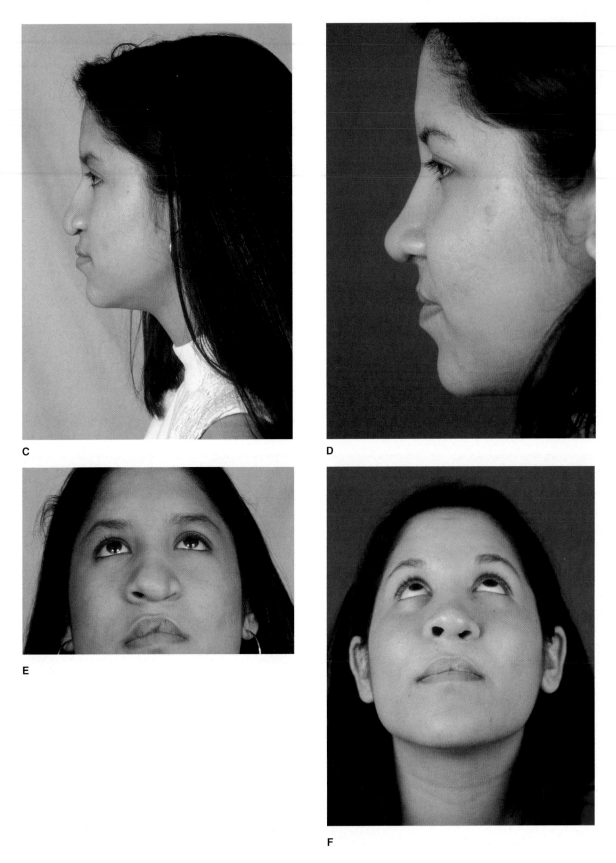

C

D

E

F

Figure 30–8. (*Continued*).

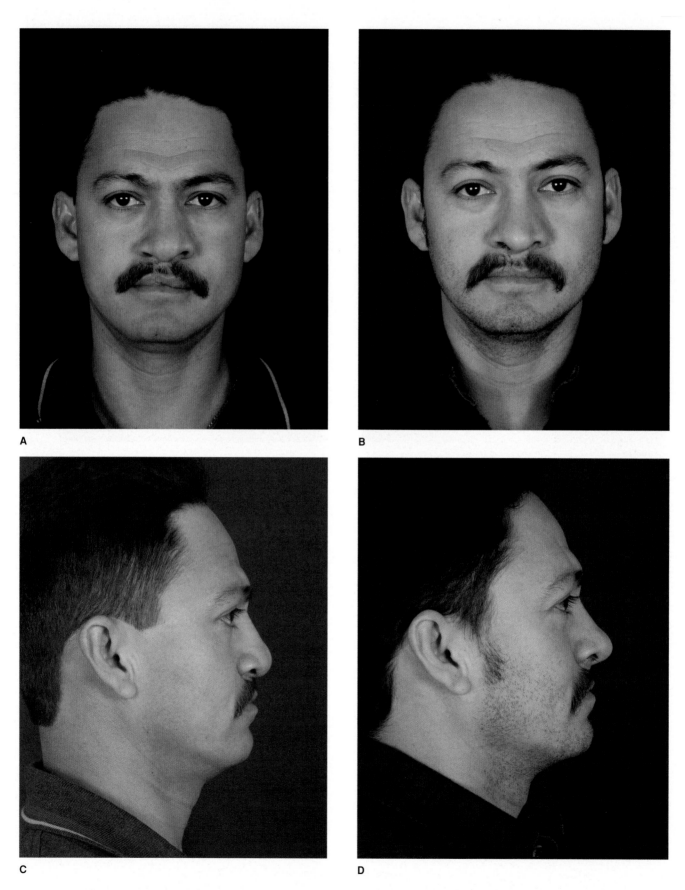

Figure 30–9. (A) Preoperative frontal view of a 35-year-old male with no primary nasal correction. (B) Postoperative frontal view, note the rib graft used for a columellar strut and septal graft for alar contour and strut. (C) Preoperative lateral view. (D) Postoperative lateral view. (E) Preoperative worms eye view. (F) Postoperative worms eye view.

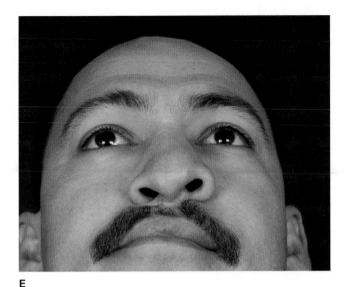

E

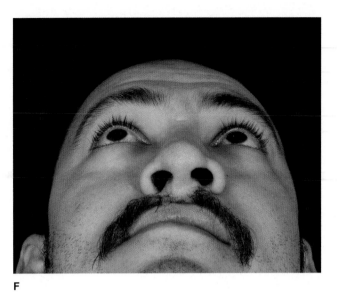

F

Figure 30–9. (*Continued*).

chain in the lateral crus remains attached to the periosteum of the pyriform, then perialar dissection is carried out mobilizing the muscle beneath the base and freeing it from the lateral cheek and lip musculature. This release goes up to the nasal lining insuring that all the attachments between the lateral crus and the pyriform periosteum have been lysed. The mobilization extends across the cleft and the sill of the nose to the midline dissection of the columella. The muscle of the alar base is then sutured to the contralateral medial footplate, thereby rotating it toward midline and bringing the muscle across the floor and sill. The divided fibrinous attachments, between the accessory chain and the pyriform, are then sutured to the muscles of the cheek, so as to float the external valve and alar base and free them from their points of anchorage along the pyriform. The dead space, from the release of the alar base, is filled by the muscle that is rotated in and toward the midline. In severe cases, cartilage augmentation of the pyriform is used.

The release of the ala from the pyriform may actually improve the tethering of the lateral crus. However, most often it is also necessary to detach the lateral crus of the lower lateral cartilage from the upper lateral cartilage along the scroll, to further mobilize the cartilage complex. If the nasal lining restricts the movement and relocation of the lateral crus, a V-Y advancement of the lining and cartilage along the nasal vestibularis is performed. Almost always, an alar strut graft, 3–4 mm in width and 28–30 mm in length, will be placed beneath the cleft lateral crus in a pocket created by elevation of the lining on the underside of the cartilage. This graft extends from the dome laterally to the alar base frequently extending beyond the point of release of the alar musculature. It can be sutured to the cheek musculature caudally, to pull a hitched, cephalically rotated ala down when necessary. The strut graft serves to stabilize external valve incompetence that can be produced by the lateral release.[45] An alar contour graft, made of residual septum, is then fashioned to span from the dome

to out beyond the alar crease.[46] These grafts essentially sandwich the abnormal alar cartilage. Domal mattress sutures are then added to further define the domes, and then the domes are sutured over the projecting rib columella strut. A slight overprojection of the cleft lateral crus and domal segment is allowed to compensate for the tight soft tissue envelope on the cleft side.

With normal soft tissue thickness, the domal tip projection is carried approximately 7–8 mm above the plane of the dorsum. Whereas in thick-skinned patients, the domal projection is increased to 10–12 mm above the plane of the dorsum.

When a Le-Fort I maxillary advancement is required, the same algorithm may be applied, but a rib graft is always used as columellar support. It is imperative that a stable maxillary segment (rigid fixation and normal dental relation) is achieved if rhinoplasty is to be combined; otherwise, malposition or displacement of the caudal columellar strut is a possible complication. Even when advancements are in the range of 6–8 mm, the advantage of the columella rib graft for control and shaping of the columella labial angle, cannot be overemphasized.

The algorithm takes a different direction if the primary nasal reconstruction accomplishes four keys: (1) adequate lining, (2) release of the lateral ala from the pyriform, (3) muscle reconstruction of the sill, and (4) dome repositioning. When these surgical steps are accomplished in the primary repair, the secondary surgical correction is frequently limited to alar contour grafting of the lateral crus, caudal septal repositioning, and other routine steps in rhinoplasty. The augmentation can frequently be done with the combination of septal and ear cartilage. Conversely, when these steps have not been taken in the primary repair, a rib cartilage columellar strut is invariably needed, allowing the entirety of the harvested sepal cartilage to be used in reshaping and controlling the deformed cleft ala. Lining release, in the form of a VY advancement of the lateral vestibule at the nasal vestibularis, release of the accessory chain from the pyriform, reconstruction of the external valve, reconstruction of the muscle ring across the sill, and septoplasty are, of course, required. Augmentation of the deficient pyriform aperture on the cleft side may be necessary in either sequence (Figs. 30–8 and 30–9).

References

1. Salyer KE, Genecov ER, Genecov DG. Unilateral cleft lip-nose repair: A 33-year experience. *J Craniofac Surg* 14:549, 2003.
2. Johnson J, Gray S. Secondary cleft lip surgery: Revision of residual cleft lip deformities. In Smith EJ, Bunstead RM (eds). *Pediatric Facial Plastic and Reconstructive Surgery*, Vol 14. New York: Raven Press, 1993, p. 197.
3. Stal S, Hollier L. Correction of secondary cleft lip deformities. *Plast Reconstr Surg* 109:1672, 2002.
4. Sadove AM, Eppley BL. Correction of secondary cleft lip and nasal deformities. Advances in management of cleft lip and palate. *Clin Plast Surg* 20:793, 1993.
5. Patel A, Hall PN. Free dermis—fat graft to correct the whistle deformity in patients with cleft lip. *Br J Plas Surg* 57:160, 2004.
6. Mulliken JB, Pensler JM, Kozakewich H. The anatomy of Cupid's bow in normal and cleft lip. *Plast Reconstr Surg* 92:395, 1993.
7. Burt JD, Byrd HS. Cleft lip: Unilateral primary deformities. *Plast Reconstr Surg* 105:1043, 2000.
8. Noordhoff MS. Reconstruction of the vermilion in unilateral and bilateral cleft lips. *Plast Reconstr Surg* 73:52, 1984.
9. Skoog T. The cleft lip. In: Skoog T (ed). *Plastic Surgery*. Philadelphia: WB Saunders, 1974, p. 107.
10. LaRossa D. Unilateral cleft repair. In Bentz M (ed). *Pediatric Plastic Surgery*. Stanford: Appleton and Lange, 1998.
11. Millard DR. The unilateral deformity. In Millard DR (ed). *Cleft Craft, The Evolution of Its Surgery*. Boston: Little Brown, 1976, p. 449.
12. Mohler LR. Unilateral cleft lip repair. *Plast Reconstr Surg* 80:511, 1987.
13. Delaire J. Theoretical principles and technique of functional closure of the lip and the nasal aperture. *J Maxillofac Surg* 6:109, 1978.
14. McComb H. Primary correction of unilateral cleft lip nasal deformity: A 10-year review. *Plast Reconstr Surg* 75:791, 1985.
15. Cronin TD, Denkler KA. Correction of unilateral cleft lip nose. *Plast Reconstr Surg* 82:419, 1988.
16. Vegter F, Hage JJ. Lack of correlation between objective and subjective evaluation of residual stigmata in cleft patients. *Ann Plast Surg* 46:625, 2001.
17. Bardach, J, Salyer KE. Correction of secondary unilateral cleft lip deformities. In Bardach J, Salyer KE (eds). *Surgical Techniques in Cleft Lip and Palate*. Chicago: Yearbook Medical Publishers, 1987.
18. Anastassov GE, Joos U. Comprehensive management of cleft lip and palate deformities. *J Oral Maxillofac Surg* 59:1062, 2001.
19. Williams HB. A method of assessing cleft lip repairs: Comparison of Le Mesurier and Millard techniques. *Plast Reconstr Surg* 41:103, 1968.
20. Assuncao G. The VLS classification for secondary deformities in the unilateral cleft lip: Clinical application. *Br J Plast Surg* 45:288, 1992.
21. Akguner M, Barutcu A, Karaca C. Adolescent growth patterns of the bony and cartilaginous framework of the nose: A cephalometric study. *Ann Plast Surg* 41:66, 1998.
22. Millard DR. Extensions of the rotation-advancement principal for wide unilateral cleft lips. *Plast Reconstr Surg* 42:535, 1968.
23. Niechajev I. Lip enhancement: Surgical alternatives and histological aspects. *Plast Reconstr Surg* 105:1173, 2000.
24. Ersek RA. Transplantation of purified autologous fat: A three-year follow up is disappointing. *Plast Reconstr Surg* 87:219, 1991.
25. de Chalain T, Black P. Secondary reconstruction of asymmetric volume deficits of the lips: A transverse twist flap technique. *Br J Plast Surg* 57:330, 2004.
26. Sadove AM, Eppley BL. Correction of secondary cleft lip and nasal deformities. Advances in management of cleft lip and palate. *Clin Plast Surg* 20:793, 1993.
27. McComb H. Primary correction of unilateral cleft lip nasal deformity: A 10-year review. *Plast Reconstr Surg* 75:791, 1985.
28. McComb H. Primary repair of unilateral cleft lip nasal deformity. *Oper Techn Plast Reconstr Surg* 2:200, 1995.
29. Wolfe SA. A pastiche for the cleft lip nose. *Plast Reconstr Surg* 114:1, 2004.
30. Huffman W, Lierle D. Studies on the pathologic anatomy of the unilateral harelip nose. *Plast Reconstr Surg* 4:225–234, 1949.
31. de Sá Nóbrega, ES. Cleft lip nose: A different approach. *J Craniofac Surg* 16:95, 2005.
32. Musgrove RH. Surgery of nasal deformities associated with cleft lip. *Plast Reconstr Surg* 28:261, 1961.
33. McComb HK, Coghlan BA. Primary repair of the unilateral cleft lip nose: Completion of a longitudinal study. *Cleft Palate Craniofac J* 33:23, 1996.
34. Stenstrom J, Oberg RH. The nasal deformity in unilateral cleft lips. *Plast Reconstr Surg* 28:295, 1961.
35. Byrd HS. Cleft lips I. Primary deformities. *Selected Readings in Plastic Surgery* 8(21):1–37, 1997.
36. Byrd HS, Salomon J. Primary correction of the unilateral cleft nasal deformity. *Plast Reconstr Surg* 106:1276, 2000.
37. Smahel Z, Mullerova Z, Nejedly A. Effect of primary repositioning of the nasal septum on facial growth in unilateral cleft lip and palate. *Cleft Palate Craniofac J* 36:310, 1999.
38. Smahel Z, Mullerova Z, Skvarilova B, et al. Differences between facial configuration and development in complete and incomplete unilateral cleft lip and palate during the prepubertal period. *Acta Chir Plast* 33:47, 1991.
39. Rifley W, Thaller SR. The residual cleft lip nasal deformity. An anatomic approach. *Clin Plast Surg* 23:81, 1996.
40. Brusse CA, Van der Werff JF, Stevens HP, et al. Symmetry and morbidity assessment of unilateral complete cleft lip nose corrected with or without primary nasal correction. *Cleft Palate Craniofac J* 36:361, 1999.
41. Trenite GJ, Paping RH, Trenning AH. Rhinoplasty in the cleft lip patient. *Cleft Palate Craniofac J* 34:63, 1997.
42. Matthews D. The nose tip. *Br J Plast Surg* 21:153, 1968.
43. Gillies H, Millard DR. *The Principles and Art of Plastic Surgery*. Boston: Little Brown & Co, 1966.
44. Cronin TD, Denkler KA. Correction of the unilateral cleft lip nose. *Plast Reconstr Surg* 82:419, 1988.
45. Rohrich RJ, Raniere J Jr, Ha RY. The alar contour graft: Correction and prevention of alar rim deformities in rhinoplasty. *Plast Reconstr Surg* 109:2495, 2002.
46. Gunter JP, Friedman RM: Lateral crural strut graft: Technique and clinical application in rhinoplasty. *Plast Reconstr Surg* 99:943, 1997.

Correction of Secondary Bilateral Cleft Lip and Nose Deformities

Terrence W. Bruner, MD, MBA • Vincent Boyd, MD • Samuel Stal, MD, FACS • Larry H. Hollier, MD, FACS

INTRODUCTION

As stated by Gillies and Kilner in 1932, "The best effort of any surgeon at primary reconstruction of a hare-lip . . . [will] usually leave some deformity."[1] Despite tremendous advances in primary bilateral cleft lip repair over the years, this statement, in many regards, still remains true. In fact, secondary deformities are the rule rather than the exception; and, in many aspects, are more difficult to repair than primary deformities.[2,3] It is the cascade of scarring, initiated by the primary repair and resultant distortion of anatomic tissue planes, which makes correction so problematic. Additionally, secondary deformities vary widely in etiology, appearance, and severity, thus further challenging any repair technique to provide excellent results consistently.

While many of the secondary procedures devised for unilateral clefts can be adapted and utilized for bilateral defects, there are some inherent characteristics in the secondary bilateral cleft lip and nose deformity that must be taken into consideration. These include paucity of tissue of the central lip, an inadequate or diminutive columella, and a limited blood supply to the prolabium, all of which affect treatment management and outcomes. As such, the techniques described herein will focus on these unique aspects of the secondary bilateral cleft lip deformity.

TIMING OF SURGERY

At its heart, the bilateral cleft lip is an anatomic insult, affecting multiple tissue components, dimensions, and layers. While parents want to have their child's deformity corrected as soon as possible,[4] the bilateral cleft lip by its nature and complexity necessitates more than one surgical procedure. The greatest consensus among cleft surgeons is that the treatment of secondary revisions starts at the primary procedure, where the impact of prevention is greatest. There is no absolute rule for the precise timing of secondary procedures; however, there is general agreement among major cleft centers with regard to revisional surgery for bilateral cleft lip and nose.[5]

The preschool years (age 4–5) are a common time to begin secondary revisions.[2,3,6–8] These include correction of the vermilion border and lip scars. While the need for early septoplasty to relieve significant airway obstruction has been documented,[9] nasal correction at this age is limited to repositioning of the lower lateral cartilages. Early adolescence is the appropriate time for correction of alveolar defects and further revision of lip scars. Cessation of facial growth is the appropriate time for definitive septorhinoplasty with osteotomies and dorsal revision, after any maxillary realignment and alveolar bone grafting have been performed.[8–14] The patient should be emotionally mature enough to participate in the decision-making process associated with the septorhinoplasty[2] as the final step in surgical correction.

SECONDARY LIP DEFORMITIES

Vermilion Deficiency

Persistent paucity of midline vermilion is primarily associated with bilateral clefts, and is the most common form of vermilion deficiency.[15] Some state that this "whistle deformity" can be adequately corrected by reapproximation of the orbicularis oris muscle.[15] The root cause of the deformity is the lack of normal musculature and mucosa in all dimensions.[16] In all but the mildest of incomplete bilateral clefts, there is a relative excess of vermilion tissue, lateral to the midline, known as "festoons" (Fig. 31–1). In mild cases, various local tissue rearrangements may compensate or camouflage the deficiency.[3,9,13] For mild deformities, a mucosal V-Y advancement can be used to augment the central vermilion deficiency, lengthen the short upper lip, and narrow the alar base[15] (Fig. 31–2). For more substantial defects, Kapetansky, in 1971, described his double pendulum island flaps—based on the orbicularis oris muscle—that facilitate transfer of lateral lip vermilion tissue to the midline. This procedure is effective in that it simultaneously corrects the lack of central muscle union, as well as the excessive lateral vermilion; and, it has been extensively utilized.[3,10,17–20] However, it does result in a scenario of multiple scars leading in some cases to a hard unnatural lip. Fat augmentation holds promise to augment the central vermilion deficiency and lengthen the lip, but it is very difficult to distend scars, and should be used for augmentation after second stage tissue rearrangement.

Abbe Flap

For more severe whistle deformities, and horizontally deficient lips, or when local measures of tissue rearrangement have been exhausted, an Abbe flap is required.[21] It was commonly used for surgical cleft lip disasters, including patients whose premaxilla and prolabium had been completely discarded at a previous operation.[14,22] Currently, the Abbe flap is used less frequently because of improvements in primary repair techniques; however, its versatility is undeniable. It is the only available procedure that can reconstruct a natural-looking philtrum, Cupid's bow, and central tubercle.[20] In addition, the donor site simultaneously corrects the relative excess vermilion projection or "pout" from the lower lip, thus restoring balance to the entire aesthetic unit. This surgical

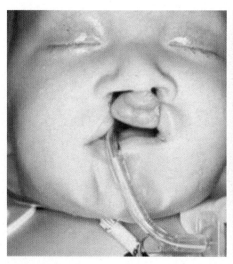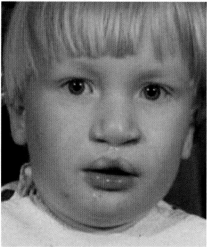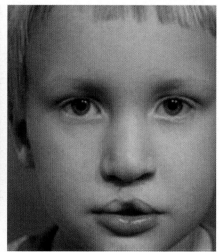

Figure 31–1. Demonstration of festooning.

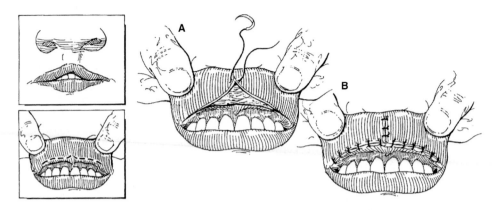

Figure 31–2. V-Y mucosal roll down for whistle lip deformity.

technique is the best available for addressing significant upper lip tissue deficiencies.

When designing the flap dimensions, emphasis should be placed on reconstructing the entire philtral unit, which will release the abnormal tightness and provide a balanced profile (Fig. 31–3). It is also advisable to harvest the flap from the center of the lower lip and place it in the aesthetic center of the upper lip.[2,20] This facilitates the appearance of a central vermilion tubercle and Cupid's bow.[20] It should also be designed slightly smaller than the intended neophiltrum, as this provides two benefits: it facilitates closure of the lower lip donor site, and allows for stretching of the flap once in

position. Most horizontally tight lips are vertically short as well. Vertical lip length should be maximized to match the neophiltrum by moving the apices of the lateral lip elements laterally. Finally, we recommend dividing the flap on postoperative day 10–14. Two assure viability, one can compress the native labial artery pedicle and check capillary refill of the inset flap.

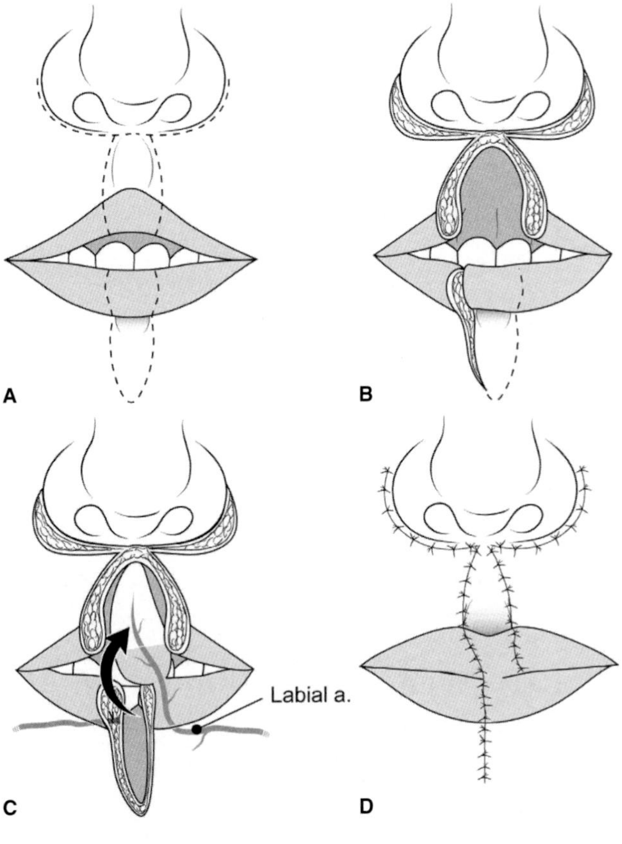

Vermilion Excess

While the bilateral complete cleft lip, at its foundation, is characterized by displacement and deficiency of tissue, it is not uncommon for the primary repair to result in relative tissue excess. In fact, the most common secondary deformity is a "relative" excess of mucosa of the lateral labial elements, or "festoons" (see Fig. 31–1).[17,18] This is nearly always caused by insufficient medial advancement of the vermilion during the primary repair, and can be corrected by re-advancement or direct excision.

Lip Scar

Often, the most noticeable and striking stigmata of a repaired bilateral cleft lip is an unsightly scar. A poor scar is one that even after 18 months remains hyperpigmented, raised, or foreshortened. Contributing factors, at the time of cleft repair, include inadequate orbicularis oris muscle continuity, a protruding premaxilla, and excessive cleft width, all resulting in a tight initial lip closure. This leads to extreme tension and subsequent widening of the lip scar over time. While some feel that the cutaneous lip should never be reopened for revision,[23,24] we advocate full thickness scar excision, from the prolabial side of the repair, and muscle reapproximation if continuity is lacking.[2] An adequate muscle repair is the basis for successful, permanent correction of widened and prominent scars.[25] It is hoped that with increasing application of presurgical alveolar molding and premaxillary repositioning, the secondary tight lip scar deformity will be seen with decreasing frequency. The desired end result is for the scars to simulate the philtral columns.[26] We have found "micro" fat grafting to be efficacious in providing soft tissue bulk, achieving more prominent and normal appearing philtral columns.

A

B

C   Labial a.   **D**

Figure 31–3. Abbe flap.

Philtrum and Cupids Bow

The philtrum truly is the keystone of the upper lip. In the bilateral cleft lip, the philtrum has a tendency to become progressively wide and convex in shape over time. The action of the orbicularis oris, combined with the persistent presence of tension from the primary repair, leads to a horizontal widening of the prolabial soft tissue, and further loss of convexity of an already abnormal philtrum.[1,2,7] While there are those who state that a child's lip should never be reopened to correct philtral size or shape,[23] we feel that surgical correction of the secondary philtral deformity is warranted. Excision of the excess philtral tissue, with reapproximation of the orbicularis to the newly redesigned philtrum, is the surgical optimum, with the resulting scars simulating the normal philtral columns.[26] Regardless of the age of the patient, the philtrum should be cut smaller than the final desired size in anticipation of this subsequent stretching.[2] To counteract the philtral convexity, a dermal suture extending to the premaxillary periosteum has been advocated.[15,27] This allows for a "dimpling" of the philtrum in most cases. Earlier reports advocated subcutaneous cartilage grafts to further accentuate the philtral columns or ridges.[15] However, we have found that a vest-over-pants dermal and muscle repair, along with a transdermal-dermal stitch, provides the best illusion of a normal philtrum (Fig. 31–4).

When considering the subtleties of the philtral subunit, one must include Cupid's bow – its peaks the upward prolongation of the superior edge of the vermilion lying beneath each philtral column.[28] While there is a tremendous anatomic variety in individuals, the presence of a Cupid's bow is an essential feature of a "normal-appearing" upper lip. This structure is so critical to the lip aesthetics; and, if there are significant Cupid's bow abnormalities, complete replacement of the philtral subunit, with an Abbe flap, is often the best option. The details of the white roll, and the geometry of Cupid's bow, are so distinct that minor skin excisions and vermilion advancements give minimal improvement. Fortunately, the lower lip, with its white roll and anatomy mimicking a philtral dimple, can be used as an Abbe flap, completely reconstructing the philtral subunit in its entirety.

Buccal Sulcus

The bilateral cleft lip often has a shallow or absent buccal sulcus and a tethering of the upper lip to the anterior aspect of the alveolus.[7,10] In fact, secondary resuspension of the mucosa in the anterior gingivolabial sulcus is one of the most commonly performed procedure for individuals with bilateral complete cleft lip.[23] An adequate sulcus, though often underemphasized, is essential for cleft lip reconstruction; and, it can be created by adequate elevation of the prolabium from the premaxilla during primary repair, and coverage of the resultant raw premaxilla with an inferiorly based mucosal flap.[15] The creation of an adequate sulcus and normal anatomy enhances proper lip function and facilitates appropriate fitting of orthodontic appliances.[15,29]

A number of surgical techniques have been described for the treatment of the shallow buccal sulcus, and fall primarily into two categories: mucosal grafts[1,2,15,22,29] and local flaps.[15,29] While mucosal grafts are not ideal, and have

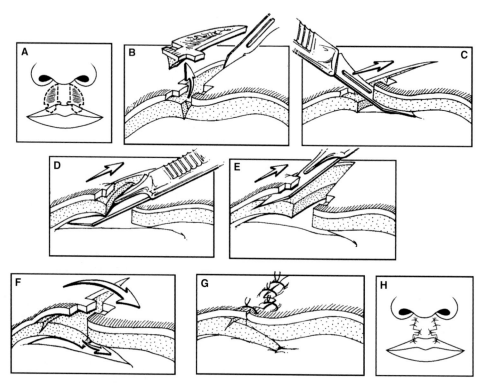

Figure 31–4. Vest over pants technique.

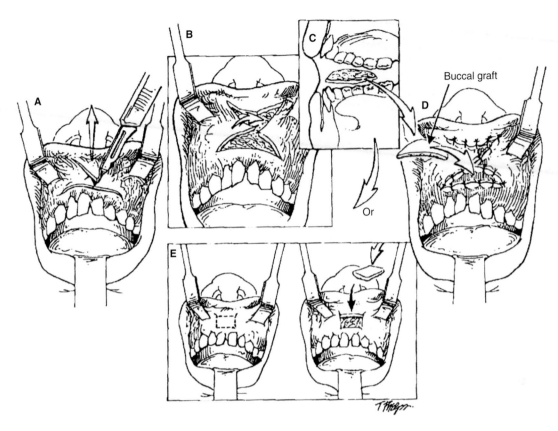

Figure 31–5. Bucal sulcus release with mucosal graft placement.

been associated with contraction, re-adhesion, and sulcus obliteration,[22,29] these complications can be minimized with the use of dental amalgam stents.[2] As such, this is the senior author's preferred method of treatment (Fig. 31–5). The first step is to release the sulcus, thereby recreating the full extent of the defect. Grafts are then taken from the buccal mucosa and stented in place to maximize graft take. Another potential long-term complication is prolapse of the posterior surface of the gingivolabial sulcus, and this necessitates resuspension of the mucosa to the premaxillary periosteum.[17]

Orbicularis Oris Muscle

The goal of primarily reconstructing the orbicularis oris sphincter and obtaining lip muscle continuity cannot be overemphasized (Fig. 31–6). The literature is replete with examples documenting its importance.[2,3,7,9,25,26,30–33] However, this was not always the case. It was previously believed that uniting the orbicularis oris would inhibit premaxillary growth.[24] It is now thought that continuity of the lip musculature reduces midfacial skeletal deformity by acting as a natural orthodontic force to further mold the premaxilla.[7,15] With regard to the soft tissues, a discontinuous orbicularis oris has been implicated in widened lip scars, wide and convex philtrums, and whistle deformities. Furthermore, failure to dissect, release, reorient, and unite the muscle fibers from the alar bases will contribute to persistent bulging of the discontinuous lateral lip musculature with attempted

animation.[2,3,9,26,30] If evaluation reveals functional abnormality of the orbicularis oris and a telltale "muscle bulge" on animation, it should be repaired.

While some have emphasized the importance of strict muscle-to-muscle union behind the prolabium,[27] we feel, *in secondary cases*, it is often sufficient to reattach the orbicularis oris to the lateral aspects of the prolabium, as seen in normal anatomy (Fig. 31–7). When undertaking orbicularis oris reorientation, the prolabial dissection should be limited to less than half of its width, to fully preserve the existing philtral dimple.

SECONDARY NASAL DEFORMITIES

Bilateral Cleft Lip Nasal Deformity

The secondary bilateral cleft lip nasal deformity includes anomalous lower lateral cartilages with deficient middle crura, a depressed nasal tip, deficient columella, lower lateral cartilage domal splay, absent or diminutive caudal septum and nasal spine, and horizontally widened alar bases (Fig. 31–8). In efforts to repair the primary anomaly, and prevent secondary deformities, a limited rhinoplasty should be performed during primary repair of the lip. Primary cleft lip rhinoplasty includes dissection and superior-medial mobilization of the lower lateral cartilages, which are then secured adjacent to each other to create a more normal appearing nasal tip.[10] Interdomal suspension sutures are then used to

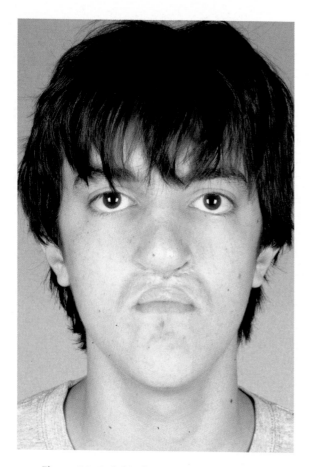

Figure 31–6. Orbicularis oris muscle deformity.

stabilize the repositioned cartilages. Fortunately, great strides have been made in the primary treatment of the cleft lip nasal deformity, most notably the advent of presurgical nasoalveolar molding[24,34,35] (Figs. 31–9 and 31–10). The nasal component of the molding process gradually reshapes the collapsed and malpositioned alae into a more normal position. This greatly facilitates primary cleft lip nasal surgery, as well as any subsequent cleft lip rhinoplasty. These advances in primary lip and nose repair will hopefully decrease the number of secondary deformities.

Nasal Tip

Correction of the alar cartilages remains a significant part of secondary nasal reconstruction.[22] Fibrofatty tissue is interposed between the laterally splayed domes of the alar cartilages; and, as well, the alar cartilages are inherently linked to the position of the premaxilla (Fig. 31–8). Therefore, the more severe the premaxillary protrusion, the greater the nasal deformity. Many methods have been used to facilitate a more anatomic positioning of the premaxilla. Early reports even described a V-shaped resection of the nasal septum to reposition or "set-back" the premaxilla.[36]

Any definitive repair of the secondary cleft lip nasal deformity depends upon restoration of nasal projection, and this is accomplished by an open rhinoplasty technique, dissecting the lower lateral cartilages, restoring domal competence with tip sutures and columellar struts or septal extension grafts, such as the extended spreader graft. Thus, the alar cartilages can then be suspended to the new septal angle, thereby augmenting and insuring tip projection.[2,9,10,18,19] While some prefer cartilage grafting over relocation of the alar cartilages to avoid surface irregularities,[26] alar cartilage

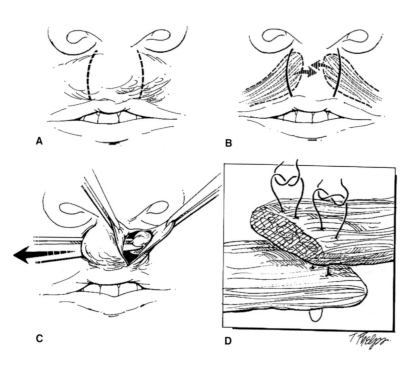

Figure 31–7. Reconstruction of orbicularis oris muscle.

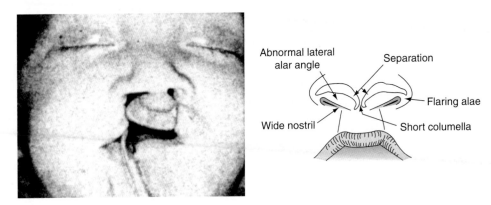

Figure 31–8. Flared nasal alae.

mobilization and suture stabilization first described by Gillies and Kilner in 1932[1] remains an essential part of the treatment of the cleft-lip nose. Often, the anomalous lower lateral cartilages are distorted and inadequate for use. This requires reconstruction of the alar cartilages with conchal cartilage grafts. While a closed rhinoplasty approach may be used for minor deformities, an open rhinoplasty is advised for more severe and asymmetric deformities typically associated with bilateral clefts.[2]

Columella

Traditionally, secondary columellar elongation has been the method of correcting the depressed nasal tip and distorted nasolabial angle in the bilateral cleft lip-nose deformity.[37,38] Secondary columellar lengthening remained the mainstay of treatment for many years, and was accomplished by various techniques including V-Y philtral or prolabial advancement,[1,7,13–15,22,28] the forked flap procedure by Millard,[7,9,15,16,20,27,37–44] and the nasal rotation-advancement by Cronin.[13,26,37,38,44,45] Unfortunately, all

these local soft tissue rearrangements result in "peculiar tertiary distortions"[17] with abnormal length with growth from extensive scarring at the lip-columella junction and abnormal columellar dimensions and appearance. Substantial criticism has been voiced with regard to these procedures.[6,13,15,17,20,34,46,47] Occasionally, soft tissue from the lip is still advocated for a small subset of patients who have persistent columellar deficiency and tethering of the nasal tip. Fortunately today, the advances in presurgical nasoalveolar molding and primary nasal correction[48] (Fig. 31–11) has changed this treatment paradigm.

Alar Base

The alar base is often excessively wide in the secondary bilateral cleft lip nasal deformity. This is from an inadequate primary correction of this defect, as well as widening and flare that can occur over time. At the time of secondary cleft lip nasal repair and alar cartilage reposition and/or reconstruction, the alar bases may be medially repositioned with nostril sill reduction and permanent suture fixation from alar-base

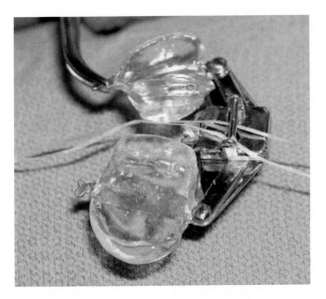

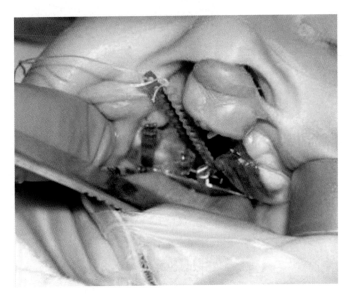

Figure 31–9. Active nasoalveolar molding device.

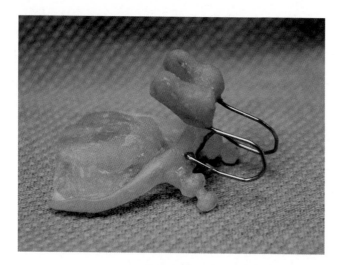

Figure 31–10. Passive nasoalveolar molding device.

to alar-base. Often, complete lower lateral cartilage release from the overlying skin and underlying mucosa is required for adequate reposition of the alar cartilages and base.

Septum

The nasal septum of the bilateral cleft is often distorted and displaced into one of the nasal vestibules. Frequently this results in the functional issue of decreased airflow. Should the septal deformity be severe enough in the growing child to result in functional concerns, such as sleep apnea, a limited septoplasty may be performed for relief of nasal obstruction. At the time of secondary septorhinoplasty, usually delayed until near complete growth of the midface has occurred, a complete submucous resection can be performed both for

improvement of the airways and harvesting of cartilage for reconstructive grafts.

SKELETAL DEFICIENCY

Maxilla and Premaxilla Development

The primary and secondary palatal structures are separated by the incisive foramen. Failure of the embryologic maxillary and frontonasal processes to fuse, results in a cleft between the pre- and lateral maxilla in both the unilateral and bilateral deformity. The central premaxilla is commonly displaced in both unilateral and bilateral alveolar clefts, and can appear in various stages of malposition. The discontinuous premaxillary segment of the bilateral cleft palate contains the tooth buds of the central and lateral incisors. Medial shift or collapse of the lateral or posterior maxillary segments causes a crowding effect, "locking-out" the premaxillary segment, resulting in difficulty reincorporating this segment into the maxillary arch. Anterior oro-nasal fistulas, at the junction of the primary and secondary palates or incisive foramen, are also a consequence of this crowded premaxillary segment in the bilateral cleft palate. Different methods of presurgical orthopedics, such as nasoalveolar molding, lip taping, early repair of the cleft lip with orbicularis approximation, and bone fixed devices such as the Latham appliance, are used to affect alignment of the premaxillary segment, facilitate lip repair, and prevent secondary maxillary arch deformities.

Studies have demonstrated that early surgical correction of the bilateral cleft lip and palate can significantly affect the morphology of the developing maxilla and mandible. Comparison of patients who underwent cleft repair with nonoperated controls demonstrate that the nonoperated

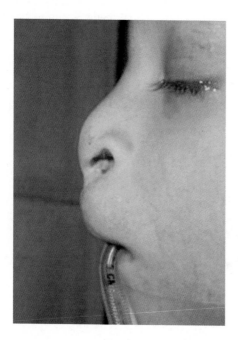

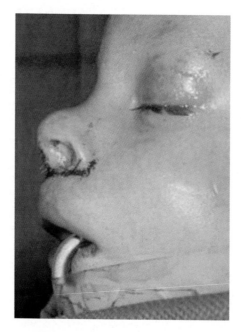

Figure 31–11. Columellar lengthening before and after.

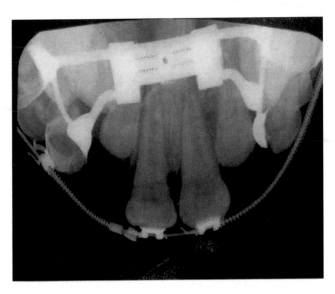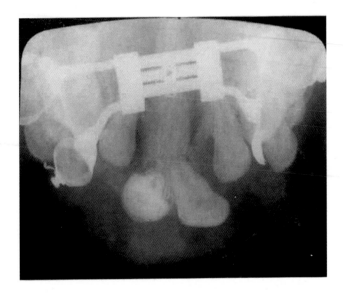

Figure 31–12. Orthodontic prealveolar segment remodeling.

patients have more normal maxillary morphology than those having had lip and palatal procedures. Patients having cleft palate repair typically demonstrate inadequate maxillary width, and typically require orthodontic intervention to achieve adequate maxillary arch width to accommodate permanent dentition and normal occlusal relationships. Occlusion difficulties including crossbite, crowding, and open bite are associated with deficient maxillary arch widths that often require future maxillary advancement (Fig. 31–12). While difficult to treat, these problems are correctable, and the main goal in surgery is to develop a functional bite, acceptable speech, and early enhanced appearance.

The Alveolar Cleft

Secondary alveolar bone grafting is indicated as part of the staged reconstruction in bilateral cleft lips where labial-nasal fistulae are present. Further rationale for their reconstruction includes stabilization of the maxillary arch, providing a bed for teeth and prostheses, and support for the alar base of the nose. Currently, bone grafting is the preferred method for alveolar repair in both unilateral and bilateral cleft palates. The timing of alveolar bone grafting should be based on dental age and orthodontic preparation of the maxillary arch. Our preferred timing is during the mixed dentition period prior to the eruption of the maxillary canine. This algorithm is based on the premise that alveolar development is nearly complete by 8 years, or about the age of first molar eruption. Grafting during this period, compared to earlier or later grafting has been shown to improve results for long-term survival of the lateral canine. It has also been shown to result in decreased late root resorption and improved implant success. With regard to closure of the oronasal fistula, bone grafting has been shown to significantly improve the chances of successful closure. Furthermore, condition of the gingiva and periosteum is an important indicator of graft survival.

Primary gingivoperiosteoplasty, at the time of primary lip and nose repair, has been used in place of alveolar bone grafting. Following nasoalveolar molding and alignment of the alveolar shelves, this technique is useful for closure of anterior fistulae. However, issues of dento-alveolar development following this procedure, as well as its long-term success, have not been adequately delineated.

Bone Graft Material

Iliac crest cancellous bone is the standard source of bone graft material with reported success rates between 70 and 95%. Pain is the primary problem with this donor material; and this issue might be lessened by placement of local anesthetic pain pumps intraoperatively. Cranial bone offers the advantage of less pain, but the quality of the specimen has shown decreased success of the graft in some studies. More recently, bone morphogenic protein, a naturally derived, synthetic human protein has been reported to have good preliminary results. This however is controversial due to the lack of indication for this process by current FDA standards.

Alveolar Bone Graft Technique

The margins of the cleft along the alveolus are incised and mucoperiosteal flaps are elevated on the anterior surface of the alveolus. The lateral mucoperiosteal flaps from the premaxillary segment are elevated along with the gingiva from the premaxillary teeth. The incision is continued laterally to the vestibule, and dissection of the maxilla anteriorly exposes the piriform aperture. The cleft lining is elevated from the lateral alveolus and the septum medially. These flaps are elevated to the posterior most aspect of the cleft, and divided on either side at the hard palate. This creates two nasal floor flaps and two palatal surface flaps. The nasal floor flaps are then approximated, and cortical bone is placed onto the nasal floor. The pyramidal shaped defect is packed with cancellous bone, and more cortical bone is used to cover the defect at the hard palate. The palatal floor and gingival flaps are closed over the bone. Bone is placed along the piriform aperture, providing support and elevating the alar base. A tension-free closure anteriorly on the lateral mucoperiosteal flap is essential, and is permitted by dividing the periosteal flap from the maxilla.

Postoperative care includes a liquid diet until healing is adequate to allow a soft diet. A soft diet is maintained for 6 weeks postoperatively. Diagnostic radiographs are not necessary for at least 6 months, and should be performed prior to any attempt at placing implants that would depend on bony fixation. If implants are anchored in the graft, this should take place after a minimum of 6 months postoperative healing time, as bone resorption is expected for 6 months to 1 year. A mobile premaxilla must be secured postoperatively through the use of an occlusal devise in conjunction with orthodontic brackets until complete consolidation of the graft material has occurred.

In the bilateral cleft, limited perfusion to the premaxilla discourages enthusiastic gingivoperiosteal and labial mucosal mobilization. The labial soft tissue of the premaxilla should be preserved anteriorly to maintain blood supply to the premaxilla. Bilateral gingivoperiosteal flaps are raised laterally and, sufficiently long flaps are created utilizing back-cuts and periosteal release that allow for medial advancement, compensating for the anteromedial paucity of premaxillary soft tissue. The surgeon should consider various options and possibly postponing the bone graft if there is less than optimal quality of the soft tissue surrounding the cleft, since adequate revascularization of graft is dependent on good quality donor tissue. This decision should be made with pediatric dental and orthodontic consultation and in coordination with the overall dento-skeletal treatment plan. Large labial-nasal fistulae, along with the presence of periodontal disease and dental caries, will decrease the chance of a successful outcome. These important issues, as well as patient and family compliance, should be considered before grafting is attempted. Finally, close apposition and meticulous closure of the gingivoperiosteal and mucoperiosteal flaps will increase the chance of successful graft outcomes. A compromise of any of these factors may result in flap compromise, bone graft loss, and recurrence of labio-nasal fistulae.

Midface Hypoplasia

The secondary bilateral cleft lip deformity often includes midface hypoplasia with skeletal and dental Class 3 relations. The LeFort I osteotomy is used most commonly in repair of maxillary deformities associated with bilateral clefts. This osteotomy extends across the anterolateral aspect of the maxilla through the pterygomaxillary junction, and is continuous through the medial septal base on either side. The maxillary (LeFort I) segment is moved in an anterior direction and can be fixed with rigid fixation and bone grafting. Maxillary or midface advancement can also be achieved using distraction osteogenesis techniques, and the results are often dramatic in improving occlusion and aesthetic balance to the face.

Pyriform Rim

The secondary bilateral cleft lip and nose deformity often includes persistent pyriform rim or naso-maxillary hypoplasia despite alveolar bone grafting and maxillary (LeFort I) advancement. Pyriform rim augmentation has been performed with autogenous only bone and/or fat grafting, as well as other forms of prosthetic augmentation such as porous polyethylene implants, bone substitutes, and fillers.

PREVENTION

Because of the severity of the primary birth insult, all bilateral clefts share a severe paucity of tissue. The paramount importance of preventing secondary cleft lip and nose deformities, with appropriate presurgical and surgical techniques when addressing the primary cleft deformity, has been emphasized.[2,22,49] It is easier to avoid a secondary deformity than it is to correct it. Therefore, the best time to prevent secondary deformities is at the time of the initial operation. While secondary deformities of the bilateral cleft lip and nose are not always the result of surgical failure at the initial operation,[7] there are certain surgical techniques that are essential for prevention of secondary stigmata. These include (1) obtaining normal alveolar arch dimension and relationships presurgically, (2) achieving muscular continuity with the primary lip repair, (3) appropriate philtral design (no greater than 4–6 mm in width at the level of the vermilion border), (4) primary domal reconstruction with repositioning of the alar cartilages, and (5) formation of the median central tubercle from the lateral labial elements. Surgical prevention is further advanced by anticipation of facial growth and soft tissue distortion that occur as the child develops. According to Mulliken, during primary repair, those nasolabial features that are programmed for rapid growth (and distortion) should be crafted on a small scale. Likewise, slow-growing features, which will fail to reach normal anatomic dimension, should be constructed on a slightly larger scale than infantile size.[23]

Most of these surgical goals are facilitated by a cleft lip, nose, and alveolus that is presurgically aligned. This is achieved with presurgical orthopedics that positions the premaxilla in alignment with the alveolar arch, and minimizes postoperative prolabial distortion and interalar widening, thereby averting secondary revisions.[17,23] The ultimate in prevention may lie in the future of fetal cleft repair, which holds the potential of scarless wound healing, thereby averting the ripple effect of postnatal scarring and midfacial growth deformity.[50]

References

1. Gillies H, Kilner TP. Hare-lip: Operations for the correction of secondary deformities. *Lancet* 2:1369–1375, 1932.
2. Stal S, Hollier LH. Secondary deformities of the cleft lip, nose, and palate. In Mathes SJ (ed). *Plastic Surgery*, 2nd edn., Vol 4, Elsevier, Philadelphia, PA, 2006, pp. 339–363.

3. Stal S, Hollier LH. Correction of secondary cleft lip deformities. *Plast Reconstr Surg* 109(5):1672–1681, 2002.

4. Huffman WC, Lierle DM. The repair of the bilateral cleft lip. *Plast Reconstr Surg* 4:489–501, 1949.

5. Weinfeld AB, Hollier LH, Spira M, Stal S. International trends in the treatment of cleft lip and palate. *Clin Plast Surg* 32:19–23, 2005.

6. Stal S, Klebuc M, Taylor T, Spira M, Edwards M. Algorithms for the treatment of cleft lip and palate. *Clin Plast Surg* 25(4):493–507, 1998.

7. Garza JR, Pessa JE, Futrell JW. Secondary deformities of the cleft lip and nose. In Bentz ML (ed). *Pediatric Plastic Surgery*. Stamford: Appleton and Lange, 1998, pp. 81–92.

8. Marsh JL. When is enough enough? Secondary surgery for cleft lip and palate patients. *Clin Plast Surg* 17(1):37–47, 1990.

9. Cohen M. Residual deformities after repair of clefts of the lip and palate. *Clin Plast Surg* 31:331–345, 2004.

10. Stal S, Hollier LH. Correction of secondary deformities of the cleft lip nose. *Plast Reconstr Surg* 109(4):1386–1392, 2002.

11. Cohen M. Secondary correction of the nasal deformity associated with cleft lip. In Cohen M (ed). *Mastery of Plastic and Reconstructive Surgery*. Boston: Little, Brown, and Company, 1994, pp. 702–719.

12. Sandove AM, Eppley BL. Correction of secondary cleft lip and nasal deformities. *Clin Plast Surg* 20(4):793–801, 1993.

13. Jackson IT. Cleft lip and palate. In Mustarde JC, Jackson IT (eds). *Plastic Surgery in Infancy and Childhood*, 3rd edn. Edinburgh: Churchill Livingstone, 1988, pp. 1–40.

14. Lamont ES. Reparative plastic surgery of secondary cleft lip and nasal deformities. *Surg Gynecol Obstet* 80:422–434, 1945.

15. Jackson IT, Fasching MC. Secondary deformities of cleft lip, nose, and cleft palate. In McCarthy JG (ed). *Plastic and Reconstructive Surgery*, Vol 4. Philadelphia: WB Saunders, 1990.

16. Viale-Gonzalez M, Barreto F, Ortiz-Monasterio. Surgical management of the bilateral cleft lip. *Plast Reconstr Surg* 51(5):530–535, 1973.

17. Mulliken JB. Primary repair of bilateral cleft lip and nasal deformity. *Plast Reconstr Surg* 108(1):181–194, 2001.

18. Mulliken JB. Primary repair of the bilateral cleft lip and nasal deformity. In Georgiade GS, Riefkohl R, Levin LS (eds). *Georgiade: Plastic, Maxillofacial, and Reconstructive Surgery*, 3rd edn. Baltimore: Williams & Wilkins, 1997.

19. Cronin TD, Upton J. Lengthening of the short columella associated with bilateral cleft lip. *Ann Plast Surg* 1:75–81, 1978.

20. Lewis MB. Secondary soft tissue procedures for cleft lip and palate. In Cohen M (ed). *Mastery of Plastic and Reconstructive Surgery*. Boston: Little, Brown, and Company, 1994, pp. 605–618.

21. Abbe, R. A new plastic operation for the relief of deformity due to double harelip. *Med Rec* 53:477–478, 1898.

22. Brown JB, McDowell F. Secondary repair of cleft lips and their nasal deformities. *Ann Surg* 114:101–117, 1941.

23. Mulliken JB, Wu JK, Padwa BL. Repair of bilateral cleft lip: Review, revisions, and reflections. *J Craniofac Surg* 14(5):609–620, 2003.

24. Mulliken JB. Bilateral cleft lip. *Clin Plast Surg* 31(2):209–220, 2004.

25. Meijer R. Secondary repair of the bilateral cleft lip deformity. *Cleft Palate J* 21(2):86–90, 1984.

26. McCarthy JG, Cutting CB. Secondary deformities of cleft lip and palate. In Georgiade GS, Riefkohl R, Levin LS (eds). *Georgiade: Plastic, Maxillofacial, and Reconstructive Surgery*, 3rd edn. Baltimore: Williams & Wilkins, 1997, pp. 247–257.

27. Millard DR. Closure of bilateral cleft lip and elongation of columella by two operations in infancy. *Plast Reconstr Surg* 47(4):324–331, 1971.

28. Brown JB, McDowell F, Byars LT. Double clefts of the lip. *Surg Gynecol Obstet* 85:20–29, 1947.

29. Erol OO, Agaoglu G. Reconstruction of the superior labial sulcus in secondary bilateral cleft lip deformities: An inverted U-shaped flap. *Plast Reconstr Surg* 108(7):1871–1873, 2001.

30. Oneal RM, Greer DM, Nobel GL. Secondary correction of bilateral cleft lip deformities with Millard's midline muscular closure. *Plast Reconstr Surg* 54(1):45–51, 1974.

31. Black PW, Scheflan M. Bilateral cleft lip repair: "Putting it all together". *Ann Plast Surg* 12(2):118–127, 1984.

32. Tessier P, Tulasne JF. Secondary repair of cleft lip deformities. *Clin Plast Surg* 11(4):747–760, 1984.

33. Rees TD, Swinyard CA, Converse JM. The prolabium in the bilateral cleft lip. *Plast Reconstr Surg* 30(6):651–662, 1962.

34. Cutting C, Grayson B, Brecht L, Santiago P, Wood R, Kwon S. Presurgical columellar elongation and primary retrograde nasal reconstruction in one-stage bilateral cleft lip and nose repair. *Plast Reconstr Surg* 101(3):630–639, 1998.

35. Rutrick R, Black PW, Jurkiewicz MJ. Bilateral cleft lip and palate: Presurgical treatment. *Ann Plast Surg* 12(2):105–117, 1984.

36. Schultz LW. Bilateral cleft lips. *Plast Reconstr Surg* 1:338–343, 1946.

37. Nakajima T, Yoshimura Y. Secondary correction of bilateral cleft lip nose deformity. *J Craniomaxillofac Surg* 18(2):63–67, 1990.

38. Wilson LF. Correction of residual deformities of the lip and nose in repaired clefts of the primary palate (lip and alveolus). *Clin Plast Surg* 12(4):719–733, 1985.

39. Millard DR. A primary compromise for bilateral cleft lip. *Surg Gynecol Obstet* 111:557–563, 1960.

40. Lehman JA. Secondary repair of bilateral cleft lip deformities: A two-stage approach. *Br J Plast Surg* 29:116–121, 1976.

41. Millard DR. Columella lengthening by a forked flap. *Plast Reconstr Surg* 22:454–457, 1958.

42. McComb H. Primary repair of the bilateral cleft lip nose. *Br J Plast Surg* 28:262–267, 1957.

43. Wray RC. Secondary correction of nasal abnormalities associated with cleft lip. *J Oral Surg* 34(2):113–117, 1976.

44. Maeda K, Ojimi H, Yoshida T. A new method of secondary correction of the bilateral cleft lip nose. *Br J Plast Surg* 40:52–60, 1987.

45. Cronin TD. Lengthening columella by use of skin from nasal floor and alae. *Plast Reconstr Surg* 21(6):417–426, 1958.

46. Trier WC. Repair of bilateral cleft lip: Millard's technique. *Clin Plast Surg* 12(4):605–625, 1985.

47. McComb H. Primary repair of the bilateral cleft lip nose: A 15-year review and a new treatment plan. *Plast Reconstr Surg* 86(5):882–889, 1990.

48. Jackson IT, Yavuzer R, Kelly C, Bu-Ali H. The central lip flap and nasal mucosal rotation advancement: Important aspects of composite correction of the bilateral cleft lip nose deformity. *J Craniofac Surg* 16(2):255–261, 2005.

49. Marcks KM, Trevaskis AE, Payne MJ, Kicos JE. The management of secondary cleft lip deformities. *Am J Surgery* 95:932–937, 1958.

50. Lorenz HP, Longaker MT. In utero surgery for cleft lip/palate: Minimizing the "ripple effect" of scarring. *J Craniofac Surg* 14(4):504–511, 2003.

32

Definitive Rhinoplasty for Adult Cleft Lip Nasal Deformity

Gary Burget, MD

INTRODUCTION

Despite primary repair of the cleft lip nasal deformity in infancy, a suboptimal aesthetic outcome often results when the child is grown. A potential reason is that the anatomy of the infant nose is rudimentary and primordial until adolescence. Until then, the lower lateral cartilages are thin and poorly formed. Only between 12–18 years of age, does the nose grow and take on its true size and form. Early surgical correction of the infant nose is hindered by its primordial anatomy and by limited surgical access and visibility. It often is not possible to give the small, paper-thin alar cartilage an aesthetically

correct shape, especially through an intranasal surgical approach. The normal adult shape of the alar cartilage, its medial, middle and lateral crura, and medial and lateral genua, are only hinted at in the first few years of life. Refined shaping with sutures often cannot be done until the cartilage has grown. Early postoperative attempts at correction of the cleft lip nasal deformity often achieves a "lift" of the alar cartilage to the septal cartilage or to the external nasal skin, as in a Tajima repair.[1] These early cartilage "lifts" require separating the alar cartilage from the nasal skin, and cutting the cartilage loose from its attachment to the upper lateral cartilage by dividing the nearly invisible infant scroll cartilage that connects the two. This dissection creates planes of contracting scar, and in some instances may do more damage to the nose than the surgery does good. Correcting the so-called "slumped" (or, posteriorly depressed) alar cartilage, by freeing and lifting it with sutures, is a desperate attempt that may fall short of the current standard guiding aesthetic open rhinoplasty.

At adolescence, the nasal bones, upper laterals, and septum begin to rapidly expand anteriorly and vertically. At the same time, the alar cartilages become increasingly convoluted, until they take on the adult dimensions and the specific, complex, mirror-image forms that make an adult nose appear normal, deformed, beautiful, or ugly. These aesthetic judgments rarely can be made until the cartilages have grown. Often, the time for definitive reshaping of the deformed cleft lip alar cartilage is after this growth is complete. Attempting to reshape or even reposition the infant's gossamer alar cartilage will succeed only when the deformity is mild.

Many articles show "before" and "after" photographs of cleft lip noses of children who are only 3–8 years after initial repair of their cleft lip nasal deformity. These comparisons are not entirely valid, as their noses are still infantile. The early "lifts" of the cleft-side alar cartilage can achieve symmetry, but only so long as the nose remains in its primordial, prepubescent state. When the nasal framework grows and assumes its mature size and shape at adolescence, nascent deformities appear.

Children with significant secondary cleft lip nasal deformities have to be reshaped or rebuilt with cartilage grafts after the adolescent growth has occurred, at 14–18 years of age. Yet these late rhinoplasties often are not performed. By the time an open rhinoplasty is indicated, a cleft lip patient has adjusted psychologically to a certain permanent facial deformity and the stigma it carries. Furthermore, the pediatric plastic surgeon that has cared for these patients since birth is not usually—with some brilliant exceptions—highly skilled at adult open rhinoplasty. Because these grownup cleft lip patients accept their deformity as "the best that can be expected," definitive correction of their twisted noses is never done.

THE CLEFT LIP ALAR CARTILAGE

It is said that the cleft lip alar cartilage (in both unilateral and bilateral deformities) is "slumped" (depressed posteriorly). In truth, it is stretched across an abnormally wide piriform aperture (Fig. 32–1). It is attached at both ends to bone, the medial end to the premaxilla and the lateral end to the maxilla via a tight leash of sesamoid cartilages. In some cases, the piriform aperture is so wide that no amount of lifting and tugging can move the alar cartilage arch anteriorly so that it projects normally. Even releasing the lateral end of the lateral crus from the maxilla by transecting the chain of sesamoid cartilages will not allow the alar arch to move foreword. The fibrocartilage of the alar arch is tightly fused to the skin that lines the nasal vestibule. Both the lining skin and the lateral crus must be cut loose from the bony edge of the piriform

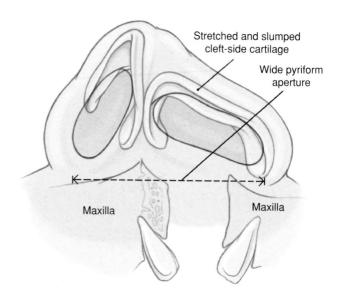

Figure 32–1. In cleft lip deformities, the alar cartilage is slumped and stretched over an abnormally wide piriform aperture.

aperture before the lateral crus can be advanced anteriorly. Yet even this radical release may not allow the alar cartilage to project anteriorly, for in many cases the alar cartilage is hypoplastic.

The alar cartilage of the cleft side often does not attain the size and form of the alar cartilage on the opposite normal side. The surface area of the alar lobule of the cleft side of the nose is often only half the surface area of the contralateral normal ala. As the nose grows at adolescence, the true magnitude of this hypoplasia becomes apparent. The middle and lateral crura are slumped and hypoplastic. The fibrofatty tissue and skin envelope of the cleft side of the nose are also hypoplastic. In many cases, no amount of lifting and release of the middle and lateral crura can make the hypoplastic alar cartilage project normally. In these cases, open rhinoplasty, performed after the nose has reached its adult proportions, allows the surgeon to construct a new alar cartilage framework over the existing hypoplastic alar cartilage—in essence, to build a new tip for the nose. Mild asymmetries can be corrected with conventional open rhinoplasty techniques used to reshape the alar cartilage with transdomal, interdomal, and lateral crural sutures. Severe deformities, in which one or both alar cartilages are hypoplastic, require reconstruction of the entire nasal tip with cartilage grafts. These grafts are harvested from the nasal septum, conchae of the ears or costal cartilages.

Early manipulations of the alar cartilage should be minimal, because such manipulations are of limited and temporary benefit, even sometimes a perfunctory exercise. The cartilage should not be cut or detached from the vestibule skin lining and probably should not be cut loose from the scroll that joins it to the upper lateral cartilage. Early lifting can fully correct only mild deformities. For major cleft lip nasal deformities, a definitive operation will be necessary around 14–18 years of age if the adult nose is to be symmetrical and of normal appearance. The operation of choice is open rhinoplasty to reshape the septal and alar cartilages under direct vision or to build a new nasal tip with cartilage grafts.

Cartilage grafts may be harvested from the nasal septum, concha of the ear, or the costal cartilages. Each donor source has advantages and detractions. The septum provides strong hyaline cartilage but in short supply. Ear cartilage is fibrocartilage and therefore weak. Septal or ear cartilage should be used only when the cleft lip nasal deformity is not severe. For the severely deformed nasal tip that needs a strong anterior projection and is covered with an inelastic nasal skin envelope stiffened by scar, costal cartilage is the material of choice. Gunter has taught that only costal cartilage has the strength to provide architectural support and aesthetic form for severely deformed noses.[2]

THE OPERATION

The Incision

The edges of a symmetric incision are easy to line up at closure. For this reason, many surgeons use a transverse columella incision with a central dentate flap. The proper position for this incision is between the anterior one-third and the posterior two-thirds of the columella (Fig. 32–2), not at the base of the columella. A normal columella has an hourglass shape when viewed from below—wider at the top and bottom than at the middle. The incision lies at the narrowest point, at about the junction of the upper and middle thirds. The belief that placing the incision at the base of the columella will somehow hide the scar in a natural, shadowed crease is not true. In truth, there is no crease at the base of a normal columella, but rather a smooth, open, obtuse angle between the lip and nose. Furthermore, the base is the most anteriorly facing part of the columella, so that a scar at the base will easily be seen on frontal view. Finally, placing the open rhinoplasty scar at the base of the columella creates an unduly long columella flap,

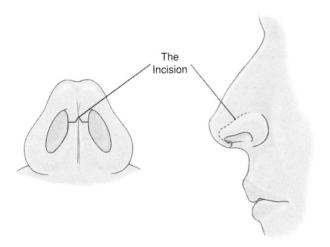

The Incision

Figure 32–2. The transverse columella incision for open rhinoplasty should be made between the anterior one-third and posterior two-thirds of the columella, not at its base.

which will then be less vascular and subject to necrosis. Many experienced, expert rhinoplasty surgeons have had cases of columella flap necrosis. Therefore, the open rhinoplasty incision should be placed anteriorly on the columella, not at its base.

The initial incision is made with a scalpel. It extends superiorly just 2.5 mm behind the lateral edges of the columella. The columella incision is then deepened to the middle crura of the alar cartilages with fine scissors. This protects the middle crura of the alar cartilages within the columella from injury, or from being elevated with the flap of skin and fat. Cutting across the columella reveals the paired columella or septal branches of the superior labial arteries; these need to be cauterized. As the flap of skin and fat is elevated off the middle and lateral crura of the alar cartilage, the internal incision is extended across the nasal vestibule following the inferior edge of the lateral crus of the alar cartilage. As the flap is elevated, the alar cartilage can be seen, and the vestibular skin can be cut with a scissors just at the inferior edge of the lateral crus. This releases the skin of the nasal tip.

If the columella incision is closed meticulously, the scar is rarely seen after a few months. Using 3.5X magnifying loupes, the incision is closed with 1–3 subcuticular 6-0 clear sutures and 9–11 7-0 monofilament skin sutures. To prevent stitch marks, the sutures should be removed within 2–4 days after surgery and are replaced with narrow (1/16-inch to 1/24-inch) tapes and held with gum mastic adhesive. The sutures should be removed with extreme gentleness. As Sir Harold Gillies said, "Do not lift the patient up by his stitches."[3]

Freeing the Deformed Alar Cartilage

When the flap of skin and fat has been elevated off the perichondrium and periosteum of the nasal cartilages and bones, one can then free the stretched and slumped lateral crus from its attachments to the maxilla. It may be impossible to reshape the alar cartilage arch on the cleft side without extensive freeing of the cartilage. There are two reasons for this: (1) The piriform aperture of the nose above the cleft maxilla is abnormally wide. The alar cartilage is stretched across this wide bony cleft between the premaxilla and the lateral maxilla. Freeing the lateral crus of the alar cartilage from the maxilla may not give the cartilage enough mobility. The tight skin lining of the vestibule must also be cut loose from the bony edge of the piriform aperture so that the nasal vestibule and alar margin may be projected anteriorly and also reshaped. This is done by cutting the vestibule skin lining free just at the anterior edge of the bony piriform aperture, or by releasing it by cutting slightly posterior to that edge so that the lining defect lies on the lateral bony sidewall of the nose and (2) The alar cartilage may be small and flimsy. In this case, attempts to give it a normal shape, size and anterior projection are futile. The cartilage should be buttressed with strong grafts of septal or costal cartilage, or replaced with a new arch of cartilage manufactured from septum, concha, or rib cartilage.

Two Techniques for Supporting the New Nasal Tip

The deformed alar cartilage is released from its posterior attachments. When it is of nearly *normal* size, it can be reshaped and braced with cartilage grafts using the techniques borrowed from cosmetic open rhinoplasty. If the alar cartilage is *hypoplastic*, then one or both alar cartilages must be reconstructed anew using cartilage graft material from the septum, ear or rib. In either case, cartilage grafts are the key to achieving a symmetric, projecting and normal-appearing nasal tip. The best donor material for reconstruction of the alar cartilage is septal or costal cartilage. Cartilage from the ear is simply too soft.

The skin of a cleft lip nose has an intrinsic form, a "memory" of the shape of the cleft lip nasal deformity. That is, if one were to remove the skin from a cleft lip nose and place it on a table, the skin would stand up—even without any cartilage support—and retain the shape of the cleft lip nose. Plastic surgeons have underestimated this intrinsic "memory of the nose" that characterizes a somewhat rigid nasal skin envelope. Furthermore, the cleft lip nose has an even more rigid form than a normal nose because of the subcutaneous layer of scar tissue from previous operations. A strong cartilage framework must be constructed in the course of open rhinoplasty to overcome the stiff skin envelope of the cleft lip nose and force the skin into a normal, natural shape.

Ear fibrocartilage is too soft for this purpose. Ear cartilage may be used for filler, or for isolated small grafts (e.g., tip grafts or alar margin grafts), but not for architectural purposes such as creating nasal tip projection. Septal hyaline cartilage is strong and easy to carve, but in short supply. Only costal cartilage from the fifth, sixth, seventh, or eighth ribs is sufficiently rigid and plentiful for creating a supportive framework for the dorsum, alae and tip of the nose, and sufficiently strong for overcoming the intrinsic cleft lip shape of the nasal skin envelope.

Cartilage Grafting When the Cleft Alar Cartilage is of *Normal* Size

When the alar cartilage on the cleft side is of nearly normal or normal size, sutures can reshape it to match the contralateral normal cartilage. Cartilage grafts harvested from the septum or rib are necessary to hold the reconstructed alar cartilage in its new, normal shape, because several strong forces will try to deform it again. As mentioned, the deformed skin envelope of the cleft lip nose has its own intrinsic shape that will force the nasal tip back to its original cleft lip shape. Also, after rhinoplasty, a sheet of contracting scar tissue will form beneath the skin envelope of the nose. This tissue will contract centripetally, further deforming the newly reconstructed nose. So, strong cartilage grafts are necessary to brace the alar cartilages and hold the nasal skin envelope in its normal dimensions and shape.

The grafts are those commonly used in cosmetic open rhinoplasty: (1) spreader grafts to straighten the dorsal sep-

tum and increase its height, (2) a columella strut to give rigidity to the medial and middle crura of the alar cartilages, (3) invisible tip grafts that stiffen and support the nasal tip framework, and visible tip grafts and cap grafts that add projection and give shape to the nasal tip, (4) lateral crural grafts to shape the lateral crura and support the vestibule airways, and (5) alar margin grafts ("battens") to correct pinching of the nasal tip or inward collapse of the alar margins and to give a pyramidal form to the nasal base.

In addition to those five types of grafts inside the nasal tip, three types of grafts outside the nasal tip can also be helpful. Dorsal onlay grafts and radix grafts may be used to raise the dorsum or radix and camouflage dorsal irregularities. Also, a premaxillary graft beneath the nasal floor can move the base of the nose forward and open an acute lip–nose angle.

Spreader Grafts

Two strips of cartilage are harvested from the nasal septum, concha or the fifth, sixth, seventh, or eighth costal cartilages. The grafts are carved to be approximately 1.7–3.0-cm long, 4-mm deep and 1.5-mm wide. These strips are used to spread the upper lateral cartilages apart and thus widen the anterior part of the nasal airway and the nasal dorsum itself (Fig. 32–3). The use of spreader grafts is the most effective way to permanently and predictably straighten a crooked nose.

When placing spreader grafts, the mucosal vaults of the nose are first separated intact from cartilaginous septum. The dorsal septum is shaved smooth and lowered, if indicated. The midline of the upper lip is marked; this will be the midline for the nose. The teeth may have a separate and different midline. If needed, the central septal cartilage is harvested for graft material. A supportive L-shaped strut 1.2–1.5-cm wide is retained for nasal support. Medial and lateral nasal osteotomies are done. The crooked septal cartilage is then compressed between the two spreader grafts to straighten the septum on anteroposterior view. When the septum is straight and in line with the midline of the upper lip, the spreader grafts are fastened in place with three No. 27 hypodermic needles that pass through the three layers of cartilage (the two spreader grafts and the septum). With the septal cartilage straight in the midline, the three layers are sutured tightly together with 4-0 monofilament mattress sutures. Spreader grafts may also be positioned anterior to the dorsum of the septal cartilage to raise the inferior end of the dorsal septum and increase the nasal facial angle (the opposite purpose of a radix graft). Finally, the upper lateral cartilages are trimmed and anchored to the straightened midline septum with 5-0 monofilament mattress sutures passed through all five layers of cartilage (the upper lateral cartilages, the spreader grafts and the dorsal septal cartilage). A crooked nose straightened in this way will remain in the midline in spite of the forces of scar contraction that act upon the nose in the postoperative period. Next, the framework for the nasal tip is constructed to project 6–8 mm above the dorsal line of the septal cartilage.

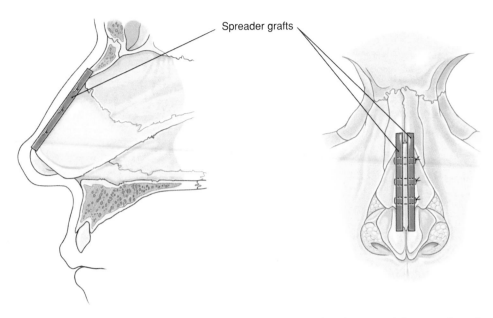

Figure 32–3. Spreader grafts permanently straighten a crooked nose. Also, they spread the upper lateral cartilages and widen the nasal airway and the nasal dorsum itself.

Columella Strut Grafts

Whenever an open rhinoplasty is performed, a strut of cartilage should be placed between the medial and middle crura of the alar cartilage. This columella strut stiffens the alar cartilage and supports the nasal tip against forces that deproject the nasal tip in the postoperative period. That is, after a rhinoplasty, a sheet of scar tissue is deposited between the nasal skin and the underlying cartilages. Starting approximately 3 weeks after surgery, myofibroblasts within the scar begin to contract with a strong force. The sheet of scar tissue tightens like a drumhead, forcing the nasal tip posteriorly against the facial plane. Tip projection can be lost. A columella strut of cartilage (or bone), as well as lateral crural grafts, form a tripod that resists the deprojecting force.[4]

A proper columella strut should have an angle to simulate Sheen's columellar–lobular angle of rotation of approximately 50 degrees.[5] If the strut is not angled, the columella may tend to be straight, giving the resulting nose a beak-like quality. Fig. 32–4 shows the columella strut and its optimal angle of rotation.

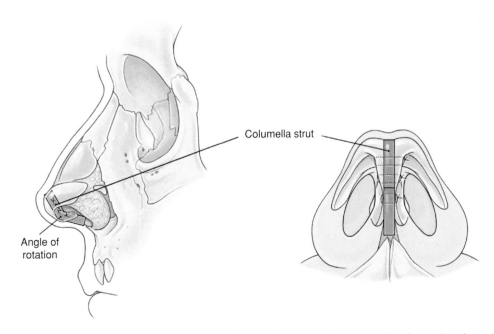

Figure 32–4. The columella strut stiffens the alar cartilages and supports the nose against forces that de-project the nasal tip after open rhinoplasty. The strut should be angled to create a normal columellar–lobular angle of rotation.

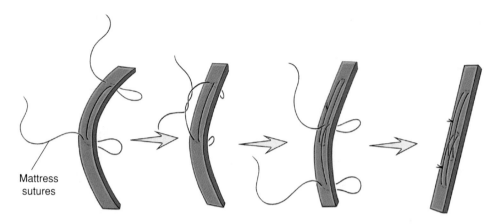

Figure 32–5. A warped columella strut can be straightened by tightening mattress sutures against the curve.

Because it is straight, septal cartilage is the best donor cartilage for a columella strut. Ear cartilage has an intrinsic curve, and costal cartilage tends to warp. However, placing mattress sutures along curved or warped strips of ear or costal cartilage, and tightening the sutures against the curve (like stringing a bow on the outside of its curve), can straighten these cartilage struts Fig. 32–5.

The columella strut is inserted into a pocket that extends deep to the feet of the existing medial crura. Some surgeons actually suture the strut to the anterior nasal spine.[6] The base of the strut is fixed to the feet of the medial crura with a gut mattress suture passed through all layers of the membranous septum. This suture fixes the height and symmetry of the alar cartilage arches. The strut is then sutured to the cephalic edges of the existing medial and middle crura of the alar cartilages with several 5-0 monofilament sutures, and this gives the new nose a stiff, strongly supported tip structure.

Visible and Invisible Tip Grafts, and Cap Grafts

Sheen (tip) grafts give strength to the alar cartilages and may add projection to the nasal tip.[7] They can be carved from septal, conchal, or costal cartilage, and even from preserved human allograft cartilage. In silhouette, the grafts look like a shield or a golf tee. A tip graft generally measures 12–16 mm in length and 9–11 mm across the top. Its edges are chamfered, or smoothed.

The tip graft is most stable when sutured to the lateral edges of the middle crura of the existing alar cartilages with a 6-0 material. The graft can be placed so its anterior end does not project above the native alar cartilage arches (an invisible tip graft or projecting 1–3 mm anterior to the alar cartilage arches (a visible tip graft)[8] (Fig. 32–6A, B). When the nasal tip skin has only a thin layer of fat, a visible tip graft may give the new nose a sharply pointed look. In these cases, a "cap" graft measuring 5–7-mm high and 9–11-mm (or more) wide is sutured cephalic to the tip graft to blunt the sharp projection

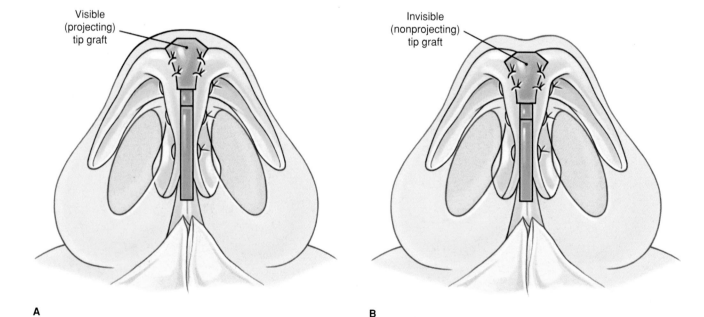

A

B

Figure 32–6. Projecting ([A]"visible") and nonprojecting ([B]"invisible") tip grafts are used to strengthen the alar cartilages.

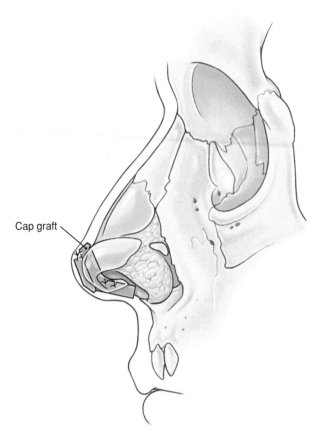

Cap graft

Figure 32–7. A cap graft can be added to soften the pointy look of a projecting tip graft when the nasal tip skin has only a thin layer of fat.

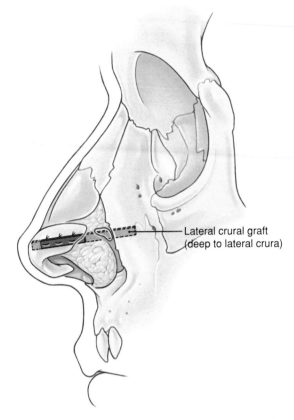

Lateral crural graft (deep to lateral crura)

Figure 32–8. A lateral crural graft (which can extend from the columella strut to the maxilla) is used to correct alar slump, straighten the lateral crus of the alar cartilage and open the airway.

and blend the nasal tip and supratip regions (Fig. 32–7). The nasal tip graft should project 6–8 mm above the dorsal line of nasal cartilages. This distance varies and is greater when the supratip fat layer is thick, and less when the supratip fat layer is thin.

Lateral Crural Grafts

Deformities of the lateral crus are best managed by inserting a straight graft under the cephalic edge of the lateral crus after cephalic trim of the lateral crus has been completed (Fig. 32–8). Lateral crural grafts may be carved from septal, conchal, or costal cartilage, or from preserved human allograft cartilage. They measure approximately 4–5-mm wide and 1–2-cm long.

If the skin of the nasal tip has a thick layer of fat, then the lateral crural graft may be inserted on top of (anterior to) the lateral crus. By fastening the lateral crura graft snugly to the lateral crus with 5-0 mattress sutures, the lateral crus can be straightened and strengthened. This procedure can correct a wide or bulbous nasal tip associated with convex (anteriorly and laterally bulging) lateral crura.

In the case of the cleft lip nasal deformity, a strong lateral crus graft will correct the alar slump, recreate a projecting alar arch and open the airway. A lateral crural graft may be extended medially and sutured to the columella strut to create

a tripod support for the nasal tip.[4] It may be extended laterally to rest on the bony edge of the piriform aperture. This stabilizes the lateral crus and prevents it from curling into the nasal vestibule in the postoperative period.

Alar Margin Grafts

These small narrow grafts (approximately 2–3-mm wide and 10–12-mm long), each approximately the size of a round toothpick, are slid into pockets along the alar margin to correct the classic pinched nasal tip deformity (Fig. 32–9). This deformity is characterized by a deep declivity between the tip subunit and the alar subunit. As a result, the tip of the nose stands out as an isolated little box on the most projecting part of the nose. After rhinoplasty, the deformity occurs as the lateral margins or the lateral ends of the alar cartilage curl into the vestibule. Cutting or removing the lateral crus can also produce a pinched tip. Alar margin grafts (battens) are effective in correcting this defect and giving the base of the nose a pyramidal shape.

Dorsal Onlay Grafts and Radix Grafts

A dorsal onlay graft can elevate the nasal dorsum and narrow the nasofacial angle (Fig. 32–10A). It also hides any bumps or divots along the dorsal edge of the cartilaginous septum, an especially important consideration for patients who will

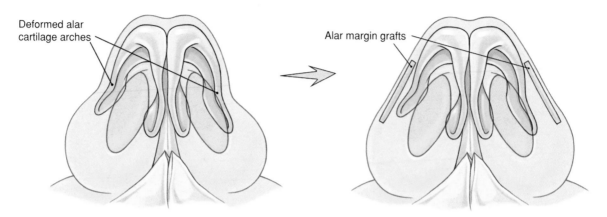

Figure 32–9. Alar margin grafts are slid into pockets along the alar margin to straighten the alar margin. They correct the classic "pinched tip" nasal deformity.

run their fingertips up and down the bridge of the nose, postoperatively. A solid dorsal graft measures 2.7–3.5 cm in length and approximately 5 mm in width. Because it seldom warps, septal cartilage with or without perpendicular plate bone is the best material for the dorsum. Place the graft with its bony portion inferior, and therefore, hidden by the thick nasal supratip skin. Ear cartilage is less suitable because of its concavo–convex qualities. Costal cartilage may be used but tends to warp. To minimize the warping of costal cartilage, one should limit carving of the graft, score the attached peri-

chondrium at 5-mm intervals, suture the graft tightly to the existing dorsal structures or pass a K-wire through the graft, as Gunter does.[9] Toriumi has said that if the costal cartilage graft is soaked in saline for 30 minutes and does not warp, it will not warp after surgery.[10] Bowstring sutures, as described above for the columella strut, may be used to straighten a dorsal onlay graft. Erol[11] and Daniel[12] have solved the warping problem by implanting diced cartilage wrapped in temporal fascia, dermis, or cellulose mesh. A radix graft narrows the nasofacial angle and straightens the dorsum (Fig. 32–10B).

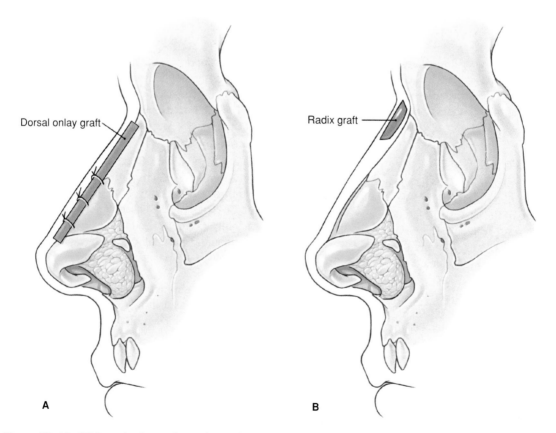

A   **B**

Figure 32–10. (A) Dorsal onlay grafts can be used to elevate and make smooth the nasal dorsum. (B) The radix graft makes the nasofacial angle more acute.

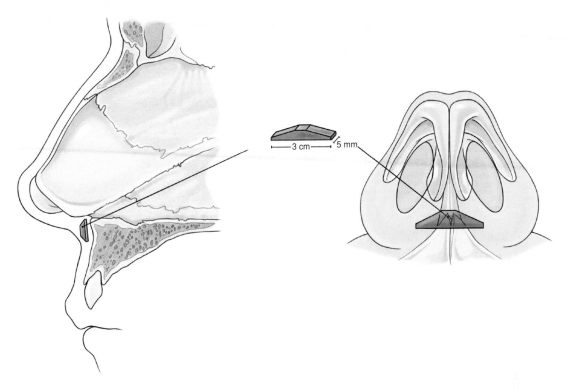

Figure 32–11. A premaxillary graft beneath the nasal floor moves the base of the nose forward.

A solid cartilage graft to the radix should be approximately 4–5-mm wide. If a wider graft is needed, it should be diced or crushed. Raising the radix allows the surgeon to create a straight dorsal line with only minimal resection of the dorsal hump. A radix graft also makes the nasofacial angle more acute and an overprotected nasal tip appear less so.

Premaxillary Grafts

The premaxillary graft advances the nasal base anteriorly and opens an acute lip–nose angle. A solid costal cartilage graft is placed through and incision in the floor of the nasal vestibule just posterior to the nostril sill and is placed in a carefully dissected pocket between the floor of the nose and the gingivolabial sulcus inferiorly. Where the maxilla and its piriform aperture are recessed and the nasolabial angle is acute, a premaxillary graft moves the nasal base and nasal tip anteriorly increasing tip projection. It also opens up an acute nasolabial angle. The premaxillary graft is shaped as a bi-taped hemispindle, measuring approximately 2.5-cm long, 10-mm high, and 7–8-mm deep (Fig. 32–11).

Cartilage Grafting When the Cleft Alar Cartilage is *Small* or *Flimsy*

When one or both alar cartilages are weak or hypoplastic, then both cartilages can be rebuilt using septal, conchal or costal cartilage grafts (Fig. 32–12). Costal cartilage is strongest and in good supply. New alar cartilage arches are constructed over and anchored to the existing alar cartilages. The new arches give symmetry, normal contour and added projection to the tip of the nose. Other useful grafts are spreader grafts

to straighten the septum, a columella strut to stiffen the medial and middle crura, and a tip graft for to add strength or projection.

FOUR CASES

The following describes open rhinoplasty for three cases of *unilateral* and one case of *bilateral* cleft lip nasal deformity.

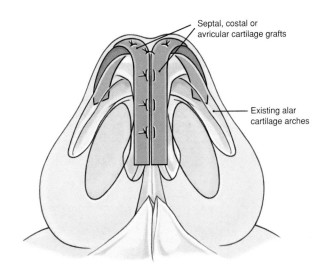

Figure 32–12. Septal, conchal, or costal cartilage can be used to reconstruct new alar cartilage arches over the existing weak or flimsy alar cartilages.

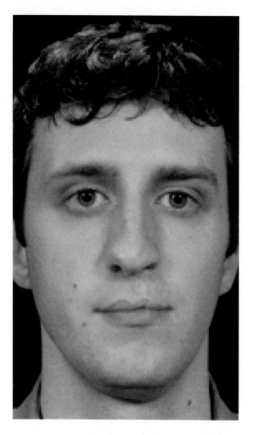 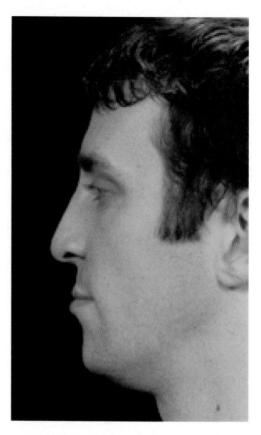

Figure 32–13. Preoperative photographs of Case 1 patient (unilateral cleft lip nasal deformity with normal-sized alar cartilage).

Case 1: Reconstruction of a Twisted Nasal Tip With a Normal-Sized Alar Cartilage

The Problem and the Plan

A 27-year-old man presented with a repaired left unilateral cleft lip (Fig. 32–13). The Millard lip repair done in the early weeks of life had produced a nearly normal result for the lip. However, the patient wanted to improve his nasal aesthetics and correct the obstructed left airway. The nasal dorsum and septum were twisted, convex to the left, with the caudal septal cartilage visible in the right nostril. The left alar cartilage was depressed posteriorly, or "slumped." The arch of the right alar cartilage also seemed to lack projection, dragged down by the slumped left cartilage. The left alar base was displaced laterally and superiorly. The central part of the septal cartilage bulged into and obstructed the left nasal airway. The right airway was obstructed by the projecting caudal edge of the septal cartilage.

Open rhinoplasty was planned. The right fifth costal cartilage was to be used to create spreader grafts to straighten the nose in the AP view, and batten grafts to straighten alar margins. Septal cartilage would be used for a columella strut and a visible Sheen tip graft, augmented by a cap graft just cephalic to the tip graft, giving symmetry and anterior projection to the nasal tip. Lateral crural grafts of septal cartilage would support the vestibule airway and give stability to the nasal tip framework.

General Techniques for Open Rhinoplasty

The general open rhinoplasty technique of Dean Toriumi, MD, described in this chapter, has evolved, and now consists of the following steps.

General anesthesia is given. Bleeding is minimized by injection of approximately 3.5 cc of 2% lidocaine with 1:500 epinephrine into the nose, and intranasal topical administration of 4% cocaine on cottonoid pledgets. Additional lidocaine is injected into the nasal septum. The nasal vestibules are cleaned and painted with iodoform solution. The vibrissae are clipped. A transverse incision with a central 4-mm-high dentate flap is incised with a scalpel between the upper one-third and lower two-thirds of the columella. The incision then runs anteriorly just 2 mm behind the lateral edges of the columella into the nasal vestibules, following the caudal borders of the normal lateral crus on the right and the slumped lateral crus on the left. The incision along the caudal edge of the lateral crus is made with a scissors as the nasal skin flap is being raised. Although the skin of the columella is incised with a scalpel, the deeper tissues are cut with a fine scissors. This technique avoids injury to the middle crura of the alar cartilages. The skin and fat flap is elevated just above the perichondrium of the alar cartilages and upper lateral cartilages alternately by sharp-scissors dissection and blunt pushing with a cotton-tip applicator. The lateral crura of the alar cartilages, the upper lateral cartilages and the thin scroll connecting the two, and the bluish dorsal edge of the septal cartilage are exposed in this manner. At the level of the nasal bones upward to the radix, a Joseph periosteal elevator is used to lift the skin and patches of periosteum off the nasal bones.

The Rhinoplasty

In Case 1, a 3-mm-thick nasal hump was removed under direct vision with a Rubin osteotome, freshly sharpened at the O.R. table with an Arkansas stone. Medial oblique osteotomies of the nasal bones were performed under direct vision using a 4-mm notched osteotome. Bilateral lateral osteotomies and infracture were done through nasal vestibule incisions just in front of the inferior turbinates. Then the dorsal edge of the septal cartilage was exposed. Mucoperichondrium along the anterior 8 mm of the dorsal nasal septum, the upper lateral cartilages and the intact mucosal vaults were separated from the septal cartilage on both sides with a perichondrial elevator. The mucosal vaults of the nose were preserved intact. Skeletonization of the nasal septum and harvest of the central septal cartilage for graft material were achieved through this dorsal approach. A piece of septal cartilage 1.3 cm × 2.2 cm was removed and reserved for graft material. An L-shaped strut of septal cartilage was retained. It was 1.0-cm wide along the dorsal septal edge and 1.5-cm wide at the anterior septal angle. The nose was then straightened. The

long, straight anterior segment of the right fifth costal cartilage was harvested through a 4-cm chest incision. The septum was fixed in the midline by two spreader grafts carved from this costal cartilage. Each spreader graft was 3.5-cm long, 1.5-mm wide and 4-mm deep. First the two spreader grafts were anchored along the dorsal edges of the septal cartilage, one on each side, with 4-0 mattress sutures, in such a way that the septum was straightened and lay in vertical line with the center of the upper lip. *Note*: the dental midline is often to the left or right of the philtral midline. If the spreader grafts warp slightly, they are placed on each side of the dorsal septum with their concave warps opposed, that is, facing each other. Next, all five layers of the nasal dorsum (the septal cartilage, two spreader grafts and both upper lateral cartilages) were fixed together with 5-0 mattress sutures. At this time, the nose was straight.

The Framework

In Case 1, cartilage grafts were added to the lower half of the nose to create a symmetric, aesthetic shape, to give strong anterior projection, and to brace the nose against collapse (Fig. 32–14). The deformed alar cartilage was of nearly normal size, so total reconstruction of the alar arches was not necessary. Instead, the existing cleft-side alar cartilage was reshaped and braced with cartilage grafts to match its normal contralateral fellow.

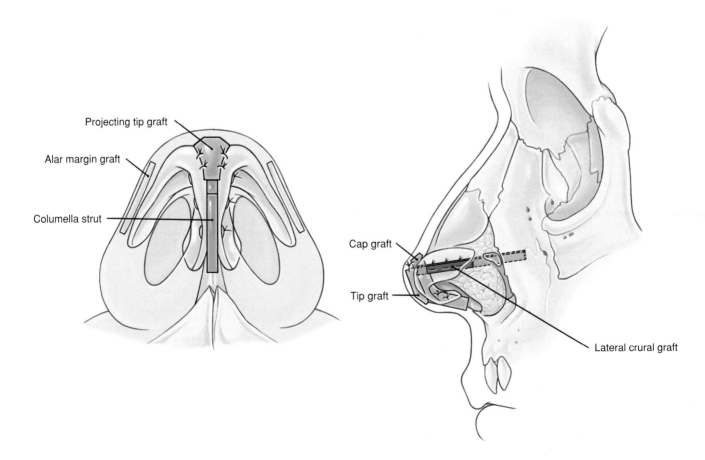

Figure 32–14. Cartilage grafts for Case 1.

The middle and medial crura of the alar cartilages were freed from one another by cutting the ligaments of Pitanguy between them.[12] The left cartilage was partially freed from its nasal mucosal lining by sharp-scissor dissection, and was freed from the maxilla by cutting the chain of sesamoid cartilages.

Next a columella strut was carved from harvested septal cartilage. The strut was 2-cm long, 3-mm wide and 5-mm deep and had an angle of 50 degrees. The angle simulated the normal columellar–lobular angle described by Sheen.[5] The columella strut was placed in a pocket between the existing paired medial crura of the alar cartilages. This pocket extended 5 mm into the upper lip. The medial and middle crura of the alar cartilages were fixed to the base of the strut with a single mattress suture of 4-0 gut. This suture was passed back and forth through the membranous septum and all the three cartilage layers (the strut and the feet of both medial crura). This suture determines the final projection of the nasal tip. The cephalic edges of the medial and middle crura were then sutured to the anterior edge of the angled strut with 5-0 monofilament sutures.

The nasal tip was made symmetrical by narrowing and shaping the alar cartilage arches. The cephalic edges of both alar cartilages were trimmed, more on the normal side than on the cleft side, so that 7-mm cartilage strips remained. Transdomal mattress sutures were placed to convert the alar domes from broad Roman arches into symmetrical narrow "McDonald's" arches. An interdomal suture stabilized and narrowed the tip complex.

The cartilage framework constructed for a cleft lip nose needs to be stronger than normal alar cartilages. Otherwise, when the nose is closed, the rigid skin envelope will collapse the new tip framework. Costal cartilage grafts are stronger than ear cartilage grafts and give the framework strength to maintain anterior nasal projection and to resist the force of a stiff nasal skin envelope. The intrinsic shape of the stiff skin envelope resists the disciplining force of the new nasal tip framework, tending to mold the nasal framework back into its preoperative asymmetric cleft-nose shape. Rib cartilage grafts are architecturally strong enough to resist the strong centripetal force of collagen contraction that occurs in the sheet of scar tissue that forms under the skin of the nose during healing.

In Case 1, a Sheen tip graft was added to further strengthen the nasal tip. This was a visible graft positioned to add projection to the nasal tip. Septal cartilage was carved with the silhouette of a golf tee and measured 9-mm wide, 3-mm thick and 15-mm long; its edges were chamfered. The graft was sutured to the middle crura of the alar cartilages with 6-0 sutures. A cap graft measuring 3 mm by 9 mm was sutured above the tip graft to smooth the contour of the nasal tip and to blend the tip with the supratip region. These grafts projected above the patient's existing alar domes by 2 mm, thus adding anterior projection to the nasal tip.

To straighten the lateral crura, a lateral crus graft was fastened with mattress sutures beneath the cut cephalic edge of the lateral crus on each side. As these sutures were tightened,

the lateral crus straightened. The lateral crural grafts were sutured also to the columella strut to further strengthen the nasal tip with the tripod configuration of Gunter.[4]

Finally, an alar margin "batten" graft was slid into a narrow pocket above the alar margin on each side. Each alar margin graft was approximately twice the diameter of an ordinary round toothpick. These grafts projected 3 mm from their pockets, and each was anchored to the soft subcutaneous tissue with a single 6-0 stitch. The nasal tip framework was complete.

Closure

The nasal skin envelope was redraped and closed in the following manner. Using strong magnification (3.5X loupes) and a very fine needle, the skin of the columella was closed with a single subcuticular suture of 6-0 clear suture plus nine skin sutures of 7-0 nylon. Great care was taken not to suture the columella flap tightly, as flap necrosis can occur from excess tension. The lateral incisions of the columella were gently closed with 6-0 gut. The nasal vestibule incisions were closed with 5-0 gut. The nasal skin was taped with half-inch and quarter-inch paper tape. Great care was taken not to compress the supratip skin with the tape, as it is here that skin necrosis most often occurs following open rhinoplasty. An Aquaplast nasal splint with the largest size perforations (the nasal skin must breathe) was placed over the nasal tape. The splint was gently conformed to the nose, not compressed against it with the fingers—again, to avoid the dread complication of nasal skin necrosis following open rhinoplasty.

The nasal cavity was not packed with gauze. A short roll of Telfa dressing 2.0-cm long, slathered in antibiotic ointment, was placed in each nostril. (The patient removed this roll 12 hours later.) A 2-inch gauze pad was taped below the nose, not against it, to avoid adherence to the columella sutures. This drip pad is meant to catch early postoperative secretions and to discourage the patient from blotting the nose with a tissue, and dislodging grafts in the process. Cold compresses were placed on the eyelids for the first 12 postoperative hours only.

Figures 32–15 and 32–16 show the patient before surgery (left side) and when he returned at 6 months just before a minor revision of the right lip border.

Case 2: Total Reconstruction of the Alar Cartilages with Conchal Cartilage Grafts

The Problem and the Plan

A 40-year-old woman presented with a repaired right unilateral cleft lip and nasal deformity (Fig. 32–17). The LeMesurier[13] lip repair, done when she was an infant, possessed a large quadrilateral flap. The upper lip was asymmetric with a redundant right vermilion border, a prominent orbicularis muscle bulge in the center of the lateral lip element, and a deeply inscribed scar through the vermilion border. At her last operation, at age 16, a Gillies-style L-shaped rib cartilage graft had been inserted into the nasal dorsum and columella. Her nose was crooked and short, with a slight over-rotation of

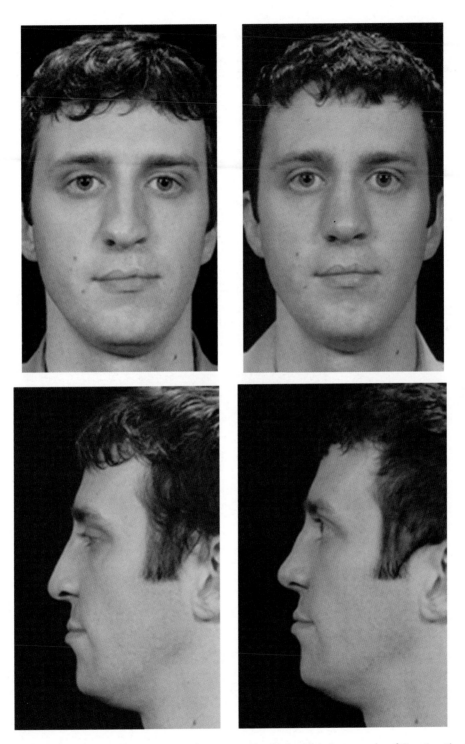

Figure 32–15. Preoperative (left side) and postoperative (right side) photographs of Case 1 patient.

the nasal tip and an overly projected bridge. The right alar base was displaced laterally and inferiorly, so that the alar base-to-white roll measurement was 1.5 cm on the deformed right side, versus 1.9 cm on the normal left side. The caudal edge of the septal cartilage was visible and partially obstructing the left nostril. The patient wanted improvement of her nasal breathing, correction of her crooked nose, a better shape and projection of the nasal tip, better proportion in the profile, and improved symmetry of the nose.

Although conchal cartilage grafts possess little architectural strength, conchal cartilage of the ear was chosen as the donor material. In this patient, Case 2, costal cartilage would have been a better choice because of its great strength and abundant supply. Because the nose was congenitally deformed and had been previously operated upon, it was covered with an envelope of rather inelastic skin. A strong framework is required to achieve anterior projection of the nasal tip and to force such a scarred and stiffened nasal skin envelope out

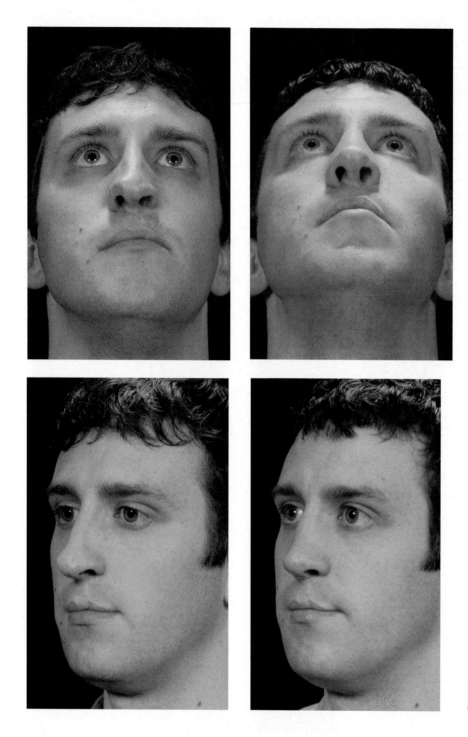

Figure 32–16. Preoperative (left side) and postoperative (right side) photographs of Case 1 patient.

of its intrinsic, deformed shape, into a normal, natural nasal shape. When relatively weak ear cartilage is used for nasal tip reconstruction, a Sheen tip graft must be added to the framework to give it necessary architectural strength. So, this graft was included in the operative plan.

The Operation

The lip repair was taken apart, realigned and closed with good apposition of the orbicularis oris muscle. In the process, the lip was lengthened using the Rose-Thompson principle[14] (in which a diamond-shaped defect in the upper lip is closed as a vertical straight line, thus lengthening the lip), the right

vermilion border was narrowed (by excision of a longitudinal strip), and the right alar base repositioned medially (by V-Y advancement). At the time of lip revision, septoplasty and harvest of the central septal cartilage were done through a caudal septal incision. The caudal edge of the septal cartilage was sutured to the foot of the medial crus of the right alar cartilage to centralize the septum and thus open the nasal airways. Then the rhinoplasty was begun.

The technique for open rhinoplasty was the same as in Case 1. The incision crossed the upper columella transversely and included a central peaked flap. Once the nasal skin was lifted off the nose, a large pencil-like costal cartilage

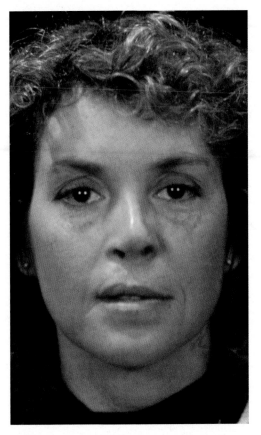
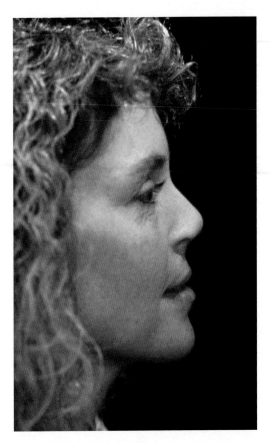

Figure 32–17. Preoperative photographs of Case 2 patient (total reconstruction of the alar cartilages with conchal cartilage grafts). (*From Burget G: Aesthetic reconstruction of the nose. In: Mathes S (ed). Plastic Surgery, Vol. 2. Philadelphia: Saunders/Elsevier, 2006, p. 611.*)

graft 7-mm wide, (placed at 16 years of age) could be seen to lie obliquely across the nasal dorsum and to be bent at a right angle into the membranous septum. The cartilage was removed and set aside for graft material. Under the old graft the nasal bones and upper lateral cartilages appeared normal but compressed. The L-shaped graft had been placed in the upper two-thirds of the nose, when, in fact, the deformity lay in the lower one-third of the nose. The existing alar cartilages, crumpled like the closed bellows of an accordion beneath the old cartilage graft, broken in several places and partly missing, were freed from their scarred bed by sharp-scissors' dissection. By themselves, the existing alar cartilages were too fragile and contracted to produce strong tip projection. A new tip framework, including new alar cartilages, was constructed over the existing alar cartilages, using graft material from the old dorsal L-strut and cartilage from the concha of the left ear.

Constructing the Framework

The technique that follows is applicable to total reconstruction of the alar cartilages for both reconstructive and cosmetic rhinoplasty.[15] The existing alar cartilages are separated from one another. Between the two, a pocket is created extending slightly deeper than the base of the columella. A columella strut 1.5–1.8-cm long and 2.5-mm wide is carved (in this case, from the old cartilage graft taken from the nasal

dorsum). The strut is inserted into the pocket and fastened in place with a 4-0 gut suture passed through the full-thickness of the membranous septum, the feet of both medial crura and the base of the strut. This suture sets the position of the columella strut and thus the entire nasal tip.

The floor and a portion of the wall of the left conchal cartilage are harvested as a single piece through a posterior incision. The graft is cut into two strips 5-mm wide and 3-cm long (Fig. 32–18). Each strip is angled 50 degrees, like a hockey stick. This angle becomes the columellar–lobular angle of rotation that gives the columella its normal upward rotation. The two ear cartilage strips are then sutured to the columella strut and the existing medial crura. When the two cartilage strips are stable in the columella, a point of anterior projection of the cartilages is chosen, so that the final alar arch projection will be approximately 24–26 mm anterior to the plane of the upper lip. At this point, the cartilage strips are weakened by stabbing them multiple times with a No. 27 hypodermic needle. The strips are then bent at the weak point and the arch is fixed with a domal spanning suture. The lateral ends of these grafts are sutured to the patient's existing lateral crura thus forming two new alar cartilage arches.

Strengthening the Framework and Adding Projection

In this Case 2, the framework was not strong. Because they are stronger, costal or septal cartilage would have been a better

Harvest of conchal cartilage grafts and creation of replacement alar cartilage arches

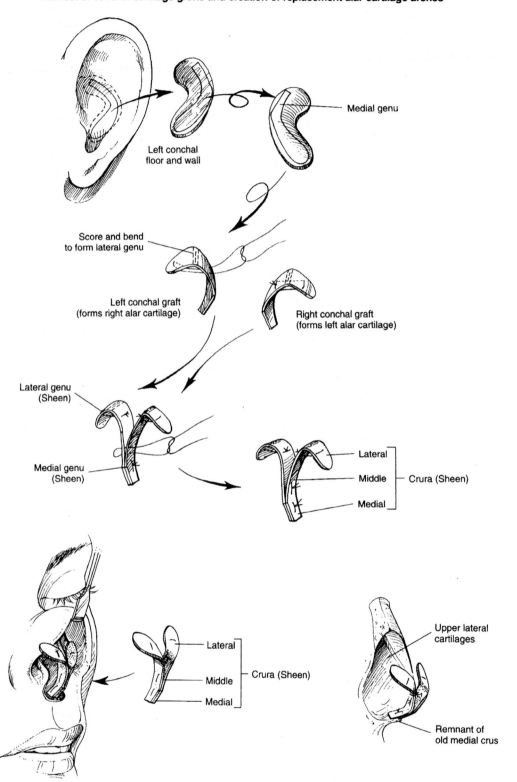

Left conchal
floor and wall

Medial genu

Score and bend
to form lateral genu

Left conchal graft
(forms right alar cartilage)

Right conchal graft
(forms left alar cartilage)

Lateral genu
(Sheen)

Medial genu
(Sheen)

Lateral

Middle

Medial

Crura (Sheen)

Lateral

Middle

Medial

Crura (Sheen)

Upper lateral
cartilages

Remnant of
old medial crus

Figure 32–18A. The first representation of how replacements for the alar cartilage arches are created from conchal cartilage grafts. (*From Burget G: Reoperative reconstruction of the nose. In: Grotting (ed). Reoperative Aesthetic & Reconstructive Plastic Surgery. St. Louis, MO: Quality Medical Publishing, 1995, p. 539.*)

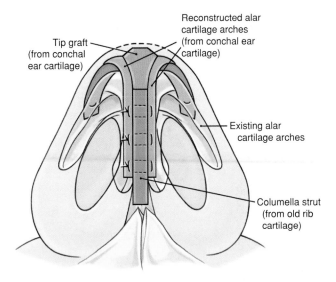

Figure 32–18B. Cartilage grafts used in Case 2, from auricular and old rib cartilages.

choice for the new alar cartilage arches. The new arches, made of auricular cartilage, were given increased strength by using 6-0 sutures to attach a tip graft, 9-mm wide across the top and 1.3-cm long, to the middle crura of the new arches (Fig. 32–19). The tip graft projected just 1 mm anterior to the tops of the new alar cartilage arches. This graft gave the tip framework extra projection and sufficient strength to resist the force of the noncompliant, inelastic nasal skin envelope that was stretched over it. The skin was redraped, the incisions

were closed, and the nose was lightly taped and covered with an Aquaplast splint.

The skin envelope of a scarred nose, such as this Case 2, has an intrinsic shape that is fixed; and the framework of cartilage, constructed during a rhinoplasty, must be sufficiently strong to force the nasal skin into a correct shape. Therefore, costal or septal cartilage is the best material for an internal nasal framework. In this case, a strong tip graft gave extra rigidity to the ear cartilage framework to compensate for its intrinsic weakness.

No further operations were done. The final photographs show the patient before the surgery and 2 years and 2 months after the surgery (Figs. 32–20 and 32–21). The nose is straight with an improved proportion of dorsal length to projection, and with a symmetric nasal tip. Alar margin and alar base symmetry are better, but the nostrils are still asymmetrical. Open rhinoplasty could not correct the congenital hypoplasia of the skin and fat of the left side of the nose.

Case 3: Reconstruction of Alar Cartilage Arches for a Hypoplastic Cleft-Side Cartilage

The Problem and the Plan

An 18-year-old female patient was born with a left unilateral cleft lip that had been repaired in infancy, revised at a later date, and finally reconstructed with a midline philtrum-Abbe flap (Fig. 32–22). Attempts at nasal correction had been done along the way; the septal cartilage had been harvested. However, the nose remained asymmetric, with the left nasal tip less projecting, and the lower half of the nose deviated to the left. The left alar lobule and the left nostril were smaller

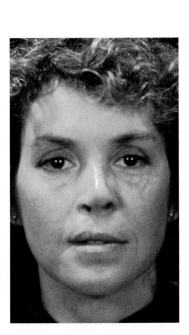

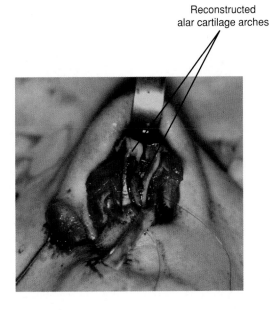

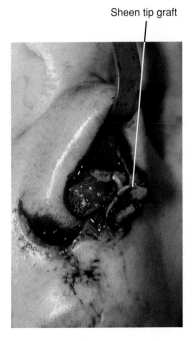

Figure 32–19. Intraoperative photographs of Case 2 patient showing reconstructed alar cartilage arches and use of a Sheen tip graft for support and projection of the nasal tip. (*From Burget G: Aesthetic reconstruction of the nose. In: Mathes S (ed). Plastic Surgery, Vol. 2. Philadelphia: Saunders/Elsevier, 2006, p. 611.*)

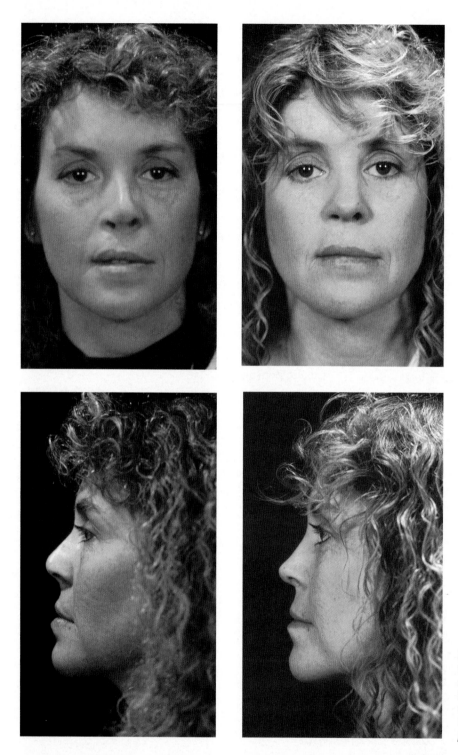

Figure 32–20. Photographs of Case 2 patient before surgery (left side) and 2 years and 2 months after surgery (right side). *(From Burget G: Aesthetic reconstruction of the nose. In: Mathes S, (ed). Plastic Surgery, Vol. 2. Philadelphia, Saunders/Elsevier, 2006, p. 611.)*

than the right. The caudal septal cartilage was deviated to the left. There were synechiae across the left nasal airway. The plan was to perform an open rhinoplasty, open the airway, centralize the caudal septum, harvest an eighth costal cartilage graft, straighten and stabilize the lower half of the nose with spreader grafts and reshape or rebuild the alar cartilage arches.

The Operation

Surgery was begun by revising the scars at the borders of the previous Abbe flap and obtaining closure of the orbicularis oris muscle across the clefts. The transverse columella incision, with its little central flap, was made; and, the nasal skin and fat were elevated off of the nose. Several old cartilage and cranial bone grafts were removed. The septum and alar cartilages were exposed. The right eighth costal cartilage was delivered through a 1.8-cm skin incision. Two spreader grafts, each measuring 4 mm × 2 mm × 17 mm, were carved from the costal cartilage and sutured to both sides of the dorsal septal cartilage to straighten the septum in line with the midline of the upper lip. The existing upper lateral cartilages were sutured to this midline nasal support.

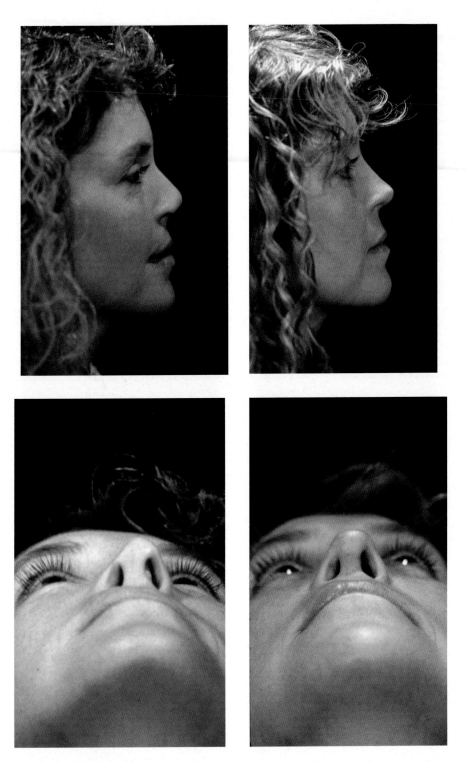

Figure 32–21. Photographs of Case 2 patient before surgery (left side) and 2 years and 2 months after surgery (right side). (*From Burget G: Aesthetic reconstruction of the nose. In: Mathes S, (ed). Plastic Surgery, Vol. 2. Philadelphia, Saunders/Elsevier, 2006, p. 611.*)

The existing alar cartilages were freed from scar. Because a segment of the right alar cartilage was missing and the left (cleft-side) alar cartilage was hypoplastic, two new alar cartilage arches were reconstructed. First, a 4 mm × 14-mm columella strut was carved from rib cartilage, inserted between the existing medial crura and fixed with a through-and-through suture of 4-0 gut. The new alar arches were cre-

ated from two costal cartilage strips, each 1.5-mm thick, 5-mm deep and 18-mm long. The strips were first sutured to the columella strut and then to the medial and middle crura of the existing alar cartilage. The two cartilage strips projected forward out of the nose. After the point of tip projection was chosen for each cartilage strip, the point was weakened by stabbing with a 27 hypodermic needle. The strips were bent

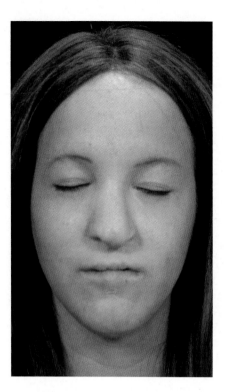

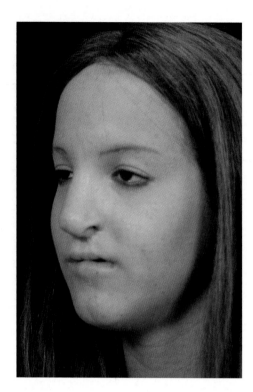

Figure 32–22. Preoperative photographs of Case 3 patient (reconstruction of alar cartilage arches for a hypoplastic cleft-side cartilage).

at these points with domal spanning sutures to form two new cartilage arches. The cephalic ends of the arches were sutured to the patient's existing lateral crura. The new alar cartilage arches were sutured to each other with intercrural and interdomal sutures.

The new tip framework was sutured to the anterior septal angle, thus shortening the nose. Finally, to increase tip projection, a Sheen tip graft (in two pieces) and a cap graft were added to the new alar cartilage arches. Septoplasty was performed, septal splints were positioned in the airways, and the nasal incisions were closed. Figure 32–23 shows the cartilage grafts used in Case 3, and Figure 32–24 provides intraoperative views of the reconstructed alar cartilage, the tip graft, and the cap graft.

Two secondary operations were done to revise lip scars, reposition the left alar base, shape the columella and infratip lobule and enlarge the left nostril. Photographs show the patient before surgery (18 years of age) and after surgery (20 years of age) (Figs. 32–25 and 32–26).

Case 4: Reconstruction of the Alar Cartilage Arches for the Bilateral Cleft Lip Nose

The Problem and the Plan

The anatomy of the bilateral cleft lip nasal deformity differs from that of unilateral deformity. Symmetry is less of a problem. Although the columella is short or missing, skin and fat in the infratip lobule of the nose can be used to make a columella. A proper nasal tip framework with a columella post can be constructed, The rather thin skin of the lowest

part of the nasal tip, called the infratip lobule, is draped about the framework to create a columella. Borrowing tissue from the upper lip to lengthen the columella is not necessary and, in truth, compounds the patient's deformity. The problem of achieving projection of the bilateral cleft lip nose, and creating a columella, becomes that of correcting the underlying nasal cartilage framework and releasing the tight lining of the nasal vestibules.

The piriform aperture of bilateral cleft patients is very wide. At open rhinoplasty, with the alar cartilages exposed, no amount of tugging can advance the alar cartilages anterior, because they are stretched tight across the abnormally wide

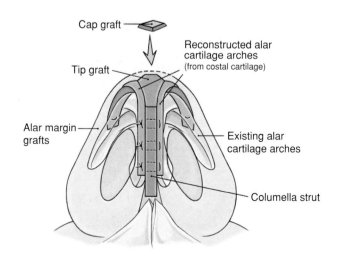

Figure 32–23. Cartilage grafts for Case 3.

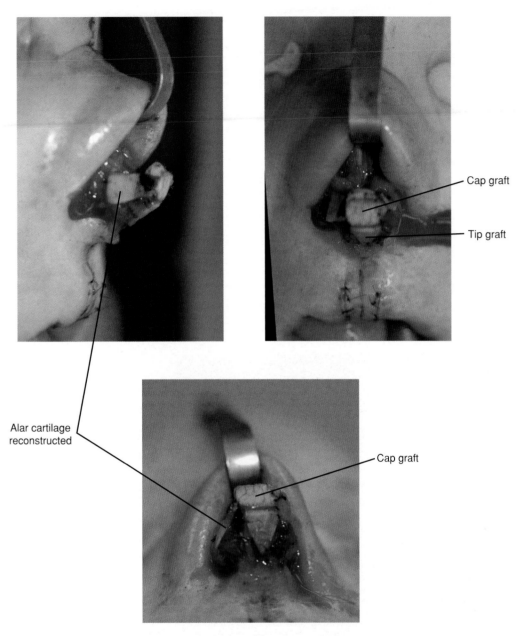

Cap graft

Tip graft

Alar cartilage
reconstructed

Cap graft

Figure 32–24. Intraoperative photographs of Case 3 patient.

piriform aperture. They are stuck to the maxilla. They must be either separated from the vestibule lining (in which case they become very flimsy free grafts) or the alar cartilages and attached nasal lining can be cut loose from their attachment to the bony edges of the piriform aperture. A third alternative is to build on top of the existing alar cartilages, new alar cartilages that project anteriorly. Then the nasal skin envelope can be redraped over this new, anteriorly projecting framework.

The patient was a 17-year-old girl born with a bilateral complete cleft lip and palate. Early repairs of the lip and palate produced good results. At age 10, cranial bone grafts were placed in the alveolar cleft, a small fistula between the primary and secondary palates was closed and lip scars were revised, all with good results. The nose, however, remained nonprojected

and the tip overhanging and hiding the very short columella from frontal view (Fig. 32–27).

The initial plan was to use an open rhinoplasty approach to mobilize the alar cartilages and to give them projection with a columella strut, lateral crural grafts, and possibly a Sheen tip graft. In practice, the tightness of the alar cartilages, which were stretched across the wide piriform aperture, and the adherence of these cartilages to the tight mucosa of the nasal vestibule made this plan impossible to carry out.

The Operation

When the nasal skin was elevated through an open rhinoplasty incision, the alar cartilages were found to be stretched across an abnormally wide piriform aperture. The wide alar

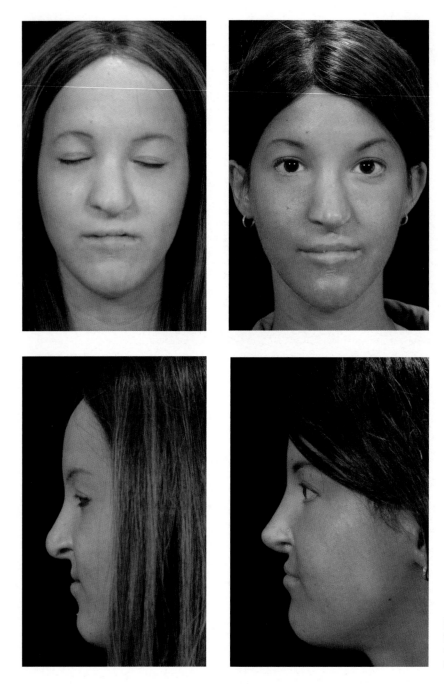

Figure 32–25. Photographs show Case 3 patient before surgery (left side: when the patient was 18 years of age) and after surgery (right side: when the patient was 20 years of age).

cartilage arches could not be advanced anteriorly or tightened into narrow "McDonald's" arches. Even cutting loose the lateral ends of the lateral crura and its skin lining from their anchorage to the borders of the piriform aperture did not allow enough movement forward to achieve normal nasal tip projection. The existing alar cartilages were weak and spread so widely across the piriform aperture that they could not alone give sufficient projection to the nasal tip. Therefore, new alar cartilages were built over the existing ones (Fig. 32–28).

For this purpose, right eighth costal cartilage was harvested through a 4-cm incision. The cartilage was then carved into several grafts. A columella strut (3 mm × 8 mm × 13 mm) was inserted into a pocket between the existing medial and middle crura. This graft was angled like a hockey stick, so that the 50-degree angle formed the columellar–lobular angle. The graft was anchored in the pocket with a single 4-0 gut suture that passed through all layers of the membranous septum at its base.

Two long thin cartilage strips were used to reconstruct the alar cartilages. Each graft measured 2.8-cm long, 5-mm wide and 1.5-mm thick. The strips were sutured to the columella strut with 4-0 monofilament sutures and to the existing medial and middle crura of the existing alar cartilages with 5-0 monofilament sutures. A point was selected on each graft at which it would be bent into an arch that

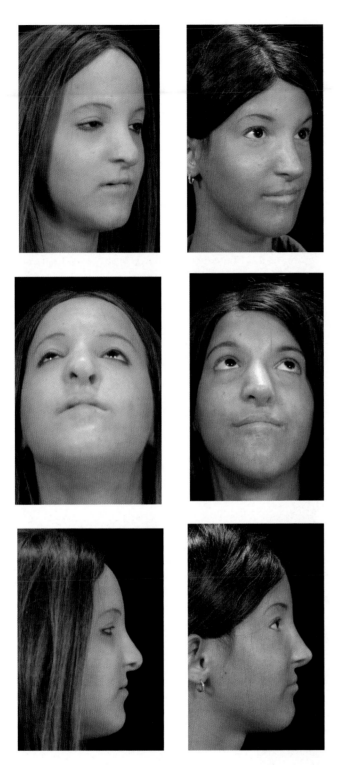

Figure 32–26. Photographs show Case 3 patient before surgery (left side: when the patient was 18 years of age) and after surgery (right side: when the patient was 20 years of age).

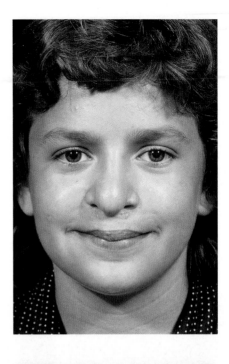

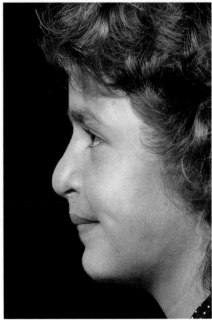

Figure 32–27. Case 4. Bilateral cleft lip nose after several closed surgical revisions.

would project 24–26 mm anterior to the plane of the upper lip. The two long grafts were then weakened at this point by multiple stabbings with a 27 hypodermic needle, and each graft was bent to form a lateral genu, or dome, of the new alar cartilages. The new arches were fixed in this shape with 5-0 transdomal sutures. The superior end of each cartilage

(the lateral crus) was anchored to the existing lateral crus. The two new alar cartilage arches were then anchored to each other with intercrural and interdomal sutures, as in cosmetic open rhinoplasty. In this case, the entire alar cartilage complex was rotated upward with a single suture placed through old and new alar cartilages and to the anterior angle of the septal cartilage.

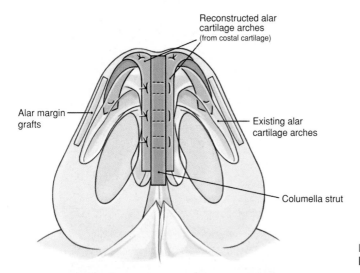

Reconstructed alar
cartilage arches
(from costal cartilage)

Alar margin
grafts

Existing alar
cartilage arches

Columella strut

Figure 32–28. Figure showing total reconstruction of alar cartilage arches for bilateral cleft lip nose.

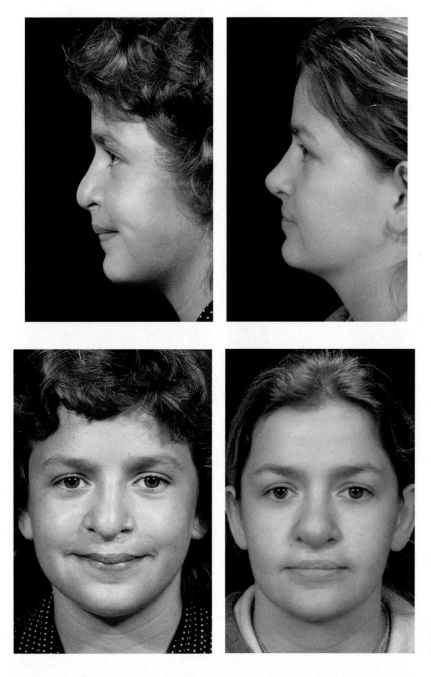

Figure 32–29. Photographs show patient before cleft lip rhinoplasty (left side) and after (right side).

A batten graft (3-mm wide by 1.5-cm long) was inserted into a pocket along each alar margin. Its purpose was to straighten the collapsed nasal alae and give a pyramidal form to the nose on basal view. The nose was closed with 5-0 gut internally, and the columella was closed with a single subcuticular 6-0 suture and nine interrupted 7-0 nylon sutures.

Healing was uneventful, and the result was acceptable, with the exception that the nasal tip remained bulbous secondary to excess subcutaneous fat. A larger nasal framework might have prevented this postoperative bulbosity. Fig. 32–29 shows the patient before and after surgery. No amount of cajoling could entice her to have another operation to give definition to her nasal tip.

SUMMARY

A child's nose is a primordium until adolescence, at which time the bag of skin and tiny cartilages rapidly enlarges to become a major projecting form with strong and well-defined anatomical parts. Attempts to correct secondary cleft lip nose deformities at an early age have limited success, because the surgeon is trying to modify, as yet, undeveloped anatomy. Patients with cleft lips, wide piriform apertures, and significant cleft lip nasal deformities will require open rhinoplasty, but only after the nose has grown to its adult size and conformation (ages of 14–19 years).

Open rhinoplasty provides the tools to restore symmetry and projection to a cleft lip nose. Because the nasal skin has a strong "memory," strong cartilage grafts are necessary to correct the deformity. Septal and conchal cartilage are best for this. The techniques of open rhinoplasty that the surgeon can use to correct a cleft lip nose include spreader grafts, a columella strut, tip and cap grafts, lateral crural grafts, alar batten grafts, dorsal onlay and radix grafts, and premaxillary grafts. When the alar cartilage arch is weak, a new arch can be reconstructed in its entirety using grafts of septal or costal cartilage.[15] Without such late surgery, performed *after* the nose has achieved its adult dimensions, an aesthetically pleasing nose may never be achieved; and, the cleft nasal deformity and the social isolation it causes may persist.

References

1. Tajima S, Maruyama M. Reverse-U incision for secondary repair of cleft lip nose. *Plast Reconstr Surg.* 60:256–261, 1977.
2. Gunter J. Frequently used grafts in rhinoplasty, nomenclature and analysis. *Plast Reconstr Surg.* 118(1):14e–29e, 2006.
3. Gilles HD, Millard Dr. *The Principles and Art of Plastic Surgery.* Boston: Little and Brown, 1957, p. 50.
4. Gunter JP, Cochran CS. Tripod concept for correcting severely deformed nasal tip cartilages. In: Gunter JP, Rohrich RJ, Adams WP (eds). *Nasal Surgery by the Masters*, 2nd edn. St. Louis, MO: Quality Medical Publishers, 2007, pp. 841–849l.
5. Sheen J, Sheen A. *Aesthetic Rhinoplasty.* St. Louis, MO: Mosby, 1987, p. 38.
6. Daniel R. Rhinoplasty: Septal saddle nose deformity and composite reconstruction. *Plast Reconstr Surg.* 119(3):1029–1043, March, 2003.
7. Sheen J, Sheen A. *Aesthetic Rhinoplasty.* St. Louis, MO: Mosby, 1987, pp. 506–530.
8. Toriumi D. The Asian nose. *Dallas Rhinoplasty: Nasal Surgery by the Masters.* 2nd edn. St. Louis, MO: Quality Medical Publishing, 2007, p. 1185.
9. Gunter J. Gunter's Approach. *Dallas Rhinoplasty: Nasal Surgery by the Masters.* 2nd edn. St. Louis, MO: Quality Medical Publishing, 2007, pp. 1331–1332.
10. Toriumi D. Toriumi's Approach. *Dallas Rhinoplasty: Nasal Surgery by the Masters.* 2nd edn. St. Louis, MO: Quality Medical Publishing, 2007, p. 1397.
11. Erol OG. Diced cartilage grafts in rhinoplasty surgery. *Plast Reconstr Surg.* 116 (4)1171–1173, 2005.
12. Daniel RK, Calvert JW. Diced cartilage frafts in rhinoplasty surgery. *Plast Reconstr Surg.* 118(10):2306, 2156–2171, 2006.
13. Millard DR. In *Cleft Craft*, Vol. 1. Boston: Little Brown, 1976, p. 129.
14. Millard DR. In *Cleft Craft*, Vol. 1. Boston: Little Brown, 1976, pp. 90–91
15. Burget GC. Reoperative surgery for nasal reconstruction. In: Grotting J, (ed). *Reoperative Aesthetic and Reconstructive Surgery.* St. Louis, MO: Quality Medical Publishing, 1995, p. 539.

33

Post-Palatoplasty Fistulae: Diagnosis, Treatment, and Prevention

Joseph E. Losee, MD • Darren M. Smith, MD • Lisa Vecchione, DMD, MDS • Ahmed M. Afifi, MD • Matthew D. Ford, MS, CCC-SLP

INTRODUCTION

Postoperative fistulae are arguably the most significant concern for palatal surgeons, second only to the patient's resultant quality of speech. Indeed, fistulae may themselves have deleterious effects on speech after palatoplasty as manifested by velopharyngeal insufficiency (VPI). Fistulae are most commonly ascribed to wound breakdown secondary to closure under tension, infection, flap trauma, hematoma, or compromise of the vascular pedicle resulting in tissue ischemia. Untreated fistulae may lead to nasal air escape, speech distortion, hearing loss, or regurgitation of fluid and food.[1] These problems are compounded by the fact that fistulae are difficult to definitively repair. The incidence of cleft palate fistulae is reported to range from 0 to 76%,[2–4] while the recurrence rate of palatal fistulae reportedly approaches 100%.[5]

The literature surrounding this complication is confusing and difficult to interpret, secondary to vague definitions and a lack of standardized language addressing fistula location and clinical significance. Ambiguous literature has impeded progress in efforts to more effectively characterize and manage post-palatoplasty fistulae. Our approach to fistula classification, detailed below, is independent of etiology and functionality, and allows one to anatomically report and consistently describe fistulae present not only after palatal repair, but also those due to other circumstances such as trauma and congenital deformities. In an effort to prospectively clarify the literature and advance the management of palatal fistulae, we recently introduced a standardized classification system for these lesions.[6] This chapter will discuss the proposed fistula classification system, and proceed to discuss palatal fistulae in terms of their etiology, repair, and prevention.

DEFINITIONS

Commenting on the confused state of the cleft palate literature, Emory et al. contended that "until a uniform definition of palatal fistula is utilized, it will be difficult to compare the results of different studies."[7] Some general definitions of palatal fistulae do exist; they have been described as an abnormal communication between two cavities,[8] or as a complication of palatoplasty, occurring along the site of a palate repair.[9] We find a definition that is both anatomically specific and independent of etiology or functionality to be most useful: "a fistula is a patency between the oral and nasal cavities."

Literature dating from the 1950s to the present offers few suggested definitions for specific types of palatal fistulae.[8,9] Folk et al. described fistulae as occurring at the level of the soft palate, junction of the hard and soft palate, hard palate, incisive foramen, or anterior to the incisive foramen.[8] In a report from the Children's Hospital of Philadelphia, Cohen et al. described fistulae as occurring at the level of the uvula, soft palate, hard–soft palate junction, hard palate, postalveolar, alveolar, and prealveolar regions.[10] Despite these isolated accounts, establishing external consistency between studies in describing fistulae is extremely difficult, as no widely accepted and regularly utilized standardized classification system for palatal fistulae has evolved. For example, one author's "alveolar fistula" might be another's "lingual alveolar-fistula," and yet another's "labial-alveolar fistula"; or, one surgeon's "hard palate fistula" may be another's "incisive foramen fistula" and yet another's "junction of the hard and soft palate fistula."

As clear nomenclature is a prerequisite to meaningful discussion, ongoing research, and evolving new treatment strategies, we recently developed a simple, logical, and anatomically based classification system to standardize fistula-related terminology.[6] The resultant Pittsburgh Fistula Classification System includes seven fistula types (Fig. 33–1). Fistulae at the uvula, or bifid uvulae, are considered type I fistulae (Fig. 33–2). Type II fistulae occur within the soft palate (Fig. 33–3). Type III fistulae are found at the junction of the soft and hard palates (Fig. 33–4). Type IV fistulae are located within the hard palate (Fig. 33–5). Type V fistulae are defined as fistulae at the incisive foramen, or junction of the primary and secondary palates; this designation is reserved for use with Veau IV clefts (Fig. 33–6). Type VI fistulae are lingual-alveolar, and type VII fistulae are labial-alveolar (Fig. 33–7). We have found the Pittsburgh Fistula Classification System to be a functional standardized scheme, whose daily clinical application in our Cleft Center has helped us to establish consistency in reporting and has thus facilitated clinical research.

A numerical classification system seems critical for several reasons. Surgeons are notoriously inadequate in routinely reporting thorough anatomical descriptions of their outcomes, especially their complications. In a recent review, our group examined over 640 charts spanning 25 years and representing 18 surgeons.[6] This study revealed that in a majority

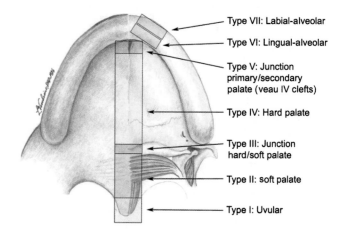

Figure 33–1. The Pittsburgh fistula classification system. Fistulae at the uvula, or bifid uvulae, are type I fistulae. Soft palate fistulae are type II. Type III fistulae are at the junction of the soft and hard palates. Hard palate fistulae are type IV. Type V fistulae are at the incisive foramen, or junction of the primary and secondary palates. This designation applies only to fistulae in the context of Veau IV clefts. Type VI fistulae are lingual-alveolar, and type VII fistulae are labial-alveolar.

Labels in figure:
- Type VII: Labial-alveolar
- Type VI: Lingual-alveolar
- Type V: Junction primary/secondary palate (veau IV clefts)
- Type IV: Hard palate
- Type III: Junction hard/soft palate
- Type II: soft palate
- Type I: Uvular

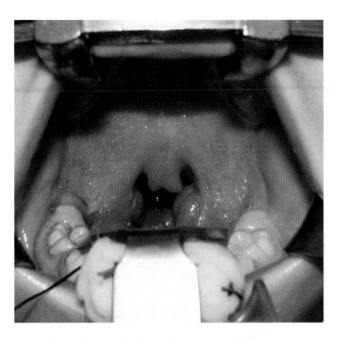

Figure 33–2. Pittsburgh fistula type I: bifid uvula.

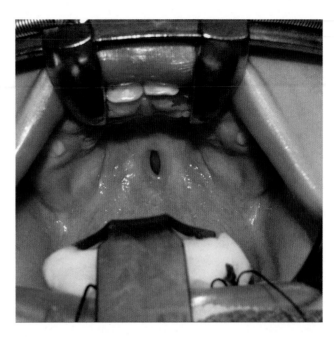

Figure 33–4. Pittsburgh fistula type III: at the junction of the hard and soft palates.

of the cases, fistulae were frequently mentioned but inadequately described. In some cases, fistulae were noted by the speech pathologist and not addressed by the treating surgeon. When a fistula was documented, the description found in the medical record was frequently vague. Rarely did these notes address the location, size, or functionality of these fistulae. As our review revealed analogous ambiguity in the literature, a lack of internal and external consistency clearly renders intercenter, surgeon-specific, and procedure-related comparisons impossible. Therefore, measures to standardize reporting, such as numerical systems, are paramount.

In addition to defining a fistula in terms of its anatomical location, it is important to recognize whether a fistula is "functional" or "symptomatic" vs. "nonfunctional" or "asymptomatic." Simply put, if a fistula is clinically significant, it is said to be "functional" or "symptomatic." Fistulae are clinically significant when they lead to nasal air escape, speech distortion, hearing loss, or regurgitation of fluid and food.[1] Clinically significant fistulae may also induce velopharyngeal insufficiency (VPI), which complicates speech management and outcome assessment.[11]

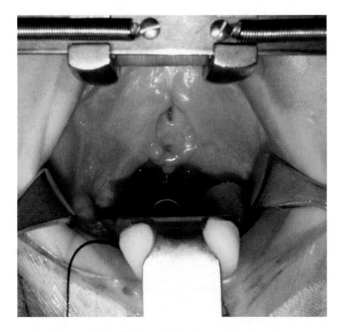

Figure 33–3. Pittsburgh fistula type II: soft palate.

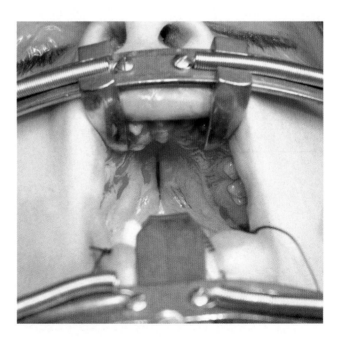

Figure 33–5. Pittsburgh fistula type IV: hard palate.

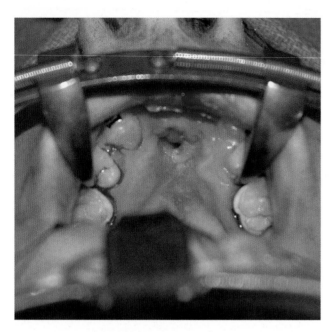

Figure 33–6. Pittsburgh fistula type V: at the incisive foramen (junction of the primary and secondary palates); this designation is reserved for Veau IV bilateral clefts.

Finally, when discussing the incidence of postoperative fistulae, it is important to determine whether the fistulae in question were intentional (such as those resulting from deliberately unrepaired alveolar clefts) or unintentional (resulting from wound breakdown secondary to closure under tension, infection, flap trauma, hematoma, or compromise of the vascular pedicle resulting in tissue ischemia). Functionality and intentionality may also be incorporated into the above-mentioned classification system.

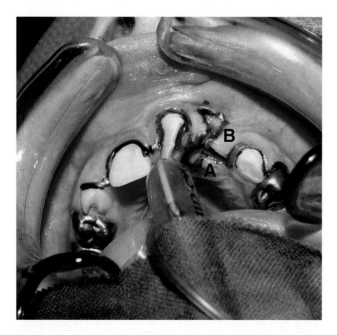

Figure 33–7. Pittsburgh fistula Types VI & VII: lingual- and labial-alveolar, A and B, respectively.

The addition of a prefix (+) or (−) could denote functionality. Fistulae resulting in nasal air escape or nasal regurgitation of liquid or food (functional, symptomatic fistulae) could be reported with a (+), while nonfunctional, asymptomatic fistulae (not clinically significant) could be noted with a (−). Thus, a (−) type V fistula would describe a "nonfunctional or asymptomatic fistula at the junction of the primary and secondary palates in a Veau IV cleft." Analogously, a suffix could be added to indicate intentionality; for example, if a gingivoperiosteoplasty was not performed, then type VI (lingual-alveolar) and type VII (labial-alveolar) fistulae would persist and the classification system would record them to be "intentional."

ETIOLOGY

Primary Fistulae or Palatal Clefts

While the primary application of the Pittsburgh Fistula Classification System is for postoperative or secondary fistulae, it may be utilized to describe primary clefts as well. Primary fistulae are by definition congenital deformities; therefore, palatal clefts can be classified as fistulae. Thus, a Veau I cleft of the soft palate may accurately be described as Pittsburgh type I–II fistula, a Veau II cleft of the soft and hard palates is a Pittsburgh I–IV fistula, a Veau III unilateral complete cleft is a Pittsburgh I–IV/VI–VII fistula, and a Veau IV bilateral complete cleft is a Pittsburgh I–VII fistula.[6]

Secondary Fistulae

Secondary fistulae are either traumatic or iatrogenic (postoperative), and the reported rates of postoperative fistulae formation range by report from 0 to 76%.[2–4] Postoperative fistulae can be described as "intentional" or "unintentional." An "intentional" fistula exists after palatoplasty if the surgeon decides to leave a portion of the primary fistula (i.e., the cleft) patent. Intentional fistulae are most likely to arise in the context of a Veau III unilateral cleft or a Veau IV bilateral cleft in which the lingual-alveolar (Pittsburgh type VI) and labial-alveolar (Pittsburgh type VII) fistulae are left unrepaired, that is, in which a gingivoperiosteoplasty is not performed. An "unintentional" fistula occurs as a complication after palatoplasty; i.e., the primary fistula, or cleft, is repaired, and a portion of the closure dehisces to produce a frank patency between the oropharynx and the nasopharynx.

While "intentional" fistulae are by definition secondary to a conscious decision on the part of the operator, "unintentional" fistulae might have multiple causes. These causes can be conceptually divided into "intrinsic" causes and "extrinsic" causes. "Intrinsic" causes are those pertaining to qualities of the patient or lesions. For instance, Emory et al. report that gender and the extent of clefting (as categorized by Veau classification) did not predict fistula formation rate.[7] In contrast, Cohen et al. found fistulae more likely to result in patients with more severe clefts by Veau classification.[10] Muzaffar et al. saw a statistically significant increase in fistula formation for patients with Veau III and IV clefts over those with Veau I and II clefts.[1] Schultz reports a positive correlation between both cleft type and width of the cleft and postoperative fistula formation.[12] Cohen et al. found that age at repair did not influence the rate of fistula formation.[10] In contrast, Emory et al. report that patients undergoing palatal repair at less than 12 months of age had a lower incidence of fistula formation than those undergoing repair between 12 and 25 months of age (7.8 vs. 19.4%, $p < 0.058$).[7] However, as reemphasized by Honnebier et al., the younger patients in this series were treated by more experienced palatal surgeons.[13] Moore's group found no association between age, sex, associated syndrome, history of otitis media, weight, preoperative hematocrit, tympanostomy tube placement, or cleft type and fistula formation.[14] Sex and age were not found to be predictive of fistulation by Muzaffar's group.[1] Schultz also found age to be insignificant in this context.[12]

"Extrinsic" causes are those more related to surgical technique and operative strategy than to patient-specific qualities. Some of the most commonly cited "extrinsic" etiologies for these lesions are tension, absent multilayer repair,[15] and poor surgical technique.[5] Cohen et al. found the individual surgeon influences fistula rate.[10] In fact, Emory et al. assert that the surgeon performing the repair was the strongest predictor of fistula formation in their experience.[7] In contrast, Muzaffar et al. saw no association between surgeon and fistula rate.[1] Interestingly, in their 1979 report on 845 palatoplasty patients, Abyholm et al. note that the rate of fistula formation was less for those patients undergoing palatal repair between 1962 and 1969 than those having the surgery between 1954 and 1961.[16] This group theorizes that progress in knowledge, surgical technique, and anesthesia are responsible for the observed improvement in surgical outcome. Moore's group noticed a similar decline in fistula rates over time, and reported no fistulae during the last 7 years of their 21-year series.[14]

Reports examining an association between surgical technique and perioperative procedures and fistula formation are disparate. Cohen reports palatoplasty technique to influence fistula rate; specifically, fistula occurrence rates were 43, 22, 10, and 0% for patients undergoing Wardill–Kilner, von Langenbeck, Furlow, and Dorrance repairs, respectively.[10] Moore and colleagues corroborate the assertion that the Wardill–Kilner repair is most prone to postoperative fistula formation, and attribute this finding to the convergence of three suture lines at one point as a result of this procedure.[14] In contrast to these reports, Schultz, Emory, and Muzaffar found that surgical technique did not influence fistula rate.[1,7,12] Intravelar veloplasty did not affect the rate of fistula formation in the Cohen or Moore series.[10,14] Moore et al. further report that intrapalatal epinephrine injection and intraoperative blood products did not affect fistula rate.[14] Perioperative antibiotics have been associated with a decreased rate of postoperative fistulation.[14] Preoperative orthodontics are not associated with fistulae: Muzaffar et al. found that palatal expansion and presurgical orthopedics did not predispose to fistulation.[1] Postoperative palatal manipulation, however, may cause fistula formation: Bardach and Schultz cite maxillary expansion and segment movement, respectively, as having an association with palatal fistulae.[2,12,17]

Tertiary Fistulae

Tertiary palatal fistulae result from the breakdown of a repaired postoperative fistula. Fistulae are extremely recalcitrant lesions, with recurrence rates reported to approach 100%.[5] This susceptibility to recurrence is not surprising given the mucosal scarring from primary palatoplasty, poor vascularization, and the lack of compliance of local tissues.[18] Rintala notes the paradoxical difficulty inherent to repairing smaller fistulae: the size of these lesions hinders the complete removal of the epithelial tract between the oral and nasal cavity.[19] Analyses of factors predisposing to tertiary fistula formation are not robust. Multivariate statistical analysis performed by Cohen et al. was able to validate only gender as predictive of fistula recurrence. This group found that cleft type, cleft repair technique, and site of the postoperative fistula were not predictive in this regard; small sample size precluded an analysis of fistula closure technique in this context.[10] Similarly, Rintala was unable to comment on the relative efficacy of fistula repair techniques.[19] In addition to breakdown and tertiary fistula formation, fistula repairs themselves can be morbid, leading to tissue loss at the donor site, hindrance of maxillary growth secondary to scar contracture, and poor aesthetic outcomes.[13]

■ DIAGNOSIS

Identification and Classification

Palatal fistulae should, for the most part, be readily diagnosed in the course of intra-oral examination. As noted earlier, fistulae can be either symptomatic or asymptomatic. In some cases, symptomatic lesions may be brought to the clinician's or parent's attention by their clinical effects. In Amaratunga's study of 346 palatoplasties with 73 resultant fistulae, nasality was identified as the most frequently occurring symptom.[20] If nasality is the most frequent symptom, few would disagree that velopharyngeal incompetence is the most significant morbidity associated with palatal fistulae. Even small palatal fistulae can have adverse effects on velopharyngeal competence and speech production.[11] Other symptoms include halitosis secondary to trapped particles of food, and an embarrassing nasal leakage of fluid.[15]

Once an unintentional fistula has been diagnosed, it should be accurately described and recorded. Important characteristics to note are location, size, and functionality. The authors employ the Pittsburgh Fistula Classification System for this purpose (see Fig. 33–1).[6] Reports on the most frequent site of fistula formation vary, but the consensus appears to be that these lesions occur most commonly at the junction of the hard and the soft palate (Pittsburgh type III) or within the hard palate (Pittsburgh type IV).[10,20,21] The frequent finding of Pittsburgh type III fistulae is logical, as palatal repair in this region is often most tenuous. At the junction of the hard and the soft palate, the surgeon is faced with atrophic friable mucosa, relative ischemia, deficient mesodermal tissues, and often the widest portion of the cleft, which together create a treacherous setting for surgical intervention.[22] The inelasticity of tissues at the hard palate leads to an intuitively difficult repair.

Indications for Treatment

It has been advocated that fistulae should be closed "in those cases when they cause problems of whatever kind,"[23] and that the "indications and timing for closure depend solely on the individual's functional needs."[5] Rosenstein et al. recommend fistula repair in the face of fluid loss, adversely affected articulation, or compromised hygiene.[24] Honnebier advocates a liberal stance on fistula repair, as fistulae are likely associated with social and developmental consequences in addition to anatomical and physiological issues.[13] Moreover, some would argue that even seemingly insignificant palatal fistulae should eventually be repaired, as lesions of any size have the potential for adverse effects on velopharyngeal competence and speech production.[11,25]

While some authors note that if left untreated, a small fistula may grow larger as the maxillary arch is expanded with orthodontic management,[16,26] others hold that fistulae should not be addressed surgically until orthodontic treatment is complete.[5] Bardach cites post-palatoplasty maxillary expansion as an etiology of palatal fistulae.[2,17] Consistent with this thinking, Cohen et al. postponed fistula repair until after maxillary arch expansion, but did not delay repair in the context of required dental arch alignment.[10] This group reports that early repair was considered in patients with large fistulae allowing for nasal air escape and resultant speech compromise; otherwise, small fistulae, and fistulae with symptoms primarily related to fluid regurgitation into the nasal cavity,

were not surgically managed until another cleft-related procedure was performed, unless the severity of an individual's symptomatology necessitated earlier intervention.[10]

TREATMENT

History

It is not surprising that this recalcitrant lesion has inspired treatment strategies spanning the reconstructive ladder. One of the most direct approaches to fistula management, chemical cauterization, was described by Obermeyer in 1967.[27] Berkman designed a continuously worn vinyl appliance designed to guide local healing of fistulae recognized early and addressed immediately with steadfast patient compliance upon discovery.[28] Local flap options for fistula repair are numerous; the origins of these procedures are encyclopedically reviewed by Millard, from von Langenbeck's 1864 turnover hinge flap to Gabka's 1964 V-Y advancement flaps.[29] Figures 33–8 to 33–12 offer historical examples.[29] Guerrero-Santos and associates popularized the tongue flap in the 1960s and 1970s.[30,31] Oshumi et al. employed free conchal cartilage grafts in this context.[32] Recent reviews describe the application of free flaps with microvascular anastomoses in fistula closure.[33–36] Despite the wealth of creativity that has been invested in approaches to the post-palatoplasty fistula, the recurrence rate of this refractory lesion has been reported to approach 100%.[5]

Nonsurgical Options

The mainstay of nonsurgical treatment is the palatal obturator. Due to local irritation and discomfort secondary to the bulk of the appliance, patient compliance is poor.[5] Moreover, as these devices are "high maintenance" with regard to their requirements for frequent adjustment and meticulous

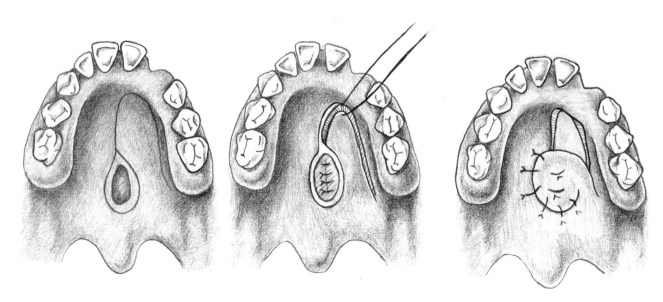

Figure 33–8. In 1964, Gabka illustrated a rotation flap for closure of a type IV (hard palate fistula).

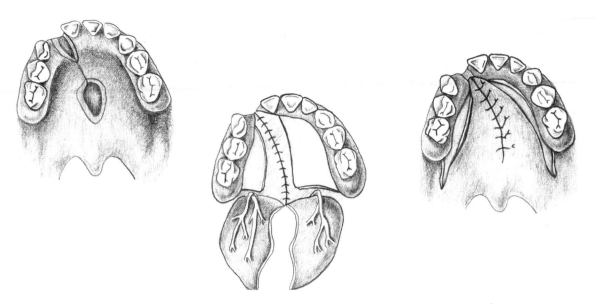

Figure 33–9. Gabka also demonstrated simultaneous closure of an alveolar (type VI/VII) fistula and a hard palate (type IV) fistula with a V-Y mucoperiosteal flap.

hygienic attention, their use should be restricted to cases in which surgery is contraindicated.[5] In a variation on the prosthetic obturator, Berkman reports that, with maximal patient compliance and identification of fistulae shortly after their appearance, a vinyl palatal appliance can be used to promote

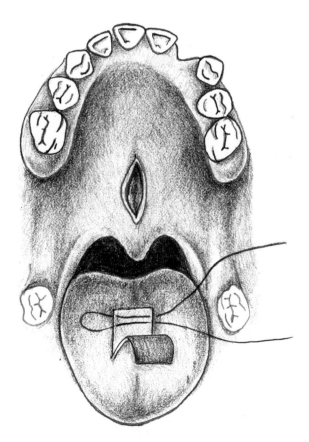

Figure 33–10. Guerrero-Santos described this distally based dorsal tongue flap in 1966.

closure of these lesions by granulation, epithelization, and fibrosis.[28] This approach, however, seems fraught with the same limitations discussed for the standard palatal obturator. Moreover, as Rintala notes, the potential of these repairs to withstand maxillary expansion is questionable.[19]

Surgical Techniques

It is clear that the surgical management of palatal fistulae can be a technically frustrating task. The surgical method chosen will depend on the fistula's location and size, the status of nearby palatal tissues, availability of flap donor sites, type of original cleft, previous methods of repair and surgeon preference. Every effort should be made to adhere to the following surgical principles in treating fistulae: closure should be performed in layers without overlapping sutures lines, well-vascularized tissues should be incorporated into the repair, tension at the suture lines must be avoided, and perfect cooptation of the wound edges must be achieved. There is no single surgical procedure that will fulfill all these criteria in treating palatal fistulae. The palate is usually heavily scarred with little to no extensibility. Moreover, larger fistulae require more tissue for closure, and less local tissue is available in the setting of a large defect. This surgical difficulty has incited surgeons to use a myriad of local, regional, and distant flaps, grafts, and alloplastic material to improve their results.

SIMPLE CLOSURE

Simple closure is probably the most common procedure used, and can adequately treat a large proportion of fistulae. This basic technique, essentially a recapitulation of the primary closure, consists of an incision at the margins of the fistula to create medial turnover flaps or "hinge flaps" for nasal lining

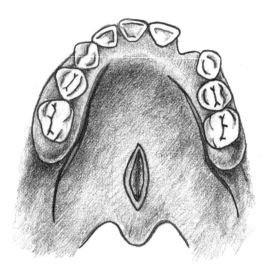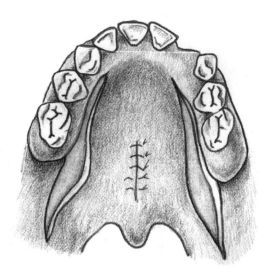

Figure 33–11. Closure of a type II (soft palate) fistula with lateral relaxing incisions for mobilization of the hard palate mucoperiosteum, as described by O'Neal in 1971. The fistula edges are turned in and three-layer closure is achieved.

closure (Fig. 33–13). These medial flaps are extended anteriorly and posteriorly along the midline palatal scar. For wide fistulae, the marginal incision around the defect may be made several millimeters away from the edge of the defect to facilitate the harvest of tissue allowing for a nasal lining repair. In addition, if the fistula is within the hard palate, vomer flaps may also be used to obtain a nasal lining closure. Lateral relaxing incisions are made at the junction of the attached gingiva and hard palate tissue, and are used to elevate palatal mucoperiosteal flaps. Alternatively, these relaxing incisions can be placed at the apex of the gingiva, removing the attached gingiva from the teeth and including it in the palatal flaps, adding a small but significant amount of length to the palatal flaps. The reported complication of gingival recession with this approach is rare in the young population.[37]

The palate is often heavily scarred and unyielding after primary palatoplasty, and the entire palate often has to be elevated with bipedicled or unipedicled flaps with mobilization of the greater palatine vessels. Underestimating the degree of palatal mobilization required is a common mistake; even in small fistulae the palatal mucoperiosteum should be widely freed to avoid tension on the closure line. In addition, wide dissection allows for complete excision of the mucosalized granulation tissue at the fistula site and proper undermining and closure of the nasal layer. Although some authors argue that closure of the nasal layer is not essential[38] and many patients can have permanent ablation of the fistula by a single-layer closure alone. However, since recurrence rates are notoriously high, it is advantageous to close both layers, especially since careful technique makes dual-layer closure practical. In fact, as mentioned in many of the techniques discussed below, a triple-layer repair is sometimes advocated.

After obtaining a nasal lining repair, it is preferable to transpose the palatal flaps laterally off to one side of the nasal suture line and avoid overlapping of the suture lines.

A helpful technique is to start the entire procedure with the lateral relaxing incisions first, elevating the oral mucoperiosteum and identifying and dissecting the fistula tract (from superficial to deep) before transecting the fistula. This sequence will allow accurate placement of the medial incision and complete excision of hypertrophied mucosa in the fistula tract.

PALATAL FLAPS

Various palatal flaps have been described in the literature to treat palatal fistulae. Hinge flaps or turnover flaps are palatal mucosal flaps from the immediate vicinity of the fistula that are based on the fistula mucosa. These flaps are hinged on their base and turned over to provide nasal layer closure.[39] Although a simple procedure with minimal donor site morbidity, hinge flaps have definite limitations: these flaps can only be used to provide nasal closure for small fistulae, are based on the original scar with questionable vascularity, and prevent complete excision of the scarred tissue in the fistula tract.

Other local flaps from the palate can be raised in a random fashion and used as transposition or rotation flaps for oral layer closure (Fig. 33–14). Despite the arc of rotation and transposition noted in illustrations, in reality these flaps are very limited in size and excursion. A variant of these flaps is the hemi-palatal island flap, in which almost an entire half of the hard palate mucosa is raised based on the greater palatine vessels.[40] After visualizing the vessels on the undersurface of the flap, a transverse cut is made in the palatal mucosa behind the vessels to completely free the flap and allow its transposition across the midline. Although this procedure will provide ample tissue for oral closure without overlapping suture lines, it involves a radical dissection, relies upon integrity of

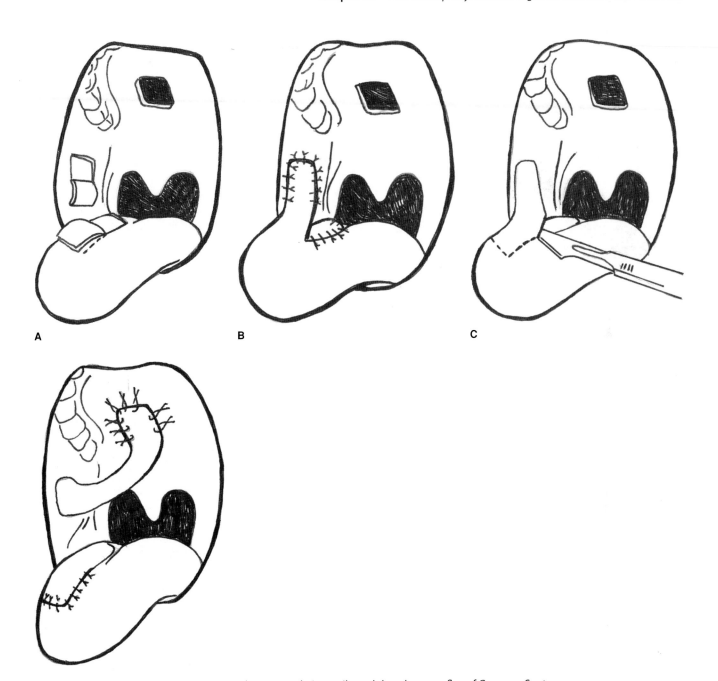

Figure 33–12. The 1973 waltzing unilateral dorsal tongue flap of Guerrero-Santos.

the greater palatine vessels after the primary repair, and leaves significant raw areas for spontaneous healing.[41]

REGIONAL FLAPS

The paucity of tissue in a scarred palate has led surgeons to design flaps using the mucosa of the cheek, tongue, and gingiva. Random flaps from the cheek or vestibular mucosa are limited in size and reach. Axial pattern flaps, however, are of controversial efficacy and are more difficult to design and elevate. In addition, axial pattern flaps have a tenuous course to the midline of the palate. The most common regional flaps described for the treatment of palatal fistulae include:

gingival flaps, the buccinator myomucosal flap, the facial artery musculomucosal (FAMM) flap, and tongue flaps. Although they can be used for closure of the nasal layer or as an interposition between the oral and nasal closures, these flaps are most commonly used for closure of the oral mucosa. This strategy allows for more oral palatal tissues to be recruited for a secure nasal layer closure, even in large fistulae.

Vestibular Mucosal Flaps

The gingival (vestibular) mucosal flaps, raised from the labial side of the alveolus, are one of the most commonly used flaps for both alveolar bone grafting and anterior palatal fistula closure.[42] Although they are random flaps, gingival mucosal

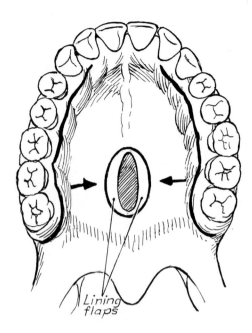

Figure 33–13. A type IV (hard palate) fistula with outline of the medial paring incision and the lateral release incisions is shown.

flaps have a reliable vascular supply. These flaps are usually raised with their width equal to the height of the alveolus and extend along the alveolar ridge (Fig. 33–15); they are transposed to the anterior palate through the alveolar defect. This technique may interfere with growth of the maxilla and future orthodontic expansion and surgery (e.g., bone grafting of the alveolar cleft). Alternatively, they can be passed through a subperiosteal tunnel at the floor of the nose to the nasal side of the fistula; however, this is a lengthy dissection and a tight tunnel. Other designs have been used, such as leaving an exteriorized pedicle for later separation, raising bilaterally based bucket handle flaps,[43] or elevating an island flap.[44] If an excessive amount of mucosa is harvested, distortion of the shape of the lip may result or, at best, the mucosa will be unavailable in future surgeries.[43]

Buccal Mucosal Flaps

Buccal flaps have been described to augment nasal layer closure both in primary clefts and in palatal fistulae.[45] They are especially helpful in type III fistulae (at the junction of the hard and soft palates), which are infamous for their paucity of local tissue; moreover, these flaps may augment palatal length. They are raised from the cheek with their base behind the upper alveolus with a width of 1.5–2 cm (Fig. 33–16). Buccal mucosal flaps are random flaps containing mucosa and submucosal tissue. In raising the flap, the surgeon must avoid the parotid duct (although this is rarely problematic) and avoid exposure of the buccal fat pad. The flap is turned over, passed in a submucosal tunnel behind the edge of the hard palate, and sutured to the edges of the nasal mucosa. The donor site is closed primarily. Alternatively, the flap can be used to close the oral layer, usually leaving an exteriorized pedicle to be separated in 2–3 weeks.

Buccinator Myomucosal Flap

The buccinator muscle has a rich arterial, venous, and nerve supply, allowing elevation of flaps that are reliable, sensate, and of variable dimensions while preserving the function of the remaining muscle.[46] The buccal artery (a branch of the internal maxillary artery) and the posterior buccal branches of the facial artery are the basis of the posteriorly based buccinator myomucosal flap.[47,48] Both arteries enter the posterior portion of the muscle, and their diameters are inversely proportional. The upper border of the flap extends from the posterior aspect of the maxilla to the oral commissure, and is 3–10 mm below the parotid duct orifice. Alternatively, the anterior limit of the flap can extend further into the lips creating a Y-shaped flap.[47] The flap's width is approximately 1–3 cm, thus allowing primary donor site closure. The mucosa and muscle are incised to create either a peninsular or island flap. The muscle is elevated and separated from the deep buccopharyngeal fascia in a loose areolar plane. Dissection in this plane should proceed rapidly and easily, preserving the integrity of the fascia and thus preventing prolapse of the buccal fat pad or injury to the facial nerve.[48] The flap's length can approach 10 cm, running posteriorly to the level of the pterygomandibular raphe.

Facial Artery Musculomucosal (FAMM) Flap

Like the buccinator myomucosal flap, the FAMM flap is raised from the cheek mucosa and includes a portion of the buccinator muscle. Although it has been argued that this flap is only a variant of the buccinator flap,[49] it is a distinct entity in its inclusion of the facial artery.[50] The flap is designed along the course of the facial artery, which can be palpated or mapped by a Doppler probe (Fig. 33–17). The flap has an oblique orientation, from the retromolar trigone to the gingivolabial sulcus at the base of the ipsilateral alar crease, with a width of 1.5–2 cm and a length up to 9–11 cm.[51] The flap is designed anterior to the orifice of the parotid duct. It is elevated to include the mucosa, part of the buccinator and orbicularis oris, and the facial artery. The venous drainage is either through the facial vein or through the random but robust venous plexuses around the facial artery. The flap can be based superiorly, to reach alveolar and hard palate fistulae (types IV–VII), or inferiorly and posteriorly to reach soft palate fistulae (types I–III). After the margins of the flap are incised, the facial artery is ligated at the distal end of the flap and dissection proceeds to include the mucosa, part of the buccinator and orbicularis oris, and the facial artery. The donor site is closed in two layers (muscle and mucosa). The flap usually requires an open dental arch for passage to the palate (e.g., through an alveolar cleft). Inferiorly based flaps can be used in a two-stage fashion, with the flap turning behind and around the maxillary tuberosity with an exteriorized pedicle for later division and insetting. This will necessitate the use of a bite block secured to the dentition for 2 weeks to prevent trauma to the flap. Other drawbacks include the bulk of the flap (which can be secondarily corrected if necessary) and initial tightness at the donor site (which usually resolves

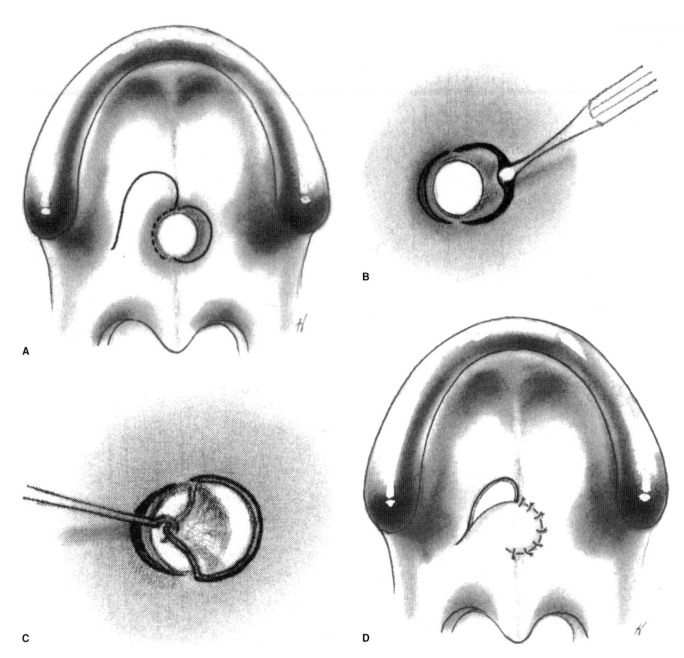

Figure 33–14. (A) Design of a transposition flap, from the palatal mucosa for oral layer closure and turn-over flaps for nasal-layer closure; (B and C) undermining of the turnover flaps to close the nasal layer; (D) the final repair.

spontaneously). Some speech therapists have discouraged the use of this flap due to possible interference with facial muscles and speech development; however, this has not been shown to be a long-term problem. The FAMM flap is fairly reliable and provides enough mucosa to cover large fistulae or create a double layer closure.[51]

Tongue Flap

Due to its efficacy in closing even large defects, the tongue flap has historically been one of the most preferred options for fistula closure in the anterior palate (Types III–V). Since

Guerrero-Santos and Altamarino published their experience using tongue flaps in 1966,[30] many authors have shown it to be highly reliable, relatively easy to perform, and to cause no deficits in lingual function.[52,53]

The paired lingual arteries run anteriorly on the ventral surface of the tongue and supply vertical branches to the dorsal tongue surface. These branches form the basis of dorsal tongue flaps. Due to its random vascular pattern, the flap can be designed in any direction on the dorsum of the tongue. The surgeon should carefully consider every possible orientation to find the design of the flap that provides the most direct and shortest path to the palatal defect while avoiding

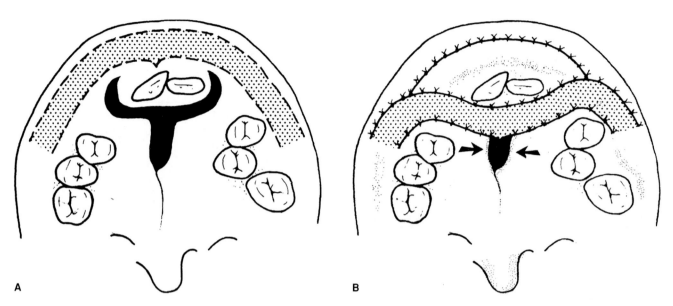

Figure 33–15. (A) Design of a bipedicled labial bucual sulcus flap; (B) transposition of bipedicled labial flap for closure of anterior hard palate fistulae.

kinking or stretching the pedicle. Tongue flaps are designed between the level of the circumvallate papillae and 1–2 cm from the tip of the tongue, and are usually 2–4 cm in width (slightly wider than the width of the fistula) and around 6 cm in length. Posteriorly based flaps are useful for type III defects, while anteriorly based flaps are employed for type V defects (Fig. 33–18). Type IV defects may be addressed with either anteriorly or posteriorly based flaps depending on the relevant anatomy in a given patient. Therefore, anteriorly based flaps are used for defects in the type IV and type V positions, while posteriorly based flaps are used for defects in the type III and type IV positions. The thickness of the flap is usually 5 mm at the tip and 7 mm at the base and includes the superficial layer of muscles with the mucosa, although some authors advocate thinner flaps (3 mm thick) containing only a thin muscle layer (the flap is based on the random submucosal plexus and not on axial muscle vessels).

The tongue flap is used to provide oral closure while the nasal layer is closed primarily or with a hinge flap. The patient is intubated with the ET tube on one side of the mouth, or via the nasal route, and a mouth block used to expose the tongue. After local injection with a vasoconstrictor, the flap is raised with a sharp knife. The donor area is directly closed in two layers after appropriate hemostasis is achieved. The oral mucosal margin surrounding the fistula is undermined slightly to create an edge for pedicled tongue flap suture-fixation.

Argamaso et al. used the tongue flap for nasal closure in conjunction with widely undermined palatal flaps for oral closure. A transverse incision is made in the palatal mucosa proximal to the fistula; the tongue flap is passed through this incision and then sutured to the nasal mucosa, with the mucosal surface of the flap facing dorsally into the nasal cavity. Argamaso et al. theorized that this indirect course would take

tension off the suture line, thus preventing separation of the flap.

Postoperative care is similar to that after primary palatoplasty: a nasopharyngeal airway for 1–2 days or longer, liquid diet for a week followed by a soft diet, arm restraints, and avoiding mechanical damage to the suture line by straws, toothbrushes, forks, etc. After 2–3 weeks, the flap is separated from the tongue. Some authors have suggested limited intermaxillary fixation, even by elastics, to decrease the chances of flap dehiscence with mouth opening, following the stage one procedure. Close postoperative monitoring of the airway is important, particularly in the younger patients. The patient may have to remain intubated for a few days until they can maintain their airway. The risk of airway compromise is magnified in patients who have had pharyngeal speech surgery.

Stage two surgery is coordinated closely with the pediatric anesthesiologist so they are aware of possible complications, as both oral and nasal intubation can disrupt the flap. Alternative options include dividing the flap under local anesthesia, or a rapid division with electrocautery before intubation.

A serious complication of tongue flaps is their potential separation from the palate. This can be caused by gravity, the thin friable palatal mucosa's inability to hold sutures, unbridled tongue movement, and movement with the mandible (e.g., yawning). This complication can be prevented by suture fixation of the tongue to the lip[31] or teeth,[54] or by maxillary mandibular immobilization.[55] However, many surgeons find that this maneuver is unnecessary, especially in older patients.

Tongue flap fistula reconstruction necessitates two visits to the operating room. In addition, the period between procedures can be trying, especially in young children. In addition, following final division and inset of the flap, the

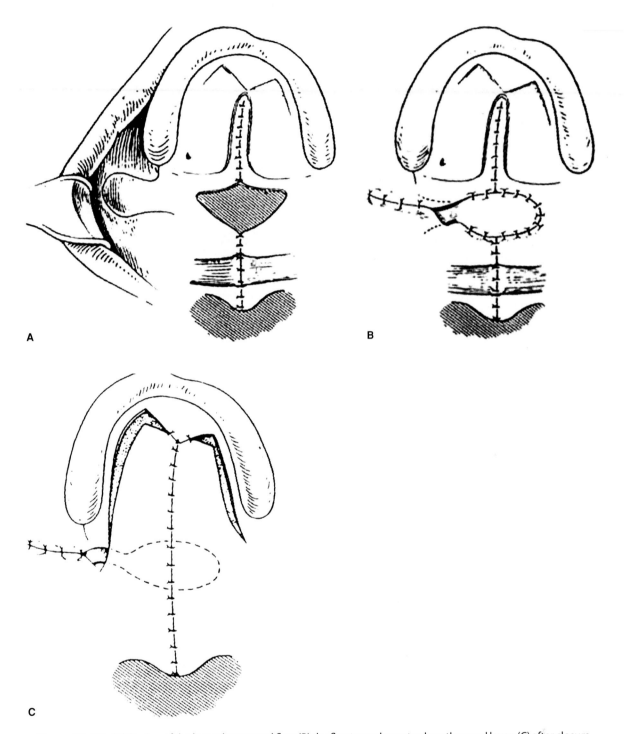

Figure 33–16. (A) Design of the buccal mucoasal flap; (B) the flap turned over to close the nasal layer; (C) after closure of the oral layer over the flap.

bulky tongue mucosa stands out from the rest of the palate, which may cause speech distortion and necessitate a third stage to debulk the flap. Simply shaving the flap flush with the surrounding mucosa and leaving the raw area to heal by secondary intention accomplishes the debulking procedure.

Despite all of its drawbacks, many surgeons consider the tongue flap their primary option for large recurrent anterior palatal fistulae, as it provides an ample amount of tissue, is

relatively easy to perform, and causes minimal donor site morbidity.

Septal Flaps

The septal mucosa is a valuable source for mucosal flaps and grafts, and can be used for closure of the nasal layer in palatal fistulae. Murrell et al. used a contralateral nasal septal flap

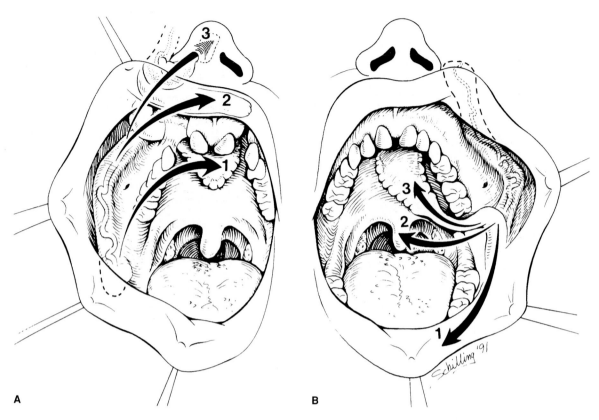

Figure 33–17. (A) Design of superiorly based FAMM flap showing its reach to the hard palate, lip, or nose; (B) design of the inferiorly based FAMM flap reaching the hard palate, soft palate, or floor of the mouth.

based on the nasal floor that hinges down into palatal fistulae in mid- and posterior hard palate defects (Pittsburgh Fistula type IV). This group cautioned against using the septal flap (1) in children, for fear of interfering with nasal growth, and (2) in anterior hard palate defects, so as not to weaken nasal support.

By raising this flap, access is gained to the septal bone and cartilage, which can be harvested as a graft for interposition between the oral and nasal layers. Although septal flaps have the advantage of replacing like tissues with like tissues, they are relatively more difficult to raise and design properly, and

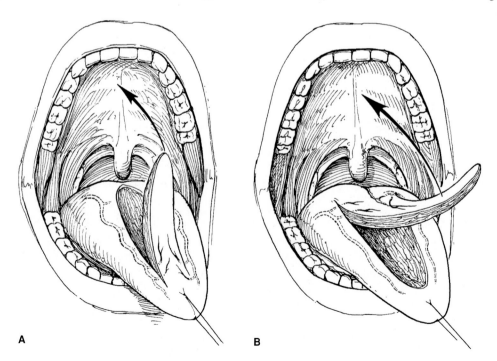

Figure 33–18. Elevation of (A) anteriorly and (B) posteriorly based tongue flaps for closure of palatal fistulae.

are limited in size. For larger fistulae, bilateral flaps can be raised, but at the risk of septal perforation.

Pharyngeal Flaps

For soft palate fistulae (type I–III) and frank palatal dehiscences, pharyngeal flaps have been described to assist the closure of fistulae as well as improving speech.

Temporalis Muscle and Temporoparietal Fascia Flap

Both the temporalis muscle and the temporoparietal fascia (TPF) flap are common options utilized in head and neck reconstruction, but they have a limited role in treating palatal fistulae, especially those secondary to clefting. This is because palatal fistulae tend to lie at the extreme limit of these flap's reach. Thus, the blood supply to the most critical portion of this flap (the distal tip) is tenuous. Utilizing these flaps for palatal fistula reconstruction requires a significant dissection to raise the flap and create a path to the palate. This dissection can require a zygomatic arch osteotomy or coronoidectomy. With the use of these flaps a risk of donor site aesthetic deformities (e.g., temporal hollowness, widened scalp scars) or injury to the frontal branch of the facial nerve exists. Due to these limitations and challenges, these flaps are rarely used in palatal fistulae correction. Although the temporalis may be used for large type II fistulae with almost total loss of the soft palate, it is often not well developed in children.

Buccal Fat Pad Flaps

Use of the buccal fat pad (BFP) has been well described in the literature for closure of maxillectomy defects, especially defects of the alveolar ridge with oro-sinus or oro-antral communication.[56] Its efficacy for use in cleft palate fistulae is debatable, however, as transposing the flap to the midline necessitates a long reach and the creation of a tunnel for the flap. The BFP is relatively larger in children, and this may facilitate its reach to the midline. It can be either used as an interposing material placed between the oral and nasal layers, or covered by a skin graft to replace the oral layer.[43] Alternatively, it can be left exposed in the oral cavity for spontaneous epithelialization.[56,57] Several studies have confirmed that mucosalization occurs within a few weeks, and biopsies have demonstrated an epithelial layer over fibrovascular connective tissue, with minimal or no remaining fat.[56–58]

The BFP is composed of a central body with four extensions: pterygoid, buccal, superficial, and deep temporal. A robust blood supply is drawn from the transverse facial branch of the superficial temporal artery, the facial artery, and the buccal and deep temporal branches of the maxillary artery. It is surrounded by a thin but definite capsule, which should be preserved during dissection of the flap. The BFP is harvested through an intraoral mucosal incision, or a gingival mucoperiosteal flap can be raised with exposure of the BFP through a periosteal incision at the base of the flap.

The BFP is then gently dissected bluntly, harvesting the part of the BFP between the buccinator and the masseter. There are several ways to transfer the BFP graft to cover the fistula in the midline, none of which is without its disadvantages. A submucosal tunnel in the soft palate is possibly the best option, but this approach can damage the soft palate musculature or create more scarring. If the flap is passed across an alveolar defect it may interfere with dentition and future orthodontic treatment. A subantral dissection is difficult and may compress the flap. Alternatively, the pedicle can be left exteriorized and divided in a second stage.

Compared to the buccinator myomucosal flap and FAMM flap, the buccal fat flap theoretically may cause less donor site morbidity as it preserves the facial musculature and the facial artery. However, the BFP flap's indistinct nature, tedious dissection, and limited reach to the midline make it a less common procedure in treating palatal fistulae.

DISTANT PEDICLED FLAPS

Distant pedicled flaps are primarily of historical interest only, due to their disadvantages and the availability of other better options. For example, tubed flaps transferred to the palate and later divided, occasionally with a preliminary delay, are unappealing due to the cumbersome high-maintenance interval between inset and pedicle division, their considerable distortion of donor sites, and bulky nature.[59] Cutaneous flaps, such as the island nasolabial flap, are likewise rarely used today.

FREE FLAPS

Reconstructive surgeons no longer strictly adhere to the reconstructive ladder for reconstructing palatal defects, but rather opt for the treatment modality with the best projected outcome. This shift in thinking has led to a dramatic increase in the utilization of free flaps in head and neck reconstruction. The value of free flaps in palatal reconstruction after oncologic resection is well documented,[60] but their role in congenital "cleft" fistulae is limited to a few studies with small patient cohorts.[61,62] In the context of congenital clefts, free flaps are usually limited to treating fistulae of considerable size for which local flaps are unavailable, and that have failed multiple attempts at repair. Free tissue transfer has the advantage of abundant tissue, allowing secure closure of the palate, and possibly even facilitating palatal lengthening. The free flap is usually used for closure of the oral layer, with the palatal tissue used for closure of the nasal lining. Alternatively, at the expense of bulk, the flap can be "double-islanded" to provide both nasal and oral closure. The vascular pedicle is commonly brought through a submucous tunnel in the palate, around the maxillary tuberosity, and through the cheek to the submandibular area for anastomosis to the facial artery. Care should be taken to create ample space for the pedicle to prevent compression, and to achieve a watertight mucosal closure to prevent salivary leakage on the anastomosis. Not only can the pedicle be compressed by a tight tunnel throughout its tortuous course, but also during mastication; subsequently, patients should be kept on a liquid diet for a few weeks postoperatively.

The radial forearm flap, due to its thin skin island and long vascular pedicle, is the most common form of free tissue transfer used for palatal defects.[63] A segment of the radius can be included in the flap to reconstruct bony defects in the hard palate. Despite increasing experience and success with free tissue transfer for reconstructive surgery, it is uncommon to see large enough palatal fistulae to justify the use of free tissue transfer in most experienced multidisciplinary cleft centers.

GRAFTS

Free tissue grafts have been used as an adjunct in the closure of palatal fistulae. However, questions remain as to the efficacy of grafts and their indications and limitations. Most studies in this area rely on historical controls. Due to the great variability in patient population, fistula site, and surgical technique, these studies provide insufficient evidence to substantiate the routine use of these grafts. Potential graft materials include cartilage, dermis, lyophilized dura, bone, and periosteum. A proposed advantage of using these grafts is that wide undermining of the palatal mucoperiosteum is not needed, theoretically decreasing the negative effect on maxillary growth.

Cartilage

Based on previous use of conchal cartilage for reconstruction of eyelids, and costal cartilage for reconstruction of the trachea, Matsuo et al. initially reported their success in closing a palatal fistula in a single patient using conchal cartilage. Further reports showed fistula closure rates of 91.7% (Ohsumi), 79% (Jeffer), and 54% (Mohanna). These reports varied in the plane of dissection (submucosal vs. submucoperiosteal) and the method of mucosal closure (primary closure over the cartilage vs. use of mucosal flaps vs. leaving the cartilage exposed, etc.). Ohsumi et al. performed an elegant experimental study in rabbits in which conchal cartilage was grafted in a submucosal pocket dissected around the fistula, leaving the cartilage exposed at the fistula site without attempting to close the overlying mucosa. Histological analysis showed that 3 weeks after surgery, the exposed cartilage in the central region of the palatal fistula had disappeared and was replaced by fibrous tissue. This fibrous tissue was gradually covered by epithelium from the periphery of the fistula, which matured over a 16-week period. Twenty of their 21 surgically created fistulae (95.2%) healed completely. The authors propose that the conchal cartilage serves as "supporting tissue" until fistula closure proceeds by fibrosis and epithelialization, with subsequent chondrocyte death and absorption of the cartilage matrix.

The use of conchal cartilage appears to assist fistula healing, especially when either the nasal or oral layer cannot

be closed or is under too much tension. If the cartilage is to be used alone for fistula closure, an incision is made around the fistula, with longitudinal extensions if necessary. A pocket of adequate size is created between the palatal mucoperiosteum and the palatine bone, and the cartilage with the overlying perichondrium is firmly fixed in position.[32] It is believed that the perichondrium plays an important role in survival of the cartilage and epithelial regeneration.[64]

Alternatively, the cartilage—acting as a barrier between two overlapping suture lines—can be used to augment closure by standard techniques. For example, one might employ a hinge flap for nasal closure and standard hard palate mucoperiosteal flaps for palatal closure, with a cartilage graft interposed between the two. Another advantage of cartilage grafts is that they allow the palate to heal without slit-like depressions, which can be difficult to differentiate from fistulae.[32] The usual donor site is the conchal bowl which can provide enough cartilage for most fistulae. Since the drawbacks of this technique (donor site morbidity and increased operative time) are relatively minor, cartilage grafts may be a good option in recalcitrant palatal fistulae.

Dermis/Mucosa Grafts

The use of skin grafts in intraoral reconstruction is an accepted technique that is relatively simple. However, the use of skin grafts in palatal fistula closure has been infrequent. Vandeput et al. used a dermal fat graft placed deep into the oral mucosa, with the fat on the nasal side and without closing the nasal layer.[65] Honnebier et al. used a mucosal graft that is sutured to the undersurface of the dissected palatal mucoperiosteal flaps so that it lies at the fistula site, again without closing the nasal layer.[13] Although these techniques are theoretically logical and relatively simple to perform with minimal increase in operative time, cost, or donor site morbidity, further studies are needed to establish their value.

Bone and Periosteal Grafts

There are scarce reports of the use of bone or periosteum grafts for closure of nonalveolar palatal fistulae.[66,67] The rationale for bone grafting is to replace lost tissues with like tissues, and therefore bone is used to induce osteogenesis in the maxillary cleft.[67] Bone graft is used to fill any dead space and act as a third layer of closure. Occasionally, bone has been used in conjunction with other flaps, such as the septal bone graft with septal mucosal flap described by Murrell et al. Although in the normal palate bone extends across the hard palate, most surgeons believe that bone is not needed in the closure of hard palate fistulae, and some feel that its inclusion can lead to a higher complication rate (Jackson, 1992).

ACELLULAR DERMAL MATRIX

In 2003, Kirschner et al. reported the use of acellular dermal matrix (ADM) in fistula closure,[18,68] in a large animal model of oral nasal fistula, followed by a clinical series demonstrating complete healing of fistulae both in the experimental and clinical series. In addition, in the experimental series, the palatal defects treated with ADM healed with no evidence of scarring but rather tissue regeneration. ADM is prepared from cadaveric skin processed to remove epidermal and dermal cells to create an immunologically inert implant. Its collagen framework, acellular vascular channels, and basement membrane act as a scaffold for migration of host fibroblasts, revascularization, and reepithelialization. It has been experimentally shown to be indistinguishable from the recipient tissues 4 weeks after implantation.[69] The basis of this therapy hinges on histological evidence of the ADM's repopulation by host cells and subsequent healing by tissue regeneration and remodeling without scarring.[18,68] Originally employed for full thickness burns, its uses have been expanded to include abdominal hernia repair,[70] dural replacement,[71] sling creation in facial reanimation,[72] and soft tissue augmentation.[73] ADM may provide a practical and effective method of palatal fistula repair as it can solve the problems of tissue insufficiency and scarring seen in most of these procedures.

The role of ADM in the repair of palatal fistulae was initially studied in a reproducible large animal porcine model of oro-nasal fistulae: fistulae were created in the hard palate of piglets and repaired by placing ADM between the bony palate and the oral mucoperiosteum.[18] No attempt was made to suture the ADM to the margins of the fistulae, or to obtain either a nasal lining or oral mucosal closure. These fistulae progressed to complete healing, with resurfacing of the oral and nasal layers by grossly and histologically normal mucosa with thick intervening fibrovascular tissue.[18] Since that time, clinical studies have demonstrated the value of acellular dermal matrix in the repair of cleft palates, palatal fistulae, and alveolar clefts (Figs. 33–19 and 33–20).[74–76] Even in instances where the mucosal suture line showed early dehiscence with exposure of the acellular dermal matrix, these fistulae went on to complete healing with mucosal regeneration over the acellular dermal matrix. In addition to its induction of tissue regeneration and ready incorporation into tissues, ADM offers further advantages over other grafts. For example, ADM eliminates donor site morbidity, is easy to handle, is available "off the shelf," and its incorporation into palatal procedures entails only a minimal increase in operative time.

Potential disadvantages of ADM could include the impairment of speech secondary to scarring of the velum and the transmission of infectious diseases. We believe these adverse outcomes are of theoretical concern only. Kirschner et al. demonstrated histological evidence that when placed in palatal defects, ADM supported the regeneration of native tissue and demonstrated scarless healing.[28,29] In addition, the ADM is placed into a relatively static portion of the velum, usually at the junction of the hard and soft palate, or on top of the hard palate, assisting in nasal lining closure. This location is at the site of the normal tensor aponeurosis, and is clear of the levator muscle reconstruction critical to speech. Finally, in a series of patients at our institution whose primary and secondary palatal procedures incorporated ADM, we have seen only positive speech outcomes, and no negative effect on speech has been demonstrated to date.[77] In terms of the transmission of infectious disease, although the ADM is of cadaveric origin, it is pretreated with a series of antipathogen measures. With its extensive applications in reconstructive surgery, ADM has never been associated with the transmission of an infectious disease.[38]

AUTHORS' PREFERRED METHOD

Regardless of the technique employed, we attempt to reach the following goals in all fistula repairs:

1. Judicious, however, complete excision of the epithelialized tract
2. Wide dissection of the nasal lining and mucosal flaps
3. A tension free, water tight, closure of the nasal lining and oral mucosa
4. Avoidance of overlapping suture lines
5. Routine use of acellular dermal matrix as a third layer of soft tissue closure, placed between the nasal lining and oral mucosal repair
6. Use of imported, well vascularized tissue (i.e., FAMM flap) if complete oral mucosal repair is not possible with palatal tissue available
7. Strict postoperative care.

What follows is a discussion of the authors' preferred techniques for closure of palatal fistulae, organized according to the Pittsburgh Fistula Classification System.

Type I (Bifid Uvula)

A postoperative bifid uvula is a common fistula frequently unreported, likely due to its questionable functional significance. The presence of an isolated cleft uvula is rarely an indication for surgery. The correction of type I fistulae is similar to the primary management of this lesion: the entire medial aspects of the uvula are demucosalized, rather than simply incised, creating a wider raw surface for healing. The uvula is repaired with multiple sutures placed closely together on both the anterior and posterior aspects of the uvula.

Type II (Soft Palate)

Fistulae within the soft palate result from either an entire dehiscence of the velum after repair, or from a lack of adequate muscle reconstruction at the time of palatoplasty. Type II fistulae usually occur only after straight-line repair of the velum. It is rare to encounter type II fistulae after Furlow double opposing z-plasty repairs as this repair utilizes a multilayer muscle reconstruction of the velum (palatopharyngeus, palatoglossus, and levator muscles).

When treating type II fistulae of the soft palate, it is our preference to perform a "conversion" Furlow palatoplasty to definitively repair the dehisced or fistulized velum.

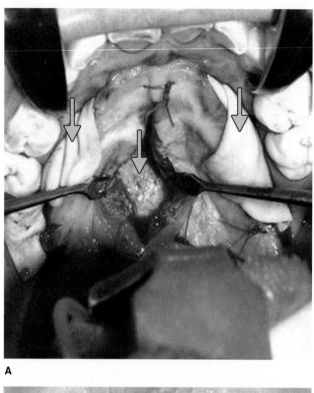

A

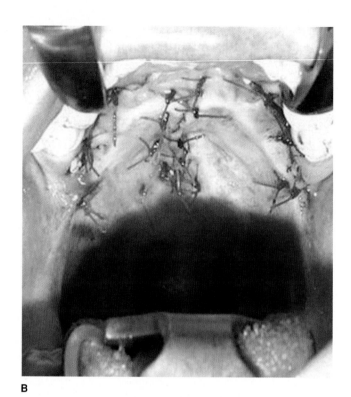

B

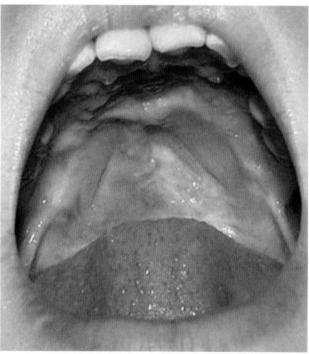

C

Figure 33–19. (A) Acellular dermal matrix (arrows) is incorporated into this repair of a type IV (hard palate fistula) as it is slipped beneath the palatal mucosa at the lateral relaxing incisions; (B) the mucosa is closed over the ADM; (C) the fistula has healed completely.

In addition, there are proven advantageous effects on palatal function and speech.[78] Although a conversion Furlow palatoplasty can be performed for even wide dehiscences of the soft palate, a pharyngeal flap can be used in this situation; however, it is a secondary option in our protocol.

Types III and IV (Junction of Hard and Soft Palate, and Hard Palate)

When encountering type III and IV postoperative, we typically avoid distant flaps for closure, and rather perform a revisionary palatoplasty of the hard and soft palates. If there

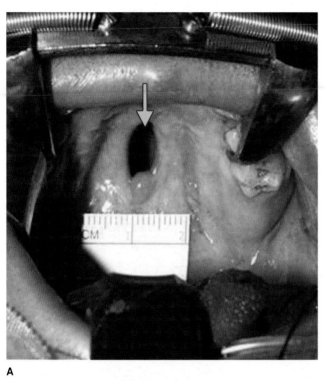

A

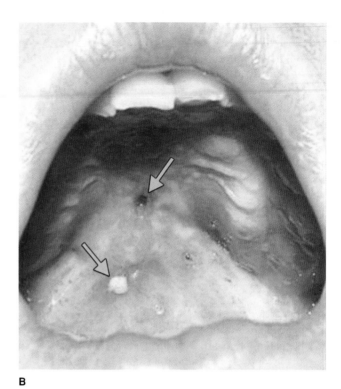

B

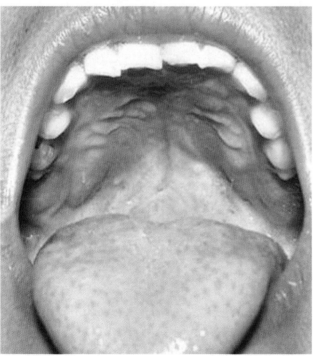

C

Figure 33–20. (A) A type IV (hard palate) fistula is indicated by the arrow. This defect was repaired with ADM, like the defect in Fig. 33–19. (B) Postoperatively there was a pinpoint dehiscence (at the arrow) to the level of the ADM. (C) The defect soon spontaneously resolved.

is any degree of velopharyngeal insufficiency with evidence of levator muscle dehiscence, there is a low threshold to perform a conversion Furlow palatoplasty. Any remaining fibers of the tensor aponeurosis are cut preforming a complete release of the levator muscle for reconstruction; this maneuver

contributes significantly to avoiding tension at the junction of the hard and soft palates which might evolve type III fistulae.

The hard palate is addressed with bilateral, unipedicled mucoperiosteal flaps. Wide dissection of the hard palate nasal lining and oral mucosa is performed to facilitate a tension-free repair of the nasal lining and oral mucosa. ADM is routinely used to augment the nasal lining repair. An ultrathin piece of ADM is laid on the nasal lining repair, just before the levator muscle reconstruction, and sewn to the lining at the junction of the hard and soft palates. It is then draped over the hard palate, and sewn to the nasal lining repair of the hard palate. The hard palate mucosal flaps are then repaired with grossly everted horizontal mattress sutures (Figs. 33–21 to 33–24).

Type V (Junction of Primary and Secondary Palates in Veau IV Bilateral Clefts)

Type V fistulae at the incisive canal, found in bilateral clefts, can be a daunting problem. A key to the decision of importing vascularized soft tissue for repair (i.e., FAMM flap, tongue flap) is whether the hard palate unipedicled mucoperiosteal flaps can be dissected well enough (i.e., island flaps based on the greater palatine vessels) to reach the free edge of the premaxillary mucosa for a stable repair. In those bilateral cleft patients with one side incomplete, the mucosa of the premaxilla can be raised with the ipsilateral hard palate flap (on the incomplete cleft side) to facilitate closure of the oral layer. If the type V fistula is very large, and/or the premaxilla is "locked out" behind the collapsed lateral maxillary segments, the decision regarding premaxillary set-back with alveolar bone grafting and/or importing free tissue to assist in the reconstruction is made.

If it appears that with adequate dissection, the hard palate flaps will reach the posterior tip of the premaxilla, the procedure is begun by creating the lateral incisions of the hard palate flaps and dissecting the hard palate flaps to the midline. Subperiosteal dissection of fistula tract and medial bony defect, extending to the nasal side of the palate as much as possible, is performed prior to making any incision of the fistula tract. This will allow for recruitment of nasal

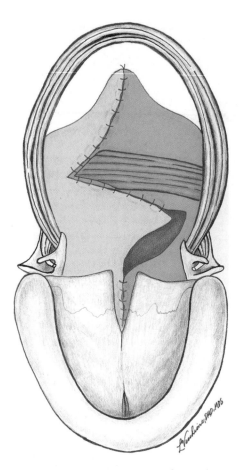

Figure 33–22. Schematic illustrating a defect in the nasal lining at the junction of the hard and soft palates during a palatoplasty.

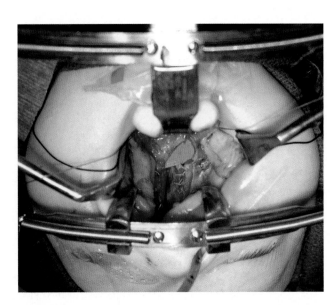

Figure 33–21. Surgical repair of a Veau III cleft with defect in nasal lining, noted by green backing.

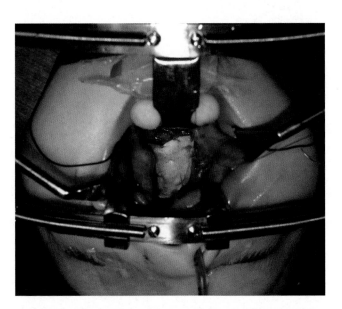

Figure 33–23. Surgical repair of a Veau III cleft with acellular dermal matrix in white, sewn onto the nasal lining, covering the junction of the soft and hard palates, draped over the hard palate, and anteriorly sewn to the alveolar gingiva.

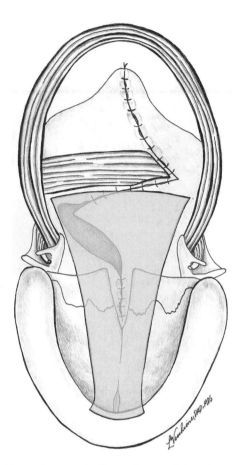

Figure 33-24. Schematic illustrating acellular dermal matrix noted in yellow, sewn to the nasal lining and covering the junction of the soft and hard palates, draped over the hard palate, and sewn to the alveolar gingiva.

lining, and adequate visualization to design "turn over" flaps for a nasal lining repair. ADM is routinely used, and is placed on top of the hard palate as an intervening layer between the nasal lining and oral mucosa repair. The ADM is placed on the hard palate, extending well beyond the fistula and covering the incisions along the cleft (Fig. 33–24).

In those severe cases when the tips of the hard palate unipedicled flaps can not reach the premaxillary mucosa, then tissue must be imported (i.e., FAMM flap, tongue flap, etc.). However, attempts at a nasal lining repair and the use of ADM as described is still recommended.

Types VI and VII (Lingual–and Labial–Alveolar)

Alveolar fistulae are often residual clefts intentionally left unrepaired at the time of the original lip and palate repairs. They are usually reconstructed at the time of alveolar bone grafting. The cleft orthodontist plays an important role in the management of these fistulae: the maxilla often needs to be expanded, and the alveolar arches aligned, before surgery, and the optimal time for bone grafting is usually determined with respect to development of the dentition.

To treat these fistulae, the lining of the alveolar cleft is subperiosteally dissected, creating flaps to be turned inwards

for nasal closure, and outwards for oral mucosal closure. Bone graft is usually placed in the alveolar cleft, between these reconstructed layers. Sometimes in cases where there are large number VI or VII fistulae, bone grafting may be postponed to a second stage, if there is concern over soft tissue coverage and the risk of incomplete closure over the bone graft.

When performing an alveolar bone graft and closure of number VI and VII fistulae, ADM can be used to reinforce either layer if necessary. If it is not possible to achieve a water tight, tension free repair of the nasal lining or oral mucosa, sufficient to protect the bone graft, ADM can be used to augment the nasal lining repair prior to the placement of bone graft, and/or be used to augment the oral mucosal repair, placed on top of the bone graft and acting as another layer of soft tissue.

PREVENTION

As evidenced by the propensity of this lesion toward recurrence, prevention is clearly the most efficacious strategy for the management of palatal fistulae. A strategy we currently utilize for the prevention of palatal fistulae grew out of Kirschner's 2003 discussion on the use of acellular dermal matrixes (ADM) in repairing palatal fistulae.[18,68] In addition to employing other strategies detailed in the following sections, our group has begun the selective use of ADM in primary cleft palate repair to decrease the incidence of postoperative fistulae.[6]

Acellular Dermal Matrix (ADM) and Primary Palate Repair

In those challenging primary palatoplasties, when unable to obtain a complete, two-layer, water-tight, and tension-free repair, ADM is utilized as an interpositional graft.[18,68,74,75,79] As often is the case, particularly when using the Furlow palatoplasty technique, a small defect in the nasal lining at the junction of the soft and hard palates is left at the conclusion of the nasal lining reconstruction. This defect, at the junction of the hard and the soft palate, is where the left-sided, anteriorly based, nasal mucosal flap cannot reach the mucosa of the right-sided posterior edge of the hard palate (Figs. 33–23 and 33–24). A thin or ultrathin 2×4 cm piece of ADM is sewn onto the nasal lining defect as a graft to complete the nasal closure. The graft is tacked down to the nasal lining around the junction of the hard and soft palate. It is then draped over the hard palate, tacked down to the hard palate nasal lining repair, and sewn anteriorly to the alveolar gingiva (Figs.33–21 and 33–24). The ADM is specifically placed in the region where the normal tensor aponeurosis would be in a nonclefted palate, and *not attached to the levator muscle repair proper*; in essence, this can be thought of as a tensor aponeurosis reconstruction. When the levator muscle sling is completely released and reconstructed, it is normally 1.5–2.0 cm away from the posterior edge of the hard palate, away from the ADM reconstruction (Fig. 33–25).

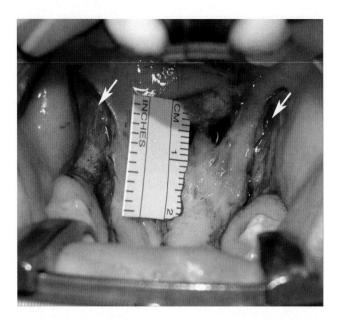

Figure 33–25. Intraoperative image with ruler demonstrating the levator muscle sling reconstruction 2 cm away from the posterior edge of the hard palate. Arrows indicate the relaxing incisions bilaterally.

Although incorporating ADM into palatoplasty has likely decreased the incidence of postoperative fistula formation in our cohort, we cannot compare our fistula outcomes to a control group not receiving ADM. We are left to judge our postoperative fistulae incidence in comparison to other comparable series utilizing similar surgical techniques. A 1999 Children's Hospital of Philadelphia (CHOP) report described a similar series of primary palatoplasties utilizing the same surgical technique—the modified Furlow double opposing z-plasty, but without ADM.[80] A comparison of CHOP's primary palatal fistula rate (6.8%) to that reported in this series (0.93%) may indicate a positive influence of ADM on postoperative fistulae incidence.

There are potential disadvantages to the use of ADM for nasal lining augmentation in primary palatoplasty; they are the same as those reviewed earlier for the use of ADM in fistula repair, including impairment of velar function and transmission of infectious disease. Again, as discussed above, these potential disadvantages are most likely of only theoretical concern.

Other Strategies to Prevent Fistulae

Type I fistulae, or bifid uvulae, can be avoided by completely demucosalizing the medial faces of the right and left components of the uvula, and making an effort to meticulously repair both the anterior and posterior surfaces of the uvula. With these maneuvers, a greater raw surface area is available for healing; and, with a more formidable connection between the two uvular halves, fistulation is less likely to occur.

Type II fistulae within the soft palate, and type III fistulae at the junction of the hard and soft palates, are inherently

prevented with the double opposing Z-plasty. The double-opposing Z-plasty incisions do not directly overlap one another, and if one incision dehisces, a layer of tissue remains intact to prevent a through-and-through defect. Several strategies facilitate a tension-free repair and prevent type II soft palate or type III soft–hard palate junction fistulae, including: (1) the liberal use of bilateral relaxing incisions, potentially extending from the retromolar region of the mandible to the anterior hard palate, allowing for the adequate mobilization of the soft palate Furlow flaps as well as the hard palate mucoperiosteal flaps, (2) a complete dissection of the neurovascular bundle and potential osteotomy of the medial aspect of the greater palatine bony foramen, (3) performing a "complete IVVP"[78] by adequately releasing the levator palatini muscle from its abnormal attachments to the posterior edge of the hard palate, the aponeurosis of the tensor veli palatini, and the superior constrictor muscle (Figs. 33–26 and 33–27), allowing for the complete mobilization of the levator muscle from its abnormal anterior–posterior orientation to an anatomically correct horizontal orientation (Fig. 33–25), (4) a complete or "total release"[81] of the tensor veli palatini muscle tendon just medial to the hamulus[82] (Figs. 33–26 and 33–27), allowing for a total release and medialization of the Z-plasty flaps with radical retroposition of the levator palatini muscle, and (5) the use of ADM for complete nasal lining reconstruction, facilitating a two-layer, tension-free repair. The ADM, placed over the junction of the hard and soft palate, provides another barrier against fistula formation (Figs. 21–24).

Type IV fistulae of the hard palate can be prevented by placing ADM, on the hard palatal shelves and over the

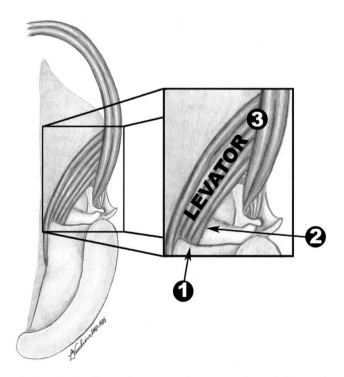

Figure 33–26. Three abnormal attachments of the cleft levator palatini muscle: (1) posterior edge of the hard palate, (2) aponeurosis of the tensor veli palatini, and (3) superior constrictor.

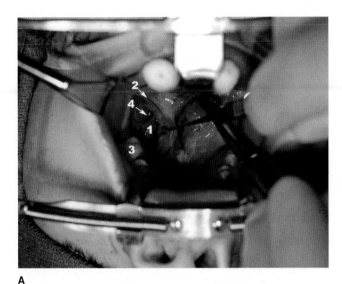 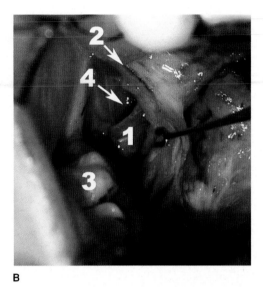

A **B**

Figure 33–27. Intraoperative dissection of the aponeurosis of the tensor veli palatini as it courses medially around the hamulus. The aponeurosis is divided to allow for a complete release of the levator muscle: (A) Operative field (1, tensor aponeurosis; 2, lateral incision; 3, molar; 4, space of Ernst). (B) Magnification of critical structures in (A).

hard palate nasal lining repair, again serving as an additional barrier against fistulae formation. In addition, the meticulously exaggerated eversion of the hard palate oral mucosa during the repair with horizontal mattress sutures is felt to assist in healing and prevent fistulae formation.

Palatal defects at the incisive canal or junction of the primary and secondary palates can be challenging to primarily repair and frequently result in type V fistulae. Type V fistulae in Veau IV bilateral clefts are exceedingly difficult to reconstruct secondary to their location and meager available tissue in the region. Multiple pedicle flaps (i.e., tongue flaps, facial artery myomucosal flaps),[30,31,51,83,84] and even free tissue transfer,[33–36,62] have been described to address this very difficult problem. Two techniques can be employed to minimize the occurrence of type V fistulae at the junction of the primary and secondary palates in Veau IV bilateral clefts. First, large palatal defects at the junction of the primary and secondary palates, secondary to the "fly away" premaxilla, can be corrected with the routine application of pre-surgical infant orthopedics in the form of naso-alveolar molding (NAM)[18,85] (Figs. 33–28 and 33–29). NAM anatomically repositions the premaxilla into the maxillary arch and facilitates a repair of the defect at the junction of the primary and secondary palates, preventing type V fistulae. In addition, if a secure reconstruction at this level is compromised, ADM may be draped over the hard palate, "tucked under," and sewn beneath the premaxillary mucosa and the gingiva of the alveolus to provide an additional soft tissue layer preventing fistulae formation.

The alveolar defects are unique in that their primary reconstruction remains highly controversial. Many believe these defects should be left patent, with resultant "intentional" type VI lingual–alveolar and type VII labial–alveolar fistulae. These intentional fistulae are left unrepaired until addressed with conventional secondary alveolar bone grafting prior to the eruption of the secondary cuspid. Alternatively, some hold

that primary closure of the alveolar clefts is appropriate. Closure of these defects and prevention of type VI and VII fistulae can be accomplished by employing NAM to align the infant's alveolar ridges, and facilitate a gingivoperiosteoplasty (GPP) or periosteal tunnel that will support bone growth.[51] Per Millard, the GPP, "gets the hole in the middle of everything closed earlier"[86] and subsequently avoids fistula formation and reduces the likelihood that secondary bone grafting will be required.[87]

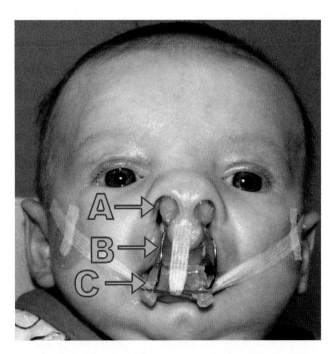

Figure 33–28. This photograph shows a nasoalveolar molding (NAM) splint in position. Note the nasal splint (A), the nasal armature (B), and the external portion of the alveolar splint (C).

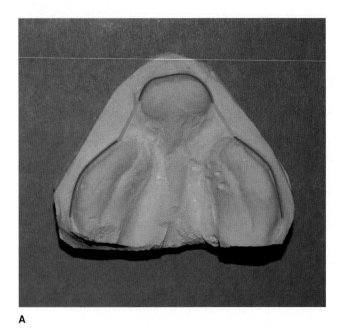

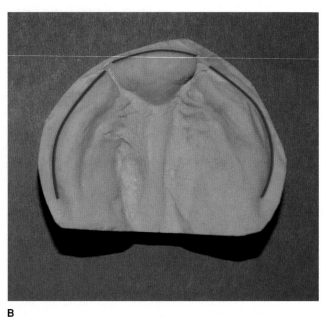

A

B

Figure 33–29. (A) A cast of a bilateral cleft alveolus. (B) The post-NAM result. Note the profile of the alveolar segments (blue) before and after NAM, with the distance to be bridged surgically indicated in red. The alveolus in B is clearly positioned for a more robust postoperative result than that in A.

Strategies common to the prevention of the full range of fistulae include the assurance of a tension-free and watertight closure at all levels of the repair, and a strict postoperative protocol employing arm restraints and allowing nothing in the mouth except a cup at the lips. Perhaps the most important strategy to prevent palatal fistulae is obsessive attention to detail.

The Pittsburgh Experience

Despite the myriad surgical approaches available, the best strategy in fistula management is avoidance. To validate the strategies for fistula prevention outlined above, we examined a large, single-surgeon, consecutive series of palatal proce-

dures (performed between 2002 and 2006) in which these strategies were implemented. Information recorded in our group's Cleft-Craniofacial Center database included Veau cleft type (Fig. 33–30), Pittsburgh Fistula type (Fig. 33–1), surgical technique, and outcomes: postoperative fistulae, Pittsburgh Weighted Speech Score (PWSS) (Table 33–1), and complications. No patients were excluded from this analysis, despite severity of cleft or complicating circumstances. This series represents consecutive palatal procedures performed by a single-surgeon as teaching cases with resident and fellow surgeons, with outcomes verified by a single surgeon and speech pathologist. As alveolar clefts were not consistently treated with gingivoperiosteoplasty during the entire study period, Pittsburgh Fistula type VI or lingual–alveolar fistulae,

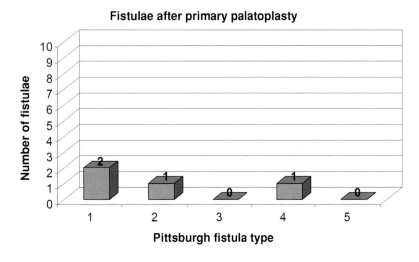

Figure 33–30. Pittsburgh fistula type following primary palatoplasty: type I = bifid uvulae, type II = soft palate, type IV = hard palate.

Table 33–1.

Pittsburgh Weighted Speech Score

Score	Interpretation
0	Competent
1–2	Borderline competent
3–6	Borderline incompetent
>7	Incompetent

as well as type VII or labial–alveolar fistulae, were not quantified in this study. Man-Whitney U tests were employed for statistical analyses of changes in PWSS with palatoplasty.

PATIENT DEMOGRAPHICS AND PROCEDURES PERFORMED

Two-hundred and thirty-nine palatal procedures (116 primary palatoplasties and 123 secondary palatal procedures) on 211 patients have been performed. 46.9% of the patients in this series were female and 53.1% were male. The average follow-up was 21.8 months (range 2.7–57.4 months). By Veau diagnosis (Fig. 33–31), the population consisted of 18.5% patients with submucous cleft palate (SMCP), 6.2% patients

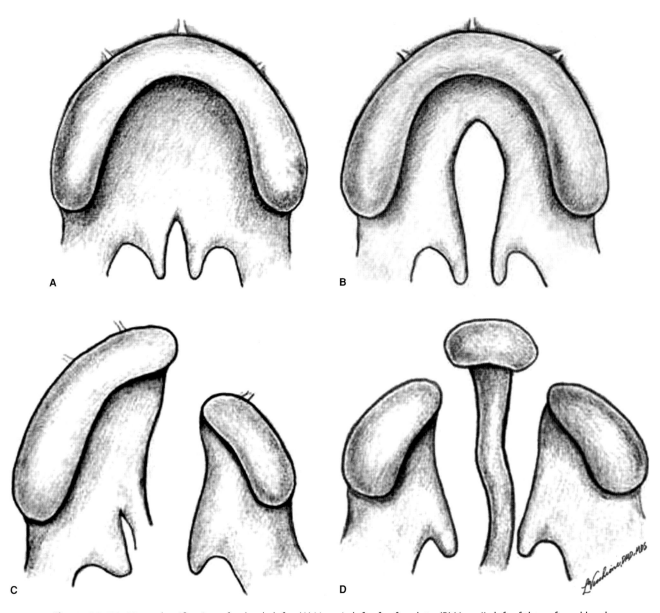

Figure 33–31. Veau classification of palatal clefts: (A) Veau I cleft of soft palate; (B) Veau II cleft of the soft and hard palates; (C) Veau III unilateral cleft; (D) Veau IV bilateral cleft.

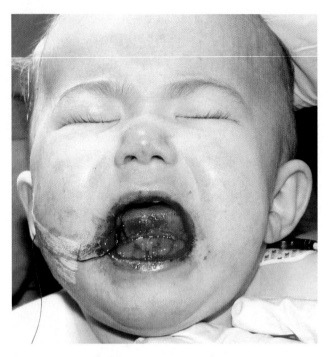

Figure 33–32. Postoperative lingual swelling can occlude the airway. Taping a "tongue stitch" to the cheek can help to emergently regain airway control and avoid re-intubation that might traumatize the palate repair.

Table 33–2.

Percent Primary Palatoplasties Incorporating Acellular Dermal Matrixes

Diagnosis	Percent with ADM
Veau I *soft palate*	0.0
Veau II *hard and soft palate*	65.0
Veau III *unilateral*	53.3
Veau IV *bilateral*	76.2
All primaries	39.7

with Veau 1 clefts of the soft palate, 22.3% patients with Veau 2 clefts of the hard and soft palate, 29.9% patients with Veau 3 clefts (unilateral cleft palate), and 22.3% patients with Veau 4 clefts (bilateral cleft palate). Palatal procedures were distributed as follows: 46.4% Furlow palatoplasties, 28.0% conversion Furlow palatoplasties (defined as secondary palatoplasties converting straight-line repairs to double opposing z-plasties), 21.8% fistula repairs, and 2.1% palatal adhesions. Patients undergoing a primary procedure for overt clefts of the palate were, on average, 1.6 years of age (range 0.6–11.5 years), and patients undergoing primary repair of SMCP were, on average, 5.2 years of age (range 2.4–18.2 years). Patients undergoing a secondary palatal procedure were, on average, 8.4 years of age (range 1.2–20.8 years). There were no mortalities in this cohort, and with the exception of postoperative fistulae, there were no major complications, such as infections or postoperative bleeding requiring a return to the operating room. One episode of postoperative tongue swelling occurred, and this resolved after re-intubation (Fig. 33–32).

Acellular Dermal Matrix (ADM)

Whenever a two-layer, water-tight, tension-free palatoplasty could not be achieved, we employed ADM. Occasionally in a Furlow palatoplasty, a defect in the nasal lining at the junction of the hard and soft palate is resistant to closure. In these instances, to achieve a complete repair of the nasal mucosa, an ultra-thin 6–12/1000th of an inch, 2×4 cm piece of ADM (AlloDerm, LifeCell, Branchburg, NJ) was sewn to the nasal lining in the region of the normal tensor aponeurosis. ADM

was employed in 39.7% of primary repairs: in no Veau 1 clefts of the soft palate, in 13 (65.0%) Veau II clefts of the soft and hard palate, in 16 (53.3%) Veau III unilateral clefts, and in 16 (76.2%) Veau IV bilateral clefts (Table 33–2). ADM was used in 48.0% of secondary cases: in 48 (94.1%) fistula repairs, 10 (14.9%) conversion Furlow palatoplasties, and a single (33.3%) Furlow palatoplasty in combination with a pharyngeal flap takedown (Table 33–3).

Fistulae after Primary Palatoplasty

Four of the 116 primary palatal procedures performed (3.5%) resulted in postoperative fistulae (Fig. 33–30). Two of these four fistulae were asymptomatic Pittsburgh type I fistulae or bifid uvulae. Two of the four fistulae in the primary palatoplasty cohort were symptomatic, resulting in a rate of symptomatic fistulae of 1.72%. One of the two symptomatic fistulae was a Pittsburgh type IV fistula of the hard palate (1×2 mm) that occurred after partial injury to a neurovascular

Table 33–3.

Percent Secondary Procedures Incorporating Acellular Dermal Matrixes

Procedure	Percent with ADM
Fistula repair	94.1
Conversion furlow palatoplasty	14.9
Furlow palatoplasty *with* pharyngeal flap take-down	33.3
All secondaries	48.0

Table 33–4.

Fistula Incidence in Primary Palatoplasty and Fistula Repair

		Pittsburgh Fistula Type						
		I	II	III	IV	V	Total	Occurrence Rate
Primary Palatoplasty	*Symptomatic*	0	1	0	1	0	2	1.72%
	Asymptomatic	2	0	0	0	0	2	1.72%
Fistula Repair	*Symptomatic*	0	0	0	0	2	2	3.9%
	Asymptomatic	0	0	0	0	4	4	7.8%

bundle during Furlow palatoplasty. The other symptomatic fistula was a Pittsburgh type II fistula of the soft palate (1 × 3 mm). This fistula occurred after a first-stage palatal adhesion without intravelar veloplasty (IVVP) in an older child adopted from Asia with a very wide Veau III unilateral cleft (Table 33–4).

Fistulae after Secondary Palatoplasty

Sixty-seven (93.1%) of the 72 secondary palatoplasties performed were conversion Furlow palatoplasties. Conversion Furlow palatoplasties were performed as secondary speech surgeries in children initially undergoing straight-line palatoplasty with incomplete IVVP and subsequent VPI. Second-stage Furlow palatoplasties following first-stage palatal adhesions and palatoplasties performed in conjunction with pharyngeal flap takedown comprised the remaining secondary palatoplasties in this cohort. No fistulae occurred after secondary palatoplasties (see Table 33–4).

Fistulae Recurring after Fistula Repair

Of the 51 fistulae repaired in this series, 6 (11.8%) recurred (Fig. 33–33). The recurrent fistulae were all Pittsburgh type V lesions, occurring at the junction of the primary and secondary palates in Veau IV bilateral clefts. These recurrent fistulae were found to occur in patients with large (1 cm or greater) fistulae just caudal to the primary palate at the incisive canal (Pittsburgh type V). Of these six recurrent fistulae, only two were symptomatic to yield a 3.9% rate of symptomatic recurrent fistulae (Table 33–4).

Speech after Primary Palatoplasty

Standardized PWSSs could not be accurately assessed for all patients in this cohort due to this study's relatively short follow up and young age of the patients receiving primary palatoplasties. Despite these limitations, 16 nonsyndromic patients have undergone standardized perceptual speech evaluation following primary palatoplasty and received PWSSs; the me-

dian value of these postoperative scores was 2 (range 0–9). It is significant that no recommendations for secondary speech surgery, at this point, have been made for any patients undergoing primary palatoplasty.

Speech after Secondary Palatoplasty

Secondary palatoplasty patients were mature enough to undergo standardized perceptual speech evaluation and could thus be assigned a formal PWSS. The PWSS is a validated tool for the assessment of velopharyngeal competence. It comprises five categories of perceptual speech symptoms: nasal emission, facial grimace, nasality, phonation, and articulation (Table 33–1).[88] While the individual components are qualitatively evaluated, the weighted, numerical composite score has prognostic value and provides a quantitative comparison between pre- and postoperative states.

Analysis of the PWSS for the 34 nonsyndromic patients undergoing conversion Furlow palatoplasties with pre- and postoperative speech data yielded a statistically significant improvement in speech with the procedure. The median preoperative PWSS was 11 (range 0–27) and the median postoperative PWSS was 1 (range 0–5) ($P < 0.01$ by Man-Whitney

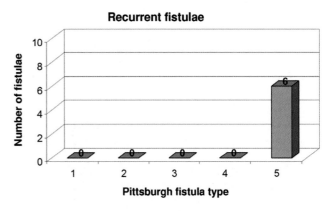

Figure 33–33. Recurrent Pittsburgh fistula type following fistula repair: type V = fistula at the junction of the primary and secondary palates or at the incisive foramen (in Veau IV clefts).

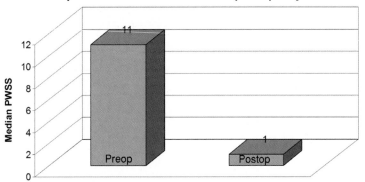

Speech with conversion Furlow palatoplasty

Figure 33–34. Pre- and postoperative Pittsburgh Weighted Speech Scores for secondary conversion Furlow palatoplasties.

U test) (Fig. 33–34). No recommendations for further speech surgery (posterior pharyngeal flap or sphincter pharyngoplasty) were made for any patients undergoing secondary Furlow palatoplasty for VPI.

We then performed a subanalysis of speech in secondary palatoplasties incorporating ADM. An improvement, although not statistically significant, was noted in PWSS for the 18 secondary palatal surgeries incorporating ADM in nonsyndromic patients with pre- and postoperative speech data. The median preoperative PWSS was 3 (range 0–27) and the median postoperative PWSS was 2 (range 0–5) (Fig. 33–35). No recommendations for secondary speech surgery were made for any patients undergoing secondary palatal procedures incorporating ADM.

CONCLUSION

Palatal fistulae are common, clinically significant, and difficult to definitively repair. Adoption of a standardized classification system will clarify the literature and advance the management of this lesion. While myriad techniques for the repair of these lesions have been developed, it is clear that prevention is the most efficacious management strategy for palatal fistulae. Key prevention strategies include (1) liberal use of relaxing incisions, (2) "complete" intravelar veloplasty,

(3) total release of the tensor tendon at the level of the hamulus, (4) complete dissection of the neurovascular bundle with optional osteotomy of the bony foramen, and (5) incorporation of ADM to achieve complete nasal lining reconstruction and adequate two-layer closure in difficult cleft repairs. In our experience, employing these strategies has resulted in the lowest incidence of postoperative symptomatic palatal fistula for primary palatoplasty seen in the literature.

References

1. Muzaffar AR, Byrd HS, Rohrich RJ, et al. Incidence of cleft palate fistula: an institutional experience with two-stage palatal repair. *Plast Reconstr Surg* 108:1515–1518, 2001.
2. Bardach J, Morris H, Olin W, McDermott-Murray J, Mooney M, Bardach E. Late results of multidisciplinary management of unilateral cleft lip and palate. *Ann Plast Surg* 12:235–242, 1984.
3. Maeda K, Ojimi H, Utsugi R, Ando S. A T-shaped musculomucosal buccal flap method for cleft palate surgery. *Plast Reconstr Surg* 79:888–896, 1987.
4. Senders CW, Sykes JM. Modifications of the Furlow palatoplasty (six- and seven-flap palatoplasties). *Arch Otolaryngol Head Neck Surg* 121:1101–1104, 1995.
5. Thaller SR. Staged repair of secondary cleft palate deformities. *J Craniofac Surg* 6:375–380; discussion 381, 1995.
6. Smith DM, Vecchione L, Jiang S, Ford MD, Deleyiannis FWB, Haralam MA, Naran S, Worrall CI, Dudas JR, Afifi AM, Marazita ML, Losee JE. The Pittsburgh fistula classification system: A standardized scheme for the description of palatal fistulas. *Cleft Palate Craniofac J* 44(6):590–594, 2007.
7. Emory RE, Jr., Clay RP, Bite U, Jackson IT. Fistula formation and repair after palatal closure: An institutional perspective. *Plast Reconstr Surg* 99:1535–1538, 1997.
8. Folk SN, D'Antonio LL, Hardesty RA. Secondary cleft deformities. *Clin Plast Surg* 24:599–611, 1997.
9. Witt PD, Marsh JL. Advances in assessing outcome of surgical repair of cleft lip and cleft palate. *Plast Reconstr Surg* 100:1907–1917, 1997.
10. Cohen SR, Kalinowski J, LaRossa D, Randall P. Cleft palate fistulas: A multivariate statistical analysis of prevalence, etiology, and surgical management. *Plast Reconstr Surg* 87:1041–1047, 1991.
11. Isberg A, Henningsson G. Influence of palatal fistulas on velopharyngeal movements: A cineradiographic study. *Plast Reconstr Surg* 79:525–530, 1987.
12. Schultz RC. Management and timing of cleft palate fistula repair. *Plast Reconstr Surg* 78:739–747, 1986.
13. Honnebier MB, Johnson DS, Parsa AA, Dorian A, Parsa FD. Closure of palatal fistula with a local mucoperiosteal flap lined with buccal mucosal graft. *Cleft Palate Craniofac J* 37:127–129, 2000.

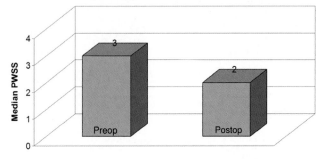

Speech with conversion Furlow palatoplasty incorporating acellular dermal matrix

Figure 33–35. Pre- and postoperative Pittsburgh Weighted Speech Scores for secondary conversion Furlow palatoplasties utilizing acellular dermal matrixes.

14. Moore MD, Lawrence WT, Ptak JJ, Trier WC. Complications of primary palatoplasty: A twenty-one-year review. *Cleft Palate J* 25:156–162, 1988.

15. Wilhelmi BJ, Appelt EA, Hill L, Blackwell SJ. Palatal fistulas: Rare with the two-flap palatoplasty repair. *Plast Reconstr Surg* 107:315–318, 2001.

16. Abyholm FE, Borchgrevink HH, Eskeland G. Palatal fistulae following cleft palate surgery. *Scand J Plast Reconstr Surg* 13:295–300, 1979.

17. Bardach J, Morris HL, Olin WH, et al. Results of multidisciplinary management of bilateral cleft lip and palate at the Iowa cleft palate center. *Plast Reconstr Surg* 89:419–432; discussion 433–415, 1992.

18. Kirschner RE, Cabiling DS, Slemp AE, Siddiqi F, LaRossa DD, Losee JE. Repair of oronasal fistulae with acellular dermal matrices. *Plast Reconstr Surg* 118:1431–1440, 2006.

19. Rintala AE. Surgical closure of palatal fistulae: Follow-up of 84 personally treated cases. *Scand J Plast Reconstr Surg* 14:235–238, 1980.

20. Amaratunga NA. Occurrence of oronasal fistulas in operated cleft palate patients. *J Oral Maxillofac Surg* 46:834–838, 1988.

21. Oneal RM. Oronasal fistulas. In Grabb WC, Rosenstein SW, Bzoch KR (eds). *Cleft Lip and Palate.* Boston: Little, Brown and Company, 1971, pp. 490–498.

22. Hayward JR. Occurence of oronasal fistulas in operated cleft palate patients: Discussion. *J Oral Maxillofac Surg* 46:838, 1988.

23. Fukuda M, Lino M, Takahashi T. Closure of large oronasal fistulas at the time of secondary bone grafting in patients with cleft lip and palate. *Scand J Plast Reconstr Surg Hand Surg* 37:339–343, 2003.

24. Rosenstein SW, Grasseschi M, Dado DV. A long-term retrospective outcome assessment of facial growth, secondary surgical need, and maxillary lateral incisor status in a surgical-orthodontic protocol for complete clefts. *Plast Reconstr Surg* 111:1–13; discussion 14–16, 2003.

25. Cosman B, Falk AS. Delayed hard palate repair and speech deficiencies: A cautionary report. *Cleft Palate J* 17:27–33, 1980.

26. Shimizu M, Shigetaka Y, Mizuki H, Okamoto A. Oronasal fistulae in repaired cleft palates. *J Craniomaxillofac Surg* 17(Suppl 1):37–38, 1989.

27. Obermeyer P. Early closure of suture dehiscence after uranoplasty by means of a conservative method. *Dtsch Stomatol* 17:168–173, 1967.

28. Berkman MD. Early non-surgical closure of postoperative palatal fistulae. *Plast Reconstr Surg* 62:537–541, 1978.

29. Millard DR. *Cleft Craft: The Evolution of its Surgery,* 1st edn. Boston: Little Brown, 1976.

30. Guerrero-Santos J, Altamirano JT. The use of lingual flaps in repair of fistulas of the hard palate. *Plast Reconstr Surg* 38:123–128, 1966.

31. Guerrero-Santos J, Fernandez JM. Further experience with tongue flap in cleft palate repair. *Cleft Palate J* 10:192–202, 1973.

32. Ohsumi N, Onizuka T, Ito Y. Use of a free conchal cartilage graft for closure of a palatal fistula: An experimental study and clinical application. *Plast Reconstr Surg* 91:433–440, 1993.

33. Batchelor AG, Palmer JH. A novel method of closing a palatal fistula: The free fascial flap. *Br J Plast Surg* 43:359–361, 1990.

34. Eufinger H, Machtens E. Microsurgical tissue transfer for rehabilitation of the patient with cleft lip and palate. *Cleft Palate Craniofac J* 39:560–567, 2002.

35. Krimmel M, Hoffmann J, Reinert S. Cleft palate fistula closure with a mucosal prelaminated lateral upper arm flap. *Plast Reconstr Surg* 116:1870–1872, 2005.

36. Ninkovic M, Hubli EH, Schwabegger A, Anderl H. Free flap closure of recurrent palatal fistula in the cleft lip and palate patient. *J Craniofac Surg* 8:491–495; discussion 496, 1997.

37. Denny AD, Amm CA. Surgical technique for the correction of post-palatoplasty fistulae of the hard palate. *Plast Reconstr Surg* 115:383–387, 2005.

38. Randall P, LaRossa D, Solomon M, Cohen M. Experience with the Furlow double-reversing Z-plasty for cleft palate repair. *Plast Reconstr Surg* 77:569–576, 1986.

39. Campbell DA. Fistulae in the hard palate following cleft palate surgery. *Br J Plast Surg* 15:377–384, 1962.

40. Henderson D. The palatal island flap in the closure of oro-antral fistulae. *Br J Oral Surg* 12:141–146, 1974.

41. Millard DR, Batstone JH, Heycock MH, Bensen JF. Ten years with the palatal island flap. *Plast Reconstr Surg* 46:540–547, 1970.

42. Stal S, Hollier L. Secondary deformities of the cleft lip nose and palate. In Mathes SJ (ed). *Plastic Surgery, Vol. IV.* Philadelphia: Elsevier, 2006.

43. Egyedi P. The bucket-handle flap for closing fistulae around the premaxilla. *J Maxillofac Surg* 4:212–214, 1976.

44. Rintala A. Labiobuccal mucosal island flap for closure of anterior palatal fistulae. Case report. *Scand J Plast Reconstr Surg* 13:480–482, 1979.

45. Jackson IT, Moreira-Gonzalez AA, Rogers A, Beal BJ. The buccal flap—A useful technique in cleft palate repair? *Cleft Palate Craniofac J* 41:144–151, 2004.

46. Licameli GR, Dolan R. Buccinator musculomucosal flap: Applications in intraoral reconstruction. *Arch Otolaryngol Head Neck Surg* 124:69–72, 1998.

47. Zhao Z, Li S, Yan Y, et al. New buccinator myomucosal island flap: Anatomic study and clinical application. *Plast Reconstr Surg* 104:55–64, 1999.

48. Bozola AR, Gasques JA, Carriquiry CE, Cardoso de Oliveira M. The buccinator musculomucosal flap: Anatomic study and clinical application. *Plast Reconstr Surg* 84:250–257, 1989.

49. Stofman GM. Facial artery musculomucosal flap. *Plast Reconstr Surg* 91:1170–1171, 1993.

50. Pribaz J, Stephens W, Crespo L, Gifford G. A new intraoral flap: Facial artery musculomucosal (FAMM) flap. *Plast Reconstr Surg* 90:421–429, 1992.

51. Ashtiani AK, Emami SA, Rasti M. Closure of complicated palatal fistula with facial artery musculomucosal flap. *Plast Reconstr Surg* 116:381–386; discussion 387–388, 2005.

52. Jackson IT. Use of tongue flaps to resurface lip defects and close palatal fistulae in children. *Plast Reconstr Surg* 49:537–541, 1972.

53. Pigott RW, Rieger FW, Moodie AF. Tongue flap repair of cleft palate fistulae. *Br J Plast Surg* 37:285–293, 1984.

54. Kruchinsky HV. A new tongue reduction method. *J Oral Maxillofac Surg* 48:756–757, 1990.

55. Steinhauser EW. Experience with dorsal tongue flaps for closure of defects of the hard palate. *J Oral Maxillofac Surg* 40:787–789, 1982.

56. Hanazawa Y, Itoh K, Mabashi T, Sato K. Closure of oroantral communications using a pedicled buccal fat pad graft. *J Oral Maxillofac Surg* 53:771–775; discussion 775–776, 1995.

57. Baumann A, Ewers R. Application of the buccal fat pad in oral reconstruction. *J Oral Maxillofac Surg* 58:389–392; discussion 392–383, 2000.

58. Samman N, Cheung LK, Tideman H. The buccal fat pad in oral reconstruction. *Int J Oral Maxillofac Surg* 22:2–6, 1993.

59. Contreras O, Gonzales M, Villalobos RA. The tongue and forehead flap in the closure of residual oronasal fistulae. *J Craniomaxillofac Surg* 17(Suppl 1):39–41, 1989.

60. Archibald S, Jackson S, Thoma A. Paranasal sinus and midfacial reconstruction. *Clin Plast Surg* 32:309–325, 2005.

61. Schwabegger AH, Hubli E, Rieger M, Gassner R, Schmidt A, Ninkovic M. Role of free-tissue transfer in the treatment of recalcitrant palatal fistulae among patients with cleft palates. *Plast Reconstr Surg* 113:1131–1139, 2004.

62. Chen HC, Ganos DL, Coessens BC, Kyutoku S, Noordhoff MS. Free forearm flap for closure of difficult oronasal fistulas in cleft palate patients. *Plast Reconstr Surg* 90:757–762, 1992.

63. MacLeod AM, Morrison WA, McCann JJ, Thistlethwaite S, Vanderkolk CA, Ryan AD. The free radial forearm flap with and without bone for closure of large palatal fistulae. *Br J Plast Surg* 40:391–395, 1987.

64. Takahashi N. Experimental study of lower eyelid reconstruction with autogenous ear cartilage and allogenic preserved sclera. *J Jap Plast Recont Surg* 10:110–126, 1990.

65. Vandeput JJ, Droogmans B, Tanner JC. Closure of palatal fistulas using a dermis-fat graft. *Plast Reconstr Surg* 95:1105–1107, 1995.

66. Lehman JA, Jr., Curtin P, Haas DG. Closure of anterior palate fistulae. *Cleft Palate J* 15:33–38, 1978.

67. Schultz RC. Cleft palate fistula repair. Improved results by the addition of bone. *J Craniomaxillofac Surg* 17(Suppl 1):34–36, 1989.

68. Kirschner RE, LaRossa D, Losee JE, Sidiqqi F, Slemp AE. *Repair of Oronasal Fistulae Using Acellular Dermal Matrices: Preclinical Study and Clinical Case Series.* Asheville, NC: American Cleft Palate-Craniofacial Association, 2003.

69. Reagan BJ, Madden MR, Huo J, Mathwich M, Staiano-Coico L. Analysis of cellular and decellular allogeneic dermal grafts for the treatment of full-thickness wounds in a porcine model. *J Trauma* 43:458–466, 1997.

70. Buinewicz B, Rosen B. Acellular cadaveric dermis (AlloDerm): A new alternative for abdominal hernia repair. *Ann Plast Surg* 52:188–194, 2004.

71. Chaplin JM, Costantino PD, Wolpoe ME, Bederson JB, Griffey ES, Zhang WX. Use of an acellular dermal allograft for dural replacement: An experimental study. *Neurosurgery* 45:320–327, 1999.

72. Fisher E, Frodel JL. Facial suspension with acellular human dermal allograft. *Arch Facial Plast Surg* 1:195–199, 1999.

73. Achauer BM, VanderKam VM, Celikoz B, Jacobson DG. Augmentation of facial soft-tissue defects with Alloderm dermal graft. *Ann Plast Surg* 41:503–507, 1998.

74. Cole P, Horn TW, Thaller S. The use of decellularized dermal grafting (AlloDerm) in persistent oro-nasal fistulas after tertiary cleft palate repair. *J Craniofac Surg* 17:636–641, 2006.

75. Steele MH, Seagle MB. Palatal fistula repair using acellular dermal matrix: The University of Florida experience. *Ann Plast Surg* 56:50–53; discussion 53, 2006.

76. Helling ER, Dev VR, Garza J, Barone C, Nelluri P, Wang PT. Low fistula rate in palatal clefts closed with the Furlow technique using decellularized dermis. *Plast Reconstr Surg* 117:2361–2365, 2006.

77. Smith DM, Vecchione L, Jiang S, et al. *Progress in Palatoplasty: Strategies to Eliminate Fistulae.* Broomfield, CO: American Cleft Palate-Craniofacial Association, 2007.

78. Noorchashm N, Dudas JR, Ford M, et al. Conversion Furlow palatoplasty: Salvage of speech after straight-line palatoplasty and "incomplete intravelar veloplasty". *Ann Plast Surg* 56:505–510, 2006.

79. Clark JM, Saffold SH, Israel JM. Decellularized dermal grafting in cleft palate repair. *Arch Facial Plast Surg* 5:40–44; discussion 45, 2003.

80. Baker SB, Kirschner R, Huang K, et al. Fistula formation with Furlow palatoplasty: Incidence and influence of variables on fistula formation in a series of 429 consecutive palatoplasties. *Plastic Surgery Forum* XXII, 1999.

81. Havlik R, Ranieri J, Young L, Coleman JJ. *"Total Release" Double-Opposing Z-Plasty in Palatal Closure in 180 Patients—An Evolution of the Palatal Repair Technique.* Baltimore, Maryland: American Association of Plastic Surgeons, 2003.

82. Dayan JH, Smith D, Oliker A, Haring J, Cutting CB. A virtual reality model of eustachian tube dilation and clinical implications for cleft palate repair. *Plast Reconstr Surg* 116:236–241, 2005.

83. Assuncao AG. The design of tongue flaps for the closure of palatal fistulas. *Plast Reconstr Surg* 91:806–810, 1993.

84. Coghlan K, O'Regan B, Carter J. Tongue flap repair of oro-nasal fistulae in cleft palate patients. A review of 20 patients. *J Craniomaxillofac Surg* 17:255–259, 1989.

85. Hayes H. *An Anthology of Plastic Surgery.* Rockville, MD: Aspen Publishers, 1986.

86. Millard DR, Latham R, Huifen X, Spiro S, Morovic C. Cleft lip and palate treated by presurgical orthopedics, gingivoperiosteoplasty, and lip adhesion (POPLA) compared with previous lip adhesion method: A preliminary study of serial dental casts. *Plast Reconstr Surg* 103:1630–1644, 1999.

87. Santiago PE, Grayson BH, Cutting CB, Gianoutsos MP, Brecht LE, Kwon SM. Reduced need for alveolar bone grafting by presurgical orthopedics and primary gingivoperiosteoplasty. *Cleft Palate Craniofac J* 35:77–80, 1998.

88. McWilliams BJ, Morris HL, Shelton RL. *Cleft Palate Speech*, 2nd edn. Philadelphia: BC Decker, 1990.

Cleft Palate Speech and Management of Velopharyngeal Dysfunction

34

Anatomy and Physiology
of the Velopharynx

David P. Kuehn, PhD • Jamie L. Perry, PhD

SURFACE STRUCTURE AND FUNCTION

The soft palate, also called the velum, and the pharyngeal walls form a three-dimensional valve to channel air and nutritional substances through the respiratory and alimentary tracts. The structure and function of the normal velopharyngeal mechanism is described in this chapter. Although the velopharynx is important in swallowing and may be involved in swallowing disorders in individuals with various disabilities, such as poststroke trauma,[1,2] individuals born with cleft palate rarely have significant difficulties in swallowing following surgical repair of the palate. In contrast, owing to grossly different velopharyngeal closure patterns for speech versus swallowing, speech difficulties may ensue even with surgical repair of the palate. The primary focus in this chapter is on the functioning of the velopharyngeal mechanism for speech purposes.

Orientation

The velopharyngeal mechanism is a muscular valve that extends from the posterior surface of the hard palate (HP) to the posterior pharyngeal wall.[3] Figure 34–1 depicts a lateral-view X-ray that demonstrates the normal velum partially elevated. It was obtained during the prolonged vowel portion of the word /maaa.../. The length, thickness, and shape of the normal velum are clearly shown. The double-headed arrow is in the center of the velopharyngeal orifice. The right arrowhead points to the velar eminence, which is the dorsal curvature that normally makes contact with the posterior pharyngeal wall during velopharyngeal closure. The left arrowhead points to the approximate location on the posterior pharyngeal wall where velar contact normally would occur. For further orientation, arrow A points to the anterior tubercle of the atlas (the first cervical vertebra), which is a major landmark that aids in identifying the approximate level of velopharyngeal

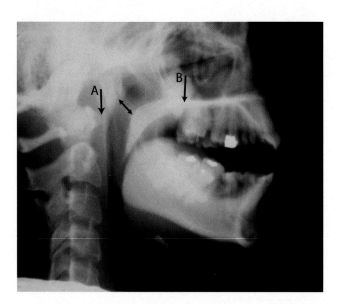

Figure 34–1. Lateral-view X-ray showing the normal soft palate (velum) partially elevated. Double-headed arrow is located in the middle of the velopharynx; right-side points to the velar eminence, left side to the posterior pharyngeal wall where velar contact would be made. Arrow A points to the anterior tubercle of the first cervical vertebra. Arrow B points to the posterior nasal spine at the junction between the hard and soft palate.

closure. Arrow B points to the posterior nasal spine, which is the posterior margin of the HP and which marks the boundary between the HP and the velum.

Velopharyngeal Closure Patterns

The overall function of the velopharyngeal mechanism is to provide separation between the oral and nasal cavities during speech and swallowing. Velopharyngeal closure is necessary during the normal production of oralized versus nasalized sounds. Only three sounds in the English language, /m,n,ng/, are normally produced with an open velopharyngeal port. At rest, the velum is suspended in the velopharynx with the tip of the velum, the uvula, pointed downward and the oral surface of the velum lying on the dorsum of the tongue. For the production of oralized sounds, such as the sound /s/, the velum is elevated and retracted to make complete contact against the posterior pharyngeal wall, an action which normally prevents the escape of air through the nasal passage. Pharyngeal wall movement also contributes to velopharyngeal closure. Lateral pharyngeal wall movement toward the midline and posterior movement of the velum create a sphincter-like closure pattern. Fig. 34–2 demonstrates the velopharyngeal closure sequence from a velar lowered position to a fully elevated position that would be observed looking down at the velopharyngeal port using nasopharyngoscopy.

Anterior movement of the posterior pharyngeal wall tends to be rather minimal in the normal mechanism. If it does contribute to velopharyngeal closure, typically in individuals with insufficient velar elevation and retraction, the anterior

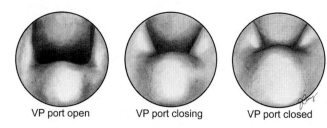

VP port open   VP port closing   VP port closed

Figure 34–2. Drawing showing the sphincteric nature of normal velopharyngeal closure (based on a similar drawing in Skolnick ML, McCall GN, Barnes M. The sphincteric mechanism of velopharyngeal closure. *Cleft Palate J* 10:286–305, 1973.). Left panel, open velopharyngeal port; middle panel, partially closed velopharyngeal port; right panel, fully closed velopharyngeal port.[47]

movement may consist of a prominent bulging forward of the posterior pharyngeal wall during closure attempts, referred to as Passavant's ridge.[4] Figure 34–3 shows an example of a patient with a repaired cleft palate who benefited from a Passavant's ridge. The velopharyngeal area is encompassed by the circle, and a Passavant's ridge can be seen bulging forward to make contact with the elevated and retracted velum.

Velopharyngeal closure may also be assisted by contact of the velum against an enlarged adenoid pad, typically found in children before adenoid involution has occurred. When adenoid involution occurs during adolescence, the velum normally adapts easily to the larger excursion that is required to achieve velopharyngeal closure. Occasionally, however, the velum may not have sufficient size or mobility to contact the adenoid pad as the adenoid tissue involutes. Figure 34–4 shows such an example in which there is a large gap between

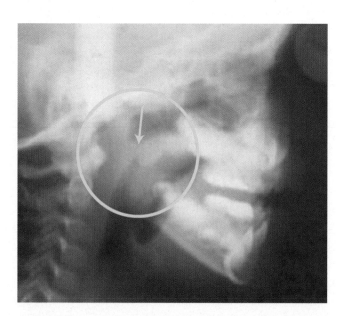

Figure 34–3. Lateral-view X-ray demonstrating velopharyngeal closure involving Passavant's ridge. Circle encloses the velopharyngeal area. Arrow points to the contact between Passavant's ridge at the left and the elevated nasal surface of the velum at the right.

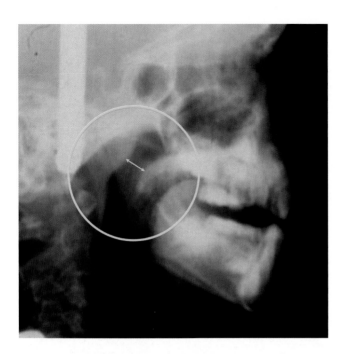

Figure 34–4. Lateral-view X-ray demonstrating lack of velopharyngeal closure between the elevated velum and the posterior pharyngeal wall. Circle encloses the velopharyngeal area. Adenoid pad along the posterior pharyngeal wall is at the left and the fully elevated velum is at the right. The abnormal velum is short and thin.

the elevated velum and the adenoid tissue, which is located along the posterior pharyngeal wall.

Several different velopharyngeal closure patterns have been identified in normal individuals and those with repaired cleft palate. The most common pattern observed in normal individuals is referred to as a "coronal" pattern because the major component of closure is the upward and backward movement of the velum, creating a coronal aperture that is eventually completely closed. Lateral pharyngeal wall movement also contributes to closure in the coronal pattern but it is a secondary component. Other closure patterns that have been reported are (1) coronal with marked medial movement of the lateral pharyngeal walls, (2) circular with equal contribution from the velum and lateral pharyngeal walls, (3) circular with Passavant's ridge, and (4) sagittal, in which lateral pharyngeal wall movement is the major component.[4]

Closure force of the velum against the posterior pharyngeal wall varies based on the type of speech sounds produced. Thus, closure force is greater for the "high" vowels /i,u/ than for the "low" vowels /a,ae/[5,6] and greater for "pressure" consonants (stops, fricatives, and affricates) such as /s,z,k,t/ than for vowels.[6] Kuehn and Moon[6] found no significant differences in the grouped closure force data in normal male subjects versus normal female subjects. However, the males exhibited a larger range and variability of closure force values, which is consistent with the reportedly more restricted range of upward velar movement by female subjects.[7,8]

Variability in velopharyngeal closure patterns observed in both male and female normal individuals cannot be accounted for solely by activity of the major muscle of velar elevation, the levator veli palatini. Other muscles likely contribute to positioning of the velum as well.[5,6,9,10]

DEEP STRUCTURE AND FUNCTION

Morphology of the Velum

The velum extends from the HP and terminates at the tip of the uvula. In normal adult males, the approximate average values for velar length, width, and thickness (at the thickest portion) are 40, 22, and 13 mm, respectively. The corresponding values for normal adult females are 37, 19, and 12 mm, respectively.[11,12] The components of the velum have been described in detail in several previous publications.[11–13] In general, the anterior two thirds of the velum is fairly consistent in its composition and organization, whereas the posterior one third is more variable.[13] This structural organization suggests that the more anterior portion of the velum is importantly related to functional requirements that are common to normal individuals, specifically, the need for fail–safe closure of the velopharyngeal port for biologic purposes. The posterior portion of the velum, including the uvula, can be more variable in composition and organization because that portion is not crucial for functional closure of the velopharyngeal port.

With regard to the components of the velum, the epithelium on the nasal side of the velum is mixed, with the more anterior portion consisting of respiratory-type pseudostratified ciliated columnar epithelium and the more posterior portion that contacts the posterior pharyngeal wall consisting of stratified squamous epithelium.[11] The oral epithelium is composed of stratified squamous epithelium and is somewhat thicker than that of the nasal side, presumably to withstand the more abrasive forces of food particles that are passed within the bolus during swallowing.[11]

The internal components in the anterior two thirds of the velum are characteristically layered. The most anterior–superior layer, just posterior to the border of the HP, consists of an aponeurosis with a prominent tendon, which winds around the hamulus and is an extension into the velum from the tensor veli palatini muscle. Also in the most anterior region and deep (i.e., inferior) to the tensor tendon is a large investment of mucous-secreting glandular tissue and pockets of adipose tissue with the latter typically displaced somewhat laterally from the midline. The most anterior portion of the normal velum contains little or no muscle tissue. Contrary to the description in many anatomy textbooks, muscle fibers do not attach to the posterior border of the HP in the normal velum.[13–15] This is an important functional aspect because any muscle fiber attachment to the HP would be counterproductive to the backward movement of the velum and would tend to inhibit stretching that normally occurs in the anterior region of the velum.[16,17] If muscle fibers are not satisfactorily dissected from the HP in the surgical repair of the cleft palate mechanism, such muscle attachment logically would tend to restrict upward and backward movement of the velum.

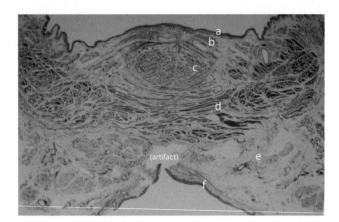

Figure 34–5. Histologic coronal section showing the layering of components within the middle portion of the velum: (a) nasal surface epithelium, (b) thin glandular layer, (c) paired musculus uvulae (MU) with a faint midline septum and the whole muscle encased within a connective tissue sheath, (d) levator veli palatini (LVP) muscle fibers intermingling and crossing the midline without an intervening septum, (e) thick layer of glandular and adipose tissue, and (f) oral surface epithelium. An artifact due to torn tissue in the oral region is indicated. *(Reprinted from Kuehn DP, Moon JB. Histologic study of intravelar structures in normal human adult specimens. Cleft Palate Craniofac J 42:481–489, 2005.)*

The middle portion of the velum contains the largest investment of muscle tissue. Figure 34–5 is a histologic coronal section of the middle part of the velum that demonstrates the layering of structures in that region. From the superior or nasal surface (at the top in the figure) to the inferior or oral surface, the following layers can be observed in sequence: (a) the relatively thin nasal epithelium, (b) a thin layer of glandular tissue, (c) the musculus uvulae (MU) with fibers cut in cross section and a faint midline septum, (d) the levator veli palatini (LVP) muscle with fibers crossing the midline and cut longitudinally in this region, (e) glandular and adipose tissue mixed (the tear in the midline is an artifact), and (f) the relatively thick oral epithelium.

In the posteroinferior regions of the velum and into the uvula proper, the layering becomes less distinct across individuals. The connective tissue capsule that typically encases the MU remains, although the muscle content of the capsule gradually diminishes and becomes sparse or totally void within the uvula.[13] The uvula proper contains a mixture of connective, glandular, adipose, and vascular tissue with little or no muscle tissue.[12]

Velopharyngeal Musculature

Levator Veli Palatini

The LVP muscle is the major muscle of velar elevation and retraction and is therefore the most important muscle of velopharyngeal closure in the normal mechanism.[18] The origin of the muscle is commonly reported to be the anterior petrous portion of the temporal bone at the base of the skull. According to Huang et al.,[19] the muscle also might have an attachment to the junction of the cartilaginous and bony parts of the auditory tube, also called the Eustachian tube. The mus-

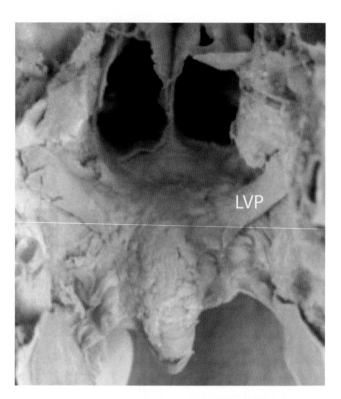

Figure 34–6. View looking down and forward on the dissected velum showing the normal sling arrangement of the levator veli palatini (LVP) muscle inserting into the middle portion of the velum from each side. Dark areas above the velum are the two nasal choanae with the nasal septum between. Uvula pointing downward. *(Dissection and figure courtesy of Jerald B. Moon, University of Iowa.)*

cle fibers course anteriorly, medially, and inferiorly along the undersurface of the Eustachian tube to insert into the middle 40% of the velum.[20] The bundles from each side course to the midline of the velum to join with each other. There is no septum or distinct separation between the two levator bundles in the midline.[13] Within the center of the velum, the fibers cross the midline and intermingle, as shown in Fig. 34–5. The paired muscle forms a muscular sling to suspend the velum from the cranial base. Figure 34–6 shows a dissection demonstrating the sling arrangement. Structures posterior to the velum and the mucosa have been removed. The viewpoint is from posterior, looking downward and forward at the nasal surface of the velum. The uvula is pointing straight downward. The levator sling can be seen entering the middle of the velum from both sides. The levator sling also can be appreciated by inspection of an oblique coronal magnetic resonance (MR) image, as that shown in Fig. 34–7. In this magnetic resonance imaging (MRI) section, which is in the same plane as the course of the levator muscle, the full extent of the levator muscle can be observed from its origin at the base of the skull on both sides to its termination in the velum. The dark area in the center of the image is the velopharyngeal airway with the velum in a lowered, relaxed position.

There is little variability in the size, shape, and location of the levator muscle amongst normal individuals. In cross section, the muscle belly has a flattened cylindrical appearance

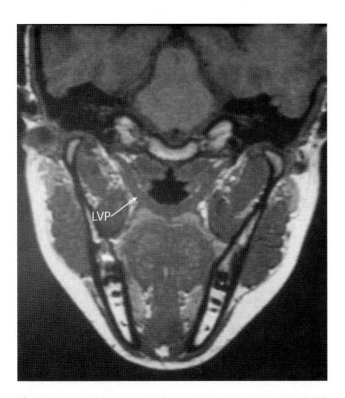

Figure 34–7. Oblique coronal magnetic resonance image (MRI) showing the levator veli palatini (LVP) muscle sling from its origin at the base of the skull to the insertion in the velum. Dark area in the center of the image is the velopharyngeal airway located just above the middle of the levator sling. *(Reprinted with permission from Ettema S, Kuehn D, Perlman A, Alperin N. Magnetic resonance imaging of the levator veli palatini muscle during speech. Cleft Palate Craniofac J 39:130–144, 2002.)*

and is nearly 1 cm in diameter in the normal adult.[15] Ettema et al.[21] used MRI to image and examine the dimensions of the levator muscle at rest and during speech. Measures included muscle length, thickness, and angle of origin. The average length, from the origin to the midline of the velum, for adult subjects was 44.7 mm for women and 45.8 mm for men. Average thickness measures, at the lateral margin of the velum, were 5.4 mm for both men and women. The average angle at the origin, between the base of the skull and the course of the muscle bundle during rest, was 64.5° for women and 60.4° for men. The angle of levator origin was found to decrease upon velar elevation, as expected, and levator length decreased by an average of 19% across all subjects, from a velar lowered position to a fully elevated position.

Although the tensor veli palatini muscle (see below) is thought to be the main Eustachian tube dilator, there still is controversy regarding the possible role of the levator in assisting in the opening of the tube.[22,23] In their study of 15 cadaver specimens, Huang et al.[19] noted that, as viewed from above, the levator crosses under the Eustachian tube anteriorly and could assist in opening the tube in that location by lifting and rotating the tube near its pharyngeal end. Because of its anatomic location, however, it is logical to assume that the levator does not open the Eustachian tube along the tube's entire length without assistance from the tensor veli palatini

muscle. If the levator were the sole dilator of the Eustachian tube, the tube would open at unwanted times, particularly during velar elevation for speech. A patent Eustachian tube during speech would allow airborne sound to travel directly to the middle ear cavities through the tube, which would be an unpleasant and undesirable activity.

Musculus Uvulae

The musculus uvulae, sometimes called the uvular muscle, is the only intrinsic velar muscle in that it is entirely contained within the velum. The muscle likely assists in velopharyngeal closure. Contrary to descriptions in many anatomy texts, probably perpetuated by the original description in Gray's anatomy, the muscle does not originate from the posterior nasal spine, but rather originates posterior to it and rather abruptly from the palatal aponeurosis at about 25% of the length of the velum.[11] As mentioned previously, and as confirmed in several studies, the most anterior region of the normal velum is devoid of muscle tissue, including that of the musculus uvulae. The muscle courses posteriorly from its origin along the midline of the velum near the nasal surface of the velum. It is in its most cohesive form in the area overlying, and cradled by, the levator sling (Fig. 34–8). The muscle becomes diffuse as it approaches the uvula, and there are few, if any, muscle fibers within the uvula proper.[13,15] Thus, the terms "uvulae" or "uvular" in association with this muscle

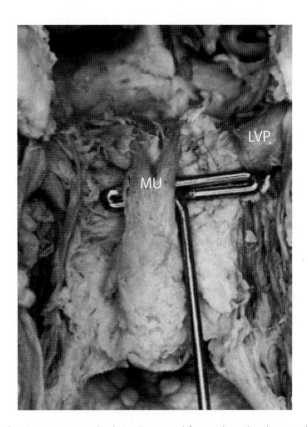

Figure 34–8. View looking down and forward on the dissected velum showing the musculus uvulae (MU) overlying the levator veli palatini (LVP) sling. T-probe separates the MU from the LVP. *(Reprinted with permission from Azzam NA, Kuehn DP. The morphology of musculus uvulae. Cleft Palate J 14:78–87, 1977.)*

are somewhat of a misnomer in that the muscle is more substantially and appropriately associated with the body of the velum rather than with the uvula.

The muscle has been described variously as a single muscle (thus the descriptor "azygos," which occasionally is used) and as a paired structure. The discrepancy is evident in comparing Figs. 34–5 and 34–8. Figure 34–8 clearly shows that, for this specimen, the muscle is paired, at least in its anterior region. On the other hand, the specimen shown in Fig. 34–5 is ambiguous with regard to the bilateral nature of the muscle. Kuehn and Moon[13] found that, in some of their normal adult specimens, the uvular muscle was clearly bilateral, as evidenced by a midline septum separating the two bundles, and in other specimens it was a single midline unpaired structure without any visible midline septum or separation. Interestingly, even in some individual specimens, the bilateral nature of the muscle was variable, i.e., singular versus paired, along the length of the velum. In functional terms, it seems to make little difference whether the muscle is single or paired because the fibers course longitudinally and are located in the midline. Thus, the force vector would be essentially the same, whether there is a single- or double-bellied muscle mass.

The uvular muscle fibers are encapsulated within a circular connective tissue sheath.[13] The capsule possibly provides greater stability and cohesiveness for the muscle along its length.[24] The capsule extends into the uvula, but the muscle fibers contained within the capsule diminish in quantity and cohesiveness such that the uvula proper is nearly devoid of muscle tissue.[11–13,15]

Kuehn et al.[24] described the functional significance of the musculus uvulae. From a structural point of view, the muscle adds bulk to the dorsal aspect of the velum, thereby helping to fill in the area between the velum and the posterior pharyngeal wall. Without such bulk, the dorsal region would be concave, rather than convex, leaving a central gap between the velum and posterior pharyngeal wall. Such a midline defect often is observed endoscopically (but not with lateral-view X-ray) in many individuals with repaired palatal clefts. This suggests that either there is a deficiency or lack of MU tissue in individuals born with cleft palate[25] or that the surgical repair in such individuals was unsatisfactory. In either case, complete velopharyngeal closure would not be achieved.

From a dynamic point of view, Kuehn et al.[24] proposed that the MU functions in a manner similar to that of the upper layer of a double-layered beam. As the upper layer (i.e., the MU) contracts, the beam (the velum) curls upward and arches posteriorly against the posterior pharyngeal wall. This action, in concert with the upward and backward pull by the levator muscle, facilitates a firm velopharyngeal seal, especially between the posterior half of the velum with the posterior pharyngeal wall.

Tensor Veli Palatini

The tensor veli palatini is a complicated muscle with several attachment sites.[26] The bulk of the muscle is located within the pterygoid fossa, between the medial and lateral pterygoid

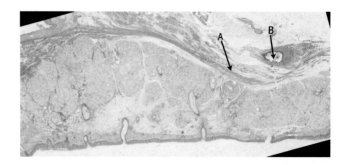

Figure 34–9. Coronal histologic section through the anterior region of the velum. Arrow A points to the tendon of the tensor veli palatini muscle. Arrow B points to a section through the hamulus. *(Reprinted with permission from Kuehn DP, Kahane JC. Histologic study of normal human adult soft palate. Cleft Palate J 27:26–34, 1990.)*

plates. The muscle courses medially and inferiorly between the pterygoid plates to end in a tendon that winds around the hamulus of the medial pterygoid plate. The tendon continues medially to form the palatal aponeurosis (Fig. 34–9). It is generally agreed that the tensor veli palatini is the primary muscle that functions to open the Eustachian tube. However, there has been much controversy and uncertainty about the details of its origin and insertion, whether it is a single-belly or a two-belly muscle, and whether it is capable of providing any force (i.e., tension) to the velum.

In their carefully controlled gross dissection and histologic study, Abe et al.[27] reported observing two adjacent origins, one from the cranial base and the other from the Eustachian tube cartilage. The cranial base origin was found to be anterior to the Eustachian tube origin in all of the specimens examined. Barsoumian et al.[26] also reported a two-belly configuration in their dissection study (Fig. 34–10). The more anterior portion of the muscle, which they referred to as the tensor veli palatini proper, was reported to be firmly attached to the hamulus. The more posterior portion of the muscle was found to originate from the Eustachian tube, and they referred to that portion of the muscle, as other authors have done, as the dilatator tubae. They suggested that the anterior portion, the tensor veli palatini, could help to provide a more stable anchoring mechanism and a stiffness gradient against which the more mobile portion, the dilatator tubae, might act to open the Eustachian tube.

As to the controversy of whether or not the tendon of the muscle is firmly attached to the hamulus, Barsoumian et al.[26] pointed out that confusion may arise if traction is placed on the more anterior portion versus the more posterior portion of the muscle. If the fibers in the anterior one third of the hamulus are pulled, this will not impart movement of the tendon around the hamulus because that portion of the muscle and tendon was found to be firmly attached to the hamulus. If the fibers in the middle one third of the hamulus are pulled, this would cause a lateral force on the velum because that portion of the muscle and tendon were found to be freely moveable around the hamulus, in agreement with the results of Abe et al.[27] Barsoumian et al.[26] further pointed

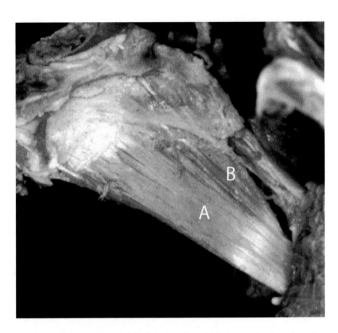

Figure 34–10. Extracted tensor veli palatini muscle showing the two-bellied arrangement of the muscle. A is the more anterior portion. B is the more posterior portion. *(Reprinted with permission from Barsoumain R, Kuehn DP, Moon JB, Canady JW. An anatomic study of the tensor veli palatini and dilator tubae muscles in relation to Eustachian tube and velar function. Cleft Palate Craniofac J 35:101–110, 1998.)*

out that a few fibers from the superior pharyngeal constrictor (SPC) muscle attach to the most posterior one third of the hamulus. These fibers might act as a curb to prevent the freely mobile portion of the tendon from slipping off the hamulus.

Although the tendon of the muscle might provide tension in the velum, as described above, it is questionable whether such tension might be useful in velopharyngeal function for speech. Any force imparted to the velum from the muscle must occur at the point of emergence into the velum from the hamulus, a point that is rather close to the posterior border of the HP and that would therefore not provide favorable leverage for either raising or lowering the bulk of the velum. By providing stiffness to the anterior portion of the velum, however, the muscle and its tendon would shift the effective pivot of the velum more posteriorly. This mechanism would logically decrease the compliance of the velum, which would aid in the rapidity of both raising and lowering movement of the velum. In addition, the tendon might act as a buffer to protect against abrasive forces during up and down movement which would otherwise occur at the abrupt boundary between the HP and the soft fleshy tissue of the velum.

There appears to be an intimate relation between the tensor veli palatini and the tensor tympani muscles both anatomically and functionally. Anatomically, the two muscles are connected to each other at a tendinous band located between them.[26,27] Therefore, it is likely that there is an interplay between the two muscles, which could be realized in adjustments for air pressure in the middle ear cavity. Opening the Eustachian tube serves to equalize air pressure across the

eardrum and, as is well known, the act of swallowing typically opens the Eustachian tube.[28] As a bolus of food passes through the oral cavity and pushes up on the velum, this could pull inward, i.e., toward the midline, on the mobile portion of the tensor tendon that is attached to the dilator portion of the tensor muscle. This activity would tend to stretch the muscle which, in turn, could activate the muscle spindles that are contained within the muscle (see later section regarding sensory innervation) causing muscle contraction via the stretch reflex mechanism. Such muscle contraction could thereby open the Eustachian tube. With regard to tensor tympani function, the muscle is attached to the malleus which, in turn, is attached to the inner aspect of the eardrum. As positive air pressure within the middle ear cavity is increased, as occurs at higher altitudes for example, the eardrum is distended outward, stretching the muscle spindles contained in the tensor tympani muscle and thereby causing the muscle to contract. Because the tensor tympani muscle is connected to the tensor veli palatini muscle, contraction of the tensor tympani muscle could, in turn, activate the muscle spindles within the tensor veli palatini, causing that muscle to contract, opening the Eustachian tube, and releasing the positive pressure in the middle ear cavity.

As mentioned previously, it is possible that the LVP muscle might assist in opening the Eustachian tube at its most medial segment during swallowing, but the tensor veli palatini muscle (specifically, the dilatator tubae portion) is directly attached to the more lateral portion of the tube and must provide the major force of opening the tube along most of its length.

Superior Pharyngeal Constrictor

The SPC muscle is a thin muscle that forms the upper lateral and posterior pharyngeal walls (Fig. 34–11). It is in a favorable position to produce inward movement of the lateral pharyngeal walls at the level of the HP.[29] The muscle has multiple sites of origin comprising distinct muscle bundles that are sometimes referred to as the pterygopharyngeus, buccopharyngeus, mylopharyngeus, and glossopharyngeus muscles. The muscle as a whole is fan-shaped, as clearly demonstrated in Fig. 34–11. The fibers from both sides diverge within the lateral pharyngeal walls and meet posteriorly in the midline to form the pharyngeal raphe (PR) along the posterior pharyngeal wall (Fig. 34–12). The fibers in the superior region attach directly to the velum, as is evident in Fig. 34–11. These fibers might aid in retraction of the velum,[30] and it is possible that they might contribute to the formation of Passavant's ridge (Fig. 34–3). These potential functions are difficult to confirm in a controlled experimental study, such as with electromyography (EMG), because of the thinness of the muscle, its overlap with other muscles, and its relative inaccessibility.

It is likely that the superior constrictor (SC) muscle contributes in a variable manner to velopharyngeal closure patterns (i.e., coronal versus circular, etc.), as described in an earlier section, especially for those individuals whose velar elevation is restricted. For normal individuals, velopharyngeal

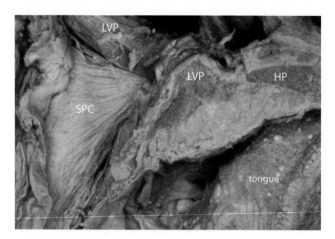

Figure 34–11. Lateral-view of the dissected velopharynx showing the superior pharyngeal constrictor (SPC) fanning out in the lateral pharyngeal wall. Midsagittal surface of the velum and posterior border of the hard palate (HP) are shown. Darker structure in the upper portion of the velum is the cut levator veli palatini (LVP) muscle sling; lighter structures in the lower half are the mixture of glandular and adipose tissue. The left levator bundle (LVP) is shown at the upper left of the figure. A portion of the tongue dorsum is shown at the lower right.

closure force patterns are very different for swallowing versus speech.[6] Maximum inward force tends to occur lower in the pharynx for swallowing than for speech, probably due to greater activity of the SC muscle for swallowing. Such greater contraction force at a lower level might be necessary to avoid nasal regurgitation of food and fluids.

Palatopharyngeus

The palatopharyngeus muscle typically is described as being contained within the posterior faucial pillar, thus consisting of vertically oriented muscle fibers. This description, however, is only partially complete because the muscle has a transverse component as well (Fig. 34–13). Cassell et al.[31] referred to the transverse fibers as the palatopharyngeus proper because the muscle fibers course posteriorly from the soft palate (the velum) and terminate along the lateral pharyngeal walls. In contrast, Cassell et al. referred to the vertically oriented fibers within the posterior faucial pillar as the palatothyroideus because those fibers continue downward along the lateral pharyngeal walls and terminate at the greater horns of the thyroid cartilage of the larynx.

Because of this complicated anatomic arrangement, it is likely that the muscle may perform different functions, depending on which portion of the muscle is contracting. Logically, the upper, transverse fibers would contribute to inward displacement of the lateral pharyngeal walls and perhaps contribute to the formation of a Passavant's ridge in a fashion similar to that of the fibers of the SPC muscle that attach to the velum. Although EMG studies of the upper pharynx have been conducted,[10] it is very difficult to separate the activity of the SC from that of the transverse fibers of the palatopharyngeus because of the overlap of the musculature and the

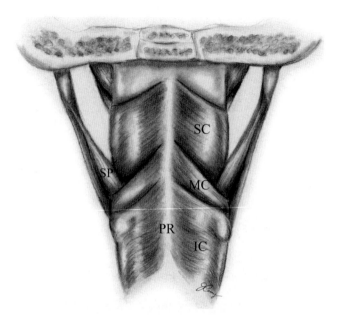

Figure 34–12. Drawing showing a posterior view of the posterior pharyngeal wall demonstrating the three pharyngeal constrictor muscles and the stylopharyngeus muscle gaining entrance into the lateral aspects of the pharynx on both sides between the superior and middle constrictor muscles. The light area above the superior constrictor muscle is the pharyngobasilar fascia that fills in the gap between the muscle and the base of the skull. SC: superior constrictor; MC: middle constrictor; IC: inferior constrictor; SP: stylopharyngeus; PR: pharyngeal raphe.

relative thinness of both muscles in that region. For practical purposes, however, it would seem to make little difference which muscle contracts to provide inward movement of the pharyngeal walls.

Given the containment of the vertical fibers of the palatopharyngeus in the posterior faucial pillars (PFP), it is much easier to examine that portion of the muscle using EMG. To examine the muscle, electrode wires are inserted into the midportion of the posterior pillar. Several EMG studies have been conducted in that fashion.[5,9,10,32] Results from these studies indicate that the vertical portion of the muscle works in concert with the LVP and the palatoglossus (PG) muscles for overall positioning of the velum. When studied apart from its interaction with other muscles, however, the palatopharyngeus demonstrates complex function. For some subjects and speech sounds, such as /a/, the vertical portion of the muscle might help to narrow the lateral pharyngeal walls and may therefore be related to velopharyngeal closure. For other speech sounds, such as /i/, it has been found to be negatively correlated with velopharyngeal closure.[5] When sphincter pharyngoplasty is performed for the management of velopharyngeal dysfunction, the muscle bundles contained within the PFP (i.e., the vertical portion of the palatopharyngeus) are rotated upward and backward to be surgically embedded in the posterior pharyngeal wall. There is some evidence that the transposed musculature is not "dynamic,"[33] that is, the transposed musculature does not actively contract during velopharyngeal closure, but rather is purely passive

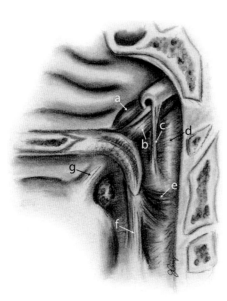

Figure 34–13. Drawing showing the velopharyngeal muscles: (a) tensor veli palatini; (b) levator veli palatini; (c) salpingopharyngeus; (d) superior pharyngeal constrictor; (e) transverse fibers of the palatopharyngeus; (f) vertical fibers of the palatopharyngeus; and (g) palatoglossus.

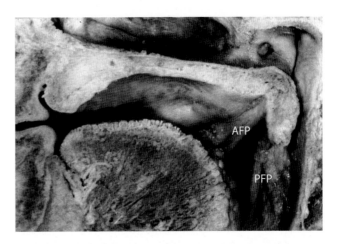

Figure 34–14. Lateral-view dissection showing the anterior (AFP) and posterior (PFP) faucial pillars. The bisected tongue is in the lower portion. The bisected velum is just above the faucial pillars. *(Reprinted with permission from Kuehn DP, Azzam NA. Anatomical characteristics of palatoglossus and the anterior faucial pillar. Cleft Palate J 15:349–359, 1978.)*

and is simply moved by other muscle activation. Further research is needed to confirm this finding. It is possible that the transposed musculature might need to be "trained" to perform a different role that is consistently related to velopharyngeal closure.

It is interesting to speculate about the possible role of the vertical fibers in relation to the singing voice, given that the fibers interconnect the velum and the larynx. It is possible that those fibers are importantly related to adjusting the timbre of the singing voice (Ingo Titze, personal communication).

Palatoglossus

The PG muscle courses from the lateral margins of the velum and extends through the anterior faucial pillar to insert into the lateral aspects of the tongue body (Fig. 34–14). It is anatomically positioned to assist in velar lowering, tongue elevation, and to constrict the faucial isthmus. In swallowing, all of these activities appear to be important in moving the bolus posteriorly and inferiorly toward the esophagus. PG activity for speech, however, is inconsistent across individuals and speech sounds.[5] With regard to velar lowering during speech, EMG studies have shown that the PG muscle is active for some, but not all, individuals, as reported by Kuehn and Azzam.[34] These authors explained this disparity by observing that the location of muscle attachment in the velum varies substantially across individuals. In some individuals, the muscle attaches quite posteriorly, which would be advantageous in velar lowering. In other individuals, the attachment is much more anterior, closer to the HP, which would be more advantageous in assisting tongue elevation and less so for velar lowering. Kuehn and Azzam[34] also observed, in histologic sections, a relatively large amount of elastic tissue along the

oral aspect of the anterior faucial pillar, which could aid in velar lowering as well as helping to keep the velopharyngeal port open during sleep. Gravity also would assist velar lowering in the upright posture. The PG muscle is rather small and not very compact. Figure 34-15 shows a histologic cross section through the anterior faucial pillar and demonstrates the sparse and diffuse nature of the PG muscle within the pillar.

Salpingopharyngeus

The salpingopharyngeus muscle is a small muscle that attaches to the posterior–inferior aspect of the pharyngeal end of the Eustachian tube.[19] It attaches to the inferior border of the torus tubarius in the velopharynx (Figs. 34–8 and 34–13). The muscle fibers course downward through the

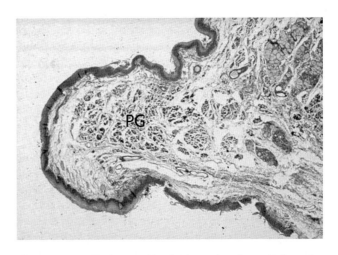

Figure 34–15. Transverse histologic section through the anterior faucial pillar showing the diffusely arranged palatoglossus (PG) muscle fibers cut in cross section. Glandular tissue can be seen on the right side.

salpingopharyngeal fold. In some individuals, this fold may consist primarily of glandular and connective tissue, being devoid of any muscle fibers.[14] The presence and size of this muscle has been reported to be variable across individuals.[35] During contraction, the salpingopharyngeus muscle may function to pull the lateral walls of the pharynx superiorly, which could assist in the downward transport of the bolus during swallowing. The functional significance of that activity for speech, however, is questionable.

INNERVATION

Motor Innervation

It is commonly agreed that the tensor veli palatini muscle is innervated by the motor root of the mandibular branch of the trigeminal nerve (cranial nerve V). It is also generally agreed that all of the other velopharyngeal muscles are innervated through the pharyngeal plexus of nerves.[36] However, there are three points of uncertainty in the literature regarding the innervation of the muscles: (1) which of the cranial nerves that make up the pharyngeal plexus actually contribute to innervation of the velopharyngeal muscles, (2) whether there is a second source of innervation (i.e., the facial nerve [cranial nerve VII], via the lesser palatine branch) to the LVP muscle and other velopharyngeal muscles, and (3) whether the facial nerve, via the lesser palatine branch, is the sole source of innervation to the musculus uvulae. Shimokawa et al.[37] shed light on the latter two issues in their carefully controlled dissection and histologic study. They observed that the levator muscle is doubly innervated through the pharyngeal plexus and also receives innervation through the lesser palatine nerve, a strand of which also innervates the palatopharyngeus and the musculus uvulae. The authors did not rule out a double innervation of the MU through the pharyngeal plexus, although they did not observe fibers from that source entering the muscle. They also pointed out uncertainty about the derivation of the lesser palatine nerve in terms of whether it actually arises from the facial motor nucleus in the brainstem.

In an early study involving rhesus monkeys, Nishio et al.[38] demonstrated that the levator, uvular, and SPC muscles are innervated by cranial nerves VII, IX, and X but not cranial nerve XI. Thus, two of the cranial nerves (IX and X) that supply the pharyngeal plexus are involved in motor innervation, but the third cranial nerve (XI) that supplies the plexus was not involved. Further research involving human subjects is needed to substantiate the results of Nishio et al.[38]

Studies in humans also are needed to determine whether there may be different neural control patterns for speech versus nonspeech activities such as swallowing. Judging from different movement patterns for speech versus nonspeech that have been well documented, it is likely that the neural control is quite different also. For example, it is possible that, given the double innervation of the levator muscle, finer control that is necessary for speech versus swallowing might benefit from innervation by an additional source, i.e., a branch from the facial nerve.

Sensory Innervation

With regard to sensory innervation, nerve supply to the palatal and pharyngeal mucosa is generally derived from branches of cranial nerves V, VII, IX, and X.[36] It has been reported that the density of cutaneous sensory innervation decreases from the anterior to the posterior oropharyngeal cavity.[39,40] Muscle spindles have been found in the tensor veli palatini and PG muscles by several investigators[41] and in the LVP muscle by Liss.[42] Although the other velopharyngeal muscles, i.e., the musculus uvulae, SPC, palatopharyngeus, and salpingopharyngeus, have been examined for the presence of spindles, they have not yet been found in these muscles.[41] Little information is available about the functional significance of muscle spindles in the velopharynx or the possibility that other sensory receptors, such as Golgi tendon organs, might be present. Much more basic research is needed in these areas.

CONCLUSION

The velopharyngeal port is normally open maximally during rest breathing to enable unencumbered flow of air through the nasal passages. During swallowing, it is important that tight velopharyngeal closure be achieved to prevent nasal regurgitation of food and fluids. For speech purposes, the velopharyngeal mechanism often is considered as functioning basically in a binary controlled fashion, i.e., open for nasal sounds and closed for nonnasal sounds. However, in practice, the mechanism is far more complicated than a simple binary system. On one hand, there are anatomic and physiologic constraints that limit the variability of control. For example, because the velopharynx must obey inertial laws of physics, the velum cannot elevate and lower instantaneously. Timing factors are therefore critical with respect to when the velum begins to lower in anticipation of nasal sounds and when it begins to elevate in relation to nonnasal sounds.[43] Given additional anatomic constraints for an individual born with cleft palate, such as those imposed by scar tissue or compromised musculature following cleft palate surgical repair, the timing of velar movements in relation to other articulatory activity might be adversely affected, leading to velopharyngeal dysfunction.[44]

Apart from anatomic and physiologic constraints, speakers do have latitude to vary velopharyngeal activity in relation to their own particular language, dialect, and grammatical requirements, and possibly to individual habit patterns. For example, the French language possesses phonemically nasalized vowels, but the English language does not. Some dialects may be characteristically more nasal than others. Speakers can and do vary nasality across different grammatical boundaries, such as phrase, clause, or sentence.[45]

Much remains to be learned about constraints that limit velopharyngeal control on the one hand versus physical and behavioral mechanisms that facilitate variability of expression on the other hand. The continued development of sophisticated imaging techniques, such as dynamic MRI,[46] will be valuable in obtaining basic information regarding how the normal mechanism functions. By knowing more about basic mechanisms of control, such information potentially could be applied to treat individuals with abnormal or compromised velopharyngeal mechanisms.

References

1. Perlman AL, Schulze-Delrieu K (eds). *Deglutition and its Disorders.* San Diego: Singular Publishing Group, 1997.
2. Logemann JA. *Evaluation and Treatment of Swallowing Disorders,* 2nd ed. Austin, TX: Pro-Ed, 1998.
3. Moon JB, Kuehn DP . Anatomy and physiology of normal and disordered velopharyngeal function for speech. In Bzoch KR (ed). *Communicative Disorders Related to Cleft Lip and Palate,* 5th ed. Austin, TX: Pro-Ed, 2004, pp. 67–98.
4. Finkelstein Y, Lerner MA, Ophir D, Nachmani A, Hauben DJ, Zohar Y. Nasopharyngeal profile and velopharyngeal valve mechanism. *Plast Reconstr Surg* 92:603–614, 1993.
5. Moon J, Smith A, Folkins J, Lemke J, Gartlan M. Coordination of velopharyngeal muscle activity during positioning of the soft palate. *Cleft Palate Craniofac J* 31:45–55, 1994.
6. Kuehn DP, Moon JB. Velopharyngeal closure force and levator veli palatini activation levels in varying phonetic contexts. *J Speech Lang Hear Res* 41:51–62, 1998.
7. McKerns D, Bzoch KR. Variations in velopharyngeal valving: The factor of sex. *Cleft Palate J* 7:652–662, 1970.
8. Kuehn DP. A cineradiographic investigation of velar movement variables in two normals. *Cleft Palate J* 13:88–103, 1976.
9. Seaver E, Kuehn D. A cineradiographic and electromyographic investigation of velar positioning in nonnasal speech. *Cleft Palate J* 17:216–226, 1980.
10. Kuehn DP, Folkins JW, Linville RN. An electromygraphic study of the musculus uvulae. *Cleft Palate J* 25:348–355, 1988.
11. Kuehn DP, Kahane JC. Histologic study of normal human adult soft palate. *Cleft Palate J* 27:26–34, 1990.
12. Ettema SL, Kuehn DP. A quantitative histologic study of the normal human adult soft palate. *J Speech Hear Res* 37:303–313, 1994.
13. Kuehn DP, Moon JB. Histologic study of intravelar structures in normal human adult specimens. *Cleft Palate Craniofac J* 42:481–489, 2005.
14. Dickson DR. Anatomy of the normal velopharyngeal mechanism. *Clin Plast Surg* 2:235–247, 1975.
15. Azzam NA, Kuehn DP. The morphology of musculus uvulae. *Cleft Palate J* 14:78–87, 1977.
16. Pruzansky S, Mason R. The stretch factor in soft palate function. *J Dent Res* 48: 972, 1969.
17. Simpson RK, Austin AA. A cephalometric investigation of velar stretch. *Cleft Palate J* 9:341–351,1972.
18. Huang MH, Lee ST, Rajendran K. Anatomic basis of cleft palate and velopharyngeal surgery: Implications from a fresh cadaveric study. *Plast Reconstr Surg* 101:613–627, 1998.
19. Huang MH, Lee ST, Rajendran K. A fresh cadaveric study of the paratubal muscles: Implications for Eustachian tube function in cleft palate. *Plast Reconstr Surg* 100:833–842, 1997.
20. Boorman JG, Sommerlad BC. Levator palati and palatal dimples: Their anatomy, relationship and clinical significance. *Br J Plast Surg* 38:326–332, 1985.
21. Ettema S, Kuehn D, Perlman A, Alperin N. Magnetic resonance imaging of the levator veli palatini muscle during speech. *Cleft Palate Craniofac J* 39:130–144, 2002.
22. Dayan JH, Smith D, Oliker A, Haring JM, Cutting CB. A virtual reality model of Eustachian tube dilation and clinical implications for cleft palate repair. *Plast Reconstr Surg* 116:236–241, 2005.
23. Kuehn DP, Moller KT. Speech and language issues in the cleft palate population: The state-of-the-art. *Cleft Palate Craniofac J* 37:348/1–35, 2000.
24. Kuehn DP, Folkins JW, Cutting CB. Relationships between muscle activity and velar positioning. *Cleft Palate J* 19:25–35, 1982.
25. Kuehn DP, Ettema SL, Goldwasser MS, Barkmeier JC, Wachtel JM. Magnetic resonance imaging in the evaluation of occult submucous cleft palate. *Cleft Palate Craniofac J* 38:421–431, 2001.
26. Barsoumain R, Kuehn DP, Moon JB, Canady JW. An anatomic study of the tensor veli palatini and dilator tubae muscles in relation to Eustachian tube and velar function. *Cleft Palate Craniofac J* 35:101–110, 1998.
27. Abe M, Murakami G, Noguchi M, Kitamura S, Shimada K, Kohama GI. Variations in the tensor veli palatini muscle with special reference to its origin and insertion. *Cleft Palate Craniofac J* 41:474–484, 2004.
28. Leider J, Hamlet S, Schwan S. The effect of swallowing bolus and head position on eustachian tube function via sonotubometry. *Otolaryngol Head Neck Surg* 109:66–70,1993.
29. Iglesias A, Kuehn DP, Morris HL. Simultaneous assessment of pharyngeal wall and velar displacement for selected speech sounds. *J Speech Hear Res* 23: 429–446, 1980.
30. Kuehn DP. Velopharyngeal anatomy and physiology. *Ear Nose Throat J* 58:316–321, 1979.
31. Cassell MD, Moon JB, Elkadi H. Anatomy and physiology of the velopharynx. *Multidisciplinary management of cleft lip and palate.* Philadelphia: Saunders, 1990.
32. Fritzell B. The velopharyngeal muscles in speech. *Acta Otolaryngol* 250(Suppl):1–81, 1969.
33. Ysunza A, Pamplona C, Molina F, Chacon E, Collado M. Velopharyngeal motion after sphincter pharyngoplasty: A videonasopharyngoscopic and electromyographic study. *Plast Reconstr Surg* 104:905–910,1999.
34. Kuehn DP, Azzam NA. Anatomical characteristics of palatoglossus and the anterior faucial pillar. *Cleft Palate J* 15:349–359, 1978.
35. Dickson DR, Dickson WM. Velopharyngeal anatomy. *J Speech Hear Res* 15:372–381, 1972.
36. Kennedy JG, Kuehn DP. Neuroanatomy of speech. In Kuehn DP, Lemme ML, Baumgartner JM (eds). *Neural Bases of Speech, Hearing, and Language.* Boston: Little, Brown, 1989.
37. Shimokawa T, Yi S, Tanaka S. Nerve supply to the soft palate muscles with special reference to the distribution of the lesser palatine nerve. *Cleft Palate Craniofac J* 42:495–500, 2005.
38. Nishio J, Matsuya T, Machida J, Miyazaki T. The motor supply of the velopharyngeal muscles. *Cleft Palate J* 13:20–30, 1976.
39. Grossman R, Hattis B. Oral mucosal sensory innervation and sensory experience. In Bosma J (ed). *First Symposium on Oral Sensation and Perception.* Springfield, IL: Charles C Thomas, 1964.
40. Kanagasuntheram R, Wong W, Chan H. Some observations on the innervation of the human nasopharynx. *J Anat* 104:361–376, 1969.
41. Kuehn DP, Templeton PJ, Maynard JA. Muscle spindles in the velopharyngeal musculature of humans. *J Speech Hear Res* 33:488–493, 1990.
42. Liss JM. Muscle spindles in the human levator veli palatini and palatoglossus muscles. *J Speech Hear Res* 33:736–746, 1990.
43. Moll KL, Daniloff RG. Investigation of the timing of velar movements during speech. *J Acoust Soc Am* 50:678–684, 1971.
44. Ha S, Sim H, Zhi M, Kuehn DP. An acoustic study of the temporal characteristics of nasalization in children with and without cleft palate. *Cleft Palate Craniofac J* 41: 535–543, 2004.
45. MacClean M. Forward coarticulation of velar movement at marked junctural boundaries. *J Speech Hear Res* 16:286–296, 1973.
46. Sutton BP, Bedoya D, Tsao J, Shinagawa H, Kuehn DP. Dynamic imaging of muscle during speech using interleaved spiral FLASH. Paper presented at the *Annual Meeting of* the *International Society for Magnetic Resonance in Medicine,* Seattle, WA, 2006.
47. Skolnick ML, McCall GN, Barnes M. The sphincteric mechanism of velopharyngeal closure. *Cleft Palate J* 10:286–305, 1973.

35

Communication Disorders Associated with Cleft Palate

Linda L. D'Antonio, PhD • Nancy J. Scherer, PhD

INTRODUCTION

Communication

The ability to communicate using speech is a distinctly human characteristic. It is, in fact, what makes us "human" and differentiates us from other species. Communication is a basic human right. It is well known that the presence of a cleft lip and palate or isolated cleft palate may negatively impact a child's ability to communicate effectively and therefore cause significant social, emotional, and educational hardship. Thus, the evaluation and management of communication disorders associated with cleft palate is a critical aspect of comprehensive cleft care.

It is also accepted that children with cleft palate are optimally cared for by an interdisciplinary team of experts working together.[1] Although no single team member can have sufficient breadth and depth of experience across the various disciplines to provide comprehensive cleft care, it is important nevertheless that team members understand and appreciate the contributions of other disciplines and have an adequate appreciation of the subject matter of related disciplines. When this is accomplished, cleft care is ideally transdisciplinary, rather than interdisciplinary or multidisciplinary.[2]

This chapter was therefore developed with the many specialists in mind and not exclusively nor principally for the speech-language pathologist. This chapter emphasizes information about the various aspects of communication that can be affected by clefting in order to facilitate a more complete understanding and exchange between disciplines. The literature and our clinical experience suggest that nonsyndromic cleft lip without cleft palate is not often likely to be associated with significant communication impairment.[3,4] Therefore, for purposes of this chapter, the discussion of communication disorders will focus on children with cleft lip and palate or isolated cleft palate.

When we think of communication disorders associated with cleft palate, we immediately think of speech production abnormalities, especially articulation and resonance. However, it is essential that we understand that communication is made up of several components including hearing, receptive language, expressive language, speech, resonance, voice, and the social use of language most commonly referred to as "pragmatic skills." All these components can be affected by the presence of a cleft. Additionally, a cleft lip and/or palate can also be associated with abnormalities in any one or combination of these communication areas. All these features of communication are mediated by overall cognitive status and a variety of psychosocial variables.

Heterogeneity

A review of the seminal texts and chapters discussing communication impairments associated with cleft lip and palate reveals many areas of agreement and disagreement. It is important to understand when we discuss communication skills in individuals with cleft lip and/or cleft palate this is an expansive topic area. As pointed out by Shprintzen,[5] it is likely that some of the apparent lack of consensus in the literature comes from the fact that this is a very heterogeneous population with one feature in common: the presence of a cleft lip and/or cleft palate. In many cases, the cleft may be an isolated abnormality, or it may be one feature of a multiple malformation syndrome. And so, any discussion of communication disorders associated with cleft lip and/or cleft palate may necessarily be misleading because of generalities. Furthermore, the cleft may be at the source of the communication differences, or it may be associated with a larger constellation of differences of which the cleft is but one feature. As listed in Table 35–1, individuals with cleft lip and palate or isolated cleft palate may present with a number of variables which are known to impact communication.

With respect to discussions of communication, it is of particular importance to differentiate between cleft types. As Shprintzen[5] notes, "Even more fundamental than diagnosing syndromes, clinicians should be aware that clefts of the palate, unilateral clefts of the lip and palate, and bilateral clefts of the lip and palate are not equivalent." The communication disorders associated with each of these cleft types can vary. In summary, there are many variables that impact the presence, type, and severity of communication disorders in individuals with cleft lip and/or cleft palate. In this chapter, we will focus on the communication impairments associated with nonsyndromic cleft palate with or without cleft lip.

Table 35–1.

Variables That May Impact Communication in Individuals with Cleft Lip and/or Palate Thus Contributing to the Heterogeneity of the Population

- Cleft type/severity
- Associated syndromes or other associated conditions
- Age at the time of palate repair
- Efficacy of the palate repair
- Unrepaired residual cleft
- Presence of a palatal fistula
- Status of velopharyngeal function
- Hearing status over time
- Timing, amount and efficacy of communication interventions
- Socioeconomic/linguistic status of the family

A Developmental Perspective

It is well accepted that cleft care is provided over a longitudinal period from birth through late adolescence and that the timing of many dental and surgical protocols are overlaid on physical growth and development. So too should cleft providers be familiar with the developmental course of speech and language. An awareness of the developmental course of normal speech and language and of communication disorders associated with cleft palate adds important information for clinicians as they make treatment plans over the long-term course of cleft care. In this chapter, we will discuss the various components of communication across the developmental continuum. For this purpose, we will divide our discussion of communication into four developmental phases:

- infant (birth to 12 months)
- toddler (12 months to 3 years)
- preschool (3 years to 5 years)
- school age and later

These categorizations correspond with phases of linguistic development that have been utilized widely in the language and developmental literature. They characterize language development in stages that are sequential and distinct from one another. There are two primary phases of communication development. The first is the *prelinguistic* phase, characterized by babbling and gestural communication. The second phase is the *linguistic* phase, characterized by the onset of true words and the development of spoken language. Such a developmental categorization across the different domains of communication is useful for identification of the aspects of communication that are emerging or of particular importance at a given age and therefore at a given time in the sequence of various forms of physical management. Such a developmental framework is also useful for considerations regarding the types of assessment protocols for evaluation of communication impairments since tests of speech and language development are routinely developed along these lines.

The Relationship between Speech and Language

As pointed out earlier, discussions of the communication characteristics of individuals with cleft palate often focus on speech and velopharyngeal function. It is easy to understand this focus. However, the velopharynx is only one part of a very complex interrelated series of valves that form the human vocal tract. Therefore, even a simple speech screening should take into consideration the structures and processes of the entire vocal tract. Furthermore, speech production and resonance are but one small portion of a larger developmental and communication process. Children with cleft palate, as all children, progress through a sequence or hierarchy of stages that are not necessarily linked to chronological age for many children with congenital anomalies. Speech and language are inextricably linked, especially during early development. This linkage is particularly complex in children with cleft palate who have limitations on oral structure during critical stages of speech and language development. For example, many children with clefts have physical limitations that result in restrictions of early sound systems which can in turn lead directly to reduced early word acquisition.

HEARING

It is well known that middle ear disease and hearing loss are common in children with cleft palate and with many of the syndromes associated with clefting.[6] The topic of hearing and audiologic concerns associated with cleft palate is discussed in detail in other chapters in this book. However, no discussion of communication disorders in children with cleft palate would be complete without reference to hearing. The literature regarding the relationship between hearing, especially otitis media with effusion (OME), and speech and language development is inconsistent. The early literature suggested a significant impact of OME on language development in young, typically developing children without cleft palate. However, a recent meta-analysis of studies on language development and OME shows that the relationship is far less conclusive and more equivocal than previously suggested.[7] Similarly, the current literature regarding the relationship between OME and speech-language development in children with cleft palate does not show a clear one-to-one relationship between middle ear disease and deficits in speech and language performance.[8] Some studies of speech and language development in children with cleft palate have

attributed communication delays to OME.[9,10] Other investigations have not shown this same association between hearing and speech and language performance in young children with cleft palate.[11,12] Despite the lack of clear research data showing a direct causal relationship between OME and communication impairment, it is critically important to closely monitor and manage hearing status as part of routine care for children with palatal clefts. Although there may be no evidence of a direct causal relationship between OME and communication impairment in children with cleft palate, it is important to consider that the child with cleft palate has numerous risk factors which are known to negatively impact speech and language development. It is likely that it is this *combination of risk factors* that is of particular concern. The search for causal links between these risk factors and later speech and language development has often revealed complex relationships between such factors, leading researchers to hypothesize a theory of "threshold for impairment." That is, a child may have one severe risk factor (such as speech impairment) or several lesser risk factors (such as OME and mild speech language delay) that push the child over the threshold of impairment. Likewise, the child's risk factors may not exceed the threshold and result in a clinically unidentified impairment. In this model, each risk factor contributes to the child's overall developmental status.[8] Because these risk factors may work together, it is important to address as many of them as possible, including aggressive management of OME.

LANGUAGE

Expressive and Receptive Language

Infant

Most clinicians experienced in the care of children with cleft palate are aware of the potential for impairments in speech production. However, there is a common assumption that there is little importance that occurs in the communication development of affected children prior to the onset of words or prior to palate repair. Anecdotally, this observation is confirmed frequently when medical professionals or families express surprise at the involvement of the speech-language pathologist in the evaluation of babies prior to the onset of speech production. This is a common misconception, one that suggests that communication development during infancy is either nonexistent or of little importance and/or not amenable to evaluation and intervention. To the contrary, however, there are important requisites to later speech and language that develop and that can be affected by the cleft during this early phase.[13]

Until recently, the focus of assessment and treatment of young children with cleft palate has emphasized speech and language problems after they appear. Currently, the focus has shifted from a rehabilitative model that addresses speech and language problems after they are established to a prevention model that addresses problems before they emerge. This recent interest in the speech and language development during infancy in children with cleft palate stems from the findings of several investigations. Studies of early language development have demonstrated differences in language skills between children with clefts and noncleft comparison groups.[9,14] However, the clinical significance and etiology of these differences is debated. Studies of early expressive language development suggest that children with clefts show delays in the onset and progression of early expressive language development prior to palate repair.[9,14] These findings have been consistent across studies and suggest the importance of the interrelationship between speech and language in early development.

While early vocalizations are the most recognizable milestone within the prelinguistic period prior to the onset of first words, other requisites of speech and language development also emerge during this stage and play a crucial role in establishing the child's interest in communication. Other milestones of early expressive language development include interactional variables, such as turn-taking, and use of gestures for communicative purposes. Although these nonlinguistic variables have not received much attention from researchers, it appears that expression of communicative intent through gestures is a relative strength for children with clefts.[15] However, when early vocalizations that accompany gestures were examined, children with clefts communicated less than noncleft peers.[16]

Another important, though often neglected, aspect of early communication development pertains to the child's understanding of speech. Receptive language development begins during the prelinguistic period and provides a foundation for joint interaction between parent and child that underlies the earliest communicative opportunities for the child. Studies of early receptive language development have shown significant differences between children with clefts and children without clefts; however, the performance of the children with clefts does not fall into a clinically significant range with the exception of children with isolated cleft palate.[9,12,17] This finding suggests a vulnerability in receptive language for some children with clefts at the earliest stages of language development.

The preventive model suggests that, given the importance of the communicative, receptive language, and speech milestones that are emerging during the prelinguistic period, intervention should begin even before palate repair.[13] Borrowing from the early intervention literature, Scherer, D'Antonio, and McGahey[18] explored the use of parent-implemented models of intervention for children with cleft palate. This approach has shown some positive outcomes for early language and speech development while reducing some of the problematic compensatory articulation errors that can persist long after palate repair.

Toddler

The time from 12 to 36 months of age is a critical period for language development. During this time, typically developing children are rapidly expanding their understanding and use of language. For example, the average 2-year-old has an expressive vocabulary of 200–300 words. Further, the size of the child's vocabulary is tied directly to the number of sounds he or she can produce. At this same age, children with cleft palate have a small inventory of consonants that they produce, leading to a cascading effect on their early language development.

Recent studies of early language development in children with cleft lip and/or cleft palate indicate that they show a delay in onset of first words and early expressive vocabulary development. It appears that children with cleft palate often choose words based on their speech sound repertoire, thus leading to limitations in vocabulary development.[9,11,14] These children produce more words beginning with nasals, vowels, and glides and fewer words beginning with oral stop consonants than children without cleft palate.[19] In an intervention study, Scherer[20] found that children with cleft palate learned words with sounds they could produce faster than words with new sounds. Together these studies suggest children with cleft palate display speech sound limitations during the first year of life that impact early vocabulary learning from the onset of first words.

While most studies of language development have focused on expressive language measures and their relationship to speech production abilities, studies of receptive language development indicate that some children with cleft palate experience delays in receptive as well as expressive language. Several studies comparing receptive language development have documented significantly poorer language scores in children with cleft lip and palate when compared to children without clefts.[9,14] However, the clinical significance of the receptive language difference is debated. While group differences reached statistical significance, the scores of the children with cleft lip and palate were often still within the normal range. A recent study[21] compared two groups of toddlers with cleft lip and palate, one with language delays and one without delays. This study showed that the language-delayed group caught up to their peers in receptive language by 3 years of age. While other studies suggest that children with cleft lip and/or cleft palate have language delays that persist into school age, there appears to be a subgroup of children with cleft lip and palate who normalize much earlier. However, these studies also suggest that some children with cleft lip and palate may have a vulnerability in receptive language development that warrants monitoring. As suggested earlier, children with clefts have a variety of risk factors that may combine to impact development. Early receptive language development should be viewed as one of those risk factors that may restrict the progression of speech and expressive language learning and, perhaps, later academic performance.

It appears that some children with cleft lip and palate do show receptive language delays, and it would be beneficial to identify those children early. Recent studies have described a play assessment that may assist in the identification of children with cleft palate who show receptive language delays. A study by Scherer and D'Antonio[22] assessed the symbolic play, language, and speech development of six toddlers between 18 and 30 months of age. They found that performance on the play measure was highly correlated with receptive language development. In a subsequent extension of this study, Snyder and Scherer[23] found that the symbolic play measure successfully predicted the children with cleft lip and palate who had receptive language delays.

While the focus of intervention for children with cleft palate is often speech development, the presence of early language delays suggests that intervention should address both speech and language development. Early intervention methods for young children often dictate a play-based approach for children under 3 years. Scherer[20] found that 2-year-old children with cleft lip and palate improved both vocabulary and speech sound production using a language intervention model. The findings of this study suggest that both language and speech improvement can be achieved simultaneously using language intervention models for young children with clefting.

Preschool

Studies of children with cleft palate continue to show receptive and expressive language differences in the 3–5 year age period when compared to children without cleft palate.[24,25] These deficits do not appear to differ based on cleft type but they do appear to be more associated with those children who demonstrate speech deficits.[25,26] These studies suggest that language impairment persists for some children with cleft palate, particularly for those children with significant speech impairments. Most studies examining language development have identified differences in expressive vocabulary and sentence complexity of children with cleft lip and palate. Scherer[25] found that preschool children with cleft lip and palate had significantly smaller vocabularies and shorter mean length utterances than children without cleft lip and palate. Further, this study determined the size of these group differences to be clinically significant. This recent study supports several older studies that documented language deficits in children with cleft lip and palate.

Some studies suggest that these expressive language deficits resolve by 5 years of age,[27] whereas other studies find that language deficits continue into the school age years. There have been few recent studies examining comprehensive assessment of language functioning in preschool or school age children with clefts.[24,25] Of the few that have provided comprehensive assessment, most include small numbers of participants.[27] While these studies each have identified some areas of language deficit, the results are often at odds with each other. For example, Eliason and Richman[24] found that 4–6-year-old children with cleft lip and palate were delayed in the ability to use verbal rehearsal strategies to mediate verbal problem-solving tasks. However, these same children did not show deficits in more traditional language measures of vocabulary and verbal analogies. On the other hand, Lowe and Scherer[27] showed deficits in some traditional language impairment measures for 5-year-old children with cleft lip palate, such as vocabulary and syntax comprehension. Al-

though these studies do not appear to be in agreement, the studies do point to a persistent language deficit for at least some children with cleft lip and palate. Given the relationship between language performance and school achievement, monitoring of language development throughout the preschool period is essential.

School Age and Later

During the school age period, language impairment may be disguised as an educational impairment. It is not uncommon to see speech and educational testing completed on children while language functioning is never addressed. The strong relationship between language performance and school achievement is well known for children with other disabilities but has not received much attention in children with cleft palate. Several studies suggest that some children with cleft lip and palate, particularly those with isolated cleft palate, continue to show poorer language performance than noncleft peers through school age and into adulthood. However, the extent, characteristics, and persistence of these differences have been debated. Many of the early studies of language performance describe general language delays that include receptive, expressive, and written language modalities extending into adolescence. However, more recent studies suggest that there may be subgroups of children within the cleft population who exhibit different profiles of language performance through school age. One subgroup of children appears to show a general language disability similar to the deficits described in the early studies.[28] These children show deficits that include broad areas of language function (e.g., verbal reasoning, categorization, abstract reasoning, use of verbal mediation for problem solving, rapid naming, and auditory sequential memory).[28,29] This general language disability profile was observed more in males with isolated cleft palate than in children with other cleft types. It should be noted that isolated cleft palate has a higher frequency of association with genetic syndromes and thus puts these children at higher risk of developmental deficits.[30] A second subgroup includes children with expressive language deficits. These children show deficits in rapid naming and auditory memory but not verbal mediation and abstract reasoning. This expressive language group included primarily children with cleft lip and palate.

These two language profiles also exhibit different degrees of risk for academic difficulties.[29,31] The children with general language disability show the greatest risk of reading and math deficits.[32] Whereas the occurrence of reading disability in the noncleft population runs between 10 and 15%, children with clefts show a 30–40% occurrence.[33] A recent study of children with clefts who had been diagnosed with attention deficit disorder found that 50% of those children had learning disabilities, and many of the children had not been previously identified.[32] The association between general language disability and academic difficulties in children with clefts underlines the importance of thorough monitoring of language and academic performance in children with clefts.[34]

Several studies have attempted to identify the source of language and academic difficulties by examining central auditory processing.[35,36] These studies have found differences between children with cleft lip and palate and isolated cleft palate that were detectable at birth and persisted into school age. The studies found poorer temporal processing and discrimination for children with isolated cleft palate than for children with cleft lip and palate and noncleft children. While these measures have been regarded as indicators of language and academic difficulties, the authors suggested that an auditory processing deficit was not the source of the language and academic differences observed in some children with clefts. It is more likely that these impairments are a reflection of the same underlying neural factor.

The persistence of language impairment in some children with cleft palate and the impact of unrecognized impairments on the child's education success indicates that language performance should be assessed thoroughly for those children with poor school performance.

Pragmatics and Social Communication

The literature describing social and pragmatic performance of children with cleft palate has not supported the presence of a pragmatic deficit but has identified aspects of pragmatic functioning that may impact social interaction. It is recognized that children must understand the basic requisites of communicative interaction in order to communicate effectively. These requisites include expressing communicative intent and interpreting social cues of conversational use. While the first requisite appears early in development, the later develops simultaneously with speech and language development. In infancy, children acquire communicative intent, which is the ability to make their communicative needs known through eye gaze, gesture, and/or vocalizations. Children with cleft palate show limitations in use of gestures when combined with vocalizations[15,16] but do not show a deficit in gestural communication alone. This information is important for determining the prognosis for persistent deficits. A child who has no words and demonstrates no communicative intent has a higher risk of slower speech and language development. A child who has no words but who has gestures and is clearly intending to communicate runs less risk of significant speech and language deficits.

During the toddler period, typically developing children begin to overlay speech onto gestural communicative intentions. It appears that children with cleft lip and palate have difficulty with the acquisition of verbal skills and with subsequent use of verbal skills in conversation. Fredrickson, Chapman, and Hardin-Jones[37] examined the communicative functions and conversational structure of children with and without cleft lip and palate. The children with clefts used fewer comments, requests, and disagreements than the children without clefts. In addition, the children with cleft palate were more passive conversational partners in that they used fewer extensions of conversational topics and more topic maintenance than children without clefts. Further, these dif-

ferences were correlated with articulation performance, suggesting that conversational differences were associated with speech difficulties. In summary, children with nonsyndromic cleft lip and palate or cleft palate do not appear to show specific deficits in pragmatic function but rather a deficit in language use associated with speech intelligibility issues.[38] However, it is important to keep in mind that children with clefts who have associated syndromic conditions may well demonstrate deficits in pragmatic function.

SPEECH

Many texts, chapters, and articles have been written on the speech disorders of individuals with cleft palate. This chapter is not intended to be a substitute for a more detailed review of the literature pertaining to the speech characteristics associated with cleft palate. Rather, in keeping with the themes and goals of this chapter as stated in the introduction, this section is written with the nonspeech pathologist in mind. Additionally, an emphasis is placed on considering speech production as one single part of the broader communication process. Our discussion of the speech patterns associated with cleft palate emphasizes the view that speech is shaped by many dynamic, linguistic processes that are active—and should be appreciated—long before the first words are present in a child's communication process.

A historical review of the literature on speech disorders associated with cleft palate shows a relatively recent move toward greater recognition of a developmental perspective regarding speech impairment. Kuehn and Moller[39] provide an excellent historical review and analysis of the literature on speech disorders associated with palatal clefting. They point out that early characterizations of speech associated with cleft palate emphasized descriptions of the types and frequency of articulation errors compared with normative data. These errors were then often related to anatomic factors such as cleft type, cleft severity, and type and timing of palatoplasty. Gradually, the literature expanded to move from an emphasis on articulation to the description of phonological patterns which acknowledged the higher linguistic processes of speech production. As Moller[40] noted, at this point, the field began to appreciate that much learning was occurring in infants and toddlers prior to age 3 which was the age that speech assessments had traditionally begun. It was acknowledged that the historical and medical propensity for delaying detailed assessments of speech production until the preschool period missed important information about ways in which the child with a cleft was both active and creative in his/her speech acquisition. In more recent years, there has been greater attention paid to how the child with a cleft develops speech sounds and then organizes those sounds into a system that is part of a larger speech and language process. This broader view has taken into account the peripheral and motor aspects of speech production while acknowledging the more central/cognitive aspects of communication. For example, in recent years we have continued to address the articulation skills of children with cleft palate while attempting to understand their phonological development as well. In this chapter, therefore, we will emphasize speech production as an active, linguistic process with patterns that are emerging from the beginning of sound development and certainly before the onset of first words. While the purpose of this chapter is not to address evaluation methods per se, our discussion of speech and the importance of considering speech production as one part of a more global linguistic/communication process has important implications regarding recommendations for when speech evaluations should be initiated in the clinical management of children with cleft palate and for what types of descriptions are useful for clinical and research purposes.

Articulation and Phonology

In linguistics and speech pathology, *articulation* is a term that describes the physical movements that are involved in shaping the vocal tract above the larynx to produce the various sounds of speech. In most languages consonants are the sounds that carry most of the information that contribute to word meaning. All sounds of any language can be described by the place in the vocal tract where the airstream is constricted and the manner in which the airstream is valved. For example, a "p" sound is made with both lips closed and is therefore called a "bilabial." When producing a "p," the air stream is temporarily held to build up intraoral air pressure and abruptly released. This is called a "stop" because of the stopping of the airstream. Therefore, "p" is a bilabial stop consonant. In contrast, the "f" sound is made with the lower lip touching the teeth, and so it is called a labiodental sound. Here, the air is valved slowly but continuously through the narrowed constriction which is referred to as "fricative." An so, "f" is a labiodental fricative.

Phonology is a branch of linguistics that studies the sound systems of languages. The study of phonology identifies the meaningful patterns of sounds in a language and how these sounds are organized in the mind. Bowen[41] explains that in clinical use, the term "phonology" refers to an individual's sounds system. The gradual process of acquiring adult speech patterns is referred to as "phonological development." Bowen points out that phonological development in children involves three components: the way a sound is stored in the child's mind; the way the sound is actually said by the child; and the rules that connect these two processes.[41]

The distinction between simple description of articulation errors and the more active, linguistically based approach to speech disorders is more than an academic distinction. It has important implications for transdisciplinary issues such as timing of palate repair and measurement of outcome variables. For example, early studies discussed the most beneficial chronological age for palate repair with respect to speech development. A more modern view would emphasize that speech and language age and phonological development are more sensitive and appropriate indicators that should be considered.[42] Similarly, many outcome stud-

ies seek to address the impact of a given surgical approach on "speech" by cataloging a variety of articulation errors while not taking into account the child's overall sound system and developmental stage.

One system for describing the speech of young children with cleft palate that can be extremely useful and is worth mentioning is described by Stoel-Gammon and Dunn.[43] This system analyzes a child's speech production capabilities using both "independent" and "relational analyses." A "relational analysis" compares the child's productions with the intended adult model. An error analysis can then examine the type of substitution or omission patterns and can be used to identify the type and frequency of errors compared with the expected adult targets. This analysis system is most similar to that discussed previously in this section whereby early descriptions of the speech of individuals with cleft palate generally were described in relation to normative data. On the other hand, an "independent analysis" documents the child's speech production inventory without comparison to the adult model. This analysis provides information regarding the diversity of sounds and syllable shapes used by children during word attempts. This measure describes the consonants that the child can produce, even though these sounds may be substituted for the correct adult sound. An independent analysis therefore allows for a description of the child's individual articulatory capability and individual sound system. This description of alternative ways of examining the speech production patterns of young children with clefts has meaningful clinical implications. For example, if the child's speech production is compared and contrasted only with the adult model it will surely appear more limited and abnormal than if we assess all of the potential sounds the child can make. It is a common observation that children with cleft palate will come into the clinical speech evaluation with reports describing the child's speech production capabilities in such a way that suggests that the child is "not speaking" or "not saying any words." An independent analysis often reveals that the child has the capability of making more sounds but they may not be using them in word attempts.

Whether conducting a relational or an independent analysis, descriptions of articulation rely primarily on the analysis of the place of articulation and manner of production of sounds and the limitations in these features. However, speech development includes more than learning the physical production of speech sounds. Children acquire a system for organizing sound use that takes into consideration the constraints of the language they are learning. In so doing, children acquire rules that guide their use of speech sounds. In the early stages of speech and language development, when speech motor production is immature, children develop rules for sound use that simplify the motor load on the speech production system. This simplification often leads to omission or substitution of sounds. For children with clefts, substituted sounds may include developmentally earlier sounds or compensatory sounds. Children then establish phonological rules to guide the use of these sounds in words and sentences. Understanding of the phonological rules that children create to guide their speech production is particularly important when determining intervention goals.

Typically developing children acquire sounds in an ordered manner and progress through well-defined stages of babbling that continue on to meaningful word use.[43] For example, children typically progress from the use of vowels and consonant-like sounds such as "w" or "y" on to the use of true consonants such as "p, t, k" etc. Between 6 and 12 months of age, the number of sounds children use shows rapid increase prior to the onset of first words. By the time typically developing children reach 2 years of age, they are generally using 12–14 different consonants in their speech sound repertoire. For children with cleft palate, the development of these consonants and the consonant sound system is often disturbed in a variety of ways.

Children with cleft palate tend to have the greatest difficulty producing high pressure consonants compared with other classes of sounds. They tend to show a high occurrence of misarticulation for the fricatives and affricates, followed by plosives, glides, and nasals.[8] In the simplest terms, children with cleft palate tend to preserve the manner of articulation while sacrificing the place. In addition to the more common substitution and omission errors, children with cleft palate commonly produce sound substitutions called compensatory articulation errors.[44] The most common and distinctive of the compensatory articulation errors that occur frequently in the speech of individuals with cleft palate is the glottal stop, the result of the child's attempt to move the primary point of articulatory constriction inferior to a malfunctioning velopharyngeal valve. However, it should be noted that compensatory articulation errors are not always a direct result of uncorrected velopharyngeal insufficiency. Such errors may be the result of previous coupling of the oral and nasal cavities that no longer exists. In fact, as pointed out by Hoch et al.,[45] dysfunction of the velopharyngeal valving mechanism can actually be the result of compensatory articulation errors, and improvement in velopharyngeal valving can actually occur through speech therapy aimed at elimination of the compensatory articulation errors. Therefore, the relationship between articulation and velopharyngeal valving is far more complex than is often discussed.[46]

Infant

A number of studies describe the composition of early vocalizations in children with cleft palate.[47,48] During the prelinguistic period, children with cleft lip and palate demonstrate deficits in the onset and composition of their babbling.[49] Their consonant inventories are limited to sounds made by coupling the nasal and oral cavities.[49] Furthermore, the effect of early vocalization deficits appears to persist despite a more normalized speech mechanism following cleft repair. Whereas the vocal limitations of children with cleft lip and/or palate prior to palate repair (at approximately 12 months) do not seem surprising, studies indicate that these limitations often still exist for 1–3 years following repair.[47,48] Additionally, these deficits are apparent regardless of cleft type or early

obturation of the palate.[50] Compensatory glottal productions are reported in the vocalizations of children prior to palate repair.[48,51] These glottal productions often take the form of growls or "ohoh" productions and may become embedded into the early sound repertoire of the children with clefts.

Longitudinal studies of the relationship between prelinguistic vocalization and later speech and language performance in children with clefts indicate that children with larger consonant inventories and higher rates of stop consonant production in babbling have better speech and language skills at 3 years of age.[11,52] Chapman et al.[11,52] demonstrated a relationship between small consonant inventories, especially limitations in the production of stop consonants, and later language measures. However, the studies did not find significant correlations between many of the prelinguistic variables and later speech and language measures. Specifically, onset and composition of canonical babbling, which differentiated prelinguistic children with cleft lip and palate from noncleft children, was not significantly correlated with later speech or language measures. While group differences are apparent in the early vocalization patterns of children with and without clefts, there are few clear predictors of later speech and language performance.

Toddler

Following palate repair, children with cleft palate often continue to show speech sound production deficits, including a preference for sounds produced at the extremes of the vocal tract (i.e., labials, velars, and glottals), limited oral stop consonants,[19,49,53] reliance on the phonological processes of backing, nasal assimilations, and use of compensatory errors.[47,48]

These limitations in sound inventory are likely responsible for the early vocabulary deficits observed in children with clefts. Such children produce more words beginning with nasals, vowels, and glides and fewer words beginning with oral stop consonants than children without clefts.[19] Scherer[20] explored the relationship between word learning and speech sound repertoire in an intervention study. She found that young children with cleft lip and palate learned words with sounds that were within their consonant inventories faster than words with sounds that were outside their inventories. Therefore, the children with cleft lip and palate used more words with nasals, glides, and glottals than words with oral consonants.

Longitudinal studies of the relationship between prelinguistic vocalization and later speech and language performance in children with cleft palate indicate that children with larger consonant inventories and higher rates of stop consonant production in babbling have better speech and language skills at 3 years of age.[11,52] Chapman et al.[11,52] demonstrated a relationship between small consonant inventories, especially limitations in the production of stop consonants, and later language measures. However, the studies did not find significant correlations between many of the prelinguistic variables and later speech and language measures. Specifically, onset and composition of canonical babbling, which differentiated children with cleft palate from children without clefts in the prelinguistic period, was not significantly correlated with later speech or language measures. Although group differences are apparent between the early vocalization patterns of children with and without clefts, there are few clear predictors of later speech and language performance.

Preschool

Children in the 3–5 year age range continue to exhibit speech impairments that are characterized by developmental errors, nasal substitutions, compensatory articulation, and persistence of phonological process errors. Hardin-Jones and Jones[54] examined the speech of 212 preschool and school-aged children with cleft lip and palate. Approximately 13% of the children used nasal substitutions and 25% used compensatory articulation errors, specifically glottal stop substitutions. The findings indicate that these error patterns persist for a substantial number of children despite the fact that 68% of the children in this study had received speech therapy.

Chapman[55] examined the use of phonological processes in 3–5-year-old children with and without cleft lip and palate. This study showed that children with cleft lip and palate use phonological processes for a protracted period of time. Phonological processes are a set of rules the children use to simplify speech production during early language development.[43] For example, young children may omit the final consonant in words (e.g., "ba" for ball) or omit the first syllable of a word (e.g., "jamas" for pajamas) in order to ease the production task. However, children also substitute sounds in predictable ways such as substituting sounds made in the back of the mouth for sounds in the front of the mouth (e.g., "gagi" for daddy). Chapman found that young children with cleft lip and/or palate used these simplification rules longer and used some processes more than children without clefts. Significant differences were found between the groups at 3 and 4 years but not by 5 years of age. The predominant processes that differentiated the groups at 3 years of age include backing (e.g., "kea" for tea), stopping (e.g., "do" for zoo), stridency deletion (e.g., "un" for sun), final consonant deletion (e.g., "ba" for ball), syllable reduction (e.g., "jammys" for pajamas), and cluster simplification (e.g., "top" for stop). The authors suggest that the first three processes may be associated with difficulty producing high pressure consonants since these processes include sounds in the stop and fricative manner categories that are problematic for children with clefts. The remaining processes are observed in the speech of children with phonological and language impairments without clefts and may result from the children's attempts to reduce speech production complexity given a limited consonant inventory.

During the preschool phase, the child's sound inventory begins to approach the adult model. Many of the developmental phonological processes are typically eliminated by this age. When speech sound errors persist, this is the age at which direct speech therapy is most likely to begin. During the preschool period the primary articulation patterns that characterize children with cleft palate include limited phonetic inventories, poor speech accuracy, and presence of compensatory articulation errors. Scherer[56] described the speech of 25 children with clefts and 25 children without clefts between 3 and 5 years of age. The children with clefts showed significantly poorer articulation scores and speech accuracy[57] than the children without clefts. A severity index associated with the speech accuracy score placed the children in the mild to moderately impaired range, an improvement over the toddler period. Although the children's speech remained behind those of age matched peers, children with clefts were making advances in speech production. The most notable category was the fricative category (e.g., /f/, /v/, /th/, /s/, /z/, /sh/, /ʒ/). Percent correct use of this category improved from 38% to 67% from 3 to 5 years.

The persistence of compensatory errors during the preschool years often provokes the onset of speech therapy for many children with clefts. Studies have suggested that approximately 25% of children with clefts use compensatory articulation errors, and glottal stops appear to be the predominant error pattern.[51,54] For children who use compensatory articulation patterns to a significant degree, speech intelligibility may be severely reduced. Further, when this pattern becomes habituated during the preschool years, it can be particularly resistant to change in therapy.[58,59]

As discussed earlier, in addition to phonetic features of speech associated with the physiologic aspects of the cleft, children with clefts show difficulty with the acquisition of the rules of the sound use. Phonological processes, or the rules used to simplify classes of sounds, are typically eliminated during the preschool period. Chapman[55] examined the use of phonological processes in children with clefts. She found that children with clefts used phonological processes for a longer period of time than children without clefts, but by 5 years of age these children had caught up to their peers. The processes that distinguished the children with clefts included processes that omitted sounds or syllables, such as final consonant deletion (e.g., "ba" for ball), syllable reduction (e.g., "jammys" for pajamas), stridency deletion (e.g., "hou" for house), or cluster simplification (e.g., "top" for stop) and processes that substituted compensatory sounds or developmentally easier sounds, such as backing (e.g., "kov" for stove), glottal replacement (e.g., "cu?" for cup), stopping (e.g., "knip" for knife), and deaffrication (e.g., "shicken" for chicken). While some of the substitution processes are more often associated with high pressure consonants that are problematic for children with clefts, the omission processes are observed frequently in the speech of other impaired groups of children, such as those with phonological and language impairments.

School Age and Later

Children with clefts continue to make progress in their speech development during the school-age years, although this progress is more rapid for the younger children than older children. As adults, individuals with clefts still are consistently judged to have poorer speech than individuals without clefts.[47,60,61] Bardach et al.[61] reported that articulation was judged to be within normal limits for 57% of adolescents with bilateral cleft and palate. This figure is similar to the 55% reported by Peterson-Falzone[62] for adolescents with a variety of cleft types. While progress is evident during the school years, a substantial number of children still do not attain normal speech production by adulthood.

The presence of unresolved compensatory articulation errors is a major concern for a subgroup of children with clefts during the school age years. Although this subgroup may be small in number, they represent a particularly challenging group of children for the speech-language pathologist. In most cases, velopharyngeal dysfunction will be addressed prior to or within the first few years of school; however, the impact of years of compensatory articulation use is often not readily overcome.[63] Further, some studies exploring the relationship between speech and language performance suggest that those children with poor speech intelligibility due to compensatory articulation errors often also have significant language impairment.[21] These findings suggest that the articulation/phonological impairments, may affect the organization of other related developmental parameters, including language and reading.

Dentition

The impact of dentition on speech production skills of children with cleft palate is a testimony to the human speech production mechanism to adapt. As we know, oral clefting can be associated with a wide range of dental and occlusal abnormalities. An excellent review of the dental/occlusal problems that can impact speech production is summarized by Peterson-Falzone, Hardin-Jones and Karnell.[8] They review the potential impact of a protrusive premaxilla, retrusive premaxilla, crossbite, low palatal vault/open bite, missing teeth, rotated anterior teeth, and ectopic teeth on articulation. While any or all of these dental abnormalities can impact speech, particularly articulation, there are few reports that show clear causal links between these features and speech articulation. Rather, the speech production system appears imminently capable of aerodynamic and acoustic compensations for most dental abnormalities.

Resonance and Velopharyngeal Function

The communication disorders most commonly associated with individuals with cleft palate are those related to velopharyngeal dysfunction or incomplete separation of the oral and nasal cavities. When this separation is disturbed, a variety of alterations in speech can occur, including hypernasality, mixed resonance, cul-de-sac resonance, weak pressure consonants, and compensatory articulation patterns. The strong relationship between palatal clefting and the presence of hypernasality is so well recognized that in the early years of the field, the presence of hypernasality in a speaker was commonly referred to as "cleft palate speech." However, it is important to know that not all individuals, nor even most individuals, with cleft palate will demonstrate hypernasality or other speech symptoms associated with faulty separation of the oral and nasal cavities. Conversely, hypernasality and symptoms of velopharyngeal dysfunction may or may not signal the presence of a cleft or submucous cleft palate.

Definitions of several of the symptoms associated with abnormal velopharyngeal valving are presented in Table 35–2. However, it is worth reiterating some important distinctions regarding some of these speech characteristics. Hypernasality is a *resonance disorder*. It refers to inordinately high nasal resonance on vowels and vocalic consonants. It is the result of abnormal coupling of the oral and nasal cavities and is a physical phenomenon that is typically assessed by perceptual means. There is wide variability across languages (and even across dialects of a given language) in terms of what is normal or acceptable nasal resonance. On the other hand, nasal emission is an *articulation disorder*. Most simply defined, it is the passage of air through the nose for high pressure consonants that should not be associated with any nasal airflow. Nasal emission may be audible or inaudible. It is often associated with reduced intra oral air pressure. Hypernasality and nasal emission may occur in the same speaker and often do coexist, but they are not the same phenomena. Additionally, both these features are the result of *supraglottal* disturbances and therefore should not be referred to as *voice disorders*, a term reserved for disorders of the larynx and phonation.

A listener does not require specialized training to hear many of the effects of abnormal oral nasal coupling on a speaker's speech quality and intelligibility. While the untrained listener might be equipped to identify the presence of a speech abnormality, it is a far more difficult and complex task to identify the cause(s) of that disorder and to develop an appropriate and effective management plan.

In particular, the role of the velopharynx in speech production and the nomenclature used to describe disturbances in this system are far more involved than is sometimes acknowledged in discussions of communication disorders associated with cleft palate. In its most simple form, the speech production process can be thought of as a large air-filled container always closed at the bottom with two openings to the atmosphere, the lips, and the nares. In this container, there are several valves that can be opened or closed to varying degrees, thus changing the shape of the container and the resistance to airflow. These valves include the larynx, the velopharynx, the tongue and lips, and the nasal passages. Airflow must move through this series of valves in a coordinated and tightly timed manner, thus creating a series of rapidly changing air pressures and airflows that we ultimately perceive as the sounds of speech. Viewed most simplistically, the role of the velopharyngeal valve is to separate the oral and nasal cavities during speech and swallowing. For speech, the velopharynx directs air from the lungs and larynx through the mouth for oral sounds and through the nose for nasal sounds. When this valving is disturbed, speech can be affected in several ways, as described above.

Table 35–2.

Resonance, Articulation, and Phonation Disorders Frequently Associated with Cleft Palate and/or Velopharyngeal Dysfunction

Hypernasality

The perception of inordinate nasal resonance during the production of *vowels*. This results from inappropriate coupling of the oral and nasal cavities. (The term *inordinate* is used because low vowels and vowels in nasal consonant contexts are normally somewhat nasalized).

Nasal emission

Nasal air escape associated with production of *consonants* requiring high oral pressure. It occurs when air is forced through an incompletely closed velopharyngeal port or a patent-oral nasal fistula. Nasal emission may be audible or not.
Note: Hypernasality and nasal emission are not synonymous, although they often occur together and are both symptoms of velopharyngeal dysfunction.

Hyponasality

A reduction in normal nasal resonance usually resulting from blockage or partial blockage of the nasal airway by any number of causes, including upper respiratory tract infection, hypertrophied turbinates, and a wide, obstructing pharyngeal flap.

Hyper-hyponasality (mixed resonance)

The simultaneous occurrence of hypernasality and hyponasality in the same speaker usually as the result of incomplete velopharyngeal closure in the presence of high nasal cavity resistance that is not sufficient to block nasal resonance completely.

Cul-de-sac resonance

A variation of hyponasality usually associated with tight anterior nasal constriction often resulting in a muffled quality.

Nasal substitution

The articulators are placed appropriately for an intended oral consonant. However, incomplete velopharyngeal closure causes the sound to be produced as a nasal consonant. For example, b becomes m and d becomes n. Such substitutions frequently are called homorganic nasals.

Compensatory articulation

The articulators are placed inappropriately so as to enable creation of the plosive or fricative characteristics of the sounds they replace. For example, if a patient cannot build up oral pressure for the fricatives (e.g., s) or plosives (e.g., p) because of velopharyngeal dysfunction, they may create those pressures below the level of the velopharyngeal port. Such substitutions include glottal stops, pharyngeal stops, and pharyngeal fricatives among others.

Sibilant distortion

Inappropriate tongue placement for the sounds /s/ and /z/.

Laryngeal/voice symptoms

A variety of phonation disorders may accompany velopharyngeal dysfunction, including hoarseness, low speaking volume, strained or strangled voice quality, and unusual pitch alternations. One theory for the co-occurrence of velopharyngeal and laryngeal symptoms is that speakers with velopharyngeal dysfunction may attempt to compensate for the inability to achieve complete closure and maintain adequate speech pressures by compensatory activity at the level of the larynx.

Modified from D'Antonio L, Scherer NJ. The evaluation of speech disorders associated with clefting. In Shprintzen RJ, Bardach J (eds). Cleft Palate Speech Management, St. Louis: Mosby Elsevier, 1995, pp. 176–220.

Historically, the velopharynx has been viewed as a simple binary valve with two positions: open or closed. However, research and clinical observations have shown that the velopharynx is a complex three-dimensional valve with a variety of shapes and patterns of activity that differ among speakers.[64] Just as the oral articulators, such as the lips and tongue, have varying degrees of shapes and movement patterns, so too does the velopharynx assume different shapes and positions for different sounds. In addition, it is not enough that the velopharyngeal valve be capable of achieving complete closure; it must do so in a tightly controlled time domain in coordination with other articulators.

As discussed earlier in this chapter, the child with a cleft, like other children, is engaged in an active process of learning the speech sounds and patterns of the ambient language. Disturbances in anatomy during early speech and language development can interact with more global linguistic processes that can impact the speech sound system of a child. Therefore, it is important for the various professionals involved in the care of children with cleft palate to be aware that the presence of symptoms of velopharyngeal valving disorders may have a variety of compound and sometimes inter-related causes that have their roots in current anatomic limitations or in earlier learning in the presence of abnormal anatomy. It is thus essential that velopharyngeal valving be appreciated with this understanding of learning and higher-level linguistic processes in mind.

Terminology

Traditionally, when symptoms were present that suggested the velopharynx was not functioning correctly, such was referred to as "velopharyngeal incompetence" or "VPI." However, hearing hypernasality or nasal emission (i.e., speech symptoms associated with VPI) does not necessarily indicate that the velopharynx cannot achieve closure. Rather, it simply means that in this instance it did not achieve closure. Such misunderstanding of the complexity of velopharyngeal function can have profound diagnostic implications. For example, the diagnosis of VPI suggests that the velopharyngeal mechanism cannot achieve closure, and for many cleft care providers it suggests that only physical management will correct the problem. In addition, this label will often bias the unfamiliar speech pathologist to believe that additional speech therapy is not warranted until physical management is completed. Therefore, it is important that our language, regarding the causes of the symptoms associated with abnormal nasal resonance and velopharyngeal valving abnormalities, be precise and based on the underlying physiology. There have been many discussions in the literature regarding the most appropriate language to use in describing velopharyngeal valving disorders.[46] There appears to be a trend in the more recent literature to use the term "VPI" (velopharyngeal incompetence or velopharyngeal insufficiency) when diagnostic studies have clearly determined a true physical limitation, whereas "velopharyngeal dysfunction" is used when it is clear that there is some malfunction, but the cause of such remains unclear.

Differential Diagnosis

There are a variety of factors that can result in speech symptoms such as hypernasality or nasal emission, i.e. symptoms most often associated with velopharyngeal dysfunction. Some of these are structural and include a true inability of the velopharyngeal port to achieve closure due to an absence of adequate tissue to allow for closure; improper muscle insertion of the levators preventing closure due to poor motion or a residual central trough in the nasal surface of the palate; the presence of an oral nasal fistula; interference from other structures such as the tonsils, adenoids, and nasal passages; or neurologic impairment. There are also a number of speech-related variables that can impact the presence of velopharyngeal symptoms, including articulation and phonologic patterns, inconsistency of speech patterns, the role of phonetic context, rate and timing of speech, and fatigue. The role of the speech-language pathologist in evaluating the speech of children with cleft palate is to determine which symptoms are the result of true physical limitations (and which therefore require physical management) and which symptoms are more related to learning or habituation of patterns (and which therefore require behavioral intervention, i.e. speech therapy).

This process of differential diagnosis can be quite difficult since speech symptoms that seem to be similar and, in fact, indistinct from one another to the casual listener may be varied in cause and, therefore, in appropriate management. For example, in patients with cleft palate, hypernasality and nasal emission may occur in the presence of a repaired cleft and a residual oronasal fistula. Casual perceptual observations may not reveal the source of these symptoms. In fact, in our experience it has been common for some team members to refer to the speech symptoms associated with a fistula as "VPI." However, it would be inappropriate to label the phenomenon as VPI without investigation. In some instances, the symptoms may be solely attributable to air escape through the fistula. In this case, the diagnosis would be hypernasality and nasal emission caused by a patent oronasal fistula, and the symptoms may thus be completely unrelated to the velopharyngeal mechanism in any way. The appropriate management would be repair or obturation of the fistula. In other cases, the symptoms may appear to be attributable to a lack of proper velopharyngeal function or to a combination of causes. For example, there are reports in the literature that have shown a relationship between temporary obturation of a patent oronasal fistula and associated improvement in velopharyngeal valving.[46,65–67] Another illustration of the need for differential diagnosis is the phenomenon of phoneme specific-VPI.[68] This is the presence of nasal emission that is isolated to specific pressure consonants, most commonly the fricatives /s/ and /z/. The inexperienced clinician often mistakes this rule-based phonological error as a sign of true VPI. Many patients with sound-specific nasal emission such as this are referred for surgical management for what is actually an articulation/phonological error pattern.

These examples emphasize the point that the resonance and velopharyngeal valving disturbances associated with cleft palate are often complex and multifactorial and require in-depth evaluation to sort out the variety of potential etiologies. Additionally, the amount of information necessary for making these differential diagnoses varies over the child's developmental course and interacts with chronologic age, developmental age, language stage, and speech development profile. In many cases, therefore, the diagnostic process must be conducted over time as the child continues to develop and in relation to other surgical, dental, and behavioral interventions.

Infant and Toddler

In the early stages of communication development, there are few insights into whether velopharyngeal valving will be adequate for speech or not. It is not possible to judge velopharyngeal function directly in these early stages of development.

However, there are some indirect links or indicators that are worth watching carefully, including phoneme repertoire and the emergence of compensatory articulation patterns, particularly the glottal stop. At this age, there is not enough speech and language development to make clear determinations regarding whether or not the velopharyngeal port is functioning or will function adequately for normal speech production.

Some young children, especially in the toddler and early preschool age range, may demonstrate inconsistent nasal emission that appears to be related more to a failure to have achieved the correct manner distinction between oral and nasal sounds. This error pattern is more related to a phonological process than to true VPI. That is, the child may not have acquired an understanding of the difference between oral and nasal sounds. In many instances, the very young child or the child with a speech and language delay may not discriminate between oral and nasal contrasts in his or her own productions or phonological system or in the models of the speech pathologist. Many young children who present with inconsistent nasal emission are stimulable for correct production of oral consonants once they recognize and understand the difference between oral and nasal airflow. It is therefore important to differentiate in such children between nasal emission due to an incompetent VP valve and nasal emission that is the result of an articulation/phonological based pattern.

Preschool

During the preschool years, resonance and velopharyngeal function can be assessed with some accuracy. As the child's sound repertoire, articulation skills, and expressive language expand, there are more opportunities to evaluate whether velopharyngeal valving is adequate for speech production. Generally, the more developed the child's speech production skills, the more accurately velopharyngeal function can be assessed. It is often difficult during the early preschool phase to sort out how much of the perceived velopharyngeal symptoms are the result of habituated patterns or phonological processes and how much are the result of true velopharyngeal insufficiency. However, careful evaluation and monitoring can result in accurate differential diagnosis.

When there are severe and consistent velopharyngeal symptoms, it is typically easy to make a determination regarding the diagnosis and therefore make appropriate treatment recommendations. Even after thorough evaluation, however, it can be very difficult in some cases to determine whether or not the velopharyngeal mechanism is adequate for speech production. In these cases of borderline or variable velopharyngeal function (or when performance appears inconsistent), it is difficult to determine whether or not the velopharyngeal mechanism is adequate for speech and therefore whether surgical management or speech therapy is the most appropriate treatment recommendation. In these complex cases, it is useful to use a circumscribed period of speech therapy to provide additional and often necessary diagnostic information.

Typically, it is during the preschool period that such diagnostic therapy becomes possible. When velopharyngeal function is variable (as it often is in young children), it is useful to attempt stimulability testing.[46,69] A cornerstone of modern speech therapy is the belief that a child's ability to be stimulated for improved speech production through auditory, visual, and in some instances tactile models and cues is a good prognostic indicator of the potential for long-term improvement. Such stimulability testing is particularly useful in the child with variable velopharyngeal function. It can provide valuable information about whether behavioral management is likely to remediate velopharyngeal symptoms or if it appears that physical management is indicated.

Morris[70] suggests that there are two major subgroups of children with marginal velopharyngeal dysfunction and that they can be most easily distinguished by their response to short-term therapeutic intervention. The first is the "almost-but-not-quite" (ABNQ) subgroup. This group tends to present with mild consistent nasalization of speech that is highly consistent among and within tasks. Morris suggests that speech therapy is not likely to be successful with this group. A brief period of therapy for the young child with inconsistent VP function should reveal whether further improvement is possible.

The second diagnostic group of marginal velopharyngeal function described by Morris is the "sometimes-but-not-always" group (SBNA). Children in this group generally show marked inconsistency in velopharyngeal function. Some children in this group will show improvement in VP function with training and some will not. It is essential to consider the children in this group who do not improve. A careful analysis of their speech errors is necessary to determine if the errors are random or if they appear to be rule-governed and part of a more encompassing phonological system. For example, it is common to see preschool children with cleft palate who can produce all or most of the stop consonants with no inappropriate nasal airflow. However, often all or most fricative and sibilant consonants are nasally emitted. In these cases it is often true that the child has developed a system where friction consonants are marked by nasal emission or substituted by a true compensatory articulation error, in particularly the posterior nasal fricative, and a thorough description of the error patterns will assist in the diagnostic process. Furthermore, a brief period of speech therapy will also provide invaluable information concerning whether velopharyngeal closure can be facilitated for the incorrectly produced sounds.

It is these children with inconsistent velopharyngeal function who present the greatest dilemma for the surgeon and speech pathologist. Especially in young preschool children, the inability to achieve consistent velopharyngeal closure is commonly related to several contributing variables. Because of the multiple, interrelated variables that can impact velopharyngeal function in these children, it is very important that decisions to provide surgical alternatives be provided only after thorough evaluation and counseling. In many instances, it is these patients who have poor surgical outcomes since the original problem was, in fact, multifactorial. It is these patients with "diagnostic dilemmas" who require intensive counseling prior to surgical intervention in order to facilitate realistic expectations for postsurgical outcomes.

It is also during the preschool stage that questions regarding whether or not a palatal fistula is symptomatic can be addressed. We know that hypernasality is the result of abnormal oral nasal coupling. As discussed above, audible nasal emission may be attributable to inadequacy of the port or to articulatory errors. However, as mentioned previously, both symptoms may also result from an oronasal fistula with or without VPI. Significant controversy exists in the literature concerning accurate identification of symptomatic fistulae, the extent of the effects of such on speech, and decisions regarding surgical repair. There are many opinions expressed in the surgical literature, and there is a common misconception that there is a relationship between the size and location of a palatal fistula and its effects on speech. A more conservative view is that the functional significance of a palatal fistula on speech must be determined for each patient individually. D'Antonio et al.[71] showed a significant improvement in perceptual judgments of hypernasality, frequency of nasal emission, perceived oral pressure, and speech quality when comparing speech ratings with fistulae unoccluded and temporarily occluded with chewing gum. However, there was no consistent relationship between the improvement in speech characteristics between the unoccluded and occluded conditions based on size or location of the fistulae. Results of the same study suggested that an important factor influencing changes in speech and aerodynamic characteristic when a palatal fistula is obturated is the individual's nasal cavity resistance. Additionally, Isberg and Henningsson[65] showed a relationship between temporary obturation of a patent oronasal fistula and concomitant improvement in velopharyngeal valving. Results from these studies concerning palatal fistuale are presented here to emphasize that a number of factors are likely to contribute to the effects of palatal fistulae on speech. Therefore, when a palatal fistula is observed, statements concerning its effect on hypernasality, nasal emission, or speech quality should be made with great caution. For many children the process of determining whether the fistula is symptomatic for speech or not begins in the preschool age range but is difficult to determine before this age when the child is capable of cooperation.

In addition to true VPI articulation and phonological-based errors, and the contribution of palatal fistulae, there is one other important yet infrequently discussed potential cause of hypernasality and nasal emission that for some clinicians is counterintuitive. In some children, hypertrophic tonsils can prevent complete VP closure, thus resulting in hypernasality and nasal emission or both.[72,73] It should be noted, however, that hypertrophic tonsils and adenoids may also impact speech by blocking the flow of air through the velopharyngeal port and may thereby also cause hyponasality or denasality. The decision to remove tonsils in a patient with a cleft palate should therefore be accompanied by a thorough perceptual and instrumental speech evaluation.

As this discussion of tonsils and adenoids suggests, and as shown in Table 35–2, individuals with cleft palate may also demonstrate hyponasal resonance, mixed hyper-hyponasal resonance, or cul-de-sac resonance. Although hypertrophic tonsils and adenoids are the most common cause of these resonance abnormalities, other factors can result in these symptoms. Patients with repaired palatal clefts frequently have structural deviations of the nasal airway that can result in a resistance to nasal airflow. Additionally, children with cleft palate are subject to the same sources of anterior nasal airway obstruction as noncleft patients, such as allergic rhinitis and other nasal airway changes. Warren[74] and Dalston and Warren[75] have suggested that the nasal cavity is an important factor affecting not only resonance, but articulation and velopharyngeal function as well. Therefore, when hyponasality is present, such should be monitored on an ongoing basis. If the symptoms persist or are reported to be chronic, then further evaluation is indicated, and referral for otolaryngologic evaluation should be considered.

School Age and Later

When velopharyngeal symptoms persist into the school age years, it is critical to establish an aggressive monitoring or management plan to normalize the child's speech as soon as possible in order to avoid social and psychological concerns. Some children continue to present with VPI into the school age years. There is significant variability in treatment protocols across centers, and with a mobile population and follow up difficulties some children may present to a new team or after a hiatus in care. They may therefore present with significant velopharyngeal symptoms that have gone undiagnosed, untreated, or incompletely treated.

The most notable risk for deterioration in velopharyngeal function during the school age years and later relates to changes in the dimensions of the pharyngeal cavity caused either by adenoid involution or maxillary advancement. As the adenoids involute, some children with cleft palate may experience difficulty achieving complete velopharyngeal closure, as the palate can no longer stretch to accommodate the increasing distance of the pharyngeal depth.[76,77]

Similarly, in patients who require advancement of the maxilla through either surgical advancement or distraction, there is a risk that movement of the maxilla and therefore the palate will result in VPI.[78–81] Following either procedure, patients may experience a temporary period of hypernasality or nasal emission. In some instances, surgery may result in permanent velopharyngeal symptoms that will require physical management.

Voice and Phonation

It is a common clinical observation that children with cleft palate have a high occurrence of voice symptoms such as hoarseness, breathiness, low intensity, and abnormal pitch.[82,83] Additionally, it has been shown that children with cleft palate demonstrate a high occurrence of laryngeal pathology including vocal nodules, vocal fold thickening, edema/inflammation, incomplete glottal closure, and hyperconstriction.[83] Although the prevalence of voice disorders in this population is unclear, the data suggest that phonation disorders are more frequent in children with cleft palate than children without clefts. The relationship between cleft palate and laryngeal dysfunction may be congenital or behavioral. For example, as mentioned previously, palatal clefting may be associated with a number of multiple malformation syndromes for which resonance and phonation disorders frequently co-occur. Also, as we have discussed previously, the vocal tract is a complex series of interrelated valves. Impairment in one valve may lead to compensatory activity or impairment in another. Specifically, speakers with impaired velopharyngeal valving may use increased respiratory effort or abnormal laryngeal valving, both of which are potentially damaging to the larynx and which may result in observable laryngeal pathology, voice symptoms, or both. D'Antonio et al.[83] reported that 41% of 85 patients with symptoms of velopharyngeal dysfunction had abnormal voice characteristics and/or observable laryngeal abnormalities. McWilliams et al.[82] reported on 32 children who were described as chronically hoarse who underwent instrumental assessment. Eighty-four percent of these children had some vocal fold pathology, and 59% had borderline velopharyngeal valving. McWilliams et al.[82] reported that alteration of velopharyngeal valving in children with velopharyngeal valving disturbances and laryngeal pathology demonstrated improvement in voice symptoms following management of velopharyngeal symptoms. These data suggest a relationship between velopharyngeal valving and laryngeal pathology. The authors further suggest that some children compensate for minimal VPI by increased laryngeal valving.

Regardless of the cause of the relationship between clefting and phonatory/laryngeal abnormalities, it is important that laryngeal/voice function be screened routinely in children with craniofacial anomalies. For infants, rapid development of laryngeal/voice function takes place in the first 12 months of life. Abnormal laryngeal voice quality in an infant may be a sign of airway obstruction, airway dysfunction, laryngeal manifestation of gastroesophageal reflux, or in some cases a more complex syndrome. Abnormalities of voice in an infant should trigger immediate referral for thorough evaluation. In later development, voice symptoms may also signal behavioral factors, such as voice abuse or compensatory strategies.

PREDICTING FUTURE SPEECH AND LANGUAGE PERFORMANCE

In this chapter, we have discussed the importance of recognizing early speech and language development in children with cleft palate. This is important for several reasons. First, babies are active learners, and a child with a cleft is developing speech and language in the presence of abnormal structure that is going to vary significantly among children. This variability will place demands that differ in type and magnitude from child to child and will therefore result in highly individualized communication strategies and communication impairments among children with clefts. Second, it is valuable to know a child's language age or stage of linguistic development for planning the timing of various forms of physical management, especially the timing of initial palatoplasty. Third, it is also valuable to be aware of early development in order to determine whether early speech and language intervention is required. Finally, with longitudinal information regarding early speech and language development important, information becomes available for attempting to predict later speech, language, and learning performance. In this era of diminishing resources, it is highly valuable to be able to identify which children we should be monitoring more intensively or which children should receive extra services with the goal of preventing some of the long-term impact on communication.

Therefore, a brief review of what is known about prediction of later speech and language characteristics in children with cleft palate is of value. Several predictors of later speech and language development have been identified in infants.[11,84] Chapman et al.[11] suggest that the presence of canonical babbling (i.e., consonant–vowel combinations) and the use of true consonants (i.e., consonants excluding /w/, /j/, and glottals) predicts better speech and language performance during the preschool period. These findings were replicated and extended in a study by Scherer et al.,[84] who found that a measure of babbling complexity known as Mean Babbling Level at 12 months predicted vocabulary size and speech accuracy at 30 months of age. These studies provide strong support for the need to consider early intervention to promote the foundation for later speech and language development. Additionally, the identification of different profiles of speech and language performance suggest that children with cleft palate, who also demonstrate receptive and expressive language delays, are at risk for later academic difficulty especially reading.[28,31] The presence of language impairment, even of a mild form, by entrance to kindergarten places the child at risk for academic delays. The association of language impairment with academic difficulties has such high predictive value that early monitoring and aggressive treatment of language impairment in the preschool period is recommended.

SPECIAL CONSIDERATIONS

As we have discussed, palatal clefting is often associated with other multiple malformation syndromes that may have communication impairment as one feature of the syndrome independent of the cleft palate and/or related to it. Cleft palate/craniofacial teams often serve as regional resource centers for complicated patients with known or suspected cleft palate and other physical impairments affecting the communication system, especially the speech production mechanism. It is not uncommon to have patients referred to specialists in cleft palate for consults regarding a variety of questions related to communication, especially to rule out cleft palate or VPI. Frequently the cleft specialist is asked to assist in differential diagnosis or in treatment planning for these children with complex or challenging impairments that may or may not be associated with cleft palate. Therefore, in this chapter we would like to mention a few of these potentially challenging populations and some of the issues that the cleft provider may encounter.

"Is there a Submucous Cleft-Palate?"

One common and challenging patient is the child who has no or very limited speech production that is referred to rule out a submucous cleft palate or other peripheral, structural abnormality that might account for the lack of speech production. This is most often a very young child in the toddler/preschool age group or an early school age child who uses very limited recognizable, meaningful speech production, or whose speech production is completely unintelligible. These children may present with limited vocalization or extensive vocalization, but their sound repertoire is severely restricted. In many cases, their speech production is characterized primarily by vowels and the nasal consonants. This pattern often results in very "nasal sounding" speech, and hence the child is often referred to the cleft palate team to rule out submucous cleft palate or VPI. In many cases, there is significant hope among family and referring clinicians that the speech delay is due to a simple structural abnormality, such as submucous cleft palate, that can be corrected surgically and rapidly. However, thorough evaluation of the more global communication system in these children often reveals subtle or sometimes more obvious impairments in receptive and expressive language. In general, it is unlikely that an overt cleft palate, a submucous cleft palate, or even severe VPI in the absence of other factors would be the sole cause of such a communication disorder.

Once again, this discussion is more than academic. This is an area with great medical–legal ramifications that impacts not only the speech-language pathologist, but often the surgeons and other medical specialists involved with children with cleft palate as well. When these complex cases are referred to cleft providers, a thorough evaluation should be conducted including an in-depth history, cognitive-academic testing (including some neuropsychometric testing), detailed speech and language evaluation, and speech motor examination.[58]

Late Repair and Communication

Another population that has received little attention in discussions regarding speech and clefting is the recent immigrant or the child of a recent immigrant who presents to the cleft team with an unrepaired or partially repaired cleft. In many cases, these children are non-English speaking or speak English as a second language. These patients can be a special challenge for cleft teams but are especially challenging with respect to speech. One question that is frequently asked about older children or adults with unrepaired cleft palate is whether surgery will improve speech for these patients.

There are few studies on the speech outcomes for palatoplasty or secondary palatal management in patients who receive very late intervention. The few studies that are available are reports from work in developing countries where there has not been long-term follow-up or rigorous speech data. One exception is a report by Sell and Grunwell,[85] who evaluated the speech of 18 patients in Sri Lanka who underwent palate repair after the age of 11 years. The authors found that speech production was usually severely impaired in patients with such late repair, and the post operative results were variable and related to cleft type. Symptoms of hypernasality and nasal emission were improved with surgery, but there was little improvement in speech articulation when surgery alone was provided without speech therapy.

A study by Hall et al.[86] evaluated the outcome of secondary palatal management in adults. These authors suggested that symptoms of hypernasality can be successfully eliminated in adults with cleft palate. The authors suggest that patients should be thoroughly assessed prior to secondary palatal management for both velopharyngeal motion (especially lateral wall motion) and stimulability for articulatory improvement.

The most salient point that warrants mention in this chapter is that the speech of individuals who present at an advanced age with unrepaired palate or severe VPI requires in-depth investigation to determine the source of their speech symptoms. It is most likely that hypernasality and some patterns of nasal emission can be eliminated directly with surgical intervention. However, other articulation errors will require aggressive speech therapy. A thorough understanding of the profile of the individual's communication impairment will allow for realistic expectations from surgical intervention.

A related case that bears mention here is the child who is an active second language learner. There are anecdotal reports that suggest that many children who learn a second language after palate repair or after normalization of velopharyngeal function will demonstrate greater deficits in their primary language. There are no evidence-based studies, however, to document this relationship. One study in the literature describes two cases wherein the speech in two bilingual children was near normal in their second language following pharyngeal flap surgery while they continued to demonstrate numerous articulation errors including compensatory articulation errors in their primary language.[87] Therefore, it is important to consider both languages and phonetic/phonological systems when evaluating and creating treatment plans for bilingual speakers with cleft palate. It is also crucial that the families of bilingual children should be questioned carefully regarding the child's speech quality and intelligibility in their first language. It is sometimes true that the child's articulation skills in English (or the second language) are far superior to those in their first language. In some cases, the child may be experiencing severe difficulties especially in being understood within the family or first-language culture while appearing only minimally impaired in the second language in which clinical speech evaluations are being conducted.

Velocardiofacial Syndrome

Another complex but common patient population often referred to cleft specialists is the child with 22q11.2 deletion syndrome, or velocardiofacial syndrome (VCFS).[88] There is a full discussion of this syndrome in this text; however, communication impairment is one of the prominent features of VCFS and therefore warrants some discussion in this chapter.

Shprintzen et al.[88] first described the speech and resonance characteristics of children with VCFS. Golding-Kushner et al.[89] identified significant language impairment in their population of children with VCFS. Gerdes et al.[90] reported on several measures of cognitive function in a group of preschoolers with VCFS and reported that 62% of the children tested were generally nonoral communicators at 24 months of age and these delays in language were beyond what would be expected for their developmental level. The early literature concerning the communication characteristics of children with VCFS has been largely composed primarily of descriptive, retrospective reports, clinical audits, case studies, and short summary statements.

Only one longitudinal study has been reported and there has been little information comparing the impairments observed in children with VCFS with other clinical populations. Scherer, D'Antonio, and Kalbfleisch[14] followed a group of children with VCFS from 6 months to 30 months of age and compared their communication development with that of comparison groups of children with cleft lip and palate, isolated cleft palate, and typically developing children. In this longitudinal study, the children with VCFS showed significant differences in receptive language, expressive language, and speech sound acquisition compared with the other three groups of children. This study suggested that the patterns of language and speech deficits in children with VCFS were not due solely to the effects of cleft palate or middle ear pathology associated with palatal clefting.

The speech patterns of children with VCFS have been described as having a predominance of glottal stop compensatory articulation substitutions. Reports suggest that 30–84% of children with VCFS have VPI.[91] Glottal stop substitutions appear particularly problematic because they occur for whole classes of sounds. Furthermore, it has been suggested that the high occurrence of glottal stop substitutions is responsible for much of the oral communication impairment in young children with VCFS. However, data from the longitudinal study reported by Scherer, D'Antonio and Kalbfleisch[14] did not support a simple relationship between the severe speech production abnormalities observed for the young children with VCFS and the presence of VPI. In fact, the VCFS group demonstrated significantly greater speech production deficits than children in the two cleft groups who also experienced VPI. The authors concluded that in young children with VCFS, the relationship between VP function and speech sound errors was not as simple and straightforward as has been suggested previously.

In a second study, D'Antonio et al.[92] compared the speech patterns of a group of children with VCFS to a group of children with speech impairment and some of the phenotypic characteristics of VCFS without a deletion at 22q11.2. The findings of this study showed that young children with VCFS had significant deficits in speech performance beyond that of the comparison group. Furthermore, the study demonstrated greater speech impairment in younger children with VCFS, such as smaller consonant inventories, greater number of developmental speech errors, greater severity of articulation disorder, and higher frequency of glottal stop substitutions, than in older children with VCFS or in the children without VCFS. As reported by Scherer et al., the relationship between ratings of velopharyngeal function and the speech variables analyzed in this study was not straightforward.

The data from these two studies has been interpreted to suggest that some children with VCFS demonstrate a communication profile that may be distinctive to this syndrome. To test this hypothesis Scherer, D'Antonio, and Rodgers[56] described the communication profiles of a group of children with VCFS compared with a group of children with Down syndrome. The profiles of the children with Down syndrome showed a flat profile, indicating all measures of communication were similarly delayed relative to chronological ages. In contrast, the children with VCFS showed vocabulary, pattern of sound types, and mean babbling length below cognitive and language age on other measures. The results suggested that communication profiles of children with VCFS differed qualitatively and quantitatively from children with Down syndrome and supported the hypothesis that some children with VCFS present with a profile of communication impairment that may be distinctive to the syndrome. The presence of this distinctive profile of communicative strengths and weaknesses points to the need for thorough assessment of cognitive and, language domains in addition to speech assessment in order to provide for adequate understanding of the disorder and for adequate intervention planning.

Finally, as discussed in the section on resonance and velopharyngeal function, there often is a pronounced need for diagnostic therapy as a means for providing information that will lead to accurate differential diagnosis for patients with VCFS. There are several sources of speech deviation in this population that can make differential diagnosis challenging. For example, it is a common clinical observation among speech clinicians experienced with the speech of children with VCFS that there is sometimes a disproportionate amount of perceived hypernasality in relation to velopharyngeal function as documented endoscopically, radiographically, and aerodynamically.[93] Especially in these cases of apparent disagreement among evaluation methods there is a greater need for stimulability testing and diagnostic therapy to assist in accurate diagnosis and treatment planning.

CONCLUSION

It is well known that the presence of a cleft palate may negatively impact an individual's ability to communicate effectively and may therefore cause significant social, emotional, and educational hardship. Thus, the evaluation and management of communication disorders associated with cleft palate is a critical component of comprehensive cleft care.

Many discussions of communication disorders associated with cleft palate focus on articulation and velopharyngeal function. In this chapter, an attempt has been made to discuss the broader components of human communication and how they are impacted by clefting. Additionally, this chapter was written with the nonspeech pathologist in mind in an attempt to facilitate a more complete understanding and exchange between disciplines.

This chapter has called attention to the developmental course of communication and communication disorders associated with cleft palate. Additionally, we have stressed the importance of considering speech and velopharyngeal function as only one part of the broader communication process. Our discussion of the speech patterns associated with cleft palate emphasizes the view that speech is shaped by many dynamic linguistic processes that are active and that should be appreciated long before the first words are present in a child's communication process.

References

1. Parameters for the evaluation and treatment of patients with cleft lip/palate or other craniofacial anomalies. *Cleft Palate-Craniofac J.* From http://www.acpa-cpf.org/teamcare/Parameters04rev.pdf

2. Martin MC, D'Antonio L. The role of the speech pathologist in the care of the patient with cleft palate. In Booth PW, Schendel S, Hausamen J (eds). *Maxillofacial Surgery,* 2nd edn. St. Louis: Elsevier, pp. 1092–1101, 2005.

3. Riski JE, DeLong E. Articulation development in children with cleft lip/palate. *Cleft Palate J* 21:57–64, 1984.

4. Haapanen ML. Cleft type and speech proficiency. *Folia Phoniatr Logop* 46:57–63, 1994.

5. Shprintzen R. A new perspective on clefting. In Shprintzen R, Bardach J (eds). *Cleft Palate Speech Management: A Multidisciplinary Approach.* St. Louis: Mosby, 1995, pp 1–15.

6. Paradise JL, Bluestone CD, Felder H. The university of otitis media in fifty infants with cleft palate. *Pediatrics* 44:35–42, 1969.

7. Casby MW: Otitis media and language development: A meta-analysis. *American J Speech-Lang Pathol* 10:65–80, 2001.

8. Peterson-Falzone S, Hardin-Jones M, Karnell M, eds. *Cleft Palate Speech,* 3rd edn. St. Louis: Mosby Elsevier, 2001.

9. Broen PA, Devers MC, Doyle SS, et al. Acquisition of linguistic and cognitive skills by children with cleft palate. *J Speech Lang Hear Res* 41:676–687, 1998.

10. Broen PA, Moller KT, Carlstrom J, et al. A comparison of the hearing histories of children with and without cleft palate. *Cleft Palate-Craniofac J* 33:127–133, 1996.

11. Chapman K, Hardin-Jones M, Halter KA. Relationship between early speech and later speech and language performance for children with cleft lip and palate. *Clin Linguist Phon* 17(3):173–197, 2003.

12. Scherer NJ, Kaiser A. Early Intervention for children with cleft palate. *Infants and Young Children* 20:355–366, 2007.

13. Hardin-Jones M, Chapman K, Scherer N. Early intervention in children with cleft palate. *ASHA Lead* 11(8):8–9, 2006.

14. Scherer NJ, D'Antonio L, Kalbfleisch J. Early speech and language development in children with velocardiofacial syndrome. *Am J Med Genet (Neuropsychiatr Genet)* 88:714–723, 1999.

15. Long NV, Dalston RM. Gestural communication in twelve-month-old cleft lip and palate children. *Cleft Palate J* 19(1):57–61, 1982.

16. Long NV, Dalston RM. Paired gestural and vocal behavior in one-year-old cleft lip and palate children. *J Speech Hear Disord* 47(4):403–406, 1982.

17. Long NV, Dalston RM. Comprehension abilities of one-year old cleft lip and palate children. *Cleft Palate J* 20(4):303–306, 1983.

18. Scherer N, D'Antonio L, McGahey H. Early intervention for speech impairments in children with cleft palate. *Cleft Palate-Craniofac J* 45:18–31, 2008.

19. Estrem T, Broen PA. Early speech production of children with cleft palate. *J Speech Hear Res* 32:12–23, 1989.

20. Scherer NJ. The speech and language status of toddlers with cleft lip and/or palate following early vocabulary intervention. *Am J Speech-Lang Pathol* 8:81–93, 1999.

21. Morris H, Ozanne A. Phonetic, phonological and language skills of children with a cleft palate. *Cleft Palate-Craniofac J* 40(5):460–470, 2003.

22. Scherer N, D'Antonio L. Language and play development in toddlers with cleft lip and/or palate. *Am J Speech-Lang Pathol* 6:48–54, 1997.

23. Snyder L, Scherer N. The development of symbolic play and language in toddlers with cleft palate. *Am J Speech-Lang Pathol* 13:66–80, 2004.

24. Eliason MJ, Richman L. Language development in preschoolers with cleft. *Dev Neuropsychol* 6:173–182, 1990.

25. Scherer N, D'Antonio L. Longitudinal study of speech and language in children with cleft palate and children with 22q11.2 deletion. *Presented at the 10th International Meeting of the Velo-cardio-facial Syndrome Educational Foundation and the Fourth International Conference for 22q11.2 Deletions.* Atlanta, GA, 2004.

26. Pamplona MC, Ysunza A, Gonzales M, et al. Linguistic development in cleft palate patients with and without compensatory articulation disorder. *Int J Pediatr Otorhinolaryngol* 54:81–91, 2000.

27. Lowe K, Scherer N. Early academic performance in children with cleft palate. *Presented at the American Speech-Language-Hearing Convention.* Altanta, GA, 2003.

28. Richman L. Cognitive patterns and learning disabilities in cleft palate children with verbal defects. *J Speech Hear Res* 23:447–456, 1980.

29. Richman L, Ryan S, Wilgenbusch T, et al. Overdiagnosis and medication for attention-deficit hyperactivity disorder in children with cleft: Diagnostic exam and follow-up. *Cleft Palate-Craniofac J* 41(4):351–354, 2004.

30. Jones M. Etiology of facial clefts: Prospective evaluation of 428 patients. *Cleft Palate J* 25:16–20, 1988.

31. Richman L, Lindgren SD. Patterns of intellectual ability in children with verbal defects. *J Abnorm Child Psychol* 85:65–81, 1980.

32. Richman L, Ryan S. Do the reading disabilities of children with cleft fit into current models of developmental dyslexia? *Cleft Palate-Craniofac J* 40(3):154–157, 2003.

33. Richman L, Eliason MJ, Lindgren SD. Reading disability in children with clefts. *Cleft Palate J* 25:21–25, 1988.

34. Richman L, Lindgren SD. Verbal mediation deficits: Relation to behavior and achievement in children. *J Abnorm Child Psychol* 90(2):99–104, 1981.

35. Ceponiene R, Hukki J, Cheiur M, et al. Dysfunction of the auditory cortex persists in infants with certain cleft types. *Dev Med Child Neurol* 42:258–265, 2000.

36. Ceponiene R, Haapanen M, Ranta R, et al. Auditory sensory impairment in children with oral clefts as indexed by auditory event-related potentials. *J Craniofac Surg* 13(4):554–566, 2002.

37. Fredrickson MS, Chapman K, Hardin-Jones M. Conversational skills of children with cleft palate: A replication and extension. *Cleft Palate-Craniofac J* 43(2):179–188, 2006.

38. Chapman K, Graham K, Gooch J, et al. Conversational skills of preschoolers and school-aged children with cleft lip and palate. *Cleft Palate-Craniofac J* 35:503–516, 1998.

39. Kuehn D, Moller K. The state of art: Speech and language issues in the cleft palate population. *Cleft Palate-Craniofac J* 37(4):348–361, 2000.

40. Moller KT. Early speech development: The interaction of learning and structure. in Bardach J, Morris HL (eds). *Multidisciplinary Management of Cleft Lip and Palate,* Philadelphia. Philadelphia: W. B. Saunders, 1990, pp. 726–731.

41. Bowen C. *Children's Speech Sound Disorders.* 1998, Retreived 7/22/2006. From http://tripod.com/Caroline_Bowen/phonol-and-artic.htm

42. Dorf DS, Curtin JW. Early cleft palate repair and speech outcome: A ten-year experience. In Bardach J, Morris HL (eds). *Multidisciplinary Management of Cleft Lip and Palate.* Philadelphia: W. B. Saunders, 1990.

43. Stoel-Gammon C, Dunn D. *Normal and Disordered Phonology in Children.* Baltimore: University Park Press, 1985.

44. Trost JE. Articulatory additions to the classical description of the speech of persons with cleft palate. *Cleft Palate J* 18:193, 1981.

45. Hoch L, Golding-Kushner K, Seigal-Sadewitz VL, et al. Speech therapy. *Semin Speech Lang* 7:313, 1986.

46. D'Antonio L. Evaluation and management of velopharyngeal dysfunction: A speech pathologist's viewpoint. *Prob Plast Reconstr Surg* 2(1), 1992.

47. Chapman K, Hardin-Jones M. Phonetic and phonologic skills of two-year-olds with cleft palate. *Cleft Palate-Craniofac J* 29(5):435–443, 1992.

48. O'Gara MM, Logemann JA. Phonetic analyses of the speech development of babies with cleft palate. *Cleft Palate J* 25(2):122–134, 1988.

49. Chapman K, Hardin-Jones M, Schulte J, et al. Vocal development of 9-month-old babies with cleft palate. *J Speech Lang Hear Res* 44:1268–1283, 2001.

50. Hardin-Jones M, Chapman K, Wright J, et al. The impact of early palatal obturation on consonant development in babies with unrepaired cleft palate. *Cleft Palate-Craniofac J* 39(2):157–163, 2002.

51. Golding-Kushner K. *Therapy Techniques for Cleft Palate Speech and Related Disorders.* San Diego: Singular, 2001.

52. Chapman K. Is presurgery and early postsurgery performance related to speech and language outcomes at 3 years of age for children with cleft palate? *Clin Linguist Phon* 18(4-5):235–257, 2004.

53. Jones CE, Chapman K, Hardin-Jones MA. Speech development of children with cleft palate before and after palatal surgery. *Cleft Palate-Craniofac J* 40(1):19–31, 2003.

54. Hardin-Jones M, Jones D. Speech production of preschoolers with cleft palate. *Cleft Palate-Craniofac J* 42:7–13, 2005.

55. Chapman K. Phonological processes in children with cleft palate. *Cleft Palate-Craniofac J* 30:60–67, 1993.

56. Scherer NJ, D'Antonio L, Rodgers JR. Profiles of communication disorder in children with velocardiofacial syndrome: Comparison to children with down syndrome. *Genet Med* 3(1):72–78, 2001.

57. Shriberg LD, Austin D, Lewis BA, et al. *The percentage of consonants correct metric: Extensions and reliability data. J Speech Lang Hear Res* 40:708–722, 1997.

58. D'Antonio L, Scherer NJ. The evaluation of speech disorders associated with clefting. In Shprintzen RJ, Bardach J (eds). *Cleft Palate Speech Management.* St. Louis, MO: Mosby Elsevier, 1995, pp. 176–220.

59. Peterson-Falzone S, Trost-Cardamone J, Karnell M, et al. *Treating Cleft Palate Speech.* St. Louis, MO: Mosby Elsevier, 2006.

60. Pannbacker M. Oral language skills in adult cleft palate speakers. *Cleft Palate J* 12:95–106, 1975.

61. Bardach J, Morris HL, Jones G. The Iowa-Hamburg Project: late results of multidisciplinary management at the Iowa Cleft Palate Center. In Bardach J, Morris HL (eds). *Multidisciplinary Management of Cleft Lip and Palate.* Philadelphia: W. B. Saunders Co., 1990, pp. 98–112.

62. Peterson-Falzone S. Speech outcomes in adolescents with cleft lip and palate. *Cleft Palate-Craniofac J* 32(2):125–128, 1995.

63. VanDemark DR, Hardin-Jones M. Effectiveness of intensive articulation therapy for children with cleft palate. *Cleft Palate J* 23(3):215–224, 1986.

64. Croft CB, Shprintzen RJ, Rakoff SJ. Patterns of velopharyngeal valving in normal and cleft palate subjects: A multi-view of videofluoroscopic and nasendoscopic study. *Laryngoscope* 91:265–271, 1981.

65. Isberg A, Henningsson G. Influence of palatal fistulas on velopharyngeal movements. A cineradiogrphic study. *Plast Reconstr Surg* 79:525–530, 1987.

66. Henningson G, Isberg A. Influence of palatal fistulae on speech and resonance. *Folia Phoniatr* 39:183–191, 1987.

67. Folk SN, D'Antonio LL, Hardesty R. Secondary cleft deformities. *Clin Plast Surg* 24(3):599–611, 1997.

68. Peterson-Falzone SJ, Graham MS. Phoneme-specific nasal emission in children with and without physical anomalies of the velopharyngeal mechanism. *J Speech Hear Disord* 55:132–139, 1990.

69. Morris HL. Clinical assessment by the speech pathologist. In Bardach J, Morris HL (eds). *Multidisciplinary Management of Cleft Lip and Palate,* Philadelphia: W. B. Saunders, 1990, pp. 757–762.

70. Morris HL. Types of velopharyngeal incompetence. In Winitz H (ed). *Treating Articulation Disorders: For Clinicians by Clinicians.* Baltimore: University Park Press, 1984, pp. 211–222.

71. D'Antonio L, Barlow SM, Warren DW. Studies of oronasal fitulae: Implications for speech motor control. *Presented at the Annual Meeting of the American Speech-Languae-Hearing Association.* San Antonio, TX: ASHA 34, 1992.

72. Shprintzen RJ, Sher AE, Croft CB. Hypernasal speech caused by tonsillar hypertrophy. *Int J Pediatr Otorhinolaryngol* 14:45–56, 1987.

73. D'Antonio L, Snyder LS, Samadani S. Tonsillectomy in children with or at risk for velopharyngeal insufficiency: Effects on speech. *Otolaryngol-Head Neck Surg* 115(4):319–323, 1996.

74. Warren DW. Compensatory speech behaviors in individuals with cleft palate: A regulation/control phenomenon? *Cleft Palate J* 23:251, 1986.

75. Dalston RM, Warren DW, Dalston ET. A preliminary study of nasal airway patency and its potential effect on speech performance. *Cleft Palate J* 2:330, 1992.

76. Mason RM, Warren DW. Adenoid involution and developing hypernasality in cleft palate. *J Speech Hear Disord* 45(4):469–480, 1980.

77. Siegel-Sadewitz VL, Shprintzen RJ. Changes in velopharyngeal valving with age. *Int J Pediatr Otorhinolaryngol* 11(2):171–182, 1986.

78. Mason R, Turvey TA, Warren DW. Speech considerations with maxillary advancement procedures. *J Oral Surg* 38(10):752–758, 1980.

79. Kummer AW, Strife JL, Grau WH, et al. The effects of Le Fort I osteotomy with maxillary movement on articulation, resonance, and velopharyngeal function. *Cleft Palate J* 26(3):193–199, 1989.

80. Guyette TW, Polley JW, Figueroa AA, et al.: Mandibular distraction osteogenesis: Effects on articulation and velopharyngeal function. *J Craniofac Surg* 7(3):186–191, 1996.

81. Haapanen ML, Kalland M, Heliovaara A, et al. Velopharyngeal function in cleft patients undergoing maxillary advancement. *Folia Phoniatr Logop* 49(1):42–47, 1997.

82. McWilliams BJ, Lavorato AS, Lavorato CD. Vocal cord abnormalities in children with velopharyngeal valving problems. *Laryngoscope* 83:1745–1753, 1973.

83. D'Antonio L, Muntz H, Province M, et al. Laryngeal/voice findings in patients with velopharyngeal dysfunction. *Laryngoscope* 98(4):432–438, 1988.

84. Scherer N, Williams AL, Proctor-Williams K: Early and later vocalization profiles of children with cleft palate. *Int J Ped Otorhinolaryngol,* 72:827–840, 2008.

85. Sell DA, Grunwell P. Speech results following late palatal surgery in previously unoperated Sri Lankan adults with cleft palate. *Cleft Palate J* 27:162–168, 1990.

86. Hall CD, Golding-Kushner KJ, Argamaso RV, et al. Pharyngeal flap surgery in adults. *Cleft Palate-Craniofac J* 28:179–183, 1991.

87. Borud LJ, Ceradini D, Eng N, et al. Second-language acquisition following pharyngeal flap surgery in non-english-speaking immigrants. *Plast Reconstr Surg* 106(3):640–644, 2000.

88. Shprintzen R, Goldberg RB, Lewin ML, et al. A new syndrome involving cleft palate, cardiac anomalies, typical facies and learning

disabilities: Velo-cardio-facial syndrome. *Cleft Palate J* 15:56–62, 1978.

89. Golding-Kushner K, Weller, Shprintzen R. Velo-cardio-facial syndrome: Language and psychological profiles. *J Craniofac Genet Dev Biol* 5:259–266, 1985.

90. Gerdes M, Solot C, Wang P, et al. Cognitive and behavior profile of preschool children with chromosome 22q11.2 deletion. *Am J Med Genet (Neuropsychiatr Genet)* 85:127–133, 1999.

91. McDonald-McGinn DM, Rossa DL, Goldmuntz E, et al. The 22q11.2 deletion: screening, diagnostic workup, and outcome of results; report on 181 patients. *Genet Test* 1:99–108, 1997.

92. D'Antonio L, Scherer NJ, Miller L, et al. Analysis of speech characteristics in children with velocardiofacial sydrome (VCFS) and children with phenotype overlap without VCFS. *Cleft Palate-Craniofac J* 38(5):455–467, 2001.

93. Riski JE, Solot C, Kirschner R, et al. Pressure flow and nasometric evaluation of velopharyngeal function in velo-cardio-facial syndrome at two centers. *Am Cleft Palate Assoc* 1999.

Assessment of Velopharyngeal Function

Ann W. Kummer, PhD, CCC-SLP, ASHA-F

INTRODUCTION

Cleft lip is an anomaly that primarily affects aesthetics, whereas cleft palate is an anomaly that primarily affects function, particularly speech. In fact, the main reason for repairing the palate is to provide adequate structure and function for normal speech production.[1] When the child is born with a cleft palate, the hard palate must be repaired to provide physical separation of the oral cavity and the nasal cavity. The velum (soft palate) is repaired to provide not only physical separation, but also to support velopharyngeal function. The velum must be able to move quickly, efficiently, and effectively in order to close and open the velopharyngeal valve for normal speech.

Despite the palatoplasty, 20–30% of children with repaired cleft palate will demonstrate some degree of velopharyngeal dysfunction (VPD) resulting in abnormal speech.[2,3] VPD is also seen in patients without a history of cleft palate for various reasons. Incomplete closure of the velopharyngeal valve, even though slight or inconsistent, will almost always affect speech production.

The purpose of this chapter is to discuss methods of assessment of velopharyngeal function for speech, using "low-tech" and "no-tech" procedures. Instrumental procedures for evaluation of velopharyngeal function are also very important, but these are discussed in another chapter.

VELOPHARYNGEAL FUNCTION AND SPEECH

In order to evaluate velopharyngeal function, the examiner must have a firm understanding of how the velopharyngeal valve contributes to normal speech production. Normal speech production requires both intraoral air pressure (for production of consonants) and sound energy (for production of some consonants and vowels). As speech is initiated, air from the lungs and sound from the vocal folds travel in a superior direction from the glottis to the oropharynx. At that point, the velopharyngeal valve must be closed completely in order to redirect all sound energy and airflow anteriorly into the oral cavity for oral sounds. The valve must then open to allow sound energy to enter the nasal cavity for the production of nasal sounds (m, n, ng). Connected speech, which includes a combination of oral and nasal sounds, requires rapid and efficient movement of the velum and pharyngeal walls.

Normal velopharyngeal function is essential for normal resonance. *Resonance*, as it relates to speech, is the balance of sound energy in the cavities of the vocal tract, which include the pharyngeal cavity, oral cavity, and nasal cavity. Because most speech sounds require oral resonance, the velopharyngeal valve is a key determinant of the resonance quality.

Normal velopharyngeal function is also very important for *articulation*, which is speech sound production. When the velopharyngeal valve is closed, the airflow is redirected anteriorly from the pharynx into the oral cavity. By closing or restricting the oral cavity with the tongue, teeth, or lips, the speaker is able to build up intraoral air pressure. The sudden or gradual release of the air results in the production of speech *phonemes* (which are speech sounds, such as /ch/, as opposed to letters which are graphemes). This is particularly important for *pressure-sensitive phonemes,* the *plosives* (p, b, t, d, k, g), *fricatives* (f, v, s, z, sh, zh), and *affricates* (ch, j).

Normal velopharyngeal function depends on three components: normal structure, normal neuromotor skills, and normal speech learning. An abnormality in any of these areas can cause VPD and a resultant speech disorder. When

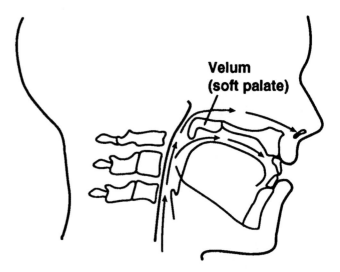

Figure 36–1. Velopharyngeal insufficiency characterized by a short velum. (*Reprinted with permission from Kummer AW. Cleft Palate and Craniofacial Anomalies: Effects on Speech and Resonance, 2nd Edition. Clifton Park, NY: Delmar, Cengage Learning, 2008.*)

evaluating velopharyngeal function, it is important to consider these three components as part of the assessment.

VPD refers to a condition wherein the velopharyngeal valve does not close consistently and completely during the production of oral speech sounds. VPD can be due to a variety of causes, which can be categorized based on the three components of normal function. Based on terminology suggested by Trost-Cardamone,[4] *velopharyngeal insufficiency (VPI)* usually refers to a defect of structure, such as a short velum, which is commonly seen following cleft palate repair (Fig. 36–1). *Velopharyngeal incompetence* (VPI) usually describes a neuromotor cause, such as velar paralysis or paresis wherein the velopharyngeal structures do not move adequately (Fig. 36–2). If there is cortical damage, the

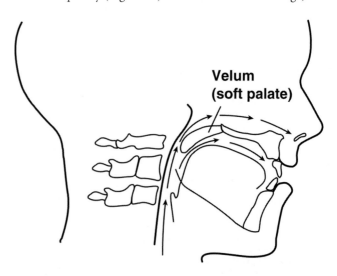

Figure 36–2. Velopharyngeal incompetence characterized by inadequate velar movement. (*Reprinted with permission from Kummer AW. Cleft Palate and Craniofacial Anomalies: Effects on Speech and Resonance, 2nd Edition. Clifton Park, NY: Delmar, Cengage Learning, 2008.*)

patient may have *dysarthria*, which is characterized by poor motor movement of all the speech articulators, including the velopharyngeal valve. VPI, therefore, refers to a medically based etiology that usually requires surgical or prosthetic intervention. In contrast, *velopharyngeal mislearning* refers to a condition where there are misarticulations that result in phoneme-specific nasal air emission or phoneme-specific hypernasality.[5] Although the speech may sound just like "cleft palate speech," this type of disorder requires speech therapy for correction. Because the symptoms of VPD have a variety of causes, a comprehensive evaluation is very important in order to make the appropriate recommendations for treatment.[1]

PATIENT HISTORY

Prior to the perceptual evaluation of velopharyngeal function, the examiner should obtain a thorough history through chart review and family (or patient) interview.[6] The family (and/or patient) should be asked about their observations and concerns regarding the patient's speech. Often, the family will report that the patient has "nasal" speech. In this case, it is best to ask if it sounds like the patient is talking through his nose (hypernasality) or if it sounds as if he is "stopped up" or has a cold (hyponasality). The time of onset can be helpful to know. For example, if hypernasality was present immediately after an adenoidectomy, the cause is likely the increase in nasopharyngeal depth. However, if speech was normal after an adenoidectomy but there was a gradual onset of nasal emission, this would suggest adenoid regrowth with an irregular surface for complete velopharyngeal closure. A history of nasal regurgitation or other feeding problems should be noted.

It is always important to determine what surgical procedures have been done in the past that could affect resonance or velopharyngeal valving. These might include palatoplasty, fistula repair, pharyngoplasty, adenoidectomy, or any other oropharyngeal procedure. Previous radiation treatment to the head or neck would shrink the normal tissues and alter velopharyngeal function. The examiner should ask about signs of upper airway obstruction (such as loud snoring, chronic open mouth posture, or mouth breathing) and signs of obstructive sleep apnea. It is important to know if the patient has any diagnoses or medical conditions that could potentially affect speech, resonance, or neurological development. If the patient has no history of cleft palate, the examiner should determine if there are any physical signs of syndromes that may present with VPD, such as velocardiofacial syndrome. If the patient is receiving speech therapy, it is helpful to know of the most recent goals and whether any recent progress has been made (Table 36–1).

Many clinics and craniofacial teams send each family a preevaluation questionnaire in order to obtain medical and development history and to determine the current concerns about speech.[7] This can save time and ensure the best accuracy of information.

SPEECH SAMPLES FOR ASSESSMENT

When assessing articulation, resonance, and velopharyngeal function, it is important to select an appropriate speech sample to obtain the information that is needed for a definitive diagnosis[5]. In addition to containing the proper types of phonemes, the speech samples sought from children should be developmentally appropriate in the areas of both speech sound production and syntax.

Getting a Reticent Child to Speak

Adults and older children are easy to test because they will cooperate with the examiner's requests. In addition, most children are naturally loquacious, and little or no effort is therefore needed to elicit connected speech. Some children, however, particularly those under the age of 5 years, are shy with strangers and therefore very reluctant to imitate sentences or even to speak during the evaluation. If this is the case, it is helpful to talk to the parents first while the child is in the room. The examiner should occasionally say something to the child, but not ask a question or require a response.

When beginning the actual examination, the examiner should first ask the child "either/or" questions (e.g., "Which do you like better, puppy dogs or kitty cats"?), as noted in Table 36–2. The child is much more likely to respond to these types of questions than to respond to open-ended questions or to requests to repeat words and sentences. Once the child starts speaking, he or she is more likely to repeat and to cooperate with the examiner's requests. If the child does not repeat, then the entire exam can be done using "either/or" questions, although the examiner must be sure that the responses contain the phonemes that need to be tested.

Formal Articulation Tests

The speech assessment should always include a test of articulation. There are two formal articulation tests that were designed to assess patients that might have VPD: the Iowa Pressure Articulation Test, a part of the Templin-Darley Tests of Articulation (Templin, 1969 #46), and the Bzoch Error Patterns Diagnostic Articulation Test (Bzoch, 1979 #54). These tests contain many words with pressure-sensitive phonemes that are particularly affected by VPD.

Although a formal articulation test with single articulatory targets is usually easiest for the novice clinician, normal speech does not usually consist of single words. In addition, velopharyngeal function (and even articulation) may be normal with single word productions but abnormal in connected speech, as such increases the demands of the oromotor system. It is therefore far better to assess articulation in connected speech, or at least with repetitive syllables.

Syllable Repetition

In order to isolate individual phonemes and eliminate the effects of other speech sounds, the examiner can ask the patient

Table 36–1.

Sample Questions for Use in a Diagnostic Interview

Current concern
- What concerns you about your child's speech?
- When did you first become concerned?
- Who referred your child for the evaluation and what was that person's concern?

Articulation
- What types of sounds does your child use during vocal play–vowels only or some consonants?
- If consonants, what are some of the consonants that you hear?
- Are they produced individually or over and over?
- Does the child jabber or use jargon?
- Does your child leave out sounds in words?
- Do you understand your child's speech all of the time, most of the time, some of the time, or hardly at all?
- How well do strangers understand your child's speech?
- Are there any particular sounds that are difficult for your child to produce?

Resonance
- Does your child sound "nasal" to you? If yes, does it sound like your child is talking through the nose, or does it sound like your child has a cold?
- When did you first notice the problem with nasality?
- If the onset was sudden, what event preceded it?
- Does it vary with the weather, allergies, fatigue, or any other factor?
- Do you ever hear air coming through the nose during speech?

Language
- Does your child communicate with gestures, single words, short phrases, incomplete sentences, or complete sentences?
- How many words does your child usually put together in an utterance?
- Does your child leave out the little words (such as "of," "to," "the," "is") in the sentence?
- Is your child communicating as well as other children of his or her age?
- Have you ever had a concern about how well your child understands the speech of others or follows directions?

Medical history
- Was your child born with any congenital problems? If so, what were they? How and when were they treated?
- Does your child have any medical problems, medical diagnoses, or conditions?
- What surgeries has your child undergone?
- Does your child take any medications on a regular basis? If so, what is it for?
- Does your child hear normally? When was the last hearing test?
- Has your child had many ear infections? If so, how were they treated?
- Does your child have any problems with vision?
- Where is your child on the growth chart?

Developmental history
- Was your child quiet, about average, or very vocal as an infant?
- Did you have any concerns about initial speech development?
- Did your child begin to use words before or after his/her first birthday?
- When your child was learning to sit up, stand and walk, did it seem normal or behind other children?
- Did your child walk before or after his/her first birthday?
- Does your child have any difficulty learning in preschool or school?

Feeding and oral–motor skills
- Does your child have any difficulty chewing, sucking, or swallowing?
- Is there a history of feeding problems?
- Does your child drool or keep the mouth open during the day?

(*continued*)

Table 36–1.
(Continued)

Airway
- Does your child snore at night?
- Does your child ever gasp for breath at night or sleep restlessly?
- Does your child like to breathe through the mouth or through the nose?
- Is your child's breathing ever noisy during the day?
- Does your child have allergies, asthma, or chronic congestion?

Treatment history
- Has your child ever had a speech evaluation or speech therapy?
- Is your child currently receiving speech therapy? If yes, what are the goals?
- Has your child's speech improved in the last 6 months? If so, in what way?

(Reprinted with permission from Kummer AW. Cleft Palate and Craniofacial Anomalies: Effects on Speech and Resonance, 2nd Edition. Clifton Park, NY: Delmar, Cengage Learning, 2008.)

to produce consonants (particularly plosives, fricatives, and affricates) in a repetitive manner (i.e., "pah, pah, pah; pee, pee, pee; tah, tah, tah; tee, tee, tee," etc.). By repeating the syllables, this speech segment has similar oromotor demands as connected speech. Each of the pressure-sensitive phonemes should be tested with both a low vowel (i.e., "ah") and then again with a high vowel (i.e., "ee"). This type of test allows the examiner to assess not only articulation, but also test for the presence of nasal emission on each individual phoneme. This procedure also makes it easy to determine if there is phoneme-specific nasal air emission (PSNAE) on sibilants (s, z, sh, ch, j) or phoneme-specific hypernasality, which usually occurs on high vowels (i.e., "ee").

Sentence Repetition

The best way to test articulation and velopharyngeal function is to use a battery of sentences that the patient can repeat, as can be found in Table 36–3. It is preferable to use sentences that contain phonemes that are similar in articulatory place-

Table 36–2.
Sample Questions and Requests in Order to Elicit Speech

What do you like best
- puppy dogs or kitty cats?
- baby dolls or teddy bears?
- cookies or cupcakes?
- chocolate chip cookies or peanut butter cookies?
- singing or dancing?
- baseball or basketball?

(Reprinted with permission from Kummer AW. Cleft Palate and Craniofacial Anomalies: Effects on Speech and Resonance, 2nd Edition. Clifton Park, NY: Delmar, Cengage Learning, 2008.)

ment (such as "Take Teddy to town."). By asking the patient to repeat certain sentences, the examiner can quickly and easily assess articulation, nasal emission, and even resonance in a connected speech environment. This is much more rapid and less expensive than a single-word articulation test. Moreover, it is, in fact, a more valid test of normal speech production than a formal articulation test.[5,6]

When evaluating for nasal emission and the other related characteristics (weak consonants or short utterance length), the sample should contain many pressure-sensitive consonants, particularly those that are voiceless (such as "Sissy sees the sun in the sky."). When testing for hypernasality, the sample should contain a high number of voiced, oral sounds. To separate out the effects of nasal air emission or compensatory errors, the examiner could use a sample with a large number of low-pressure consonants (such as "How are you? Where are you? Why are you here"?). Sample sentences with low-pressure sounds can be found in Table 36–4. To test for hyponasality, the examiner should use sentences with a high frequency of nasal phonemes (such as "My mama made lemonade for me."). Sample sentences loaded with nasal sounds can be found in Table 36–5.

Rote Speech and Counting

Connected speech can be difficult to elicit when testing young children. However, they are often more willing to produce rote speech, such as counting from 1 to 10 or reciting the alphabet. Even producing common rhymes or word games (i.e., "Patty Cake") can help to elicit connected speech.

Counting can also provide the examiner with a very fast, easy, and reliable screening test. To test velopharyngeal function, the patient can either count from 60 to 70, or simply repeat "60, 60, 60, 60" or "66, 66, 66." The word "sixty-six" is a great screening word because it contains several /s/ sounds and the high vowel ("ee"), which are particularly sensitive to VPD. In addition, it contains several /s/ blends ("kst" and "ks"), which further tax the velopharyngeal mechanism and

Table 36–3.

Sample Sentences for Assessment Articulation and Resonance

Have the patient repeat the following sentences while noting articulation errors

p	Popeye plays in the pool
b	Buy baby a bib
m	My mommy makes lemonade
w	Wade in the water
y	You have a yellow yo yo
h	He has a big horse
t	Take teddy to town
d	Do it for daddy
n	Nancy is not here
k	I like cookies and cream
g	Go get the wagon
ng	Put the ring on the finger
f	I have five fingers
v	Drive a van
l	I like yellow lollipops
s	I see the sun in the sky
z	Zip up your zipper
sh	She went shopping
ch	I ride a choo choo train
j	John told a joke to Jim
r	Randy has a red fire truck
er	The teacher and the doctor are here
th	Thank you for the toothbrush
blends	Splash, sprinkle, street

(Reprinted with permission from Kummer AW. Cleft Palate and Craniofacial Anomalies: Effects on Speech and Resonance, 2nd Edition. Clifton Park, NY: Delmar, Cengage Learning, 2008.)

Table 36–4.

Sample of Low-Pressure Sentences for Evaluation of Resonance Without the Complication of Nasal Air Emission

How are you?
Who are you?
Where are you?
Why are you here?
You are here.
They are here.
Where are they?
They are where you are.

(Reprinted with permission from Kummer AW. Cleft Palate and Craniofacial Anomalies: Effects on Speech and Resonance, 2nd Edition. Clifton Park, NY: Delmar, Cengage Learning, 2008.)

Spontaneous Connected Speech

Although the syllable and sentence repetition tests help the examiner to isolate the production of individual phonemes, it is helpful to assess articulation, and particularly resonance, in spontaneous connected speech. Connected speech increases the demands on the velopharyngeal valving system to achieve and maintain closure. As a result, hypernasality and nasal emission will be more apparent in connected speech than in

Table 36–5.

Sentences for Evaluation of Hyponasality, Denasality or Cul-de-Sac Resonance

My mama made lemonade for me.
My name is Amy Minor.
My mama makes so much money.
Many men are at the mine.
Ned made nine points in the game.
My nanny is not mean.
Nan needs a dime to call home.
My home is many miles from her.
Many men are needed to move the piano.

(Reprinted with permission from Kummer AW. Cleft Palate and Craniofacial Anomalies: Effects on Speech and Resonance, 2nd Edition. Clifton Park, NY: Delmar, Cengage Learning, 2008.)

will overwhelm a tenuous velopharyngeal valve. Counting from 70 to 79 can be diagnostic as this series contains a nasal phoneme followed by an alveolar plosive. If there are timing difficulties, this may become apparent in this speech sample as assimilated hypernasality. If there are concerns regarding possible hyponasality, counting from 90 to 99 allows the examiner to assess the production of the nasal /n/ in connected speech.

2. Rintala AE, Haapanen ML. The correlation between training and skill of the surgeon and reoperation rate for persistent cleft palate speech. *Br J Oral Maxillofac Surg* 33:295–298; discussion 297–298, 1995.

3. Witt PD, Wahlen JC, Marsh JL, Grames LM, Pilgram TK. The effect of surgeon experience on velopharyngeal functional outcome following palatoplasty: Is there a learning curve? *Plast Reconstr Surg* 102:1375–1384, 1998.

4. Trost-Cardamone JE. Coming to terms with VPI: A response to Loney and Bloem. *Cleft Palate J* 26:68–70, 1989.

5. Kummer AW. *Cleft Palate and Craniofacial Anomalies: The Effects on Speech and Resonance.* Clifton Park, NY: Thomson Delmar Learning, 2001.

6. Hirschberg J, Van Demark DR. A proposal for standardization of speech and hearing evaluations to assess velopharyngeal function. *Folia Phoniatr Logop* 49:158–167, 1997.

7. Scherer NJ, D'Antonio LL. Parent questionnaire for screening early language development in children with cleft palate. *Cleft Palate Craniofac J* 32:7–13, 1995.

8. Schneider E, Shprintzen RJ. A survey of speech pathologists: Current trends in the diagnosis and management of velopharyngeal insufficiency. *Cleft Palate J* 17:249–253, 1980.

9. Sell D. Issues in perceptual speech analysis in cleft palate and related disorders: A review. *Int J Lang Commun Disord* 40:103–121, 2005.

10. McWilliams BJ, Morris HL, Shelton R. *Cleft palate speech,* 2nd ed. Philadelphia, BC Decker Inc., 1990.

11. Peterson-Falzone SJ, Hardin-Jones MA, Karnell MP. *Cleft palate speech,* 3rd ed. St. Louis: Mosby, Inc., 2001.

12. Zraick RI, Liss JM, Dorman MF, Case JL, LaPointe LL, Beals SP. Multidimensional scaling of nasal voice quality. *J Speech Lang Hear Res* 43:989–996, 2000.

13. Zraick RI, Liss JM. A comparison of equal-appearing interval scaling and direct magnitude estimation of nasal voice quality. *J Speech Lang Hear Res* 43:979–988, 2000.

14. Whitehill TL, Lee AS, Chun JC. Direct magnitude estimation and interval scaling of hypernasality. *J Speech Lang Hear Res* 45:80–88, 2002.

15. Kummer AW, Curtis C, Wiggs M, Lee L, Strife JL. Comparison of velopharyngeal gap size in patients with hypernasality, hypernasality and nasal emission, or nasal turbulence (rustle) as the primary speech characteristic. *Cleft Palate Craniofac J* 29:152–156, 1992.

16. Kummer AW, Briggs M, Lee L. The relationship between the characteristics of speech and velopharyngeal gap size. *Cleft Palate Craniofac J* 40:590–596, 2003.

17. Trost JE. Articulatory additions to the classical description of the speech of persons with cleft palate. *Cleft Palate J* 18:193–203, 1981.

18. Wang NM, Yeung KW, Chen TA, Chen YR. Voice disorders in children with velopharyngeal valving problems. *Changgeng Yi Xue Za Zhi* 13:48–53, 1990.

19. Lewis JR, Andreassen ML, Leeper HA, Macrae DL, Thomas J. Vocal characteristics of children with cleft lip/palate and associated velopharyngeal incompetence. *J Otolaryngol* 22:113–117, 1993.

20. D'Antonio LL, Muntz HR, Province MA, Marsh JL. Laryngeal/voice findings in patients with velopharyngeal dysfunction. *Laryngoscope* 98:432–438, 1988.

21. Kummer AW, Marsh JH. Pediatric voice and resonance disorders. In Johnson AF, Jacobson BH (eds). *Medical speech-language pathology: A practitioner's guide, Vol 613–633.* New York: Thieme, 1998.

22. Paal S, Reulbach U, Strobel-Schwarthoff K, Nkenke E, Schuster M. Evaluation of speech disorders in children with cleft lip and palate. *J Orofac Orthop* 66:270–278, 2005

23. See Scape, Super Duper Publications, Greenville, SC.

24. Bzoch KR. Clinical assessment, evaluation and management of 11 categorical aspects of cleft palate speech. In Bzoch KR (ed). *Communicative Disorders Related to Cleft Lip and Palate, Vol 4.* Austin, TX: Pro-Ed, 1997, pp. 261–311.

25. Haapanen ML. A simple clinical method of evaluating perceived hypernasality.[Erratum appears in Folia Phoniatr (Basel) 1991;43(4):following 203]. *Folia Phoniatrica* 43:122–132, 1991.

26. Johns DF, Rohrich RJ, Awada M. Velopharyngeal incompetence: A guide for clinical evaluation. *Plast Reconstr Surg* 112:1890–1897; quiz 1898, 1982, 2003.

27. Garrett JD, Deal RE, Prathanee B. Velopharyngeal assessment procedures for the Thai cleft palate population. *J Med Assoc Thai* 85:682–692, 2002.

28. Middendorf J. Use of fruit roll ups in occlusion of a fistula during speech assessment. Personal communication, 2005.

29. Moller KT. An approach to evaluation of velopharyngeal adequacy for speech. *Clin Commun Disord* 1:61–75, 1991.

30. Smith B, Guyette TW. Evaluation of cleft palate speech. *Clin Plast Surg* 31:251–260, 2004.

31. Beste DJ. Special considerations in the assessment of the pediatric otolaryngology patient. In Cotton RT, Myer CM III (eds). *Practical Pediatric Otolaryngology.* Philadelphia: Lippincott-Raven, 1999, pp. 3–14.

32. Boorman JG, Sommerlad BC. Levator palati and palatal dimples: Their anatomy, relationship and clinical significance. *Br J Plast Surg* 38:326–332, 1985.

33. Chen KT, Wu J, Noordhoff SM. Submucous cleft palate. *Changgeng Yi Xue Za Zhi* 17:131–137, 1994.

34. Finkelstein Y, Hauben DJ, Talmi YP, Nachmani A, Zohar Y. Occult and overt submucous cleft palate: From peroral examination to nasendoscopy and back again. *Int J Pediatr Otorhinolaryngol* 23:25–34, 1992.

35. Gosain AK, Conley SF, Marks S, Larson DL. Submucous cleft palate: Diagnostic methods and outcomes of surgical treatment. *Plast Reconstr Surg* 97:1497–1509, 1996.

36. Golding-Kushner KJ, Argamaso RV, Cotton RT, et al. Standardization for the reporting of nasopharyngoscopy and multiview videofluoroscopy: A report from an International Working Group. *Cleft Palate J* 27:337–347; discussion 347–348, 1990.

37. Sell D, Harding A, Grunwell P. A screening assessment of cleft palate speech (Great Ormond Street Speech Assessment). *Eur J Disord Commun* 29:1–15, 1994.

38. Sell D, Harding A, Grunwell P. GOS.SP.ASS.'98: An assessment for speech disorders associated with cleft palate and/or velopharyngeal dysfunction (revised). *Int J Lang Commun Disord* 34:17–33, 1999.

37

Instrumental Measures of Velopharyngeal Function

Virginia A. Hinton, MA, PhD, CCC-SLP

INTRODUCTION

As noted in the previous chapter, an experienced speech-language pathologist can make reliable perceptual judgments of velopharyngeal function during speech production. However, the velopharynx is complex and variable, and the ability to obtain objective measures of its function has been a long-standing concern for professionals who are responsible for the treatment of individuals with cleft palate. To that end, many instruments have been used to assess palatal function, either directly or indirectly. The goals of these instrumental assessments have been to provide information that allows for the development of appropriate treatment plans, to assess the effectiveness of treatment and to determine the efficacy of various surgical and/or prosthetic techniques. In addition, instrumental assessment has been used to increase under-

standing of variations in palatal anatomy and physiology in normal and/or dysfunctional velopharyngeal mechanisms.

Generally, if speech is judged to be normal by an experienced speech-language pathologist, instrumental assessment is not necessary. However, if speech characteristics associated with velopharyngeal dysfunction (e.g., hypernasality, nasal emission, or weak-pressure consonants) are observed, instrumental assessment can be used to determine the source and nature of the velopharyngeal deficit or dysfunction. Consequently, the American Cleft Palate Craniofacial Association has stated that "careful evaluation of velopharyngeal function is required for many patients. Procedures include in-depth analysis of articulatory performance, aerodynamic measures, videofluoroscopy, nasopharyngoscopy, and nasometric studies, all of which should be conducted with the participation of the team speech-language pathologist."[1] Multiview videoflouroscopy, nasoendoscopy, and nasometry are the most frequently used instruments for assessing velopharyngeal function[2,3]; however, no universally accepted guidelines are available regarding the type of measures obtained or reporting of that data.

Instrumental techniques can be divided into direct or indirect measures. Direct measures, primarily radiography and endoscopy, allow the examiner to visualize structures used in velopharyngeal closure and the manner in which the structures move during speech. Indirect procedures provide information concerning the results of velopharyngeal function during speech, such as aerodynamic or acoustic events. Both types of assessment have strengths and weaknesses, and no single instrument is sufficient for treatment planning or determining the effectiveness or efficacy of treatment. Combined data from different instruments can be used to provide clinicians with information pertaining to the size, location, and shape of the velopharyngeal port, the nature of the movement and interactions of the velum and pharyngeal walls, and some functional outcomes of velopharyngeal function during speech.[4] Although a thorough assessment should include a combination of instruments as well as perceptual ratings,[5] there are inconsistent correlations between instrumental measures and perceptual judgments,[6] and the acoustic analog of instrumental measurements may vary by speaker and context, suggesting that the resonance characteristics of speech are not solely dependent on the function of the velopharyngeal mechanism.[7] Therefore, data obtained from all instrumental measures must be interpreted relative to perceptual speech performance.

DIRECT MEASURES

Direct instrumental measures allow the examiner to observe one or more components of the velopharyngeal mechanism at rest and during functional activities. Frequently reported techniques include lateral-view cephalometric radiographs, multiview videofluorography, and nasoendoscopy. Additional direct measures that are used for research or are in various stages of development for clinical use include magnetic resonance imaging (MRI), electromyography (EMG), and electromagnetic articulography (EMA). Each type of direct assessment has advantages and disadvantages related to use, interpretation of data, and application to clinical practice.

Radiography

Lateral Cephalometric Radiographs

Lateral cephalometry was one of the techniques originally used to assess velopharyngeal function.[4] It produces still radiographic images obtained at a constant magnification factor, while the velopharynx is at rest and while the patient produces a sustained speech sound, typically /ee/ or /s/. Successful production of either of these sounds requires tight velopharyngeal closure and thus, should provide images that can be compared to rest position images to determine maximum velar excursion and degree of contact against the posterior pharyngeal wall (Fig. 37–1). The use of barium, injected through the nose, can improve the view of the margins of the structures and allow more accurate measurement of a velopharyngeal gap in the sagittal plane. Although lateral cephalometry is a relatively simple procedure, and is quantifiable and reliable

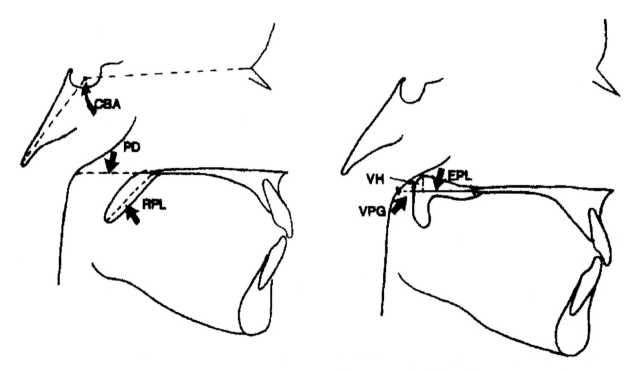

Figure 37–1. (A) Lateral cephalometric roentgenogram during breathing at rest. (B) Lateral cephalometric roentgenogram during production of sustained [s]. (*From Smith & Guyette, 2004, Evaluation of Cleft Palate Speech, Clinics in Plastic Surgery, 31 (1), page 254.*)

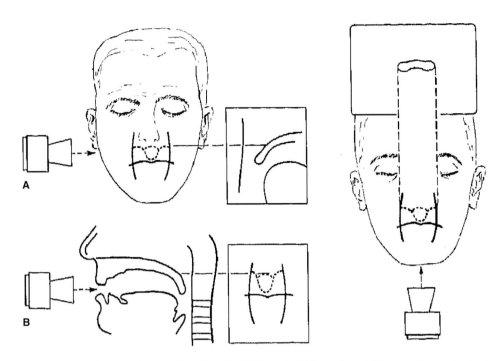

Figure 37–2. Radiographic positioning of patient for (A) lateral, (B) frontal, and (C) base views of velopharyngeal portal. (*From Skolnick, 1975, Velopharyngeal Function in Cleft Palate Speech, Clinics in Plastic Surgery, 2(2), page 287.*)

method for assessing velopharyngeal function, it produces only a two-dimensional static image in sagittal plane of complex three-dimensional dynamic structures. As such, it provides no information pertaining to lateral pharyngeal wall movement or the degree of closure at the midline of the velum. Further, the amount of radiation exposure from this method is typically judged to be too high for the limited amount of information that is obtained.[4] For these reasons, lateral cephalometry is rarely used in assessing velopharyngeal function at this time, but was the source of data for many research studies until the early 1990s. Therefore, caution should be exercised in comparing data from early studies using lateral cephalometrics to data from more recent studies that use current techniques.

Multiview Videofluorsocopy

Improved radiographic technology led to the development of videofluoroscopy. This technique allows examiners to view velopharyngeal function during a variety of speech tasks, with less radiation exposure (approximately one tenth) than lateral still cephalometrics.[8] Videofluorography, which is performed by a radiologist, provides moving radiographic images that allow for measurement of degree and timing of movement of the velum and pharyngeal walls.[8] Barium, instilled through the nose, provides improved visualization of the margins of the velopharyngeal structures. Videofluoroscopy can provide accurate and reliable data if the patient's head remains in a stable position; a consistent speech sample is used that includes the full range of phonemic possibilities in a language, the inherent nonlinearities of the equipment are minimized by frequent calibration, and inter- and

intrajudge reliability for all measures is established at each center.[2,8–11] Radiographic exposure from videofluoroscopy should be minimized by using a narrow radiographic field and limiting the entire process to 2 minutes or less.[10]

Although videofluoroscopy has been used for many years, the types and number of images to be obtained remains controversial. Images may be obtained in lateral (sagittal), frontal, en-face (basal and Towne) views, or in any combination of these views (Fig. 37–2). Lateral views show the extent of velar movement superiorly and posteriorly, as well as the contribution of the posterior wall. However, a lateral view does not provide visualization of the velum in the transverse plane and thus, may lead to an assumption of complete closure when a persistent gap exists at midline or in the area of the lateral ports. Frontal views can be used to visualize the degree, symmetry, and location of lateral pharyngeal wall movement, but do not provide a view of the velopharyngeal gap. En-face views are the least frequently used videofluoroscopic image because of the potential for distortion of the velopharyngeal structures during positioning, thus, artificially increasing the anterior–posterior dimension of the velopharyngeal gap. Despite this limitation, basal or Towne views can be used to obtain information pertaining to the degree of velar and pharyngeal wall movement, and the location, shape, and extent of the velopharyngeal gap during speech.[2,8,10,11] Since no single view provides complete information regarding velopharyngeal closure, multiple views should be used to fully assess degree of movement, coordination of velar and lateral pharyngeal wall movement, size of the velopharyngeal port, and depth of the nasopharynx.[11] The combined information from frontal, lateral, basal, and/or Towne projections provides information about the velopharyngeal port in three dimensions

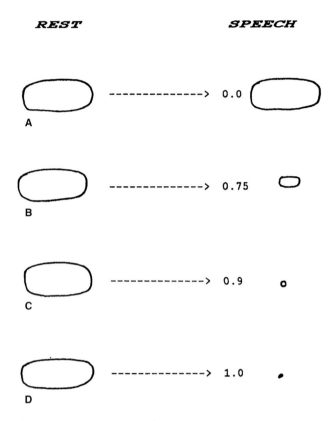

Figure 37–3. Nasopharyngoscopy or en face videoflouroscopy: velopharyngeal gap size as estimated compared to the size of the velopharyngeal valve at rest. The gap may be estimated or calculated by computer programs that compute surface area. (*From Golding-Kushner, et al, 1990, Standardization for Reporting of Nasopharyngoscopy and Multiview Videofluoroscopy: A Report from an International Working Group. Cleft Palate Journal, 27(4), page 341.*)

and provides a more accurate representation of function than any single view.[2]

After videofluorographic images have been obtained, they must be analyzed and reported in a standardized manner to achieve optimal patient care. Anecdotal evidence suggests that during routine clinical evaluations, some professionals simply examine the images visually and make decisions without formal measurements. However, most research studies report the use of absolute measures (e.g., length or angle) or ratios obtained from structures at rest and at maximum excursion. Golding-Kushner[10] reported that videofluorographic standardization should be based on ratios rather than absolute values to eliminate the effects of differences in anatomy and size. Ratios can be computed for the structure being analyzed relative to the resting position of the structure located on the opposite side of the port. In this system of analysis, a ratio of 1 is equal to 100% closure and a ratio of 0 represents rest position or the absence of movement (Fig. 37–3). The use of ratios in this manner can minimize errors related to image distortion and allow for comparison between patients with different sized structures or for individual patients across time. More recently, Johns et al.[4] recommended use of a scale for rating movement of specific structures and velopharyngeal closure. On this scale, 0 represents rest or no movement and

5 represents maximum movement relative to rest position.[3,4] To date, neither of these methods has been shown to be more valid or reliable than the other and both should only be used by well-trained professionals who have established inter- and intrajudge reliability to prevent examiner bias.

Nasoendoscopy

Recent literature suggests that many cleft palate–craniofacial teams in the United States have decided that the use of radiation is no longer essential for evaluation of velopharyngeal function and have chosen nasoendoscopy as their primary instrumental assessment tool.[12] This technique involves the insertion of a flexible endoscope through the nose. It is positioned above the level of the soft palate and allows for visualization of the nasal surface of the velum, as well as the lateral and posterior pharyngeal walls at that level, without interfering with speech production.[8] Unlike videofluorography, which requires participation of a radiologist, valid and reliable measures of velopharyngeal function can be obtained from nasoendoscopy when performed by any well-trained professional of the team, usually the surgeon or speech-language pathologist.[7,11] In addition to a well-trained examiner, patient cooperation is essential for the successful use of nasoendoscopy in children and adults. While most adults can comply with the examiner's instructions to remain still and produce the required speech sample, nasoendoscopy may be difficult in young children because of movement during the procedure, crying, and subsequent irritation of the mucosa.[4,8]

Proponents of nasoendoscopy report that this technique provides substantial information about patterns of velopharyngeal closure (Fig. 37–4), the relative contributions of velum and pharyngeal walls,[2,13] and the symmetry of palatal and pharyngeal wall movement during velopharyngeal closure.[11] In addition, nasoendoscopy has been shown to be the most appropriate instrumental measure for diagnosing an occult submucous cleft[14] and for assessing velopharyngeal closure when a pharyngeal flap has been constructed.[8] Alternatively, nasoendoscopy may not allow for the identification of small velopharyngeal gaps or of the exact position of the gap in three-dimensional space.[4] Additional reported limitations to this technique include wide angle distortion of the lateral pharyngeal walls, difficulty viewing both lateral pharyngeal walls simultaneously, obliquity of view, poor visualization due to glare from the light source, and interference form adenoidal tissue.[8,10]

As with videofluoroscopy, nasoendoscopic images must be measured and reported in a standardized manner to determine the most effective treatment for patients with palatal clefts.[4,10] Golding-Kushner[10] recommends the use of a ratio scale that compares the position of one structure relative to the position of the structure on the opposite side of the mechanism. More recently, Poppelreuter et al.[13] have recommended the use of a transverse sagittal quotient that is calculated by dividing the transverse diameter of the velopharyngeal port by the sagittal diameter (Fig. 37–5). This method provides a quantifiable measure that can be compared across patients or across time.

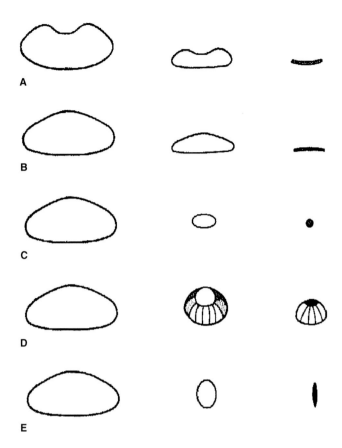

Figure 37–4. Schematic representation of sphincteric patterns of velopharyngeal competence, base view. Left column – contour of portal at rest; middle column – partial closure; right column – full closure. A, Normal subject. B, Repaired cleft palate subject. C, Circular closure pattern, repaired cleft palate. D, Circular pattern with Passavant's ridge, repaired cleft palate. E, Sagittal closure pattern, repaired cleft palate. (*From Skolnick, 1975, Velopharyngeal Function in Cleft Palate Speech, Clinics in Plastic Surgery, 2(2), page 289.*)

Combining Nasoendoscopy and Videofluorography

Limitations to the data available from nasoendoscopy and videofluorography have some cleft palate–craniofacial teams to use both instruments when assessing velopharyngeal closure.

A combined instrumental assessment may include frontal and lateral videofluoroscopic views, as well as en-face videofluoroscopy or nasoendoscopy[10] or, more simply, lateral-view videofluorography then nasoendoscopy when further information is needed.[8,11] Pigott[15] recommends simultaneous recording of videofluorography and nasoendoscopy, so that the endoscopic views can be used to assist in interpretation of complex shadows on the videofluoroscopic image.

Magnetic Resonance Imaging

MRI is a more recent technique for visualizing velopharyngeal function. It has advantages over videofluoroscopy in that it is noninvasive and does not require the use of radiation,[16] and it is superior to other radiographic techniques in terms of visualizing soft tissues, such as muscles.[17] Specifically, MRI can provide clear views of muscle origin, insertion, course, and volume[14] and has been used successfully to provide quantifiable information regarding temporal changes in articulatory structures,[16] to detect the presence of occult submucous clefts,[18] to assess changes in infant anatomy before and after surgery,[19] and to examine the characteristics of levator muscle function during velopharyngeal closure.[17] This information has provided a more complete understanding of the complex biomechanical characteristics of the velopharynx for research purposes and may lead to improved surgical procedures in the future.[20]

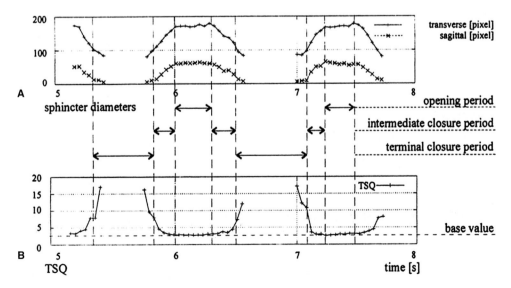

Figure 37–5. The time series plots of the video-endoscopic analysis. A: sphincter dimension. B: TSQ (transverse sagittal quotient) with the base value. (*From Poppelreuter, Engelke, & Bruns, 2000, Quantitative Analysis of the Velopharyngeal Sphincter during Speech, Cleft Palate Craniofacial Journal, 37(2), page 162.*)

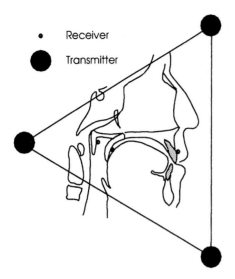

Figure 37–6. Display of transducer positions in the midsagittal plane. (*From Engelke, Bruns, Striebeck & Hoch, 1996, Midsagittal Velar Kinematics during Production of VCV Sequences, Cleft Palate Craniofacial Journal, 33(3), page 237.*)

Despite the advantages of MRI over other radiographic techniques in terms of some types of images, it has limited clinical utility at this time. MRI requires a substantial degree of patient cooperation that is possible for most adults, but many children require a level of sedation that may interfere with their ability to produce adequate speech samples.[14] In addition, MRI is expensive, requires substantially more time to complete that videofluorography,[17] and may distort tissues in the velopharyngeal mechanism due to use in a supine position.[4]

Electromagnetic Articulography

EMA is a relatively recent technique for direct assessment of velopharyngeal function.[13] It is based on the use of alternating magnetic fields that induce voltages in small transducers placed on a speaker's head (Fig. 37–6). One transducer is placed in the midsagittal plane on the oral surface of the velum under local anesthesia. A reference transducer is attached superiorly to the central incisors. The output voltages from the transducers are processed to produce data reflecting transducer positions as a function of time (Articulograph AG 100™, Carstens, Bovender, Germany) and represent degree and direction of velar movement. Poppelreuter et al.[13] state that EMA is an appropriate technique for assessing velopharyngeal function during speech because the velum moves only in the sagittal vertical direction. They suggest further that EMA be conducted simultaneously with nasoendoscopy to obtain a more complete assessment of velopharyngeal function in three dimensions. However, at this time, EMA has limited clinical applications because of the invasive nature of the transducer placement, the time required to complete the assessment, and the limited amount of information obtained.

Electromyography

EMG has been used extensively, experimentally and clinically, to observe muscle activity in many parts of the body. Through surface or hooked-wire electrodes, bioelectric activity resulting from muscle activation can be recorded and analyzed relative to structural movement. Due to the location and complexity of the velar and pharyngeal muscles, hooked-wire electrodes rather than surface electrodes must be used for EMG studies of velopharyngeal function.[4] To date, this direct technique has been used exclusively in research and has provided detailed information regarding levator veli palatini function in relative to intraoral pressure variations,[21] the effect of speech prostheses on muscle function,[22] and muscle reserve in the prior to maxillary advancement.[23] In the future, these data may prove to be important in predicting some surgical outcomes, but clinical use of EMG is limited at this time because of the invasive nature of the procedure,[23] discomfort from placement of electrodes, difficulty in electrode placement due to the small size of the velar muscles, and the variability of muscle location in patients with clefts.[4]

Summary of Direct Measures

Nasoendoscopy and videofluorography are the preferred instruments for directly visualizing the velopharyngeal mechanism during speech production.[3] Other direct methods for assessing velopharyngeal closure, such as MRI and EMG, can provide valuable information related to the biomechanical characteristics of the velopharynx for research purposes, but have limited clinical utility at this time. Both nasoendoscopy and videofluorography present problems in terms of standardization of measurements, clinically and in research, and the use of ratios or scales may improve consistency of reporting across patients and teams. Problems with consistent positioning of a nasoendoscope and distortion of the visual field has led to the description of videofluoroscopy as a more quantitative technique and nasoendoscopy as more qualitative.[15,24] However, some professionals prefer to use nasoendoscopy rather than videofluoroscopy because it does not require the use of radiation.[14] Until more definitive information is available regarding the efficacy of these techniques, either may be used successfully if results are interpreted relative to speech performance. In addition, only well-trained practitioners should perform these procedures and cleft palate-craniofacial teams should use standardized protocols that ensure minimal discomfort and radiation exposure, reliability of the data, and, thus, optimal patient care.

INDIRECT MEASURES

Indirect measures of velopharyngeal function do not provide visualization of the velopharyngeal structures, but they do provide information about the functional outcome of those structures as observed in aerodynamic and acoustic speech events. This information allows the examiner to make inferences about velopharyngeal competence but does not provide information about the movement or relative contribution of the velum and pharyngeal walls to velopharyngeal sufficiency or insufficiency. Most indirect assessment techniques focus on measurement of pressure and airflow patterns or acoustic energy that occurs during speech production. Other indirect techniques include photo-optic transduction and accelerometry. As with the direct instrumental assessments, all indirect assessment methods have strengths and weaknesses that have an impact on their applicability for clinical use. Consequently, indirect measures should never be used in isolation to make decisions regarding patient care, but should be interpreted relative to data from perceptual evaluation by a trained speech-language pathologist, as well as direct measures of velopharyngeal function.

Nasometry

Nasometry is the most commonly used indirect method for assessing velopharyngeal function.[2,3] An early version of nasometry instrumentation was first described by Fletcher in 1970 as an easy, noninvasive method for assessing the adequacy of the velopharyngeal port during speech. Since that time, multiple studies have demonstrated the validity and reliability of this technique.[25–29] Currently, many types of equipment are available for obtaining this measure, including the Nasometer™ (Kay Elemetrics), NasalView™ (Tiger Electronics, Inc.), OralNasal System™ (Glottal Enterprises, Inc.), SNORS™,[30] Aerophonoscope™ (SOREFAC, France), and Nasal resonometer.[31] In general, all of these instruments calculate nasalance, a ratio of acoustic energy output from the nasal and oral cavities during connected speech. To obtain this measure, directional microphones located on either side of a sound separator transduce acoustic energy that is then converted to a nasalance score reported as a percentage. Specifically, nasal energy/nasal energy + oral energy × 100 = nasalance. Higher percentages of nasalance are associated with increased amounts of hypernasality[32] and normative data are available for many languages.[26,33–35]

Different research methodologies have led to widely varying correlations of nasalance scores with perception of hypernasality, ranging from 0.02[36] to 0.82.[25] Despite these reported differences, nasalance is typically more highly correlated to perceptual ratings of hypernasality when nonnasal sentences are used as the speech sample and to hyponasality when sentences loaded with nasal consonants are used. More recently, derived nasalance measures have been reported as useful for routine clinical application. These are nasalance distance (maximum nasalance–minimum nasalance) and a nasalance ratio (minimum nasalance/maximum nasalance).[37] Reportedly, these derived measures allow for a more detailed interpretation of an individual patient's scores, across different contexts and across time.

Variations in nasalance data may occur for reasons other than a change in velopharyngeal function, including the phonetic characteristics of the speech stimulus used during assessment,[35] inconsistencies in positioning the sound separator,[38] differing microphone sensitivities,[39] and the patient's degree of nasal congestion.[40] Further, because of variations in computational algorithms and equipment construction, nasalance scores should not be compared directly when obtained from machines produced by different manufacturers[41] or from different versions of machines produced by the same manufacturer.[42]

Aerodynamics

Because speech is produced on an exhaled airstream that is characterized by varying airflows and a series of pressure waves, measuring the aerodynamic events associated with speech output will provide information about the status of the structures used during speech productions. Specifically, studies of pressure and airflow characteristics during speech can assist in determining the presence and magnitude of velopharyngeal dysfunction.

Pressure and Airflow

Warren and Dubois reported the first use of aerodynamics for assessing velopharyngeal function in 1964.[43] Since that time, many investigators have examined the reliability and validity of these measures for research and clinical purposes.[44–47] Currently, the PERCI-SARS™ (MicroTronics Corporation, Chapel Hill, NC, 27415) is the most commonly used commercially available equipment for assessing velopharyngeal function based on the aerodynamic formula developed by Warren and Dubois.[43] The technique involves placement of one catheter in the oral cavity and one in a nostril held in place by a cork that occludes the nostril. Both catheters measured static air pressures that are transmitted to differential pressure transducers. Nasal airflow was measured by a pneumotachograph attached by tubing or a mask to the unoccluded nostril (Fig. 37–7). The pressure and flow measures are then used by the system to calculate velopharyngeal port size. During the production of bilabial sounds, an area of 0–5 mm^2 indicates adequate velopharyngeal closure for speech, 5–10 mm^2 represents borderline adequate closure, 10–19 mm^2 indicates borderline inadequate, and closure greater than 20 mm^2 represents gross velopharyngeal inadequacy for speech.[48] These values represent the physiologic status of the velopharyngeal port during connected speech, but the actual acoustic analogs are dependent on other characteristics including articulatory behaviors, degree of mouth opening, rate and laryngeal muscle tension, as well as level of nasal resistance.[49]

Like most other instrumental assessments of velopharyngeal function, obtaining aerodynamic measures requires a degree of patient cooperation and a facility with speech production that may not be possible for very young children or patients with cognitive or motor deficits. In addition, modification of the standard procedures may be necessary to obtain accurate in young children.[50] These modifications can include the collection of only differential oral–nasal pressure data, use of nasal mask to obtain pressure and flow data, and use of a nasal mask to collect airflow data only.

Nasal Airflow

As an alternative to a system that incorporates both air pressures and flows in determining velopharyngeal function for speech, some clinicians and researchers have used measures such as nasal airflow only as a means of indirect assessment.[51–53] The use of nasal airflow as an indicator of velopharyngeal function is based on reports of a positive correlation between increased nasal air emission during articulation of nonnasal consonants and perceived hypernasal speech

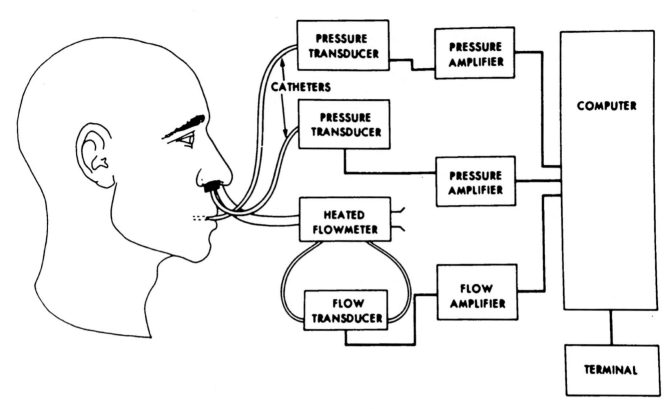

Figure 37–7. Diagrammatic representation of the pressure-flow system used to measure airflow and pressure during production of /mp/ in the word "hamper". (*From Dalston, Warren & Smith, 1990, The Aerodynamic Characteristics of Speech Produced by Normal Speakers and Cleft Palate Speakers with Adequate Velopharyngeal Function. Cleft Palate Journal, 27(4), page 395.*)

resonance.[54,55] In addition, temporal measures of nasal airflow appear to be sensitive to distinguishing between varying degrees of velopharyngeal adequacy in children with clefts.[52] Measures of nasal airflow during speech are obtained from a pneumotachograph attached to a commercially available nasal continuous positive airway pressure mask.[52] A speech sample is recorded simultaneously through a head mounted microphone that is placed in front of the patient's mouth. Measuring nasal airflow appears to be a safe, relatively easy method of indirect assessment that yields a useful and reliable indicator of velopharyngeal function even in small children.[51–53] However, the technique is limited in that it does not quantify the size of the velopharyngeal port during speech or any pressure and airflow characteristics related to velopharyngeal closure.

Accelerometry

Accelerometry indirectly assesses velopharyngeal function by transducing vibration of nasal and laryngeal tissue during speech production. The relative intensities of these signals reflect the relationship between the oral and nasal components of a speech signal.[56] Accelerometry is noninvasive and can provide a valid representation of nasalization associated with velopharyngeal function during speech.[57] The vibrations are transduced by accelerometers or contact microphones that are used in a variety of equipment configurations, including HONC,[6] NORAM,[58,59] and NAVI.[56] All of these systems use similar procedures for obtaining data. However, variations in signal processing and the mechanical characteristics of the equipment result in limitations in comparison of data acquired from different systems.

Typically, accelerometric assessment of velopharyngeal function is accomplished by attaching one contact microphone or accelerometer to the nasal ala on most patent side and another on the thyroid lamina.[6] In young children, an airborne microphone may used for an oral signal to eliminate potential difficulty in attaching an accelerometer to thyroid lamina.[57] Signals from the accelerometers are amplified, low-pass filtered, and rectified.[56,59] The processed data are used to calculate the metric or index that represents the degree of nasalization. Accelerometric data have been used to supplement direct techniques,[6] and have been shown to reliably discriminate different degrees of hypernasality when compared to judgments made by experienced listeners.[59]

Acoustic Analysis

Acoustic analysis is used to describe the intensity, frequency, and temporal characteristics of a speech signal. These characteristics may be displayed and analyzed in the form of a sound wave (pressure as a function of time), spectrum (frequency as a function of amplitude), or spectrograph (amplitude and frequency changes as a function of time). Many commercially available systems are designed for this purpose. When used as an indirect assessment of velopharyngeal function, acoustic analysis has focused on the relative amplitudes of formant frequencies in vowels[60–62] and the temporal characteristics of nasalization.[63] In general, acoustic analyses of speech in individuals with palatal clefts reveal decreased amplitude of the first formant (F1), increased width of formant bandwidths, and increased amplitude between the first two formants (F1 and F2) in the region of 1000 Hz as well as decrease in amplitude at or above F2.[62] In addition, acoustic studies have reported that children with palatal clefts produce longer nasal onset intervals, nasal offset intervals, and total nasalization times than children without clefts.[63] Although there is limited published data relating to the acoustic analysis of speech in individuals with velopharyngeal dysfunction, this indirect technique is noninvasive, relatively easy-to-use with most patients and is, therefore, suitable for clinical use.[60] However, additional investigation is needed to more clearly establish the relationships between velopharyngeal function and the measurable characteristics of an acoustic speech signal.

Phototransduction

Phototransduction involves the use of light transmission to obtain relative information on change in the size of the velopharyngeal port during speech.[4] As described by Dalston,[64] a light source coupled to an electronic detector is passed through the nasal cavity until the light source is below the velopharyngeal port and the detector fiber is above the velopharyngeal port. Changes in the amount of light recorded by the sensor provide quantifiable data that are directly related to the opening and closing movements of the port. This technique provides data that are similar to those provided by aerodynamic measures,[64] but is more invasive and generates a higher level of discomfort.

In order to obtain direct as well as indirect measures of velopharyngeal function, the standard phototransduction system can be combined with nasoendoscopic procedures.[65] Specifically, the phototransduction fibers can be placed through internal instrument channel of a pediatric bronchoscope. Data from this combined system are linear, but measurement errors can occur as a result of variations in positioning.[24]

■ SUMMARY AND RECOMMENDATIONS

In summary, instrumental measures do not evaluate speech performance as perceived by the listener, and recommendations for surgery or prosthetic management should never be made on the basis of instruments alone. Rather, treatment recommendations should be based on information from multiple sources, both perceptual and instrumental. Experienced clinicians from different disciplines can obtain valid and reliable information from a variety of instruments regarding the physical nature of a velopharyngeal deficit or dysfunction that can be used to supplement perceptual speech evaluations. Simply stated, a diagnosis of velopharyngeal

dysfunction is determined by a perceptual speech evaluation and the characteristics of the velopharyngeal mechanism that contribute the dysfunction are described by instrumental assessment. The information obtained from visual, aerodynamic, or acoustics studies can improve surgical planning and provide objective evidence of treatment outcomes. Currently, multiview videofluoroscopy, nasoendoscopy, and nasometry are the most frequently reported methods of instrumental assessment. However, there is no literature that provides the definitive conclusion that any one instrumental method is better than any other method. In many cases, it appears that the personal preference of one or more team members is a major factor in selecting the instruments that are used to assess velopharyngeal function. In light of these findings and because instrumental assessment is only as valid as the instrument used and only as reliable as the user recommendations for optimal use of instruments in assessing velopharyngeal function in patients with clefts include:

1. Input from all team members regarding the type of instrumentation that will facilitate best treatment practices;
2. Consideration of the training, experience, and expertise of those individuals who will be performing the assessments;
3. Individualized assessment for each patient;
4. Understanding the specific purpose of the evaluation (i.e., the need for surgery vs. the type of surgery);
5. The use of direct and indirect measures to ensure complete diagnostic information;
6. Assessment of the trade-off between the desire to obtain accurate and complete information and the risks of discomfort, increased expense, and the potential for cumulative radiation exposure;
7. Ongoing training in current and new techniques through professional development courses, professional meetings, or mentorship by an experienced user;
8. Development of intra and inter.observer reliability ratings for all equipment to ensure collection and reporting of accurate measures; and
9. Compilation of patient outcome data, since the usefulness of any instrumental technique can only be evaluated by measuring the outcomes of whatever treatment recommendation is made.

References

1. American Cleft Palate Craniofacial Association (ACPCA). *Parameters for Evaluation and Treatment of Patients with Cleft Lip/Palate or Other Craniofacial Anomalies,* revised ed. Chapel Hill, NC: ACPCA, 2004, p. 24.
2. Gosain AK, Conley SF, Marks S, Larson DL. Submucous cleft palate: Diagnostic methods and outcomes of surgical treatment. *Plast Reconstr Surg* 97(7):1497–1509, 1996.
3. Kuehn DP, Moller KT. Speech and language issues in the cleft palate population: The state of the art. *Cleft Palate Craniofac J,* 37(4), 348–1,348–35, 2000.
4. Johns DF, Rohrich RJ, Awada M. Velopharyngeal Incompetence: A guide for clinical evaluation. *Plast Reconstr Surg* 112(7):1890–1898, 2003.
5. Chanchareonsook N, Samman N, Whitehall TL. The effect of craniomaxillofacial osteotomies and distraction osteogenesis on speech

and velopharyngeal status: A critical review. *Cleft Palate Craniofac J* 43(4):477–487, 2006.

6. Laczi E, Sussman JE, Stathopoulos ET, Huber J. Perceptual evaluation of hypernasality compared to HONC measures: The role of experience. *Cleft Palate Craniofac J* 42(2):202–211, 2005.

7. Paal S, Reulbach U, Strobel-Schwarthoff K, Nkenke E, Schuster M. Evaluation of speech disorders in children with cleft lip and palate. *J Orofac Orthop* 66(4):270–278, 2005.

8. Havstam C, Lohmander A, Persson C, Dovetall H, Lith A, Lilija J. Evaluation of VPI-assessment with videofluoroscopy and nasoendoscopy. *Br J Plast Surg* 58(7):922–931, 2005.

9. Birch MJ, Sommerlad BC, Fenn C, Butterworth M. A study of measurement errors associated with the analysis of velar movements assessed from lateral videofluoroscopic investigations. *Cleft Palate Craniofac J* 36(6):499–507, 1999.

10. Golding-Kushner KJ. Standardization for reporting of nasopharyngoscopy and multiview videofluoroscopy: A report from an international working group. *Cleft Palate Craniofac J* 27(4):337–348, 1990.

11. Seagle MB, Mazaheri MK, Dixon-Wood VL, Williams W. Evaluation and treatment of velopharyngeal insufficiency: The University of Florida experience. *Ann Plast Surg* 48(5):464–470, 2005.

12. Sommerlad BC. Commentary: Evaluation off VPI-assessment with videofluoroscopy and nasoendoscopy. *Br J Plast Surg* 58(7):932–933, 2005.

13. Poppelreuter S, Engelke W, Bruns T. Quantitative analysis of the velopharyngeal function during speech. *Cleft Palate Craniofac J* 37(2): 157–165, 2000.

14. Rowe MR, D'Antonio LL. Velopharyngeal dysfunction: Evolving developments in evaluation. *Curr Opin Otolaryngol Head Neck Surg,* 13:366–370, 2005.

15. Pigott RW. An analysis of the strengths and weaknesses of endoscopic and radiological investigations of velopharyngeal incompetence based on a 20 year experience of simultaneous recording. *Br J Plast Surg* 55(1):32–34, 2002.

16. Shinagawa H, Ono H, Honda E, et al. Dynamic analysis of articulatory movement using magnetic resonance imaging movies: Methods and implications in cleft lip and palate. *Cleft Palate Craniofac J* 42(3):225–230, 2005.

17. Yamawaki Y, Nishimura Y, Suzuki Y, Sawada M, Yamawaki S. Rapid magnetic imaging for assessment of velopharyngeal muscle movement of phonation. *Am J Otolaryngol* 18(3):210–213, 1997.

18. Kuehn DP, Ettema SL, Goldwasser MS, Barkmeier JC, Wachtel JM. Magnetic resonance imaging in the evaluation of occult submucous cleft palates. *Cleft Palate Craniofac J* 38(5):421–431, 2001.

19. Kuehn DP, Ettema SL, Goldwasser MS, Barkmeier JC. Magnetic resonance imaging of the levator palatini muscle before and after primary palatoplasty. *Cleft Palate Craniofac J* 41(6):584–592, 2004.

20. Ettema SL, Kuehn DP, Perlman AL, Alperin N. Magnetic resonance imaging of the levator veli palatini muscle during speech. *Cleft Palate Craniofac J* 39(2):130–144, 2002.

21. Kuehn DP, Moon JB. Levator veli palatini muscle activity in relation to intraoral air pressure variation in cleft palate subjects. *Cleft Palate Craniofac J* 32(3):376–381, 1995.

22. Tachimura T, Nohara K, Fujita Y, Wada T. Change in levator veli palatini muscle activity for patients with cleft palate in association with placement of a speech-aid prosthesis. *Cleft Palate Craniofac J* 39(4):503–508, 2002.

23. Nohara K, Tachimura T, Wada T. Prediction of deterioration of velopharyngeal function associated with maxillary advancement using electromyography of levator veli palatini muscle. *Cleft Palate Craniofac J* 43(2):174–178, 2006.

24. Karnell MP, Seaver E. Measurement problems in estimating velopharyngeal function. In Bardach J, Morris HL (eds). *Multidisciplinary Management of Cleft Lip and Palate.* Philadelphia: WB Saunders, 1990, pp. 776–786.

25. Dalston RM, Warren DW, Dalston ET. Use of nasometry as a diagnostic tool for identifying patients with velopharyngeal impairment. *Cleft Palate Craniofac J* 28(2):184–188, 1991.

26. Dalston RM, Neiman GS, Gonzalez-Landa G. Nasometric sensitivity and specificity: A cross-dialect and cross-cultural study. *Cleft Palate Craniofac J* 30(3):285–291, 1993.

27. Karnell MP. Nasometric discrimination of hypernasality and turbulent nasal airflow. *Cleft Palate Craniofac J* 32(1):145–148, 1995.

28. Lewis K, Watterson T, Quint T. The effects of vowels on nasalance scores. *Cleft Palate Craniofac J* 32(1):145–148, 2000.

29. Watterson T, Lewis K, Deutsch C. Nasalance and nasality in low pressure and high pressure speech. *Cleft Palate Craniofac J* 35(2):293–298, 1998.

30. Main A, Kelly S, Manley G. Instrumental assessment and treatment of hypernasality, following maxillofacial surgery, using SNORS: A single case study. *Int J Lang Commun Disord* 34(2):223–238, 1999.

31. Birch M, Humphries C, Stock C. Nasal resonometer: An instrument for the assessment and treatment of hypernasality. *J Biomed Eng* 13(5):429–432, 1991.

32. Smith BE, Guyette TW. Evaluation of cleft palate speech. *Clin Plast Surg* 31(2):251–260, 2004.

33. Tachimura T, Mori C, Hirata S, Wada T. Nasalance score variation in normal adult Japanese speakers of mid-west Japanese dialect. *Cleft Palate Craniofac J* 37(5):463–467, 2000.

34. Whitehall TL. Nasalance measures in Cantonese-speaking women. *Cleft Palate Craniofac J* 38(2):119–125, 2001.

35. Sweeney T, Sell D, O'Regan M. Nasalance scores for normal-speaking Irish children. *Cleft Palate Craniofac J* 41(2):168–174, 2004.

36. Nellis JL, Neiman GS, Lehman JA. Comparison of nasometry and listener judgments of nasality in assessment of velopharyngeal function after pharyngeal flap surgery. *Cleft Palate Craniofac J* 29(1):157–163, 1992.

37. Bressman T, Sader R, Whitehall TL, Awan SN, Zeilhoffer HF, Horch HH. Nasalance distance and ratio: Two new measures. *Cleft Palate Craniofac J* 37(3):248–256, 2000.

38. Watterson T, Lewis KE. Test-retest nasalance score variability in hypernasal speakers. *Cleft Palate Craniofac J* 43(4):415–419, 2006.

39. Zajac DJ, Lutz R, Mayo R. Microphone sensitivity as a source of variation in nasalance scores. *J Speech Hear Lang Res* 39(6):1228–1231, 1996.

40. Pegoraro-Krook MI, Dutka-Souza JCR, Williams WN, Magalhães LCT, Rossetto PC, Riski JE. Effect of nasal decongestion on nasalance measures. *Cleft Palate Craniofac J* 43(3):289–294, 2005.

41. Bressman T. Comparison of nasalance scores obtained with the nasometer, the nasalview, and the oronasal system. *Cleft Palate Craniofac J* 42(4):423–434, 2005.

42. Watterson T, Lewis K, Brancamp T. Comparison of nasalance scores obtained with the Nasometer 6200 and the Nasometer II 6400. *Cleft Palate Craniofac J* 42(5):574–579, 2005.

43. Warren DW, Dubois AB. A pressure-flow technique for measuring velopharyngeal orifice area during continuous speech. *Cleft Palate Craniofac J* 1(1):52–71, 1964.

44. Zajac DJ. Pressure-flow characteristics of /m/ and /p/ production in speakers without cleft palate: Developmental findings. *Cleft Palate Craniofac J* 37(5):486–477, 2000.

45. Liu H, Warren DW, Dalston RM. Increased nasal resistance induced by the pressure-flow technique and its effects on pressure and airflow during speech. *Cleft Palate Craniofac J* 28(3):261–265, 1991.

46. Zajac DJ, Hackett AM. Temporal characteristics of aerodynamic segments in the speech of children and adults. *Cleft Palate Craniofac J* 39(4):432–438, 2002.

47. Smith BE, Guyette TW, Patil Y, Brannan TS. Pressure flow measurements for selected nasal sounds produced by normal children and adolescents. *Cleft Palate Craniofac J* 40(2):158–64, 2003.

48. Warren DW, Dalston RM, Trier WC, Holder MB. A pressure-flow technique for quantifying temporal patterns of palatopharyngeal closure. *Cleft Palate Craniofac J* 22(1):11–19, 1985.

49. Kummer AW, Briggs M, Lee L. The relationship between the characteristics of speech and velopharyngeal gap size. *Cleft Palate Craniofac J* 40(6):590–596, 2003.

50. Zajac DJ. Maximizing clinical acquisition and interpretation of aerodynamic and acoustic speech data with velopharyngeal dysfunction. *Perspect Speech Sci Orofacial Disord* 15(2):11–14, 2005.

51. Realica RM, Smith MK, Glover AL, Yu JC. A simplified pneumotachometer for the quantitative assessment of velopharyngeal incompetence. *Annals of Plastic Surgery* 44(2):163–166, 2000.

52. Dovetall H, Ejnell H, Bake B. Nasal airflow patterns during the velopharyngeal closing phase in speech in children with and without cleft palate. *Cleft Palate Craniofac J* 38(4):358–373, 2001.

53. Dovetall H, Lohmander-Agerskov A, Ejnell H, Bake B. Perceptual evaluation of speech and velopharyngeal function in children with and without cleft palate and the relationship to nasal airflow patterns. *Cleft Palate Craniofac J* 39(4):409–424, 2002.

54. Warren DW, Dalston RM, Mayo R. Hypernasality and velopharyngeal impairment. *Cleft Palate Craniofac J* 32(3):257–262, 1994.

55. Lohmander-Agerskov A, Söderpalm E, Friede H, Lilja J. A longitudinal study of speech in 15 children with cleft lip and palate treated with late repair of the hard palate. *Scand J Plast Surg* 29(1):21–31, 1995.

56. Jones DL. The relationship between temporal aspects of oral–nasal balance and classification of velopharyngeal status in speakers with cleft palate. *Cleft Palate Craniofac J* 37(2):363–369, 2000.

57. Jones DL, Morris HL, Van Demark DR. A comparison of oral–nasal balance in speakers who are categorized as "almost be not quite" and "sometimes but not always." *Cleft Palate Craniofac J* 41(5):526–534, 2004.

58. Karling J, Lohmander A, De Serpa-Leitâo A, Galyas K, Larson O. NORAM: Calibration and operational advice for measuring nasality in cleft palate patients. *Scand J Plast Surg* 9(1):261–267, 1985.

59. Karling J, Larson O, Leanderson R, Galyas K, De Serpa-Leitâo A. NORAM—An instrument used in the assessment of hypernasality: A clinical investigation. *Cleft Palate Craniofac J* 30(2):135–140, 1993.

60. Kataoka R, Zajac D, Mayo R, Lutz RW. The influence of acoustic and perceptual factors on perceived hypernasality in the vowel [i]: A preliminary study. *Folia Phoniatr Logop* 53(3):198–212, 2001.

61. Casal C, Dominquez C, Fernández A, et al. Spectrographic measures of speech of young children with cleft lip and cleft palate. *Folia Phoniatr Logop* 54(5):247–256, 2002.

62. Lee A, S-Y, Ciocca V, Whitehall TL. Acoustic correlates of hypernasality. *Clin Linguist Phon* 17(4):259–264, 2003.

63. Ha S, Hyunsub S, Minje Z, Kuehn DP. An acoustic study of the temporal characteristics of nasalization in children with and without cleft palate. *Cleft Palate Craniofac J* 41(5):535–543, 2004.

64. Dalston RM. Photodetector assessment of velopharyngeal activity. *Cleft Palate Craniofac J* 19(1):1–8, 1982.

65. Covello LV, Karnell MP, Seaver EJ. Videoendoscopy and photodetection: Linearity of a new integrated system. *Cleft Palate Craniofac J* 29(2):168–173, 1992.

38

Speech Therapy for the Child with Cleft Palate

Lynn Marty Grames, MA, CCC-SLP

▮ INTRODUCTION

Speech therapy techniques for children with cleft palate are among the best kept secrets in the world of communication sciences and disorders in the United States. Course work in cleft palate is not mandated by the association that certifies training programs for speech-language pathologists. Those programs that do not offer a complete course in cleft palate speech include some relevant material within other courses, perhaps a few lectures. The course instructor may have limited experience with individuals who are cleft-affected. By the time the overview of anatomy, physiology, genetics, communication morbidity, diagnostics, and surgery is complete, there remains little time for discussion of speech therapy techniques. The therapeutic skills of problem analysis, prioritization of objectives, task analysis, and skill training are relegated to the clinical practicum experience.

However, owing to the low population density of individuals with cleft compared with individuals having other forms of communication disorder, many training programs do not have a substantial practicum in cleft palate speech to offer their students. The occasional child affected with a cleft in the clinic may be the best that many programs can offer. But only one clinician can treat that child at a time, and that particular child's disorder may not be representative of larger numbers of children affected with clefts communication disorders. As a result, many fully certified, excellent, practicing speech-language pathologists and academicians in the United States have little to no background and experience with cleft palate-related communication disorders.

This issue was apparent as late as 2004, when an invited tutorial concerning therapy for cleft palate and velopharyngeal dysfunction was published in a journal for school-based speech-language pathologists.[1] The tutorial contained much information that was erroneous or that did not reflect current practice or concepts in cleft palate care. There was much consternation in the community of speech-language pathologists who care for children with clefts. Several groups mobilized to produce lengthy and detailed refutations to the tutorial, and these were published by the same journal in 2006.[2,3] The incident serves to illustrate the depth of unintentional misconception regarding cleft palate speech therapy that pervades the speech pathology profession and training programs in the United States today.

Speech-language pathologists who serve on cleft palate and craniofacial teams have long been concerned about the appropriateness of some therapy techniques used by their colleagues in the community and also with the amount of therapy a child receives in the community. Techniques that have been documented to be ineffective[4,5] continue to be used. Children with cleft palate and/or lip may be grouped with other children with different types of communication disorders, although the program that is effective for the others in the group may not be effective for the child with a cleft.

Books and articles on cleft palate speech therapy have existed under the radar of most practicing clinicians for several decades. Since the turn of the twenty-first century, two books have been published that have received some good attention in the field and that may be effective tools in improving clinical attention to cleft palate speech therapy techniques. In 2001, Golding-Kushner published *Therapy Techniques for Cleft Palate Speech and Related Disorders*.[6] Then, in 2006, Peterson-Falzone et al. produced *The Clinician's Guide to Treating Cleft Palate Speech*.[7] Both provide rationale and techniques for cleft palate speech therapy. Thorough background information is present in each text, and each gives step-by-step instructions for the clinician who is unfamiliar with cleft palate speech therapy techniques. Each has been appreciated and recommended by team clinicians giving guidance to the community clinician.

Can one describe in a single book chapter the essence of cleft palate speech therapy? Of course not. If it was as simple as that, cleft palate speech therapy techniques would be widely known by all clinicians. One can summarize some overarching concepts of cleft palate speech therapy; however, these are the concepts from which a practicing clinician can organize his thought processes when confronted with a child with a cleft.

GENERAL CONCEPTS IN CLEFT PALATE SPEECH THERAPY

1. Not all children born with clefts need speech therapy. The child born with a cleft has a much higher risk for needing speech therapy than the child born without a cleft,[8] but the risk is not 100%. This suggests that the eventual expected outcome for all children with clefts without concomitant neurologic disorder is normal speech.

2. Children with clefts have multiple risks for communication disorder, and the nature of the communication disorder varies widely across children affected with clefts. Therefore, communication diagnostics in children with clefts should be as comprehensive as they are for any child.

3. There may be interaction of multiple systems (phonatory, resonatory, articulatory, linguistic, and auditory) in the child with a cleft palate a communication disorder that should be considered in the diagnostic and therapeutic processes.

4. Cleft–related sound system disorders do not, in most cases, result from muscular weakness or sound-sequencing problems.

5. The most frequently observed disorder is one of articulation, in which the child substitutes one consonant for another. Some of the consonants used by the child may be unusual or atypical. Some may be glottal stops, which may be mistaken for consonant deletions, rather than consonant substitutions. This disorder is described as being a phonetic disorder, as opposed to a phonemic disorder or a phonologic disorder. The error is one of motor output, rather than of linguistic output.[9]

6. Cleft-related articulation disorders respond most readily to a type of therapy that has been described by several terms in the literature: "traditional articulatory approach,"[10] "conventional articulation therapy,"[11] "hierarchical phonetic approach,"[7] "traditional placement procedures,"[5] and "motor skill learning approach."[9] These approaches assume that the child has, as Ruscello[9] explains, "the underlying representation of the sound . . . but has not learned the physical movements or is using incorrect movements . . . to produce the sound."

7. Blowing and sucking exercises, as well as other non-speech or "oral motor" exercises, are not useful. Children with cleft palate do not typically have deficient muscle strength. Nonspeech tasks differ physiologically from speech tasks, so that change resulting from nonspeech exercise does not typically carry over into speech.[12]

8. Resonance disorders resulting from a truly dysfunctional velopharynx will usually not respond to either blowing or sucking exercises or to the behavioral therapy techniques listed in point 6 above. Some forms of articulation disorder can mimic a resonance disorder, and some resonance deviations can have a behavioral or functional overlay. These situations are relatively infrequent, however, and they are the only type that may respond to behavioral therapy techniques.

9. Although normal speech is the expected therapy outcome for children with cleft palate, it is not usually achieved quickly. Therapy resulting in normalization may take several years and a level of intensity not usually available in current medical and educational models. Insurance benefits providing 20 visits a year or 60 consecutive calendar days of therapy, or school programs providing 60 minutes per week in a group of 4, are rarely adequate to meet the needs of the child with a cleft.

10. Since many practicing clinicians do not have a great deal of training or coursework in cleft palate speech therapy,

it becomes necessary for the community-based clinician and the team-based clinician to develop a collaborative relationship when treating a child with a cleft.[13] The team-based clinician usually has the expertise in cleft palate medical, diagnostic, and therapeutic care. The community-based clinician has the knowledge of the child's day-to-day environment and the most frequent contact with the child. Each has a part of what the child needs, and only in partnership can the best possible treatment be provided.

These general principles constitute a very broad, current consensus of cleft palate speech therapy in the United States. There is still a great deal that needs to be done to advance the evidence base in the realm of cleft palate speech therapy, and there is newer research that must be further explored and considered by those concerned with the care of the child with a cleft palate. These issues will be considered next.

PHYSIOLOGIC FORMS OF THERAPY

Two forms of speech therapy hypothesized to improve velopharyngeal function for speech were developed from studies of physiologic theories and principles. In each case, hypotheses were formed around how physiologic function could be improved, and a therapy technique was devised to test the hypotheses. Each uses speech functions, rather than nonspeech functions, to treat speech disorder. In each case, pilot study and data collection occurred before the techniques were published. Although still more information is needed about each technique, each merits further examination and consideration by the community of professionals caring for individuals with cleft palate and velopharyngeal dysfunction.

The first therapy (CPAP therapy)[14] uses Continuous Positive Airway Pressure to provide resistive muscular exercise for the velopharyngeal mechanism during speech tasks. This therapy is carried out as a home program, conducted 6 days per week over a period of 8 weeks. A CPAP machine, normally used to treat obstructive sleep apnea, is used to force air into the nose and through the velopharynx, while the individual articulates syllables and phrases containing both nasal and oral pressure consonants, working to close the velopharynx against the positive air pressure. Gradually, over the 8-week period, the intensity of the air pressure and the length of the session are increased in accordance with exercise physiology principles. CPAP therapy does not treat articulation disorder; it is designed to treat resonance disorder.

Kuehn et al.[14] reported mixed results in a multicenter trial, and indicated that subjects with smaller velopharyngeal air leaks tended to show better improvement than subjects with larger air leaks. Clearly, some subjects do better with CPAP therapy than others, and further study is needed to clarify the best candidates for CPAP therapy. It is important to note that CPAP may only be effective if the individual has oral pressure consonants to be used in the therapy sessions.

Since nasal and glottal stops, nasal fricatives, and pharyngeal fricatives may cause the velopharynx to open inappropriately with speech, their production with CPAP therapy will not yield any useful effect. Only those oral consonants that are appropriately articulated, even if air leakage occurs, should be used in the CPAP regimen.

A second form of therapy is referred to as PiNCH, which stands for "Prolonged Nasal Cul-de-Sac with High Pressure Speech Acts".[15] Following seven principles are cited by Fisher as the basis for PiNCH therapy:

1. Increasing intraoral pressure simulates normal homeostasis and therefore neural programming for normal VP function.
2. Occluding the nares increases intraoral pressure.
3. Using speech acts facilitates carryover into speech.
4. Use of high-pressure speech acts increases intraoral pressure.
5. Adducting the vocal folds, as with voicing, increases velopharyngeal activity.
6. Extinguishing sounds backed to pharynx and glottis reduces velopharyngeal inactivity.
7. Motor learning is achieved through drill, drill, and drill.

The technique involves production of appropriately-articulated, voiced oral pressure consonants with the nose occluded. Intensive (40-minute) sessions at least twice per week were initially piloted, and some subjects showed positive changes. As with CPAP, PiNCH is designed to treat resonance disorder, not articulation disorder, but can be conducted in addition to articulation therapy. More data with additional subjects was reported more recently,[16] also showing promise. A multicenter study involving a larger subject pool is now needed to provide broader and deeper analysis of the technique.

These two techniques are good examples of how the study of theories and principles of speech production drives the formulation of hypotheses, which in turn spur creative treatment techniques for testing. Other translational research is needed to support best practices in cleft palate speech therapy. This direction will be critical to cleft care in the next decade. Other existing treatment issues need to be examined as well.

TECHNOLOGY

Technological advances in the last several decades have rapidly advanced speech diagnostics in cleft palate care, but less advancement has been seen in cleft palate speech therapy. The most prominent instances are biofeedback techniques for velopharyngeal function using videonasopharyngoscopy or nasometry.[17] Case studies have reported various degrees of success in facilitating improved velopharyngeal closure for speech with these instrumental techniques. However, technology has been used less often in the advancement of articulation therapy for individuals affected with clefts.

The exception to this has been in the use of electropalatography, or EPG.[18–21] In EPG, a custom-fitted device, looking much like an orthodontic retainer with carefully placed electronic sensors, can be placed in the subject's mouth. The device records tongue placement during articulation of speech sounds on a video screen schematic. The subject and therapist can use the visual feedback to observe correct and incorrect articulation and to train and habituate correct articulation placements. As with the velopharyngeal biofeedback techniques, case studies have yielded promising results in some individuals.

While interesting and of value, all of these high-tech techniques share the significant drawback of high equipment costs and need for specialized training for the therapist using the equipment. At present, cost restraints within educational and practice systems seldom allow for such equipment or expertise outside of a medical center, and the medical centers are usually not close enough to the patients' homes to allow for regular use of such therapies. In one interesting exception, a program funded to allow use of portable EPG units in schools in Scotland yielded good results in changing abnormal articulation patterns in school-aged children with cleft palate.[11] Other reports of similar programs are absent, however, suggesting that funding for such programs may be difficult to obtain.

Low-tech or no-tech techniques continue to be the standard in most cleft palate speech therapy, and it can be argued that the clinician's and client's ears are the best training tools in the clinician's armamentarium. Intensity of the therapy is one element that may be manipulated and tested for results.

SUMMER CAMPS

Summer camp therapy has existed for many years, and is based on the notion that residential programming offers an opportunity for high intensity that is difficult to replicate in any other program. Various programs have been tried over the years.[22–24] Some summer camps are primarily speech camps, designed to provide an intensive speech articulation training experience. Other camps are more generalized, focusing on educational and psychosocial experiences but also offering speech therapy. Good results in articulation improvement are commonly reported, but long-term stability of the improvement is not consistently seen. There are several factors that may contribute to suboptimal long-term stability. One factor may be differences in the follow-up care available in the community. If one therapist uses very different techniques or approaches than another, the child may lose ground in the adjustment needed to apply new motor skills in a different setting or approach. Secondly, a hiatus in therapy between the summer camp, and the reinitiation of the community therapy (e.g., in the public schools during the school calendar year) may cause a regression that may not occur if the therapy continued without hiatus. A third factor may be the improvement level achieved during the camp experience in combination with the above-noted factors. Good

skills lacking stability, that is, those that are still in need of regular practice and reinforcement in order to be used successfully, are not likely to remain stable without the regular practice and reinforcement. The motor patterns that have fully stabilized in connected speech will be the patterns more likely to withstand a therapeutic hiatus or a change in therapeutic approach.

The summer camp approach is an appealing one, especially if functional bridges between the summer camp therapy and the follow-up therapy in the community can be developed. The disadvantages to a summer camp program are related primarily to labor and facility expenses, which are high. Few centers can afford to provide such programs despite the efficacies that have been reported. In addition, summer camps are generally not seen as ideal environments for the youngest of children, who may not be emotionally equipped to benefit from a lengthy experience away from home and family. It is a frustration that the youngest of children, those who would benefit most from the greatest intensity, are the least able to receive treatment in an intensive setting such as a camp. The risk, then, is that the summer camp becomes a "last ditch" program for the older child with significant communication disorder that should have been corrected years before, had adequate services been provided.

It is clear that, in the ideal world, the young child with cleft palate communication disorder would benefit from intensive and appropriate therapy that would mitigate the need for residential experiences later in childhood. How can this be delivered?

GROUP VERSUS INDIVIDUAL THERAPY

Experienced clinicians often feel that one-on-one therapy offers the best chance to facilitate change in a child. In an individualized situation, the clinician can address specific needs, react immediately to behaviors, and experiment to find the most effective cue or reinforcement without having to accommodate a group of children with disparate needs. This is particularly true when one is trying to alter a motor pattern, which requires constant vigilance over the child's efforts, to be certain that an incorrect pattern is not unintentionally practiced, and which also requires frequent repetitions in a practice session to achieve stability. Motor patterns will likely stabilize more slowly if the therapist must turn away from one child's practice to attend to another's or if the practice time is limited by the clinician's need to attend to another child in a given session. In one study of speech normalization histories in children with cleft palate,[25] the total length of a child's therapy course was increased as the amount of group therapy increased as a percentage of the total time in therapy. This suggests that individual therapy is more likely to result in more rapid normalization of speech articulation.

But what if the child is grouped with his or her own parent or with another child with a similar disorder? Pamplona and Ysunza[26,27] studied two groups of preschool-aged, cleft-affected, Spanish-speaking children. Group language therapy was provided to both groups. In the control group, children were seen in groups of two, with just the speech-language pathologist present. In the experimental condition, children were also seen in pairs, but with their mothers participating in each session. The therapy was conducted three times per week for 1 hour for an entire year. All of the children made gains, but those in the experimental group with mothers participating made the largest gains. The authors posited that the presence of the mothers in the group accelerated language development in the mother–child mode of daily-life interaction. The gains measured were only language skills, not specific articulation skills. It should be noted that Pamplona's and Ysunza's subjects had additional advantages not consistently available in therapy programs in the United States: The subjects were all children with cleft palates, closely similar in age. This type of grouping is seldom available to U.S. children in school programs. The intensity was thrice weekly for 1 year. Even if there were only 40 weeks of the 52 in which therapy was conducted (the article doesn't give the number of sessions), that would mean that each child could have attended 120, quite possibly more, sessions per year. That is far more than the most insurance plans offer an individual in a year in the United States.

ARTICULATION–MOTOR LEARNING OR PHONOLOGIC CYCLE THERAPY

The majority of U.S. texts and articles on cleft palate speech therapy support a traditional, motor-learning based articulation approach to therapy and are skeptical of the phonologic cycle approaches that were designed to teach sound rule use in a fully linguistic context. This preference is based upon the notion that the cleft-affected child has no difficulty with the underlying sound-rule representations, but is applying the incorrect motor pattern to the rule system.

Hodson et al.[28] reported a single subject case study of the phonologic cycle approach with a 5-year-old boy having cleft secondary palate. The child had a functional velopharynx, and the pattern that was judged to be the most deviant was his omission of prevocalic voiceless obstruents. Some might consider this child atypical of the larger population of children with clefts who need speech therapy, since he articulated and used tip-alveolar consonants frequently and substituted them for other consonants. However, his speech intelligibility was reported to be significantly impaired at the beginning of the therapy course, and the authors reported significant improvements after 65 hours of phonologic remediation.

In the 1980s and 1990s, many training programs for speech-language pathologists in the United States taught phonologic cycle therapy techniques and abandoned teaching the older motor learning or phonetic placement approach. The therapy techniques are quite different, and there now exists a generation of speech pathologists for whom the motor learning approach is often an unfamiliar territory.

Pamplona and Ysunza[10] raised questions about the preference for the motor learning approach and undertook to study therapeutic progress of children with cleft palate sound system disorders. In a prospective trial of two matched groups of Spanish-speaking children with cleft palate described as having compensatory articulation disorders, they studied the progress that children made in therapy using a phonologic cycle approach versus a traditional articulation approach. They reported that the total time of speech intervention was significantly reduced when a phonologic approach was used. It was the authors' belief that "speech sound production as an integral component of higher levels of language organization" facilitates more rapid phonetic integration than "traditional treatments which practice execution of gestures in meaningless syllables."

Proponents of the articulation-based motor learning approach will argue that if the child's underlying representations on a linguistic level are intact but the child is applying an incorrect motor pattern, then a linguistic approach will have little effect. The child needs to learn to be able to apply a rapid, automatic motor pattern to the already established linguistic rule system.

Both camps have theories of merit. Prospective studies such as that of Pamplona et al. cannot be dismissed outright. In the process of establishing a comprehensive evidence base for speech therapy in children with cleft palate, additional studies should be conducted to evaluate the merits of the two approaches and to determine the patient characteristics that may cause one approach to be more effective than another in particular circumstances.

THE CHALLENGES AHEAD

There is still much to be learned about the most effective therapies for children with cleft-related speech disorder. Examination of the literature on cleft palate speech therapy yields important information about the level of intensity required for a child to achieve full normalization (Table 38–1). Despite this information, children with cleft palate seem to be routinely underserved in the United States. Educational systems assign a certain number of minutes of service per week, or per school calendar year, to a child, and quite often the therapy is carried out in a group of children who are dissimilar with respect to the etiology and nature of their disorder. The risk of these groupings is that the service is significantly diluted and therefore less effective, even if the therapist is knowledgeable and experienced in cleft palate speech therapy (which is often not the case). In more recent years, school systems have stepped up demands for documentation of adverse educational impact in order to provide service, with the result that children with adequate academic achievement may be denied therapy for sound system disorder.

Therapists in medical and private practice settings are dependent on third-party payor authorization and payment. Allowable levels of intensity are dictated by the particular

Table 38–1.

An Analysis of Amount of Therapy Subjects with Cleft Palate Received in Course of Study, and Outcome Achieved

Study	Number of Cleft-Affected Subjects	Number of Sessions or Total Time in Speech Therapy	Therapeutic Outcome
Hodson et al. [28]	1 (case study)	65 hours	Markedly improved intelligibility
Albery and Enderby [22]	46 (controlled trial)	Once weekly over 2 years vs. 90 sessions in 6 weeks	Significant improvement in intensive course vs. slight improvement in weekly course
Van Demark and Hardin [23]	13 (residential camp)	4 hours per day for 6 weeks	Improved articulatory performance immediately and 9 months after therapy
Pamplona, Ysunza, et al. [10]	30 (controlled trial)	Mean 30.07 months articulation group, mean 14.5 months phonologic group	Elimination of compensatory articulation disorder
Pamplona and Ysunza [26]	41 (controlled trial)	3 hours per week for 1 year	Improvements in language development, greater in group with mothers present for therapy
Grames et al. [25]	173 (retrospective review of controlled surgical trial)	8–1117 sessions; mean 239 sessions over 4.5 years	Complete normalization
Van Lierde et al. [29]	14 (population outcome)	Two to three times per week for 2 years	Near-normal speech
Pamplona et al. [30]	30 (controlled trial)	Small group, 1-hour sessions two times per week, range of 4–27 months in therapy	Complete elimination of compensatory articulation disorder
Brunner et al. [17]	11 pre–post comparison study of biofeedback method	2–16 sessions (two feedback sessions per target sound)	Improved velopharyngeal closure on target sounds

plan under which the patient receives coverage. Plan benefits of 20–60 visits per calendar year are common and may need to be shared with physical and/or occupational therapy. Some plans offer a benefit of 60 consecutive calendar days only after a qualifying surgical procedure; some offer a lifetime benefit of just 60 consecutive calendar days.

Neither the educational nor medical system is providing adequate frequency and intensity of therapy for the child with a cleft-related speech disorder. Until research identifies universally effective means for prevention of cleft-related communication disorders, the challenges ahead for speech-language pathologists who treat children with cleft-related speech disorder are these: (1) To amass further evidence regarding the most effective therapy techniques for particular patterns of symptoms, and (2) To develop educational and medical systems that can deliver the appropriate intensity of service delivery.

References

1. Dworkin JP, Marunick MT, Krouse JH. Velopharyngeal dysfunction: Speech characteristics, variable etiologies, evaluation techniques, and differential treatments. *Lang Speech Hear Serv Sch* 35:333, 2004.
2. Kummer AW, Grames LM, Jones, DL, et al. Response to velopharyngeal dysfunction. *Lang Speech Hear Serv Sch* 37:236, 2006.
3. Bayliss A, Cordero KN, Thurmes A, et al. Response to Dworkin et al. (2004). *Lang Speech Hear Serv Sch* 37:239, 2006.
4. Schneider E, Shprintzen RJ. A survey of speech pathologists: Current trends in the diagnosis and management of velopharyngeal insufficiency. *Cleft Palate J* 17:249, 1980.
5. Hardin MA. Intervention. *Clin Commun Disord* 1(3):12, 1991.

6. Golding-Kushner KJ. *Therapy Techniques for Cleft Palate Speech and Related Disorders.* San Diego: Singular, 2001.

7. Peterson-Falzone SJ, Trost-Cardamone J, Karnell M, et al. *The Clinician's Guide to Treating Cleft Palate Speech.* St. Louis: Mosby, 2006.

8. Peterson-Falzone SJ, Hardin-Jones MA, Karnell MP. *Cleft Palate Speech,* 3rd ed. St. Louis: Mosby, 2001.

9. Ruscello D. Treatment of sound system disorders via motor skill learning. Presented at *American Speech-Language-Hearing Association Convention,* Philadelphia, 2003.

10. Pamplona MC, Ysunza A, Espinosa J. A comparative trial of two modalities of speech intervention for compensatory articulation in cleft palate children, phonologic approach versus articulatory approach. *Int J Pediatr Otorhinolaryngol* 49:21, 1999.

11. Gibbon F, Crampin L, Hardcastle B, et al. Cleftnet (Scotland): A network for the treatment of cleft palate speech using EPG. *Int J Commun Disord* 33:44, 1998.

12. Clark HM. Neuromuscular treatments for speech and swallowing: A tutorial. *Am J Speech Lang Pathol* 12:400, 2003.

13. Grames LM. Implementing treatment recommendations: The role of the craniofacial team speech-language pathologist in working with the client's speech-language pathologist. *Perspect Speech Sci Orofacial Anomalies* 14:6–8, 2004.

14. Kuehn DP, Imrey PB, Tomes L, et al. Efficacy of continuous positive airway pressure of treatment of hypernasality. *Cleft Palate Craniofac J* 39:267, 2002.

15. Fisher HR. Preliminary studies on efficacy of prolonged nasal cul-de-sac with high pressure speech acts (P.i.N.C.H.) on hypernasality. *Internet JAllied Health Sci Prac* 12:2004.

16. Fisher HR. Prolonged nasal cul-de-sac with high pressure speech acts. Presented at the *Annual Meeting of the American Cleft Palate and Craniofacial Association,* Vancouver, BC, 2006.

17. Brunner M, Stellzig-Eisenhauer A, Proschel U, et al. The effect of nasopharyngoscopic biofeedback in patients with cleft palate and velopharyngeal dysfunction. *Cleft Palate Craniofac J* 42:649, 2005.

18. Michi K, Suzuki N, Yamashita Y, et al. Visual training and correction of articulation disorders by use of dynamic palatography: Serial observation in a case of cleft palate. *J Speech Hear Disord* 51:226, 1986.

19. Michi K, Yamashita Y, Imai S, et al. Role of visual feedback treatment for defective [s] sounds in patients with cleft palate. *J Speech Hear Res* 36:277, 1993.

20. Whitehill T, Stokes SF, Yonnie, MYH. Electropalatography treatment in an adult with late repair of cleft palate. *Cleft Palate Craniofac J* 33:160, 1996.

21. Scobbie JM, Wood SE, Wrench AA. Advances in EPG for treatment and research: An illustrative case study. *Clin Linguist Phon* 18:373, 2004.

22. Albery L, Enderby P. Intensive speech therapy for cleft palate children. *Br J Disord Commun* 19:115, 1984.

23. Van Demark DR, Hardin MA. Effectiveness of intensive articulation therapy for children with cleft palate. *Cleft Palate J* 23:215, 1986.

24. Pamplona C, Ysunza A, Patino C, et al. Speech summer camp for treating articulation disorders in cleft palate patients. *Int J Pediatr Otorhinolaryngol* 69:351, 2005.

25. Grames LM, Marsh JL, Pilgram T. Predictive factors for the length of therapy course in children with cleft palate with or without cleft lip. Presented at the *Meeting of the American Cleft Palate-Craniofacial Association,* Minneapolis, MN, 2001.

26. Pamplona C, Ysunza A. Active participation of mothers during speech therapy improved language development of children with cleft palate. *Scand J Plast Reconstr Hand Surg* 34:231, 2000.

27. Pamplona MC, Ysunza A, Jimenez-Murat Y. Mothers of children with cleft palate undergoing speech intervention change communicative interaction. *Int J Otorhinolaryngol* 59:173, 2001.

28. Hodson BW, Chin L, Redmond B, et al. Phonological evaluation and remediation of speech deviations of a child with a repaired cleft palate: A case study. *J Speech Hear Disord* 48:93, 1983.

29. Van Lierde KM, De Bodt M, Baetens I, et al. Outcome of treatment regarding articulation, resonance and voice in flemish adults with unilateral and bilateral cleft palate. *Folia phoniatrica et Logopaedica* 55: 80, 2003.

30. Pamplona MC, Ysunza A, Ramirez P. Naturalistic intervention in cleft palate children. *Int J Pediatr Otorhinolaryngol* 68:75, 2004.

Velopharyngeal Dysfunction

Peter D. Witt, MD

Velopharyngeal dysfunction (VPD) is the constellation of speech production disorders that includes velopharyngeal insufficiency, incompetence, and incorrect learning. Anomalous velopharyngeal closure prevents appropriate speech production. Patients with VPD may present with hypernasality, nasal emission, or facial grimacing. Affected patients often develop compensatory maladaptive articulations that are very difficult to reverse if left untreated. Many times, this failure of the velopharyngeal mechanism is the result of a structural defect of the pharyngeal walls or the velum (soft palate) at the level of the nasopharynx.

Increasingly, speech pathologists and surgeons have converted to using the term VPD in place of the older and more entrenched term, VPI.[1,2] In common parlance, VPI generally means that there is incomplete velopharyngeal valve closure during production of oral speech sounds. Use of the term VPI is confusing, however, because various authors use it to connote "insufficiency," "incompetence," "inadequacy," or "incorrect learning." Although such descriptors are used synonymously, they are not necessarily equivalent. In contrast, the term VPD does not assume or exclude any possible origin of speech symptoms. Anatomic, myoneuronal, behavioral, or combinations of disorders are all possible causes of the dysfunction. VPD occurs in approximately 20% of children who undergo palatoplasty.[3] In-depth evaluation of symptoms, causes, and treatment outcomes are critical aspects of managing patients with VPD.

Patients with VPD should be managed within the context of multidisciplinary team care. In 1988, an international working group convened to standardize definitions and assessment methodologies.[4] The working group strongly recommended implementing a multidisciplinary team approach and using multimodal instruments to evaluate preoperative and postoperative speech outcomes. The group asserted that comprehensive analysis of specific causes of speech production disorders, through perceptual and instrumental measures of velopharyngeal function, allows for customized treatment algorithms for specific patients. Surgical management of velopharyngeal dysfunction combined with postoperative speech therapy is an effective means of normalizing VP function in children after palatoplasty.

ROLE OF THE SPEECH PATHOLOGIST

The surgeon, speech pathologist, and other health care providers work closely together to achieve the goal of optimal patient management. These practitioners collaborate in their review of the in-depth diagnostic assessment results and the individual patient's medical history. Consensus evaluation usually provides an appropriate course of management for affected individuals and allows differential diagnosis to lead to differential management.[5] Ideally, such an approach allows care providers to attempt to match gap size, shape, and velopharyngeal closure pattern to the most appropriate intervention.[6]

Surgeons, as well as lay people, are usually capable of recognizing speech "differences." Perception of "difference" doesn't require a sophisticated understanding of speech physiology, whereas discrimination of the causes and severity/magnitude of that difference and subsequent treatment planning do. Speech and language pathologists are particularly adept at sorting out the components of a communication disorder and their respective weights, frequently dictating *what* receives surgical attention and not *whether* it receives attention.

An example of how the speech pathologist understands the complex and subtle nuances of VPD is the speculative relation between the size of the VP gap and degree of hypernasality.[7] This lack of relation may be due to the fact that the ratio of oral and nasal cavity impedances can affect the perception of hypernasality, and this impedance relationship changes with effort, articulatory configuration, and size of the vocal tract relative to the degree of oral–nasal coupling. Timing of VP closure is also a variable that can affect the perception of hypernasality, especially because the timing of VP opening and closure can be complex in connected speech. Speech pathologists may predict information regarding the VP gap size from the speech assessment alone. Confidence in the prediction is strongest if the patient has a nasal rustle, suggesting a small gap, or if the patient has moderate to severe hypernasality, which is more commonly associated with a large opening. The speech pathologist's understanding of these complex phenomena is both a skill and a talent that surgeons and lay people rarely possess.

The Relationship between Speech Pathologist and Surgeon

It is important to make the critical distinction between velopharyngeal valve function (structural defect) and speech function. The answer to this question is basic to the investigational algorithm, determining not only what to do next, but who is to do it. Treatment may involve repairing the velopharyngeal valve (surgeon) or teaching the speaker (speech and language pathologists). Examining the velopharyngeal valve should be quite straightforward. Can the patient eliminate nasal escape? This is fairly easy to determine by simple mirror test at the bedside. Diagnosis of hypernasality is much more difficult and complex. Using vocal, nonverbal testing can obviate such problems as phoneme-specific velopharyngeal insufficiency. An astute speech and language pathologist should be able to make the determination despite the confounding glottal stops, fistulae, and so forth. Surgeons should emphasize to parents, patients, and other providers that surgical success can be anticipated with respect to nasal escape and hypernasality. The speech and language pathologist's battle for speech and language success (articulation, and so forth) follows.

ANATOMY

The anatomy of the velopharynx (palate, posterior pharyngneal wall, airway) is depicted in Fig. 39–1.

The composite movements of the lateral pharyngeal walls, the velum, and posterior pharyngeal walls, close the velopharyngeal port in deglutition and during oral speech sounds and open the port for breathing and some nasalized articulations. Patterns of closure observed on preoperative instrumental assessments include coronal, sagittal, bow tie, circular, and Passavant's ridge formation (Fig. 39–2).

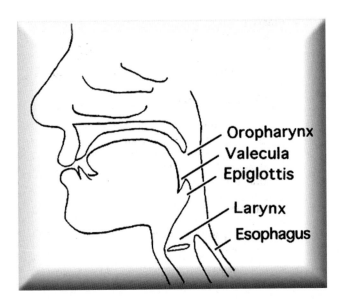

Figure 39–1. Schematic lateral view of the velopharynx illustrating anatomy.

DIFFERENTIAL DIAGNOSIS AND DIFFERENTIAL MANAGEMENT

Several treatment options are available for management of VPD. Once it is documented by perceptual and instrumental measures that speech symptoms are due to a structural limitation that is amenable to physical management, options include prosthetic management, posterior pharyngeal wall augmentation, palatal lengthening and/or re-repair, and velopharyngeal narrowing.

The concept of differential management based on differential diagnosis of VPD has become vogue. The pairings of residual gap size/shape and secondary procedures advocated in this chapter are based on 17 years of experience with intramural outcome assessment. These pairings are made with the

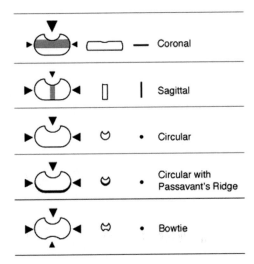

Figure 39–2. Schematic "bird's eye" view of the velopharynx, illustrating directional movements of the representative closure patterns.

assumption that the representative speech sample was made with maximal effort on properly articulated phonemes that require VP closure:

1. If the gap is small and central, the status of the uvula is assessed. If an elevated bulge is present in the midline of the nasal surface of the velum, the muscle is assumed to be intact and functional, and a pharyngeal flap is recommended.
2. If a bulge in the midline is not present, a radical intravelar veloplasty, or a double opposing Z-plasty is recommended.
3. If there is a large central gap or coronal gap with bow tie or without midline contact to posterior pharyngeal wall or hypodynamic, a sphincter pharyngoplasty is recommended.

BASIC SPEECH TERMINOLOGY FOR THE SURGEON

Presumably, care providers representing the various disciplines of the cleft team use the same nomenclature so that they may organize and communicate their knowledge effectively. Trost–Cardamone[8] developed a useful taxonomy to classify possible causative factors of VPD.

In velopharyngeal insufficiency, there is insufficient tissue to accomplish closure of the velopharyngeal sphincter. Additionally, velopharyngeal insufficiency occurs when structural etiologies exist, such as mechanical interferences with closure (including excessively large tonsils and/or webbing of the posterior tonsillar pillars).[9]

Velopharyngeal incompetence occurs with neurogenic etiologies, such as motor disorders.

Velopharyngeal incorrect learning may be the result of phoneme-specific nasal emission and deafness or hearing impairment.

Hypernasality and hyponasality are resonance types. Hypernasality is excessive resonance in the nasal cavity that is usually related to VPD because of a lack of barrier between oral and nasal cavities. Whereas hypernasality usually refers to velopharyngeal function, it may be secondary to a fistula or unrepaired cleft palate. Hyponasality refers to diminished resonance in the nasal cavity and is usually due to anatomic obstruction of the nasopharyngeal airway.

A lexicon of additional terms used to describe some elements of cleft palate speech dysfunction is provided in Table 39–1.[10,11]

HISTORY AND PHYSICAL EXAMINATION: FOCUS OF THE INITIAL CONSULTATION

When a patient is referred for surgical treatment of VPD, the surgeon should elicit specific information germane to speech problems and/or cleft palate:

Questions: Has the speech production disorder caused psychosocial stigmatization, peer teasing, or frustration in

Table 39–1.

Some Characteristics of Cleft Palate Speech

Nasalance	An acoustic correlate of nasal resonance, calculated as ratio of nasal to nasal plus oral acoustic energy
Nasal emission	Different from nasal acoustic energy; nasal air escape associated with hypernasality. Nasal emission and turbulence are disturbances of airflow mostly on production of pressure consonants
Nasal rustle, or turbulence	Nasal rustle or turbulence is distracting, accompanies consonant production. Generally, small constriction in the nasopharynx produces a distinctive fricative sound. On the voiced pressure consonants b, d, and g
Hypernasality	Nasally escaping air reverberating in a confined postnasal space
Grimace	Aberrant facial muscle movement, subconscious attempt to inhibit the abnormal nasal airflow by constricting the nares
Hyponasality	Blocked up tone; may occur with nasal obstruction; enlarged adenoids, deviated septum, inadequate nasal airway, or chronic catarrh

not being able to communicate with others? Are nasal regurgitation of liquids or solids and associated hygiene problems a source of social embarrassment?

Findings: During intraoral inspection, the surgeon should look for palatal fistulae, enlarged tonsils, visibly aberrant carotid pulsations along the posterior pharyngeal wall, a prominent adenoid pad, a palatal zona pellucidum, a palpable notch at the junction of the hard and soft palate, and a bifid uvula. Assessment of velar mobility (elevation) and levator muscle orientation during speech tasks indirectly assesses levator muscle status.

Provocative tests: There are simple bedside maneuvers that can help define the speech problem. A pocket-sized handheld mirror may be placed beneath the patient's nares in order to observe nasal airflow (visible nasal air emission).

It may be difficult to distinguish hypernasality from hyponasality. To help make the distinction, one may use the bedside "pinch test," alternately occluding the nares while asking the patient to recite the same word. Patients with denasal speech will exhibit little change in the speech sound while pinching the nostrils, whereas patients with hypernasal speech will exhibit significant change in the nasal quality of the speech sound. Another provocative bedside maneuver is the straw test. A straw may be placed at the corner of the patient's mouth while he/she recites a speech task. The listener at the other end of the straw perceives amplified air sound and/or unmasked hypernasality.

It is useful to listen to both spontaneous speech and structured provocative samples. Provocative samples of speech are designed to elicit phonemes requiring velopharyngeal closure. A representative sequence might include the following words or phrases: "ma, ma, ma," "puppy," "puffy," "muffin," "pamper," "sissy," "go get a big egg," "bye-bye

Bobby," "Katy likes cookies," "Sally sees the sky." Production of voiceless consonants such as 'p,' 't,' 'k,' 's,' 'f,' 'sh' require maximal pulmonary pressures and are thus a brief screen for integrity of plosive sounds. One should try to ascertain overall intelligibility in running, spontaneous, connected speech. Patients with suspected velopharyngeal dysfunction are incapable of achieving velopharyngeal closure on maximum effort, when producing properly articulated phonemes that require closure.

It should be emphasized that errors in these sequences of sounds should serve only as a "red flag" for the surgeon; interpretive significance of the errors should be left to the qualified speech and language pathologist. Most physicians are unfamiliar with the behavioral variables that can affect velopharyngeal function, such as oronasal discrimination proficiency, the presence of maladaptive articulations, the effects of co-articulation, range of articulatory motion, and the contribution of speaking effort. The speech evaluation should include attention to error types and "stimulability" of performance during visualization of dynamic speech activity. Arguably, it is the speech pathologist who best understands and interprets the movements and the use of the articulatory and vocal structures.

AIRWAY EVALUATION

Lymphoid hyperplasia is not in itself an indication for tonsillectomy, but it may have consequences that warrant surgery. The tonsils and adenoids are often important components of the velopharyngeal closure mechanism. Occasionally, hypertrophic tonsils may herniate into the velopharyngeal port, so that lymphoid obstruction may actually be a source of speech dysfunction or chronic obstructive sleep apnea.[12] At other times, enlarged tonsils may limit the technical placement of pharyngoplasty flaps, or their sheer size may efface the myomucosal pillars, making flap elevation difficult. Similarly, enlarged, friable, and hemorrhagic adenoids may inhibit performance of velopharyngeal surgery, and their presence may even compromise intervention outcome. In these circumstances, preoperative tonsillectomy and/or adenoidectomy may be indicated.

This decision, however, must be made cautiously, in conjunction with the team otolaryngologist and speech pathologist. Tonsillectomy and particularly adenoidectomy should be avoided in any patient with symptoms of velopharyngeal dysfunction until a differential diagnosis is established and a management plan is formulated by care providers and accepted by the patient and family. Clinical manifestations of velopharyngeal dysfunction are likely to worsen after adenoidectomy. If it is necessary to perform adenoidectomy to facilitate technical execution of velopharyngeal surgery, the patient and family need to be duly warned about this predictable deterioration. The surgeon should wait 3 months or more after adenoidectomy before proceeding with velopharyngeal surgery. It is wise to *personally* communicate with the team otolaryngologist to be certain he/she preserves the precious posterior tonsillar pillar tissue for later construction of the port.

Historically, otolaryngologists, plastic surgeons, and speech pathologists have been reluctant to recommend adenotonsillectomy for patients with cleft palate. This reluctance is based on the experience of having the procedure unmask VPD which was not present preoperatively, or of having the procedure exacerbate preexisting VPD. In reality, it is the adenoids rather than the tonsils that are more frequently the culprit of the iatrogeny. The tonsils and adenoids have very different potentials for impairing normal speech. On the other hand, it is known that in some cases, tonsillectomy alone may be curative of VPD. Tonsils may interfere with palatal motion by intruding into the velopharynx, producing a muffled speech effect (the potato-in-mouth phenomenon). These differences in structure and function account for differences in the perception of hypernasal acoustic resonance.

INSTRUMENTAL ASSESSMENT OF SPEECH

Several diagnostic modalities assess speech production in patients who demonstrate symptoms of VPD. Detailed descriptions of these modalities are found in published articles[13] and in other chapters of this text. These modalities include video-recorded standard perceptual speech screenings (acoustic evaluation of sounds or listener judgments), nasendoscopy, nasometry, aerodynamics, and/or fluoroscopic speech evaluations. The studies have the advantage of being readily archived on digital media for review, study, strobe analysis, and so forth. Usually, test results are reviewed by the interdisciplinary staff of velopharyngeal specialists, including a speech and language pathologist, otolaryngologist, prostho-

dontist, and plastic surgeon. The composite data gathered about velopharyngeal closure pattern size of gap, symmetry, activity of pharyngeal walls, and soft palate allow clinicians to distinguish different patterns of VPD.

If cephalometric evaluations are available, they can facilitate diagnosis. Tracings can quantitatively assess the ratio of velar length to velopharyngeal depth, often a good predictor of which patients will require physical management of the velopharynx.

MANAGING VPD

Nonsurgical and Treatment Options

In a small number of cases, prosthetic management may be the best solution for treatment of velopharyngeal dysfunction. Prostheses include:

- Palatal lift: Good for patients with adequate tissue but poor control of coordination and timing of velopharyngeal movements (Figs. 39–3 and 39–4).
- Speech bulb/obturator: An acrylic mass used for closing residual velopharyngeal gaps to achieve closure when there is inadequate tissue.

Prostheses may be used as a temporary "reversible trial," by providing diagnostic information in patients with variable VPD in whom it is unclear whether surgery alone will provide significant improvement in speech quality. A prosthesis may

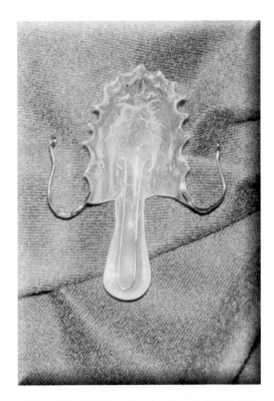

Figure 39–3. Palatal lift, showing hard and soft palatal components.

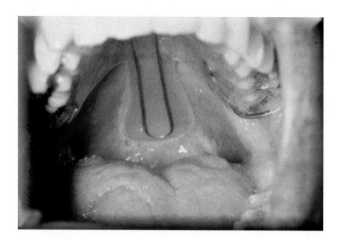

Figure 39–4. Palatal lift in situ.

be useful in some patients with a short, scarred velum; or in other patients with a long supple paretic velum. Some authors have hypothesized that prostheses may stimulate neuromuscular activity,[14] although definitive proof for this is lacking.[15]

Contraindications to Surgery

Velopharyngeal narrowing procedures are not appropriate for patients who meet the following criteria:

- Patient declines surgical management by choice.
- Patient has known or suspected risk for airway obstruction.
- Patient has intermittent or inconsistent closure that responds well to speech therapy.
- Patient has incomplete diagnostic results. With further studies and improvements in diagnostic technologies, speech production disorders should be more accurately assessed and individually managed to achieve optimal results.

Visible pulsations on the posterior pharyngeal wall, indicating aberrant carotid arteries, should not be an absolute contraindication to surgery.[16]

What about aberrant carotid arteries? Anomalous internal carotid arteries have been shown to be a frequent feature of 22q11.2 (velocardiofacial) syndrome. These vessels pose a potential risk for iatrogenic injury and hemorrhage during velopharyngeal narrowing procedures. Cervical vascular imaging studies, such as magnetic resonance imaging, computerized tomography, or angiography, have been advocated as aids to surgery by defining the preoperative vascular anatomy. Nevertheless, it remains unclear whether these studies alter either the conduct or the outcome of operations on the velopharynx. Iatrogenic injuries to the carotid artery during velopharyngeal surgery are strikingly absent in the extant literature. Occasionally, transmission of vascular pulsations through "floppy" redundant mucosa may artificially masquerade as an ominous vessel. Additionally, tortuous and medially displaced vessels observed at one point in time have been shown to straighten and lateralize on later studies.

How should the surgeon approach the problem of aberrantly located carotid vessels? This is a provocative and controversial question that deserves clear answers from each participating surgeon. In the end, safety must prevail as the first priority. When displaced vessels are identified, surgeons are faced with a few options: (1) the surgeon may abandon the procedure; (2) the surgeon may "operate around" the vessels; (3) the surgeon may choose to perform one procedure instead of another, i.e., sphincter pharyngoplasty instead of pharyngeal flap (theoretically, performance of the latter procedure could expose a vessel over the full length of the flap).

It is certainly possible to operate safely in the presence of aberrant vessels, provided that the flap(s) can be repositioned so as not to interfere with their presence, expose them to oropharyngeal secretions, or compromise the execution of the procedure. The author does not routinely obtain preoperative vascular imaging studies on all patients, although many surgeons do. In performing more than 150 velopharyngeal narrowing procedures, the author has not been compelled to abort a single procedure because of concern about injury to aberrantly placed carotid vessels. Awareness of their presence comes from careful inspection of the small operative field, palpation of aberrant vessels intraoperatively, and cautious surgery.

Surgical Procedures for VPD

Partial obstruction, either temporary or permanent, of the velopharyngeal port is the unifying feature of most current operative management of VPD. There are two broad categories of options for VPD management, selection of which depends upon the patient's specific diagnosis: (1) lengthening the palate by retropositioning the velum (this is purported to result from a V-Y pushback procedure, an intravelar veloplasty[17] or double opposing Z-plasty[18]) and palatal re-repair[19] and (2) reduction of the static opening between the nasal and oral pharynges.[20,21] Reduction of the velopharyngeal port may be accomplished with a pharyngeal flap or sphincter pharyngoplasty. The pharyngeal flap creates a single subtotal central obstruction of the velopharyngeal port, leaving two open ports laterally. Alternatively, sphincter pharyngoplasty may be performed to diminish the cross-sectional area of the central port. Posterior pharyngeal wall augmentation is another method of treating resonance disorders, and this procedure is used in various centers around the world with variable success. This chapter focuses primarily on pharyngeal flap and sphincter pharyngoplasty procedures.

Timing of Surgical Intervention

It is often assumed that young patients are better candidates for VP surgery than older ones. However, data on the effect of timing of surgery for velopharyngeal dysfunction on speech do not support the suggestion that delaying surgical management will increase the amount of speech therapy necessary to achieve normalization of the speech impairments secondary to VPD after such management.[22] The data suggest instead

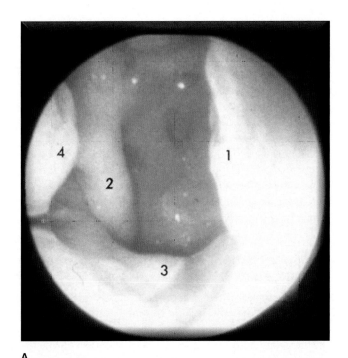

A

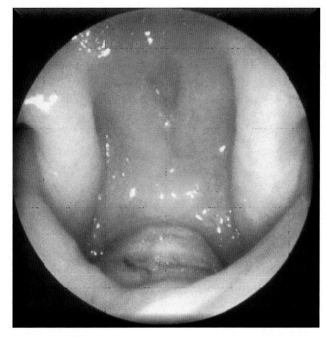

B

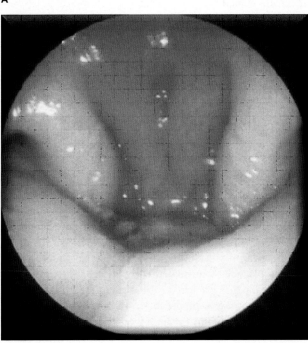

C

Figure 39–5. A. Preoperative nasoendoscopic view of the velopharynx. 1 = lateral pharyngeal wall; 2 = velum; 3 = tonsil; 4 = tonsil. **B**. Postoperative nasendoscopic view of velopharynx, indicating open pharyngeal flap as central subtotal midline obstruction; two patent velopharyngeal ports are visible laterally. **C**. Postoperative nasendoscopic view of velopharynx, indicating two lateral pharyngeal walls opposed against pharyngeal flap to affect complete velopharyngeal closure.

that there is *no* relation between age of the patient at the time of VPD surgery and amount of speech therapy needed subsequently. The timing of surgery for VPD management does not affect the length of postoperative speech therapy required to achieve normalization of VP function. Thus, VPD surgery should not be denied to older individuals on the assumption that they cannot benefit from it because of their age.

Candidates for Pharyngeal Flap Surgery

It is known that lateral wall motion is important for effective valving after pharyngeal flap surgery.[23] Creation of a pharyn-

geal flap is most effective in patients with satisfactory lateral pharyngeal wall movement and sagittal or circular velopharyngeal closure patterns.

The objective of the pharyngeal flap is to create a central static obstruction and to leave two lateral ports or openings (Fig. 39–5). The lateral openings should remain patent during breathing and nasal consonant speech production and closed during the production of oral consonants. Schoenborn originally published a description of this procedure in 1876.[24] The pharyngeal flap was widely adopted in the 1950s and has been studied fairly extensively.

Different Kinds of Pharyngeal Flaps

The pharyngeal flap has been modified to a great extent, and variations in specific techniques abound. Key questions stimulating the development of these modifications include the following: What is the appropriate width of the pharyngeal flap? Is a superiorly or inferiorly based flap more effective in achieving the ideal outcome? Should the flap be lined with mucous membrane to prevent postoperative contraction/attenuation of the flap?

What is the Appropriate Level and Width of Pharyngeal Flap?

Determination of level of insertion and flap width may influence proper closure of the new lateral ports during speech. An excessively wide, nearly obstructive flap may induce untoward secondary consequences (i.e., mouth breathing, hyponasality, sleep disturbances ranging from snoring to sleep apnea, and retention of nasal secretions and mucous). Hypernasality may persist if the flap is too long and thin. Historically, flap width has been determined at the time of surgery by the surgeon's experience or preference. Many surgeons attempt to create a flap as wide as the field allows.

Lining the Pharyngeal Flap

If the flap is unlined, a broad, raw surface of pharyngeal tissue is left exposed after its elevation. Subsequent contraction may narrow the flap and diminish its efficacy. Thus, initial postoperative results may indicate improvement in velopharyngeal function, and yet symptoms of the dysfunction may recur gradually thereafter. To reduce the tendency for contraction, "book flap" linings usually are raised from the nasal surface of the posterior velum and folded over to cover the unfulfilled surface of the flap (Figs. 39–6A–I).

Level of Flap Inset Affects Outcome

The level of flap insertion is linked to surgical success. Ideally, the flap should be placed (and should remain) at the level of attempted velopharyngeal closure. Insertion of a short, wide flap along the free margin of the soft palate may reduce the contraction of unlined flaps and limit flap displacement during the healing process. This method narrows the gaps between the base of the flap and the attached tonsillar folds where they merge with the pharyngeal wall. Port size may be varied by varying either flap width and/or the width of flap insertion along the posterior soft palate and posterior tonsillar pillars. By creating a very wide flap with a broad insertion, one may create a velopharynx that is nearly completely obstructed and that requires little contribution from the lateral pharyngeal walls to achieve closure.

Can Lateral Port Size be Controlled?

Hogan[25] devised a surgical technique to modulate the postoperative port size. He introduced the concept of lateral port control in the 1970s, using indirect information of the size of the velopharyngeal port from differential nasal and oral airflow. Studies by Ishiki and Warren, Warren, and Devereau corroborated this hypothesis and demonstrated that port size is related to the perception of nasal resonance.[26,27] Kummer et al. have recently extended this concept.[7]

Hogan's technique involves placement of 10 mm^2 catheters that he assumed to be the crucial variable for anticipated normal resonance. Although this technique may seem intuitive and logical, uncontrolled variables such as the vagaries of wound healing, scarring, and postoperative migration of the flap must lead one to believe that port size cannot always be rigorously and reliably controlled.

Can Specifications of Pharyngeal Flap be Tailored to Patient's Needs?

It remains unclear whether appropriate flap width can be determined intraoperatively on a routine basis. In most cases of post-palatoplasty velopharyngeal dysfunction, control of the flap width based on the morphology observed during the operation is ineffective. However, it seems logical in cases of grossly asymmetric closure patterns to focus on correcting that asymmetry.[28,29] For example, patients with VPD secondary to hemifacial microsomia, stroke, or tumor resection may need specific skewing (tailoring) of flaps to affect closure.

Basing the Flap Superiorly or Inferiorly

Whether the flap is inferiorly or superiorly based has been the subject of lively debate among surgeons over the years; however, proof of significant differences between the two types is lacking.[30] Currently, most surgeons favor a superiorly based flap. The disadvantages of an inferiorly based flap include limitation of flap length and inferior tethering of the flap below the level of velopharyngeal closure.[31] Extrapolating from the information on failed sphincter pharyngoplasties, in which low flap placement correlated with failure, superiorly based pharyngeal flap is preferred.[32]

A fairly recent modification of the pharyngeal flap is the so-called lined pull-through procedure.[33] This procedure involves de-mucosalization of the oral surface of the posterior soft palate which juxtaposes with the raw surface of the elevated pharyngeal flap. In the present author's experience, however, this procedure results in substantial downward migration and tethering, thus antagonizing normal velopharyngeal movement.

Sphincter Pharyngoplasty

The goal of sphincter pharyngoplasty is to narrow the central velopharyngeal orifice, thereby minimizing airflow through the nose during speech. Sphincter pharyngoplasty tightens the central orifice without creating lateral ports, resulting in a configuration of the velopharynx that is the opposite of that produced by pharyngeal flap.

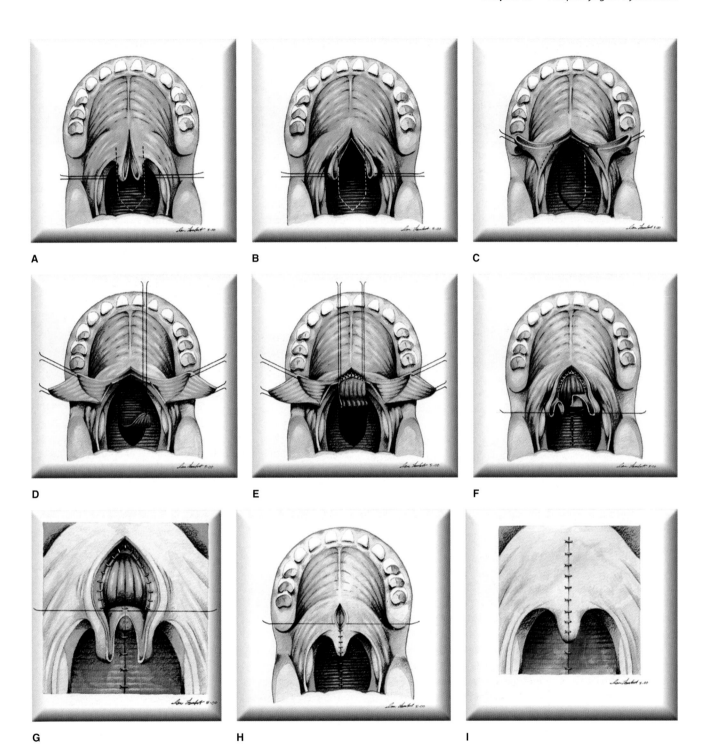

A   B   C

D   E   F

G   H   I

Figure 39–6. Posterior pharyngeal flap. **A**. Sutures are placed bilaterally in the soft palate to enhance visualization. A midline incision divides the soft palate to the posterior nasal spine. **B**. Soft palate flaps are retracted. **C**. An incision is made along the dotted line on the posterior pharyngeal wall down to the prevertebral fascia. A pharyngeal flap is created. A book flap incision that will line the lateral ports with mucous membrane is then made bilaterally on the nasal surface of the soft palate. **D**. Pharyngeal flap is plotted with indelible ink and elevated to the prevertebral fascia. Two soft palate flaps are opened laterally. **E**. Free inferior edge of pharyngeal flap is sutured to the posterior edge soft palate. **F**. Sutures are placed between the pharyngeal flap and the nasal edges of the soft palate. The raw surfaces arising from the origin of the pharyngeal flap are closed by simple approximation of tissue. **G**. Two flaps from the soft palate used to cover the raw tissue of the pharyngeal flap are sutured to the base of the pharyngeal flap. **H** and **I**. Oral side of the soft palate is sealed to conceal the pharyngeal flap. **J**. Immediate postoperative view from oral cavity.

Sphincter pharyngoplasty was first described more than 50 years ago, and yet only recently has it become a procedure of choice amongst many surgeons. Because of insufficient collation of data, a detailed description of risks, benefits, and long-term outcomes has not been confirmed. The original concept of sphincter pharyngoplasty was described by Hynes[34] and has been modified by others, including Orticochea.[35] The procedure rearranges palatopharyngeus myomucosal flaps raised from the posterior tonsillar pillars, transposing them to the posterior pharyngeal wall and to each other. This procedure may result in less airway morbidity than the pharyngeal flap[36] and is conceptually more physiologic, although these impressions reflect the author's personal bias and remain unproven.

Candidates for Sphincter Pharyngoplasty

Sphincter pharyngoplasty may be an appropriate management option for patients with velopharyngeal dysfunction whose nasendoscopic evaluations indicate a large-gap, coronal, circular, or bow-tie pattern of closure. Essentially, patients who demonstrate good velar elevation but poor lateral wall motion are good candidates for sphincter pharyngoplasty.

Operative Technique

A red rubber catheter is passed transnasally and sutured to the uvula. The catheter may then be used to reflect the velum into the nasopharynx in order to achieve exposure of the posterior pharyngeal wall (Fig. 39–7A). The posterior pharyngeal wall is palpated for the pulsations of aberrant carotid arteries. Next, the lines of incision are marked with indelible ink on both the anterior and, with the aid of a retractor, the posterior aspects of the posterior tonsillar pillars, identifying the proposed myomucosal flaps (Fig. 39–7B). An epinephrine-containing solution is infiltrated for hemostatic purposes.

Beginning on the right and then repeating the same maneuver on the left, the posterior tonsillar pillars are elevated as myomucosal flaps, based cephalad (Fig. 39–7C). The flaps are elevated to the height of attempted velopharyngeal closure as documented on the preoperative speech video fluoroscopy.

The posterior pharyngeal wall is incised transversely at the proposed level of insertion, corresponding to the cephalad extent of flap elevation. The continuous cut extends from the superior end of the posterior limb of one lateral flap to the other, allowing the lateral flaps to be transposed and fully inset. This design eliminates the bilateral fistulae inherent in Orticochea's original construction. All sutures are placed in sequence and subsequently secured from cephalad to caudad. The red rubber catheter is removed before securing knots.

Using 4-0 polyglactin sutures, the superior mucosal edge of the left flap is attached to the mucosa at the superior edge of the incision on the posterior pharyngeal wall. The caudal mucosal edge of the left flap is sutured to the superior mucosal edge of the right flap, overlapping the two flaps as described by Hynes. The caudal mucosal edge of the right flap is sutured to the mucosa at the inferior edge of the incision on the posterior pharyngeal wall (Fig. 39–7D).

The integrity of the newly created sphincter may be ensured by suturing the lateral flaps securely to one another and to the superior constrictor and pharyngobasilar membrane. Each stitch should capture the mucosa, submucosa, and epimysium in order to maximize its holding power. The tissues are approximated without tension, and the donor sites closed. After construction of the sphincter pharyngoplasty, an orogastric tube is passed to aspirate the gastric contents, then removed.

The central orifice of the sphincter pharyngoplasty port at the conclusion of the procedure should admit a small finger breadth (about 1 cm in diameter). A "tight" sphincter pharyngoplasty port usually measures approximately 0.5 cm in diameter, and a "loose" sphincter pharyngoplasty port usually measures approximately 1.5 cm in diameter.

Long-Term Outcome of Sphincter Pharyngoplasty

Riski demonstrated that the height of insertion appears to be a critical factor for success and emphasized the importance of inset height for placement of the myomucosal flaps. In a follow-up study, he reported results in a large number of patients over a 15-year period.[37] There was a high success rate amongst patients who underwent sphincter pharyngoplasty before speech dysfunction developed fully. Success also seemed to correlate with patients who were younger than 6 years at the time of operation.

Witt[38] published a report in which preoperative speech and instrumental assessments were separated to provide perceptual information and physiologic relationships. Only 18% of the patients in the study showed 100% resolution of hypernasality and nasal emission. Approximately 30% of the patients developed hyponasality and/or obstructed speech and breathing patterns. Sphincter pharyngoplasty remains an effective treatment modality for VPD; however, the study emphasizes the need for further comparative data.

Postoperative Care

Patients are monitored overnight with pulse oximetry. They may resume a soft or liquid diet immediately. Most patients are discharged from the hospital after one night, although patients with 22q11.2 deletion often require at least two nights in the hospital. Patients return 3 weeks after surgery for follow-up. In the meantime, parents are given information about sleep apnea and instructed to watch for and report signs of upper airway obstruction. Speech therapy usually resumes 3–6 weeks after surgical VPD intervention.

Complications

Risks associated with the surgical management of VPD include obstructive sleep apnea, dehiscence, and bleeding. Sleep disturbance as a consequence of sphincter pharyngoplasty

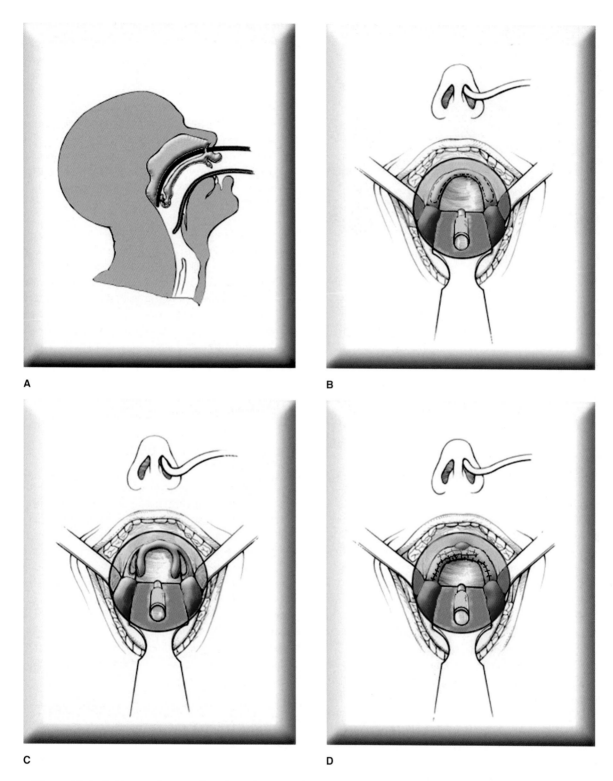

Figure 39–7. Sphincter phayngoplasty. **A**. Schematic of lateral view. Catheter has been passed transnasally and attached to uvula. **B**. Schematic showing proposed incisions (dashed lines). **C**. Schematic showing elevation of both tonsillar pillar flaps. **D**. Schematic showing completed sphincter pharyngoplasty. Flaps are overlapped, sutured to each other and posterior pharyngeal wall.

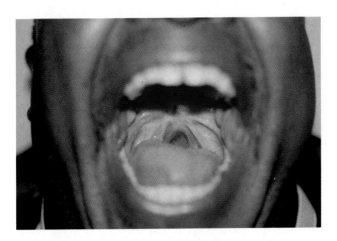

Figure 39–8. Complete nasopharyngeal stenosis.

may range from simple snoring to acute obstructive sleep apnea. Rarely is sleep apnea so severe as to require hospitalization. This adverse effect appears to occur in a substantial percentage of patients surgically managed for VPD, as suggested in a preliminary report by Witt in which the incidence was 13% of 58 patients observed.[39]

Complete nasopharyngeal obstruction should be a rare complication, assuming that all raw surfaces were properly lined at the time of primary pharyngoplasty. Misguided surgery, however, may lead to nasopharyngeal stenosis and the unfortunate triad of sleep apnea/snoring, hyponasal resonance, and retained secretions/maxillary sinusitis (Fig. 39–8).

Velopharyngeal surgery is still more of an art than a science. The goal is to create a subtotal obstruction that improves resonance but that avoids airway morbidity. Still, in about 10% of cases, re-operation is necessary to treat residual hypernasality or nasal emission.

Postoperative Assessment

Postsurgical speech therapy, if necessary, should be based on the same comprehensive process of evaluation utilized before the surgery. It should not be assumed that the patient has been given an adequate velopharyngeal mechanism that he/she must simply learn to use effectively. It is still unclear whether different surgical procedures work better for patients having different patterns of VPD; cleft palate teams have an obligation to study long-term intervention outcomes using a variety of perceptual and instrumental techniques in order that the validity and efficacy of these procedures can be established.

Complex Problems Associated with VPD Research

Several studies have been published in support of each of the available options for the management of velopharyngeal insufficiency; however, most of the data have not been validated by large numbers of patients, nor have these re-sults been subjected to critical analysis. Most of these studies lack a multidisciplinary evaluation, standardized evaluation/treatment criteria, and methods for assessing surgical outcome.

For example, several different types of sphincter pharyngoplasties have been described, although they have often been grouped together as though they were the same. These procedures differ with respect to the transposition of the flaps, the use of muscle tissue, the levels of insertion, and the use of a synchronous pharyngeal flap. The status of tonsils represents an uncontrolled variable in most studies. This heterogeneity explains some of the difficulty in describing postoperative outcomes.

There is inherent instability of cleft palate populations, migratory patterns of treating physicians, and dogmatism among surgeons regarding the "best technique." Additionally, study designs often do not include rigorous documentation of the methodology used for evaluation of the intervention. It is an arduous task to achieve a high compliance rate from a patient population stratified for age, sex, socioeconomic factors, and number of surgical interventions. The outcome assessment instrument must be designed to allow for analysis of intra- and inter-rater reliabilities of all the extramural raters and at the same time not be so cumbersome or burdensome so as to reduce compliance.

Outcome Assessment: How Do You Define Success?

Improvement in clinical symptomatology may be interpreted as success, but cleft care providers must define success precisely and inform patients and their families of what surgery can realistically accomplish. Outcome assessment between cleft surgeons and independent raters may reflect the lack of a standardized definition of success for the former or the unbiased objective assessments of the latter. Does "success" mean that the patient has no hyponasality? Is the operation successful if the resonance improves but the patient develops obstructive sleep apnea? Randomized studies, with results judged by independent raters whose reliabilities are known, should determine the efficacy of specific interventions.

FUTURE DIAGNOSTIC/ASSESSMENT/ TREATMENT MODALITIES

There are exciting new technologies on the horizon, such as dynamic magnetic resonance imaging of the velopharynx, that may soon be available for clinical use. Magnetic resonance data can be reformatted to simulate endoscopy. Planar images may be converted to three dimensional volumes. Although still in its infancy, this technology may someday allow clinicians view the anatomic structures they have scanned with "fly-throughs," focusing on specific regions. This has the potential of evolving into a form of "noninvasive endoscopy," assuming that it can meet or exceed the gold standards currently available.[40]

AXIOMS

- A finite number of patients will develop VPD, regardless of surgeon experience, palatoplasty technique, timing of operation, early speech therapy intervention.[41,42,43]
- Patients with VPD should be managed by a team of specialists.
- Midface advancement may affect velopharyngeal function, particularly those with borderline function.
- Patients with 22q11.2 microdeletion (velocardiofacial syndrome) are notoriously difficult to manage[44,45]; parents need to be counseled carefully, usually on repeat occasions preoperatively, to temper their expectations about intervention outcomes.
- Removing enlarged tonsils 3 months prior to velopharyngeal surgery may facilitate the procedure and reduce the risk of postoperative sleep apnea.
- Pharyngoplasty flaps should be inset at least as high as the atlas (C1), corresponding to the level of attempted velopharyngeal contact as noted on preoperative speech videofluoroscopy.

References

1. Looney RW, Bloem TJ. Velopharyngeal dysfunction: Recommendations for use of nomenclature. *Cleft Palate J* 24(4):334–335, 1987.
2. Folkins JW. Velopharyngeal nomenclature: Incompetence, inadequacy, insufficiency, and dysfunction. *Cleft Palate J* 25(4):413–416, 1988.
3. Witt PD, D'Antonio LL. Velopharyngeal insufficiency and secondary palatal management: A new look at an old problem. *Clin Plast Surg* 20(4):707–721, 1993.
4. Golding-Kushner KJ, Argamaso RV, Cotton RT, et al. Standardization for the reporting of nasopharyngoscopy and multiview videofluoroscopy: A report from an International Working Group. *Cleft Palate J* 27(4):337–347, 1990; discussion 347–348.
5. Becker DB, Grames LM, Pilgrim T, Kane AA, Marsh JL. Differential diagnosis for differential management of velopharyngeal dysfunction. *J Craniofac Surg* 15(5):804–809, 2004.
6. Armour S, Fschbach S, Klaiman P, Fisher DM. Does velopharyngeal closure pattern affect the success of pharyngeal flap pharyngoplasty? *Plast Reconstr Surg* 115(1):45–52, 2005; discussion 53.
7. Kummer AW, Briggs M, Lee ML. The relationship between the characteristics of speech and velopharyngeal gap size. *Cleft Palate Craniofac J* 40(6):590–596, 2003.
8. Trost-Cardamone JE. Coming to terms with VPI: A response to Loney and Bloem. *Cleft Palate J* 26(1):68–70, 1989.
9. D'Antonio LL, Synder LS, Samadani S. Tonsillectomy in children with or at risk for velopharyngeal insufficiency: Effects of speech. *Otolaryngol Head Neck Surg* 115(4):319–323, 1996.
10. Kummer AW. *Cleft Palate and Craniofacial Anomalies: The Effects on Speech and Resonance.* San Diego, CA: Singular Press, 2001.
11. Wyatt R, Sell D, Russel J, Hardings A, Harland K, Albery E. Cleft palate speech dissected: A review of current knowledge and analysis. *Br J Plast Surg* 49(3):143–149, 1996 (Review).
12. Shprintzen RJ, Sher AE, Croft CB. Hypernasal speech caused by tonsillar hypertrophy. *Int J Pediatric Otorhinolaryngol* 14(1):45–46, 1987.
13. Witt PD, Marsh JL, McFarland EG, Riski J. Evolution of velopharyngeal imaging. *Ann Plast Surg* 45(6):665–673, 2000.
14. Tachimura T, Nohara K, Fujita Y, Wada T. Change in levator veli palatini muscle activity for patients with cleft palate in association with placement of a speech-aid prosthesis. *Cleft Palate Craniofac J* 39(5):503–508, 2002.
15. Witt PD, Rozzelle A, Marsh JL, et al. Do palatal lift prostheses stimulate velopharyngeal neuromuscular activity? *Cleft Palate Craniofac J* 32(6):469–475, 1995.
16. Witt PD, Miller DC, Marsh JL, Grames LM, Muntz HR. The limited value of preoperative cervical vascular imaging in patients with velocardiofacial syndrome. *Plast Reconstr Surg* 101(5):1184–1195, 1998; discussion 1196–1199.
17. Marsh JL. Intravelar veloplasty. *Cleft Palate J* 26(1):46–50, 1989.
18. D'Antonio LL. Correction of velopharyngeal insufficiency using the Furlow double-opposing Z-plasty. *West J Med* 167(2):101–102, 1997.
19. Sommerlad BC, Mehendale FV, Birch MJ, Sell D, Hattee C, Harland K. Palate re-repair revisited. *Cleft Palate Craniofac J* 39(3):295–307, 2002.
20. LaRossa D. The state of the art in cleft palate surgery. *Cleft Palate Craniofac J* 37(3):225–228, 2000.
21. Sloan GM. Posterior pharyngeal flap and sphincter pharyngoplasty: The state of the art. *Cleft Palate Craniofac J* 37(2):112–122, 2000.
22. Becker DB, Grames LM, Pilgram T, Kane AA, Marsh JL. The effect of timing of surgery for velopharyngeal dysfunction on speech. *J Craniofac Surg* 15(5):804–809, 2004.
23. Argamaso RV, Shprintzen RJ, Strauch B, et al. The role of lateral pharyngeal wall movement in pharyngeal flap surgery. *Plast Reconstr Surg* 66(2):214–219, 1980.
24. Schoenborn D. Uber eine neue methode der staphylorraphies. *Arch F Klin Chir* 19:528–531, 1876.
25. Hogan VM. A clarification of the surgical goals in cleft palate speech and the introduction of the lateral port control (l.p.c.) pharyngeal flap. *Cleft Palate J* 10:331–345, 1973.
26. Warren DW. Velopharyngeal orifice size and upper pharyngeal pressure flow patterns in normal speech. *Plast Reconstr Surg* 33:148–162, 1964.
27. Warren DW, Devereux JL. An analog study of cleft palate speech. *Cleft Palate J* 3:103–114, 1966.
28. Mehendale FV, Sommerlad BC. Gross unilateral abnormalities of the velum and pharynx. *Cleft Palate Craniofac J* 39(4):461–468, 2002.
29. Argamaso RV, Levandowski GJ, Golding-Kushner KJ, Shprintzen RJ. Treatment of asymmetric velopharyngeal insufficiency with skewed pharyngeal flap. *Cleft Palate Craniofac J* 31(4):287–294, 1994.
30. Whitaker LA, Randall P, Graham WP III, et al. A prospective and randomized series comparing superiorly and inferiorly based posterior pharyngeal flaps. *Cleft Palate J* 9:304–311, 1972.
31. Trier WC. Pharyngeal flap. *Clin Plast Surg* 12(4):659–675, 1985.
32. Riski JE, Serafin D, Riefkohl R, et al. A rationale for modifying the site of insertion of the Orticochea pharyngoplasty. *Plast Reconstr Surg* 73(6):882–894, 1984.
33. Johns DF, Cannito MP, Rohrich RJ, Tebbetts JB. The self-lined superiorly based pull-through velopharyngoplasty: Plastic surgery–speech pathology interaction in the management of velopharyngeal insufficiency. *Plast Reconstr Surg* 94(3):436–445, 1994.
34. Hynes W. Pharyngoplasty by muscle transplantation. *Br J Plast Surg* 3(2):128–135, 1950.
35. Orticochea M. Construction of a dynamic muscle sphincter in cleft palates. *Plast Reconstr Surg* 41(4):323–327, 1968.
36. Witt PD, Marsh JL, Muntz HR, et al. Acute obstructive sleep apnea as a complication of sphincter pharyngoplasty. *Cleft Palate Craniofac J* 33(3):183–189, 1996.
37. Riski JE, Ruff GL, Georgiade GS, et al. Evaluation of the sphincter pharyngoplasty. *Cleft Palate Craniofac J* 29(3):254–261, 1992.
38. Witt PD, D'Antonio LL, Zimmerman GJ, et al. Sphincter pharyngoplasty: A preoperative and postoperative analysis of perceptual speech characteristics and endoscopic studies of velopharyngeal function. *Plast Reconstr Surg* 93(6):1154–1168, 1994.
39. Marsh JL, ed. The evaluation and management of velopharyngeal dysfunction. *Clin Plastic Surg* 31(2):261–269, 2004.

40. Kuehn D, Ettema SL, Goldwasser MS, Barkmeier JC, Wachtel JM. Magnetic resonance imaging in the evaluation of occult submucous cleft palate. *Cleft Palate Craniofac J* 38(5):421–431, 2001.

41. Sell D, Ma L. A model of practice for the management of velopharyngeal dysfunction. *Br J Oral Maxillofac Surg* 34(5):357–363, 1996.

42. Witt PD, Wahlen JC, Marsh JL, Grames LM, Pilgram TK. Effect of surgeon experience on velopharygeal functional outcome following palatoplasty. Is there a learning curve? *Plast Reconstr Surg* 102(5):1375–1384, 1998.

43. Witt PD, Marsh JL, Grames LM, Muntz HR, Gay WD. Management of the hypodynamic velopharynx. *Cleft Palate Craniofac J* 32(3):179-187, 1995.

44. Witt PD, Cohen DT, Grames LM, Marsh JL. Sphincter pharyngoplasty for the surgical management of speech dysfunction associated with velocardiofacial syndrome. *Br J Plast Surg* 52(8):613–618, 1999.

45. Mehendale FV, Birch MJ, Birkett L, Sell D, Sommerlad BC. Surgical management of velopharyngeal incompetence in velocardiofacial syndrome. *Cleft Palate Craniofac J* 41(2):124–135, 2004.

Correction of Velopharyngeal Insufficiency by Double-Opposing Z-Plasty

Leonard T. Furlow, Jr., MD

I. INTRODUCTION

II. PROCEDURE

▮ INTRODUCTION

Double-opposing Z-plasty is a method for primary repair of cleft palate,[1–4] and is applicable as a secondary procedure for velopharyngeal insufficiency (VPI).[5,6] The velar Z-plasties reposition the palatal muscles transversely, construct a functioning palatal muscle sling by overlapping them, and in addition, add velar length. Because the velopharyngeal (VP) anatomy is rearranged toward normal, rather than being narrowed by the interposition of flaps, the incidence of nasal airway obstruction and obstructive sleep apnea (OSA) seems to be lower than after pharyngeal flap[7] or sphincter pharyngoplasty.

On nasendoscopy, Witt and D'Antonio[8] found that when a sagittal groove in the dorsum of the velum was present preoperatively, it was obliterated by secondary double-opposing Z-plasty.

In 12 patients with VPI, D'Antonio et al.[9] showed that, when the operation produced marked increases in velar length or thickness, in some cases greater than matched norms, or moderate increases in both, VP competence resulted.

However, when increases in both velar length and thickness were minimal, VPI persisted. Six of the 8 (75%) operated on for VPI after palatoplasty demonstrated VP competence. In 13 consecutive patients with VPI after cleft palate repair, Hudson et al.[10] achieved VP competence in 11 (85%) with a secondary double-opposing Z-plasty. In these two series, in which preoperative closure measurements were not given, 17 of 21 (81%) developed VP competence.

In several series, the preoperative measurement of a residual VP gap in millimeters (mm) has been used as a criterion for selecting double-opposing Z-plasty as a treatment for postoperative VPI. In a study by Chen et al.,[11] VP competence was attained in 16 of 18 (89%) patients with VPI after secondary double-opposing Z-plasty. All 15 patients with preoperative residual VP gaps on videofluoroscopy of 5 mm or less achieved VP competence after secondary double-opposing Z-plasty. Although no patients in the study had residual gaps of 6–10 mm, three patients with residual gaps greater than 10 mm were selected for secondary double-opposing Z-plasty because of anteriorly directed unrepaired levator muscles. One of the three achieved VP competence, and the other two improved to marginal VPI. In this series, age did not predict failure; both patients over 20 years old achieved VP competence.

Lindsey and Davis[12] produced VP competence by secondary double-opposing Z-plasty in 7 of 8 patients (88%) whose preoperative VP gap was estimated on nasendoscopy to be 6–8 mm.

In the author's private practice experience, the two patients for whom I used a secondary double-opposing Z-plasty for VPI after primary palate repair developed VP competence postoperatively.[2] The criteria for selection were primary repair other than by double-opposing Z-plasty, good palatal motion, a residual gap of 5 mm or less on videofluoroscopy, velar muscles still in the anteriorly directed cleft orientation, and an absence of compensatory articulation; good lateral pharyngeal sidewall motion was not a requirement.

In the reports herein reviewed, the overall rate of VP competence achieved by secondary double-opposing Z-plasty was 25 of 28 patients (89%). When stratifying these 25 patients achieving VP competence according to VP gap size prior to secondary surgery, we find that: 1 of 3 patients (33%) with residual gaps over 10 mm, 7 of 8 (87%) with gaps of 5–10 mm, and 17 of 17 (100%) with gaps of 0–5 mm, obtained VP competence. Thus, when palatal morphology was measured in mm, secondary double-opposing Z-plasty seemed to be effective (96%) for residual gaps up to between 8 and 10 mm.

Three studies[13–15] provided pre- and postoperative nasendoscopy data to evaluate secondary double-opposing Z-plasty. These studies reported closing ratios, defined as the percent of the open VP port that can be closed by the elevated velum.[16,17] Using a ratio, rather than a measurement, avoids two problems: the variation in size among patients of different ages, and the inability to measure through the nasendoscope. The ratio between the "resting gap," or VP port size at rest, and the "residual gap," or size of the VP port gap upon attempt at closure, describes what remains open. Pre- and postoperative closing ratios were reported as less than 50% (large residual gap), 50–80% (moderate gap), 80–99% (small gap), and in one of the studies,[15] 100% (complete closure).

Perkins et al.[14] reported on 148 patients with VPI treated with secondary double-opposing Z-plasty. Each patient on preoperative nasendoscopy was found to have a sagittal velar groove, indicating that the velar muscles were in the cleft orientation. The report did not distinguish between the 98 patients with secondary VPI after palatoplasty and the 50 patients with submucous cleft palate (SMCP) and primary VPI. 64 of the patients had a syndrome or associated condition, including 16 with velocardiofacial syndrome (VCFS) and 8 with Pierre Robin sequence (PRS). The diagnosis of VPI was based on perceptual evaluation of hypernasality and nasal escape. Postoperatively, only 73 (49.3%) had normal resonance, and only 47 (31.8%) had no nasal emission, yet 83 (56%) "had no VPI".

Both preoperative closing ratios and VPI ratings predicted the rate of postoperative VPI. 73% of the 52 patients with preoperative closing ratios of 80–100%, 51% of the 51 with preoperative closing ratios of 50–80% and only 13% of the 31 with closing ratios below 50% had no or minimal VPI postoperatively. Except for the 16 patients with VCFS, syndromic patients did as well as nonsyndromic.

These results prompted the authors to change their protocol by adding a sphincter pharyngoplasty at the time of double-opposing Z-plasty for patients with closing ratios less than 50%. However, a VP competence rate of 51% for patients with closing ratios of 50–80% suggests that the double-opposing Z-plasty be reserved for patients with closing ratios above 80%.

Deren et al.[15,18] conducted a prospective study of 27 nonsyndromic children with VPI whose cleft palates had been repaired after age 3 by pushback palatoplasty. At the time of secondary double-opposing Z-plasty for the treatment of their VPI, the patients' ages ranged from 4 to 13 years. This publication is particularly instructive because data are provided on each individual patient.

Preoperative and 1-year postoperative evaluations categorized nasal emission, nasality, articulation and intelligibility into four categories: none/normal, mild, moderate or severe. Nasendoscopy was also performed preoperatively and one-year postoperative after double-opposing Z-plasty. Closing ratios were classified into four categories: less than 50% (large residual gap), 50–80% (moderate gap), 80–100% or almost complete closure (small gap), and 100% or complete closure (no gap).

For the purposes of outcomes discussion, nasal emission and hypernasality, the primary consequences of an incompetent velopharyngeal valve, will be called the "valve tests", and articulation and intelligibility, secondary characteristics due to compensatory articulations related to the learning of speech, will be called the "speech tests".[18]

Preoperatively, all 27 children had moderate to severe grades of nasal escape, hypernasality, articulation and intelligibility, with closing ratios < 80% (either large or moderate gaps). Preoperative closing ratios correlated with postoperative VP function. 18 of the 27 patients had preoperative closing ratios less than 50% (large gaps), one year postoperatively, only four had neither hypernasality nor nasal escape, one-third had no test indicating closure, and only one-half had evidence of closure on nasendoscopy (Fig. 40–1). All nine patients with preoperative closing ratios of 50–80% (moderate gaps) had evidence of valve competency one year after surgery; four had neither hypernasality nor nasal escape, and the remaining five had either no nasal escape or no hypernasality. Two-thirds demonstrated closure on nasendoscopy, and all 27 tests of postoperative VP competency were either normal or mild (Fig. 40–2).

There was a high correlation among the three measures of VP valve function (nasal escape, nasal resonance, and nasendoscopy); in only two patients (#'s 8, 27) was there more than one grade difference between scores (Figs. 40–1 and 40–2). Postoperative outcome was not related to the patient's age (Fig. 40–3).

Comparison between scores on the valve tests (nasal escape and hypernasality) and the speech tests (articulation

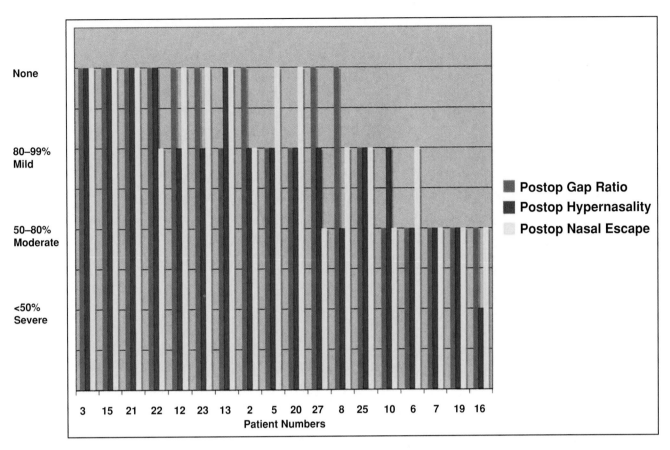

Figure 40–1. Of 18 patients with preoperative closing ratios less than 50% (large gaps), four developed VP competence (neither nasal escape nor hypernasality), five had either no nasal escape or no hypernasality, and seven had moderate nasal escape and/or hypernasality.

and intelligibility) showed that the speech grade equaled or lagged behind the valve grade, exceeding the valve grade in only one of the 27 children, patient #16, who had the worst result. This demonstrated that the children could speak no better than their VP mechanism would permit (Fig. 40–4). Intelligibility and articulation improved to normal or mild only when there was evidence of capability for valve closure. However, evidence of capability for valve closure did not ensure speech improvement. *Normal speech depends on, but is not ensured by, normal valve function.*

Some studies report that double-opposing Z-plasty is ineffective for correction of VPI in patients with VCFS.[14,19] Sphincter pharyngoplasty has been found to be a far better choice.[20,21]

Except for two cases performed in private practice, my experience with double opposing Z-plasty as a secondary procedure for VPI after palate repair has consisted of several dozen cases performed without benefit of preoperative videofluoroscopy or nasendoscopy on volunteer surgery trips such as Interplast or Rotaplast. As the incidence of airway obstruction and OSA appears to be lower in secondary palatoplasty when compared to pharyngeal flap or sphincter pharyngoplasty; and because follow-up in surgical mission trips is often a problem, I have felt that double-opposing

Z-plasty would be less likely to leave rural patients with OSA, with little understanding and no treatment.

PROCEDURE

Before utilizing double-opposing Z-plasty for correction of postpalatoplasty VPI, one should be experienced and successful with the technique for primary repair. Although the operation is usually easier in secondary cases because one begins with no cleft to close, scarring from the primary palatoplasty can shorten and stiffen the tissues, particularly along the cleft, making secondary palatoplasty a challenging procedure. Fistula repair can be done at the same time.

The operation[5,6] is little different from the velar portion of primary repair and can be seen in greater detail in chapter 23 on the double-opposing Z-plasty in this text. The design of the Z-plasties is based on the anatomy of the palate, not geometry; the angle of one Z-plasty flap may well not match the other. Attention to the anatomic landmarks and proper design of the Z-plasty, in my experience, eliminates the need for soft palate lateral relaxing incisions, and precisely aligns and overlaps the levator muscles.

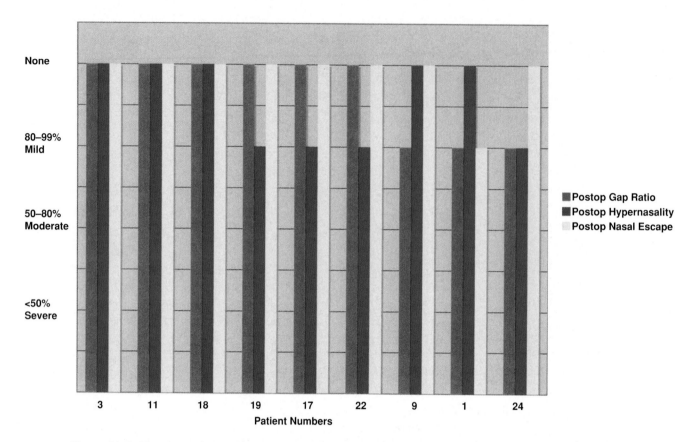

Figure 40–2. The nine patients with preoperative closing ratios of 50–80% (moderate gaps) had evidence of valve competency one year after surgery. Four had neither hypernasality nor nasal escape, and the remaining five had either no nasal escape or no hypernasality. Closure was seen on videonasendoscopy in two-thirds, and every test of postoperative VP competency was either normal or mild.

When marking the palate for double-opposing Z-plasty, landmarks on the oral-side include the hamuli, the base of the uvular halves, and the posterior edge of the hard palate; these determine the angles and size of the oral Z-plasties. The hamuli should be found and marked prior to the injection of local anesthesia. The midline velar scar, which may be quite thick, is incised through the uvula to the back of the hard palate. The fourth landmark, the Eustachian tube orifice, can now be located by putting a Freer elevator through the cleft and running it back and forth laterally under the hamulus area. It will drop into the Eustachian orifice.

I next incise the posteriorly-based oral flap's lateral limb to a point just posterior to the hamulus, detach the scarred levator muscle from its hard palate attachment with scissors, and carefully elevate the muscle with the oral mucosal flap from the nasal mucosa. Scar may complicate the medial aspect of this dissection; however, using the Freer elevator or the closed scissors, placed through the cleft to identify the undersurface of the nasal mucosa, will help to avoid perforating it. In my entire experience, completely elevating the muscle from the nasal mucosa along the entire lateral limb dissection *automatically* divides the tensor aponeurosis, which has made lateral relaxing incisions, hamular fracture, tensor tendon release and dissection in the space of Ernst unnecessary.

When the lateral extent of the dissection nears the hamulus, one should stop cutting and begin to bluntly push the palate muscles posteriorly, not laterally, from the superior constrictor. The levator will appear as a distinct muscle bundle coming into the flap from between the nasal mucosa and the superior constrictor at the posterior margin of the Eustachian orifice, where it normally enters to run directly medially into the velum. When the dissection is complete, the flap is retracted with a suture, which exposes the nasal mucosa beneath.

On the same side, I next make the nasal mucosal Z-plasty lateral limb incision from the base of the uvula to the superior constrictor at the point of entry of the levator, which will be immediately behind the Eustachian orifice. *It is important that this point be precise, because it determines both the anterior-posterior and transverse position of the tip of the opposite side nasal myomucosal flap. The exact transverse orientation and adequate tension of the opposite side's levator muscle depends on proper positioning of the lateral end of this nasal mucosal incision.*

The lateral limb incision for the oral mucosal flap on the other side is now made from the base of the uvula to just lateral to the hamulus. Along the cleft margin and posteriorly along the lateral limb, the incision should be shallow to expose

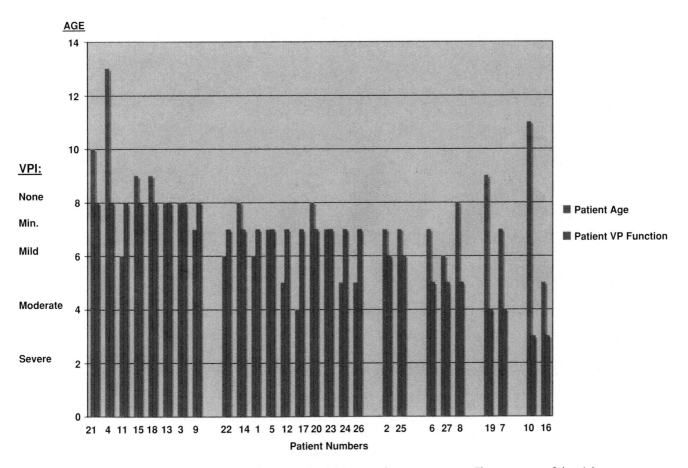

Figure 40–3. Patient age at operation had no relationship to VP function outcome. The mean age of the eight patients with VP competence was 8.8 years, of the 10 patients with either no nasal escape or no hypernasality 6.1 years, and of the nine patients with both nasal escape and hypernasality, 7.4 years.

but not cut the muscles. As the flap elevation approaches the base of the flap along the posterior edge of the hard palate, the plane should be deepened to the back of the hard palate and carefully detached from it, without damaging the greater palatine vessels. Transverse traction on the flap tip will tell whether a backcut around the back of the alveolus will be necessary to free the flap adequately.

The fourth lateral limb incision, for the nasal myomucosal flap, is made from 3 or 4 mm from the posterior edge of the hard palate toward the Eustachian orifice for about a centimeter. With the tip of the flap pulled transversely, the levator is found with a Freer elevator where it lies against the nasal mucosa, and is pushed posteriorly from the superior constrictor The levator muscle is carefully released from the new free margin of the nasal mucosal incision, and the lateral limb incision extended if necessary, until the tip of the flap will reach the end of the contralateral nasal mucosal flap lateral limb incision. This brings the distal end of the levator muscle against the contralateral superior constrictor, immediately under the contralateral levator.

The nasal myomucosal flap is then inset from tip to uvula, beginning with a suture bringing the tip of the flap into the notch at the lateral end of the contralateral mucosal

flap. This brings the tip of the levator muscle to the contralateral superior constrictor. Take care not to include any of the contralateral levator muscle, which should be immediately above the flap tip. Insetting the nasal mucosal flap completes the nasal side.

With a generous suture, the tip of the oral myomucosal flap is positioned at the point along the lateral limb incision over the contralateral levator muscle belly, just posterior to the hamulus. This orients the levator transversely to complete the overlapping levator sling. Note that this may not be at the end of the lateral limb incision, and will not be if a backcut around the maxillary tuberosity has been necessary. Insetting the oral mucosal flap completes closure.

If the incisions have extended anteriorly onto the hard palate, particularly if fistula repair has been a part of the procedure, the mucoperiosteal flaps should be closed with mattress sutures to ensure raw to raw tissue apposition.

One Should Consider Double-Opposing Z-Plasty for Surgical Treatment of VPI When:

1. The surgeon is experienced and successful with double-opposing z-plasty as a technique of primary repair for cleft palate.

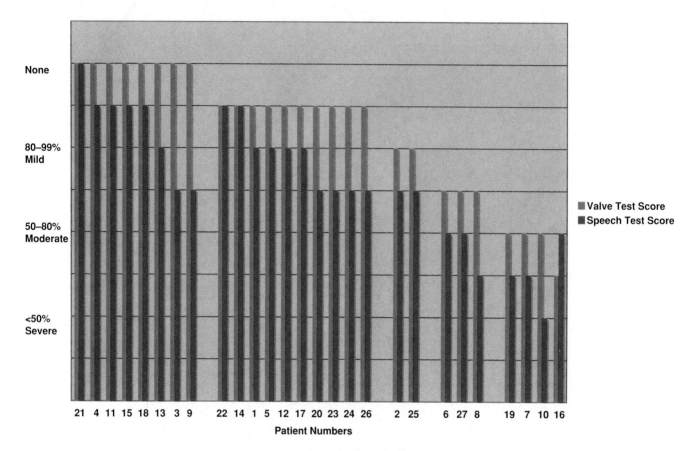

Figure 40–4. Intelligibility and articulation improved to normal or mild only when there was evidence of capability for VP valve closure (either no nasal escape or no hypernasality [10 patients], or neither nasal escape nor hypernasality [8 patients]), although evidence of capability for valve closure did not ensure speech improvement. Valve capability was the limiting factor in speech outcome; the children could speak no better than their VP mechanism would permit.

2. Double-opposing Z-plasty is as likely to succeed as would other methods because it is less likely to result in airway obstruction and OSA.

3. On videofluoroscopy the residual VP gap is less than 8–10 mm.

4. On nasendoscopy the velar closing ratio is 80–99%, or the surgeon has had consistent success at lesser closing ratios (larger gaps).

5. The patient's diagnosis suggests a higher risk of airway obstruction and OSA, such as Pierre Robin or Stickler Syndrome.

6. When a fistula is to be closed and nasal escape and hypernasality have persisted when speech was tested with the fistula plugged with gum or tissue.

7. In circumstances such as third world sites where nasendoscopy or videofluoroscopy is not available to help in selection of a VPI operation, because double opposing z-plasty is less likely to leave a patient with OSA and no follow-up.

Consider Another Procedure Than Double Opposing Z-plasty When:

1. The patient has VCFS.

2. The residual gap on videofluoroscopy is greater than 10 mm.

3. The closing ratio on nasendoscopy is less than 80%, unless the surgeon has had consistent success at lesser closing ratios (larger gaps).

4. The palate is anatomically normal, or the velar muscles have been well overlapped in previous surgery such as a double-opposing Z-plasty, because the Z-plasties will disorient an optimally-aligned levator sling.

5. The surgeon's previous experience with the procedure has been a less than 75% VP competency rate.

When nasal escape and hypernasality remain after double-opposing Z-plasty has been performed for VPI, a trial of speech therapy for a specific length of time may be warranted. If VPI persists at the end of the trial of speech therapy, videofluoroscopy and/or nasendoscopy should be repeated to assist in selection of another surgical procedure. The procedure selected should not divide the velum sagittally, which would cut the overlapped velar muscles.

My first choice for secondary speech surgery following a double-opposing Z-plasty is usually a sphincter pharyngoplasty. My second choice would be a palatal pushback with pharyngeal flap for nasal lining. If the residual gap is 2 mm or smaller, or the closing ratio larger than 70%, one might consider re-elevating and posteriorly advancing the oral-side myomucosal flap, as Chen et al.[22] described. This reportedly produced VP competence in all six patients undergoing the procedure. A pharyngeal flap, with transverse (fishmouth) posterior velar inset, should be reserved for patients who still have large residual gaps and good lateral pharyngeal "sidewall" motion.

References

1. Furlow LT, Jr. Cleft palate repair by double opposing Z-plasty. *Plast Reconstr Surg* 78:724, 1986.
2. Furlow LT, Jr. Cleft palate. In Vistnes LM (ed). *Procedures in Plastic and Reconstructive Surgery: How They Do It.* Boston, Little, Brown, 1991, pp. 351.
3. Furlow LT, Jr. The double opposing Z-plasty for palate closure—Part I. In Jackson IT, Sommerlad BC, (eds). *Recent Advances in Plastic Surgery 4.* Edinburgh, Scotland, Churchill Livingston, 1992, pp. 29.
4. Randall P, LaRossa D, Cohen SR, Cohen MA. The double opposing Z-plasty for palate closure—Part II. In Jackson IT, Sommerlad BC, (eds). *Recent Advances in Plastic Surgery 4.* Edinburgh, Scotland, Churchill Livingston, 1992, pp. 41.
5. Furlow LT, Jr. Secondary cleft palate surgery. In Grotting J (ed). *Reoperative Aesthetic and Reconstructive Plastic Surgery.* St. Louis, MO, Quality Medical Publishers, 1995.
6. Furlow LT. Cleft palate repair by double opposing Z-plasty. *Oper Tech Plast Reconstr Surg* 2:223, 1995.
7. Liao YF, Noordhoff MS, Huang CS, et al. Comparison of obstructive sleep apnea syndrome in children with cleft palate following Furlow palatoplasty or pharyngeal flap for velopharyngeal insufficiency. *Cleft Palate Craniofac J* 41:152, 2004.
8. Witt PB, D'Antonio LL. Velopharyngeal insufficiency and secondary palatal management. *Clin Plast Surg* 20:707, 1993.
9. D'Antonio LL, Eichenberg BJ, Zimmerman GJ, et al. Radiographic and dynamic measures of velopharyngeal anatomy and function following Furlow Z-plasty. *Plast Reconstr Surg* 106:539, 2000.
10. Hudson DA, Grobbelaar AO, Fernandes DB, Lentin R. Treatment of velopharyngeal incompetence by Furlow Z-plasty. *Ann Plast Surg* 34:23, 1995.
11. Chen KT, Wu J, Chen YR, Noordhoff MS. Correction of secondary velopharyngeal insufficiency in cleft palate patients with Furlow palatoplasty. *Plast Reconstr Surg* 94:933, 1994.
12. Lindsey WH, Davis PT. Correction of velopharyngeal insufficiency with Furlow palatoplasty. *Arch Otolaryngol Head Neck Surg* 122:881, 1996.
13. Sie KC, Tampakopoulou DA, Sorom J, Gruss JS, Eblen LE. Results with Furlow palatoplasty in management of velopharyngeal insufficiency. *Plast Reconstr Surg* 108:17, 2001. Discussion, Furlow LT. *Plast Reconstr Surg* 108:26, 2001.
14. Perkins JA, Lewis CW, Gruss JS, Eblen LE, Sie KC. Furlow palatoplasty for management of velopharyngeal insufficiency: A prospective study of 148 consecutive patients. *Plast Reconstr Surg* 116:72, 2005. Discussion, Furlow LT. *Plast Reconstr Surg* 116:81, 2005.
15. Deren O, Ayhan M, Tuncel A, et al. The correction of velopharyngeal insufficiency by Furlow palatoplasty in patients older than 3 years undergoing Veau-Wardill-Kilner palatoplasty: A prospective clinical study. *Plast Reconstr Surg* 116:85, 2005.
16. Golding-Kushner KJ, et al. Standardization for the reporting of nasopharyngoscopy and multiview videofluoroscopy: A report from an international working group. *Cleft Palate J* 27:337, 1990.
17. Perkins JA, et al. Furlow palatoplasty for management of velopharyngeal insufficiency: A prospective study of 148 consecutive patients. *Plast Reconstr Surg* 116:81, 2005.
18. Furlow LT. Discussion of: Deren O, Ayhan M, Tuncel A, et al. The correction of velopharyngeal insufficiency by Furlow palatoplasty in patients older than 3 years undergoing Veau-Wardill-Kilner palatoplasty: A prospective clinical study. *Plast Reconstr Surg* 116:94, 2005.
19. D'Antonio L, Davio M, Zoller K, Punjabi A, Hardesty RA. Results of furlow Z-plasty in patients with velocardiofacial syndrome. *Plast Reconstr Surg* 107:1077, 2001.
20. Witt P, Cohen D, Grames LM, Marsh J. Sphincter pharyngoplasty for the surgical management of speech dysfunction associated with velocardiofacial syndrome. *Brit J Plast Surg* 52:613, 1999.
21. Losken A, Williams JK, Burstein FD, Malick DN, Riski JE. Surgical correction of velopharyngeal insufficiency in children with velocardiofacial syndrome. *Plast Reconstr Surg* 117:1493, 2006.
22. Chen PKT, Wang R, Yun C, Chen YR. Re-repair for salvaging unsatisfied Furlow palatoplasty in managing secondary velopharyngeal insufficiency in cleft patients. Presented at the *American Cleft Palate-Craniofacial Association Annual Meeting*, Minneapolis, MN, April 25–28, 2001, Abstract 128.

41

Posterior Pharyngeal Flaps

Christopher R. Forrest, MD, MSc, FRCSC, FACS • Paula M. Klaiman, MCISc,
Reg CASLPO • Aaron C. Mason, MD, FAAP

INTRODUCTION

The inability to articulate and speak well may severely stigmatize a child and carry significant psychosocial implications. It is estimated that between 10% and 36% of children following cleft palate repair suffer from velopharyngeal dysfunction.[1–6]

The inability of the velopharyngeal sphincter to isolate the nasopharynx from the oropharynx leads to velopharyngeal insufficiency (VPI). The characteristics of VPI may include hypernasal resonance, nasal air emission, nasal/facial grimacing, nasal turbulence, inadequate intraoral air pressure resulting in weak, nasalized or absent consonants, and compensatory articulation substitutions. Compensatory articulations develop as the result of consonants produced at the level of the pharynx or larynx in an attempt to shape the airstream more posterior in the vocal tract. The speech sequelae of VPI can have a profound effect on an individual's ability to be understood (speech intelligibility) jeopardizing social integration and peer acceptance. Fortunately, a combined approach of surgery and speech therapy can produce an excellent prognosis for most patients.

Surgical techniques for correction of VPI may be characterized as static (flaps) or dynamic (sphincter techniques). As a static procedure, the posterior pharyngeal flap represents the most common surgical technique used to treat VPI following cleft palate repair.[1,2] However, the correction of speech problems using this technique is one of the least physiologic surgical procedures performed in the cleft armamentarium and can incur significant morbidity.

This chapter will specifically describe the technique and application of posterior pharyngeal flaps in the management of VPI in cleft patients. Previous chapters have specifically addressed the anatomical concerns, speech evaluation and other surgical techniques for VPI correction, and this information will not be repeated here. In general, it is safe to say that a single operation is not likely to correct all cases of VPI—as a result of a heterogeneity of underlying medical conditions, intellectual capacity, degree and type of attempted closure patterns in patients with this condition. Optimal results are obtained by customizing the procedure to fit the patients needs, based upon careful preoperative assessment.

EVOLUTION OF POSTERIOR PHARYNGEAL FLAPS

Gustav Passavant[7] in 1865, is credited as being the first to attempt surgical correction of VPI by suturing the posterior border of the soft palate to the posterior pharyngeal wall. The inferiorly-based pharyngeal flap was originally described by Karl Schoenborn[8] in 1875 and was first performed on a 17-year-old female with an un-repaired cleft of the hard and soft palate. A fistula that developed between the left side of the flap and the palate required a second von Langenbeck procedure for complete healing, but Schoenborn was impressed that the patient's speech was clear and understandable as soon as healing had taken place. Schoenborn eventually switched to a superiorly-based flap as he felt that suturing the inferiorly-based flap was technically difficult because of the presence of fragile adenoid tissue. He also advocated dividing the flap if the patient maintained acceptable speech for some years but is not known if this was common practice. In 1924, Wolfgang Rosenthal[9] combined the inferiorly-based pharyngeal flap with a von Langenbeck cleft palate closure for the first time and claimed perfect speech results.

The pharyngeal flap was popularized in the United States by Padgett[10] in the 1930s, and has been modified by many authors. Length and width of the flap, donor site closure, and techniques of attachment and insetting have all

undergone various degrees of adjustment in the 1950s and 1960s. However, it is our belief that the key contributions to improving the superior pharyngeal flap technique have consisted of lining the raw surface of the flap, lateral port control, and tailoring the flap size to suit the patient's needs, by utilizing data collected from preoperative videofluoroscopy and nasendoscopy.

According to Millard[11], splitting the soft palate in order to improve exposure and reflecting nasal mucosal flaps to cover the raw undersurface of the pharyngeal flap was presented by Blackfield in 1963. Further attempts to provide lining to the superiorly-based flap included, in 1975, Isshiki and Morimoto's[12] technique of folding it back on itself in the hopes that it would minimize postoperative scar contracture and shrinkage. However, it was Michael Hogan's[13] concept of attempting to provide control of the lateral port size initially in 1971 that led to the most commonly used method for flap lining (Fig. 41–1). Previous work had demonstrated that oropharyngeal pressure began to decrease when the size of the lateral pharyngeal port was greater than 10 mm^2 and was greatly impaired when the port size was 20 mm^2 leading to significant nasal air emission and hypernasality. Hogan concluded that the 20 mm^2 area represented the threshold of velopharyngeal incompetence, and decided to modify the superior pharyngeal flap in an attempt to improve control of the lateral port size by using a catheter with an external diameter of 4 mm^2 to establish the port size during insetting of the flap. In his 1973 publication, Hogan reported his belief of creating a total surface area of the 2 ports of approximately

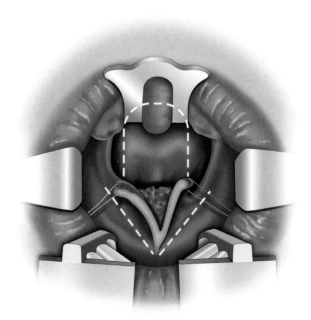

Figure 41–1. Set-up for the Hogan modification of the superior flap technique. The soft palate has been split down the middle and retraction sutures placed. Nasal flaps are marked out and may be triangular or rectangular in shape. The superior flap is marked out on the posterior pharyngeal wall with the upper extent at the adenoid pad allowing for insetting at the level of the soft palate.

25 mm², and claimed a success rate of 97% in a series of 93 patients. However, he was aware of the risk of creating significant hyponasality with absence of nasal respiration, snoring, and increased mucous production, and therefore recommended reopening of the ports in adults, and caution when doing so in the growing child. He describes lining the pharyngeal flap with nasal mucosal flaps in an attempt to maintain flap size and prevent shrinkage. His innovative modifications continue to receive wide acceptance to this very day.

Shprintzen et al.[14] and several others have contributed in important ways to improving the success and decreasing morbidity by suggesting that the flap be tailored to the needs of the patient based upon preoperative nasendoscopy and videofluoroscopy.[1] Modifications of this versatile flap continue.

CLASSIFICATION OF POSTERIOR PHARYNGEAL FLAPS

The posterior pharyngeal wall is an ideal donor site and represents unscarred, well vascularized, nonviolated expendable tissue with minimal long-term donor site morbidity. The donor site consists of the region of the pharynx bounded superiorly by the adenoid pads and extending inferiorly to the region of the third cervical body. The lateral pharyngeal walls determine the lateral extent of the donor area.

Posterior pharyngeal flaps may be classified as static or dynamic, inferiorly based, superiorly based, or laterally based (Table 41–1). This chapter will deal with static flaps, and these are musculomucosal flaps incorporating segments of the palatopharyngeus and superior constrictor muscles. Flaps that are based superiorly have the advantage that they can be made longer than inferiorly-based flaps where the length is limited by the presence of the adenoid pad. Regardless of the location of the flap base, the aim of the pharyngeal flap procedure is to create a central subtotal velopharyngeal obstruction with 2 small lateral ports remaining for nasal airflow.

Table 41–1.
Classification of Pharyngeal Flaps
Static
Posteriorly based
Inferior base
Superior base
Laterally based
Dynamic
Sphincter techniques
Hynes
Orticochea
Jackson-modification

ANATOMY

Although anatomy of the nasopharynx has been covered in previous chapters, some specific points are worth noting. The muscles of the posterior pharyngeal wall consist of the superior pharyngeal constrictor, a curved quadrilateral sheet of muscle encompassing the nasopharynx and upper oropharynx, and the thinnest of the three constrictor muscles. It originates from the posterior pharyngeal raphe and runs laterally and anteriorly to insert into the palate and hamulus superiorly, and the pterygomandibular raphe and mandible inferiorly. It is innervated by the cranial division of the accessory nerve, originating from the pharyngeal plexus. Contraction of the superior constrictor muscle results in the medial and anterior movement of the lateral pharyngeal walls.

The palatopharyngeus muscle forms part of the palatopharyngeal arch and is composed of two fasciculi that lie in the same plane but are separated by the levator veli palatini. These two layers unite at the posterolateral border of the soft palate and run downwards and lateral to form an internal incomplete muscle layer in the pharyngeal wall. It is also innervated by the cranial part of the accessory nerve from the pharyngeal plexus.

Passavant's ridge is a thickened band of muscle on the posterior pharyngeal wall, seen at the level of the soft palate when the soft palate is elevated. Controversy exists as to whether this represents a separate distinct muscle (Passavant's muscle), or whether it is a part of the superior constrictor and palatopharyngeus muscle.[15] This is also the site of the change from columnar ciliated respiratory epithelium of the nasopharynx to the stratified squamous epithelium of the oropharynx.

Lateral wall movement of the pharynx results from contraction of the superior constrictor and palatopharyngeus muscles that form hemi-sphincters; this causes medial displacement of the lateral pharyngeal walls. Creation and elevation of a pharyngeal flap may have an impact upon lateral pharyngeal wall function caused by the disruption of the transverse fibers of both these muscles with the vertical incisions of the flap. While Zwitman documented reduced lateral wall movement following posterior-pharyngeal-flap surgery, this finding was not born out in subsequent studies suggesting that there exists considerable ability to compensate.[14,16,17]

Anatomical studies of the blood supply to inferiorly- and superiorly-based pharyngeal flaps were performed by Mercer and McCarthy using radio-opaque injection techniques in cadavers.[18] The study primarily documented the anatomy of the ascending pharyngeal artery, arising as a branch of the external carotid artery, as the primary blood supply to the pharynx. Several interesting findings were documented. The first was that there exists a midline dehiscence of the superior constrictor over a distance of 8 mm from the cranial base. This is the region of the arch of the first cervical vertebrae (C1), or the lower pole of the adenoid pad, and implies that the mucosa is attached directly to the pharyngobasilar fascia. Therefore, a superiorly-based flap would not be likely to have functional muscle in its base unless the base was placed lower than the first cervical vertebrae.

Secondly, raising a superiorly-based flap divides the pharyngeal branches of the ascending pharyngeal artery that run under the prevertebral fascia and supply the overlying muscle and mucosa. No axial vessels were detected in the flap. This would suggest that the superiorly-based flap is a random pattern one, and the laws of length to width ratios should be recognized. Ischemia may therefore be an additional reason why these flaps are known to shrink and form tubes over time, although muscle denervation is also a recognized factor. Flap shrinkage has been documented to be approximately 50% of its original width.[19] Ischemia may also contribute to flap dehiscence, which has been reported in up to 7% of cases.[18,20,21]

Finally, inferiorly-based and laterally-based flaps are likely to contain axial vessels which allow flaps to be elevated with a length to width ratio greater than 2:1. The popularity of such flaps has been limited because of the limitations in the flap length and tethering of the palate low in the pharynx.

INDICATIONS FOR POSTERIOR–PHARYNGEAL–FLAP SURGERY

Indications for treatment of VPI should be derived from both subjective and objective data. Subjective speech assessments should document speech intelligibility, resonance, articulation and nasal air escape. Objective measures of nasality, using various speech stimuli, include the nasalance score, which is a ratio of the nasal acoustic output relative to oral plus nasal acoustic output, and is expressed as a percentage. This score is matched against age and dialect appropriate normal values. Nasendoscopy provides direct visualization of the soft palate and surrounding velopharyngeal structures during speech and nonspeech activities. The type of closure pattern, symmetry of movement, degree of closure, palatal morphology, presence of tonsils and adenoids, and pharyngeal pulsations should all be documented. Velopharyngeal closure rating (out of 1.0 in 0.1 increments) is based upon the fraction of the diameter of the velopharyngeal port that is closed off during attempted sphincter closing. Multiview videofluoroscopy may also be used for determining the defect size and closure pattern but carries the risk of radiation exposure. At the Hospital for Sick Children, Toronto, Canada, videofluoroscopy is reserved for the child who is unable to tolerate nasendoscopy, or when lateral-view imaging (which cannot be obtained using nasendoscopy) is needed.

Armour et al.[22] from the Hospital for Sick Children, Toronto, Canada hypothesized that the closure pattern of the velopharyngeal sphincter was an important determinant in selecting the proper operation for children with VPI. Closure patterns may be classified into coronal (good velar movement), sagittal (good lateral wall movement), circular (good velar and lateral wall movement), plus or minus a contribution from Passavant's ridge[22,23] (Table 41–2). In a retrospective correlation, they demonstrated that preoperative

velopharyngeal closure pattern was a significant factor in predicting the effectiveness of superiorly-based pharyngeal flaps in correcting the hypernasality associated with VPI. As a static procedure, success of the superiorly-based flap is dependent upon lateral port closure as result of medial movement of the lateral pharyngeal walls. This study nicely demonstrated that noncoronal (sagittal and circular) closure patterns were satisfactorily addressed by the superiorly-based flap technique. Coronal-closure patterns, associated with poor lateral pharyngeal wall movement, resulted in a lower success rate, and may be better managed in selected patients with a sphincter pharyngoplasty.

The decision to treat VPI is dependent upon many factors including: patient age, length of time VPI has been present, etiology of VPI (congenital versus acquired, structural versus idiopathic, neuromuscular) severity of VPI, intellectual capacity of the patient, comorbidities, and the presence of mitigating factors such as obstructive sleep apnea, to mention a few. Nonsurgical therapies include prosthetic management with speech bulbs and palatal lift devices; but, in general, these are not well tolerated in children. At the Hospital for Sick Children, Toronto, Canada, the spectrum of surgical management of VPI consists of superiorly-based pharyngeal flaps, sphincter pharyngoplasty, and palatal lengthening (double opposing Z-plasty Furlow or pushback palatoplasty) techniques. Inferiorly and transversely based flaps are not routinely performed.

We believe the indications for treating VPI with superiorly-based pharyngeal flaps include, VPI associated with poor palatal motion, a velopharyngeal gap detected upon nasendoscopy, and the presence of some lateral wall movement (i.e., a noncoronal closure pattern). Palatal lengthening techniques may be applied when velopharyngeal closure is marginal, an overt or occult submucous cleft palate has been detected, or when the presence of aberrant vessels in the posterior pharyngeal wall precludes safe elevation of a pharyngeal flap. Poor lateral wall movement seen with a predominate coronal closure pattern, is an indication for sphincter pharyngoplasty (Table 41–3).

Regardless of the surgical technique, the successful management of VPI depends upon the patient and families understanding of the limitations of surgery and the fact that postoperative speech therapy may very well be required.

INFERIOR–VERSUS SUPERIORLY–BASED FLAPS

It has not been incontrovertibly proven that one flap type is superior to the other. The inferiorly-based flap may have an advantage in terms of vascularity, but has limitations with its length, ability to inset the flap secondary to incorporated adenoid tissue at the tip, and the low position of the base in the pharynx. The superiorly-based flap may be lengthened and inset at the level of the soft palate, but may be lacking as robust a vasculature. Previous studies by Skoog[24] (1965), Hamlen[25] (1970), Whitaker et al.[26] (1972), and Karling et al.[27]

Table 41–2.

Velopharyngeal Closure Patterns*

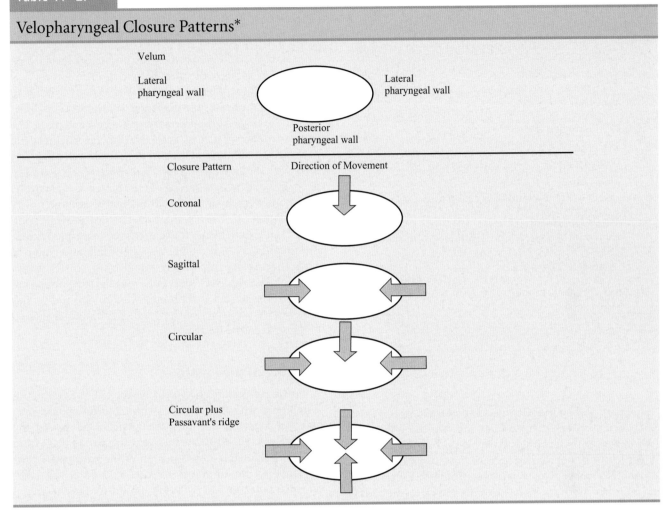

Anatomy of the velopharyngeal port and closure patterns.
After Skolnick, M, McCall G, Barnes. M. The sphincteric mechanism of velopharyngeal closure. Cleft Palate J 10:286, 1973; Armour et al. Does velopharyngeal closure pattern affect the success of pharyngeal flap pharyngoplasty? Plast Reconstr Surg 115:45, 2005.

(1999) found no significant differences in postoperative speech, hearing, complications, or length of stay between those patients who had a superiorly-based; compared to an inferiorly-based flap.

TIMING OF SURGERY

The diagnosis of VPI is not usually established until the child is around 4 years of age. This allows the language and articulation systems a chance to mature and to benefit from speech therapy, which should be instituted as soon as speech disorder is detected. In some cases, improvements in velopharyngeal valving occur as articulation skills improve. This is particularly true when compensatory articulation substitutions can be remediated. Correction of the hypernasality component is ideally performed once these issues have been addressed. In addition, patient cooperation for visualization techniques (nasendoscopy and multiview videofluoroscopy) needs to be considered. Once all necessary data has been obtained, ideally, surgery should be performed around age 5 years. Although some studies have suggested that surgery before age 6 years may be associated with improved outcomes,[28,29] others have not shown such an advantage.[30]

SURGICAL TECHNIQUE

Preoperative Assessment

All patients in the Cleft Lip and Palate Program at the Hospital for Sick Children, Toronto, Canada are seen in a multidisciplinary setting and undergo regular team assessments including Otolaryngology, Pediatric Dentistry, Orthodontics, Plastic Surgery, Speech and Language Pathology, Social Work, Psychiatry and Audiology at 1, 3, 5 and 9 years, and more frequently depending on the treatment plan for the individual child. Prior to pharyngeal-flap surgery, appropriate medical, behavioral, and family history is obtained. Preoperative

Table 41–3.

Treatment Indications for VPI Based Upon Findings at Nasendoscopy

Superior Pharyngeal Flap
- good lateral wall movement
- moderate to large defect

Sphincter Pharyngoplasty
- poor lateral wall movement

Furlow (double opposing Z-plasty) Palatoplasty
- small defect
- occult or small submucous cleft palate

Pushback Palatoplasty
- moderate to large defect if combined with superior flap
- small defect if isolated procedure

Nonsurgical (palatal lift device)
- surgical contraindication
- patient request
- training device for borderline/marginal VPI

audiograms are important to rule out conductive hearing loss; and, when necessary, myringotomy and ventilation tube insertion may be performed with the pharyngeal-flap surgery. When felt to be appropriate, preoperative cervical vascular imaging is obtained. This issue of preoperative vascular imaging is further addressed in the following section on the 22q11 Microdeletion Syndrome. Physical examination of all patients includes an oral examination, perceptual judgment of resonance, acoustic analysis (nasometry), and visualization of the velopharyngeal mechanism (multiview videofluoroscopy, or nasopharyngoscopy).

Patient Preparation

The patient is placed supine on a headrest, with bolsters placed under the shoulders, and the neck is extended. A general anesthesia is delivered via oral RAE endotracheal tube that is placed in the midline and taped. A Dingman mouth gag with the largest possible tongue blade is inserted and care is taken not to compress the endotracheal tube when opening the gag, or encroach upon the posterior pharyngeal wall. A small throat pack may be useful. Direct visualization of the pharynx is accompanied by finger palpation in order to detect aberrant vasculature. A headlight worn by the operating surgeon improves visualization. Prophylactic antibiotics are not routinely administered unless cardiac or other medical issues dictate. Excessive neck extension is to be avoided because of the rare but documented occurrence of spontaneous cervical dislocation. Trendelenburg positioning may assist in

visualization and improve comfort for the surgeon, however, this will increase venous bleeding.

Flap Marking

The flap is marked out with its base located at the adenoid pad and correlating to the anterior tubercle of the first cervical vertebrae (Fig. 41–1). Flap width may be varied according to need as determined by the preoperative investigations, however, the average flap width ranges between 2 and 3 cm. The width of the flap needed will depend upon the patients lateral pharyngeal wall movement; but, in general, wider flaps are used when the lateral pharyngeal wall movement is poor. The flap may be skewed to one side in the presence of abnormal pulsations, or preoperative determination of asymmetric lateral wall motion. The length of the flap is dependent upon access and requirements for tension-free insetting. Average flap length is 2.5–3 cm, but it may extend inferiorly for up to 4 cm. The tip of the flap has been found to often correlate with the second cervical vertebrae. Following marking, the posterior pharyngeal wall is infiltrated with Xylocaine 1% with 1:200,000 epinephrine, and a period of 7 minutes is allowed to elapse to ensure vasoconstriction.

Splitting of the Palate

If the Hogan modification is to be applied, the soft palate is infiltrated with Xylocaine 1% with 1:200,000 epinephrine, and after adequate time for vasoconstriction has passed, the soft palate is split down the middle with a No. 11 blade from the tip of the uvula to the margin of the hard palate (Fig. 41–1). Retraction on the uvula with 4–0 sutures will facilitate this maneuver. This will aid exposure for the pharyngeal flap significantly. Triangular or rectangular flaps of nasal mucosa based along the free posterior edge of the soft palate are marked out and raised at a submucosal level using a No. 15 blade or fine dissecting scissors (Fig. 41–2). The posterolateral extent of these nasal-lining flaps determines the size of the lateral ports, and is critical to the success of the procedure. The length of these flaps should be similar to the depth of the palate. Once these flaps have been elevated, traction sutures are used to keep them out of the field.

Posterior-Pharyngeal-Flap Elevation

The lateral incisions of the flap are made with either diathermy or a No. 15 blade and then blunt scissors are used to dissect through the superior constrictor and palatopharyngeus muscles to expose the prevertebral fascia. This is easily identifiable by its white avascular appearance. It is simple to undermine the flap in a bipedicle fashion; and, then with retraction of the flap in a cranial fashion, sharp cutting scissors or diathermy may be used to cut the distal end of the flap at the appropriate length. The flap is mobilized completely to its base to allow for a tension free inset (Fig. 41–3). Posterior pharyngeal veins represent the most common site for bleeding and are visible on the prevertebral fascia.

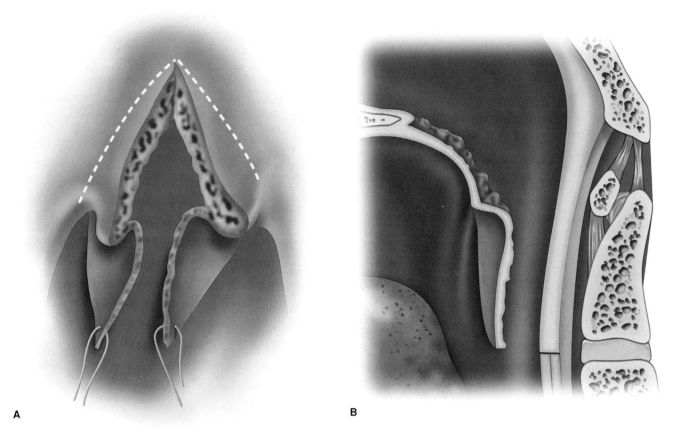

Figure 41–2. Nasal flaps have been elevated at a submucosal level and may be retracted away out of the field. (**A**) Incisions for the nasal side lining flaps noted by dotted lines, sutures retracting the raised nasal mucosal flaps. (**B**) Sagittal view of nasal flaps raised.

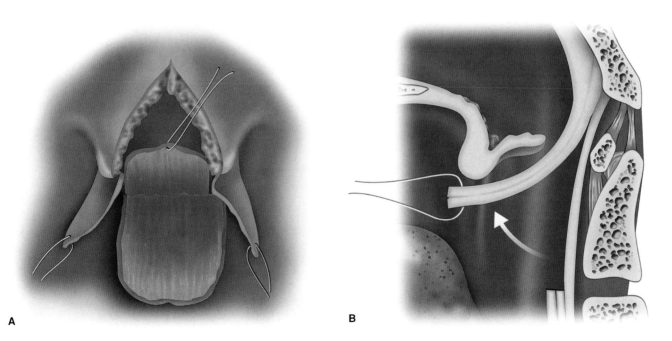

Figure 41–3. A superiorly-based flap has been raised at the level of the prevertebral fascia. The flap incorporates the muscle of the posterior pharyngeal wall. (**A**) superior suture retracting the posterior flap cephalad, and two lower sutures retracting the nasal lining flaps. Raw surface of the donor site on posterior pharyngeal wall noted. (**B**) Sagittal view of the posterior pharyngeal flap raised cephalad and noted by arrow.

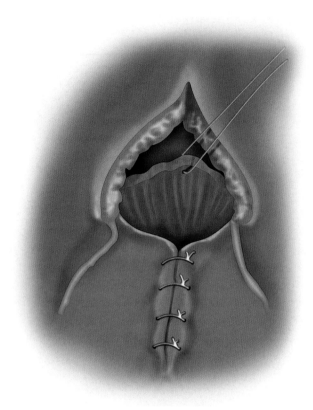

Figure 41–4. Closure of the posterior pharyngeal wall flap donor site with care taken to incorporate bites of the prevertebral fascia to eliminate webbing and close the dead space.

Donor Site Management

Donor site closure should always be performed, as closure is better for patient comfort and reduces the risk of postoperative hemorrhage and infection. The lateral free edges of muscle and mucosa of the posterior pharyngeal wall donor site are sutured together with 3–0 absorbable sutures as one layer (Fig. 41–4). Care must be taken to pick up a bite of the prevertebral fascia in the closure as this prevents webbing and narrowing of the pharynx and may also prevent hematoma formation by eliminating dead space. Care must be taken at the cranial end of the donor site not to constrict the flap base during closure.

Flap Insetting

Several methods of flap insetting may be employed. A 5-point suture technique may be used where one stitch is placed to position the lateral extent of each side of the flap, one stitch in the midline, and bilateral sutures placed in between these points (Fig. 41–5). Obtaining the appropriate size of the lateral ports may be facilitated using a catheter placed nasally. Delayed tying of these sutures is recommended.

If nasal lining flaps are used, once the pharyngeal flap has been sutured, the two nasal flaps are sutured in the midline with 4–0 absorbable suture (Fig. 41–6). The tips of these flaps are then sutured to the prevertebral fascia in the midline at the base of the pharyngeal flap. This lines the raw surface of the underside of the pharyngeal flap. A suture is placed through the lateral margin to facilitate creation of the lateral port.

If lining flaps are not to be utilized, insetting the pharyngeal flap may be performed using a "fish-mouth" technique. An incision is performed along the posterior free margin of the soft palate, and scissor dissection is used to create a pocket for the flap. Using 4–0 absorbable sutures introduced into the pocket from the lingual side of the palate, a midline suture is then placed using a mattress technique through the flap tip in the depth of the velar pocket, and brought out and tied on the lingual side of the palate a few millimeters from the first suture pass. Variations on this method have included insetting the flap in a "pull-through" manner in the mid-portion of the soft palate.

Regardless of the technique of insetting, it is important that the base of the flap be established at the level of the palatal plane, as inferior displacement of the flap base has been shown to develop over time and may be associated with recurrence of VPI.[31,32]

Postoperative Care

At the end of the procedure, the pharynx is carefully examined for hemostasis and a soft nasopharyngeal tube is placed through one of the nostrils and through one of the lateral ports (Fig. 41–7). It is sutured to the membranous septum of the nose for security. It is designed to act as a suction conduit and temporary airway aid. It is usually removed on the second day following surgery. When the Dingman mouth gag is removed, care must be taken to disengage the endotracheal tube from the groove in the tongue retractor to prevent accidental extubation. Prior to reversing the general anaesthetic, the surgeon should check that both temporomandibular joints are seated within the fossa as subluxation may occur when the mouth gag is opened. Throat packs should be removed prior to extubation.

All patients are managed in an observation unit postoperatively for 24 hours. Analgesia and mouth care is administered. Moisturized air or oxygen may be administered by facemask. Pulse oximetry is routinely used during the length of hospital stay. Suctioning may be performed using a soft catheter through the nasopharyngeal tube or in the cheek vestibules, away from the surgical site. Patients are maintained on clear liquids for 24 hours followed by a soft diet. Patients are discharged home when drinking well and pain is well controlled. Complications such as airway compromise or hemorrhage are most likely to occur within the first 24 hours postoperatively, and patients should be carefully monitored during this time.

INFERIORLY-BASED FLAPS

The inferiorly-based flap is used infrequently today. The technique is similar to that described above. Important technical details of flap elevation include elevation as necessary to inset the flap into the soft palate in a tension free manner.

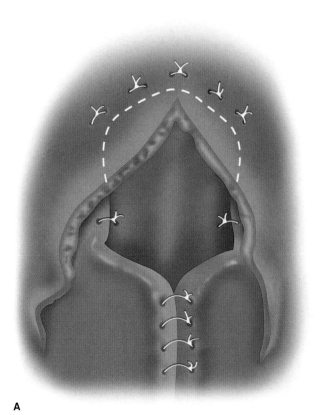

A

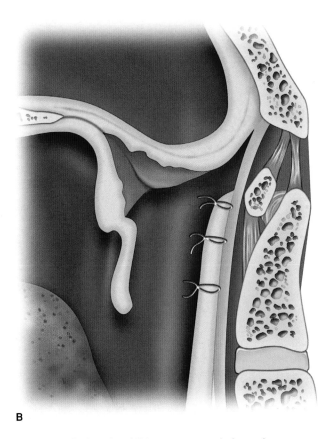

B

Figure 41–5. (**A**) Insetting of the pharyngeal flap with a 5-point suture technique in addition to suture to help establish the lateral port size. This may be aided with then introduction of a nasal catheter. (**B**) Sagittal view of superiorly-based posterior pharyngeal flap inset and nasal palatal lining flaps yet to be sewn in place.

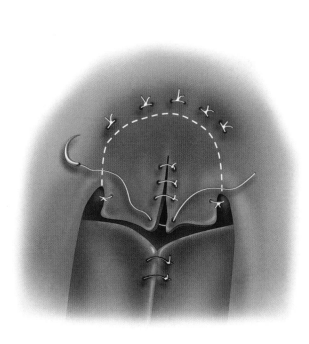

A

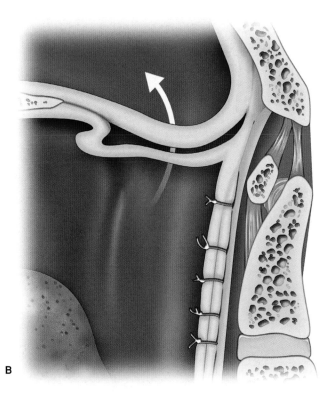

B

Figure 41–6. (**A**) Closure of the soft palate followed by approximation of the nasal mucosal lining flaps in the midline. These flaps are attached to the prevertebral fascia at the base of the pharyngeal flap. (**B**) Sagittal view of the inset and closure of the nasal mucosal lining flaps.

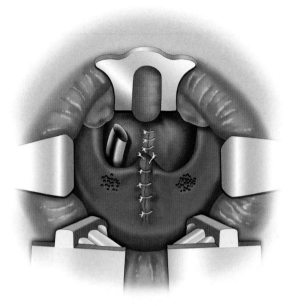

Figure 41–7. Final result at closure. The stippled areas represent the lateral pharyngeal ports. A nasopharyngeal tube has been placed to secure the airway and allow for suctioning.

Unfortunately, this pulls the soft palate inferiorly and posteriorly and will impede its mobility.

LATERALLY-BASED FLAPS

In 1975, Donald Kapetansky described bilateral transverse flaps based laterally created by making a wide S-shaped incision on the posterior wall of the pharynx.[33] Each flap was described to have a base of 15–20 mm with a length of 30 mm (Fig. 41–8). They are sutured together to cover the posterior 15–20 mm of the mid-portion of the soft palate with one flap sutured on the nasal side and the other on the oral side (Fig. 41–9). The donor site is closed. Strictly speaking, these may be also considered as dynamic flaps as the intention was to preserve the nerve supply. Kapetansky believed that this also prevented denervation atrophy of the flap and maintained the bulk over time. These flaps are not commonly used, and this technique has been supplanted by dynamic sphincter techniques described in another chapter.

RESULTS

There are many studies assessing the efficacy of pharyngeal-flap surgery for the correction of VPI. In general, success rates of 63–98% have been quoted following superiorly-based pharyngeal flap correction of VPI.[1–6,34–36] Only a few randomized trials have been performed, and most of the literature on the subject is retrospectively based. No single study has clearly documented strong advantages of one technique over the next.

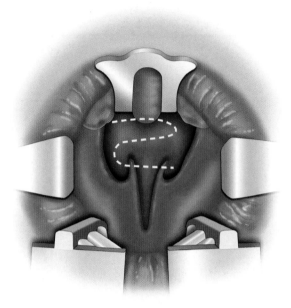

Figure 41–8. Kapetansky's modification using laterally-based flaps in an S-shaped incision made on the posterior pharyngeal wall. The base of each flap is approximately 15–20 mm wide with a length of 30–35 mm.

Canady detailed the experience from the University of Iowa in 87 patients (53 cleft lip and palate; 8 cleft palate; 26 submucous cleft palate) over a 10-year span with a minimum 2-year follow-up noted in 44 patients.[34] Success was reported in 78% of patients as defined by near-normal nasality and by the lack of hypernasality and hyponasality.

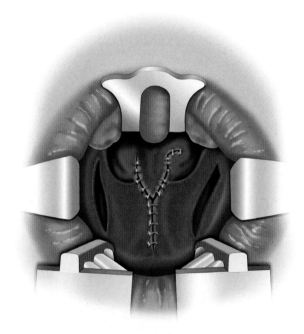

Figure 41–9. Kapetansky's flaps elevated and inset at the time of palatoplasty. The flaps are elevated at the level of the prevertebral fascia to incorporate muscle and nerve supply.

Peat et al.[28] (1994) compared different techniques for VPI correction and found that a superiorly-based flap combined with a pushback palatoplasty (Honig operation) and a modified Hynes dynamic sphincteroplasty had identical results with 81% acceptable nasal resonance compared with 63% following a superiorly-based flap alone. However, 51% of patients complained of snoring postoperatively, and 9% required revision of their pharyngoplasty as a results of the onset of sleep apnea in the Honig and Hynes groups. Pensler and Reich[37] (1991) found no difference in speech outcome between pharyngeal flaps and dynamic sphincteroplasty, but noted a 4% incidence of sleep apnea in the flap group. Ysunza et al.[38] (2002) documented the experience from Mexico City and compared 25 pharyngeal flaps and 25 sphincter pharyngoplasties post-cleft palate repair and found no difference in outcome with success rates between 84–88% in children between ages 4 and 8 years. Consideration was made to ensure that articulation problems were eliminated prior to surgery. No cases of sleep apnea were noted in either group.

In a rare international multicenter randomized trial, no statistically significant difference between pharyngeal flap and sphincter pharyngoplasty was detected at 12 months postoperatively, although results were much better in the flap group at 3 months postoperatively. Both techniques demonstrated elimination of hypernasality in 85% of patients.[39] Furthermore, sleep apnea was rarely seen in either group. Tailoring the flap according to preoperative lateral pharyngeal wall motion and palatal movement, as seen on instrumental evaluation, was initially suggested by Shprintzen et al.[14] and appears to make intuitive sense. Interestingly, however, as all patients were randomly assigned to either a flap or sphincter group, this study did not support preoperative technique selection, and casts some doubt upon the validity of endoscopic preoperative assessment.

Hathaway[40] (1980) found no difference between vertically based and transversely based flaps. Skoog[24] (1965) and Whitaker et al.[26] (1972) found no difference comparing superiorly and inferiorly-based flaps. Karling et al.[27] (1999) found no difference in speech outcome when comparing two methods (longitudinal versus transverse splitting) of insetting superior pharyngeal flaps into the soft palate. Marsh[4] (2003) stated a preference for superior pharyngeal flaps when a sagittal gap with good lateral wall motion was present, and applied the technique of sphincter pharyngoplasty when there was poor movement of the velopharyngeal mechanism. He found no difference in speech outcome between the two groups (74% and 72%, respectively, after primary surgery, 92% and 85%, respectively, following secondary revision), and reinforced the important concept that the technique should be tailored to meet the needs of the patient.

The effectiveness of the superiorly-based pharyngeal flap, in relation to the type of palatal defect and timing of the operation, was investigated by Seyfer at al.[30] (1988). While 100% of patients under age 6 were noted to have improvement, compared to only 74% of those over 6 years, this difference was not found to be statistically significant when assessing improvement scores in the two groups. The length of

time that VPI was present before surgery was also found not to be important. Demark and Hardin[41] (1985) had had similar results, stating that age at time of pharyngeal surgery was not a critical factor in speech outcome. However, Leanderson et al.[42] from the Karolinska Institute in Stockholm (1974), as well as Riski[43] (1979), had previously reported that the best results for speech improvement were seen in children younger than 6.4 years of age. This philosophy is shared by our team at the Hospital for Sick Children, Toronto, Canada.

It must be kept in mind that outcome assessment of pharyngeal-flap surgery may likely suffer from reviewer bias, lack of objective data, lack of agreement in what constitutes success, and the evolutionary changes in the status of speech over time as child grows and the pharynx and flap change. However, the diligent long-term application of objective measures such as nasalance scores, and a high level of experience of a dedicated multidisciplinary team, will ensure that the highest quality of care is met.

22q11 DELETION SYNDROME

The 22q11 Deletion Syndrome (22q11 DS), also known as 22q11 Microdeletion Syndrome, Shprintzen Syndrome, and Velocardiofacial Syndrome, is an autosomal dominant condition associated with conotruncal heart anomalies, learning disabilities, immunodeficiency, characteristic facies, and communicative issues, and requires special mention in the context of the surgical correction of VPI. Three-quarters of patients diagnosed with the 22q11 DS may have a palatal anomaly, and the vast majority has significant speech and language impairments that may include hypernasal resonance. It is the most common syndrome to be associated with cleft palate and comprises 8% of all cases of isolated cleft palate (overt and submucous).[44] It deserves special mention as a challenge to the cleft team.

The management of speech and articulation disorders in 22q11 DS patients can be challenging depending upon the age at first presentation, wide variability of expression, cognitive and behavioral profile, expertise of the Speech and Language Pathologist, and compliance with speech therapy. The experience of our institution involves the management of these children with a specialized team to address medical issues (cardiac, immunologic, hematologic, renal and endocrine) and early assessment by the cleft surgeon and Speech/Language Pathologist.

In a recent evaluation of 135 patients with 22q11 DS seen at the Hospital for Sick Children, Toronto, Canada, 63 underwent the following surgical techniques specifically to address issues of nasal hyper-resonance: superiorly-based pharyngeal flap (51 patients), sphincter pharyngoplasty (3 patients), primary Furlow palatoplasty (6 patients) and revision pharyngoplasty (2 patients).[45] Pharyngeal flaps were successful in 50% of cases reviewed 2 years postoperatively with no evidence of sleep apnea, while some improvement was noted in 35% of patients. A modest improvement in resonance was noted in 35% of patient's whereas 15% of

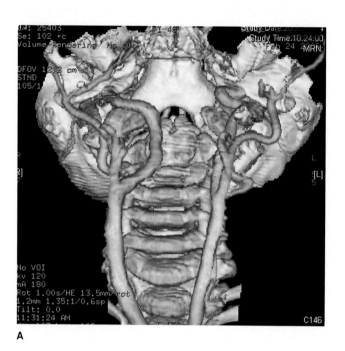

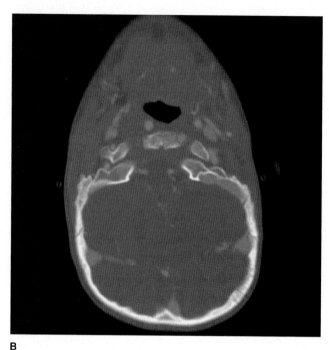

A   B

Figure 41–10. (A) CT angiogram in a patient with 22q11 microdeletion showing a 3-D rendering demonstrating the aberrant course of the right internal carotid artery with marked deviation to the midline. **(B)** Noted on the axial view.

patients had no or minimal improvement whatsoever, despite a technically satisfactory procedure. A Furlow palatoplasty procedure was reserved for those cases in which a posterior flap was not anatomically possible and parents were anxious to pursue surgical management, or in those with a submucous cleft palate. In our series, all of these patients undergoing Furlow palatoplasty had submucous cleft palates, and although the number of patients reviewed is small, 33% were successful, and 33% showed some improvement after this procedure. One patient had a concurrent diagnosis of cleft lip and palate in addition to deviation of the carotid arteries and had a successful outcome 2 years after undergoing a secondary Furlow palatoplasty (palate re-repair). The treatment philosophy of our institution dictates that superiorly-based pharyngeal flaps are useful in up to 85% of cases, and Furlow palatal lengthening procedures may be beneficial for those with unrepaired submucous cleft palates and small velopharyngeal gaps or defects. It is felt that the earlier the age of surgery, the better the prognosis for improved speech. This experience was mirrored by Great Ormond Street Hospital for Children in London, demonstrating significant improvement in nasal air emission following a Hynes pharyngoplasty in 42 children with the 22q11 DS, however, suggested that, depending on velopharyngeal anatomy and function, there is a role for multiple procedures in order to achieve improvements in speech.[46]

An association between the 22q11 DS and medial displacement of the internal carotid arteries was established in 1987, and concerns were voiced regarding the suitability of pharyngeal-flap surgery in the management of VPI in

these cases (Fig. 41–10).[47] It is crucial to assess all patients preoperatively with nasendoscopy to document pulsations along the posterior pharyngeal wall. In patients with the 22q11 DS, CT angiogram or magnetic resonance angiography have been recommended to document the anatomy and course of the internal carotid vessels. This is a somewhat controversial topic as "cautious surgery" was recommended by Witt et al.[44] after 10 patients with documented pulsations on endoscopy underwent uncomplicated pharyngeal-flap surgery without preoperative radiologic imaging. Witt and his group performed uneventful pharyngeal-flap surgery on 10 patients with known 22q11 DS, using nasendoscopy as a screening tool. In a questionnaire sent to 30 individuals at 28 cleft-craniofacial centers, 55% of surgeons did not routinely order cervical vascular imaging studies on such patients. The authors carefully point out the need for careful intraoperative search for abnormal pharyngeal vasculature prior to dissecting a flap, but conclude that preoperative cervical vascular imaging may have limited value in this group of patients.

Spontaneous straightening and lateral displacement of the internal carotid arteries has been described in 2 patients who underwent repeat imaging 4 years after originally being turned down for surgery on the basis of their CT scans.[48] Although both underwent successful unmodified superiorly-based pharyngeal-flap surgery, this was performed many years later, and one could question whether the wait was justified. While the role of presurgical imaging has been the source of some debate, it is paramount that the issue of displacement of the arteries be respected. Modified or skewed superiorly-based flaps may be possible in most patients with medially deviated carotid arteries, and the senior author routinely makes a decision to operate on such patients based upon intraoperative examination under anaesthesia with the neck appropriately extended following preoperative assessment with nasendoscopy. Nasendoscopy is vital in assessing these patients for pulsations, but a careful intraoperative assessment is just as good as a preoperative CT. Nasendoscopy has been demonstrated by Ross et al. to have a high degree of accuracy in the detection of carotid artery variants.[49] Ross et al.[49] performed CT angiography on 25 patients with the 22q11 DS to document the course of the internal carotid vessels. All 25 children showed some degree of carotid artery deviation (bilateral in 44%, right sided in 24% and left sided in 32%) with a high degree of variability and severity. No constant pattern of anomaly was demonstrated, but the study did show that in 18 of 25 children, the abnormally positioned vessel was 3 mm from the surface of the pharyngeal mucosa. This study also demonstrated that the flap did not extend caudal to the disc space between C2 and C3 vertebrae. The majority of the anomalies were found to have corrected themselves by the time the vessels got in to the region where the flap was to be raised. Of the children assessed, 52% were felt to be safe to proceed as planned, as the deviation was located below the surgical site, 28% of patients required some degree of flap modification, but alternate forms of treatment were offered to 20% of patients caused by the severity and position of the abnormal vessels which impacted on the site of the pharyngeal flap.

COMPLICATIONS

Pharyngoplasty is a serious and potentially morbid operation, and full disclosure of the risks should be given to the patient and families prior to undertaking such treatment (Table 41–4). A fine balance exists between obstructing a patient's nasopharynx sufficiently enough to eliminate nasal air emission, but not too much to produce nasal obstruction. A patient's death in 1990 prompted two comprehensive reviews of complication rates in 386 patients undergoing superiorly-based pharyngeal-flap surgery at the Hospital for Sick Children, Toronto, Canada by Valnicek et al.[50] (1994) and Fraulin et al.[51] (1998). The first review, based upon data collected between 1985–1992, demonstrated that the operation carried an overall risk of 19.4%, and a 16.4% acute risk in the perioperative period, including an 8.2% risk of bleeding and a 9.1% risk of airway obstruction. The majority of these complications occurred within the first 24 hours postoperatively.[50] A follow-up study, several years later at the same institution by Fraulein et al., demonstrated a decrease in the overall complication rate from 19.5 to 6.3%, a decrease in bleeding rate to 1.4%, and a decrease in airway obstruction rate to 3.2%, in patients operated upon after the mortality in 1990.[51] Increased awareness of the staff, an improved rigor in patient selection, adequate preoperative investigation of obstructive sleep apnea, the use of preoperative CT angiograms to assess internal carotid artery position, improved hemostasis, fewer operating surgeons, slower reversal of anaesthesia, donor site closure, use of postoperative nasopharyngeal airways, and decreased incidence of ancillary procedures were the factors felt to contribute to the decrease in complication rate. These studies highlight the importance and necessity of internal audits and critical reviews.

Rare complications include spontaneous atlantoaxial subluxation with torticollis entitled "la maladie de Grisel".[52] Care must be exercised when extending the neck during initial preparation of the patient.

Hyponasality

Hyponasality may be a common finding following surgery. As documented by Seagle et al.[2], who demonstrated a 91% success rate in 80 patients and a hyponasality rate of 18.2%, this complication can easily overlooked unless it is manifest as part of a sleep apnea problem.

Residual VPI

Residual postoperative VPI may result from a flap being too narrow or placed too low, either by faulty design, or as a result of postoperative shrinkage. Secondary treatment may involve revision of the lateral ports, or performing a second flap, however, this should depend upon the findings from nasendoscopy. Barone et al.[31] (1994) reported on 21 patients with residual VPI following pharyngeal-flap surgery, who had successful salvage procedures either by creation of a new superiorly-based flap elevated from a scarred bed, or a localized superiorly-based patch-flap, created to manage unilateral port insufficiency. Witt et al.[32] (1998) found that 20% of patients following pharyngeal flap or sphincter pharyngoplasty required revisionary surgery for residual VPI occurring primarily as the result of flap dehiscence. While the majority of patients in each group were managed successfully with a single

Table 41–4.

Complications of Pharyngoplasty

Early
  Airway compromise
  Hemorrhage
  Infection
  Aspiration/Pneumonia
  Flap dehiscence
  Cervical subluxation

Late
  Sleep apnea
  Hyponasality
  Residual VPI

revisional procedure, a sizeable minority of those originally treated with a flap, required a second revisional operation.

Infection

Fortunately, postoperative infection is a rare occurrence. Cervical osteomyelitis has been reported, however, following a pharyngeal flap operation in which the donor site was left open.[53] Antibiotic prophylaxis is not routinely recommended unless cardiac issues are present.

Aspiration/Pneumonia

Following pharyngeal-flap surgery, the airway is relatively unprotected immediately following extubation, and aspiration of blood should be watched for. Judicious suctioning, head elevation, and careful observation are indicated in the first 24 hours following surgery.

Flap Dehiscence

Partial or complete separation of the flap from the palate has been reported in up to 7% of cases by Graham et al.[21] Pharyngeal flap dehiscence has been more commonly observed following inferiorly-based flaps, and may be associated with infection. Possible ischemic factors in flap design have also been alluded to in the etiology of flap dehiscence. The initial treatment for flap dehiscence is usually conservative and followed by a salvage procedure several months later, once the wound has had a chance to mature.

Obstructive Sleep Apnea

Virtually all patients snore following the placement of a superior pharyngeal flap. Obstructive sleep apnea, however, is a recognized problem occurring in up to 38% of cases immediately following pharyngoplasty surgery.[54] Obstructive sleep apnea (OSA) may occur following any type of surgery for VPI, but in one study was more likely to be experienced following superiorly-based flap pharyngoplasty.[55]

Apnea may be a problem in the acute perioperative period because of swelling, alteration of airway physiology, and bleeding—such that all patients should receive appropriate monitoring. However, the obturating effect of the flap may result in significant obstructive sleep apnea, which may worsen as scar contracture of the lateral ports occurs. There is considerable variability to the long-term incidence of OSA following pharyngeal-flap surgery, ranging from 1–20%, however, the numbers of patients are limited in these studies.

Sirois et al.[56] (1994) performed sleep studies in 41 children undergoing pharyngeal flap operations, and demonstrated the presence of sleep apnea in 35% of patients in the early postoperative period, but this resolved in all patients over the ensuing months. Similar findings were reported by Lesavoy et al.[54] (1996), with 38% of patients showing symptoms of upper airway obstruction, that resolved in all but 2 of 29 patients by 5 months postoperatively. In addition, neither of these patients with upper airway obstructive symptoms was severe enough to require surgical revision. The Mexico City experience was not so forgiving in a study of 585 patients treated for VPI, where sleep apnea was confirmed by sleep study in 2.6% of patients, and all required secondary surgical management.[38]

The preoperative identification of potential risk factors for sleep apnea mandates a preoperative sleep study. These potential risk factors include snoring, the history of Pierre Robin Sequence, and noncleft (neuromuscular) causes of VPI. Postoperative OSA may be managed by nasal continuous positive airway pressure, but may require takedown or modification of the flap. Interestingly, the speech benefits achieved by the flap may be maintained after the flap has been divided, and the correction of the OSA achieved.[57] Agarwal et al.[58] (2003) felt this was due to the residual bulk left in the posterior pharyngeal wall, or perhaps to adaptive speech mechanisms developed while the flap was in situ.

CONCLUSIONS

There are many ways to address VPI in the cleft and noncleft patient. As one technique, superiorly-based-pharyngeal flaps are associated with good results in eliminating the hypernasality associated with cleft speech in children. Many modifications have been described. Complications may be minimized by careful patient selection and experience.

References

1. Sloan GM. Posterior pharyngeal flap and sphincter pharyngoplasty: The state of the art. *Cleft Palate Craniofac J* 37(2):112–122, 2000.
2. Seagle MB, Mazaheri MK, Dixon-Wood VL, et al. Evaluation and treatment of velopharyngeal insufficiency: The University of Florida experience. *Ann Plast Surg* 48(5):464–470, 2002.
3. Albery EH, Bennett JA, Pigott RW, et al. The results of 100 operations for velopharyngeal incompetence–selected on the findings of endoscopic and radiological examination. *Br J Plast Surg* 35(2):118–126, 1982.
4. Marsh JL. Management of velopharyngeal dysfunction: differential diagnosis for differential management. *J Craniofac Surg* 14(5):621–628, 2003.
5. Cable BB, Canady JW, Karnell MP, et al. Pharyngeal flap surgery: long-term outcomes at the University of Iowa. *Plast Reconstr Surg* 113(2):475–478, 2004.
6. Schmelzeisen R, Hausamen JE, Loebell E, et al. Long-term results following velopharyngoplasty with a cranially based pharyngeal flap. *Plast Reconstr Surg* 90(5):774–778, 1992.
7. Passavant G. Ueber die Beseitigung der naselnden Sprache bei angeborenen Splaten des harten und weichen Gaumens (Gaumensegel-Schlundnacht und Rucklagerung des Gaumensegels). *Arch Klin Chir* 6:333–349, 1865.
8. Schoenborn K. Ueber eine neue. Methode der staphylorrhaphie. *Verh Dtsch Ges Chir* 4:235–239, 1875.
9. Rosenthal W. Pathologie und therapie der Gaumendefekte. *Fortschr Zahnheilk* 4:55, 1928.
10. Padgett EC. The repair of cleft palates after unsuccessful operations with special reference to cases with an extensive loss of palatal tissue. *Arch Surg* 20:453–472, 1930.

11. Millard DR, Jr. Velopharyngeal synechiae with various pharyngeal flaps. In Millard DR, Jr. (ed). *Cleft Craft: The Evolution of its Surgery III. Alveolar and Palatal Deformities.* Boston: Little, Brown and Company, 1980, pp. 605.

12. Isshiki N, Morimoto M. A new folded pharyngeal flap: Preliminary report. *Plast Reconstr Surg* 55:461–465, 1975.

13. Hogan VM. A clarification of the surgical goals in cleft palate speech and the introduction of the lateral port control (l.p.c.) pharyngeal flap. *Cleft Palate J* 10:331–345, 1973.

14. Shprintzen RJ, McCall GN, Skolnick ML. The effect of pharyngeal flap surgery on the movements of the lateral pharyngeal walls. *Plast Reconstr Surg* 66(4):570–573, 1980.

15. Gray's Anatomy: The anatomical basis of clinical practice. In Standring S (ed).(Editor in Chief). Neck and Upper Aerodigestive Tract: Pharynx. Toronto, Canada: Elsevier Churchill Livingstone, 2005; p. 619.

16. Zwitman DH. Oral endoscopic comparison of velopharyngeal closure before and after pharyngeal flap surgery. *Cleft Palate J* 19:40–46, 1982.

17. Lewis MB, Pashayan HM. The effects of pharyngeal flap surgery on lateral wall pharyngeal motion: A videographic evaluation. *Cleft Palate J* 17:301–308, 1980.

18. Mercer NS, MacCarthy P. The arterial basis of pharyngeal flaps. *Plast Reconstr Surg* 96(5):1026–1037, 1995.

19. Vandevoort MJ, Mercer NS, Albery EH. Superiorly based flap pharyngoplasty: The degree of postoperative "tubing" and its effect on speech. *Br J Plast Surg* 54(3):192–196, 2001.

20. Tharanon W, Stella JP, Epker BN. The modified superior based pharyngeal flap. Part III. A retrospective study. *Oral Surg Oral Med Oral Pathol* 70(3):256–267, 1990.

21. Graham WP, III, Hamilton R, Randall P, et al. Complications following posterior pharyngeal flap surgery. *Cleft Palate J* 10:176–180, 1973.

22. Armour A, Fischbach S, Klaiman P, et al. Does velopharyngeal closure pattern affect the success of pharyngeal flap pharyngoplasty? *Plast Reconstr Surg* 115(1):45–52, 2005.

23. Skolnick M, McCall G, Barnes M. The sphincteric mechanism of velopharyngeal closure. *Cleft Palate J* 10:286–305, 1973.

24. Skoog T. The pharyngeal flap operation in cleft palate. *Br J Plast Surg* 18:265–282, 1965.

25. Hamlen M. Speech changes after pharyngeal flap surgery. *Plast Reconstr Surg* 46(5):437–444, 1970.

26. Whitaker LA, Randall P, Graham WP, III, Hamilton RW, Winchester R. A prospective and randomized series comparing superiorly and inferiorly based posterior pharyngeal flaps. *Cleft Palate J* 9:304–311, 1972.

27. Karling J, Henningsson G, Larson O, et al. Comparison between two types of pharyngeal flap with regard to configuration at rest and function and speech outcome. *Cleft Palate Craniofac J* 36(2):154–165, 1999.

28. Peat BG, Albery EH, Jones K, Pigott RW. Tailoring velopharyngeal surgery: The influence of etiology and type of operation. *Plast Reconstr Surg* 93(5):948–953, 1994.

29. Meek MF, Coert JH, Hofer SO, et al. Short-term and long-term results of speech improvement after surgery for velopharyngeal insufficiency with pharyngeal flaps in patients younger and older than 6 years old: 10-year experience. *Ann Plast Surg* 50(1):13–17, 2003.

30. Seyfer AE, Prohazka D, Leahy E. The effectiveness of the superiorly based pharyngeal flap in relation to the type of palatal defect and timing of the operation. *Plast Reconstr Surg* 82(5):760–764, 1988.

31. Barone CM, Shprintzen RJ, Strauch B, et al. Pharyngeal flap revisions: Flap elevation from a scarred posterior pharynx. *Plast Reconstr Surg* 93(2):279–284, 1994.

32. Witt PD, Myckatyn T, Marsh JL. Salvaging the failed pharyngoplasty: Intervention outcome. *Cleft Palate Craniofac J* 35(5):447–453, 1998.

33. Kapetansky DL. Transverse pharyngeal flaps: A dynamic repair for velopharyngeal insufficiency. *Cleft Palate J* 12(00):44–50, 1975.

34. Canady JW, Cable BB, Karnell MP, et al. Pharyngeal flap surgery: protocols, complications, and outcomes at the University of Iowa. *Otolaryngol Head Neck Surg* 129(4):321–326, 2003.

35. Morris HL, Bardach J, Jones D, Christiansen JL, Gray SD. Clinical results of pharyngeal flap surgery: The Iowa experience. *Plast Reconstr Surg* 95(4):652–662, 1995.

36. Johns DF, Cannito MP, Rohrich RJ, et al. The self-lined superiorly based pull-through velopharyngoplasty: Plastic surgery-speech pathology interaction in the management of velopharyngeal insufficiency. *Plast Reconstr Surg.* 94(3):436–445, 1994.

37. Pensler JM, Reich DS. A comparison of speech results after the pharyngeal flap and the dynamic sphincteroplasty procedures. *Ann Plast Surg* 26(5):441–443, 1991.

38. Ysunza A, Pamplona C, Ramirez E, et al. Velopharyngeal surgery: a prospective randomized study of pharyngeal flaps and sphincter pharyngoplasties. *Plast Reconstr Surg* 110(6):1401–1407, 2002.

39. Abyholm F, D'Antonio L, Davidson Ward SL, et al. VPI Surgical Group. Pharyngeal flap and sphincterplasty for velopharyngeal insufficiency have equal outcome at 1 year postoperatively: Results of a randomized trial. *Cleft Palate Craniofac J* 42(5):501–511, 2005.

40. Hathaway RR. A comparison of transverse and vertical pharyngeal faps using electromyography and judgments of nasality. *Cleft Palate J* 17(4):305–308, 1980.

41. Van Demark DR, Hardin MA. Longitudinal evaluation of articulation and velopharyngeal competence of patients with pharyngeal flaps. *Cleft Palate J* 22(3):163–172, 1985.

42. Leanderson R, Korlof B, Nylen B, et al. The age factor and reduction of open nasality following superiorly based velo-pharyngeal flap operation in 124 cases. *Scand J Plast Reconstr Surg* 8(1–2):156–160, 1974.

43. Riski JE. Articulation skills and oral-nasal resonance in children with pharyngeal flaps. *Cleft Palate J* (16(4):421–428, 1979 Oct.

44. Witt PD, Miller DC, Marsh JL, et al. Limited value of preoperative cervical vascular imaging in patients with velocardiofacial syndrome. *Plast Reconstr Surg* 101(5):1184–1195, 1998.

45. Klaiman P. Speech/Language Pathologist, The Hospital for Sick Children, Toronto, Canada, personal communication.

46. Mehendale FV, Birch MJ, Birkett L, et al. Surgical management of velopharyngeal incompetence in velocardiofacial syndrome. *Cleft Palate Craniofac J* 41(2):124–135, 2004.

47. MacKenzie-Stepner K, Witzel MA, Stringer DA, et al. Abnormal carotid arteries in the velocardiofacial syndrome: a report of three cases. *Plast Reconstr Surg* 80:347–351, 1987.

48. Hopper RA, Armstrong DC, Clarke HM. Straightening of aberrant carotid arteries with age in velocardiofacial syndrome. *Plast Reconstr Surg* 104(6):1744–1747, 1999.

49. Ross DA, Witzel MA, Armstrong DC, Thomson HG. Is pharyngoplasty a risk in velocardiofacial syndrome? An assessment of medially displaced carotid arteries. *Plast Reconstr Surg* 98(7):1182–1190, 1996.

50. Valnicek SM, Zuker RM, Halpern LM, Roy WL. Perioperative complications of superior pharyngeal flap surgery in children. *Plast Reconstr Surg* 93(5):954–958, 1994.

51. Fraulin FO, Valnicek SM, Zuker RM. Decreasing the perioperative complications associated with the superior pharyngeal flap operation. *Plast Reconstr Surg* 102(1):10–18, 1998.

52. Robinson PH, de Boer A. La maladie de Grisel: A rare occurrence of "spontaneous" atlanto-axial subluxation after pharyngoplasty. *Br J Plast Surg* 34:319–321, 1981.

53. Bardach J, Salyer KE, Jackson IT. Pharyngoplasty. In Bardach J, Salyer KE (ed). *Surgical Techniques in Cleft Lip and Palate*, 2nd ed. Toronto, Mosby Year Book, 1991, pp. 274.

54. Lesavoy MA, Borud LJ, Thorson T, et al. Upper airway obstruction after pharyngeal flap surgery. *Ann Plast Surg* 36(1):26–30, 1996.

55. Liao YF, Noordhoff MS, Huang CS, et al. Comparison of obstructive sleep apnea syndrome in children with cleft palate following Furlow

palatoplasty or pharyngeal flap for velopharyngeal insufficiency. *Cleft Palate Craniofac J* 41(2):152–156, 2004.

56. Sirois M, Caouette-Laberge L, Spier S, et al. Sleep apnea following a pharyngeal flap: a feared complication. *Plast Reconstr Surg* 93(5):943–947, 1994.

57. Caouette-Laberge L, Egerszegi EP, de Remont AM, et al. Long-term follow-up after division of a pharyngeal flap for severe nasal obstruction. *Cleft Palate Craniofac J* 29(1):27–31, 1992.

58. Agarwal T, Sloan GM, Zajac D, et al. Speech benefits of posterior pharyngeal flap are preserved after surgical flap division for obstructive sleep apnea: Experience with division of 12 flaps. *J Craniofac Surg* 14(5):630–6, 2003.

Sphincter Pharyngoplasty

Jeffrey L. Marsh, MD

INTRODUCTION

An individual who lacks the ability to completely separate the nasal cavity from the oral cavity for required speech tasks (velopharyngeal dysfunction) has a verbal communication impairment that can range from minor speech distortion to unintelligibility.[1] Once such an impairment is recognized, evaluation and management may involve speech/language pathologists, endoscopists, radiologists, prosthodontists, surgeons, and geneticists, usually in the context of a cleft palate team.[2] These health care disciplines may even work as an interdisciplinary velopharyngeal team. While the discussion of an holistic approach to velopharyngeal dysfunction evaluation and management is the subject of other chapters in this text, this chapter will review velopharyngeal anatomy and hypotheses regarding velopharyngeal dysfunction manage-

ment, in an effort to facilitate the discussion of one specific surgical procedure to treat velopharyngeal dysfunction—sphincter pharyngoplasty.

ANATOMY OF THE VELOPHARYNX

The velopharynx is space bounded in the axial plane (horizontally) by soft tissues, which usually are capable of approaching each other through the dynamism of underlying muscles, and in the sagittal plane (superiorly/inferiorly) by spaces. The axial plane soft tissues are anteriorly, the velum (soft palate); posteriorly, the posterior pharyngeal wall; and laterally, the right and left lateral pharyngeal walls. The superior/inferior spaces are superiorly, the nasopharynx and inferiorly, the oropharynx. The velopharynx is often referred to as either a *sphincter*, thereby emphasizing the normal dynamism of the surrounding myomucosal tissues, or a *port*, emphasizing the space connecting the nasal and oral pharynges. The normally functioning velopharynx is usually fully patent, allowing unencumbered airflow between the nasal and oral cavities, and free drainage of nasal secretions into the throat, except during swallowing and specific speech tasks when contraction of its surrounding muscles separates the nasal cavity from the oral cavity. The malfunctioning velopharynx is characterized by one or more of the following: hypernasality (excessive and/or inappropriate nasal resonance), nasal turbulence, and facial grimacing. Velopharyngeal function is initially assessed by auditory perceptual speech evaluation, and secondarily by instrumental-assisted standardized speech sample assessments of oronasal airflow, nasal sound emission, and/or dynamic anatomic visualization using endoscopy or fluoroscopy.

VELOPHARYNGEAL DYSFUNCTION MANAGEMENT: BASIC HYPOTHESIS

The basic hypothesis regarding velopharyngeal dysfunction management is that modification of the velopharyngeal port will improve velopharyngeal function for speech. Specifically, velopharyngeal dysfunction management will normalize resonance, permitting the secondary elimination of velopharyngeal dysfunction associated compensatory misarticulations through speech therapy. In addition, velopharyngeal dysfunction management will eliminate nasal turbulence and facial grimacing. Of note, maintenance of nasal airway patency, for breathing and secretion control, generally has not been a component of the basic management hypothesis.

HYPOTHESES REGARDING CLEFT PALATE REPAIR AND VELOPHARYNGEAL FUNCTION

The major morbidity of an unrepaired cleft palate is impaired speech intelligibility. While not affecting physical existence, this impairment usually compromises self-image, education, employment, and socialization. At the onset of the modern surgical era in the mid-nineteenth century, it was hypothesized that elimination of the overt palatal defect would resolve the functional problems associated with cleft palate. However, the inability of successful static anatomic repair of cleft palate to consistently eliminate speech impairment was appreciated by at least the first quarter of the twentieth century.

This led to the second major cleft palate repair hypothesis—increased velar length will improve speech intelligibility. Surgical techniques designed to lengthen the palate can be grouped as follows: (1) those that include dorsal displacement of the mucoperiosteum of the hard palate in an attempt to dorsally displace the soft palate (often referred to as "palatal pushback") and (2) those that only attempt to directly increase the length of the soft palate. While rigorous validation of either of these types of operations to consistently im-

prove velopharyngeal function is lacking, multiple purported validations have been published over the past several decades.

By the 1920s, some cleft surgeons hypothesized the importance of dynamism, rather than the amount of physical palatal tissue present, as the critical variable in velopharyngeal function. Two categories of operations were proposed to optimize such function: (1) reconstruction of the intravelar muscular sling with an intravelar veloplasty and (2) reorientation of the lateral pharyngeal wall musculature, specifically the palatopharyngeus muscles. Intravelar veloplasty, the generic name of the first of these categories, initially became a standard component of primary palatoplasty by the 1970s, and subsequently has been advocated by some as the preferred initial technique for postpalatoplasty velopharyngeal dysfunction management.[3] More recently, increasing velar length and velar muscle reorientation have been combined in the double-opposing Z-plasty of Furlow.[4]

An alternative approach to velopharyngeal dysfunction management focuses on obstruction of the excessively patent velopharyngeal port during physiologic tasks when it fails to close sufficiently. Obstruction of the velopharyngeal port can either be (1) completely reversible, using a prosthetic device such as a palatal lift, obturator, or "lift orator,"[5,6] that is only worn during the day for speech or (2) a permanent, and hopefully, subtotal surgical obstruction that can only be reversed with another operation. Such obstructive operations either result in a diminished single central velopharyngeal port (posterior pharyngeal wall augmentation and sphincter pharyngoplasty) or two laterally placed ports (pharyngeal flap). However, diminution of the cross-sectional area of the velopharyngeal port can introduce a new morbidity not associated with other attempts at eliminating velopharyngeal dysfunction: sufficient obstruction of the nasal airway to impair both breathing (causing mouth breathing and/or obstructive sleep apnea) and hygiene (nasal secretion retention and stasis).[7-9]

No operation, whether a component of primary palatoplasty or a specific intervention for velopharyngeal dysfunction, can normalize velopharyngeal function for speech, swallowing, and breathing in all patients. Some surgeons have applied differential treatment for velopharyngeal dysfunction based upon differential diagnosis. This approach assumes that one specific intervention will not be successful in normalizing resonance and maintaining a patent nasal airway for all patients regardless of the etiology of the velopharyngeal dysfunction. Rather, it assumes that specific etiologies of velopharyngeal dysfunction require specific matched interventions. Some studies have attempted to test this hypothesis.[10-12]

INDICATIONS FOR SPHINCTER PHARYNGOPLASTY

As already noted, the author subscribes to the philosophy of utilizing the differential diagnosis of velopharyngeal dysfunction to determine the specific treatment offered to an individual patient. Whereas auditory perceptual speech evaluation

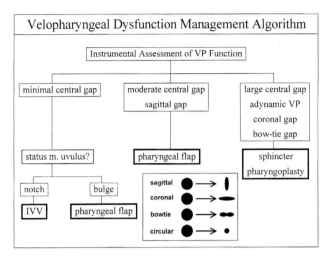

Figure 42–1. Personal algorithm for management of velopharyngeal dysfunction with differential management based upon differential diagnosis of velopharyngeal port dysfunction, (i.e., residual gap).

can identify velopharyngeal dysfunction and document-associated speech impairments, listening to speech cannot identify the pathophysiology of the velopharyngeal dysfunction, even when the listener is a speech/language pathologist who is well experienced in velopharyngeal dysfunction. Furthermore, instrumental velopharyngeal assessments that indirectly measure changes in the velopharyngeal port during function (aerodynamics, nasalance) also cannot delineate the pathophysiologic basis of velopharyngeal dysfunction so quantified. Imaging of velopharyngeal function, either with nasendoscopy or videofluoroscopy, can define which of the velopharyngeal components is malfunctioning.[13] Based upon the author's 29 years of clinical experience with velopharyngeal management, sphincter pharyngoplasty is specifically utilized for the surgical treatment of those patients whose velopharyngeal dysfunction is secondary to markedly impaired or absent lateral pharyngeal wall motion.[14] (Fig. 42–1) The sphincter pharyngoplasty is employed for patients who would otherwise require a wide obstructive pharyngeal flap, which is usually associated with significant impairment of the nasal airway. In the author's experience, while the sphincter pharyngoplasty also can impair the nasal airway,[7,8] the magnitude of morbidity has been less than with wide-obstructive pharyngeal flaps.

PERSONAL TECHNIQUE OF SPHINCTER PHARYNGOPLASTY

Presurgical

Prior to surgical intervention for velopharyngeal management, the patient will have undergone auditory perceptual and instrumental evaluations of velopharyngeal function.[15] All of these examinations are video recorded for review by treatment providers not present during the examination, and for longitudinal comparative outcome analysis. Based

on that review, a velopharyngeal treatment plan is formulated and communicated to the parents and/or the patient directly when they are of sufficient age for empowerment or consent. This communication includes the proposed interventions, expected benefits, possible complications, and alternative managements.

It should be noted that the posterior pharyngeal wall is carefully examined during the nasendoscopy for aberrant pulsations that could indicate an ectopic carotid artery. If no such pulsations are seen, which is almost always the case, no vascular imaging is performed, even when the patient has a positive diagnosis of the 22q.11 deletion of velocardiofacial syndrome or DiGeorge syndrome.[16] When aberrant pulsations are observed, a magnetic resonance arteriogram of the head and neck is obtained to determine the possibility of performing a sphincter pharyngoplasty without carotid injury. Using this approach for the past 18 years, the author has not witnessed any vascular complications with the sphincter pharyngoplasty, nor has this finding resulted in the inability to treat such a patient surgically.[17] Sphincter pharyngoplasty is a safe and effective means of managing velopharyngeal dysfunction in patients with velocardiofacial syndrome (DiGeorge syndrome).

Once it has been determined that the patient requires a sphincter pharyngoplasty, based on a combination of speech impairment and anatomic pattern of velopharyngeal dysfunction, adenoidectomy and tonsillectomy, if not already done, these are performed in a separate preliminary operation. The preliminary removal of adenoid tissue allows for the positioning and insertion of the reoriented posterior tonsillar pillars high enough on the posterior pharyngeal wall, and into stable scar tissue, to prevent failure from either too-low insertion or dehiscence.[18] The tonsils are removed to facilitate harvest of the posterior tonsillar pillars (palatopharyngeus muscles), and to avoid subsequent obstruction of the markedly narrowed velopharyngeal port by tonsillar tissue, also a benefit of adenoidectomy. Sphincter pharyngoplasty is scheduled for a minimum of 3 months after the tonsillectomy and adenoidectomy to allow for healing of the ablative sites. It is important for the ENT surgeon who will perform the tonsillectomy and adenoidectomy to understand the importance of preservation of the tonsillar pillars for the performance of the subsequent sphincter pharyngoplasty and not either to obliterate them or cause them to fuse into a single tissue mass. In patients with some pretonsillectomy and adenoidectomy lateral pharyngeal wall mesial motion, imaging of velopharyngeal function is then repeated 6–8 weeks after the tonsillectomy and adenoidectomy to confirm the pattern of velopharyngeal dynamism. In patients with no lateral pharyngeal wall mesial motion, imaging is not repeated posttonsillectomy and adenoidectomy prior to sphincter pharyngoplasty.

Operative Technique

The author's preferred technique is essentially the one reported by Jackson.[19] The patient is admitted to hospital on the day of surgery through the same day surgery unit. After the induction of general endotracheal anesthesia and sterile draping, the patient's head is lowered by placing the operating room table into Trendelenburg position and then slid into the surgeon's lap, who performs the operation while sitting. The first assistant is positioned facing the surgeon on their left side, and the surgical scrub technician is at the right side of the surgeon. For those left-handed surgeons, the scrub may be positioned on the left side. A Dingman mouth gag is inserted, opened for adequate exposure of the surgical field, and compliance of ventilation is checked verbally with the anesthesiologist since the Dingman's tongue blade can excessively compress the endotracheal tube. The palate is inspected for a bifid uvula, and when present is repaired. The presence or absence of aberrant pulsations on the posterior pharyngeal wall is reconfirmed under direct vision. A 14 French red rubber catheter (or latex-free Foley catheter if the patient is latex-sensitive) is inserted into one nare, passed posteriorly until seen in the posterior pharynx, and then the tip clamped and passed ventrally beneath the bar of the mouth gag where it is secured. This catheter displaces the velum ventrally, exposing the velopharynx and inferior nasopharynx. As determined preoperatively from videofluoroscopy, the optimum level on the posterior pharyngeal wall for insertion of the palatopharyngeus myomucosal flaps is identified with respect to the digitally palpated ventral ring of C-1. (Fig. 42–2) The posterior pharyngeal wall mucosa, at the proposed insertion site, is infiltrated with 1 cc of 0.25% Marcaine with 1/200,000

epinephrine. Traction sutures of 4–0 silk are placed in each posterior tonsillar pillar, and the overlying mucosa is infiltrated with 1 cc per side of 0.25% Marcaine with 1/200,000 epinephrine. Five minutes are allowed for vasoconstriction to be optimum. Attention is first directed to the junction of the ventral surface of the posterior tonsillar pillar and the tonsillar bed. The traction silk suture is placed on tension, improving exposure and the junctional mucosa is incised with the #12 blade. A Metzenbaum scissor is inserted into the mucosal incision and spread separating the palatopharyngeus muscle from the tonsillar bed in continuity with the overlying mucosa of the posterior tonsillar pillar. A unipedicled, superiorly based, myomucosal flap is developed, whose length is equal to the transverse width of the insertion site. The superior aspect of the flap is preserved as its base, at the level of the pharyngeal wall insertion site, and the inferior aspect divided with the scissors. A curved right-angled scissor is then used to transect the flap mucosa where the posterior aspect of the pillar joins the posterior pharyngeal wall. The flap is then elevated until the level of the transverse posterior pharyngeal wall insertion site is reached. The same procedure is then repeated for the opposite posterior tonsillar pillar. (Fig. 42–3) Any persistent bleeding is managed with bipolar cauterization. Then, the mucosa of the transverse posterior pharyngeal wall insertion site is cut, using a #12 blade. This transverse posterior pharyngeal wall insertion site incision is connected to the superior aspects of each lateral posterior pillar myomucosal flap donor site incisions, resulting in a final incision shape of a "**U**." Care is taken to only cut the mucosa with a minimum of the underlying muscle. A full division of the underlying superior

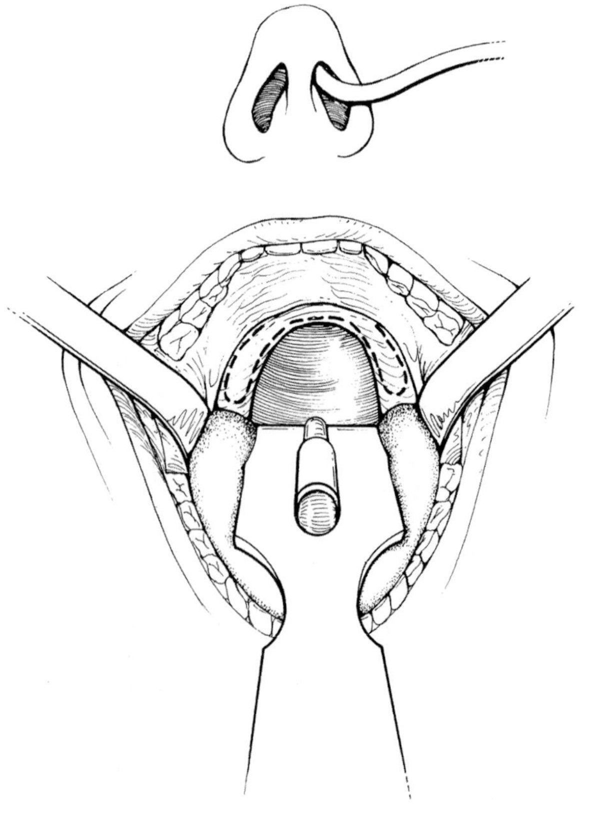

Figure 42–2. Preoperative markings for the sphincter pharyngoplasty.

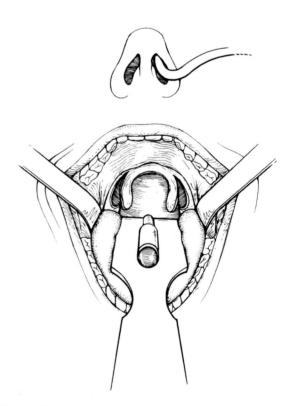

Figure 42–3. Sphincter pharyngoplasty incised and elevated.

constrictor muscle, as is done when raising a pharyngeal flap off the prevertebral fascia, often results in an inferior migration of the sphincter pharyngoplasty impairing the long-term result.

The posterior pillar flaps are then rotated 90° and inset into the posterior pharyngeal wall mucosa defect and to each other in an overlapping **Z** pattern. Based on my handedness and training with this operation, I prefer to use the left pillar as the superior sphincter flap and the right as the inferior but this is simply a matter of individual preference. 4–0 Vicryl on **J** needles (Ethicon # PS-4C, J656G) on a Straite needle holder is used for all sutures. The medial myomucosal edge of the left pillar flap is sutured to the superior myomucosal edge of the posterior pharyngeal wall incision; the lateral myomucosal edge of the left pillar flap is sutured to the medial myomucosal edge of the right pillarflap; and then the lateral myomucosal edge of the right pillar flap is sutured to the inferior myomucosal edge of the posterior wall incision. All sutures are placed in sequence and arranged using the retention springs on the Dingman mouth gag. After all sutures have been placed, the tension on the catheter displacing the velum is released and then the sutures are tied in sequence from cephalad to caudad following a **Z** pattern. The lateral pharyngeal wall donor sites are then repaired with several 4–0 Vicryl on each side so that no raw areas remain. (Fig. 42–4.) The velar traction catheter is removed. An orogastric tube is placed under direct vision, the gastric contents emptied, and the tube removed. The patient is returned to the supine position, the Dingman mouth gag is removed, and the patient is then extubated in the operating room prior to transfer to the postanesthetic recovery room.

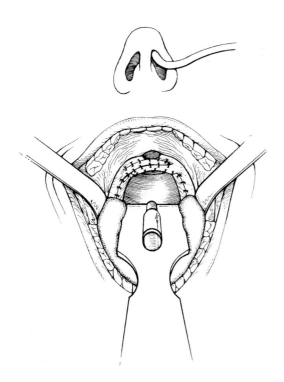

Figure 42–4. Sphincter pharyngoplasty inset into posterior pharyngeal wall with reconstructed nasopharyngeal port.

Postoperative Care

Postoperatively, the patient is positioned prone or lateral decubitus until there is no active bleeding and fully awake and recovered. Positioning then is the patient's preference. Following postanesthesia recovery, the patient is preferentially monitored overnight in the Pediatric Intensive Care Unit; however, any bed with adequate pulse oximetry and electrocardiography monitoring, as well as adequate nurse/patient ratio will suffice. Intravenous maintenance fluids are administered until the patient is able to take sufficient oral fluids; a soft diet is offered. Parenteral morphine and enteral Tylenol with codeine elixir are used for pain control as needed. The patient is discharge from hospital when taking adequate oral fluids and comfortable on oral pain medication, usually the day after surgery. Unlimited physical activity is permitted when the patient's energy level has returned to presurgical status. Speech therapy is resumed 3 weeks after the operation. The patient returns for an auditory perceptual speech evaluation 3 months after surgery. If there remains residual symptomatic velopharyngeal dysfunction or nasal airway obstructive symptoms, repeat diagnostic nasendoscopic and/or fluoroscopic velopharyngeal visualization. If symptomatic velopharyngeal dysfunction persists, the sphincter pharyngoplasty can be revised.[20,21] Many patients will have some initial problems with retained nasal secretions following sphincter pharyngoplasty. Should these symptoms become a concern, nasal saline spray and, if necessary, nasal steroids are prescribed.

SPHINCTER PHARYNGOPLASTY OUTCOME DATA

The author's experience with the sphincter pharyngoplasty can be separated into two time periods, reflecting two different practice locations. However, during both time periods, there was no injury to the carotid arteries, need for blood transfusions, or mortalities. Morbidity in both periods consisted of persistent velopharyngeal dysfunction, impaired nasal secretion drainage, and obstructive sleep apnea.

The first period was 1989–2003. A review of sphincter pharyngoplasties from that period, reported in 2002,[22] documented resolution of symptomatic velopharyngeal dysfunction in 72% of 162 patients differentially selected and treated. The resolution of symptomatic velopharyngeal dysfunction increased to 85% with secondary surgical tightening of the incompletely closed central velopharyngeal port, as documented on postsphincter pharyngoplasty nasendoscopy. For the 11 of 162 patients with residual symptomatic velopharyngeal insufficiency following secondary tightening of the sphincter, tertiary surgical revision of the sphincter pharyngoplasty, with tightening of the velopharyngeal port was performed; or, a narrow pharyngeal flap was placed in the center of the sphincter pharyngoplasty port. For all 162 patients, significant hyponasality was noted in only 10%. During this initial period, a separate study of 20 patients, who underwent sphincter pharyngoplasty having pre- and postoperative basilar fluoroscopic images suitable for quantification, documented sphincter dynamism. This study demonstrated at least a 10% reduction in velopharyngeal port diameter in 100% of cases at the 3-month postoperative nasendoscopic and fluoroscopic evaluations (which were routine for all postsphincter pharyngoplasty patients at that time).[23] The average amount of sphincter pharyngoplasty orifice closure on speech tasks requiring velopharyngeal port closure was 61% (range: 37–80%). This documents the true dynamism of this operation, even though the procedure was used almost exclusively for those patients with markedly impaired velopharyngeal function.

The second clinical period covered 2003–2006. During this time, the author performed 29 sphincter pharyngoplasties and 6 pharyngeal flaps, based on the differential treatment for differential diagnosis, as described above. Of the 29 patients who underwent sphincter pharyngoplasty, 83% had resolution of velopharyngeal dysfunction and did not experience symptomatic nasal airway obstruction. Five patients required secondary surgical modification of the sphincter to resolve residual velopharyngeal dysfunction: three with direct port tightening and two with tertiary modified pharyngeal flap for port narrowing after failure of secondary port tightening. However, all of these patients, requiring secondary or tertiary surgery, had correction of hypernasality at the cost of hyponasal resonance and moderate nasal airway obstruction without obstructive sleep apnea. Eight of the primary sphincter pharyngoplasty patients (28%) had difficulty managing nasal secretions, and were initially managed by nasal saline and/or nasal steroid sprays. A resolution of symptoms occurred in three patients, and in the rest, it is "too soon to know." One patient experienced postsurgery obstructive sleep symptoms, and benefited from nocturnal CPAP; one patient required secondary sphincter port surgical widening for the resolution of the nasal obstructive symptoms without regression of velopharyngeal function. In this series, one patient has persistent postsphincter obstructive sleep apnea per abnormal sleep study, despite lack of clinical symptoms. The patient has been managed by nocturnal CPAP for over $2^{1}/_{2}$ years, and demonstrates a visually patent port by direct oral and nasal evaluation. In addition, the patient has the ability to breathe through his nose with lips closed when awake, and his velopharyngeal port calibration to at least 28 French, while under anesthesia for an unrelated operation, has been documented. The patient's parents are considering the recommendation for surgical port widening.

Several outcome studies of sphincter pharyngoplasty alone, and compared to pharyngeal flap, have been reported with similar results.[12,24−29]

CONCLUSION

In the author's experience, the sphincter pharyngoplasty has been an effective means of managing velopharyngeal dysfunction without significant upper airway morbidity, for patients with limited to absent lateral pharyngeal wall motion.

References

1. Folkins JW. Velopharyngeal nomenclature: Incompetence, inadequacy, insufficiency, and dysfunction. *Cleft Palate J* 25:413–416, 1988.
2. Sell D, Ma L. A model of practice for the management of velopharyngeal dysfunction. *Br J Oral Maxillofac Surg* 34:357–363, 1996.
3. Sommerlad BC, Mehendale FV, Birch MJ, et al. Palate re-repair revisited. *Cleft Palate Craniofac J* 39:295–307, 2002.
4. D'Antonio L, Eichenberg B, Zimmerman G, et al. Radiographic and aerodynamic measures of velopharyngeal anatomy and function following Furlow Z-plasty. *Plast Reconstr Surg* 106:550–553, 2000.
5. Marsh JL, Wray RC. Speech prosthesis versus pharyngeal flap: A randomized evaluation of the management of velopharyngeal incompetency. *Plast Reconstr Surg* 65:592–594, 1980.
6. Riski JE, Gordon D. Prosthetic management of neurogenic velopharyngeal incompetency. *N Carolina Dent J* 62:24–26, 1979.
7. Witt PD, Marsh JL, Muntz HR, Marty-Grames L, Watchmaker GP. Acute obstructive sleep apnea as a complication of sphincter pharyngoplasty. *Cleft Palate Craniofac J* 33:183–189, 1996.
8. Saint Raymond C, Bettega G, Deschaux C, et al. Sphincter pharyngoplasty as a treatment of velopharyngeal incompetence in young people: A prospective evaluation of effects on sleep structure and sleep respiratory disturbances. *Chest* 125:864–871, 2004.
9. Kravath RE, et al. Obstructive sleep apnea and death associated with surgical correction of velopharyngeal incompetence. *J Ped* 96:645–648, 1980.
10. Peat BG, Albery EH, Jones K, et al. Tailoring velopharyngeal surgery: The influence of etiology and type of operation. *Plast Reconstr Surg* 93:948–953, 1994.
11. Marsh JL. Management of velopharyngeal dysfunction: Differential diagnosis for differential management. *J Craniofac Surg* 14:621–628, 2003.
12. Seagle MB, Mazaheri MK, Dixon-Wood VL, Williams WN. Evaluation and treatment of velopharyngeal insufficiency: The University of Florida experience. *Ann Plast Surg* 48:464–470, 2002.
13. Golding-Kushner KJ, Argamaso RV, Cotton RT, et al. Standardization for the reporting of nasopharyngoscopy and multiview videofluoroscopy: A report from an International Working Group. *Cleft Palate J* 27:337–348, 1990.
14. Witt PD, Marsh JL, Marty-Grames L, et al. Management of the hypodynamic velopharynx. *Cleft Palate Craniofac J* 32:179–187, 1995.
15. Witt PD, D'Antonio LL, Zimmerman GJ, et al. Sphincter pharyngoplasty: A preoperative and postoperative analysis of perceptual speech characteristics and endoscopic studies of velopharyngeal function. *Plast Reconstr Surg* 93:1154–1168, 1994.
16. Witt P, Cohen D, Grames LM, et al. Sphincter pharyngoplasty for the surgical management of speech dysfunction associated with velocardiofacial syndrome. *Br J Plast Surg* 52:613–618, 1999.
17. Witt PD, Miller DC, Marsh JL, Muntz HR, Grames LM. Limited value of preoperative cervical vascular imaging in patients with velocardiofacial syndrome. *Plast Reconstr Surg* 101:1184–1195, 1998.
18. Riski JE, Serafin D, Riefkohl R, et al. A rationale for modifying the site of insertion of the orticochea pharyngoplasty. *Plast Reconstr Surg* 73:882–894, 1984.
19. Jackson IT. Sphincter pharyngoplasty. *Clin Plast Surg* 12:711, 1985.
20. Witt PD, Marsh JL, Grames LM, Muntz HR. Revision of the failed sphincter pharyngoplasty: An outcome assessment. *Plast Reconstr Surg* 96:129–138, 1995.
21. Riski JE, Ruff GL, Georgaide GS, Barwick WJ. Evaluation of failed sphincter pharyngoplasties. *Ann Plast Surg* 28:545–553, 1992.
22. Mount D, Marsh J. Sphincter pharyngoplasty. Presented at the *Annual Meeting of the American Association of Plastic Surgeons*, Seattle, Washington; 2002.

23. Witt PD, Marsh JL, Arlis H, et al. Quantification of dynamic velopharyngeal port excursion following sphincter pharyngoplasty. *Plast Reconstr Surg* 101:1205–1211, 1998.

24. Losken A, Williams JK, Burstein FD, Malick D, Riski JE. An outcome evaluation of sphincter pharyngoplasty for the management of velopharyngeal insufficiency. *Plast Reconstr Surg* 112:1755–1761, 2003.

25. Ysunza A, Pamplona C, Ramirez E, Molina F, Mendoza M, Silva A. Velopharyngeal surgery: A prospective randomized study of pharyngeal flaps and sphincter pharyngoplasties. *Plast Reconstr Surg* 110:1401–1407, 2002.

26. Riski JE, Ruff GL, Georgaide GS, Barwick WJ, Edwards PD. Evaluation of the sphincter pharyngoplasty. *Cleft Palate J* 29:254–261, 1992.

27. Abyholm F, D'Antonio L, Davidson Ward SL, et al. Pharyngeal flap and sphincterplasty for velopharyngeal insufficiency have equal outcomes at 1 year postoperatively: Results of a randomized trial. *Cleft Palate Craniofac J* 42:501–511, 2005.

28. de Serres LM, Deleyiannis FW, Eblen LE, Gruss JS, Richardson MA, Sie KC. Results with sphincter pharyngoplasty and pharyngeal flap. *Internl J Ped Otolaryngol* 48:17–25, 1999.

29. Sie KC, Tampakopoulou DA, De Serres LM, Gruss JS, Eblen LE, Yonick T, Sphincter pahryngoplasty: Speech outcome and complications. *Laryngocope* 108:1211–1217, 1998.

Prosthetic Management of Velopharyngeal Insufficiency

M. Mazaheri, MDD, DDS, MSc • Lawrence E. Brecht, DDS

SPEECH AID APPLIANCES AND PROSTHODONTIC CLEFT PALATE MANAGEMENT

Since the early 16th century, dentists have been making appliances designed to close defects in the hard palate. Like their predecessors, prosthodontists today are also vitally involved in helping the individual with an oral cleft. As surgical techniques have improved, surgeons have been enabled to successfully repair the cleft palate deformity and

to treat velopharyngeal insufficiency in most cases, thereby diminishing the need for prosthesis, to separate the oral and nasal cavities. The use of a speech appliance simply as a last resort is a poor method of cleft management. A prosthetic speech aid appliance should be used when it is clearly indicated, just as the pharyngeal flap or other types of pharyngoplasty procedures should be used only when they are indicated. Prosthetic speech appliances fabricated by dentists and prosthodontists are still recommended as a primary or secondary treatment for many patients with cleft palate. The decision for prosthetic cleft palate rehabilitation is made based on the individual patient's needs, motivation for improvement, and the availability of the suggested rehabilitation program.[1]

As knowledge and experience in the cleft palate field has increased, those responsible for providing prosthetic care have recognized the importance of establishing better prosthodontic concepts and principles regarding treatment. In order to render the best service to the effected patients, the prosthodontist should first follow the rules and accepted principles, governing the fabrication and use of a fixed or removable partial denture prosthesis. Secondly, a sound understanding of the anatomy involved, and of how the cleft deformity alters this anatomy, should remove any fear of causing harm because of existing anatomic, functional, and physiologic deviation.[2]

The terms *obturator, speech aid appliance,* and *speech bulb appliance* are frequently used synonymously, but it has become customary to apply the term *obturator* to a device used to treat acquired defects, such as those resulting from trauma or tumor removal surgery, whereas *speech aid appliance* is employed to describe a prosthesis designed to treat congenital oral clefts. The design and construction of speech appliances and obturators has changed much in the last 20 years.[3] This has been due primarily to the development of improved materials and methods, as well as to the use of osseointegrated implants for appliance support and retention of the prosthesis. A speech aid prosthesis (Fig. 43–1) has three components: (1) a *maxillary* component that is positioned in the oral cavity, and that is retained by the patient's teeth (or

by the residual alveolar ridges if the patient is edentulous). Osseointegrated implants may be placed in patients that are partially or totally edentulous for additional retention of the maxillary portion of the prosthesis, (2) A *velar* section that connects the maxillary portion of the appliance with the functional bulb, and (3) the *pharyngeal* portion of the appliance that extends posteriorly from the maxillary component and that serves to obturate the pharyngeal defect. The *pharyngeal* portion is more commonly referred to as the "bulb" portion.

There are five primary goals associated with speech aid prosthesis fabrication for a cleft palate patient:

1. Socially acceptable speech,
2. Prevention of food and fluids from leaking through the nose,
3. Restoration of the masticatory structures,
4. Esthetic facial and dental harmony,
5. Successful psychological adjustment of the patient to the prosthesis.

The use of cineradiography studies, nasal endoscopy, serial cephalometric films, maxillary and mandibular casts, speech recordings made before and after surgery, sound spectrographic analysis, measurements of nasal and oral air pressure and flow, and speech and audiometric evaluations may all be of use in assessing the success of any prosthetic speech appliance fabrication.

REQUIREMENTS OF SPEECH AID PROSTHESIS

1. The prosthesis must be designed for an individual patient in relation to the oral and facial balance, masticatory function, and speech.
2. Appropriate knowledge of removable partial and complete denture prostheses should be used in designing the maxillary portion of the cleft palate prosthesis. Preservation of the remaining dentition and of the surrounding soft and hard tissues in cleft palate patients is of utmost importance. Improperly designed cleft palate appliances can result in premature loss of both hard and soft tissues, further complicating prosthetic habilitation.
3. The prosthetic speech appliance should have more retention and support than most other removable prostheses. The crowning and splinting of the abutment teeth in adult patients may increase retention and support of the prosthesis and may extend the life expectancy of abutment teeth and/or osseointegrated implants.
4. Oral and dental preparations should be completed before making final impressions. In situations where lateral and vertical growth of the maxilla is incomplete and partial eruption of the deciduous and permanent teeth is evident, careful mouth preparations should be made. To provide support for the prosthesis, these preparations may include gingivectomy procedures to expose clinical crowns (to make them usable) and the placement of copings on remaining teeth to prevent decalcification and caries.

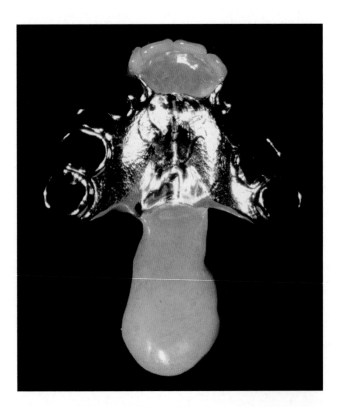

Figure 43–1.

Osseointegrated implants have been a great help in gaining adequate retention for speech aid prostheses.

5. The weight and size of the prosthetic speech appliance should be kept to a minimum.

6. The materials used should lend themselves easily to repair, modification, extension, and reduction.

7. Soft tissue displacement in the velar and nasopharyngeal areas by the prosthesis should be avoided.

8. Movements of the lateral and posterior pharyngeal wall muscles or the tongue during swallowing and speech should never displace the velar and pharyngeal sections of the prosthesis.

9. The superior portion of the pharyngeal section should be sloped laterally to eliminate the collection of nasal secretions. The inferior portion of the pharyngeal section should be slightly concave to allow freedom of tongue movement.

10. The location and the changes of the speech bulb should include consideration of the following factors:

    a. The speech bulb should be positioned in the location of the greatest posterior and lateral pharyngeal wall activity because voice quality is judged best when the speech bulb is at these positions.

    b. The inferior–superior dimension and weight of the speech bulb may be reduced without apparent effect on nasal resonance. (The lateral dimension of the bulb does not change significantly as the position is varied).

    c. The speech bulb should be placed at or above the palatal plane in cases where posterior and lateral pharyngeal wall activities are not present or where visual observation of the bulb is not possible due to a long soft palate.

    d. The anterior tubercle of the atlas bone can be used as a reference point, however, investigation has shown that the relative position of the tubercle of the atlas varies amongst individuals and that the position of the velopharyngeal structures changes in relation to the tubercle as the individual moves his or her head. Therefore, the atlas is no longer used as the definitive reference point for positioning the pharyngeal section of the bulb, but it should serve only as a relative reference point in determining the final position of the pharyngeal section.

INDICATIONS FOR PROSTHESIS: PATIENTS WITH AN UNREPAIRED CLEFT PALATE

The majority of palatal clefts can be surgically repaired, enabling the patient to develop acceptable velopharyngeal function without the need for a speech aid prosthesis. In some rare situations, however, a prosthesis is the restoration of choice. The entire cleft palate team is charged with caring for the patient, and no one individual team member—the surgeon, the prosthodontist, or the speech pathologist—should make this decision alone. The prosthodontist can assist both the

surgeon and the patient, and a mutual understanding among the specialists of a well-organized team is of great benefit to the patient. Following are the situations where a removable speech aid prosthesis may be indicated over a surgical treatment option:

A Wide Cleft with a Deficient Soft Palate

Clefts of this type, rarely do not lend themselves to surgical repair. In unusual cases, a prosthesis may be preferable to complex surgical intervention. Many patients need a prosthesis to restore missing dental units, and a prosthesis provides an economical method to do so, while serving to provide pharyngeal habilitation at the same time.

Neuromuscular Deficiency of the Soft Palate and Pharynx

It is often difficult to create and maintain a pharyngeal flap large enough to produce competent palatopharyngeal valving without inducing upper airway obstruction in the presence of neurogenic velopharyngeal dysfunction. A pharyngeal flap functions best when surrounded by dynamic musculature. When such does not exist, the pharyngeal section of a speech-aid prosthesis may serve better to reduce hypernasality and nasal emission. The prosthesis can also act as a physical therapy modality, providing a resistive mass against which the muscles to act. Should muscle function improve, definitive surgical measures may then be considered.

DELAYED SURGERY

When surgery is delayed for medical reasons, or when the surgeon prefers to repair the palate when the patient is older, the palatal cleft may be temporarily obturated with a prosthetic speech aid.

SPEECH AID PROSTHESIS: CONTRADICTIONS

1. Patients with reduced mental capacity are not good candidates for prostheses because they frequently are not capable of giving the appliance the care it requires.

2. Speech aid prosthesis is not recommended for an uncooperative patient or for a child with uncooperative parents.

3. If caries are rampant and not controlled, the prosthesis will require unusual care, often with the need for frequent replacement. Therefore, in the patient with a high caries index, regularly scheduled dental examinations are important.

4. The edentulous condition is not a contraindication to a speech aid prosthesis, however, the lack of teeth for retention will severely compromise the stability and retention and, as a result, the efficiency of the prosthesis.

Osseointegrated implants may be used to improve retention for these patients.

5. Because construction of a functional prosthesis requires the services of a dentist who has had training in cleft palate prosthodontics, it would be better to resort to surgical ingenuity when experienced prosthodontic help is not available.

FABRICATION OF SPEECH AID PROSTHESIS: PEDIATRIC AND ADULT PATIENTS

For pediatric or adolescent patients with deciduous, mixed, or permanent dentition that has not fully erupted, all three sections of the prosthetic speech appliance are made of acrylic resin, and wrought wire clasps are used for retention. In adult patients whose permanent teeth are fully erupted, the anterior or maxillary section of the prosthetic speech appliance should be made of cast metal or a combination of cast metal and acrylic resin.

Preliminary Impression

A stock tray of adequate dimensions is selected. If a registration of the entire cleft is desirable, the stock tray is modified with modeling compound extending posteriorly to the posterior pharyngeal wall. The added section is under-extended approximately 4–5 mm in all directions, leaving adequate space for impression material. Fast-setting, irreversible hydrocolloid is used for registering the preliminary impression. The following suggestions should be kept in mind when the preliminary impression is made:

- The anatomy of the cleft defect should be closely examined and any small fistulae should be identified. All oral perforations should be packed with gauze that has been saturated with petroleum jelly to prevent lodging impression material in them.
- If the patient is a child, he or she should be given the opportunity to examine the tray; in some cases the child may be permitted to try the tray in his mouth. Children should be told that their cooperation is needed; otherwise, it will be necessary to make several impressions. Talking to children throughout the procedure is helpful.
- The patient should have an early morning appointment.
- The patient should have an empty stomach.
- A topical anesthetic should be used on a child who has a severe gag reflex.
- The tray should not be overloaded with impression material. Excess material in the nasopharynx will increase the difficulty of removing the impression without tearing the impression material.

Deciduous Teeth Preparation for Retention

Most deciduous teeth do not have sufficient undercuts for retention of the prosthesis. However, a small degree of bilateral undercuts can provide adequate retention. The following recommendations will help to produce retention when deciduous teeth are present:

1. Carefully extend the clasp arms into interproximal areas of the teeth.
2. Place bands with soldered retention lugs on the teeth.
3. Use metal crowns with retention lugs for teeth with extensive carious lesions or areas of decalcification.
4. Apply a small amount of composite material to the buccal surface of the tooth to create a slight undercut for retention.

After the clasp design has been determined on the diagnostic casts and the teeth have been prepared for retention, the final impression is made. If adequate retention is not available in the permanent dentition, crowning of the molars or metal-to-tooth bonding might be desirable to provide proper retentive areas.

Final Impression

A custom tray is constructed over the diagnostic cast with adequate relief to allow for a uniform thickness of impression material. The patient is prepared in the same manner as for the preliminary impression, and the final impression is then made with an irreversible hydrocolloid or elastomeric impression material. The master cast is made of dental stone.

Maxillomandibular Relation Records

Maxillomandibular relation records such as vertical dimension, centric relation, and protrusive relation are determined and used in the adjustment of the articulator.

DESIGN AND FABRICATION OF THE PROSTHESIS

The master casts are surveyed, and the prosthesis is designed. For patients with severely constricted maxillary and mandibular arches, teeth are arranged outside the remaining natural teeth to establish the proper aesthetics, lip support and occlusion. In such situations, the anterior flange region that retains the prosthetic teeth may be fashioned to provide increased maxillary lip support and improve lip aesthetics. Such and addition to the prosthesis is commonly termed a *lip plumper appliance.*

The prosthetic speech appliance is constructed in three sections. The design of the anterior (maxillary) portion is similar to that of a partial or complete removable denture. After this section is completed, the patient is instructed to wear it for at least 1 week. The length of this adjustment period depends on the ability of the patient to adapt to this part of the prosthesis. The construction of the middle part, or velar section, varies for operated and nonoperated clefts. In operated palates that are short and require prosthesis, the position of the velar section is marked on the posterior margin of the prosthesis. The velar section extends approximately

3 mm behind the posterior margin of the soft palate. The width of the velar section is approximately 5 mm, and its reinforced thickness should be at least 1.5 mm.

Velar Section: Construction

A piece of shellac baseplate material of the required width and length is used as a tray. It is securely attached to the posterior part of the prosthesis with approximately 2-mm relief. This assemblage is examined in the patient's mouth for proper extension. The tissue side of the tray is filled with irreversible hydrocolloid impression material, and the appliance is inserted into the mouth. The patient is instructed to hold his or her head in a vertical position to prevent escape of the impression material into the nasopharynx. The head is held in this position for 1 minute, and then the patient is instructed to swallow a little water so that the muscular movement of the soft palate will be registered in the impression. After the material has hardened, the prosthesis is removed from the mouth, and the velar section is processed with self-curing acrylic resin. The denture portion with the finished velar section is placed in the mouth for testing. Swallowing of small amounts of water will stimulate muscle action along the lateral edge of the velar section. If the velar section is overextended laterally, undue muscle displacement and eventual tissue soreness will occur.

Pharyngeal Section or Speech Bulb: Construction

Two holes are drilled in the posterior part of the tailpiece. A piece of separating wire is drawn through the holes to form a loop that extends superioposteriorly beyond the superior part of the tailpiece. The ends of the wire are twisted together inferiorly (oral side), and secured to the appliance by sticky wax. The wire loop that is extended into the nasal pharyngeal area is manipulated into an oval form, and the appliance is inserted into the mouth. The patient is asked to swallow, and the wire is adjusted so that it will not contact the pharyngeal walls at any time. Spraying those tissues with water can stimulate posterior and lateral pharyngeal wall activity. The desired position of the wire is in the area of the maximum posterior and lateral pharyngeal constriction. Green modeling compound is added around the wire loop to reinforce it and its attachment to the velar section. The appliance is inserted into the patient's mouth, and is asked to swallow a little water. Adaptol™, softened in water at 150–160°F for 4–5 minutes, is added over the green compound, and the appliance is inserted into the mouth. Again, the patient is instructed to swallow a little water to produce muscle activity, and thus the impression material is molded.

The prosthesis is reinserted a number of times, and the patient is instructed to swallow each time when additions of Adaptol™ are made to the mass on the wire loop. These steps are repeated until a functional impression of the lateral and posterior pharyngeal walls are made. Instructing the patient to place the chin against the chest and move the head from side to side molds the impression material.

In the rest position, the patient swallows water and talks to allow further molding of the impression material by muscular activity. If the mass is overextended, the patient will feel it during these actions. Reheating the bulb on the exterior surface and reinserting it into the patient's mouth easily adjust the over-extended bulb impression. While the material is soft, the patient is instructed to produce the desired muscular activities. The completed speech bulb impression is chilled thoroughly in ice water. To check the position of the bulb, water is injected again, and the position of the bulb is examined in the mouth for its relation to the posterior and lateral pharyngeal wall activities. A spray of water onto the tissue will again stimulate these activities. In non-operated clefts, muscle function along the speech bulb during swallowing can be observed directly when the mouth is wide open and water is being sprayed onto the tissues. When the posterior pharyngeal wall activity is not present or direct visualization is not possible due to the length of the soft palate, a lateral cephalometric radiograph will reveal the position of the bulb in relation to the nasopharyngeal structures. Caution should be exercised to avoid blocking or extending the speech bulb into the Eustachian tube. Ideally, the final position of the bulb portion of the prosthesis should be assessed with the aid of a nasendoscopic examination to directly visualize the relationship of the bulb to the surrounding soft tissues both at rest and in function. When nasendoscopy or a lateral cephalometric examination is not available, the bulb is placed in the area of the palatal plane as a general guideline. When the bulb form has been perfected, the bulb and velar section are processed onto the denture portion of the appliance. A clear, heat-cured acrylic resin is used for making these parts.

For patients with unusually sensitive posterior and lateral pharyngeal walls (i.e., when the gag reflex is easily triggered), the making of a final impression for the speech bulb on the initial try is delayed until the patient is properly prepared for the impression. In such cases, it is helpful to construct an under-extended bulb in self-curing acrylic resin, and to allow the patient to become adjusted to this small bulb for 2 or 3 weeks. After the patient has become accustomed to the undersized bulb, adding Adaptol™ to the bulb following the procedures previously outlined makes a final impression. The final impression of the speech bulb is processed in a heat-curing type of acrylic resin and given a high polish after processing.

To prevent the patient from swallowing the bulb in case the velar section is fractured, the appliance should be reinforced by incorporating a piece of No. 11 gauge half-round wire in the anterior body of the appliance and extending the wire into the bulb. If the anterior part of the appliance is made of cast metal, the frame should be extended posteriorly to strengthen the velar and pharyngeal section.

Insertion of the Appliance

The finished speech aid prosthesis is inserted into the mouth and examined for muscle adaptation to the speech bulb during swallowing and phonation, excessive pressure against the posterior and lateral walls of the pharynx, stability of the appliance during function, and improvement of the quality of the speech.

Position of the Speech Bulb

If the bulb is positioned too far inferiorly, the following undesirable effects are seen in most patients:

1. It has a tendency to be displaced by the dorsal part of the tongue during tongue movements.
2. It fails to relate to the normal region for making adequate velopharyngeal closure.
3. It has a detrimental acoustical effect on the quality of the speech.

Following delivery of the completed speech aid prosthesis, the patient should be able to demonstrate comfortable palatopharyngeal function that allows for normal speech and deglutition. Excessive palatopharyngeal tissue contact from the bulb may result in painful swallowing and well as hyponasal speech, as the excessive contact will prevent sufficient airflow and actively displace soft (and possibly hard) tissues when the appliance is in place. Insufficient bulb contact with the palatopharyngeal tissues will result in hypernasal speech, as too much air will be allowed to flow around the appliance. Similarly, food and fluids may be expressed from the patient's nose if there is insufficient contact between the appliance and the palatopharyngeal tissues during swallowing. Although the experienced prosthodontist may be able to subjectively discern the modifications required to remedy a deficient speech bulb appliance, more objective assessment tools may make the adjustment process much more efficient. Of all the methods available to assess the fit of the bulb in relationship to the palatopharyngeal tissues, direct visualization of the bulb-tissue relationship by nasoendoscopic examination is the most useful.

■ SUMMARY

As surgical techniques have improved, surgeons have become better able to successfully treat velopharyngeal dysfunction in most cases. Use of a prosthetic speech aid appliance may be clearly indicated in some cases, however, just as specific surgical procedures may be indicated in others. The prosthodontist is, therefore, an integral part of the multidisciplinary management of cleft palate speech.

References

1. Conley S, Gosain A, Marks S, Lawson, D. Identification and assessment of velopharyngeal inadequacy. *Am J Otolaryngol* 18:38, 1997.
2. Tachimura T, Nohara K, Wada T. Effect of a speech appliance on levator veli palatini muscle activity during speech. *Cleft Palate Craniofac J* 37(5):478–482, 2000.
3. Mazaheri M. Prosthodontic aspects of palatal elevation and palatopharyngeal stimulation. *J Prosthet Dent* 35:319–326, 1976.

Dental and Orthodontic Management

Pediatric Dentistry

Donald V. Huebener, DDS, MS, MAEd

Contemporary management of patients with cleft lip and palate requires a coordinated effort by many care providers to achieve the most desirable outcome. Such a multidisciplinary approach to habilitation is necessary due to the complexity and multiple issues involved in the clefting process. In the past, individual care providers managed patients with cleft lip/palate in respective offices, clinics, and hospitals with collaboration as appropriate and necessary. However, it has become apparent that a more coordinated effort by a team of specialists evaluating each patient and formulating an individual treatment plan is more appropriate. Furthermore, team coordination of not only of the evaluation process but also of the specialty providers' interventions streamlines cleft care and promotes efficiency. For example, palatoplasty and myringotomy with ventilating tubes can be scheduled during the same hospital stay and under the same general anesthetic. Likewise, coordination of regular recall examinations by the pediatric dentist and adjustments for braces by the orthodon-

tist can minimize trips to urban centers and reduce the total time for care.

Current management protocols have been developed by cleft/craniofacial teams of health care individuals involving many disciplines. Team care should be based on a philosophy developed by its members guided by the principles of the American Cleft Palate/Craniofacial Association Standards of Team Care.[1] Team members comprise the medical specialties (plastic surgery, otolaryngology, and pediatrics), the dental specialties (oral surgery, orthodontics, pediatric dentistry, and prosthodontics), and the allied health professionals (audiology, speech pathology, nursing, care coordinators, and social workers). With the more complex cleft/craniofacial syndromic diagnoses, additional specialties are necessary, such as anesthesiology, genetics, ophthalmology, and radiology.

The pediatric dentist is unique among the many team providers involved in caring for cleft patients because of the scope of practice. Pediatric dental care begins in infancy[2] with the Infant Oral Health Care Program and continues thought adolescence. The routine periodicity of dental visits[3] provides an unparalleled opportunity for cleft patients and their dental treatment to be monitored longitudinally. Whereas all other cleft team care providers examine and provide services to cleft patients at certain intervals (orthodontists), episodically (oral surgeons), interventionally (speech pathologists), and surgically (plastic surgeons), the pediatric dentist evaluates and observes the developing dentition and monitors overall oral health at 6-month intervals. Among the services provided by the pediatric dentist are preventive dental care, which begins early with the establishment of the "dental home"[4]; caries risk assessment[5]; restorative dental services; space management; nutritional counseling; and trauma management.

The purpose of this chapter is to provide the insight and rationale for pediatric dental intervention during the course of cleft lip/palate care. Principles of the American Cleft Palate/Craniofacial Association have been incorporated into an endorsement by the American Academy of Pediatric Dentistry for care of cleft lip/palate patients.[6] This dental care is a continuum with similar needs of preventive and restorative dentistry as are required in healthy patients, but with unique procedures and collaboration with specialists for cleft lip/palate management. The location of specific services also may be unique in that many dental procedures are performed in a hospital in conjunction with other specialists on the team.

SEQUENCING OF DENTAL CARE IN CLEFT PATIENTS

In general, the timing of dental intervention in the cleft habilitation process is correlated to odontogenic and oral facial development. Four classical stages related to the patient's age have been established which roughly correspond to tooth eruption time and to the establishment of the occlusion.[7] The dental cleft team members—oral surgeons, orthodontists, pediatric dentists, and prosthodontists—perform specialty procedures on cleft infants, children, and adolescents based on dental maturity, age, and patient behavior/cooperation in coordination with other care providers. Usually, interventions proceed in an orderly fashion in stepwise manner with defined treatment objectives and a timetable for completion. That is not to say, however, that planned, sequential intervention cannot be adjusted. For example, maxillary expansion in the early mixed dentition is normally performed prior to bone grafting. If the eruption of the maxillary permanent first molars is delayed, it may be necessary to postpone this procedure because these teeth are necessary for placement of the expansion appliance. Likewise, if the patient is uncooperative for this early phase of orthodontic therapy, the orthodontist may elect to defer treatment until more maturity is attained.

Stage I: Initial Management/Maxillary Appliance Stage (Birth to 24 Months)

Initial cleft management in Stage I begins with addressing the immediate issue of infant nutrition and feeding. Because of

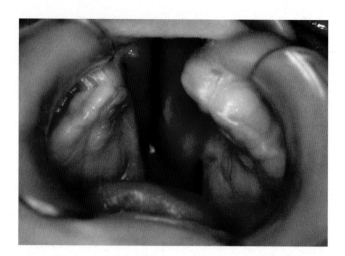

Figure 44–1. A 4-week-old infant with unilateral cleft lip and palate (UCLP).

the nature of the clefting process, infants with either unilateral cleft lip and palate (UCLP) (Fig. 44–1) or bilateral cleft lip and palate (BCLP) (Fig. 44–2) have unique feeding issues. Adequate nutrition is of utmost importance. The team clinical nurse specialist or the feeding specialist instructs parents in the methods of cleft infant feeding. Various types of infant cleft nipples have been advocated for use in feeding as well as many feeding techniques.[8] Most of the time, adequate infant nutrition can be achieved with assisted feeding with a compressible or squeezable bottle.[9] In a few special instances (syndromic infants, severe facial clefts, etc.), it may be necessary for the pediatric dentist to fabricate a feeding appliance to assist with oral intake. These appliances are constructed on plaster casts made from impressions of the cleft infant's maxilla. Usually, they are designed to obturate the entire cleft defect and to allow food and liquids to enter the digestive tract properly.

The second major consideration at Stage 1 is the use of maxillary appliances, active or passive; extraoral or intraoral. The sequencing of appliance usage must be coordinated

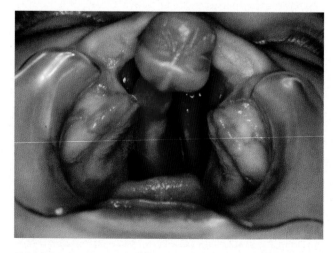

Figure 44–2. A 4-week-old infant with bilateral cleft lip and palate (BCLP).

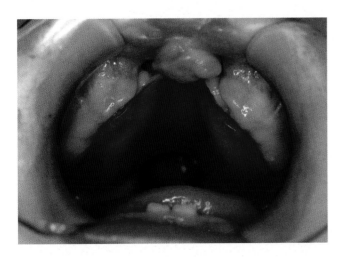

Figure 44–3. Bilateral cleft lip/palate infant with an alveolar molding appliance in place.

with the initial lip closure. Depending on team protocols and care provider availability, both orthodontists and pediatric dentists (and sometimes prosthodontists) perform these procedures and coordinate such care with the plastic surgeon. Active appliances are designed to provide a force to alter relationships of the hard and soft tissues. Such appliances can be either extraoral (e.g., head cap/bonnet with tape/straps applied to a projecting premaxilla) or intraoral (e.g., acrylic with springs). Passive appliances utilize the forces created by lip adhesion/definitive lip repair to stabilize the posterior maxillary alveolar segments while allowing the anterior cleft segments to rotate or "mold" about an acrylic framework (Fig. 44–3).

The timing of appliance usage is related to the intent and outcome. True "presurgical" maxillary appliances (i.e., tape across the premaxilla or nasoalveolar molding appliances) are performed prior to initial cheiloplasty and either adjust alveolar segment position or alter tissue form. Presurgical benefits include the adjustment of the cleft tissues to a more ideal relationship before initial surgery in order to enhance surgical outcome. Passive appliances (e.g., alveolar molding appliances) utilize the forces created by either lip adhesion or definitive lip repair to provide a force over time and mold the alveolar segments. These appliances allow controlled anterior alveolar segment rotation and reorientation of the maxillary frenum toward the midsaggital plane while maintaining posterior cleft segment position.

There is considerable controversy among clinicians and researchers as to the purpose and short and long-term outcomes with the use of early infant maxillary appliances. In the past, clinicians utilized "presurgical appliances," "presurgical orthodontics," "neonate orthopedics" with the intent of reducing the magnitude of the cleft deformity and to help to eliminate the need for extensive orthodontics in the future. Many surgeons noted that successful initial lip surgery was easier to attain, but researchers studying the long-term effect of presurgical orthopedics on the growth of the nasomaxillary complex saw little change with the use of early infant appliances. Currently, there is a renewed interest in the use of early

cleft appliances to assist in "normalizing" the cleft lip and alar cartilage and providing better soft tissue relationships prior to initial cleft surgery.[10] Most researchers agree that the absence of sufficient evidence either for or against the use of presurgical maxillary appliances is due to small treatment populations in cleft teams, lack of longitudinal studies utilizing randomized clinical trials, the length of time necessary to fully evaluate a particular technique or philosophy of treatment, and variables associated with multi-center studies.

When using infant cleft appliances, it is necessary to consider the increased patient and care provider time and the increased costs associated with the appliance and multiple visits for adjustment. More complex cleft procedures tend to be performed in urban cleft centers where many of the team specialists are located. Many cleft patients and their families and must travel long distances for such specific interventions. In addition, the increased financial burden may impact on the family's ability to receive care. As a result, care providers must evaluate the benefits of early cleft appliance usage and the additional time and increased costs of the procedure when considering early maxillary appliances.

In Stage I, the pediatric dentist begins infant oral health care. During this first "age one" dental visit, the pediatric dentist examines the oral cavity, notes any abnormalities in the hard or soft tissues, and provides anticipatory guidance to parents regarding dental care. Dietary intake of fluoride and the benefits of fluoride are discussed. The problem of early childhood caries and its relationship to prolonged nursing or bottle-feeding and to the frequency of intake of cariogenic foodstuffs is addressed. Finally, common injuries to the erupting primary teeth are discussed, and instructions are given to the parents for use should an unfortunate traumatic event occur.

One of the major components of the age one dental visit is a review of oral hygiene practices for the infant. Proper toothbrushing and flossing are essential in removing plaque and cariogenic bacteria from tooth surfaces. Instruction for parents by the pediatric dental team begins as soon as the first incisors erupt. Using a moistened cloth or gauze square, the parent or caregiver wipes each tooth surface including those in the cleft area daily. This can be accomplished while holding the child or lying the child down. Soon after the first primary molars erupt, it is advisable to begin brushing the occlusal surfaces of these teeth using a soft-bristled infant toothbrush. At this early age, parents may begin using a nonfluoridated toothpaste if the texture and flavor is agreeable to the child. Routine use of toothpaste with fluoride should be delayed until the child can expectorate because of the concern of fluoride ingestion. Parents may begin flossing when the contacts between the teeth begin to close.

At this stage, the pediatric dentist begins to answer some of the many questions parents have regarding the cleft deformity. These concerns relate in part to congenitally missing teeth in the cleft area, timing of orthodontics, bone grafting, and replacement of missing teeth in primary school-age children and in the teen years. The pediatric dentist reassures the parents that all of their questions and concerns are priorities in team care and, as a member of the team, explains the procedures and treatment benchmarks at each stage. In some instances, the team members will not only be the diagnostic and treatment planning group but also the providers of the cleft care. In other instances, the team will direct the overall care and provide some of the more complex services with more routine services provided by local care providers. In all cases, the cleft team will monitor the progress of individual services through regular team visits and make appropriate recommendations for subsequent interventions.

Stage II: The Primary Dentition Stage (2.5–6 Years of age)

The primary dentition stage is marked by the complete eruption of all primary teeth and continues until the beginning of mixed dentition with the eruption of the mandibular permanent incisors and permanent molars. The process of tooth eruption in the primary dentition normally begins in the mandibular arch with the eruption of the central incisor at 8 months of age (6–10 months ± 1 SD) and in the maxillary arch with the eruption of the central incisor at 10 months of age (8–12 months ± 1 SD).[11] The normal sequence of primary tooth eruption in both the maxilla and the mandible begins with the central incisor followed by the lateral incisor, first molar, canine, and second molar.

In cleft lip and palate infants and children, there is delay of eruption of the primary teeth on the cleft side in both the maxilla and mandible when compared to the homologues on the noncleft side. This delay is statistically significant for the maxillary lateral incisor, the maxillary cuspid, and the mandibular lateral incisor.[12] The sequence of primary tooth eruption on the maxillary cleft side is altered with the lateral incisor erupting last.[12,13] There is an increased incidence of natal teeth (teeth present at birth) and neonatal teeth (those teeth which erupt during the first 30 days) in infants with cleft lip and palate and in syndromic conditions.[14]

The major emphasis during Stage II is the establishment of the primary occlusion and the promotion of good oral hygiene. Pediatric dental concerns at this time are focused on a good oral health care program at home, prevention of dental caries, restoration of carious teeth, preparation of the teeth for any necessary maxillary appliances, and routine periodic visits to the dental office. During this time, there are continued questions from parents and caregivers regarding the cleft defect and its effect on the primary and permanent teeth. As the primary teeth erupt, parents soon notice that the teeth in the cleft area may appear to be out of position, rotated, tipped into the cleft defect, malformed and/or discolored, or missing. Many times, they may see anterior–posterior malalignment of the dental arches with the mandible in anterior crossbite. Likewise, they may be aware of a "tipping in" of an alveolar segment resulting in a posterior malocclusion, and they may become cognizant of supernumerary teeth erupting in or around the cleft site. Some of these issues may be addressed during this stage; others will be deferred until further development of the dentition.

Oral Hygiene for Cleft Children

The promotion of good oral hygiene that began in infancy is reinforced in Stage II as the primary dentition matures children with unilateral and bilateral cleft lip/palate have abnormal alveolar segment relationships with rotation and tipping of the teeth near the cleft defect and in the cleft alveolar segments. Crowding can occur and restrict the ability of the toothbrush to reach difficult areas. In addition, there may be supernumerary teeth, missing teeth, abnormal tooth morphology and hypoplastic enamel, severely protruding maxilla, etc., all of which may affect the ability to properly brush and remove bacteria and plaque from the tooth surfaces. Because of these factors, cleft lip/palate children are at higher risk for the development of caries when compared to the normal population and require a personalized program of preventive dental care.

Cleft Lip/Palate and Dental Caries

Streptococcous mutans, one of the most virulent of the caries-producing microorganisms, begins to colonize in the oral cavity around 15.7 months and by the age of 24 months, 84% of young children harbor the bacteria.[15] In an earlier study, positive cultures of *S. mutans* appeared at the mean age of 15.3 months, with a positive correlation between the time of acquisition of the bacterium and the number of erupted teeth.[16] Most likely, the mode of transmission of *S. mutans* is oral, from the parent (mother) to the infant.[15,16] These microorganisms metabolize carbohydrates, and byproducts of this metabolism then reduce the pH of the oral cavity and initiate the process of caries formation. Most experts agree that the earlier the transmission, the more likely the infant will be at risk for caries.

Researchers have long documented that children with cleft lip/palate have a higher incidence of dental caries.[17–19] Recent studies have confirmed this observation.[20] However, researchers have also noted that there are no differences in the proportion of caries-producing microorganisms at the cleft site when compared to unaffected sites.[21] This would seem to indicate that there would not be more carious activity than normal at cleft sites, but conventional wisdom notes that teeth tipped into the cleft area and supernumerary teeth present there collect plaque and frequently become carious.

In general, any caries risk factor that may contribute to the caries process in normal infants and children may also be applied to special patients, such as those with cleft lip and palate. Some of these factors are previous caries, salivary disease, presence of orthodontic appliances, between-meal sugar exposure, intake of carbonated beverages, inadequate fluoride exposure, poor toothbrushing habits, and lack of regular dental visits. In addition, there are certain factors that may contribute to the apparent increase in dental caries in cleft infants and children, such as the position of teeth in the dental arch, crowding of teeth in the cleft area, difficulty in brushing in the altered alveolar segments, and oral hygiene and dietary habits. Recently, researchers have developed new strategies for the prevention of caries in cleft lip/palate patients that can

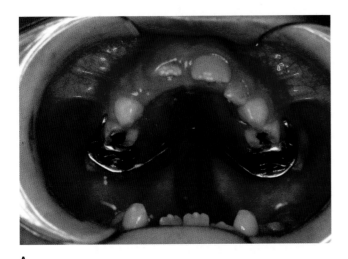

A

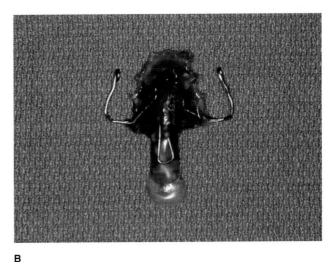

B

Figure 44–4. Speech aid for velopharyngeal dysfunction. (*Courtesy of Dr. Donald Gay.*)

assist cleft teams and their oral health care programs for their patients.[22]

Maxillary Appliances

Maxillary appliances may be indicated in the primary dentition stage in order to assist specialty providers in the course of cleft habilitation. In selected patients, for example, obturators or palatal lift prostheses may be utilized for management of velopharyngeal dysfunction (Fig. 44–4). In other patients, appliances may be used to obdurate oronasal fistulae. The pediatric dentist or the prosthodontist will utilize a stone cast made from an impression of the cleft maxilla to construct these palatal appliances. Wire clasps for retention are placed posteriorly to surround the molar tooth and hold the appliance in place.

The retention of maxillary appliances in the primary dentition presents unique problems. This issue may be partially overcome by the use of stainless steel crowns with soldered buccal lugs on the maxillary first and/or second primary molars (Fig. 44–5). Stainless steel crowns provide excellent retention but necessitate alteration of tooth structure for proper adaptation. Certainly, this becomes a moot issue if the teeth used for retention are carious and require stainless steel crowns in the course of treatment. If, however, no caries are present, two alternative retentive procedures are possible. First, orthodontic bands with soldered buccal lugs can be used (Fig. 44–6). The bands are adapted to the appropriate teeth in the maxilla and then carefully removed. In the lab, round 0.045 gauge orthodontic wire is tack-welded to the buccal side of the band, keeping the wire parallel to the superior and inferior edges of the band. Solder is then flowed over the wire and buccal surface of the band taking care not to allow solder to flow inside of the band. A 90-degree ledge on the gingival side of the band is created utilizing an abrasive rotating disc. This ledge allows for a secure retentive area for the wire clasp following placement of the maxillary appliance. The finished band/lug is smoothed and polished prior to cementation.

Bands with soldered lugs as described above are very useful when utilizing second primary molars and first permanent molars. When it is necessary to utilize first primary molars for retention, regular orthodontic bands do not fit properly, and an alternative method may become necessary due to their unique anatomical morphology. In this instance, a precrimped primary molar stainless steel crown is selected for size and the crown's occlusal portion is removed, leaving the proximal surfaces intact. The crown is then placed on the first primary molar and adjusted occlusally–gingivally for fit. The anatomical contour of the precrimped crowns will allow them to act as well-adapted orthodontic bands. Lugs are added and soldered in a fashion similar to that used for standard bands. Finally, if added retention is necessary for any maxillary appliances, the buccal and lingual surfaces of the tooth can be etched prior to cementation of the band.

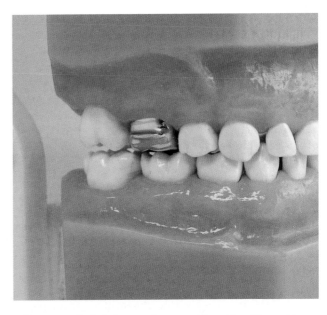

Figure 44–5. Stainless steel crown with soldered buccal lug.

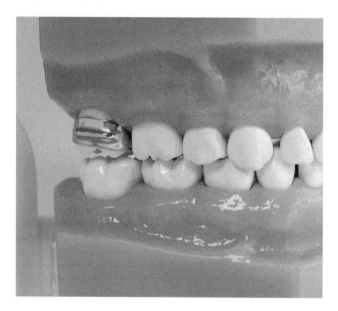

Figure 44–6. Orthodontic band with soldered buccal lug.

Ectopic Eruption and Supernumerary Teeth

During Stage II, ectopic eruption of teeth and eruption of supernumerary teeth are common in the area surrounding the cleft defect. The abnormal number of teeth and tooth buds, as well as the location of these odontogenic structures, may be understood as a function of the clefting process, for during embryological development, the facial processes (medial nasal process and the maxillary process) and the dental lamina, the precursor of the primary and permanent tooth buds, arise as adjacent structures.

It is reasonable to assume that any factor that interferes with the normal union of the medial and maxillary processes may also interfere with normal odontogenic development. The medial nasal and maxillary processes contact and fuse during the sixth week of development. Palatogenesis occurs somewhat later (7–9 wk), and fusion of the palatal processes is complete by the twelfth week of development.[23] The dental lamina, the precursor of both the primary teeth and permanent teeth, develops during the sixth week of gestation.[24] First, the dental lamina produces the primary tooth bud. Then, the leading edge of the dental lamina continues to grow, forming the permanent tooth bud. Both incisor primary and permanent buds mature in stages and develop near the borders of the cleft. Evidence of dental enamel defects and enamel hypoplasia in both the primary and permanent incisors in cleft children can be correlated with the mechanism of cleft lip/palate development.[25]

Common clinical manifestations of disruption of normal tooth development in cleft children are congenital absence of primary and/or permanent teeth (annihilation of the tooth bud), supernumerary teeth (splitting or "twinning" of the tooth bud), disturbance during the enamel matrix formation (abnormal morphology of teeth), disturbance during the calcification stage of tooth development (enamel hypoplasia), rotations, malpositions and tipping of teeth (distortion

of the normal alveolar segment relationships during the clefting process). In general, decisions regarding supernumerary teeth and congenitally missing teeth in the cleft site are deferred until Stage III when odontogenic structures in the cleft alveolar are more developed and calcified.

Crossbites in the Primary Dentition

As the primary teeth erupt and interdigitate in cleft patients, there is frequently an abnormal occlusal relationship in either the anterior or posterior alveolar segment areas. When the maxillary incisor/s are lingual to the mandibular incisors when the teeth are in occlusion, an anterior crossbite exists. This relationship may be either the result of the axial inclination of the primary teeth, considered "dental," or the manifestation of cleft maxillary hypoplasia, or "skeletal." When the cusps of the maxillary posterior teeth occlude lingual to the mandibular teeth, a posterior crossbite exists. This may be either partial (involving one or two teeth) or complete (involving the entire quadrant).

There are many factors that should be considered when addressing crossbite correction in the primary dentition stage. These factors include: (1) age and cooperation of the child, (2) dental or skeletal crossbite manifestation, (3) caries risk, (4) long-term maintenance with space maintainers, (5) oral hygiene, (6) timing of bone grafting to consolidate the alveolar segments, and (7) parental interest. Whereas care providers may be eager to habilitate the cleft child as early as possible, it may be more appropriate to delay crossbite intervention until Stage III when the permanent incisors and first permanent molars have erupted.

Dental Radiographs

Dental radiographs for cleft patients should follow the American Dental Association/U.S. Food and Drug Administration/American Academy of Pediatric Dentistry guidelines.[26] These should be based on risk assessment, occlusal development, and the "need-to-know" prior to any dental intervention. Bitewing radiographs are necessary after the contacts in the posterior area are closed to detect interproximal caries. Anterior periapical radiographs are useful in evaluating for caries and enamel hypoplasia in and around the cleft area. The routine use of panoramic radiology very early in the primary dentition stage is not indicated because of the immaturity of dental structures in the anterior area, the inherent distortion in the panoramic radiographic view, the cooperation of the child, and the delay for most dental intervention until later.

The risk of exposing the cleft child to radiation should be weighed against the benefits and knowledge gained. Certainly, toward the late stage of primary dentition or the beginning of mixed dentition, a panoramic radiograph becomes very useful in diagnosis and treatment planning (Fig. 44–7). Cephalometric and panoramic radiographs by the orthodontist are part of the diagnostic protocol for Phase I maxillary expansion in preparation for alveolar bone grafting. Postoperative maxillary periapical radiographs of the bone-grafted site/s are useful in determining success of the surgical

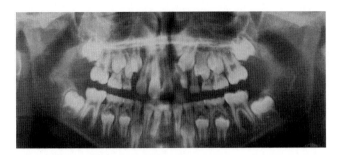

Figure 44–7. Panoramic radiograph of the mixed dentition of left UCLP. (*Courtesy of Dr. Richard Nissen.*)

procedure. Radiographs (bitewing and periapical) for caries detection may be necessary based upon the clinical examination and the risk factors present (Fig. 44–8). Finally, additional radiographs in preparation for Phase II full-banded orthodontics are indicated when the dentition reaches maturity.

Stage III: The Mixed Dentition Stage (6–12 Years of Age)

Stage III begins with the eruption of the permanent teeth, notably the mandibular central incisors and the first permanent molars. This stage continues until the eruption of the maxillary permanent canine, usually the last permanent tooth to erupt, with the exception of the permanent third molars or "wisdom teeth." During this time, the central incisors (most notably the central incisor adjacent to the cleft defect in unilateral cleft lip/palate and both right and left central incisors in bilateral cleft lip/palate) erupt ectopically. These teeth can be rotated, inclined labially or lingually, and sometimes tipped into the cleft area. In the molar region, crossbites involving the posterior alveolar segments are common. In unilateral cleft lip/palate, for example, the lesser alveolar segment on the cleft side is frequently in crossbite; in bilateral cleft lip/palate, both lateral cleft segments may be in crossbite.

It is during this time that many dental interventions occur. The timing of treatment is usually dependent on eruption of teeth and maturation of the dentition. For example, correction of posterior crossbite may begin after complete eruption of the maxillary first molars when orthodontic band placement on these is possible. If eruption of the first molars is delayed, crossbite correction in preparation for secondary alveolar bone grafting may occur later. Many care providers will defer posterior crossbite correction until not only the maxillary first molars are completely erupted but also the maxillary central incisors. This will allow simultaneous correction of the posterior crossbite as well as the anterior tooth rotations and help to eliminate the psychological effects associated with the cleft deformity.

Congenitally Missing Lateral Incisors, Supernumerary Teeth, and Enamel Defects

During Stage III, a panoramic radiograph of a cleft patient will provide much diagnostic information regarding the dentition. The permanent lateral incisor is the most commonly affected tooth in the area of the cleft and is affected in most instances.[27] Frequently, this tooth is congenitally missing. When present, the maxillary lateral incisor on the cleft side cleft erupts at a later age than its homologue on the noncleft side.[28] In addition, radiographs may reveal the presence of a supernumerary tooth or teeth that developed due to a developmental disturbance in the dental lamina. The lateral incisor may be hypoplastic, or it may exhibit a significant delay in root development when compared to noncleft lateral incisor.[29] Finally, cleft lip/palate individuals exhibit a significant delay in formation and mineralization of the second premolars.[30]

Clinically, there is a higher prevalence of enamel alterations affecting incisors adjacent to the cleft when compared to the noncleft side, and the permanent central incisor is affected more than the primary incisor.[31] These affected enamel may be hypoplastic (change in morphology), or it may exhibit

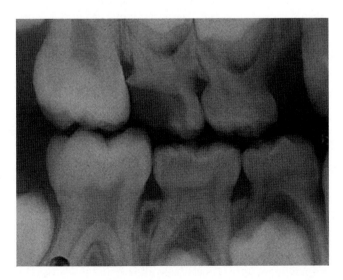

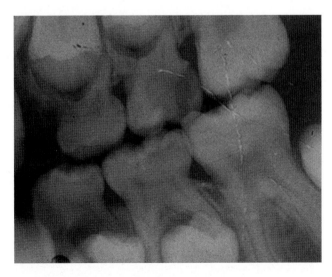

Figure 44–8. Bite wing radiographs of the mixed dentition with dental caries.

yellow or brown spots (change in mineralization). In addition, cleft individuals have a higher occurrence of hypodontia and asymmetric dental development when compared to non-cleft individuals.[32]

Treatment decisions are made jointly be members of the dental team. The oral surgeon, orthodontist, and the pediatric dentist review the radiographs and determine the appropriate intervention, timing, and sequence.

Anterior and Posterior Crossbite Correction

During Stage III, the issue of anterior and posterior crossbites is usually addressed. Anteriorly, eruption of the permanent central incisors often occurs with traumatic occlusion. This is due in part to the maxillary hypoplasia that may be associated with cleft lip/palate, with resultant incisor edge-to-edge occlusion and the rotation, tipping, and abnormal inclination of the incisors due to the abnormal maxillary-mandibular alveolar segment relationship. A similar situation often occurs posteriorly, where the maxillary lateral segment is in malalignment. Usually, team protocols advocate correction of these abnormal segmental relationships prior to and in preparation for secondary alveolar bone grafting. Correction at this time diminishes the possibility of abnormal incisal and enamel wear from traumatic occlusion, lessens the psychological impact of severely rotated and tipped incisors, provides for an unobstructed operating field during secondary bone grafting surgery, and allows for favorable and secure closure of the surgical graft site.

The pediatric dentist and the orthodontist are in frequent consultation during Stage III because of the numerous decisions in cleft habilitation. First, if the maxillary lateral incisor in the cleft area is congenitally missing, a decision must be made regarding the lateral space. This decision should be based on the patient's growth prediction, skeletal pattern, tooth size, tooth position near the cleft site, knowledge of additional congenitally missing teeth, and parental desires. Two options exist: (1) maintaining a lateral incisor space and (2) closure of the normal lateral incisor space. If the lateral incisor space is closed orthodontically, the maxillary canine moved into the space is reshaped to appear similar to the contralateral incisor. If the lateral space is maintained, treatment options include the immediate need for tooth replacement following expansion and secondary bone grafting. A discussion of the final tooth replacement options includes a fixed bridge replacing the missing tooth, a bonded bridge ("Maryland Bridge"), an intraosseous implant, or a removable appliance to replace the missing lateral incisor.

Prior to maxillary expansion, a thorough oral examination, including bitewing radiographs, prophylaxis, and fluoride treatment should be performed. All restorative needs should be addressed before any orthodontic appliances are inserted into the oral cavity. This is especially true for the maxillary central incisors because of the frequent maxillary hypoplasia and the need for restorative dentistry (Fig. 44–9).[31] Consideration should be given to the placement of sealants, if necessary, on the first permanent molars to aid in caries prevention during Phase I of orthodontic treatment.

As discussed for Stage II, a personalized program of preventive dental care may be necessary to minimize the possibility of enamel decalcification and the development of caries. During Stage III, regular recall examinations with prophylaxis/fluoride treatments are necessary. Maxillary arch wires should be removed before dental recall visits to enable thorough cleaning interproximally and, based on the patient's risk assessment, molar bands removed followed by bite wing radiographs if necessary. Close monitoring of the cleft patient's oral hygiene both by the pediatric dentist and the orthodontist is essential. If the patient's risk factors change, more frequent recall examinations with prophylaxis/fluoride treatments and oral hygiene instructions may become necessary. Both care providers should demonstrate proper tooth brushing techniques during office visits, evaluate whether these procedures are being followed, and intervene when necessary.

The emphasis of Phase I orthodontic treatment in Stage III centers on correction of the posterior alveolar segment alignment in both unilateral and bilateral complete clefts. In addition, in either cleft type, it is desirable to move the tipped maxillary central incisors away from the cleft site toward the midline. Care must be taken not to torque the roots of the incisors into the cleft area (Fig. 44–10). Most commonly, a "W" arch wire or quadhelix appliance is utilized. Tissue borne acrylic jackscrew appliances have limited use since there is no midpalatal suture in complete cleft lip/palate individuals.

Following complete posterior segment correction, a transpalatal holding appliance with lateral lingual canine extensions is preferable to a maxillary lingual holding arch wire. The latter may interfere with the surgical approach to secondary alveolar bone grafting. The holding appliance is worn continuously from correction until 3 months after secondary alveolar bone grafting. At this time, the fixed transpalatal appliance is removed, and a maxillary Hawley retainer is placed with a fixed "dummy" tooth replacing the maxillary lateral incisor, if necessary. Postoperative maxillary radiographs at appropriate intervals are helpful in monitoring the progress of the bone-grafted site. The orthodontic retainer is worn until later full orthodontic treatment.

Stage IV: The Permanent Dentition Stage (13–18 Years of Age)

Stage IV begins with the complete eruption of the premolars and maxillary canines. At this time, the second permanent molars may or may not be fully erupted and in occlusion, while the third molars are still in the process of formation. During this stage, the orthodontist revaluates facial growth and malocclusion. In general, the majority of cleft lip and palate individuals can be treated with conventional orthodontics to place their teeth in a desirable occlusion. This active tooth movement is accomplished approximately a period of 21–24 months and is followed by orthodontic retainers. When the lateral incisor is congenitally missing and the lateral incisor space is maintained, a "dummy' tooth is placed on the

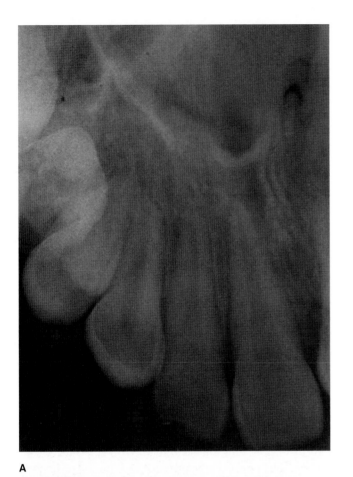

A

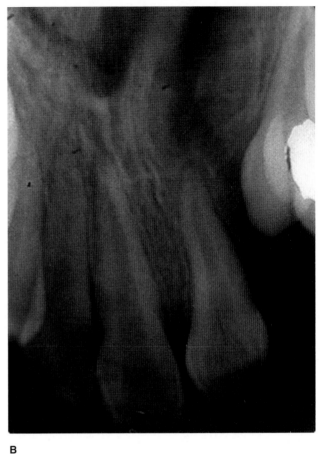

B

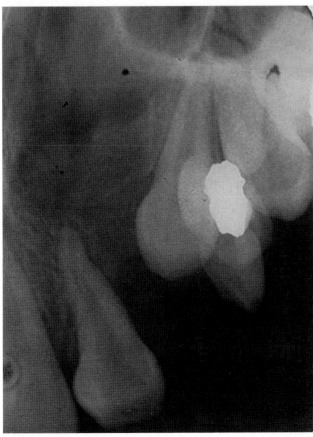

C

Figure 44–9. Anterior periapical radiographs of (A) nonaffected side, (B) midline, and (C) cleft side showing enamel hypoplasia of the central incisor near the cleft side and congenitally missing lateral incisor.

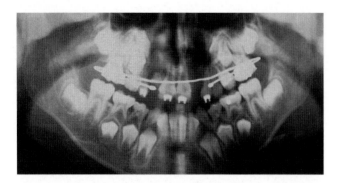

Figure 44–10. Panoramic radiograph of Phase I orthodontic treatment. BCLP with maxillary "W" arch wire in place. (*Courtesy of Dr. Richard Nissen.*)

maxillary retainer for aesthetics and space management. A final restoration in the lateral incisor cleft site is deferred until completion of facial growth and the full maturation of the dentition.

Some individuals with cleft lip and palate will require a surgical–orthodontic approach to place their teeth in a proper occlusion. Maxillary deficiency, genetic and environmental factors, and the overall pattern of facial growth may contribute to a Class III malocclusion that cannot be corrected by orthodontics alone. In these cases, close collaboration by team members is necessary. A first phase of orthodontics is necessary to properly align the dental arches prior to any surgical procedure. When the first phase of orthodontics is complete, the surgeon performs the necessary osteotomies to place the maxilla and mandible in the proper relationship. These surgical procedures are performed after facial growth is complete. This occurs at approximately 18 years of age in males and at approximately 15–16 years in females. The orthodontist makes final adjustments with appliances following surgery. Orthodontic retainers are worn after removal of appliances to stabilize the dentition.

Orthodontic Appliances and Caries

Much has been written about oral hygiene and dental care during the course of full orthodontic therapy. Orthodontic appliances provide harboring areas for microorganisms to colonize in plaques and to adhere to the surrounding tooth surfaces. Following the ingestion of fermentable substrates, caries-producing microorganisms metabolize these substrates and produce a lowered pH, which contributes to "white spot" formation. This is particularly evident on the labial and buccal surfaces of teeth between the brackets and wires and the free gingival margin. If the integrity of the tooth surface disintegrates or cavitates, a dental restoration becomes necessary.

It is very important that the orthodontist and the pediatric dentist communicate on a regular basis during the Stage IV. A complete recall examination including bitewing radiographs and fluoride treatment should be performed prior to the placement of orthodontic bands and/or brackets. Orthodontic treatment should begin at the appropriate time to

minimize the length of therapy because of the caries risk. The patient's oral hygiene practices should be reevaluated, and any deficiencies addressed.[33] During the course of orthodontic treatment, the use of topical fluorides in addition to fluoride toothpaste can reduce the incidence of decalcification.[34,35] Additional caries preventive measures during orthodontic therapy that may be helpful in preventing white spot lesions include chlorhexidine mouth rinses, sealants, and fluoride-releasing bonding materials.[36] Should clinical caries be detected during active orthodontic treatment, radiographs must be obtained and appropriate restorative measures performed.

Team Care and Access Issues

It is widely accepted that multidisciplinary team care for cleft individuals provides the most desirable outcomes. There are, however, several issues that may affect the ability of the team's recommendations to be implemented. One such issue is that of access to care. Whereas team recommendations may stipulate the appropriate time for Phase I orthodontic intervention (maxillary expansion prior to secondary alveolar bone grafting), care providers may be unavailable because of restrictive dental insurance plans, low reimbursement provided by of third party payors, or complete lack of funding for specific dental procedures. Even when care providers are available, the financial "cap" on the specific dental intervention cost is often far below the actual fee. In such instances, many families must look to other funding sources to augment their resources. The same problem exists in the planning for Phase II orthodontics in the permanent dentition. Finally, some families may not have any insurance coverage for dental or other procedures and, as a result, must bear the entire cost of care. All of these issues hinder the patients' ability to receive the necessary services recommended by teams.

Another issue is that of utilization of financial resources. Often, more advanced interventional procedures may seem to benefit the child with a cleft, but such services may be considered optional by insurance plans. Parents may therefore elect to forgo additional or very expensive treatments because of limited insurance coverage or financial means.

Finally, geographical distance may affect the ability of affected children to access care. Many families live far from cleft treatment centers and must travel long distances because cleft services do not exist in their local communities. In doing so, parents spend considerable time away from their employment to keep appointments for their children. Likewise, children often miss school instruction in order to visit the cleft specialty providers. In some instances, local care providers may assist teams in metropolitan centers. This helps to ease the travel burden and time away from work and school.

SUMMARY

Pediatric dentists on cleft teams should help to ensure that every cleft individual receives the appropriate level of dental care to ensure the most optimal outcome. This care should begin in infancy and continue throughout adolescence. Sequencing of dental care is based an orderly timetable of intervention that is related in part to the chronological age of the patient. During all stages, the pediatric dentist performs specific treatment regimes in coordination with other dental, medical, and allied specialists. The overall objective of cleft lip/palate care is to habilitate a cleft individual to normalcy in society. This requires a team approach with all caregivers providing services according to a defined treatment plan with measurable outcomes.

References

1. Team Standards Committee, American Cleft Palate-Craniofacial Association. *The Cleft and Craniofacial Team*. Chapel Hill, NC: American Cleft Palate-Craniofacial Association, 1996.

2. American Academy of Pediatric Dentistry. *Guideline on Infant Oral Health Care*. Chicago, IL: American Academy of Pediatric Dentistry, Reference Manual, 2006–2007, pp. 73–76.

3. American Academy of Pediatric Dentistry. *Guideline on Periodicity of Examination, Preventive Dental Services, Anticipatory Guidance, and Oral Treatment for Children*. Chicago, IL: American Academy of Pediatric Dentistry; Reference Manual, 2005–2007, pp. 89–101.

4. American Academy of Pediatric Dentistry. *Policy on the Dental Home*. Chicago, IL; American Academy of Pediatric Dentistry, Reference Manual, 2006–2007, pp. 17–18.

5. American Academy of Pediatric Dentistry. *Use of a Caries-risk Assessment Tool (CAT) for Infants, Children, and Adolescents*. Chicago, IL: American Academy of Pediatric Dentistry, Reference Manual, 2005–2007, pp. 24–28.

6. American Academy of Pediatric Dentistry. *Policy on Management of Patients with Cleft Lip/Palate and Other Craniofacial Anomalies*. Chicago, IL: American Academy of Pediatric Dentistry, Reference Manual, 2006–2007, pp. 202–203.

7. Jones JE, Sadove AM, Dean JA, Huebener DV. Multidisciplinary team approach to cleft lip and palate management. In: McDonald RE, Avery DR, and Dean JA (eds). *Dentistry for the Child and Adolescent*, 8th edn. St. Louis, MO: Mosby/Elsevier, 2004, pp. 684–711.

8. Reid J. A review of feeding interventions for infants with cleft palate. *Cleft Palate Craniofacial J* 41(3):268–278, 2004.

9. Shaw WC, Bannister RP, Roberts CT. Assisted feeding is more reliable for infants with clefts—a randomized trail. *Cleft Palate Craniofacial J* 36(3):262–268, 1999.

10. Grayson BH, Santiago PE, Brecht LE, Cutting CB. Presurgical nasoalveolar molding in infants with cleft lip and palate. *Cleft Palate Craniofac J* 36(6):486–498, 1999.

11. McDonald RE, Avery DR, Dean JA. Eruption of the teeth: Local, systemic, and congenital factors that in the process. In McDonald RE, Avery DR, and Dean JA (eds). *Dentistry for the Child and Adolescent*, 8th edn, St. Louis, MO: Mosby/Elsevier, 2004, p. 178.

12. Duque C, Dalben GS, Aranha AM, Carrara CF, Gomide MR. Chronology of deciduous tooth eruption in children with cleft lip and palate. *Cleft Palate Craniofacial J* 41(3):285–289, 2004.

13. Peterka M, Tvrdek M. Tooth eruption in patients with cleft lip and palate. *Acta Chir Plastic* 35(3–4):154–158, 1993.

14. Baumgart M, Lussi A. Natal and neonatal teeth. *Schweiz Monatsschr Zahnmed* 116(9):884–909, 2006.

15. Careletto KA, Irber FO, Cornejo LS, Gimaznez MG. Early acquisition of *Streptococcus mutans* for children. *Acta Odontol Latinoam* 18(2):69–74, 2005.

16. Berkowitz RJ, Mutans streptococci: Acquisition and transmission. *Pediatr Dent* 28(2):106–109, 2006.

17. Bokhout B, Hofman FX, van Limbeek J, Kramer GJ, Prahl-Anderson B. Incidence of dental caries in the primary dentition in children with a cleft lip and/or palate. *Caries Research* 31(1):8–12, 1997.

18. Chapple JR, and Nunn JH. The oral health of children with clefts of the lip, palate, or both. *Cleft Palate Craniofacial J* 38(5):525–528, 2001.

19. Ahluwalia M, Brailsford SR, Tarelli E, Gilbert SC, Clark DT, Bernard K, et al. Dental caries, oral hygiene, and oral clearance in children with craniofacial disorders. *J Den Res* 83(2):175–179, 2004.

20. Kirchberg A, Treide A, Hemprich A. Investigation of caries prevalencein children with cleft lip, alveolus, and palate. *J Craniomaxillofacial Surg* 32(4):215–219, 2004.

21. Lucas VS, Gupta R, Ololade O, Gelbier M, Roberts GJ, Dental health indices and caries associated microflora in children with unilateral cleft lip and palate. *Cleft Palate Craniofacial J* 37(5):447–452, 2000.

22. Cheng LL, Moor SL, Ho CT, Predisposing factors to dental caries in children with cleft lip and palate: A review and strategies for early prevention. *Cleft Palate Craniofac J* 44(1):67–72, 2007.

23. Berkovitz BKB, Holland GR, Moxham BJ. *Oral Anatomy, Histology and Embryology*, 3rd edn. Edinburgh: Mosby, 2002, p. 273.

24. Avery JK, Chiego DJ, *Essentials of Oral Histology and Embryology, A Clinical Approach*. St. Louis, MO: Mosby/Elsevier, 2006, p. 65.

25. Malanczuk T, Opitz C, Retzlaff R, Structural changes of dental enamel in both dentitions of cleft lip and palate patients. *J Orafac Orthop* 60(4):259–268, 1999.

26. American Academy of Pediatric Dentistry. *Guideline on Prescribing Dental Radiographs for Infants, Children, Adolescents, and Persons with Special Health Care Needs*. Chicago, IL. American Academy of Pediatric Dentistry, Reference Manual, 2006–2007, pp. 200–201.

27. Ranta R. A review of tooth formation in children with cleft lip/palate. *Am J Orthod Dentofacial Orthop* 1:11–18, 1986.

28. deCaravalho Carrara CF, deOliveira Lima JE, Carrara, CE, Gonalez VB, Chronology and sequence of eruption of the permanent teeth in patients with complete unilateral cleft lip and palate. *Cleft Palate Craniofac J* 41(6):642–645, 2004.

29. Ribeiro LL, dasNeves LT, Costa B, Gomide MR. Dental development of permanent lateral incisor in complete unilateral cleft lip and palate. *Cleft Palate Craniofacial J*, 39(2):193–196, 2002.

30. Mitsea AG, and Spyropoulos MN, Premolar development in Greek children with cleft lip and palate. *Quintessence Int* 32(8):639–646, 2001.

31. Maciel SP, Costa B, Gomide MR, The difference in enamel alterations affecting central incisors of children with complete unilateral cleft lip and palate. *Cleft Palate Craniofac J* 42(40):392–295, 2005.

32. Eerens K, Vlietinck R, Heidbuchel K, Van Olmen A, Derom C, Willems G, et al. Hypodontia and tooth formation in groups of children with cleft, siblings without cleft, and nonrelated controls, *Cleft Palate Craniofac J* 38(4):374–378, 2001.

33. Travess H, Roberts-harry D, Sandy J. Orthodontics. Part 6: Risks in orthodontic treatment, *B Dental J* 196(2):71–77.

34. Bensen PE, Shah AA, Millett DT, Dyer F, Parkin N, Vine RS. Fluorides, orthodontics and demineralization: A systematic review. *J Orthods* 32(2):102–114, 2005.

35. Kalha AS, Topical fluorides and decalcification around fixed orthodontic appliances. *Evid Based Dent* 7(2):38–39, 2006.

36. Derks A, Katsaros C, Frencken JE, van'tHof MA, Kuijpers-Jagtman AM. Caries-inhibiting effect of preventive measures during orthodontic treatment with fixed appliances. A systematic review. *Caries Res* 38(5):413–420, 2004.

45

Presurgical Orthopedics

Mohammad Mazaheri, MDD, DDS, MSc • Lawrence E. Brecht, DDS

■ REVIEW OF LITERATURE

Since the early 1950s, many investigative clinicians have shown a great deal of interest in the management of patients with unilateral or bilateral clefts utilizing presurgical orthopedics with or without primary bone grafting of the dental alveolus. This chapter outlines our own philosophy regarding presurgical orthopedics in patients with cleft lip and palate.

McNeil,[1–3] a prosthodontist from Scotland, first advocated the use of presurgical orthopedics (PSOT). He theorized that more favorable maxillary, nasal, and lip growth would occur after using PSOT to mold palatal segments into a more appropriate position. As a result of this process, the maxillary retrusion often seen in cleft lip and palate patients could be prevented. It was expected that this improved maxillofacial growth would allow for concurrent symmetric growth of the mandible,[4] allowing for a more stable correction of the dental malocclusion. In situations where there was a bilateral cleft, the appliance provided mechanical traction to direct a posterior force on the premaxilla, eventually providing a better anatomical position to facilitate surgery.

The philosophy of PSOT gained acceptance, but it was not until its use in conjunction with primary alveolar bone grafting[5–8] that interest became widespread. Shortly thereafter, this approach rapidly became the standard of care among clinicians worldwide, and several favorable reviews were published.[9–11] Burston,[12–14] an orthodontist from England, was an early proponent of PSOT and primary bone grafting and cited additional benefits, including the facilitation of normal respiration and improved feeding, occlusion, speech, and middle ear function. Additional potential benefits claimed were the reduced need for prosthetic replacement of missing lateral incisors and improved bony architecture of the alveolar ridge. A presurgical orthopedic ward at Children's Hospital in Haswell, England, was eventually established under his direction. The primary rationale for this practice was to prevent the collapse of maxillary hard and soft tissues.

Other names for PSOT and its variations include *neonatal maxillary orthopedics*, *presurgical infant orthopedics* (PSIO), and most recently, *nasoalveolar molding* (NAM). Appliance design and function has varied considerably, with examples including the Rosenstein,[15] the Millard,[16] and the Latham[11] appliances. Generally, appliances can be divided into three categories: active, semi-active, and passive. Designs include pin-retained[16] with activation screws, extraoral straps,[1,12] or simple plates held through adhesion and suction.[8] Depending on the PSOT technique being used, the appliance may be inserted before, during, or after surgery.

Controversy over the use of PSOT arose in the mid-1960s and continues to the current day. Pruzansky[17,18] criticized the use of PSOT, claiming that proponents of this procedure did not rely on a critical review of the literature, but rather on speculation and opinion. In a 1977 "State of the Art" report, an international committee concluded that most of the claimed benefits of PSOT were not supported by solid evidence in the literature.[19]

There is, however, some evidence to support the claim that PSOT is able to realign the maxillary segments, thereby reducing the cleft size before surgery. Mishima[20,21] conducted a study evaluating PSOT and found that the maxillary segments were placed closer toward the midline prior to surgery in the PSOT group than in the control group. At 18 months of age, the curvature of the palatal shelves was less steep, and there was decreased arch collapse than in the control group. At 4 years of age the distance between the canines and second molars (deciduous) was greater in the PSOT group. Rosenstein[15,22] published a long-term retrospective outcomes assessment of facial growth, secondary surgical need, and maxillary lateral incisor status following his center's surgical/orthodontic protocol. He concluded that this protocol, which included early maxillary orthopedics and primary osteoplasty in a planned sequence with lip and palate closure, had a positive influence on the above-mentioned measures. However, many have found that, after repair of the lip, these effects disappear over time. Kujipers-Jagtman and Prahl,[23–25] in an ongoing three-center randomized prospective clinical trial in the Netherlands, conducted a study investigating maxillary arch dimensions. They found significant differences in maxillary dimensions between the PSOT and non-PSOT groups prior to lip surgery at 15 weeks of age. However, this difference was no longer found at 12 months of age. Prahl[26] published a prospective two-arm randomized controlled trial specifically to study the effects of PSOT on maxillary arch form. The authors found that PSOT in patients with UCLP did not facilitate initial contact between the maxillary segments, nor did it prevent collapse of the alveolar segments. There was no positive effect on the severity of collapse from birth until 18

months, and they therefore concluded that PSOT has no use in preventing maxillary collapse. Pickrell[27] found similar results after the use of PSOT and concluded that primary alveolar bone grafts did not grow adequately to maintain the height of the alveolar process and that the dentition was unable to migrate into the graft site.

Weil[28] reported that palatal surgery could be delayed as a result of a stimulating orthopedic plate inserted immediately after birth. Although he did not provide data to support the claim of growth stimulation in terms of cleft size and growth of the palatal shelves, he reported a decrease in crossbite in the mixed dentition. Many, including Pruzansky[29] and Bishara,[30] agree that closure of the cleft space is part of the "catch up growth" phenomenon observed in the cleft lip and palate population. This means that the developing palate will reach its inherent growth potential, regardless of any stimulus. This growth can be negatively affected by nonphysiological or traumatic surgery, and therefore midfacial is not due to an intrinsic growth deficiency, but rather to the effects of surgery. Berkowitz[31] also found that midfacial growth could not be stimulated and stated that the cost/benefit ratio further invalidates the use of PSOT. Skoog[32] suggested that a well-performed lip repair procedure, without PSOT, is sufficient to mold and reposition the maxillary segments into proper alignment.

Mazaheri's studies on changes in arch form and dimensions of cleft patients[33–37] found that the greater and lesser segments undergo favorable change with growth and eruption of the deciduous dentition, provided the growth is not retarded by traumatic surgical intervention and scar tissue. Surgical closure of the lip had a significant effect upon reduction of the alveolar and palatal cleft and upon maxillary segmental relationships and positioning. The reduction of the palatal cleft after lip surgery was attributed to segmental repositioning, downward growth and changes in angulation of the palatal shelves, and medial growth of the palatal shelves. After lip repair, the following changes were observed: an intact circumoral muscular complex that resulted in a molding action on the dental arches, thereby reducing the size of the cleft, and growth of the palatal shelves.

The practice of performing primary alveolar bone grafting in conjunction with PSOT has been suggested by some. Autologous bone has been grafted into the alveolar cleft with the expectation that the resulting increased osteogenic activity would result in bone and tooth migration. However, negative experiences with this technique have been well documented. Notably, Jolleys and Roberton[38,39] found that PSOT in conjunction with primary alveolar bone grafting had a detrimental effect on anterior posterior maxillary development, resulting in an increase in the number of patients with cross-bite. Berkowitz's report on neonatal maxillary orthopedics concluded that PSOT in conjunction with primary bone grafting was detrimental to midfacial growth.[19] Although primary bone grafting has been discontinued in the majority of craniofacial centers, some, including Kernahan and Rosenstein,[40] still advocate its use. Skoog[32] described an alternative to primary bone grafting through the use of periosteal flaps (periosteoplasty). Although this practice was not widely accepted, a variation (gingivoperioplasty) was more recently introduced.[16,41] While short-term bone formation[42] and growth[43] have been documented, studies of the long-term effects of this approach on maxillofacial growth are still underway.

There is still no clear evidence to support or reject the use of PSOT. Winters and Hurwitz[44] concluded that "not one research paper has even been published investigating the possible benefits to cleft surgery resulting from PSOT." The authors stated that no significant orthodontic benefits from PSOT have been documented, nor has there been any evidence to support the claim of reduced need for complex orthodontic treatment post-PSOT. However, newer methods, including NAM, do show clear promise. Nasoalveolar molding was introduced in the 1990s by Grayson at the NYU Medical Center in order to correct the deformity of the nasal cartilages and the deficiency of columella tissue in unilateral and bilateral cleft patients.[45] A recent study[46] revealed that a NAM appliance utilized in a newborn with UCLP for 4 months followed by a one-stage lip, nose, and alveolus repair statistically increased the symmetry of the nose into early childhood. For the infant with a bilateral cleft, the nasoalveolar molding technique may eliminate the need for surgical lengthening of the columella.[47] Modifications to this technique have been made and found to be promising, and the technique continues to evolve.[48,49] Recent studies demonstrate very favorable cost/benefit considerations when NAM is employed.[50]

PRESURGICAL ORTHOPEDICS AT THE LANCASTER CLEFT PALATE CLINIC

Mmohammad Mazaheri, MDD, DDS, MSc

At the Lancaster Cleft Palate Clinic we do not utilize presurgical orthopedics or primary bone grafting in any type of unilateral cleft of the lip and palate. In patients with a bilateral cleft and a protruded premaxilla, we sometimes utilize an extraoral orthopedic appliance. Our treatment rationale is based on our detailed and controlled longitudinal growth studies on more than 500 patients with unilateral and bilateral cleft lip and palate and on cross-sectional analysis of hundreds of patients.

To date, we have observed hundreds of patients with constricted arches, scarred palates, and severe malocclusion. These patients have had extensive surgical procedures that appear to have resulted in maxillary growth restriction. Many of these patients were treated by unqualified or unskilled surgeons. Such patients are often presented by the advocates of presurgical orthopedics (with or without primary bone grafting) as examples why presurgical orthopedics is indicated. Often, the proponents of presurgical orthopedics present patients with severe arch collapse, palatal scarring, and malocclusion, noting that such unfavorable results would not have occurred if presurgical orthopedics had been utilized. In the past, many of us had the courage to state that the

most important variable in the development of arch collapse and malocclusion is simply the competency of the surgeon and quality of his surgical skills. Surgical results vary significantly from surgeon to surgeon. Some centers demonstrate excellent results, while others demonstrate severe maxillary growth inhibition, arch collapse, and malocclusion. Most of these unfavorable conditions are caused by radical and traumatic surgery. The best dental specialist, with all of his gadgetries of presurgical orthopedics, cannot prevent arch collapse and malocclusion unless the surgeon performs his surgical procedure with the utmost proficiency and skill and without creating excessive scar tissue. A well-controlled longitudinal study is needed to support presurgical orthopedics, with or without primary bone grafting, as an effective means of guiding growth processes to maintain normal structural relations. In 1964, Pruzansky[18] expressed an opinion that many still hold: "Their proposal to make things right and whole as early as possible seems sensible and has emotional appeal. Regrettably, and despite all these enthusiasms, what has been offered so far is a prolonged and costly manipulation, and a surgery that is needless and sometimes barbaric."

It has been stated that the primary goal of presurgical orthopedics is to achieve optimal alignment of the maxillary segments prior to lip and palate surgery. It has been claimed that doing so will decrease the incidence of maxillary arch constriction and subsequent cross-bite malocclusion. In our studies, however, a constant change was observed in the relationship between the greater and the lesser segments during various states of arch development. In most patients in whom there was an overlap of the greater segment over the lesser segment, the segmental relationships began to change prior to the age of 3 years and assumed an end-to-end relationship after the eruption of the deciduous dentition. Surgical repair of the lip resulted in significant reduction in the width of the alveolar and palatal clefts and significantly altered maxillary segmental positioning and relationships. Reduction of cleft width after lip surgery was the result of segmental repositioning, changes in palatal shelf angulation, and downward and medial growth of the palatal shelves. Indeed, there have been no studies reported illustrating a more satisfactory arch form and dental occlusion than those reported by Pruzansky, Aduss and Mazaheri, et al.

These findings suggest that it may not be necessary to treat the arch in early infancy with a holding or an expansion appliance, since it appears that the arch and the segmental relationship will undergo favorable change with growth and with eruption of the deciduous dentition, provided that growth is not restricted by traumatic surgical intervention and scar tissue formation. It is our opinion that the segments are able to assume a more favorable position when they were not locked in within the region of the alveolar cleft by any type of surgical intervention.

The most critical period of maxillary growth is between birth and one year. This is the time when one should not interfere with the growth of the maxilla with any form of orthopedic appliances or bone grafting procedures. Some have claimed that presurgical orthopedics (with or without primary bone grafting) minimizes the need for orthodontic treatment. To date, however, the results reported by the proponents of this technique do not substantiate their claim. The prevalence of arch collapse and malocclusion in our series of patients appears to be less than in those treated orthopedically.

Those patients with cross-bite requiring orthodontic treatment can be treated with a simple expansion appliance during primary, mixed, or permanent dentition, which will correct the deformity in a short period of time. Final orthodontic treatment is performed after the eruption of the permanent dentition, followed if needed, by prosthetic replacement of the missing dental elements. The prosthesis will also act as a splint for the stability of the segments.

Summary and Conclusion

A slight constriction of the arch or a simple cross-bite can be corrected by the age of 4 or 5 years using a simple orthodontic appliance. The use of early orthopedics and bone grafting to prevent a slight cross-bite does not seem to be justified. Many patients travel long distances to cleft palate clinics. Parents often lose a day of work to make the visit. The care and adjustment of an orthopedic appliance may require more frequent visits, further increasing the burden of care.

We have not supported the opinion that primary bone grafting at an early age serves a useful purpose. The mobilization of soft tissue flaps to cover bone grafts creates scar tissue, which has a limiting effect on growth. We believe that secondary bone grafts are useful in all patients with unilateral and bilateral cleft lip and palate before or after eruption of the teeth in the line of cleft.

No consensus will be achieved without properly designed controlled research that allows for treatment outcomes assessment.

NASOALVEOLAR MOLDING (NAM) AT THE INSTITUTE OF RECONSTRUCTIVE PLASTIC SURGERY AT NEW YORK UNIVERSITY MEDICAL CENTER

Lawrence E. Brecht, DDS

It is important to note that there are a number of different variations of PSIO that have vastly different designs and efficacy. Perhaps the greatest disservice done to the debate on the advantages and disadvantages of PSIO in general, is to lump *all techniques* into one general category and then make equally generalized claims regarding *all* PSIO techniques. To read the literature on PSIO and think that claims or refutations may be applied across all techniques is simply erroneous. The Cleft Palate Service at the Institute of Reconstructive Plastic Surgery (IRPS) at New York University Medical Center (NYU) has successfully employed the *nasoalveolar molding (NAM)* variation of the PSIO technique for more than 15 years for over 400 infants. Multiple studies from our center objectively document our experiences with this form of PSIO and support the claim that it is a successful technique.

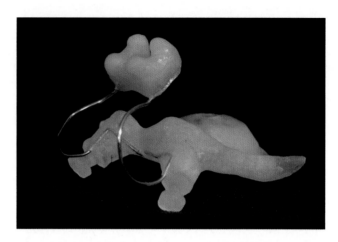

Figure 45–1. Bilateral nasoalveolar molding appliance consists of an acrylic oral molding appliance and two wire and acrylic nasal stents.

Nasoalveolar molding (NAM) consists of an alveolar oral molding appliance (i.e., Hotz plate, "passive" molding plate, Zurich appliance, etc.), with one nasal stent for unilateral clefts and two nasal stents when the cleft is bilateral (Fig. 45–1). To evaluate any positive and/or negative treatment effects of NAM, each component of the appliance should be considered separately. NAM differs significantly from other forms of PSIO in that nasal molding occurs independently of oral alveolar molding.

There is no biologic rationale to support the contention that nasal molding imparts any negative impact on alveolar molding. These two components (nasal and alveolar) will be examined separately. Additionally, the variable of gingivoperiosteoplasty (GPP) will be addressed.

The Alveolar Component of NAM

The intraoral portion of the nasoalveolar molding appliance consists of the standard presurgical orthopedic molding plate, in use for many decades throughout Europe and North America. We agree with Ross[51] and his carefully documented study which stated, "presurgical orthopedics in the neonatal period has no apparent long-term effect on facial growth in height and depth." By comparison, no such statement regarding the long-term effects of the Latham device has been made. Berkowitz has convincingly shown that the Latham apparatus followed by a Millard GPP *is* harmful to facial growth. There are no growth studies on Latham appliance therapy alone, *without* an associated gingivoperiosteoplasty.

An alveolar molding appliance is *not* the same as the Latham device. When we compare the two different presurgical orthopedic techniques, Latham and NAM, we see considerable differences between them. The intraoral portion of the NAM appliance is a simple molding plate, which has already been shown to have no effect on skeletal facial growth. Alveolar molding results in a much gentler retraction of the cleft premaxilla in BCLP or molding of the alveolar segments in UCLP. This retraction or molding is done slowly and gently over a period of 3–5 months. In contrast, rapid and forceful physical retraction of the premaxilla and repositioning of alveolar segments occur with the Latham appliance over a period of only several days. Here, the rate of physical movement and level of orthopedic force on the sutures of the nasal septum may have differing levels of impact on facial growth.

A number of cleft units, such as The Lancaster Cleft Palate Clinic, feel strongly that presurgical alveolar molding should never be performed, but these units often resort to the use of a lip adhesion surgery. Lip repair or lip adhesion is one of the most aggressive alveolar molding devices that may be employed. Within weeks of lip surgery, the gap between the alveolar segments may be dramatically narrowed. It is difficult to imagine how a gentle, guided alveolar approximation performed by a molding plate over a period of 4–6 months could be more detrimental than lip adhesion or repair. Alveolar molding and the resulting closure of the cleft gap have been blamed for eliminating the lateral incisor space. Our experience (as well as that of many other centers) has shown that this space is closed following the primary lip repair or lip adhesion. However, the manner in which it closes can be predictably controlled through alveolar molding. Such is not the case with lip repair alone without molding.

Most of us have come to believe that patients with clefts show varying amounts of inherent maxillary, dentoalveolar, and soft tissue deficiency. Following closure of the alveolar gap (by lip adhesion or oral molding plate therapy with or without a GPP), the maxillary alveolar arch circumference can be restored by performing orthodontic maxillary mid-palatal suture expansion (i.e., RPE) therapy. As many experienced orthodontists and pediatric dentists are aware, maxillary expansion is associated with the development of a diastema that forms between the maxillary central incisors, *not* between the lateral and canine incisors. The suture that responds to rapid palatal expansion and results in opening of space between the maxillary central incisors is not impacted by the carefully performed GPP (which occurs in the cleft site, between central and canine). Our team at NYU routinely achieves maxillary expansion with the expected expansion occurring at the suture, between the maxillary central incisors, not in the region of the cleft.

The Nasal Component of NAM

The Eurocleft and Dutchcleft studies have shown that presurgical infant orthopedics with alveolar molding plates has no positive or negative effect on feeding, speech, facial growth, or occlusion. As a result, many cleft centers abandoned presurgical infant orthopedics. Although the intraoral portion of the NAM device is consistent with that used in the European studies, the similarities stop there. The treatment goals of NAM therapy are markedly different to those goals set out in the above-referenced studies, and therefore NAM needs to be evaluated by distinctly different criteria. The treatment goals of NAM include presurgical molding of the nasal cartilages, elongation of the nasal mucosal lining, and an increase in length of columella, all leading to observable improvements in the esthetic outcome of the one-stage primary lip and nasal repair (Fig. 45–2).

Those opposed to NAM point out that long-term data has not shown the benefits of the technique. Our cleft unit at The Institute of Reconstructive Plastic Surgery at NYU has consistently studied our NAM patient population in an

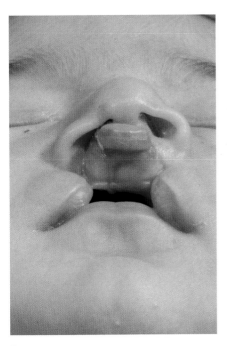
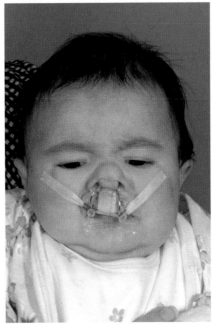
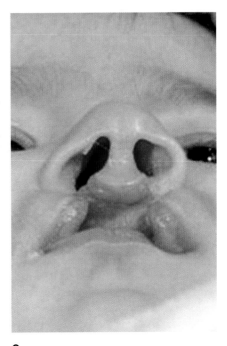

A   B   C

Figure 45–2. (a) Bilateral cleft lip, alveolus and palate prior to NAM treatment. (b) Infant with bilateral NAM appliance in place. (c) Bilateral cleft lip, alveolus, and palate following several weeks of NAM appliance therapy demonstrating retraction of premaxilla, nonsurgical columella elongation, nasal dome elevation and more normalized nasal anatomy.

attempt to objectively assess the technique and its long-term benefits and drawbacks. These published studies support the positive esthetic nasal benefits of NAM up to the age of 6 years.

Presurgical columellar lengthening in the bilateral cleft cannot be achieved without NAM (or surgery). Another major (and unique) advantage to NAM is its ability to stretch the nasal lining. This minimizes the need for lateral or columellar incisions during surgery and allows the nasal domes to be brought up and into correct approximation without tension. Stretching of the nasal mucosal lining is every bit as important as the presurgical lengthening of the columellar skin. No prior method of PSIO addressed these issues and, as a result, these treatment goals were never even considered for evaluation in any study in the cleft literature prior to 1995.

We believe that the proper repositioning of the lower lateral cartilages through NAM, followed by modified surgery, will result in more ideal nasal growth over time, diminishing the need for surgical revisions. The reduced need for nasal revision surgery has been clearly documented in our unit.[46]

Evaluation of GPP

It is important to note that NAM can be performed without a GPP, still affording the patient the nasal esthetic benefits of this technique. However, at NYU-IRPS, we usually choose to perform GPP when successful alveolar alignment is achieved. The close (1 mm) approximation of cleft segments necessitates only minimal undermining of the periosteum proximate to the cleft gap in order to be able to perform the GPP. The GPP is a technique-sensitive procedure that has been shown to negatively impact maxillary growth, but only when more extensive undermining of the surrounding periosteum is necessitated by having widely spaced alveolar segments that have not been brought into approximation through NAM or some other form of PSIO.[32]

To consider the impact of our very conservative Millard Cutting type GPP on maxillary growth, we compared a group of our earliest treated patients with complete unilateral cleft lip and palate that received presurgical infant orthopedics (alveolar oral molding or pin-retained appliances) alone to a group receiving PSIO plus a GPP. We found no significant differences between the horizontal or vertical position of the maxilla between these two groups at an average age of 18 years. Both groups were treated by the same orthodontist and surgeon.[43,52] Whereas both the treatment groups showed the expected shift of the bell curve in the direction of midface hypoplasia, GPP as an isolated variable did *not* show a negative effect on growth of the midface.

Patients with UCLP enjoy at least a 60–80% success rate with GPP.[42] Even if a secondary alveolar bone graft becomes necessary later in life following primary GPP, our research has shown that this subsequent bone graft is clinically more successful.[53] Most patients with bilateral clefts treated with GPP will still require secondary alveolar bone grafting (60% of patients with bilateral clefts needed bone grafts in our series). If a GPP is performed on at least one side, however, major orthodontic advantages ensue. Stabilizing the other-

wise mobile premaxilla enables the child to use his/her incisor teeth during mastication. This functional loading of the premaxilla serves to maintain its bone mass rather than having the bone thin out to its usual atrophic dimension. Also, once the premaxilla has an osseous connection to one of the lateral alveolar segments, the premaxilla will not descend vertically, eliminating the need for a subsequent premaxillary repositioning procedure.

Although patients with bilateral clefts treated without PSIO, NAM, or GPP may have good anterior projection of their premaxilla on lateral cephalograms, they often have large fistulae located immediately behind the premaxilla, effecting speech and resulting in chronic nasal inflammation of the nasal mucosa. In addition, such patients often have difficulty controlling the passage of food and liquids from the oral cavity into the nose. The large size of these palatal defects may require either segmental LeFort I osteotomies to achieve adequate soft tissue closure or the long-term use of a removable prosthesis to obturate the oronasal fistula. The combined treatment effect of alveolar molding and GPP has all but eliminated the occurrence of these fistulae. It should also be noted that the treatment of infants with unilateral clefts with nasoalveolar molding and GPP has resulted in a significant cost savings when compared to that without NAM and with secondary alveolar bone grafting later in childhood.[50]

We agree with Dr. Mazaheri and the Lancaster Cleft Palate Team that the skill of the surgeon has a great deal of influence on the quality of the cleft repair result. We propose, however, that NAM improves the anatomic relationships of both the alveolar segments and the nasal structures prior to surgery, thus necessitating less radical and more atraumatic surgery. It is imperative that the surgeon learn a modified surgical approach to optimize the foundational anatomic relationships provided to the surgeon through NAM. Often, less than optimal results are seen even after NAM when the surgeon has failed to change his/her technique to take into consideration the changes in underlying structures provided by NAM.

There have been many sincere attempts to study and explain the advantages and disadvantages of various cleft treatment protocols. Endless contradictions and confusion have prevailed in the published literature, largely due to poor study design and to lack of agreement on the definition of both common terminology and the ultimate treatment goals. It is only through continued effort to better articulate and understand one another's research and clinical outcomes that we will be in a position to offer our patients care that more fully meets their needs while optimizing outcomes and minimizing the total number of surgical procedures required to complete their care.

Summary

1. When considering the efficacy of the NAM variation of PSIO, it is imperative to be aware that all forms of PSIO are not the same.

2. The nasal and alveolar molding components of NAM can be considered separately.

3. Alveolar molding has been shown to have no impact on maxillary growth.

4. Bilateral NAM provides early correction of the cleft nasal deformity, provides nonsurgical elongation of columellar tissues, and increases the surface area of nasal mucosal lining, all of which enables the surgeon to achieve a better primary nasal repair with no scar at the lip–columella junction.

5. The lateral incisor space is always lost, either through the uncontrolled forces resulting from lip repair or through the gentle controlled forces of alveolar molding.

6. A conservative GPP does not negatively impact the growth of the maxilla when used in combination with gentle alveolar molding.

7. Clinical research from multiple cleft centers demonstrates the positive treatment effects of NAM on nasal form, at least up to the age of 6 years.

8. Surgeons must alter the surgical technique utilized in the cleft repair to optimize the advantages provided by NAM.

References

1. McNeil CK. Orthodontic procedures in the treatment of congenital cleft palate. *Dental Record* 70:126–132, 1950.
2. McNeil CK. *Oral and Facial Deformity.* London: Sir Isaac Pitman and Sons, 1954.
3. McNeil CK. Congenital oral deformities. *Brit Dent J* 101:191–198, 1956.
4. Jones JE. Cleft orthotics and obturation. *Oral Maxillofac Surg Clin North Am* 3:517–529, 1991.
5. Huddart AG. Presurgical dental orthopedics. *Trans BR Soc Orthod* 107–117, 1961.
6. Huddart AG. Treatment procedures in cleft lip and palate cases. *Brit Dent J* 122:185–192, 1970.
7. Huddart AG. An analysis of the maxillary changes following presurgical dental orthopedic treatment in unilateral cleft lip and palate cases. In *European Orthodontic Society Report of Congress,* 1967, pp. 299–314.
8. Hotz MM. Pre- and early post-operative growth guidance in cleft lip and palate cases by maxillary orthopedics (an alternative procedure to primary bone grafting). *Cleft Palate J* 6:368–372, 1969.
9. Brauer RO, Cronin TD, Reaves EL. Early maxillary orthopedics, orthodontia and alveolar bone grafting in complete clefts of the palate. *Plast Reconstr Surg* 29:625–641, 1962.
10. Georigade N, Pickrell K, and Quinn G. Varying concepts in bone grafting of alveolar palatal defects. *Cleft Palate J* 1:43–51, 1964.
11. Latham RA. Orthopedic advancement of the cleft maxillary segment: A preliminary report. *Cleft Palate J* 17:227, 1980.
12. Burston WR. The pre-surgical orthopaedic correction of the maxillary deformity in clefts of both primary and secondary palate. In Wallace AB (ed.). *Transactions of the International Society of Plastic Surgeons,* Second Congress, London, 1959. Edinburgh and London: E&S Livingston Ltd, 1960, pp. 28–36.
13. Burston WR. The early orthodontic treatment of alveolar clefts. *Proc R Soc Med* 58:676–771, 1965.
14. Burston WR. Treatment of the cleft palate. *Ann R Coll Surg Engl* 25:225, 1967.
15. Rosenstein SW. A new concept in the early orthopedic treatment of cleft lip and palate. *Am J Orthod* 55:765–775, 1969.
16. Millard DR Jr, Latham R, Huifen X, Spiro S, Morovic C. Cleft lip and palate treated by presurgical orthopedics, gingivoperioplasty, and lip adhesion (POPLA) compared with previous lip adhesion method: A preliminary study of serial dental casts. *Plast Reconstr Surg* 103:1630–1644, 1999.
17. Pruzansky S. Factors determining arch form in clefts of the lip and palate. *Am J Orthod* 41:827–851, 1955.
18. Pruzansky S. Presurgical orthopedics and bone grafting for infants with cleft lip and palate: A dissent. *Cleft Palate J* 1:164–187, 1964.
19. Fletcher S, Berkowitz S, Bradley DP, Burdi AR, Koch L, Mave-Dickson W. Cleft lip and palate research: An updated state of the art. *Cleft Palate J* 14:261–321, 1977.
20. Mishima K, Sugahara T, Mori Y, Sakuda M. Comparison of palatal forms in complete unilateral lip and palate infants with and without a Hotz plate. In Lee ST, Huang M (eds). *Transactions of the 8th International Congress on Cleft Palate and Related Craniofacial Anomalies.* Singapore: Stamford Press, 1997, pp. 394–397.
21. Mishima K, Sugahara T, Mori Y, Sakuda M. Three-dimensional comparison between the palatal forms in infants with complete unilateral cleft lip, alveolus, and palate with and without Hotz' plaste. *Cleft Palate Craniofac J* 33:312–317, 1996.
22. Rosenstein SW, Jacobson BN. Early maxillary orthopedics: A sequence of events. *Cleft Palate J* 4:197–204, 1967.
23. Kujipers-Jagtman AM, Prahl C. A study into the effects of presurgical orthopedic treatment in complete unilateral cleft lip and palate patients. A three-center prospective clinical trial in Nijmegen, Amsterdam and Rotterdam. Interim analysis. Nijmegen: University Press, 1996.
24. Kujipers-Jagtman AM, Long RE. The influence of surgery and orthopedic treatment on maxillofacial growth and maxillary arch development in patients treated for orofacial clefts. *Cleft Palate Craniofac J* 37:527, 2000.
25. Prahl C, Kujipers-Jagtman AM, Prahl-Anderson B. Effect of presurgical infant orthopedics on maxillary arch dimensions. In Lee ST, Huang M (eds). *Transactions 8th International Congress on Cleft Palate and Related Craniofacial Anomalies.* Singapore: Stamford Press, 1997, p. 1026.
26. Prahl C, Kuijpers-Jagtman AM, van't Hof MA, Prahl-Anderson B. A randomized prospective clinical trial of infant orthopedics in unilateral cleft lip and palate: Prevention of collapse of the alveolar segments (Dutchcleft). *Cleft Palate Craniofac J* 40:337–342, 2003.
27. Pickrell K, Quinn G, Massengill R. Primary bone grafting of the maxilla in clefts of the lip and palate: A four year study. *Plast Reconstr Surg* 41:438–443, 1968.
28. Weil J. Orthopedic growth guidance and stimulation for patients with cleft lip and palate. *Scand J Plast Reconstr Surg* 21:57–63, 1987.
29. Pruzansky S, Aduss H. Prevalence of arch collapse and malocclusion in complete unilateral cleft lip and palate. *Eur Orth Society Report of Congress,* 1967, pp. 365–382.
30. Bishara SB. Effects of palatoplasty and cleft palate on facial and dental relations. *Int J Oral Surg* 3:65–70, 1974.
31. Berkowitz S. Section III: Orofacial growth and dentistry: A state of the art report on neonatal maxillary orthopedics. *Cleft Palate J* 14:288–301, 1977.
32. Skoog T. The use of periosteal flaps in the repair of clefts of the primary palate. *Cleft Palate J* 2:332–339, 1965.
33. Mazaheri M, Harding RL, Nanda S. The effect of surgery on maxillary growth and cleft width. *Plast Reconstr Surg* 40:22–30, 1967.
34. Mazaheri M, Sahni PP. Techniques of cephalometry, photography, and oral impressions for infants. *J Prosthet Dent* 21:315–323, 1969.
35. Mazaheri M, Krogman WM, Harding RL, Millard RT, Mehta S. Longitudinal analysis of growth of the soft palate and nasopharynx from six months to six years. *Cleft Palate J* 14:52–62, 1977.
36. Mazaheri M, Harding RL, Cooper JA, Meier JA. Changes in arch form and dimensions of cleft patients. *Am J Orthod* 60:19–32, 1971.
37. Mazaheri M, Nanda S, Sassouni V. Comparison of midfacial development of children with clefts with their siblings. *Cleft Palate J* 4:334–341, 1967.
38. Jolleys A, Robertson NRE. A study of the effects of early bone grafting in compete clefts of the lip and palate—five-year study. *Br J Plast Surg* 25:229–237, 1972.
39. Robertson NRE. Recent trends in the early treatment of cleft lip and palate. *Dent Pract Dent Rec* 21:326–338, 1971.

40. Kernahan DA, Rosenstein SW (eds). *Cleft Lip and Palate: A System of Management.* Baltimore, MD: Williams and Wilkins, 1990.

41. Delaire J. Premiers resultants de la gingivo-peristo-plastie primaire (avac ou sans osteoplastie). In II trattamento chirurgico ed ortodontico della labio—palatoschisi. Liricostruzione dell'equilibrio funzionale. Vol. II. Milan ACPS Magnta, 1989, p. 121.

42. Santiago PE, Grayson BH, Gianoutsis ME, Brecht LE, Kwon SM, Cutting CB. Reduced need for alveolar bone grafting by presurgical orthopedics and primary gingivoperioplasty. *Cleft Palate Craniofac J* 35:77–81, 1998.

43. Wood RJ, Grayson BH, Cutting CB. Gingivoperioplasty and midfacial growth. *Cleft Palate Craniofac J* 34:17–20, 1997.

44. Winters JC, Hurwitz DJ. Presurgical orthopedics in the surgical management of unilateral cleft lip and palate. *Plast Reconstr Surg* 95:755–764, 1995.

45. Grayson BH, Santiago PE, Brecht LE, Cutting CB. Presurgical nasoalveolar molding in infants with cleft lip and palate. *Cleft Palate Craniofac* 36:486–498, 1999.

46. Maull DJ, Grayson BH, Cutting CB, et al. Long-term effects of nasoalveolar molding on three-dimensional nasal shape in unilateral clefts. *Cleft Palate Craniofac J* 36:391–397, 1999.

47. Cutting CB, Grayson BH, Brecht LE, Santiago PE, Wood R, Kwon SM. Presurgical columellar elongation and retrograde nasal reconstruction in one-stage bilateral cleft lip and nose repair. *Plast Reconstr Surg* 101:630–639, 1998.

48. Da Silveira AC, Oliveira N, Gonzalez S, et al. Modified nasal alveolar molding appliance for management of cleft lip defect. *J Craniofac Surg* 14:700–703, 2003.

49. Liou EJ, Subramanian M, Chen PK. Progressive changes of columella length and nasal growth after nasoalveolar molding in bilateral cleft patients: A 3-year follow-up study. *Plast Reconstr Surg* 119:642–648, 2007.

50. Pfeifer TM, Grayson BH, Cutting CB. Nasoalveolar molding and gingivoperiosteoplasty versus alveolar bone graft: An outcome analysis of costs in the treatment of unilateral cleft alveolus. *Cleft Palate Craniofac J* 39:26–29, 2002.

51. Ross RB. Treatment variables affecting facial growth in complete unilateral cleft lip and palate. Part 1: Treatment affecting growth. *Cleft Palate J* 24:5–23, 1987.

52. Garfinkle J, Grayson BH, Brecht LE, Cutting CB. Long-term effect of midface growth of gingivoperiosteoplasty with presurgical infant orthopedics in unilateral cleft lip and palate. American Cleft Palate-Craniofac Assn, 63rd Annual Scientific Session, April 2006.

53. Sato Y, Grayson BH, Garfinkle J, Barillas I, Cutting CB. The success rate of gingivoperiosteoplasty with and without secondary bone grafts, compared to secondary alveolar bone grafts alone. *Plast Reconstr Surg* 2008 (in press).

46

Nasoalveolar Molding and Columella Elongation in Preparation for the Primary Repair of Unilateral and Bilateral Cleft Lip and Palate

Barry H. Grayson, DDS • Judah S. Garfinkle, DMD, MS

INTRODUCTION

The focus of this chapter is primarily on the role of the or-thodontist (or other dental professional) during the presur-gical management of an infant born with clefts of the lip, alveolus, and palate. This chapter will begin with a general description of clefting and its early clinical management so as to provide a foundation for the presurgical orthopedic treat-ment intervention. A historical perspective on presurgical in-fant orthopedics (PSIO) will be offered that introduces the rationale for nasoalveolar molding (NAM). The remainder of the chapter will focus on the specific clinical procedures, com-plications, and benefits of NAM. An evidence based approach will be offered whenever possible.

While every member of the interdisciplinary cleft palate team has a specialized role, the team functions best when each clinician becomes an informed novice in the other team members' specialties. By the conclusion of this chapter, it is our desire that the theory and technique of NAM have been adequately explained so that each team member could better integrate this component into their overall understanding of the management of patients with clefts.

BACKGROUND

Demographics

Clefts of the lip, alveolus, and palate represent a group of the most common congenital anomalies of the craniofacial skele-ton. The incidence ranges from approximately one in 500 to one in 1000 births depending on the specific condition as well as on racial and ethnic circumstances. Although the physi-cal impact of a cleft appears well localized, there are many seemingly different (but ultimately connected) anatomical systems affected. To satisfactorily address the constellation of treatment issues, the expertise and care of an interdisciplinary cleft palate team is required. In this way, the most favorable treatment sequence can be developed and implemented for each individual patient based both on their specific physical and psychosocial needs and their respective stage of growth and development. The treatment for a patient with an orofa-cial cleft often spans the first two decades of life and involves intervention by every member of the cleft team.

Etiology

Although the phenotypic aberration resulting in cleft lip and palate has been well characterized, the ultimate cause is still being investigated. Currently, both genetic and environmen-tal factors have been implicated in the etiology of clefting disorders. In regards to the physical disturbance to normal growth and development, cleft lip results when the medial nasal and maxillary processes fail to fuse during the fifth week of embryonic development. Between the eighth and 12th week of fetal development, failure of the right and left palatal processes to assume the proper horizontal orientation

and fuse results in the palatal defect. Even though all cleft anomalies are a product of similar alterations to normal fetal development, there is great variability in clinical presentation.

Presentation of the Cleft Deformity

A cleft lip can range from a slight soft tissue notch to a pro-found absence of both hard and soft tissue involving the lip, alveolus and anterior maxilla. Clefting of the palate can in-clude the hard palate, the soft palate, and/or the uvula. The further anterior the palatal clefting begins, the more struc-tures will be involved. Both lip and palatal clefts will occur to a variable extent on one (unilateral) or both sides (bilateral).

The clinical hallmark of unilateral cleft lip and palate (UCLP) includes not only clefting of the upper lip and alve-olus, but a distorted nasal form as well. Absence of the tissue at the base of the nose that normally tethers the medial and lateral aspects of the nostril aperture together results in a widened and flattened nostril. The tip of the nose loses its sagittal projection and the columella deviates to the noncleft side with the greater lip and alveolar segments. The medial as-pect of the greater alveolar segment is often displaced slightly superiorly. The nasal septum deviates to the noncleft side (Fig. 46–1A, B, and C).

Complete bilateral cleft lip and palate (BCLP) is char-acterized by some amount of dorsi-flexion or rotation of the premaxillary segment, which is tethered to the tip of the nose, absent of any distinguishable columella. The nose is deficient in sagittal projection and widened due to the connection of the lateral aspects of the nasal cartilages to the remaining lat-eral lip segments. There is a prolabial tissue patch, attached to the tip of the nose, which often appears reduced in overall volume (Fig. 46–2A, B, C, D, and E).

OBJECTIVES OF PSIO

Lip, Nose, and Alveolus

The ultimate treatment goal in the management of clefting disorders is to restore both normal function and esthetics. A challenging component in the esthetic repair of UCLP is in recreating normal lip and nasal anatomy. Proper approx-imation of the vermillion border and reconstruction of the philtral column, without the formation of excessive scar tis-sue, is the primary objective for lip reconstruction. Obtaining greater sagittal projection and symmetric nasal anatomy, both in size and shape of the nasal apertures, are the primary objec-tives for the nose. Due to the symmetry inherent in the BCLP anomaly, attainment of a symmetric lip and nose repair is common. The challenge in BCLP is obtaining normal nasal anatomical relationships, specifically an esthetic columella, adequate nasal tip projection, and appropriate narrowing of the nasal tip and base. An additional objective of NAM is the presurgical alignment of the alveolar segments, including the premaxilla in BLCP. This often enables closer approximation of the overlying soft tissues, as well as the performance of

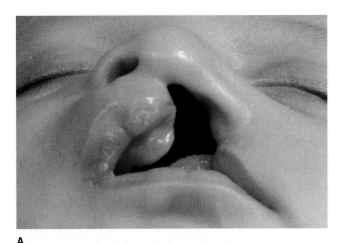

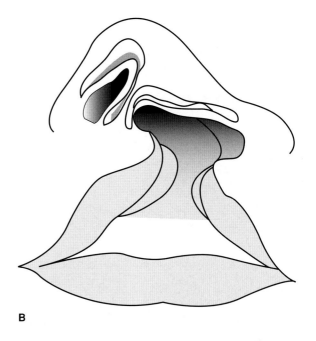

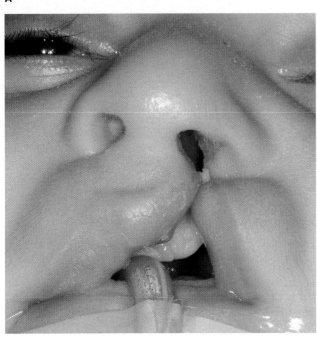

Figure 46–1. A: Initial presentation of patient with complete UCLP. **B:** Diagram illustrating deformity of complete UCLP. Note absence of the tissue at the base of the nose that normally tethers the medial and lateral aspects of the nostril aperture together results in a widened and flattened nostril. The tip of the nose loses its sagittal projection and the columella deviates to the noncleft side with the greater lip and alveolar segments. The lower lateral alar cartilage on the cleft side drops down at the nostril apex and often takes on a concave form. The medial aspect of the greater alveolar segment is often displaced slightly superiorly. The nasal septum deviates to the noncleft side. **C:** Patient with UCLP following NAM treatment. Note the increase in nasal tip projection and columella length on the cleft side. Improved nasal symmetry and approximation of the lip segments at rest has been achieved. In addition, the alveolar cleft gap has been closed with the alveolar segments in passive contact. The increased surface area (following NAM therapy) of nasal mucosal lining, facilitates surgical repositioning and retention of the nasal tip cartilage.

a gingivoperiosteoplasty (GPP) with minimal tissue undermining.

Reducing the Severity of the Deformity Prior to Surgery

The desired outcome for the lip and nose are more accessible from a surgical perspective when the initial deformity is mild rather than severe. In the mild deformity, the wounds heal under less tension, there is less tissue deficiency, and the anatomical foundation underlying the cleft more closely resembles the structures in normal configuration. While variability in clinical presentation of clefting often results in some mild cases, most are of a moderate to severe nature. Clinicians have been grappling with cleft severity for hundreds of years, and have come up with some creative attempts to reduce the severity of deformity prior to the primary surgical repair.

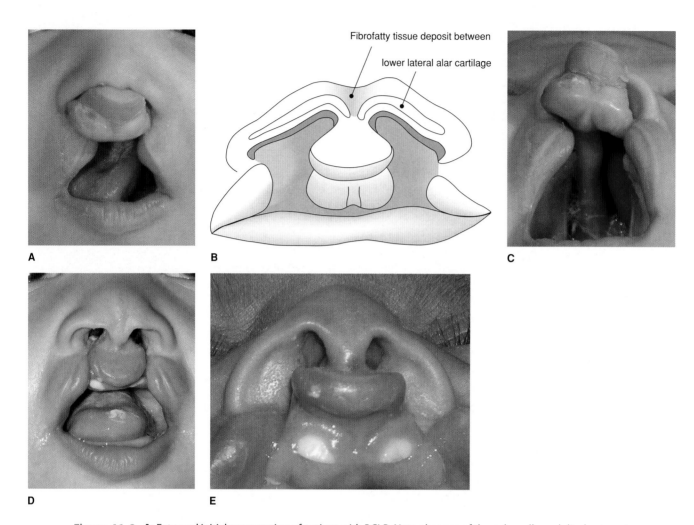

Figure 46–2. A: Extraoral initial presentation of patient with BCLP. Note absence of the columella and displacement of premaxilla and prolabium. **B:** Diagram illustrating bilateral anatomical deformity, specifically showing displacement of lower lateral alar cartilage and subsequent deposition of fibrofatty tissue between the nasal tip cartilage. In addition, it demonstrates deficiency of the columella and displacement of the premaxilla. **C:** Intraoral initial presentation of patient with BCLP. Note extraoral position of the rotated premaxilla and prolabium, discontinuity of the lip and alveolar segments, and complete bilateral palatal clefts. **D:** Patient with BCLP following NAM therapy and nonsurgical columella elongation. Note the change in columella length, repositioning of the premaxilla, and approximation of the lip segments at rest. **E:** Patient with BCLP following NAM therapy. Note the increased length of the columella, reduction in width of the nasal tip, and increased nasal tip projection.

■ HISTORICAL PERSPECTIVE ON PSIO

Inherent in the term "presurgical infant orthopedics" is the concept of altering the position and/or the shape of the cleft maxillary alveolar ridges prior to surgery. While the alveolar segments were the primary target of such treatment, the overlying soft tissues were affected by treatment as well, resulting in closer proximity of the lip segments and to a lesser extent, the base of the nose.

Evolution of PSIO

Generating the necessary force system for efficient PSIO presented a biomechanical challenge. Originally, force was generated from an extraoral appliance system. In the late 17th century, Hoffman described the use of an appliance to retract

the premaxilla, which was anchored to a head cap. Since then, various advancements have been made to extraoral anchorage devices, some of which are still used today, primarily in bilateral cleft cases. In the 1950s, McNeil described an intraoral molding plate[1] to achieve, "Preoperative reduction of the width of the palate cleft by nonsurgical means".[2] Obtaining adequate retention and generating the desired force system proved challenging. In 1975, Georgiade and Latham proposed the use of a pin-retained intraoral appliance to achieve presurgical maxillary arch alignment in patients with bilateral clefts.[3] This device promised to offer three-dimensional control. A few years later, Latham introduced a pin-retained appliance to align the alveolar segments in patients with unilateral clefts as well.[4] The pin-retained appliance has gained much attention and is still in use today, although there are as many opponents as proponents. During this time Hotz continued his work with "passive" molding plates, referred to as the Zurich appliance, and reported successful treatment outcomes.[5–7] For the last 20 years, most of the above techniques, with some modifications, are still being used in cleft centers all over the world. In addition to the devices described above, the use of a lip adhesion surgery[8] and lip taping[9] have been shown to reliably produce orthopedic movement of the alveolar segments and are currently advocated at some cleft centers.

All of the above PSIO techniques that span the last 300 years share at least one thing in common. The collective element is that the desired effect was ultimately a better treatment outcome for patients with cleft lip and palate. Had the first attempt achieved this goal, it is likely that no others would have followed.

Controversy of PSIO

Multiple PSIO strategies have been proposed over the years, because no one solution has proved completely satisfactory. Part of the difficulty in establishing consensus is due to inconsistency in clinical terminology (e.g., active versus passive appliances) and in the definition of clinical success itself. Further, clinical research in cleft lip and palate is challenging due to the multiple treatment interventions and variables that need to be accounted for over a long period of time. Another variable, often unaccounted for in setting up research populations, is the variation in severity of the cleft tissue deficiency among patients. Thus, patients with severe tissue deficiency may not be expected to respond to a given treatment protocol in the same way as a patient with a minimal amount of tissue deficiency.

Various assertions have been offered regarding the potential benefits of PSIO. These claims range from improved speech and feeding, to optimized dental relationships, and overall facial esthetics.

As a consequence of the above challenges, both the type and application of PSIO remains controversial. The only way to traverse the confusion is to identify the clinical variables in cleft palate patients, and clearly define the parameters for treatment success. In this way, the outcome studies regarding PSIO will be more meaningful. Furthermore, once the clinical variables and definitions of success are agreed upon, scientific discourse will be greatly facilitated. Although it is generally a positive thing that clinicians and investigators, in the field of cleft lip and palate treatment, are charged with emotion and passion, at times, this blurs the lines between beliefs and science.

Take, for example, the Dutchcleft studies that have produced a wealth of information about PSIO in UCLP, in regards to maxillary arch form,[10] speech,[11–13] deciduous dental relationships,[14] and nutritional status.[15] Consider that the focus of these reports failed to address outcomes in terms of nasal esthetics or the frequency and type of secondary surgical procedures. For those patients who underwent PSIO, the resulting cleft gap distance present at lip closure, or the performance of GPP, was not mentioned. Other significant clinical variables were not accounted for, such as, the specific type of molding plate adjustments, or the severity of the tissue deficiency within the study population.

This analysis is not being offered has a rebuke of the Dutchcleft study, just the opposite; the study is a model for cleft research and has been very well received. The hazard lies in careless interpretation of the data. The Dutchcleft studies concluded that PSIO did not have a significant impact on maxillary arch form, speech, nutritional status, and deciduous dental status. Many wrongly interpret these results to mean that the entire concept of PSIO should be abandoned. Alternatively, if these studies had measured and reported treatment outcomes such as nasal and labial esthetics, or the number of secondary lip, nose and fistula repairs, then PSIO may have been viewed as an efficacious treatment modality. As is so often the case in cleft research, the truth is rarely obtained, but only gradually approximated with time. The scientific and professional debate on many of these issues will continue until we more precisely define the variables inherent in this heterogeneous patient population, and define the variables of successful treatment.

Neonatal Tissue Plasticity

Although it had been well appreciated that the esthetic restoration of the cleft nose deformity was one of the greatest surgical challenges, limited clinical attention had been directed to address this problem presurgically. Drawing on their experience and success with malformed auricular cartilage molding, Matuso et al.[16] in 1988 described a technique for molding the nasal cartilage following initial lip repair at approximately one week of age through insertion of a custom made nasal stent. The stent was to remain in the nose for 3 months. This technique depended on the surgical construction of a nasal floor for retention of the nasal stent. The proposed biologic foundation enabling effective molding of the nasal cartilage (and auricular cartilage) was the elevated level of maternal estrogen in the newborn infant resulting in an increased level of circulating hyaluronic acid that ensures cartilaginous plasticity. In 1991, Matsuo et al.[17] demonstrated a technique of presurgically molding nasal cartilage in cleft patients that had a Simonart's band present which served as the nasal floor necessary for stent retention. While the work by Matsuo et al.[17] finally addressed the nasal deformity presurgically, there were many drawbacks. The technique could only be used on unilateral cleft cases with Simonart's bands; and, the alveolar defect, which is primarily responsible for the overlying soft tissue asymmetry, was not addressed. The treatment challenge to incorporate both nasal cartilage and alveolar segment molding in unilateral and bilateral cleft cases remained unsolved.

A Novel Approach to PSIO

In 1993, Grayson et al.[18] described a technique of PSIO that not only addressed the alveolar and lip segment approximation prior to surgery, but established specific presurgical

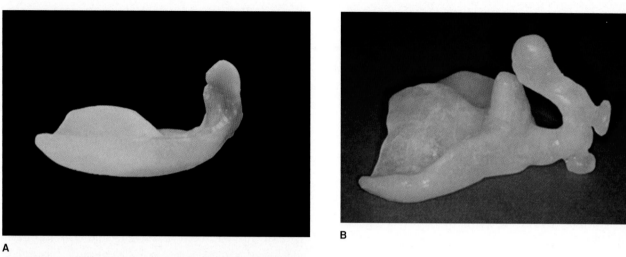

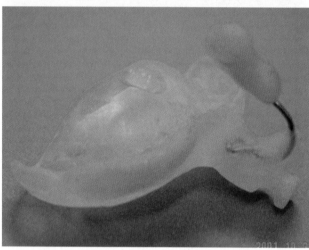

Figure 46–3. Evolution of the unilateral NAM appliance. **A:** Initial NAM appliance that was retained by palatal undercuts and tissue adhesive. Note absence of retention button. The intranasal portion lacked the bilobed form which is currently in use. **B:** Note addition of retention buttons to acrylic nasal stent that entered the nose from an extraoral approach. **C:** Current version of the NAM appliance. Note the nasal stent is fabricated out of wire and acrylic, only one retention button is utilized, there is a hole in the middle of the palatal acrylic, and the intranasal portion of the nasal stent is bilobed.

treatment goals regarding correction of the nasal cartilage asymmetry and increasing the length of the deficient or usually absent columella. The treatment modality was refined and illustrated further by Grayson et al. in 1999[19] and 2001[20] and termed NAM (Figs. 46–3A, B, and C and 46–4A, B, and C) As discussed above, the plausibility and rationale for this treatment approach was borne out of the work of Matsuo et al. involving infant auricular and nasal cartilage plasticity, as well as an appreciation of the principles underlying tissue expansion, and the previous PSIO strategies.

Over the past 15 years, the technique of NAM has been widely accepted around the world. Many investigators have published their clinical experiences and various treatment modifications[21–27] Although some controversy remains surrounding the long-term benefits versus costs of NAM (and PSIO in general), the discussion is a healthy one, allowing clinicians and families to more specifically de-

fine treatment outcome, based on their particular treatment goals.

TREATMENT OBJECTIVES OF NAM

NAM is focused on reducing the severity of the cleft deformity prior to surgery. This process includes reduction in the size of the alveolar gap, the lip gap, and the distance between the medial and lateral aspects of the alar cartilages, as well as increasing nasal tip projection, and obtaining symmetry and definition of the nasal cartilages and nasal apertures. Presurgical elongation of the columella is a treatment goal specific to bilateral cleft cases. If these presurgical goals are achieved, then the esthetic and functional outcome of the primary lip and nose repair should be enhanced. Realizing also, that the hallmark of these clefting disorders is some degree of tissue

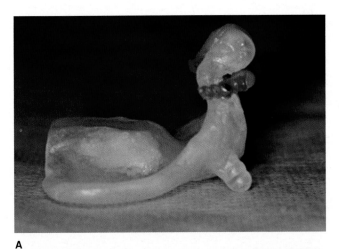

A

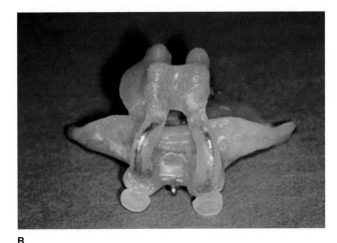

B

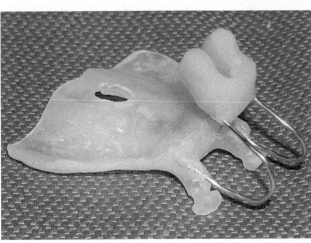

C

Figure 46–4. Evolution of the bilateral NAM appliance. **A:** Initial BCLP NAM appliance. Note that the intranasal portion of the nasal stent is not bilobed. The armature of the nasal stent is made of acrylic. The horizontal columella band is fabricated on an elastic chain and secured with steel buttons. **B:** Transitional period when the horizontal columella band was fabricated with acrylic and the nasal stent armature was being fabricated out of wire. **C:** Current version of the BCLP NAM appliance. Note the nasal stent armature is fabricated out of wire and the intranasal portion of the nasal stent is bilobed. There is a hole in the middle of the palatal acrylic.

deficiency, the more that the missing tissues are replaced with the patients own tissues, the better. A further discussion of the definition of success with NAM is discussed in the Section "Benefits of NAM" below.

The Nose

The NAM appliance consists of an intraoral molding plate and a nasal stent. The nasal stent serves to increase nasal tip projection, establish proper curvature of the alar cartilage through molding, and to increase the internal surface area of the nasal mucosal lining through tissue expansion. An attempt is made to overcorrect the anterior projection of the nasal tip in anticipation of some degree of relapse associated with postsurgical scar contracture. The apex of the nasal aperture in UCLP, on the affected side of the nose, is adjusted to a similar position as the unaffected side. In unilateral cases, approximation of the alveolar ridges and lip segments facilitates up righting of the tipped columella. To aid in this process, the cleft lip segments are taped together, simulating a surgical lip adhesion. An additional benefit to nasal stenting is the increased nasal airflow through the cleft nostril, reported by many parents.

The Columella

The vast majority of bilateral cleft patients are born with no columella. Instead, the displaced prolabium, and premaxilla, emerges directly from the tip of the nose. The traditional surgical procedures used to create a functional columella result in a scarred and tethered nose with limited anterior or superior projection of the nasal tip.[28] Long term, this results in an acute nasolabial angle and a broad and retrusive nasal tip. The surgically-constructed columella is also unusually wide with noticeable scarring. Utilization of the bilateral nasal stents of the NAM appliance, as well as a combination of taping techniques, provide for nonsurgical columella elongation prior to primary lip and nose surgery. This process results in improved nasal esthetics, including a scar-free columella,

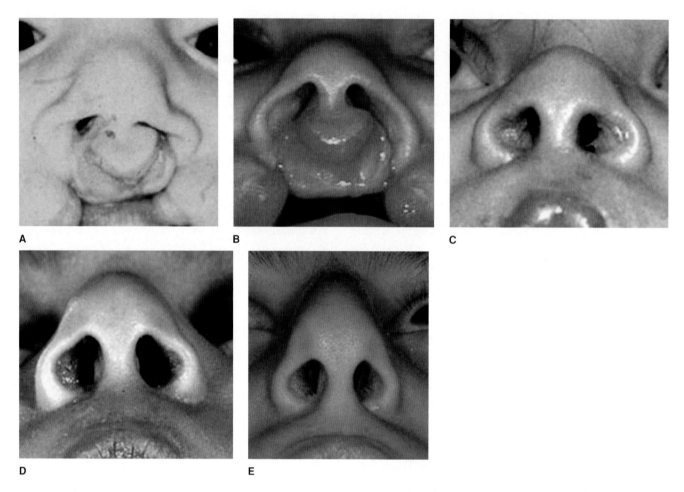

Figure 46–5. Long term follow up nasal morphology, including columella length and nasal tip projection, following NAM treatment of this patient with BCLP **A:** Initial presentation at 2 weeks of age, prior to NAM therapy. **B:** At 1.5 months of age during NAM therapy. **C:** At 2 years of age. **D:** At 10 years of age. **E:** At 12 years of age. No labial or nasal revisions were performed.

enhanced nasal tip projection, and narrowing of the alar base, which has long term benefits for nasal growth and development (Fig. 46–5A, B, C, D, and E).

The Lips

The relationship of the lip segments, and the medial and lateral aspects of the alar base, improve as the alveolar segments come into alignment. The objective is to have nearly passive contact of the lip segments and improved nasal symmetry prior to the primary surgical repair of the lip and nose (Figs. 46–1C and D and 46–2D and E). In this way, the surgeon is able to approximate the soft tissues with less tension and more precision, resulting in a superior esthetic outcome. In support of this surgical maxim regarding the benefits of reducing the tension in healing surgical wounds, Burgess et al.[29] illustrated that tissues healing under less tension produce narrower scars.

Gingivoperiosteoplasty

If the alveolar gap distance is reduced to less than 1 mm, a Millard-type GPP can be performed at initial lip closure.

There are many advantages to this type of GPP, which will be discussed in more detail in the Section "Benefits of NAM" below.

The Premaxilla

An additional objective of NAM in infants with BCLP is the presurgical alignment of the premaxilla. This not only enables performance of the GPP and reduction in the tension of the lip scars, but it eliminates the circumstance of an anteriorly displaced or "blocked-out" premaxillary segment.

CLINICAL TECHNIQUE OF NAM

Diagnosis

The primary step in preparation for NAM is obtaining the proper diagnosis. It is estimated that 10% of clefts are associated with one of more than the 300 possible syndromes, many of which may be associated with the medical conditions that require treatment. While NAM is an important step in the initial therapy of these infants, sometimes there are more pressing health issues that should be addressed immediately following birth. Once the infant's health status has been confirmed and stabilized, it is important to assess the family and their social support structure.

Family Support

NAM therapy requires considerable time and effort on behalf of both the family and clinical staff. The parents must be committed to making weekly or bi-monthly appointments for the serial NAM adjustments. In addition, the process of applying face tapes, and cleaning the appliance, requires hours of dedication at home during the time immediately following the birth of the infant through its first 3–5 months of life. A high level of parent cooperation is required to attain success with this technique. Successful treatment outcomes do not correlate with socioeconomic status or traditional family structures.

Intraoral Examination

The final step prior to initiation of treatment is the performance of a comprehensive intraoral examination. This is best accomplished with the surgeon and orthodontist examining the infant together. The specific anatomical cleft variation needs to be documented and its implications for treatment considered. A precise description of the nasal, labial, alveolar, and cleft anomalies should be noted in the patient record and photographed. The presence of Simonart's bands, ectopic neonatal tooth buds, and any other remarkable findings should be recorded. This step is essential for proper treatment planning, as it will establish the specific treatment goals. For example, if the palate is noncleft, and the alveolar segments are in good alignment, then the NAM treatment will be focused on nasal stenting alone. Closure of an alveolar gap is a more significant challenge if the palate is intact or if the infant presents at an older age (4–5 months). These variables in the presentation of clefting help to delineate the specific treatment goals. The clinical examination, a specific diagnosis, and a comprehensive treatment plan, informs the clinician and parents of the possible treatment outcomes, costs, risks and benefits of the procedures, before initiating treatment. This enables obtaining the proper informed consent.

Maxillary Impression

A maxillary impression and medical photographs are among the first clinical steps taken. This is accomplished in a hospital setting with the surgeon, orthodontist, and a dental assistant working together. It is essential to have the proper emergency airway and resuscitation protocols worked out, as well as the appropriate equipment assembled in advance, should they become necessary. First, an impression tray is fit to the maxillary arch, ensuring adequate transverse and sagittal extensions. The infant's hands and feet are restrained, while the tray is fit. The surgeon turns the baby upside down while the impression is performed (Fig. 46–6A). The infant's

airway is maintained with a dental mirror handle gently applied to the dorsum of the tongue. The inside of the infant's oral cavity is well illuminated during the procedure, which enables the clinician to see the functioning airway back to the posterior pharyngeal wall. It is important to eliminate excessive impression material in the posterior aspect of the tray to minimize the risk of material breaking off in the infant's mouth. A generous amount of material is needed in the anterior portion of the impression tray in order to manipulate it around the alveolar segments and the premaxilla. The more accurately the impression characterizes the anatomy, the more exact the fit can be with the appliance. Once the impression material is set, the tray is removed and the oral cavity examined for any excess impression material that may have remained in the nose or cleft. The maxillary impression is taken with a Polysiloxane putty material (type 0). We also regularly obtain a nasal impression with a light-body Vinyl Polysiloxane material as part of the initial record set (Fig. 46–6B).

Appliance Fabrication

The maxillary impression is poured up with dental stone. Undercuts are blocked out with utility wax. Self-curing acrylic is then used to fabricate the intraoral molding plate. Once set, the gross acrylic excess is removed, the vestibular extensions are reduced 2–3 mm from the height of the vestibular fold, and relief is made for the frenal attachments. A 6-mm diameter hole is placed through the plate in the midline approximately 10 mm from the posterior border. This hole would maintain a patent airway should the NAM appliance drop down onto the tongue and possibly be pushed forward into an upright position. The appliance is then polished and ready for the delivery appointment.

Appliance Delivery

Extra time is scheduled for the delivery appointment. In this visit, there is much to be accomplished. The tray needs to be adjusted for fit and the retention button(s) attached. The parents need to be instructed in the care and use of the NAM appliance including retention taping procedures, oral hygiene, and how to perform an intraoral examination. Time needs to be budgeted for questions that the parents will have.

Before placing the NAM appliance in the infant's mouth, the clinician should run his or her finger over all the surfaces to ensure a smooth finish and that no sharp angles exist anywhere on the plate. View the plate on the stone cast to verify that the necessary reduction has been made in the vestibular extensions and for the frenal attachments. The plate is now ready to be inserted in the mouth. It can be helpful to have a parent hold the infant's hands next to its ears. In this way, the head can be held still at the same time the hands are restrained. For intraoral examination, we find long cotton tip applicator sticks and a pen-light to be very effective. With the plate in the mouth, apply gentle occlusal pressure to the undersurface. Retract the lips and view the relationship of the

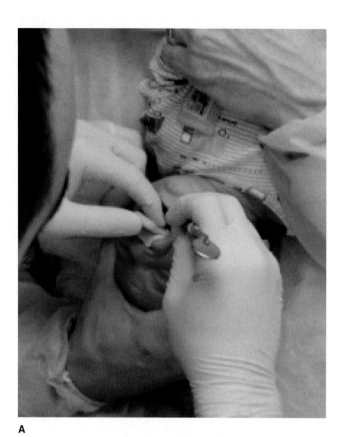

A

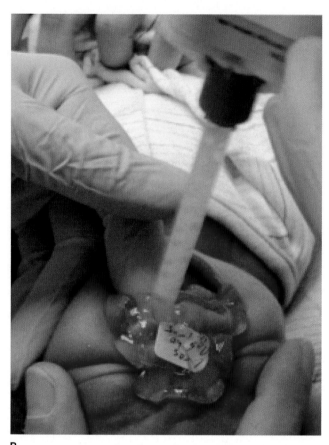

B

Figure 46–6. A: Maxillary impression technique. Note the baby is held upside down and a patent airway is actively maintained with the handle of a dental mirror. **B:** Nasal impression technique. Note the capture of the medial canthi in the impression to later serve as a source of anatomical orientation.

plate's margins to the surrounding tissues. Remove the plate and make any necessary adjustments with a low speed hand drill and acrylic bur.

Retention Button

The retention button should be placed on the anterior surface of the molding plate, midway between the cleft lip segments. In this way, the button will not impede approximation of the lips as they are brought together. The button should be placed at a 30–40 degree angle to the occlusal surface of the alveolar ridges in order to achieve proper retention and to avoid unseating of the appliance from the palate. To determine the length of the button, measure the distance from the most anterior aspect of the plate to approximately 3–5 mm past the lips. Create an indentation on the plate, at the point that the button will be attached. Make an acrylic mix of self-curing resin and fix the button in place. Immersing the appliance in a hot water bath can greatly decrease the setting time of the self-curing resin. Refine the new addition of acrylic, ensuring that it is smooth and that retention of the button is adequate. Remember to rinse the appliance prior to placing it in the mouth after making additions or adjustments. Try the appliance in again, this time with the retention tapes attached. The

measure of proper retention is that the appliance remains adherent to the palate. Also, confirm that the optimal positions for the button and tapes have been achieved (Fig. 46–7).

Face Tapes

Proper taping technique should provide adequate retention for the NAM appliance with a minimum of discomfort to the skin of the infant. Since the "active" tapes, that provide for retraction and molding force via elastic rubber bands, need to be changed one time per day, a "base" tape is placed on each cheek. This base tape is usually replaced one time per week, allowing more frequent placement and removal of the active retraction tape, without causing excessive skin irritations. The active retraction tape is fabricated by taking a 0.25-inch steri-strip and doubling it back on itself at one end, around an elastic orthodontic rubber band. The elastic, measuring 0.1875 inch, is calibrated to deliver approximately 4 ounces of force when stretched 20–30 mm (Fig. 46–8A). The parents are shown where to position the base and active tapes to optimize NAM appliance retention. The parents are instructed to clean the appliance at least one time per day with warm water. Although it may seem traumatic to be applying tapes to the infant's cheeks, the alternative approaches for

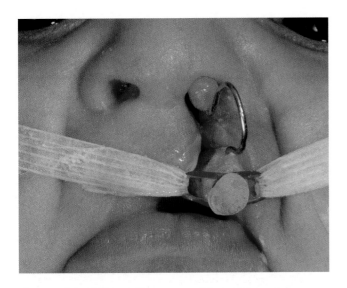

Figure 46-7. NAM appliance seated in mouth and nose, retained by well positioned elastics and tapes. The shaft of the button has been gradually reduced in width to allow approximation of the lip segments. The nasal stent is elevating the nostril apex and nasal tip, resulting in improved nasal symmetry.

appliance retention (an extraoral cap, placement of retention pins into the alveolar ridges, or considerable amounts of a denture adhesive) are in most cases inferior alternatives to cheek taping (Fig. 46–8B and C).

Parent Education

Parents need to learn about the anatomy of the cleft and how to assess the infant's oral cavity for sores. This simple technical ability and new vocabulary facilitates a more meaningful exchange with the parents. An understanding of the cleft anatomy removes some of the parental fear or anxiety in manipulating the oral tissues, enabling them to more intimately care for their child. We provide the parents with labeled anatomical diagrams and reinforce these by demonstrating the equivalent structures in their baby's mouth.

The final objective to be accomplished during the initial appliance delivery appointment is to instruct the parents on the proper use and care of the NAM appliance. The appliance should be worn 24 hours per day except for cleaning and when the base tapes are being changed. Prior to the end of the first visit, the parents remaining questions are answered. They are encouraged to write down questions that come up while at home, to be discussed at the next visit.

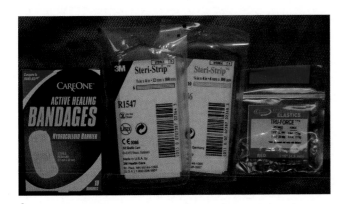

A

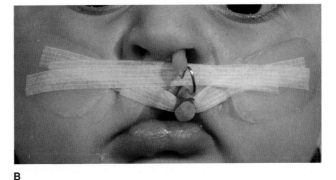

B

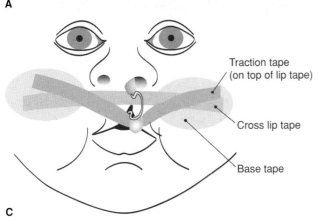

C

Figure 46-8. A: Taping supplies for NAM include (from left to right): base tapes, Steri-Strips, and orthodontic elastics. **B:** Taping technique. Base tapes are directly applied to the cheek. Steri-Strips with orthodontic elastics are adhered to the base tapes. Note the additional use of a cross-lip tape aiding the approximation of lip and alveolar segments, uprighting the columella, and narrowing of the alar base. **C:** Taping diagram.

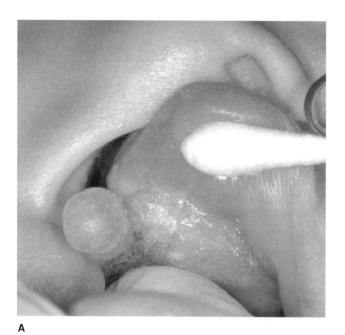

A

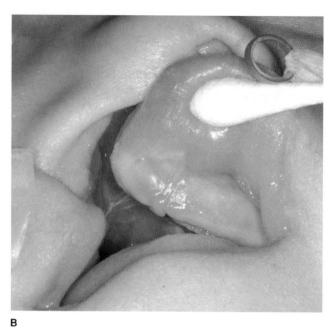

B

Figure 46–9. A: Note the overextended vestibular portion of the NAM appliance under the maxillary frenum. **B:** Intraoral sore around maxillary frenum. The proper clinical course of action is to reduce the vestibular extension of the NAM appliance under the irritated tissue.

Appliance Adjustments

Serial visits should be set up for the baby to return every 7–14 days for adjustments to the NAM appliance. These appointments begin by viewing the orientation of the appliance and the surrounding tissues with the tapes and elastics in place. In this way, an assessment can be made about remaining activity in the device and how the tapes have been worn at home. Parental reinforcement may be provided, or changes in appliance placement and taping technique can be suggested.

The plate is then removed from the mouth and cleaned. An intraoral examination is performed. Request that a parent or assistant hold the hands of the infant against the infants' own ears. Elevate each cheek away from the alveolar ridge, using the cotton tip applicator stick, checking for sores in the labial vestibule and on the alveolar ridge, and verify that there are no sores on the palatal aspects of the alveolar ridges. Examine the internal surface of each nostril in which there is a nasal stent present. Sores can either look white and ulcerous, or red and inflamed (Fig. 46–9A and B). In either case, the position of the sore should be noted in the chart for reevaluation at the next visit, and the etiology should be addressed. Pressure sores are treated by relieving the pressure created by the plate or nasal stent. The pressure applied to these delicate tissues may be reduced by carefully relieving the acrylic molding plate at the point of contact with the sore or irritation.

As part of the intraoral examination, the alveolar gap distance should be measured. We accomplish this with an indirect measurement. A block of soft and malleable wax, the approximate size of the gap, is formed and inserted repeatedly into the gap, with necessary alterations made, until the fit is passive. The block of wax is then measured with a boley gauge caliper. The measurement can be taken more than once to increase precision. The vertical position of the medial aspect of the alveolar ridge is assessed, the interarch relationships (both sagittal and transverse) noted, and the position of the lip and nose segments observed. It is from these observations, and an appreciation of the specific treatment goals, that the treatment objectives for the adjustment become apparent.

Biomechanics of NAM

There are three primary ways that molding force is generated with the NAM appliance. One, the application of the elastic retention tapes results in a posteriorly directed force to tissue surfaces contacting the leading edge of the NAM device. To achieve closure of a unilateral alveolar gap, the greater alveolar segment needs to be retracted or molded posteriorly while allowing the lesser segment to remain in place. To attain this goal, acrylic is removed from the inside of the molding plate that is in contact with the leading edge of the lesser alveolar segment. The plate then contacts the leading edge of the greater alveolar segment first and applies a vector of posteriorly directed force. As the alveolar gap closes, the plate literally translates and subtlety rotates posteriorly. For this reason, the back edge of the plate should be reduced at each visit to avoid eliciting a gagging reflex and irritation in the back of the mouth (Fig. 46–10A and B). Once the alveolar gap is closed, tension in the elastic bands can be reduced to a level that is meant to simply retain the plate and position of the alveolar

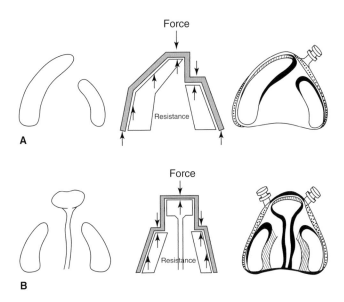

A

B

Figure 46–10. A: UCLP and **B:** BLCP—There are three primary ways that molding forces are generated. One, application of the elastic retention tapes results in a posteriorly directed force to tissue surfaces contacting the inside of the NAM device. Two, when reciprocal additions and subtractions of acrylic are made to the NAM appliance. Three, the reaction to pushing forward on the nasal tip is pushing back on the projecting alveolar processes. Note the black areas indicate hard acrylic relief, the lined areas indicate soft acrylic additions, and the dotted areas indicate hard acrylic additions.

ridges. The elastic retention tapes do not contribute to nasal molding.

The second contributing force in NAM is applied to the oral and nasal tissues, when reciprocal additions and subtractions of acrylic are made to the NAM appliance. In this way, force is applied in one area on the alveolar ridges, and is relieved in another, facilitating gradual and gentle molding of the alveolar ridges, as well as the nose. For example, in addition to the elastic forces described above, some soft acrylic would be added to the plate on the anterior inner surface (facing the anterior labial aspect of the greater segment). In concert with this soft acrylic addition there would be removal of the same volume of hard acrylic from the anteriorly facing palatal surface of the plate (behind the anterior greater alveolar segment). In this way, the labiopalatal dimension of the greater alveolar segment is maintained as it is molded posteriorly (Fig. 46–10A and B). This force system is activated with the normal function of the infant through eating and sucking. These movements lift the plate into the nose and onto the alveolar ridges more actively. In addition, the plate eliminates tongue and bottle access to the cleft.

The third force that is utilized in NAM comes from the active lifting and forward projection of the nasal tip by the nasal stent. In this process, the nasal stent, in combination with elastic tapes, becomes an additional source of anchorage for the molding plate, pushing backward on the projecting edge of the greater alveolar segment in unilateral cases, and

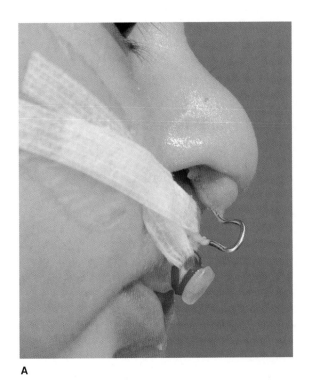

A

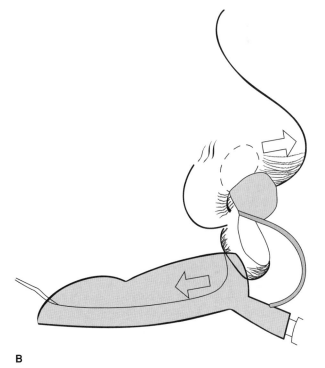

B

Figure 46–11. A: Lateral view of UCLP NAM appliance in place. **B:** Illustration of NAM appliance delivering superior and anterior forces to the nasal tip and nostril apex. This delivers an equal but opposite force to the greater segment in UCLP and premaxilla in BLCP.

for retraction of the premaxilla in bilateral cases. The reaction to pushing forward on the nasal tip, is pushing back on the projecting alveolar processes (Fig. 46–11A and B).

Addition of Nasal Stent

The nasal sent is added to the intraoral molding plate when the alveolar gap is reduced to approximately 5 mm (Fig. 46–12A). It is desirable to reduce the width of the alveolar gap prior to introduction of the nasal stent in order to achieve some degree of approximation of the lateral and mesial aspects of the nasal aperture. This prevents overexpansion of the nasal alar base and creation of a "mega-nostril".

The nasal stent is fabricated out of a 0.036-inch stainless steel wire that is embedded with acrylic into the molding plate. A channel is carved out of the plate in order to achieve a secure joining of this wire and the molding plate. The wire is custom bent to extend from the bottom of the plate, around the side of the retention button, gradually curving back towards the plate in a "swan neck" like arch, and ending in a "R" pattern set of bends (Fig. 46–12B). Hard acrylic is added to create a "kidney bean" structure to provide a strong and secure foundation for nasal molding (Fig. 46–12C). Soft acrylic is progressively added to the "kidney-bean" shaped nasal stent. Activation of the superior lobe, which defines the nasal tip projection, can be accomplished via addition of material or by bending the wire armature resulting in a superior and forward movement of the nasal stent (Fig. 46–12D). The inferior lobe of the nasal stent prevents over insertion of the nasal stent into the nostril and is responsible for lifting the nostril aperture at the nostril apex. The space between the lobes rests firmly against the nostril apex. It should be directed medially and superiorly, mirroring the noncleft side (Fig. 46–12E).

Maintenance Adjustments

To optimize the molding effects of the NAM appliance, there are several adjustments that should be periodically repeated. Hard acrylic located in the alveolar gap should be systematically eliminated to facilitate reduction of the alveolar gap width. Since the greater alveolar segment is often displaced vertically into the nose, maintaining adequate vertical dimension of the molding plate should facilitate leveling of the occlusal plane. If the greater segment remains displaced vertically into the nose, a foot-plate of soft acrylic can be added to the under surface of the nasal stent to apply an inferiorly directed molding force. Directly under the greater segment, it will be necessary to add hard acrylic on the undersurface of the plate to facilitate removal from the inner surface. In this way, the critical molding plate thickness of approximately 1.5 mm will be maintained. If the plate gets thinner than this, it may be prone to fracture. A boley gauge caliper is indispensable for the evaluation of the plate thickness at every visit and after every adjustment that is made to the plate.

During the course of treatment, the NAM appliance should be periodically expanded to accommodate normal growth and development of the infant maxilla. A 0.5–1 mm

addition of hard acrylic is added to the external lateral borders of the appliance bilaterally, ensuring smooth, even additions. An equal amount of hard acrylic is then removed from the inner surface of the molding plate walls all along the buccal alveolar segments. This should be done approximately one time per month to keep up with the expected increase in transverse width of the infant's maxillary arch.

As the cleft gap is reduced through alveolar molding, the posterior aspect of the NAM plate is continuously reduced to prevent gagging or sores from developing. This reduced anteroposterior dimension enables some babies to extrude the plate by getting the tongue behind the posterior border of the NAM appliance. To prevent this from occurring, a "bell-shaped curve" acrylic extension of only 3–4 mm can be placed on the posterior aspect of the plate with the highest portion in the midline.

The overall shape of the NAM appliance undergoes a gradual metamorphosis during the course of treatment. As the alveolar segments are brought into closer approximation and ultimately into contact, the initial irregular shape of the maxillary arch and NAM appliance, is replaced by a normal and symmetric arch form. As the lip segments come into closer resting approximation, it may be necessary to gradually thin the retention buttons (Fig. 46–13A and C).

Bilateral NAM Cases

The description of NAM treatment thus far offered was based primarily on the UCLP deformity. The majority of these principles apply directly to the treatment of BCLP patients as well. Several topics unique to bilateral cleft care require special attention. Specifically, we will discuss adjustments to the molding plate and nasal stents in regard to presurgical repositioning of the premaxilla and nonsurgical columella elongation.

A bilateral NAM plate requires two retention buttons oriented in a similar fashion as in the unilateral appliance, but positioned between the prolabium and the lateral lip segments on each side. Instead of a greater and lesser alveolar segment represented by two depressions in the plate, there are three areas that contain the two lateral alveolar segments and the premaxilla. Serial modifications are made in the hard acrylic plate to reduce the size of both cleft defects, facilitating premaxillary retraction. Adjustments may need to be made in the midline of the molding plate to prevent irritation to the exposed vomer. An attempt should be made to first center the premaxilla and then to proceed with its retraction. If the premaxilla is very protrusive and mobile at the beginning of treatment, it can be grossly repositioned and retracted several millimeters prior to fabricating the NAM appliance. This can be accomplished by use of a Bonnet with elastic traction, or broad elastic adhesive bands applied directly to the face and the premaxilla.

Two nasal stents are added to the anterior surface of the molding plate once the alveolar cleft gaps are reduced to approximately 5 mm on each side. When several millimeters (2–3) of columella have been produced, the two nasal stents

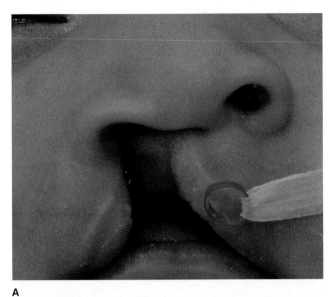

A

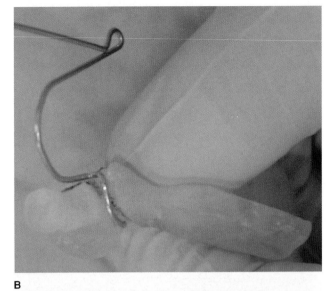

B

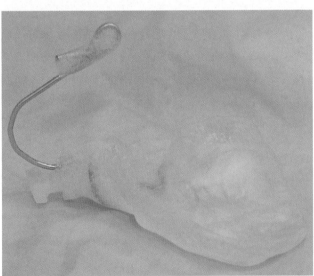

C

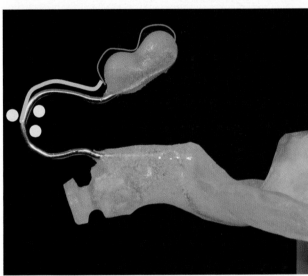

D

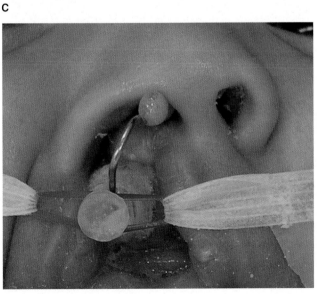

E

Figure 46–12. A: UCLP demonstrating a prolapsed alar carti-lage and deviated columella. The alveolar gap has been reduced to 5 mm. **B:** Wire fabrication of nasal stent bent out of 0.036-inch stainless steel wire that is embedded with acrylic into the mold-ing plate. A channel is carved out of the plate in order to achieve a secure joining of this wire and the molding plate. The wire is custom bent to extend from the bottom of the plate, around the side of the retention button, gradually curving back towards the plate in a "swan neck" like arch, and ending in a "R" pattern set of bends. **C:** Nasal stent added to molding plate and base layer of hard acrylic added to bilobed intranasal portion of stent. **D:** Soft acrylic is progressively added to the intranasal portion of the nasal stent. Activation of the superior lobe, which results in nasal tip projection, can be accomplished via addition of mate-rial or by bending the wire armature resulting in a superior and forward movement of the nasal stent. **E:** Nasal stent upon deliv-ery. A cradle is created by the inferior lobe and the space between the lobes to elevate the nostril apex, mirroring the noncleft side. Note the improved nasal symmetry upon insertion of the nasal stent.

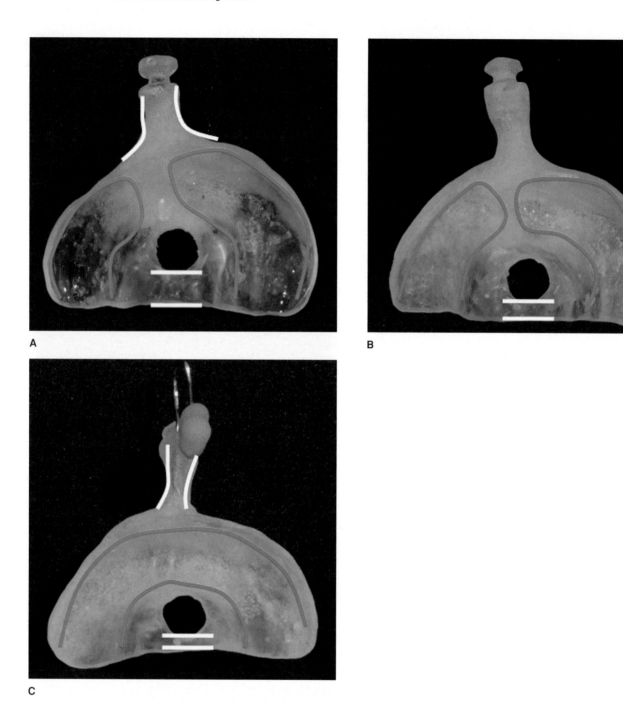

Figure 46–13. A: UCLP NAM appliance goes through a gradual metamorphosis during the treatment. Device at delivery. **B:** Six weeks of treatment. Note the approximation of the alveolar segments and the trimming of the posterior border, which has resulted in decreased distance between the hole and the posterior edge of the appliance. **C:** Twelve weeks of treatment. Note the continuity and symmetry of the space provided for the alveolar ridge and further reduction in the distance between the hole and the posterior border of the molding plate. In addition, the shaft of the retention button has been reduced in width and the nasal stent had been added.

are connected by a band of soft acrylic. This "horizontal prolabial band" crossing over the base of the columella, in combination with the active portions of the nasal stents and taping of the prolabium, will provide the necessary force system for nonsurgical columella elongation (Fig. 46–14).

It is helpful if the infant is a little hungry during the adjustment appointments, so that after the NAM appliance has been adjusted, the parents can attempt a feeding while still at the clinic to ensure that the baby is comfortable before returning home.

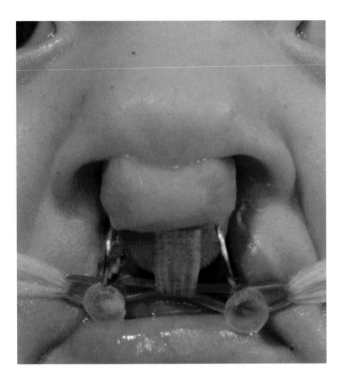

Figure 46–14. Bilateral NAM appliance in place with prolabial taping and horizontal band connecting the two nasal stents. The resulting force system is responsible for achieving nonsurgical columella elongation.

COMPLICATIONS

The process of NAM is not without its complications. All risks and benefits of treatment are important to consider and should be communicated to prospective parents as part of the process of obtaining informed consent.

Intraoral/Intranasal Sores

The most frequent complication of NAM is the development of intraoral and intranasal pressure sores (Fig. 46–9). These sores arise primarily due to either excessive or improper activations of the plate or nasal stent. Excessive activations result in pressure ulcers at the point of contact. The sores will begin to heal within hours upon reduction of acrylic from the walls of the molding plate or nasal stent. It is mandatory that there are no sharp edges anywhere on the plate. It is also important to reduce the vestibular acrylic border under the maxillary frenal attachments, which are the most frequent points of irritation. Occasionally, the vomer develops a sore from excessive superior extension of the plate.

Even with seemingly appropriate activation and trimming of the appliance in the clinic, problems can still arise at home. Through prolonged functional activation (sucking) by the baby, and treatment related anatomical changes occurring in the infant's mouth, the resting position of the plate may change and sores can develop. The occurrence of intraoral sores highlights the utility of training the parents to perform intraoral examinations, and of providing accurate anatomical descriptions of what they see. In this way, triage over the phone is greatly facilitated. Due to the fact that most of the sores heal in a few hours with the plate removed (or following adjustment of the plate), we request that the parent ensure that the plate is in place for a few hours prior to bringing the baby in for an adjustment. In this way the sore is visible to the clinician and an appropriate adjustment can be made to the appliance.

Taping Issues

Difficulty with taping is commonly encountered at least at the beginning of the NAM process. Inadequate or excessive elastic forces and cheek irritations are the most frequent events. To achieve active movement of the alveolar segments, a 0.1875-inch elastic should be stretched approximately two times its resting length. Alternatively, the elastics could be applied passively just to ensure stability and retention of the plate. Cheek irritations arise when the base tapes are removed abruptly or removed and replaced too often. Some babies have hypersensitive skin that is prone to developing irritations. When skin irritations arise, the taping procedures are reviewed and corrected or modified to relieve the problem. Application of skin moisturizer may be recommended. Sometimes it may be necessary to change the base tape material or to alter the position of the base tapes in order to periodically give the skin some relief. If necessary, a referral to a pediatric dermatologist is made.

Ectopic Neonatal Teeth

Occasionally, infants will present with a soft tissue sack filled with fluid and a primary tooth bud on the margin of an alveolar cleft (Fig. 46–15). Due to its position external to

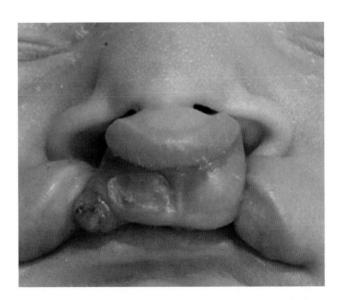

Figure 46–15. An ectopic tooth bud at the right margin of the premaxilla. This is removed to allow approximation of the alveolar segments and to prevent the possibility of the baby aspirating the tooth bud.

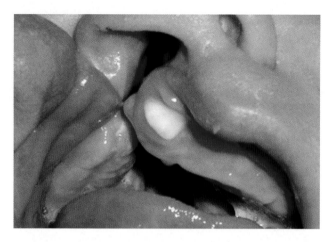

Figure 46–16. Premature eruption of a maxillary primary central. NAM treatment should continue following reduction of acrylic from the inside of the molding plate in the corresponding area.

the alveolar bone and surrounded by soft tissue, these teeth will not develop into a functional tooth and may prevent the alveolar segments from coming into direct contact during the molding process. The ectopic neonatal tooth sack does not respond well to the application of molding force from the NAM appliance. For these reasons, the ectopic neonatal tooth should be removed. This can be accomplished either before or after the maxillary impression; but, if it is done after, the NAM study model should be altered to represent this anatomical change prior to appliance fabrication. The removal of the neonatal tooth is tolerated well by the infant and takes only a couple of minutes. Under local anesthesia, a small incision is made in the soft tissue sack, the tooth bud removed, and one or two sutures are placed. The molding plate can be inserted immediately after this procedure, ensuring adequate relief in the molding plate around the surgical site.

Due to premature eruption or exposure from the direct surface pressure, a maxillary primary central incisor occasionally is uncovered. A combination of pressure on the anterior aspect of the alveolar ridge, in the absence of relief from the palatal aspect, essentially thins the alveolus, exposing the facial aspect of the primary incisor. Advancing patient age makes this situation more likely to occur. These teeth should not be extracted. Rather, the plate around the teeth should be adequately relieved and treatment can continue. The eruption of mandibular teeth should not impact NAM treatment appreciably (Figs. 46–16 and 46–2D and E).

Interarch Relationship

In some instances, a Class III interarch relationship may develop as the alveolar segments achieve alignment. This often represents the inherent tissue deficiency of the maxilla associated with the cleft deformity. It would be desirable to maintain the maxillary arch circumference and position in normal relationship to the intact mandibular arch; unfortu-

nately, this is not always possible based on the maxillary tissue deficiency. In many cases treated without PSIO, shortly after primary lip repair or lip adhesion, tension from the reconstructed oral aperture delivers an orthopedic force, molding the maxillary arch and closing the cleft gap in an uncontrolled manner. This is often responsible for creating a Class III interarch relationship and often an irregular arch form. For this reason, we currently advocate closing the cleft gap in a controlled manner, resulting in acceptable maxillary arch form and facilitating the performance of a GPP if desired.

BENEFITS OF NAM

The benefits of NAM are numerous although still controversial in some clinical settings. The foundation of this controversy resides in the fundamental differences in the definition of "successful" PSIO cleft treatment. As the definition of success can vary considerably among clinicians, controversy is not unexpected.

Definition of Success

The clinical success of NAM is manifested as an improved surgical esthetic outcome of the primary lip and nose repair; both, in the immediate postoperative period, and through continued growth and development of the child. In bilateral patients, success is further defined by having a scar-free columella of normal dimension, achieved through presurgical columellar elongation using the NAM appliance. Successful NAM treatment should reduce the number of surgical revisions of lip, nose, and fistula closures, prior to the final cosmetic and functional surgical intervention. This reduction, in the number of secondary surgical interventions, reduces the number of hospital admissions, morbidity, and cost of care over the many years of cleft patient care. Further, establishing a more normal appearance early in a child's life, provides the opportunity for psychosocial development without some of the stigma related to clefting disorders.

Traditional outcome studies of PSIO (e.g., Eurocleft and Dutchcleft) have defined PSIO success in terms of a superior ability for the infant to feed with a bottle, improved early weight gain, better speech outcome, improved occlusion (Goslon Yardstick) and improved growth of the midface skeleton. These traditional outcome studies have satisfactorily demonstrated that PSIO alone, without nasal molding and columella elongation, does not achieve the traditional definition of success. When these traditional studies examine facial esthetics, the asymmetry of the primary nasal repair often overshadows any improvement in the lip esthetics achieved by the presurgical alignment of the alveolar ridges. Presurgical correction of the nasal cartilage deformity and augmentation of the nasal lining and elongation of the columella, combined with the alignment of alveolar segments, has been shown to have measurable esthetic benefits in terms of the primary labial, nasal, and alveolar repair.

Lip and Nose Esthetics

There is little debate among surgeons that the clinical outcome following repair of a mild or minimal cleft deformity is superior to that of a severe cleft deformity. However, an important question is whether the esthetic benefit of surgical repair following NAM therapy is retained over time. In addition, does NAM reduce the need for the expected, multiple surgical revisions of the lip and nose deformity during early childhood?

Lee et al.[30] investigated the effects of NAM on bilateral cleft columella length, as well as the need for surgical revisions through the ages of 7–9 years. In this study, the length of the columella at age 3 was not significantly different when comparing the bilateral cleft group treated with NAM, to the noncleft control group of Farkas.[31] The cleft group, not treated with NAM, had significantly shorter columella length and an increased need for surgical revisions by the age of 7–9 years.

Maull et al.[32] studied the nasal symmetry obtained in unilateral cleft patients treated with NAM versus patients who had alveolar molding alone. This study was performed on a group of consecutively treated patients, and was based upon nasal casts that were scanned by a three-dimensional camera. The age of the study and control population was 5 years. A Procrustes analysis of the nasal casts showed that the NAM treated patients had significantly greater nasal symmetry at the age of 5 years than the control group.

The esthetic benefits of NAM to nasal shape and the lip repair are difficult to deny when comparing children who's PSIO did not address the nasal deformity. The literature supports the finding that these esthetic benefits are maintained until the ages of 5–9 years. Anecdotal experience and our initial pilot studies have shown that the beneficial esthetic effects last through early adulthood. As a sufficient study population comes of age, the data will be collected, studied and reported.

GPP

There are many significant benefits to the patient from the performance of a GPP. Research has shown that GPP does not attenuate growth of the midface through the age of 18 years.[33–35] At least 60% of the time, patients avoid the need for a secondary alveolar bone graft.[36] Adequate bone in the site of the former cleft defect allows for more normal eruption of teeth into the alveolus. A GPP secures the arch form achieved via NAM, making it possible to more accurately control the ultimate shape of the maxillary arch form. Even when the GPP "fails", the outcome from secondary bone grafting is superior to that following no GPP.[37] The frequency of patent fistulas has been shown to be greatly reduced following GPP, and this decreases the need for surgical fistula repairs. The absence of oronasal fistulas has a positive impact on the speech of many patients. Our treatment regimen including GPP has been shown to reduce the burden of cost on the medical system.[38] GPP remains a controversial topic, due to the inherent difficulty of isolating the "procedure effect" from the myriad of other variables influencing outcomes in long-term studies. It is, however, possible to utilize NAM and not perform a GPP.

The successful outcome of NAM, as well as the cleft surgical repair itself, is quite technique sensitive. The more clinical training and experience that one has delivering these procedures and techniques, the more predictable and refined the treatment outcome could be. Reducing the severity of the cleft nasal and alveolar deformities, as well as the presurgical elongation of the columella prior to the primary surgical repair, are undeniable benefits of carefully performed NAM. While there is a cost to the patient and family for this form of presurgical treatment, the physical and psychosocial benefits well out weigh the effort involved.

Psychosocial

The birth of a baby is a time of much excitement, intense feelings, and gratitude. The new parents are immediately thrust into the role of caregiver, and essentially need to have or find all of the answers necessary to ensure that their baby thrives. When a baby is born with a cleft deformity, an additional level of complexity to parenthood is introduced that very few parents are ready to provide. This creates additional anxiety and disorientation during an already challenging time. During the course of presurgical NAM treatment, the parents receive an education about the cleft deformity, are able to see tangible reduction in the severity of the cleft, and are put in touch with other families that are at various stages of the same treatment program. This type of institutional and parent-to-parent support should not be discounted, as it is a meaningful and valuable service to the families. A great number of parents network with other families to answer questions, provide support, and volunteer or raise money for local and national cleft organizations. Successful bonding of parents and their infants to the staff, physicians, and peer support group, is evidenced by their return for care to the same Institution and cleft palate team through the first two decades of life and beyond.

It is well appreciated that parents, teachers, doctors, and other children react differently to people with craniofacial differences, even if subconsciously. These sometimes subtle alterations in normal social interactions can have profoundly destructive repercussions on the emotional status of the developing child. Restoring optimal facial esthetics and function, to children with clefts during the preschool and elementary years, allows them to grow up as ordinary children, normalizing their view and experience of the world around them.

References

1. McNeil CK. Congenital Oral Deformities. *Br Dent J* 18:191–198, 1956.
2. McNeil CK. Orthopaedic principles in the treatment of lip and palate clefts. In Hotz R (ed). *Early Treatment of Cleft Lip and Palate.* Bern, Switzerland, Huber and Company, 1964, pp. 59–67.

3. Georgiade NG, Latham RA. Maxillary arch alignment in the bilateral cleft lip and palate infant, using pinned coaxial screw appliance. *Plast Reconstr Surg* 56(1):52–60, 1975.

4. Latham RA. Orthopedic advancement of the cleft maxillary segment: A preliminary report. *Cleft Palate J* 17(3):227–233, 1980.

5. Hotz MM. Pre- and early postoperative growth-guidance in cleft lip and palate cases by maxillary orthopedics (an alternative procedure to primary bone-grafting). *Cleft Palate J* 6:368–372, 1969.

6. Hotz MM. Aims and possibilities of pre- and postsurgical orthopedic treatment in uni- and bilateral clefts. *Trans Eur Orthod Soc* 553–558, 1973.

7. Hotz M, Gnoinski W. Comprehensive care of cleft lip and palate children at Zurich university: A preliminary report. *Am J Orthod* 70(5):481–504, 1976.

8. Meijer R. Lip adhesion and its effect on the maxillofacial complex in complete unilateral clefts of the lip and palate. *Cleft Palate J* 15(1):39–43, 1978.

9. Pool R, Farnworth TK. Preoperative lip taping in the cleft lip. *Ann Plast Surg* 32(3):243–249, 1994.

10. Prahl C, Kuijpers-Jagtman AM, van't Hof MA, Prahl-Andersen B. A randomised prospective clinical trial into the effect of infant orthopaedics on maxillary arch dimensions in unilateral cleft lip and palate (Dutchcleft). *Eur J Oral Sci* 109(5):297–305, 2001.

11. Konst EM, Rietveld T, Peters HF, Kuijpers-Jagtman AM. Language skills of young children with unilateral cleft lip and palate following infant orthopedics: A randomized clinical trial. *Cleft Palate Craniofac J* 40(4):356–362, 2003.

12. Konst EM, Rietveld T, Peters HF, Weersink-Braks H. Use of a perceptual evaluation instrument to assess the effects of infant orthopedics on the speech of toddlers with cleft lip and palate. *Cleft Palate Craniofac J* 40(6):597–605, 2003.

13. Konst EM, Rietveld T, Peters HF, Prahl-Andersen B. Phonological development of toddlers with unilateral cleft lip and palate who were treated with and without infant orthopedics: A randomized clinical trial. *Cleft Palate Craniofac J* 40(1):32–39, 2003.

14. Bongaarts CA, Kuijpers-Jagtman AM, van 't Hof MA, Prahl-Andersen B. The effect of infant orthopedics on the occlusion of the deciduous dentition in children with complete unilateral cleft lip and palate (Dutchcleft). *Cleft Palate Craniofac J* 41(6):633–641, 2004.

15. Prahl C, Kuijpers-Jagtman AM, Van 't Hof MA, Prahl-Andersen B. Infant orthopedics in UCLP: Effect on feeding, weight, and length: A randomized clinical trial (Dutchcleft). *Cleft Palate Craniofac J.* 42(2):171–177, 2005.

16. Matsuo K, Hirose T. Nonsurgical correction of cleft lip nasal deformity in the early neonate. *Ann Acad Med Singapore* 17(3):358–365, 1988.

17. Matsuo K, Hirose T. Preoperative non-surgical over-correction of cleft lip nasal deformity. *Br J Plast Surg* 44(1):5–11, 1991.

18. Grayson BH, Cutting C, Wood R. Preoperative columella lengthening in bilateral cleft lip and palate. *Plast Reconstr Surg* 92(7):1422–1423, 1993.

19. Grayson BH, Santiago PE, Brecht LE, Cutting CB. Presurgical nasoalveolar molding in infants with cleft lip and palate. *Cleft Palate Craniofac J* 36(6):486–498, 1999.

20. Grayson BH, Cutting CB. Presurgical nasoalveolar orthopedic molding in primary correction of the nose, lip, and alveolus of infants born with unilateral and bilateral clefts. *Cleft Palate Craniofac J* 38(3):193–198, 2001.

21. Chavarria C, Chen JW, Teichgraeber JF. Use of presurgical nasal alveolar molding appliance in treating cleft lip and palate patients. *Tex Dent J* 121(10):976–981, 2004.

22. Da Silveira AC, Oliveira N, Gonzalez S, et al. Modified nasal alveolar molding appliance for management of cleft lip defect. *J Craniofac Surg* 14(5):700–703, 2003.

23. Mitsuyoshi I, Masahiko W, Masayuki F. Simple modified preoperative nasoalveolar moulding in infants with unilateral cleft lip and palate. *Br J Oral Maxillofac Surg* 42(6):578–580, 2004.

24. Pai BC, Ko EW, Huang CS, Liou EJ. Symmetry of the nose after presurgical nasoalveolar molding in infants with unilateral cleft lip and palate: A preliminary study. *Cleft Palate Craniofac J* 42(6):658–663, 2005.

25. Singh GD, Levy-Bercowski D, Santiago PE. Three-dimensional nasal changes following nasoalveolar molding in patients with unilateral cleft lip and palate: Geometric morphometrics. *Cleft Palate Craniofac J* 42(4):403–409, 2005.

26. Suri S, Tompson BD. A modified muscle-activated maxillary orthopedic appliance for presurgical nasoalveolar molding in infants with unilateral cleft lip and palate. *Cleft Palate Craniofac J* 41(3):225–229, 2004.

27. Bennun RD, Figueroa AA. Dynamic presurgical nasal remodeling in patients with unilateral and bilateral cleft lip and palate: Modification to the original technique. *Cleft Palate Craniofac J* 43(6):639–648, 2006.

28. McComb HK, Coghlan BA. Primary repair of the unilateral cleft lip nose: Completion of a longitudinal study. *Cleft Palate Craniofac J* 33(1):23–30; discussion 30–21, 1996.

29. Burgess LP, Morin GV, Rand M, Vossoughi J, Hollinger JO. Wound healing. Relationship of wound closing tension to scar width in rats. *Arch Otolaryngol Head Neck Surg* 116(7):798–802, 1990.

30. Lee CTH, Garfinkle JS, Warren SM, Brecht LE, Cuting CB, Grayson BH. Nasoalveolar molding improves appearance in children with bilateral cleft lip/palate. Plastic Reconstructive Surgery. In Press.

31. Farkas LG. *Anthropometry of the Head and Face*, 2nd ed. New York: Raven Press, 1994.

32. Maull DJ, Grayson BH, Cutting CB, et al. Long-term effects of nasoalveolar molding on three-dimensional nasal shape in unilateral clefts. *Cleft Palate Craniofac J* 36(5):391–397, 1999.

33. Wood RJ, Grayson BH, Cutting CB. Gingivoperiosteoplasty and mid-facial growth. *Cleft Palate Craniofac J* 34(1):17–20, 1997.

34. Lee CT, Grayson BH, Cutting CB, Brecht LE, Lin WY. Prepubertal midface growth in unilateral cleft lip and palate following alveolar molding and gingivoperiosteoplasty. *Cleft Palate Craniofac J* 41(4):375–380, 2004.

35. Garfinkle JS, Grayson BH, Cutting C, Brecht LE. Maxillary growth following gingivoperiosteoplasty in unilateral cleft lip and palate: 18 year follow-up. Paper presented at the *American Cleft Palate–Craniofacial Association*, Vancouver, BC, 2006.

36. Santiago PE, Grayson BH, Cutting CB, Gianoutsos MP, Brecht LE, Kwon SM. Reduced need for alveolar bone grafting by presurgical orthopedics and primary gingivoperiosteoplasty. *Cleft Palate Craniofac J* 35(1):77–80, 1998.

37. Sato Y, Grayson BH, Barillas I, Cutting C. The effect of gingivoperiosteoplasty on the outcome of secondary alveolar bone graft. Paper presented at the *American Cleft Palate–Craniofacial Association*, Seattle, WA, 2002.

38. Pfeifer TM, Grayson BH, Cutting CB. Nasoalveolar molding and gingivoperiosteoplasty versus alveolar bone graft: An outcome analysis of costs in the treatment of unilateral cleft alveolus. *Cleft Palate Craniofac J* 39(1):26–29, 2002.

Orthodontic Principles in the Management of Orofacial Clefts

Ana M. Mercado, DMD, MS, PhD • Katherine W.L. Vig, BDS, MS, DOrth, FDS.RCS

Since the mid-1940s, the management of patients born with facial clefts and craniofacial anomalies has progressed from specialists providing care independently to the concept of a team approach. Previously, the care of this special group of patients was delivered during independent evaluations and hospitalizations by medical, dental, and paramedical specialists without a comprehensive, systematic, and collaborative approach. The team concept was fostered by the establishment of the American Cleft Palate-Craniofacial Association (ACPA) in 1943. The mission of ACPA is to be an advocate for the patient and parent while promoting the team approach and supporting research.

The document "Parameters for Evaluation and Treatment of Patients with Cleft Lip/Palate or other Craniofacial Anomalies," developed by the ACPA in 1992[1] and later revised in 2007, has provided clinicians and third-party payors with guidelines to the timing and sequencing of treatment for patients with cleft lip and/or palate. The role of the orthodontist is therein defined as a collaborative effort with other dental, medical, and allied-health professionals. Emphasis is given to monitoring of craniofacial growth and development and to providing treatment when necessary to achieve optimal function and appearance. It is recommended that orthodontic treatment be delivered in discrete stages of skeletodental development of the craniofacial complex, avoiding continuous treatment from the early mixed dentition to the permanent dentition. These concepts are further explained in texts outlining the role of the orthodontist in the management of cleft lip/palate.[2,3]

The purpose of this chapter is to discuss the orthodontic principles involved in the contemporary management of the patient with an orofacial cleft, from diagnostic considerations to issues of timing and sequencing of treatment.

THE TEAM APPROACH

The team approach to the comprehensive care of children born with orofacial clefts requires collaboration of the orthodontist with the other members of the team (Fig. 47–1). The timing and sequencing of orthodontic interventions requires prioritization of the patient's other health care needs in

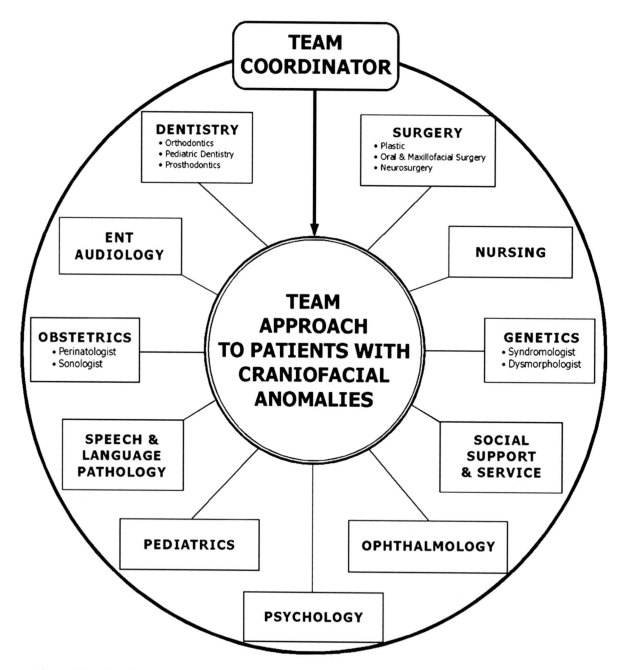

Figure 47–1. Members in the team approach to patients with craniofacial anomalies. (*Modified from Vig KWL, Mercado AM. The orthodontist's role in a cleft palate-craniofacial team. In Graber TM, Vanarsdall RL, Vig KWL (eds). Orthodontics: Current Principles and Techniques, pp. 1097–1121. Copyright 2005, with permission from Elsevier.*)

the context of an integrated treatment plan. Although the orthodontist's role is primarily in the postnatal care of these patients, the diagnosis of an orofacial cleft may be made during prenatal ultrasound examination.

PRENATAL DIAGNOSIS OF OROFACIAL CLEFTS

High-resolution ultrasonography may detect many clefts in utero (Fig. 47–2).[4] By 20 weeks gestation, fetal cleft lip may be diagnosed with detection rates as high as 73%.[5] Clefts of the palate are somewhat more difficult to detect sonographically. Although prenatal diagnosis of orofacial clefts has the advantages of preparing and educating the parents, it may also induce maternal anxiety and emotional distress. Prenatal diagnosis is important for the clinical geneticist and syndromologist, as orofacial clefting is associated with over 300 syndromes. A diagnosis of nonsyndromic cleft of the lip/palate as opposed to syndromic orofacial clefting has consequences in both the management and outcome of treatment.

The timing and sequencing of orthodontic care may be conveniently divided into four distinct periods defined by age and dental development: neonatal period, primary dentition, mixed dentition, and permanent dentition.

NEONATAL MAXILLARY ORTHOPEDICS

Neonatal orthopedics occurs during the early postnatal period, usually in the first postnatal month unless contraindicated by other congenital anomalies or birth defects. This intervention was introduced in the 1960s by Burston and McNeil[6,7] with the intention that early alignment of the maxillary segments would allow the dentition to erupt into a more normal occlusion and eliminate the need for orthodontic correction. As this intervention gained popularity, so too did the complexity of the appliances, the least invasive of which was simple extraoral lip taping (Fig. 47–3). The benefit of this early intervention was challenged in the 1970s. At that time, however, the literature included protocols in which infants underwent primary bone grafting at the time of primary lip repair. The outcome of the presurgical neonatal orthopedics was therefore unclear since the cephalometric measures also included those patients with primary bone grafts. By the 1980s, neonatal maxillary orthopedics had fallen into disrepute as an intervention for orthodontic alignment of the maxillary segments. Such treatment was nevertheless espoused by surgeons as an adjunctive method to reduce the gap between the lip segments, hence providing the benefits of reduced operating time and reduced dehiscence of the primary lip repair. The 1990s brought an increased enthusiasm for neonatal maxillary orthopedics with the addition of presurgical nasoalveolar molding.[8] These treatment interventions have been well described in the preceding chapters.

The 1990s also brought advances in clinical trials design and intercenter studies. The Dutch Intercenter prospective two-arm randomized clinical trial (RCT) was designed to study the outcome of neonatal maxillary orthopedics. It had been reported previously by Shaw et al.[9] in the Eurocleft study that 54% of the 201 European centers were using infant

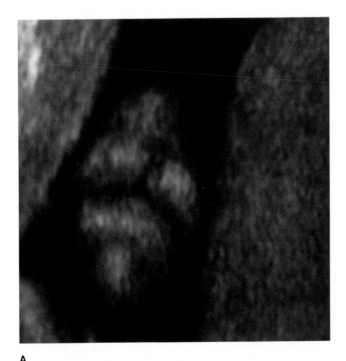

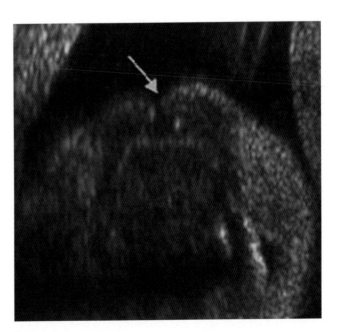

A   **B**

Figure 47–2. Transabdominal ultrasonography images of the midface of a fetus with unilateral cleft lip. (A) Coronal view at 21 weeks gestational age: the defect on the left side extends into the nostril. (B) Axial view at 29 weeks gestational age: discontinuity in the upper lip skin and muscle is evident.

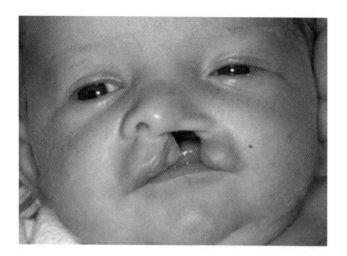

A

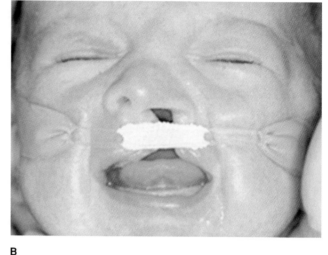

B

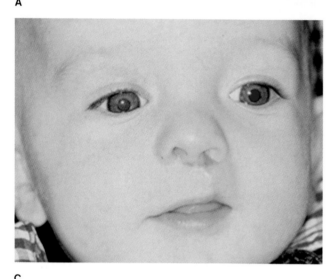

C

Figure 47–3. Infant with complete unilateral left cleft lip and palate. (A) Defect prior to orthopedic intervention. (B) Presurgical orthopedics with lip taping to approximate the segments. (C) Postsurgical result of definitive lip repair.

orthopedics as part of comprehensive team management of infants born with clefts of the lip and palate. The study compared the effect of infant orthopedics on maxillary arch dimensions, demonstrating that infant orthopedics only had a temporary effect.[10] A later report on the effect of infant orthopedics on feeding, weight, and length indicated that no significant effect could be found between the two randomized groups on feeding, nutritional status, or somatic growth.[11] This RCT is continuing to follow these infants longitudinally to comprehensively evaluate outcome variables such as facial and dental development, speech outcome, and cost effectiveness.

If neonatal orthopedics is recommended, it is completed in the first few months after birth so that definitive surgical lip repair can be achieved in the first 6 months of life. Palate repair is usually delayed until the infant is 12–18 months of age. There remains some controversy with respect to the balance between restoration of palatal anatomy, so as to optimize palatal function for speech, and the effects of postsurgical scar tissue formation on the growth and development of the nasomaxillary complex. Ross[12] evaluated the outcome of both active and passive presurgical appliances in

children with unilateral cleft lip and palate (UCLP) at age 10. Results in these two groups were compared to those of age-matched untreated subjects with UCLP. This cephalometric study of facial growth reported no beneficial long-term effect of neonatal orthopedics. Indeed, there were some negative effects observed in those children who had received extraoral strapping.

PRIMARY DENTITION

The primary dentition has usually fully erupted by the time the child is 2½ to 3 years of age. At this age, the facial soft tissues may mask an underlying skeletal deficiency (Fig. 47–4). As the toddler grows into a young child, growth of the nasomaxillary complex lags behind that of the mandible, resulting in increased relative midface deficiency. This may be reflected in the dentition by inevitable crossbites, both anterior and/or posterior. Cases of bilateral cleft lip and palate may present severe constriction of the posterior segments and protrusion/extrusion of the premaxillary segment (Fig. 47–5). The unilateral or bilateral crossbite may be associated

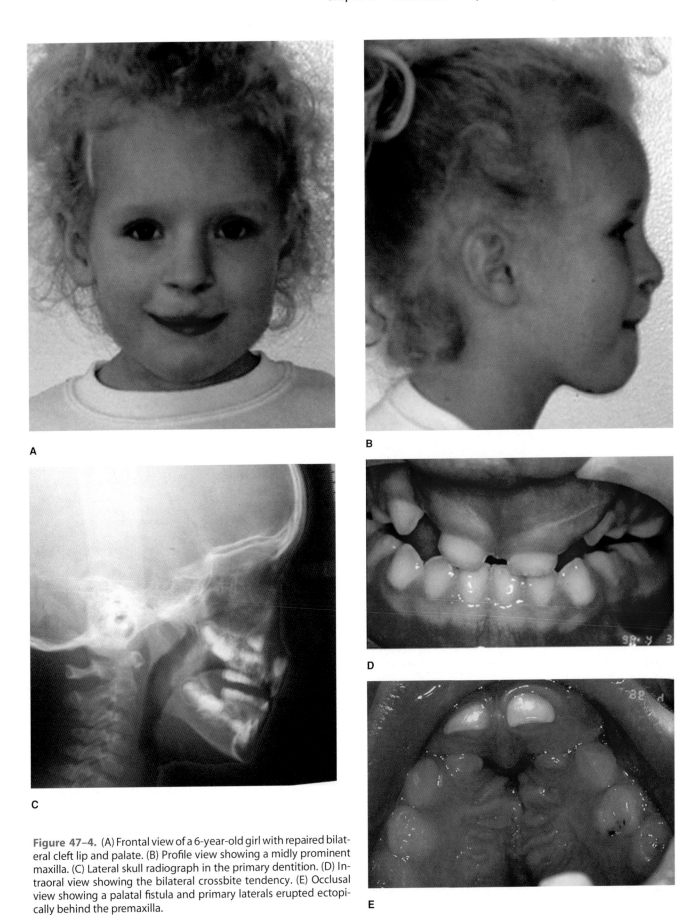

Figure 47–4. (A) Frontal view of a 6-year-old girl with repaired bilateral cleft lip and palate. (B) Profile view showing a midly prominent maxilla. (C) Lateral skull radiograph in the primary dentition. (D) Intraoral view showing the bilateral crossbite tendency. (E) Occlusal view showing a palatal fistula and primary laterals erupted ectopically behind the premaxilla.

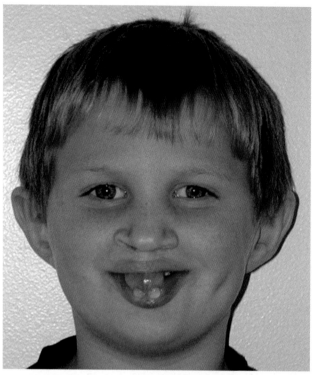

A

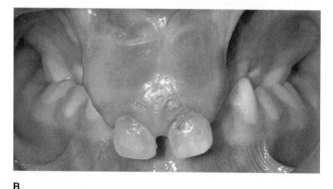

B

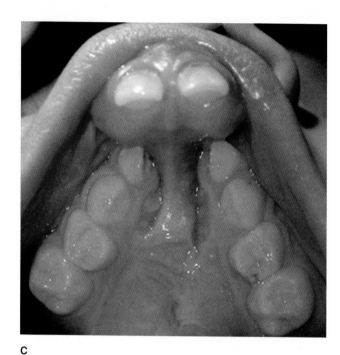

C

Figure 47–5. (A) Five-year-old boy with repaired complete bilateral cleft lip and palate and severe extrusion of the premaxillary segment. (B) Frontal intraoral view showing premaxillary segment out of the vertical plane of occlusion. (C) Maxillary occlusal view showing severe constriction of posterior segments and extrusion of the premaxillary segment. (*Reprinted from Vig KWL, Mercado AM. The orthodontist's role in a cleft palate-craniofacial team. In Graber TM, Vanarsdall RL, Vig KWL (eds). Orthodontics: Current Principles and Techniques, pp. 1097–1121. Copyright 2005, with permission from Elsevier.*)

with a functional mandibular shift, which is an early indicator for orthodontic treatment in the primary dentition. However, as the crossbite is likely to recur with the eruption of the permanent successors, a decision may be made to postpone orthodontic intervention until the mixed dentition.

Constriction of the dental arch is manifested in both the transverse and sagittal dimensions of the maxilla. Early skeletal midface deficiency has been treated with some success in the primary or early mixed dentition by a protraction face mask (Figs. 47–6 and 47–7). Whereas the occlusal correction includes dentoalveolar proclination of the incisors, the modification and redirection of the skeletal midface deficiency may be transitory. Continued poor growth of the nasomaxillary complex results in failure of the midface to keep up with normal mandibular growth. Consequently, malocclusion is re-established during the late mixed dentition and into the early permanent dentition. Long-term follow up[13] indicates that there is a biological variability in response to the protraction facemask. The most logical time for the in-

tervention is before 10 years of age, a time during which the circum-maxillary sutures are more responsive. However, a severe malocclusion in the primary or early mixed dentition is unlikely to be corrected with growth modification, and may then simply become a costly and unnecessary burden to the patient, one with questionable and often transient benefit. In such severe malocclusions, skeletal correction should be delayed until the permanent dentition stage, a time when comprehensive orthodontics in combination with orthognathic surgery or distraction osteogenesis may be a more predictable option.

MIXED DENTITION

The transition in the child's dental development occurs between 6 and 12 years of age as the primary dentition is exfoliated and the permanent teeth erupt. Eruption of the permanent teeth coincides with a period of psychosocial transition

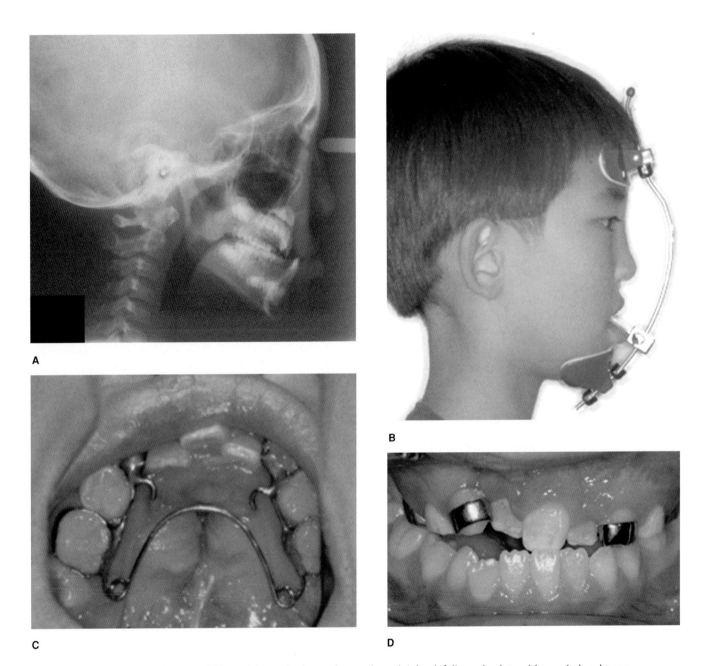

Figure 47–6. Eight-year-old boy with repaired complete unilateral right cleft lip and palate with saggital and transverse maxillary deficiency. (A) Lateral skull radiograph – note the 7 mm reverse overjet. (B) Protraction facemask with elastics attached to palatal hooks on expander. (C) Palatal expander with bands cemented on the maxillary second primary molars and canines with palatal hooks to attach elastics. (D) Lateral and anterior crossbites improving with palatal expansion and maxillary and dental protraction. (*Reprinted from Vig KWL, Mercado AM. The orthodontist's role in a cleft palate-craniofacial team. In Graber TM, Vanarsdall RL, Vig KWL (eds). Orthodontics: Current Principles and Techniques, pp. 1097–1121. Copyright 2005, with permission from Elsevier.*)

during preadolescence when the degree of friendship intimacy intensifies and independence from parents increases.[14] In preadolescents with craniofacial anomalies, the dissatisfaction with appearance is related to social withdrawal, social anxiety, and self-consciousness.[15] This is also the period when the greatest advances have been made in restoring bone in the cleft site with secondary alveolar bone grafts, treatment which improves the periodontal support of teeth adjacent to the cleft site, thus eliminating the need for extraction and prosthetic replacement of compromised teeth.

The orofacial cleft disrupts the dental lamina in the cleft site so that the developing permanent teeth may be missing, malformed, or supernumerary. The incisors adjacent to the cleft site may be misplaced, rotated, malformed, or hypoplastic, with an absence of bone in the cleft site for the permanent lateral incisor and canine to erupt (Figs. 47–8 and 47–9). Alveolar bone grafts restore the continuity of the alveolar ridge and allow closure of oronasal fistulae. Transverse maxillary constriction is a consequence of scar tissue following surgical repair of the secondary palate, resulting in a characteristic

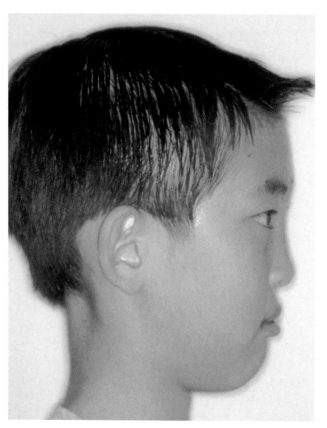

A

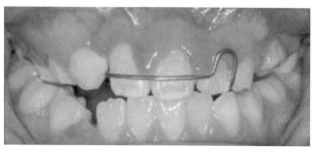

B

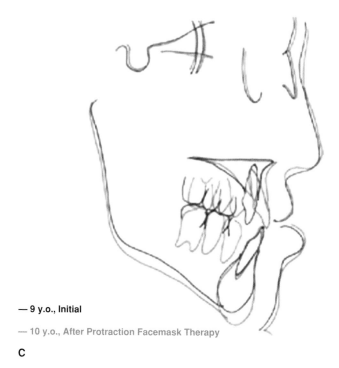

— **9 y.o., Initial**

— 10 y.o., After Protraction Facemask Therapy

C

Figure 47–7. (A) Facial profile of same patient as Figure 47–6, after 9 months of protraction facemask therapy and palatal expansion. (B) Intraoral view with correction of anterior and posterior crossbite, maxillary retainer in place. (C) Superimposition of initial and post-protraction lateral cephalogram tracings showing correction of reverse overjet by incisor proclination and mild maxillary advancement. (*Reprinted from Vig KWL, Mercado AM. The orthodontist's role in a cleft palate-craniofacial team. In Graber TM, Vanarsdall RL, Vig KWL (eds). Orthodontics: Current Principles and Techniques, pp. 1097–1121. Copyright 2005, with permission from Elsevier.*)

omega or V-shaped arch form which is reflected in anterior and posterior dental crossbites (Fig. 47–8D). With the eruption of the first permanent molars and incisors, a maxillary expansion appliance is often recommended. Collaboration between the surgeon and the orthodontist in the mixed dentition is aimed to coordinate the treatment sequence that will ultimately result in a successful alveolar bone graft with healthy adjacent teeth.

■ ALVEOLAR BONE GRAFTING

Primary Bone Grafting

Primary grafting typically involves the placing of bone in the neonatal cleft site at the time of primary surgical lip repair and, thus, before eruption of the primary incisors. Although some teams in the US are advocates of early bone grafting,[16]

most cleft palate teams prefer to delay bone graft placement until further maxillary growth and development has occurred.[17]

Secondary Bone Grafting

Secondary, or delayed, alveolar bone grafting is performed after primary lip repair and is classified according to the age at which the bone graft is placed: *early* secondary bone grafting (2–5 years), *intermediate secondary* bone grafting (6–15 years), or *late* secondary bone grafting (adolescence to adulthood). The principles of secondary bone grafting were first introduced by Boyne and Sands.[18,19] In 1986, Bergland and coworkers studied 378 consecutive patients who had undergone secondary alveolar bone grafting, noting that the best outcomes were achieved in cases wherein the bone graft was performed prior to the eruption of the maxillary canine.[20] This report was followed by a cephalometric study from the same

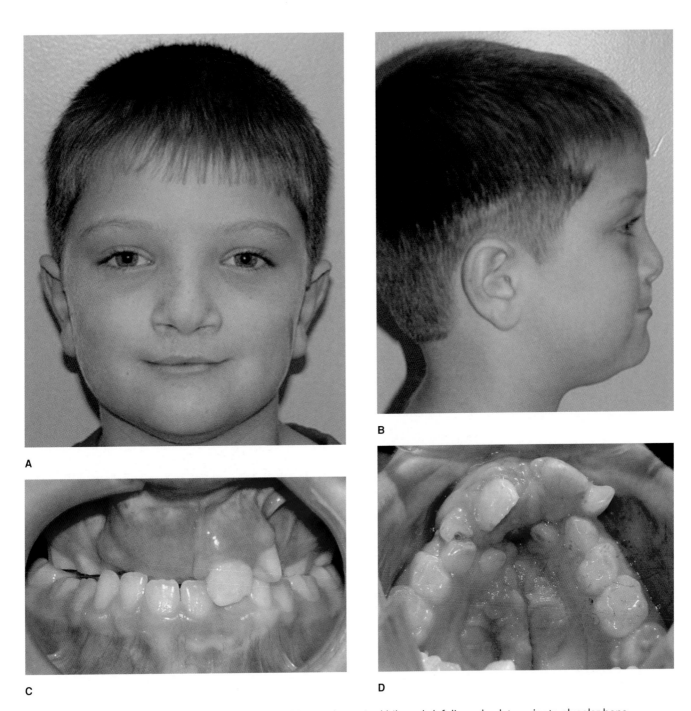

Figure 47–8. (A) Frontal view of a 7-year-old boy with repaired bilateral cleft lip and palate, prior to alveolar bone grafting. (B) Profile view showing straight profile. (C) Intraoral view in occlusion, showing partial anterior crossbite, posterior crossbites, and rotated incisor. (D) Maxillary occlusal view showing constricted posterior segments, prominent premaxilla, supernumerary lateral incisors located palatally, and decayed primary incisors. Patient needs maxillary expansion prior to bone grafting to improve the alignment of posterior segments with the premaxilla, selected extractions, restorative care, and a bite plane to relief traumatic occlusion on the premaxilla.

center that compared maxillary growth in children who received secondary alveolar bone grafting between the ages of 8 and 12 years to the maxillary growth in nongrafted children.[21] The study demonstrated no adverse effect of bone grafting on anteroposterior or vertical maxillary growth, a finding attributed to the postponement of grafting until most of the growth of the anterior maxilla had ceased and to the ability

of the grafted tissue to develop vertically with the alveolus.[21] Since these landmark articles, current opinion supports the *intermediate* period as the most appropriate time for grafting. This practice has the greatest benefits and least risk for interfering with midfacial and skeletodental growth and development. Current research also supports the above contentions. Levitt et al. (1999)[22] demonstrated that there were no

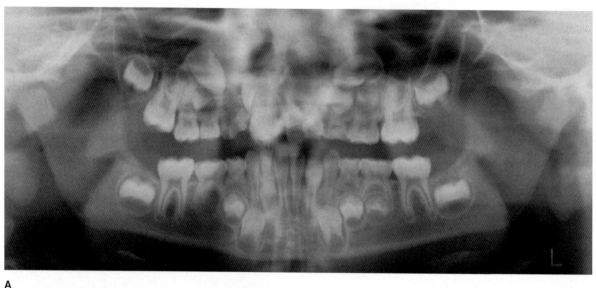

A

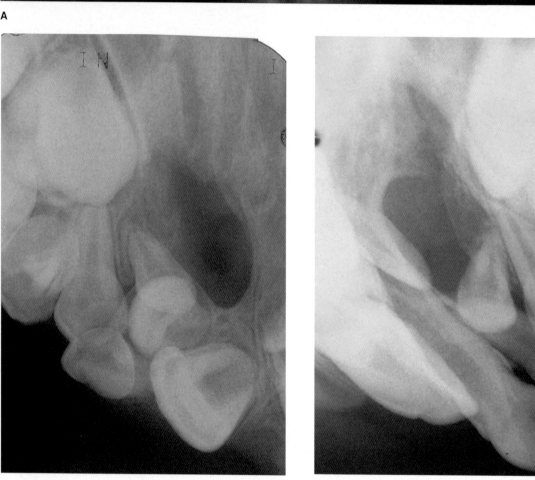

B   C

Figure 47–9. (A) Panoramic radiograph of the same child as Figure 47–8. Maxillary and mandibular right second premolars are missing. (B) Right oblique occlusal radiograph (through the cleft) shows the bony defect and a permanent lateral incisor developing in the premaxilla. (C) Left oblique occlusal radiograph shows the bony defect and contralateral lateral incisor. The left permanent lateral incisor is missing.

significant differences in maxillary sagittal or vertical growth following secondary bone grafting in patients with complete unilateral cleft lip and palate when compared to nongrafted patients with similar clefts. The multicenter Eurocleft study of treatment outcomes in patients with complete cleft lip and palate compared craniofacial form in individuals treated at five European centers.[23] The only center performing primary bone grafting obtained less favorable results in vertical maxillary growth, soft tissue sagittal relationships, and soft tissue facial proportions than the centers performing secondary bone

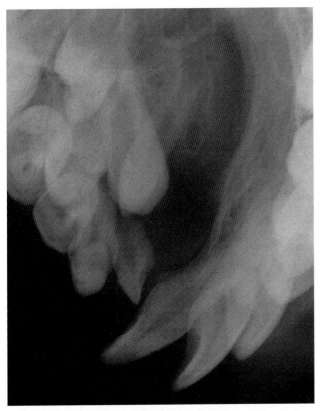

A

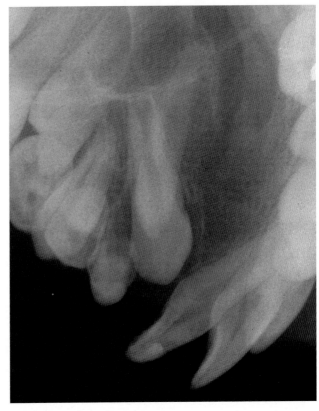

B

Figure 47–10. Periapical radiograph of bone defect at the cleft site prior to alveolar bone grafting. Transposed lateral incisor and canine have more than two-thirds of the roots developed (close to eruption). Note the thin layer of bone covering the adjacent central incisor. No orthodontic incisor alignment is planned. (B) Periapical radiograph taken 4 months after alveolar bone grafting, showing excellent fill of cleft defect with cancellous bone. Canine is erupting through the grafted bone.

grafting between the ages of 8 and 11. Moreover, the center performing primary bone grafting obtained the least favorable dental arch relationships, with almost 50% of the patients requiring surgical correction of Class III malocclusion at 17 years of age.[24] In light of these reports, it is not surprising that a recent survey of alveolar bone grafting among ACPA teams across North America revealed that most of the centers perform intermediate or secondary alveolar bone grafting.[17] The following discussion will therefore focus on intermediate or secondary alveolar bone grafting.

Benefits of Secondary Alveolar Bone Grafting

i) *Provision of bone for eruption of teeth in the line of the cleft.* A bone graft placed before the eruption of the teeth adjacent to the cleft (especially the lateral or canine when located on the posterior segment) provides a bony matrix to enable the eruption of these teeth into a continuous alveolar ridge, generating additional alveolar bone in the area[20] (Fig. 47–10). Generally, grafting is done prior to the eruption of the permanent maxillary canine on the cleft side, which is usually located in the maxillary segment posterior to the cleft.

ii) *Provision of bone for teeth adjacent to the cleft.* Teeth directly adjacent to the cleft, particularly maxillary central

or lateral incisors located on the proximal (mesial) segment, erupt into unfavorable positions. They are often ectopic, rotated, or unfavorably inclined. This malposition is usually a reflection of the anatomy of the alveolar cleft, which is usually narrower on the occlusal side and wider on the nasal aspect, thus limiting the amount of bone support of the teeth, especially on their distal aspects (directly facing the bony defect). Radiographs of these teeth show a thin layer of cortical bone along their distal surface (see Fig. 47–10), which may be at risk of resorption if nonjudicious presurgical orthodontic alignment is done. If a bone graft is placed before extensive orthodontic alignment of erupted teeth adjacent to the cleft, crestal bone heights are preserved, and postsurgical orthodontic alignment can be accomplished with minimal risk of bone resorption while ensuring adequate bony coverage of the roots.

iii) *Closure of oro-nasal fistulae.* Oronasal fistulae can lead to nasal air escape with speech and can contribute to velopharyngeal dysfunction in patients with cleft lip and palate.[25] Moreover, unrepaired fistulae may allow for chronic nasal leakage of food and fluids and thereby to chronic nasal irritation. Surgical closure of oronasal fistulae at the time of secondary alveolar bone grafting eliminates this problem and can result in a significant improvement of speech, manifested as decreased nasality and nasal emission postoperatively.[26]

iv) *Provision of alar base support and elevation on the cleft side.* Alveolar bone grafting contributes to improved nasal and lip symmetry by providing a stable platform upon which the nasal structures rest.[27]

v) *Re-establishment of maxillary alveolar ridge continuity.* Following successful bone grafting, the orthodontist can move the teeth bodily and upright roots into the cleft site without risk of compromising their periodontal support.[20,28] In addition, the prosthodontist can create a more esthetic and hygienic prosthesis to replace missing teeth in the cleft area.[28] Insertion of endosseous implants into the grafted cleft is possible and provides functional stimulation to the transplanted bone.[3,29]

vi) *Stabilization of maxillary segments.* Patients with bilateral clefts present with varying degrees of mobility of the premaxilla, which usually remains unstable throughout life.[20] In such cases, secondary alveolar bone grafting stabilizes the premaxilla, allowing patients to have functional incisors with adequate stability to serve as abutments for fixed prostheses.[20,28]

Dental/Orthodontic Considerations Associated with Secondary Bone Grafting

Timing

The time to perform secondary alveolar bone grafting can be established according to the chronological age of the patient or, alternatively, according to dental development as defined by the stage of root development.

- *Chronological age.* By definition, secondary bone grafting is performed in the mixed dentition prior to the eruption of the maxillary canine (or lateral, if located in the posterior segment). Once teeth have erupted into the cleft site, their limited periodontal support will not improve with a graft since the transplanted bone will not adhere to the tooth surface.[30] The height of the crest of alveolar bone eventually resorbs to its original level. It is therefore essential to complete grafting prior to eruption of the permanent teeth adjacent to the cleft. This period may encompass a range of several years, from ages 6 to 15, and it is during this period that bone grafting has a high success rate. It has been shown, however, that the older the patient at the time of surgery, the poorer the outcomes of secondary bone grafting.[31] Therefore, the available evidence supports an optimum age at which patients should receive bone grafts. Using chronological age alone for defining the optimum age for grafting may not be clinically valid, since patients with cleft lip and/or palate have delayed development of the teeth compared to individuals with no clefts.[32] Moreover, teeth adjacent to the cleft side demonstrate more developmental delay than the contralateral teeth of the same patient.[32] Dental development represents a more accurate indicator of the optimum timing for the bone grafting procedure rather than chronological age alone.

- *Maxillary canine development.* One developmental indicator that has been proposed for establishing the optimum timing for grafting is the extent of root formation of the permanent maxillary canine on the cleft side. It has been recommended that the optimal timing for secondary grafting is when the maxillary canine has developed 1/2 to 2/3 of its final length, which generally occurs between the ages of 8 and 11 years (see Fig. 47–10).[28,33] When the root has developed 2/3 of its expected full length, there is accelerated eruption of the canine. The tooth can then erupt spontaneously through the graft, bringing additional alveolar bone into the area. In a retrospective study of patients with nonsyndromic unilateral cleft lip and palate, Mercado et al. (2006) demonstrated that there is a significant positive correlation between stage of canine root development at the time of surgery and the outcome of alveolar bone grafting.[34]

- *Maxillary lateral incisor development.* A recent study of patients with unilateral cleft lip and palate demonstrated that the cleft-side permanent lateral incisor was present in 50.2% of patients.[35] Of these patients, 76.5% had the permanent lateral incisor located on the posterior segment, distal to the cleft.[35] When the maxillary lateral incisor is located in the posterior segment, there is generally insufficient alveolar bone adjacent to the cleft to support the lateral incisor as it drifts anteriorly and occlusally along its eruptive path into the arch. In such cases, it may be advisable to graft prior to the eruption of the lateral incisor in order to improve the prognosis for this tooth.[36,37] The developmental indicator of 1/2 to 2/3 canine root formation for timing of an alveolar bone graft may prove to be too late when the aim is to preserve an existing lateral incisor. Lilja et al. (2000) discourage the use of root formation as an indicator for bone graft placement, proposing the assessment of the thickness of bone covering the crown (of the lateral incisor or canine) to determine timing of bone grafting.[38] They advocate that bone grafting be completed when there is a thin layer of bone covering the tooth distal to the cleft. Other studies have reported no significant relationship between the degree of radiographic canine eruption through the alveolar cleft and the outcome of secondary bone grafting.[39,40]

Sequencing

The sequencing of procedures associated with alveolar bone grafting requires interdisciplinary communication and cooperation for a successful outcome. Orthodontists, general/pediatric dentists, oral and plastic surgeons intervene at coordinated times to ensure that one discipline's efforts do not interfere, delay, or jeopardize those of the others. Parents and caregivers may be concerned about teeth (often supernumerary) that have erupted near the cleft either palatally or high in the labial vestibule. Ectopic teeth present a challenge for the parents and patient to maintain in good hygiene due to their location and limited accessibility. The role of the general or pediatric dentist is to ensure that patient and parents are aware of the ectopic teeth and instructed on good oral hygiene practices in order to maintain them free of decay, to keep

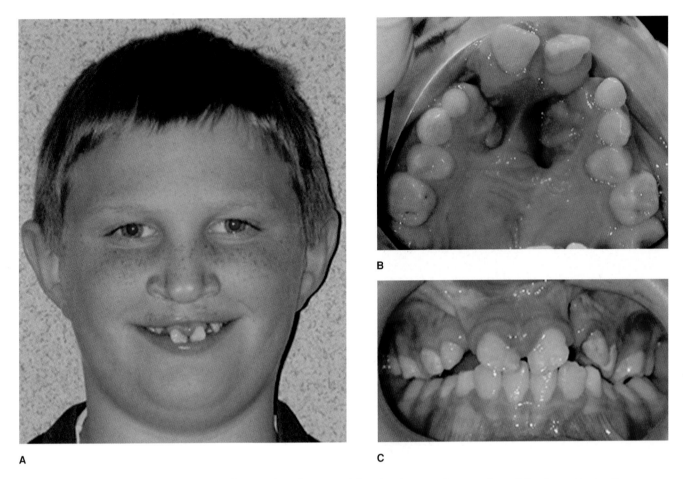

Figure 47–11. (A) Same patient illustrated in Figure 47–5, hereby shown at 9 years of age following orthodontic treatment to expand maxilla and intrude premaxilla. Note the improved facial esthetics. (B) Maxillary occlusal view showing adequate expansion of posterior segments in alignment with the premaxilla. Patient is ready for alveolar bone grafting. (C) Frontal intraoral view showing improved vertical alignment of premaxilla with posterior segments. Permanent lateral incisors are congenitally missing.

them out of traumatic occlusion, and to prevent them from contributing to traumatic ulcerations of the surrounding mucosa. Preservation of these teeth prior to surgery maintains the supporting alveolus. The general or pediatric dentist should restore any decayed teeth adjacent to the cleft prior to the grafting procedure. On the other hand, erupted teeth adjacent to the cleft that have poor periodontal or restorative prognosis should be extracted at least 2 months prior to surgery in order to allow the soft tissues to heal (see Fig. 47–8). Healthy ectopic primary or supernumerary teeth that have erupted along the line of the cleft should also be removed at least 2 months prior to surgery so that intact mucosal flaps may be reflected, positioned, and sutured over the graft. Orthodontic treatment may be required presurgically to reposition maxillary teeth that are in traumatic occlusion or to expand a severely constricted maxilla, thereby providing the surgeon better access to the cleft defect. In bilateral cases, a mobile premaxilla with anterior traumatic occlusion may need to be relieved with a posterior bite plane to minimize mobility during the healing period, as such may compromise the success of the grafts.[30] A severely extruded maxilla may need to be intruded to level it with the posterior segments (Figs. 47–5, 47–11). Other sur-

gical procedures, such as minor esthetic revisions of the nose and lip, as well as the insertion of tympanostomy tubes, can be undertaken at the time of the alveolar bone grafting.

The Transverse Dimension

A maxillary expansion appliance is often recommended before alveolar bone graft placement in order to improve the alignment of the posterior segments with the premaxillary segment (Figs. 47–8, 47–12). Care should be taken not to expand the maxillary arch to correct the dental crossbite relationship without prior consultation with the surgeon who will be placing the secondary alveolar bone graft, as adequate soft tissue will be required to close the site. Although some clinicians favor presurgical maxillary expansion for better access to the cleft and for improved hygiene of adjacent teeth, overexpansion to achieve complete correction of posterior crossbite may be counterproductive, especially in patients with large cleft defects. If the orthodontist expands the dental arch to eliminate the crossbite, the width of the alveolar cleft may increase as well, as may the size of the oronasal fistula. As a result, the patient may face an increased risk of postoperative wound dehiscence, compromised healing, and graft loss, as

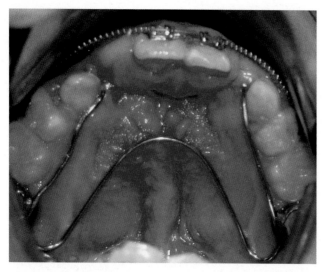

A

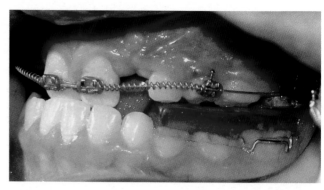

B

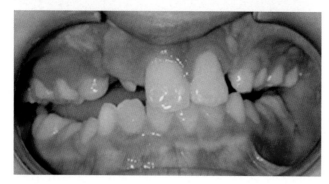

C

Figure 47–12. (A) Occlusal view of the same patient as Figures 47–8 and 47–9, after maxillary expansion and successful alveolar bone grafting. (B) Buccal view showing limited orthodontic treatment to procline maxillary incisors and correct the anterior crossbite. Posterior bite plane is in place. (C) Frontal view after orthodontic treatment. Hawley retainer was delivered and the use of bite plane was discontinued to allow eruption of posterior teeth. Maxillary right lateral incisor is erupting.

well as relapse of the transverse maxillary collapse and resulting posterior crossbite.

When maxillary expansion is needed in the mixed dentition prior to alveolar bone grafting, a Quad Helix or W-arch appliance is cemented to the first permanent molars (Fig. 47–6C). The appliance has lateral arms that extend anteriorly and that can be adjusted for differential expansion along the arch. Finger springs can be added to move incisors out of traumatic occlusion while simultaneously expanding the posterior segments. These appliances provide a slow and continuous force that is often sufficient to achieve expansion of the maxillary segments, since the main resistance to expansion is the scar tissue within the secondary palate. Palatal scar tissue is allowed to gradually stretch and reorganize as the slow expansion proceeds. Separation of the maxillary segments will occur at the point of least resistance, which pre-surgically is located at the cleft alveolus and palate. Following placement of the alveolar bone graft, a passive maxillary expander, palatal arch, or heavy labial archwire ligated to brackets should be placed in order to retain the expansion during the healing period. If more expansion is needed in the young permanent dentition after bone grafting, a rapid maxillary expander with a palatal jackscrew can be used (Fig. 47–13). Cavassan et al. (2004) have shown that rapid maxillary expansion after secondary bone grafting of the maxilla obtains separation of the intermaxillary suture.[41] This has been confirmed both clinically

by the opening of a diastema between the maxillary central incisors and radiographically by the sagittal opening of the intermaxillary suture anterior to the cleft secondary palate.

Incisor Alignment

The position of the incisors adjacent to the cleft, characterized clinically by rotations and tipping, is a reflection of the limited amount of bone covering their roots, as seen radiographically. When the malposition of incisors results in traumatic occlusion or in limited access for surgical manipulation of the cleft, the orthodontist in consultation with the surgeon may decide to perform some degree of orthodontic alignment of such teeth. Another indication for performing limited, controlled incisor alignment prior to grafting is to address the patient's esthetic concerns related to the display of rotated or tipped teeth when smiling. Orthodontic alignment of incisors must be limited by the available bone into which the teeth can be moved. Uprighting of tipped incisors in the mesio-distal dimension should be kept to a minimum to prevent moving the apical portion of the root into the cleft site.[30] Similarly, rotating a crown into its ideal orientation will increase the mesio-distal dimension of bone that it occupies, resulting in loss of alveolar bone height at the level of the cemento–enamel junction.[30] If the erupted teeth adjacent to the cleft have low levels of crestal bone support prior to surgery, the alveolar bone graft will quickly resorb to the level of the pre-existing

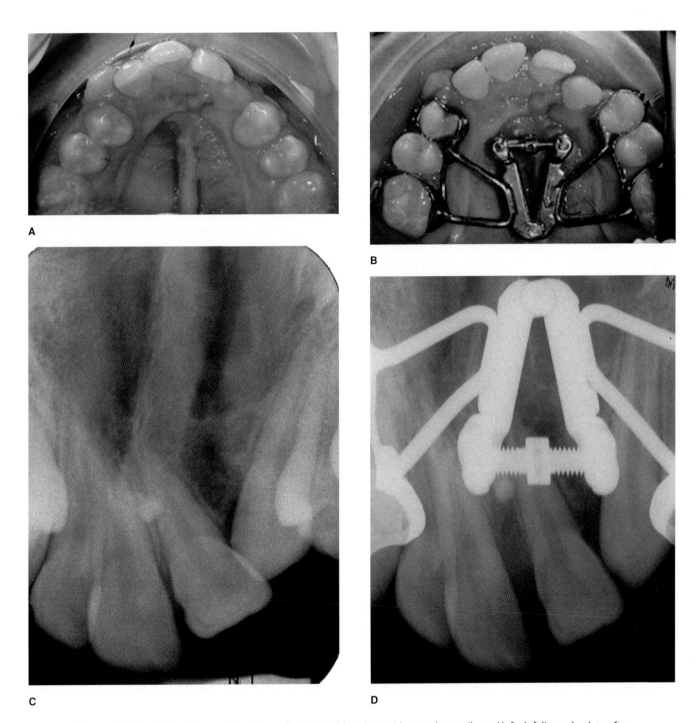

Figure 47–13. (A) Maxillary occlusal view of 10-year-old patient with complete unilateral left cleft lip and palate after alveolar bone grafting. Note constriction of premolar regions. (B) Palatal Spider¤ (Leone S.P.A. Orthodontic Products, Oxnard, CA) cemented: activation of the screw system produces differential expansion in the premolar and canine regions while pivoting around a posterior hinge next to the molars. Note the midline diastema between maxillary central incisors. (C) Periapical radiograph prior to expansion. Note excellent bony fill of left alveolar cleft. (D) Periapical radiograph during rapid maxillary expansion showing evidence of opening of the intermaxillary suture and intact grafted area.

crest without improving its height. It has been demonstrated that presurgical levels of bone on the dental surfaces directly adjacent to the cleft are correlated with the outcome of the secondary alveolar bone graft.[42] Following evidence of successful consolidation of the graft, which should be visible radiographically within 8 weeks, orthodontic movement of

teeth adjacent to the cleft is resumed.[30] Early movement of the roots into the grafted bone appears clinically to consolidate the alveolar bone and improve the crestal height.[29] Alignment of malposed incisors shortly after successful healing of the bone graft contributes to improved oral hygiene and a positive patient's self-perception.

Eruption of the Maxillary Canine

Following surgery, the maxillary canine erupts through the grafted bone (Fig. 47–10). Removal of unerupted supernumerary teeth is usually performed at the time that the bone graft is placed in order to create an unobstructed path for eruption for the canine. With orthodontic movement, enough space is created in the arch to allow the canines to erupt after bone grafting. Often the canine will erupt spontaneously following the bone graft, and there are many reports of eruption rates as high as 80–97%.[18,20,28,43] In the late mixed dentition and when more than 2/3 of the root length has developed, a canine that does not show signs of spontaneous eruption over a reasonable period of time (4–6 months) will need to be surgically uncovered. This will facilitate its eruption, with or without orthodontic traction, into the arch.

Absence of the Maxillary Lateral Incisor

Numerous studies have shown that there is a high incidence of congenitally missing lateral incisors in patients with cleft lip and palate. Even when the lateral incisors are present, they may need to be extracted early in cases of nonrestorable decay, severe crown/root malformations, or poor periodontal support. Therefore, many children reach the age of secondary bone grafting with an absence of the maxillary lateral incisor next to the cleft. In these cases, the canine is allowed to erupt adjacent to the central incisors following bone grafting. The canine brings more alveolar bone into the area, consolidating the graft and preserving the width of the alveolar ridge. Several studies[29,44] have demonstrated that patients with cleft lip and palate who had secondary alveolar bone grafting followed by orthodontic gap closure had better bone height of the grafted area and improved osseous support of the cleft-adjacent teeth compared to patients whose space was preserved for insertion of a prosthetic bridge. This is likely due to functional stress on the grafted bone exerted by the teeth located in the grafted area as well as by the adjacent teeth, preventing progressive resorption of the graft. Closing the edentulous space with mesial eruption of the canine, mesial movement of posterior teeth, and cosmetic "re-shaping" of the canine precludes the need for a prosthetic replacement of the absent lateral incisor. Other functional and cosmetic considerations related to "canine substitution" of the lateral incisor will be addressed below.

Assessing the Outcome of Secondary Bone Grafting

As with any other health care intervention, the results of secondary alveolar bone grafting require systematic evaluation of outcome in the context of the risk, benefit, and cost. In the assessment of success or failure of an alveolar bone graft, it is imperative to have objective measures or scales to accurately and consistently evaluate the volume of bone in the cleft and the amount of bone coverage for the adjacent teeth and the teeth migrating into the cleft. Several assessments have been reported in an effort to quantitatively describe the bone available following a bone graft. Current methods include conventional radiography, conventional computer-assisted tomography (CT scans), and cone beam computerized tomography (CBCT scans).

Radiographic Appearance of the Bone

Occlusal and periapical radiographs are similarly reproducible for assessing the quality of alveolar bone grafts.[45] However, there are limitations and inconsistencies on the information that can be derived from such radiographs. First, the radiographic method relies on a two-dimensional representation of the three-dimensional cleft area. The anteroposterior depth of the alveolus is not captured, making assessment of surfaces or structures along the bucco-palatal plane impossible. In the horizontal plane, medio-lateral assessments are limited by the superimposition of adjacent structures along the curvature of the arch. In the vertical plane, there are often size errors and distortions due to elongation or foreshortening of the exposed structures. Additionally, variations in the technique of exposure and/or chemical developing of the film may affect the contrast of the resultant radiograph, making it difficult to locate landmarks and to assess the density of bone. Nevertheless, the use of dental radiographs is considered a standard of care because it is a relatively noninvasive, circumscribed, efficient, and economical method. Several outcome scales have been proposed for radiographic evaluation of alveolar bone grafting. The original method described by Bergland et al. in 1986 relies on semi-quantitative evaluation of the height of the interalveolar septum achieved in relation to the CEJ of adjacent teeth.[20] Four outcome groups are described, including Type I (approximately normal), Type II (height at least $3/4$ of normal), Type III (height less than $3/4$ of normal), and Type IV (failure). A prerequisite of this technique is the presence of the canine (or lateral incisor) adjacent to the cleft brought into its final position in the maxillary arch. The Bergland scale produces categorical data that can be analyzed using nonparametric statistical methods. However, defects in the bone fill at the level of the root apex are not assessed. Other semi-quantitative radiographic scales have been developed which allow the evaluation of the bone on the nasal aspect of the graft[31,46–48] and which can be used both in the mixed and permanent dentition. Long et al. (1995) developed a quantitative method in which a direct measurement is taken from the radiograph and all measurements are converted to ratios using the various measures of alveolar bone height and root length.[43] The resultant ratios are suitable for parametric statistical analysis. It is possible to establish the bony coverage of the root of the teeth adjacent to the cleft, including coverage at the apical level.

Computer-Assisted Tomography (CT Scans)

The primary advantage of CT assessment is its ability to delineate the bone graft in three dimensions, thereby allowing the evaluation of bone volumes. It provides information on the amount of bone in the buccopalatal direction at different axial levels. Moreover, the size of the defect and the position of teeth next to the cleft can be assessed more accurately than with conventional radiography. This information is valuable for diagnostic assessment prior to orthodontic movement of adjacent teeth into the cleft, eruption of an unerupted canine through the graft, or insertion of dental implants in the grafted area. The major disadvantage of using CT scans is the high amount of radiation exposure to the patient. Other disadvantages include the cost of the procedure, considerable physical space required for the apparatus, and more limited accessibility. The technique is also time consuming, since the multiple slices captured by the detector screens need to be stacked to obtain a complete image.[49]

Cone Beam Computerized Tomography (CBCT)

This technology is different from conventional CT devices in that a single rotation of the radiation source is able to capture an entire region of interest without having to stack multiple slices. The advantages include a much lower radiation dose and higher resolution compared to conventional, spiral CT scans due to a more focused beam and less scatter radiation.[50] The total radiation delivered is approximately 20% of conventional CT scans and is comparable to a full mouth periapical radiographic exposure.[51] The apparatus is less expensive and occupies a smaller space than conventional CT apparatus. Wörtche et al. (2006) demonstrated that CBCT can also be used prior to alveolar bone grafting, rendering two-dimensional sections through the cleft area in both the axial and coronal planes, as well as a three-dimensional reconstruction to delineate the anatomy of the alveolus, facial bones, and palate.[52] Preliminary studies by Hamada et al. (2005) have shown that limited cone beam CT apparatus are also suitable for clinical assessment of alveolar bone grafting.[50] Their CBCT apparatus (Dental 3D-CT) made it possible to measure the vertical and buccal-palatal width of the bone bridge from the images using a millimeter ruler on the film. These measurements were helpful in determining the optimal size of the dental implant and the need for additional alveolar ridge augmentation. CBCT is therefore a very promising tool for the three-dimensional evaluation of the cleft, the alveolar bone graft, and the adjacent structures. Certainly, further investigation is needed to develop valid and reproducible quantitative measures that would justify application of CBCT to the assessment of outcomes of alveolar bone grafting.

PERMANENT DENTITION

The permanent dentition is established with the eruption of the canines and premolars. Generally, the establishment of the young permanent dentition coincides with the somatic changes of puberty. Secondary sexual characteristics are noticeable, such as facial hair and voice changes in males and breast development in females. A growth spurt occurs, characterized by an acceleration followed by a deceleration in height, with growth of the long bones as well as many internal organs. Craniofacial growth includes an increase in

mandibular growth, which accentuates the skeletal discrepancy and compromises both facial appearance and occlusal relationships (Fig. 47–14). With such changes in facial appearance, many patients have a special need for early intervention by the surgeons and orthodontists.

Increased self-consciousness is normal during adolescence, but it may become more intense when a teen has a visible facial difference.[53] Facial scars, asymmetry, and maxillo/mandibular discrepancies may affect the way that the adolescent perceives him/herself and may influence social interactions. Decisions related to the surgical and orthodontic care of the cleft may create additional tensions for teens at a time when they are dealing with issues of self esteem, identity, independence, and sociability, all of which contribute to their quality of life.

Management of Maxillo/Mandibular Discrepancies

Skeletal-Facial Considerations in Esthetics

It is critical to examine the patient's facial balance and proportions when developing a treatment plan that will potentially combine surgery and orthodontics. A systematic clinical evaluation is superior to two-dimensional photographs and should be carried out with the patient standing so that the overall stature and posture can be taken into consideration. Full-face and profile assessments will provide the clinician with information in all three dimensions, both in the resting position and in occlusion. Further information is derived from cephalometric analysis and prediction tracings, helping to determine whether a patient can be treated by orthodontics alone to camouflage a mild skeletal discrepancy or by an orthognathic surgical procedure in more severe cases.

Patients with unilateral complete clefts of the lip and palate typically develop increased maxillary deficiency and relative mandibular prognathism as they reach adolescence and into adulthood. This is a result of a deficiency in sagittal maxillary growth, resulting in a concave facial profile (Figs. 47–14 and 47–15). As vertical maxillary growth is also deficient, the resulting overclosure of the mandible to achieve occlusion of the teeth accentuates the Class III malocclusion. The clinician should evaluate the extent of overclosure contributing to the Class III relationship by measuring the interocclusal clearance at the premolar region with the patient at rest. Maxillary deficiency in the sagittal plane may accentuate discrepancies in the transverse plane, resulting in posterior crossbites. Plaster study models provide three-dimensional information to evaluate the dentition and to allow differentiation between a crossbite due to maxillary constriction, to maxillary retrusion, or to a combination of both.

Patients with mild skeletal discrepancies and minimal esthetic concerns may benefit from dental compensation by orthodontic treatment alone. A change in axial inclination of the teeth (proclination of maxillary incisors, retraction or retroclination of mandibular incisors) may adequately camouflage the skeletal discrepancy. However, dental compensation for the skeletal discrepancy in children whose growth

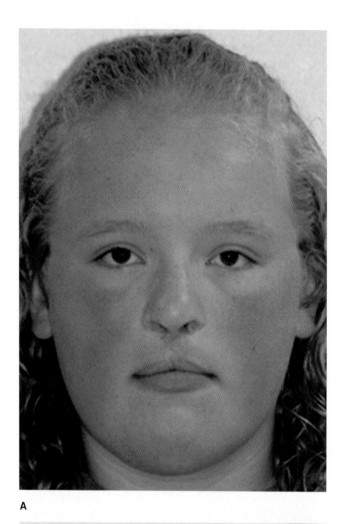

A

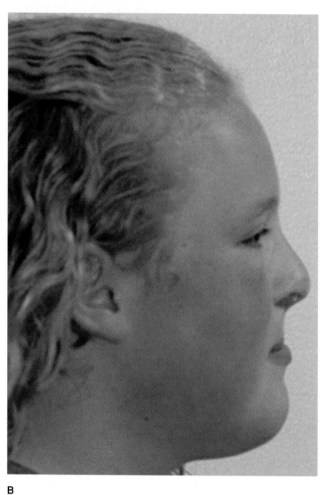

B

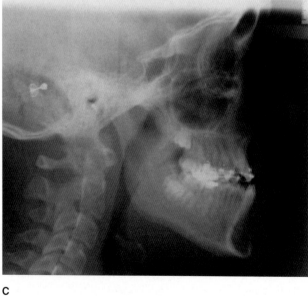

C

Figure 47–14. (A) Same patient illustrated in Figure 47–4; at 15 years of age. Alveolar bone grafting has been done and patient underwent limited orthodontic alignment. (B) Profile view showing concave profile and midface deficiency. (C) Lateral skull radiograph showing maxillary retrusion, proclined maxillary incisors, and reverse overjet. The need for orthognathic surgery (maxillary advancement) is foreseen.

has not stabilized may result in the correction being outgrown and, ultimately, to a recommendation for orthognathic surgery.

Patients with severe skeletal discrepancies and significant esthetic concerns are candidates for orthodontic treatment combined with orthognathic surgery. Presurgical orthodontic treatment prepares the patient for surgical advancement of the maxilla. In the past, conventional surgical correction of severe maxillary hypoplasia (greater than 10 mm) commonly involved the advancement of the maxilla as

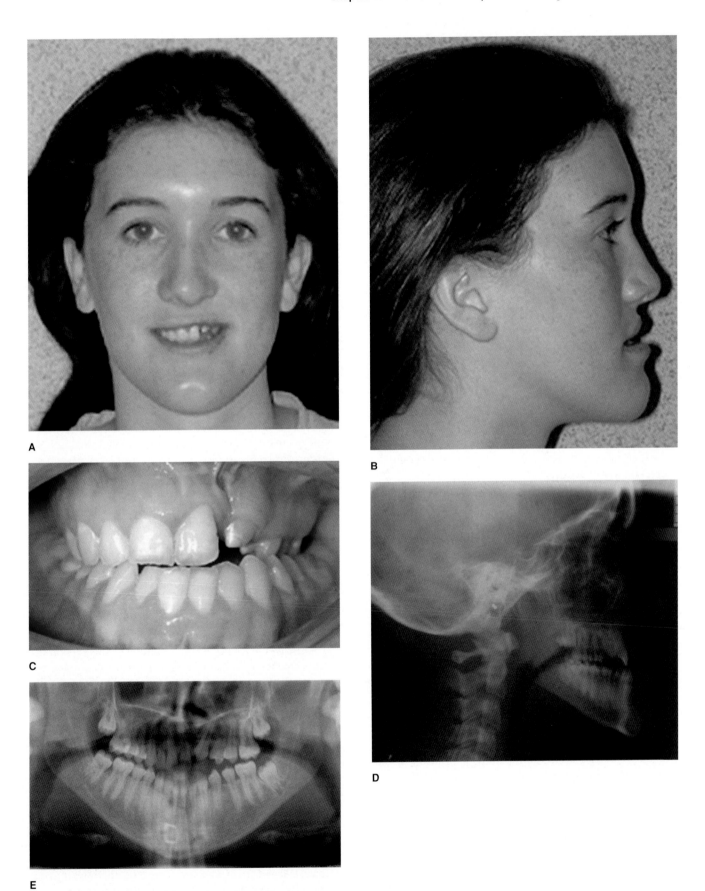

Figure 47–15. (A) Frontal view of a 15-year-old female with complete unilateral left cleft lip and palate. (B) Profile view showing concave profile, midface retrusion, and malar deficiency. (C) Intraoral view showing repaired alveolar cleft, left posterior crossbite, and midline discrepancy. (D) Lateral skull radiograph. Note reverse overjet, upright mandibular incisors, and prominent pogonium. (E) Panoramic radiograph. Note absence of maxillary left lateral incisor and dilacerated root on maxillary left central.

much as possible within the constraints of the scar tissue from the lip and palate repairs. The amount of sagittal maxillary advancement was often not sufficient to correct the skeletal discrepancy. Simultaneous setback of the mandible was done to correct the remaining skeletal discrepancy. This approach can be considered as a surgical camouflage to correct the severe maxillary hypoplasia (Figs. 47–16 and 47–17). The disadvantage of this two-jaw approach in patients with clefts is that facial balance and proportions may be compromised when a small and retrognathic mandible exists or even in those patients with mandibles of normal size and position.[54]

Orthognathic Surgery

Timing and Sequencing

The timing and sequencing of treatment requires close collaboration between the members of the cleft/craniofacial team. In patients with severe skeletal discrepancies, the decision to delay surgical orthodontic treatment until growth has stabilized may be sound judgment, for the stability of the outcome. If psychosocial concerns exist, the timing should be reconsidered. In such instances, presurgical orthodontics can be started during early adolescence in the young permanent dentition, delaying skeletal surgery until after the pubertal growth spurt has occurred. This decision should be made jointly with the parent and patient, emphasizing the possibility that an additional procedure may be indicated should the correction be outgrown.

Secondary lip and nose revisions are typically postponed until after orthognathic surgery and prosthetic rehabilitation of the dentition are complete. Correction of the jaw relationship and dental occlusion influences the lip support and nasal contour. If alveolar bone grafting is indicated to augment an edentulous space in the maxilla, especially at the cleft area, it is often postponed until after orthognathic surgery. This will ensure adequate blood supply to the grafted bone, thus improving the probability of successful graft vascularization and healing.

Role of the Orthodontist

Coordination between the orthodontist and the oral/craniofacial surgeon is indicated during treatment planning and also during the presurgical phase of orthodontic treatment. The *presurgical phase* of orthodontic treatment takes approximately 12–18 months, with the goals of aligning and decompensating the teeth, coordination of the dental arches, and distribution of space for prosthetic replacement of missing teeth. This may result in accentuating the malocclusion as the maxillary and mandibular dentitions are placed in their correct relationship to the underlying skeletal bases (Fig. 47–16). Following surgical correction of the jaw discrepancy, the occlusion should be optimal if the goals of the presurgical orthodontic treatment have been attained. If a segmental osteotomy is planned, adequate space for the surgical cuts is a prerequisite of the presurgical orthodontic tooth movements between both the crown and the roots of adjacent teeth. When the above objectives are attained, the patient

is referred to the surgeon for a presurgical consultation. The surgeon models the surgical movements on mounted dental casts and cephalometric tracings and communicates to the orthodontist whether occlusal discrepancies are encountered that prevent adequate coordination of arches. Once the orthodontist and the surgeon agree that the presurgical setup is acceptable, the orthodontist places full-size rectangular surgical arch wires with crimped or soldered lugs to provide a means of intermaxillary fixation at the time rigid internal fixation is performed. During the postsurgical period, the surgeon continues to manage the patient for several weeks to ensure no complications occur during the healing phase. Once the patient is stable and able to tolerate a soft diet, the *postsurgical phase* of orthodontics treatment can proceed. This phase, which should be completed within 4–6 months, is aimed to fine detail the occlusion and finalize the preparations for prosthetic replacement of any missing teeth (Fig. 47–17).

Upon removal of orthodontic appliances, fixed retainers in the form of a wire bonded to the lingual aspect of the incisors are indicated to maintain the alignment of the incisors. The orthodontist may find, however, that the corrected transverse dimension of posterior segments is prone to relapse if not retained after the archwires are removed. This is likely due to the tension of palatal scar tissue. A maxillary acrylic plate or a Hawley retainer may be indicated to hold the transverse dimension and also for prosthetic replacement of missing teeth.

Distraction Osteogenesis

With the advent of distraction osteogenesis, it may be possible to correct a severe cleft maxillary hypoplasia solely by advancing the cleft maxilla (Fig. 47–18). With this technique, the extent of maxillary advancement can be greater than the 10 mm possible within the range of stability of a conventional LeFort I osteotomy. This is accomplished by gradual traction of the mobilized maxilla and expansion of the scarred palatal tissues during the slow distraction protocol.

Briefly, the technique of rigid external distraction involves cementation of an intraoral splint with extraoral extensions (hooks) for traction,[54] frequently done by the orthodontist. A complete LeFort I osteotomy is performed, and a rigid external distraction (RED) device is placed at the time of surgery. The vector of the anterior force can be customized to each patient and also altered during the course of distraction. Distraction is done at home by patients/parents turning the activation screw at a rate of 1 mm per day. After the desired advancement is achieved, the RED device is left in place for 2–3 weeks to permit bone consolidation, followed by a retention period with an orthodontic face mask. Internal distractors, which rely on fixation of the rigid component to the facial bones and alveolus, have also been used in patients with maxillary clefts.[55] The distractor rod penetrates into the oral cavity, making activation of the system possible via an intraoral approach. Long consolidation periods (3 months) are possible by removing the turning arms, leaving the submucosal components in place.

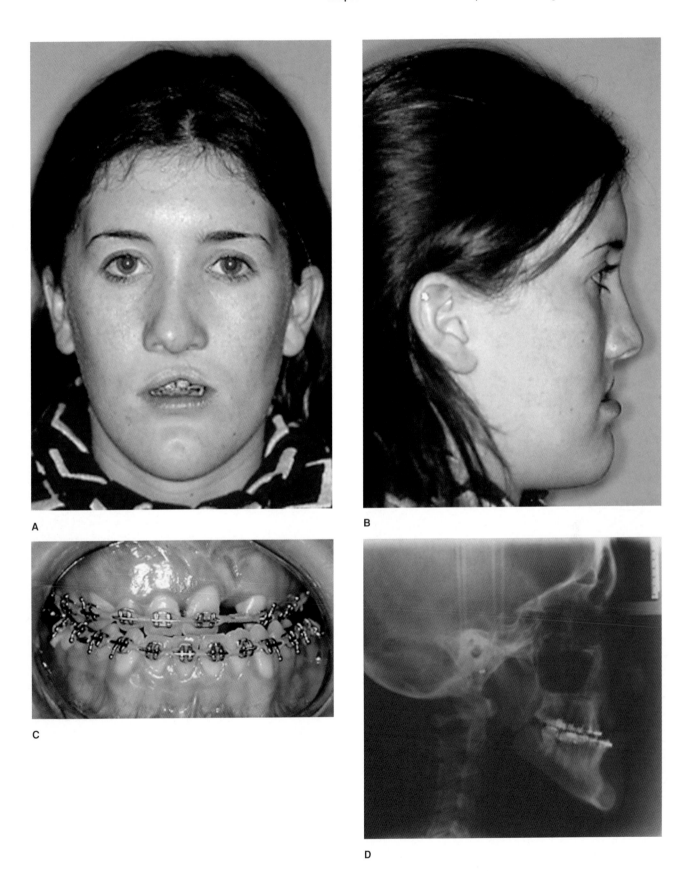

Figure 47–16. (A) Frontal view of same patient illustrated in Figure 47–15; shown at 17 years of age during presurgical orthodontic treatment for dental decompensation. (B) Profile view shows marked maxillary deficiency. (C) Frontal intraoral view shows leveled and aligned arches. Space has been preserved for replacement of the maxillary left lateral incisor. (D) Lateral skull radiograph shows the Class III skeletal pattern with maxillary and mandibular incisors in corrected angulation within their respective apical bases.

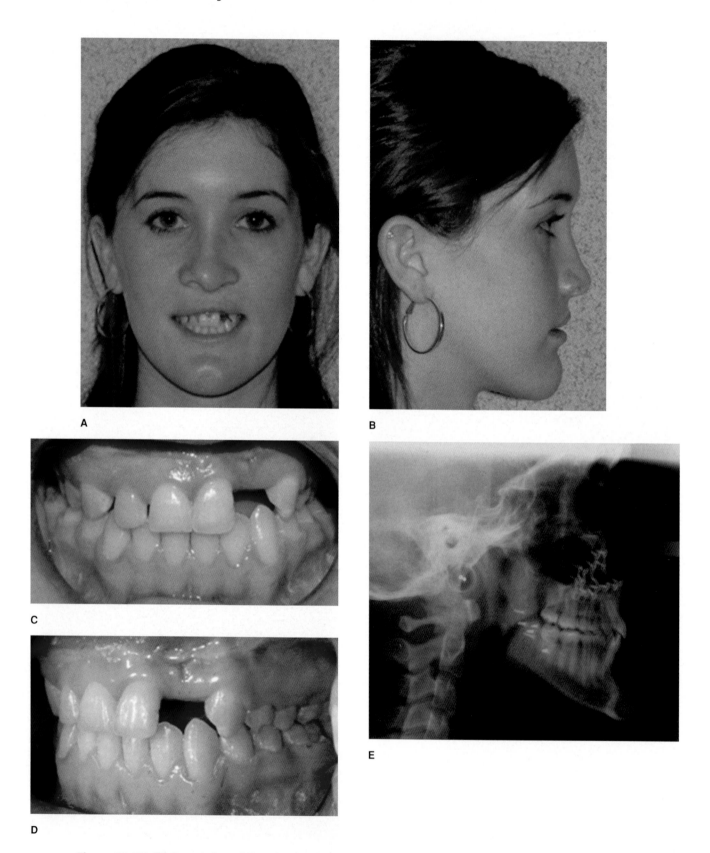

Figure 47–17. (A) Frontal view of same patient illustrated in Figures 47–15 and 47–16; shown at 18 years of age following maxillary advancement, asymmetric mandibular set-back surgery, and postsurgical orthodontic treatment. (B) Profile view shows a balanced profile and good upper lip support. (C) Frontal intraoral view shows coincident midlines. (D) Left intraoral view shows adequate overbite and overjet with Class I occlusion. Patient is ready for cosmetic bonding and has opted for a fixed partial denture to restore tooth #10. (E) Lateral skull radiograph shows adequate relationship of maxilla and madible.

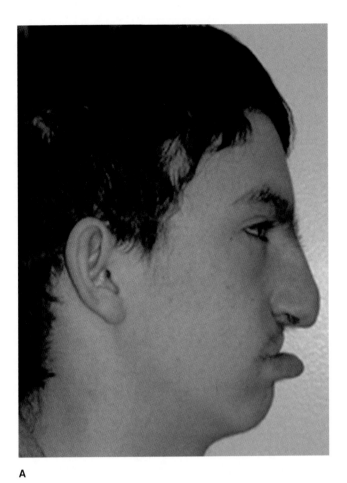

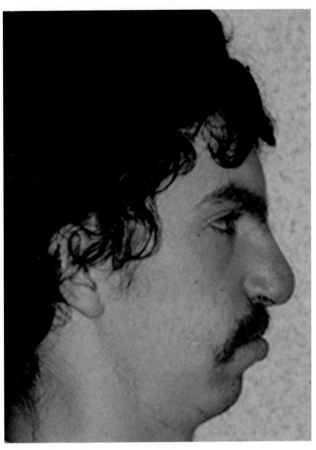

A   B

Figure 47–18. (A) Profile view of a 17-year-old male with repaired complete bilateral cleft lip and palate. Note bimaxillary retrusion with severe maxillary deficiency. (B) Profile view after distraction osteogenesis to advance the maxilla. Note improved position of maxilla. Patient may benefit from mandibular advancement.

Few studies on the long-term stability of distraction osteogenesis have been published. Figueroa et al. (2004) found that the advancement achieved by distraction was stable when followed up to 3 years. They attributed this stability to autologous bone formation in the pterygomaxillary area, posterior to the maxillary tuberosity.[56] Kumar et al. (2006) reported that patients with severe cleft maxillary deficiency (greater than 10 mm) who underwent distraction osteogenesis had a lower relapse rate after 1 year compared to patients of similar severity who underwent conventional LeFort I advancement.[55] More long-term follow-up studies are needed to determine the predictability of the results when maxillary distraction is performed in growing children. Some of these patients will still require additional surgical procedures (for maxillary advancement, impaction, or mandibular set-back) in the postadolescent period to detail the occlusion. The orthodontist and the oral surgeon should counsel patients and their families presurgically on the potential need for such additional surgery (Fig. 47–18).

The impact of distraction osteogenesis on speech has been subject of increased interest in the literature. Hyponasality improves in patients who have preoperative hyponasality.[57,58] Improvements in articulation are due to more favorable labio-lingual relationships.[57,58] Most studies show increased hypernasality after distraction osteogenesis with the greatest effect in cases of borderline velopharyngeal insufficiency.[57] However, the incidence of increased hypernasality after distraction osteogenesis in patients with cleft palate compares favorably with that reported after conventional LeFort I maxillary advancement in patients with cleft palate.[58] The theoretical benefit of distraction osteogenesis is that, with gradual advancement of the palate, the velopharyngeal mechanism has time to adapt. Nevertheless, candidates for distraction osteogenesis should be counseled prior to the procedure on the risks and benefits to speech, especially patients with borderline velopharyngeal function.[58]

The End Game of Treatment: Management of the Missing Lateral Incisor

In patients with an edentulous ridge in the region of the cleft, either due to congenital agenesis or previous extraction of teeth, several options are available for the management of the space. These include space closure, fixed or removable prostheses, osseointegrated implants, and autotransplantation.

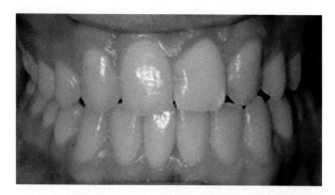

Figure 47–19. Young adult patient with complete unilateral left cleft lip and palate who has been orthodontically treated with bilateral maxillary canine substitution. Canines should be recontoured to resemble lateral incisors. It was difficult to achieve adequate palatal root torque of #11, which also has a high gingival margin in relation to the central incisors.

Space Closure

The edentulous space can be closed by allowing mesial eruption of the canine, moving the posterior teeth anteriorly with orthodontics and cosmetically "re-shaping" the canine. This approach precludes the need for a prosthetic replacement of the absent lateral incisor (Fig. 47–19). Studies in patients without clefts have shown that patients with closed maxillary lateral incisor spaces are periodontally healthier than patients with fixed prostheses.[59,60] Use of "canine substitution" for patients with alveolar clefts, however, needs to be considered in light of several factors:

- *The position of the maxilla in relation to the mandible.* In patients with maxillary deficiency, space closure by moving the canine adjacent to the central incisor may accentuate the maxillary retrusion due to the aligning and uprighting of incisors into a smaller arch perimeter. If the skeletal discrepancy is managed with orthodontic camouflage, consideration should be given to preserve the lateral incisor space and restore it prosthetically. This will facilitate the attainment of positive overjet and adequate support for the upper lip. If the skeletal discrepancy is managed with a combined orthodontic/surgical approach, space closure via canine substitution can be an acceptable strategy to manage the lateral incisor space.
- *The existing posterior occlusion on the cleft side.* In a patient with stable, well interdigitated posterior occlusion, it may be difficult, time-consuming, and unnecessary to move all the posterior teeth forward. Preserving the existing posterior occlusion and restoring the lateral incisor space prosthetically may be a simpler and more time-efficient option for the patient.
- *Aesthetic limitations of the canine in the lateral incisor position.* When positioned anteriorly, the crown of the maxillary canine needs to be recontoured to resemble the narrow, rectangular, and flatter shape of the lateral incisor (Fig. 47–19). This can be done with enamel re-contouring, composite build-up, or porcelain veneer. The heights of

the gingival margins among the maxillary incisors need to be evaluated. A high gingival margin on the canine crown may look unaesthetic next to the lower gingival level on the central incisor. Orthodontic extrusion and/or periodontal surgery may be needed to harmonize the gingival heights among incisors. This may not be an issue if the patient's lip does not elevate significantly upon animation, which is often the case in patients with repaired cleft lip.

Fixed versus Removable Prostheses

In patients with cleft lip and palate, there are several considerations in the choice of fixed versus removable prostheses for the replacement of missing teeth at the cleft. Fixed prostheses are recommended for nongrowing patients with a single tooth missing in the cleft area, patients who need rigid permanent stabilization of the maxillary segments (cases of failed or nonexistent alveolar bone grafts), and patients whose adjacent teeth are malformed and could benefit from crowns. Resin-retained bridges (Maryland bridges) have been used in patients with cleft lip and palate, with a stabilizing effect achieved by including more teeth in the design than the conventional cantilever bridge. On the other hand, removable prostheses are indicated for replacement of multiple teeth along the arch, restoration of long edentulous spans, simultaneous obturation of large palatal fistulae, addition of flange acrylic to improve lip support/gingival esthetics in cases of severe alveolar defects, and for transitional replacement of teeth in young patients prior to fixed prosthesis placement. For both fixed and removable options, the orthodontist should work in consultation with the prosthodontist to determine the alignment/angulation of teeth that will provide optimal space distribution between teeth, favor an unrestricted path of insertion for the prosthesis, and result in adequate occlusion of both natural and prosthetic teeth.

Osseointegrated Implants

It is feasible to restore the edentulous cleft area with endosseus implants.[61–63] An indication for this approach is the restoration of a single missing tooth without the need to reduce healthy adjacent teeth. Another indication is the stabilization and retention of fixed or removable dentures, with or without obturators. An adequate volume of alveolar bone at the cleft area is essential prior to implant placement. In children whose lateral incisor space is preserved for future implant placement, the edentulous grafted area may show radiographic evidence of resorption over several years. An interval of several years is often inevitable if the team of orthodontist, oral surgeon, and prosthodontist has postponed implant placement until the patient has completed both sagittal and vertical growth, which is the current guideline.[64] Studies by Kearns et al. (1997) suggest that the greater the interval between bone graft and implant, the more likely it is that there will be insufficient bone volume for an implant and that the residual graft will need to be further augmented with additional bone.[62] The recommendation stipulates that patients who receive secondary bone grafts in the mixed dentition should be re-grafted between 15 and 17 years of age with autogenous bone followed by implant placement within 4 months post-regrafting.

When planning placement of osseointegrated implants in the area of the cleft, the orthodontist works in concert with the oral surgeon and the prosthodontist. After a diagnostic setup has been done in plaster study models and reviewed among all specialists, orthodontic treatment can be instituted to distribute the spaces between the teeth. It is important for the orthodontist to ensure that roots of teeth adjacent to the edentulous area are parallel, as can be assessed with periapical radiographs. This will allow the surgeon to place the endosteal implant fixture without risk of damaging adjacent roots. In the young postadolescent patient, the orthodontist determines when the patient has completed his/her facial growth. This is done by superimposing cephalometric radiographs taken 6 months apart and comparing the changes over time in the antero-posterior and vertical dimensions. When completion of facial growth has been confirmed, the oral surgeon places the implants, followed by restoration by the prosthodontist.

Autotransplantation

Some patients with clefts of the lip and palate have a malformed, ectopic, or severely hypoplastic central incisor adjacent to the cleft, one which often needs to be extracted due to its poor prognosis. If these patients are also missing a lateral incisor, as frequently occurs, their orthodontic management becomes more challenging. Simple orthodontic space closure cannot be obtained in such patients, and prosthetic restoration is therefore required. Autotransplantation of premolars into or adjacent to the grafted cleft has been advocated by some as an alternative to prosthetic restoration in such cases. This method provides a means by which to restore missing teeth in the growing patient, since the premolar needs to be transplanted with partially formed roots. The transplanted tooth provides functional stimulation to the grafted bone shortly after the bony bridge has established,[65] preventing the bone atrophy that occurs while waiting for growth to cease prior to inserting implants or fixed prosthesis. The guidelines stipulate that transplantation should occur 4 months after alveolar bone grafting, when the bony bridge has established but bone remodeling is still underway.[66–68] Premolars should have half to three-fourths of final root length at the time of surgery. Orthodontic movement, including the transplanted teeth, should not be initiated prior to 6 months post-transplantation.[66] Upon completion of treatment, a bonded palatal retainer is recommended, including two teeth on each side of the cleft.

Follow-up studies of transplanted teeth in or near the cleft area have shown no increased mobility, periodontal pockets, signs of progressive root pathology, or periodontal attachment loss.[66] These studies have also demonstrated regeneration of the periodontal space and lamina dura and favorable crown-to-root ratios.[66] To date, however, the available studies are primarily case reports,[65–67] underscoring the need for prospective, controlled clinical studies on the risks and benefits of autotransplantation in patients with cleft lip and palate.

FUTURE CONSIDERATIONS

The direction of future advances in orthodontic treatment and for the development of parameters for infants born with cleft lip and/or palate relates primarily to advances in technology, economic considerations, and measured outcomes. The emergence of evidence-based clinical practice in the 1990s emphasized the need to evaluate and compare alternative interventions by their risks, benefits, and costs, including their associated burden of care. Some of our current practice information is generated from the Eurocleft longitudinal intercenter cohort study that compared orthodontic records of 9-year-old children with UCLP centers and considered how the burden of care related to clinical outcomes and to patient/parent satisfaction. The complexity of measuring patient-centered outcomes includes addressing patient satisfaction in the context of psychological adjustment and the contemporary and complex quality of life measures. Collaboration of multiple teams allows for the development of "good practice archives" to be assembled, as has occurred with Eurocran (www.eurocran.org) and in North America with the craniofacial outcomes registry (www.cfregistry.org) for diagnostic and outcomes data. The establishment of a multicenter database allows individual teams to anonymously compare their results with the aggregate.[9,24]

SUMMARY

Diagnostic, timing, and sequencing considerations in the orthodontic treatment of the patient with cleft lip and/or palate have been described. Four discrete periods of skeleto-dental development have been discussed: (1) neonatal or infant maxillary orthopedics; (2) interventions in the primary dentition; (3) mixed dentition including presurgical considerations prior to alveolar bone grafting; and (4) comprehensive treatment in the permanent dentition with or without orthognathic surgery. The role of the orthodontist in facilitating any necessary prosthodontic treatment has also been discussed. Other aspects that influence the patient's quality of life need to be taken into consideration when planning the appropriate timing and sequencing for orthodontic intervention. These include psychosocial dynamics, speech considerations, soft tissue facial appearance, and the burden of care for the family. Patients and their families should be empowered to make informed decisions on treatment after being provided with evidence-based analysis of outcome probability estimates. It is the duty of the orthodontist and other team members, in a single center or in a multi-center context, to evaluate what works and what does not based upon a prospective approach using valid and reliable outcome measures. The mission of the orthodontist as a clinician, in collaboration with all other team members, is to help patients with clefts reach their full rehabilitation and attain satisfaction from both the functional and esthetic results.

ACKNOWLEDGMENTS

We are grateful to Dr. Jack Lude for permission to publish Figure 47–3 (neonatal orthopedics) and to the members of the Cleft Palate Team at Children's Hospital, Columbus, for their collaboration in the treatment of the cases illustrated in this chapter. We also thank Ms. Pamela Foy (sonographer) at The Ohio State University Department of OB/GYN for permission to publish Figure 47–2. Figures 47–1, 47–5, 47–6, and 47–7 were modified with permission from Vig KWL & Mercado AM: The orthodontist's role in a cleft palate-craniofacial team. In Graber TM, Vanarsdall RL, Vig KWL (eds). *Orthodontics: Current Principles and Techniques*. Saint Louis: Elsevier, 2005.

References

1. Parameters for the evaluation and treatment of patients with cleft lip/palate or other craniofacial anomalies. American Cleft Lip and Palate Association. *Cleft Palate Craniofac J* 30(Suppl 1) pp. 1–30, 1993.
2. Lidral AC, Vig KWL. The role of the orthodontist in the management of patients with cleft lip and/or palate. In Wyszynski D (eds). *Cleft Lip & Palate: From Origin to Treatment*, 1st edn. New York: Oxford University Press, 2002, p. 381.
3. Vig KWL, Mercado AM. The orthodontist's role in a cleft palate-craniofacial team. In Graber TM, Vanarsdall RL, Vig KWL (eds). *Orthodontics: Current Principles and Techniques*, 4th edn. Saint Louis: Elsevier, 2005, p. 1097.
4. Davalbhakta A, Hall PH. The impact of antenatal diagnosis on the effectiveness and timing of counseling for cleft lip and palate. *Br J Plastic Surg* 53:298, 2000.
5. Robinson JN, McElrath TF, Benson CB, et al. Prenatal ultrasonography and the diagnosis of fetal cleft lip. *J Ultrasound Med* 20:1165, 2001.
6. Burston WR. The early treatment of cleft palate conditions. *Dent Pract* 9:41, 1958.
7. McNeil CK. Orthopedic principles in the treatment of lip and palate clefts. In *International Symposium on Early Treatment of Cleft Lip and Palate*. Berne: Hans Huber, 1961.
8. Grayson BH, Santiago PE, Brecht LE, et al. Presurgical nasoalveolar molding in infants with cleft lip and palate. *Cleft Palate Craniofac J* 36:486, 1999.
9. Shaw B, Semb G, Nelson P, et al. *The Eurocleft Project 1996-2000*. Amsterdam: IOS Press, 2000.
10. Prahl C, Kuijpers-Jagtman AM, A VtHM, et al. A randomised prospective clinical trial into the effect of infant orthopedics on maxillary arch dimensions in unilateral cleft lip and palate. *Eur J Oral Sci* 109:297, 2001.
11. Prahl C, Kuijpers-Jagtman AM, A VtHM, et al. Infant orthopedics in UCLP: Effect on feeding, weight and length. A randomised clinical trial (Dutchcleft). *Cleft Palate Craniofac J* 42:171, 2005.
12. Ross RB. Treatment variables affecting facial growth in unilateral cleft lip and palate. Part 2: Presurgical orthopedics. *Cleft Palate Craniofac J* 24:24, 1987.
13. Tindlund RS. Skeletal response to maxillary protraction in patients with cleft lip and palate before age 10 years. *Cleft Palate Craniofac J* 31:295, 1994.
14. Berndt TJ. The features and effects of friendship in early adolescence. *Child Dev* 53:1447, 1982.
15. Pope AW, Ward J. Factors associated with peer social competence in preadolescents with craniofacial anomalies. *J Pediatric Psychol* 22:455, 1997.
16. Rosenstein SW, Monroe CW, Kernahan DA, et al. The case for early bone grafting in cleft lip and cleft palate. *Plast Reconstr Surg* 70:297, 1982.
17. Murthy AS, Lehman JA. Evaluation of alveolar bone grafting: A survey of ACPA teams. *Cleft Palate Craniofac J* 42:99, 2005.
18. Boyne PJ, Sands NR. Secondary bone grafting of residual alveolar and palatal clefts. *J Oral Surg* 30:87, 1972.
19. Boyne PJ, Sands NR. Combined orthodontic-surgical management of residual palato-alveolar cleft defect. *Am J Orthod Dentofacial Orthop* 70:20, 1976.
20. Bergland O, Semb G, Abyholm FE. Elimination of the residual alveolar cleft by secondary bone grafting and subsequent orthodontic treatment. *Cleft Palate Craniofac J* 23:175, 1986.
21. Semb G. Effect of alveolar bone grafting on maxillary growth in unilateral cleft lip and palate patients. *Cleft Palate Craniofac J* 25:288, 1988.
22. Levitt T, Long RE, Trotman C-A. Maxillary growth in patients with clefts following secondary alveolar bone grafting. *Cleft Palate Craniofac J* 36:398, 1999.
23. Brattstrom V, Molsted K, Prahl-Andersen B, et al. The Eurocleft study: Intercenter study of treatment outcomes in patients with complete cleft lip and palate. Part 2: Craniofacial form and nasolabial appearance. *Cleft Palate Craniofac J* 42:69, 2005.
24. Semb G, Brattstrom V, Molsted K, et al. The Eurocleft study: Intercenter study of treatment outcome in patients with complete cleft lip and palate. Part 1: Introduction and treatment experience. *Cleft Palate Craniofac J* 42:64, 2005.
25. Karling J. Oronasal fistulae in cleft palate patients and their influence on speech. *Scand J Plast Reconstr Surg Hand Surg* 27:193, 1993.
26. Bureau S, Penko M, McFadden L. Speech outcome after closure of oronasal fistulae with bone grafts. *J Oral Maxillofac Surg* 59:1408, 2001.
27. Brattstrom V, McWilliam J, Larson O, et al. Craniofacial development in children with unilateral clefts of the lip, alveolus, and palate treated according to three different regimes. Assessment of nasolabial appearance. *Scand J Plast Reconstr Surg Hand Surg* 26:313, 1992.
28. Turvey TA, Vig KWL, Moriarty J, et al. Delayed bone grafting in the cleft maxilla and palate: A retrospective multidisciplinary analysis. *Am J Orthod Dentofacial Orthop* 86:3, 1984.
29. Dempf R, Telztrow T, Kramer F-J, et al. Alveolar bone grafting in patients with complete clefts: A comparative study between secondary and tertiary bone grafting. *Cleft Palate Craniofac J* 39:18, 2002.
30. Larsen PE. Reconstruction of the alveolar cleft. In Miloro M, et al. (eds). *Peterson's Principles of Oral and Maxillofacial Surgery*, 2nd edn. Hamilton: BC Decker, 2004.
31. Williams A, Semb G, Bearn D, et al. Prediction of outcomes of secondary alveolar bone grafting in children born with unilateral cleft lip and palate. *Eur J Orthod* 25:205, 2003.
32. Solis A, Figueroa AA, Cohen M, et al. Maxillary dental development in complete unilateral alveolar clefts. *Cleft Palate Craniofac J* 35:320, 1998.
33. Vig KWL. Alveolar bone grafts: The surgical/orthodontic management of the cleft maxilla. *Ann Acad Med Singapore* 28:721, 1999.
34. Mercado AM, Lubitz K, Halderman J, et al. Root development and bone grafting in patients with alveolar clefts. *J Dent Res* 85:Abstract No. 0124, 2006.
35. Ribeiro LL, Das Neves LL, Costa B, et al. Dental anomalies of the permanent lateral incisors and prevalence of hypodontia outside the cleft area in complete unilateral cleft lip and palate. *Cleft Palate Craniofac J* 40:172, 2003.
36. Boyne PJ. Bone grafting in the osseous reconstruction of alveolar and palatal clefts. *Oral Maxillofac Clin North Am* 3:589, 1991.
37. Vig KWL, Turvey TA, Fonseca RJ. Orthodontic and surgical considerations in bone grafting the cleft maxilla and palate. In Turvey TA, Vig KWL, Fonseca RJ (eds). *Facial Clefts and Craniosynostosis:*

Principles and Management, 1st edn. Philadelphia: WB Saunders, 1996, p. 396.

38. Lilja J, Kalaaji A, Friede H, et al. Combined gone grafting and delayed closure of the hard palate in patients with unilateral cleft lip and palate: Facilitation of lateral incisor eruption and evaluation of indicators for timing of the procedure. *Cleft Palate Craniofac J* 37:98, 2000.

39. Long RE, Paterno M, Vinson B. Effect of cuspid positioning in the cleft at the time of secondary alveolar bone grafting on eventual graft success. *Cleft Palate Craniofac J* 33:225, 1996.

40. Halderman J, Lubitz K, Premaraj S, et al. Canine eruption and alveolar bone grafting in UCLP patients. *J Dent Res* 84:Abstract No. 3690, 2005.

41. Cavassan AO, DeAlbuquerque MD, Filho LC. Rapid maxillary expansion after secondary alveolar bone graft in a patient with bilateral cleft lip and palate. *Cleft Palate Craniofac J* 41:332, 2004.

42. Aurouze C, Moller KT, Bevis RR, et al. The presurgical status of the alveolar cleft and success of secondary bone grafting. *Cleft Palate Craniofac J* 37:179, 2000.

43. Long RE, Spangler BE, Yow M. Cleft width and secondary alveolar bone graft success. *Cleft Palate Craniofac J* 32:420, 1995.

44. Schultze-Mosgau S, Nkenke E, Schlegel AK, et al. Analysis of bone resorption after secondary alveolar cleft bone grafts before and after canine eruption in connection with orthodontic gap closure or prosthodontic treatment. *J Oral Maxillofac Surg* 61:1245, 2003.

45. Nightingale C, Witherow H, Reid FDA, et al. Comparative reproducibility of three methods of radiographic assessment of alveolar bone grafting. *Eur J Orthod* 25:35, 2003.

46. Premaraj S, Larsen PE, Vig KWL. Alveolar bone graft outcomes using a modified Bergland scale. *J Dent Res* 81:Abstract No. 2949, 2002.

47. Kindelan JD, Nashed RR, Bromige MR. Radiographic assessment of secondary autogenous alveolar bone grafting in cleft lip and palate patients. *Cleft Palate Craniofac J* 34:195, 1997.

48. Witherow H, Cox S, Jones E, et al. A new scale to assess radiographic success of secondary alveolar bone grafts. *Cleft Palate Craniofac J* 39:255, 2002.

49. Kau CH, Richmond S, Palomo JM, et al. Current products and practice: Three dimensional cone beam computerized tomography in orthodontics. *J Orthod* 32:282, 2005.

50. Hamada Y, Kondoh T, Noguchi K, et al. Application of limited cone beam computed tomography to clinical assessment of alveolar bone grafting: A preliminary report. *Cleft Palate Craniofac J* 42:128, 2005.

51. Mah JK, Danforth RA, Bumann A, et al. Radiation absorbed in maxillofacial imaging with a new dental computed tomography device. *Oral Surg Oral Med Oral Path Oral Radiol Endod* 96:508, 2003.

52. Wortche R, Hassfeld S, Lux CJ, et al. Clinical application of cone beam digital volume tomography in children with cleft lip and palate. *Dentomaxillofac Radiol* 35:88, 2006.

53. Kapp-Simon KA. Psychological issues in cleft lip and palate. *Clin Plast Surg* 31:347, 2004.

54. Figueroa AA, Polley JW. Management of severe cleft maxillary deficiency with distraction osteogenesis: Procedure and results. *Am J Orthod Dentofacial Orthop* 115:1, 1999.

55. Kumar A, Gabbay JS, Nikjoo R, et al. Improved outcomes in cleft patients with severe maxillary deficiency after Le Fort I internal distraction. *Plast Reconstr Surg* 117:1499, 2006.

56. Figueroa AA, Polley JW, Friede H, et al. Long-term stability after maxillary advancement with distraction osteogenesis using a rigid external distraction device in cleft maxillary deformities. *Plast Reconstr Surg* 114:1382, 2004.

57. Chanchareonsook N, Samman N, Whitehill TL. The effect of craniomaxillofacial osteotomies and distraction osteogenesis on speech and velopharyngeal status: A critical review. *Cleft Palate Craniofac J* 43:477, 2006.

58. Guyette T, Polley JW, Figueroa AA, et al. Changes in speech following maxillary distraction osteogenesis. *Cleft Palate Craniofac J* 38:199, 2001.

59. Robertsson S, Mohlin B. The congenitally missing upper lateral incisor. A retrospective study of orthodontic space closure versus restorative treatment. *Eur J Orthod* 22:697, 2000.

60. Nordquist GG, McNeill RW. Orthodontic vs. restorative treatment of the congenitally absent lateral incisor—long term periodontal and occlusal evaluation. *J Periodontol* 46:139, 1975.

61. Takahashi T, Fukuda M, Yamaguchi T, et al. Use of endosseous implants for dental reconstruction of patients with grafted alveolar clefts. *J Oral Maxillofac Surg* 55:576, 1997.

62. Kearns G, Perrott DH, Sharma AB, et al. Placement of endosseous implants in grafted alveolar clefts. *Cleft Palate Craniofac J* 34:520, 1997.

63. Kramer FJ, Baethge C, Bremer B, et al. Dental implants in patients with orofacial clefts: A long-term follow-up study. *Int J Oral Maxillofac Surg* 34:715, 2005.

64. Brugnolo E, Mazzocco C, Cordioll G, et al. Clinical and radiographic findings following placement of single-tooth implants in young patients—case reports. *Int J Periodon & Rest Dent* 16:421, 1996.

65. Hillerup S, Dahl E, Schwartz O, et al. Tooth transplantation to bone graft in cleft alveolus. *Cleft Palate Craniofac J* 24:137, 1987.

66. Czochorowska EM, Semb G, Stenvik A. Nonprosthodontic management of alveolar clefts with 2 incisors missing on the cleft side: A report of 5 patients. *Am J Orthod Dentofacial Orthop* 122:587, 2002.

67. Hamamoto N, Hamamoto Y, Kobayashi T. Tooth autotransplantation into the bone-grafted alveolar cleft: Report of two cases with histologic findings. *J Oral Maxillofac Surg* 56:1451, 1998.

68. Stenvik A, Semb G, Bergland O, et al. Experimental transplantation of teeth to simulated maxillary alveolar clefts. *Scand J Plast Reconstr Surg Hand Surg* 23:105, 1989.

Facial Growth and Development in Cleft Children

Sven Kreiborg, DDS, PhD, Dr. Odont • Nuno V. Hermann, DDS, PhD • Tron A. Darvann, MSc, PhD

INTRODUCTION

"Knowledge concerning the development of the face and the dentition in individuals with congenital clefts of the lip and palate is of the utmost importance in planning treatment of the clefts"

Erik Dahl.

"Whoever sees things from their beginning will have the most advantageous view of them"

Samuel Pruzansky.

Since the introduction of roentgencephalometry 75 years ago,[1] numerous studies, including both unoperated and operated cleft individuals have suggested that some facial deviations are directly caused by the anomaly, whereas others are caused by the surgical interventions and the following dysplastic and compensatory growth of the facial skeleton.

However, the relative importance of the intrinsic factors, the iatrogenic factors (surgery), and the functional or adaptive factors for the facial development is still unclear.[2,3] The reason for this is that comprehensive knowledge of craniofacial morphology in newborns with cleft is very scarce. Only very few studies have employed infant cephalometry, and, of these, most have been limited to the lateral cephalometric projection, the method of analysis has been limited to relatively few reference prints, and, most importantly, the samples have been small and selected.

In these authors' opinion, the incomplete knowledge about the initial state ("the beginning") has lead to excessive emphasis in the literature on the importance of iatrogenic and functional or adaptive factors in facial growth and development of cleft children in the literature.[3]

The aim of this chapter is, based on comprehensive three-projection cephalometric studies of a large consecutive sample of cleft individuals, to:

- describe the facial morphology in newborns with various types of clefts,
- describe the early facial growth in unoperated children with isolated cleft palate (ICP) from 0–2 years of age, and
- describe the effect of lip surgery on facial growth in the first two years of life in individuals with unilateral complete cleft lip palate.

BACKGROUND

During the period 1976–1981, there were 359,027 live births in Denmark and among these 678 Caucasian children were born with a nonsyndromic cleft lip and/or palate. About 90% of these children were studied with three-projection cephalometry at both 2 and 22 months of age.[4] All children were unoperated at 2 months of age. The children with cleft lip, with or without cleft palate, were operated at 2–3 months of age by the same surgeon (Dr. Poul Fogh-Andersen) using a Tennison procedure. The classification of the children according to cleft type was previously presented by Jensen et al.[4] The method of three-projection cephalometry and the comprehensive cephalometric analysis employed were described by Kreiborg et al.[5] Heller et al.[6] and Hermann et al.[7]

FACIAL MORPHOLOGY IN NEWBORNS WITH CLEFTS

This description will be limited to the following patient categories:

- ICP
- Unilateral complete cleft lip and palate (UCCLP)
- Bilateral complete cleft lip and palate (BCCLP)

The description is based on previously published data.[8–10] All the patients were examined at about 2 months of age, before any surgical treatment of the cleft anomaly had been carried out. The control group consisted of an age-matched group of children with unilateral incomplete cleft lip (UCCLP) without involvement of the alveolus, since a previous study by Dahl[11] had shown that the average facial morphology of adult individuals with isolated cleft lip is very close to that of normal individuals except for minor localized changes in the region of the cleft and a somewhat increased interorbital distance (Fig. 48–1). For ethical reasons, no attempt was made to collect cephalometric data for normal Danish newborns. Since it was shown that there was no gender difference in craniofacial morphology between any of the cleft groups at 2 months of age, data for the two genders were pooled within all groups. The sample sizes were as follows:

- Control group: N = 45
- ICP: N = 53

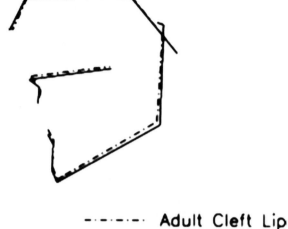

- - - - - - **Adult Cleft Lip**
—————— **Adult Control**

Figure 48–1. Mean plot of the facial morphology in adult males with ICP (N = 62) superimposed on a mean plot of an adult male control group (N = 102). (*Based on data from Dahl E. Craniofacial morphology in congenital clefts of the lip and palate. Acta Odontol Scand 28(Suppl. 57):1–167, 1970.*)

- UCCLP: N = 48
- BCCLP: N = 19

For each diagnosis, the data will be presented as mean plots (lateral, frontal, and axial projections) superimposed on the respective mean plots for the control group. Only variables with differences between the means significant at the 1% level will be mentioned.

Isolated Cleft Palate

The mean plots of the ICP-group are presented in Fig. 48–2. The most striking findings in the ICP-group were: receding soft tissue profile in relation to the anterior cranial base, especially for the chin; short maxilla; reduced posterior maxillary height; increased posterior maxillary width; short mandible; reduced posterior height of the mandible; bimaxillary retrognathia; and reduced pharyngeal depth and height.

Unilateral Complete Cleft Lip and Palate

The mean plots of the UCCLP-group are presented in Fig. 48–3. The most striking findings in the UCCLP-group were: receding soft tissue profile in relation to the anterior cranial base, except for a relative protrusion of the upper lip; relative protrusion of the premaxilla which deviated to the noncleft side; decreased length of the basal part of the maxilla; reduced posterior maxillary height; increased posterior maxillary width; short mandible; bimaxillary retrognathia (except for the relative protrusion of the premaxilla); and reduced pharyngeal depth and height.

Bilateral Complete Cleft Lip and Palate

The mean plots of the BCCLP-group are presented in Fig. 48–4. The most striking findings in the BCCLP-group were:

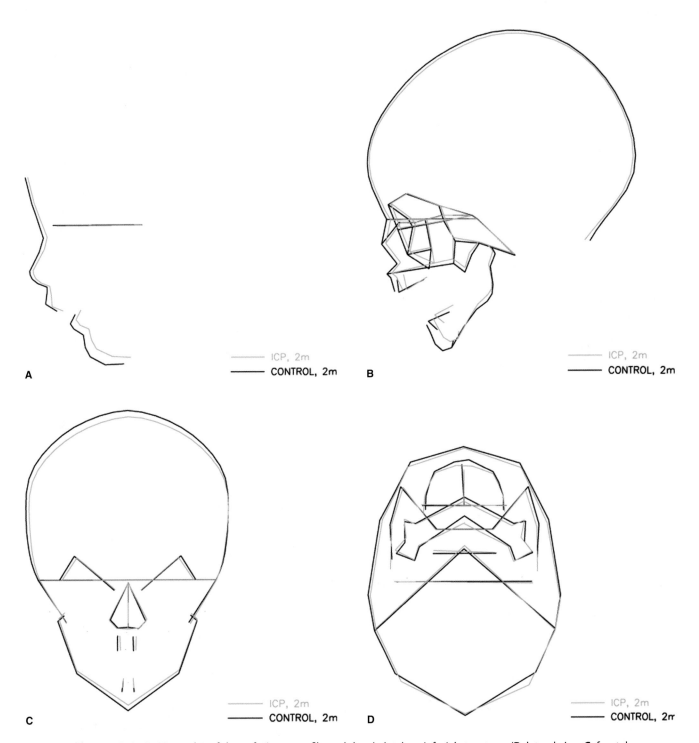

Figure 48–2. A: Mean plot of the soft tissue profile and the skeletal caniofacial structures (**B:** lateral view **C:** frontal view, and **D:** axial view) in 2-month-old infants with ICP (*N* = 53) superimposed on mean plots of an age-matched control group (*N* = 45). (*Modified from Hermann NV, Kreiborg S, Darvann TA, Jensen BL, Dahl E, Bolund S. Early craniofacial morphology and growth in children with unoperated isolated cleft palate. Cleft Palate Craniofac J. 39:604–622, 2002.*)

receding soft tissue profile in relation to the anterior cranial base, except for protrusion of the upper lip; an extremely protruding premaxilla; decreased length of the basal part of the maxilla; reduced posterior maxillary height; increased posterior maxillary width; short mandible; bimaxillary retrognathia (except for the protruding premaxilla); and reduced pharyngeal depth and height.

Discussion and Conclusion

Newborn infants with clefts of the palate, with or without cleft lip, share a number of craniofacial characteristics when compared to a control group without cleft palate: the soft tissue profile is, in general, receding in relation to the anterior cranial base; the basal part of the maxilla is short; the posterior maxillary height is reduced; maxillary width is increased;

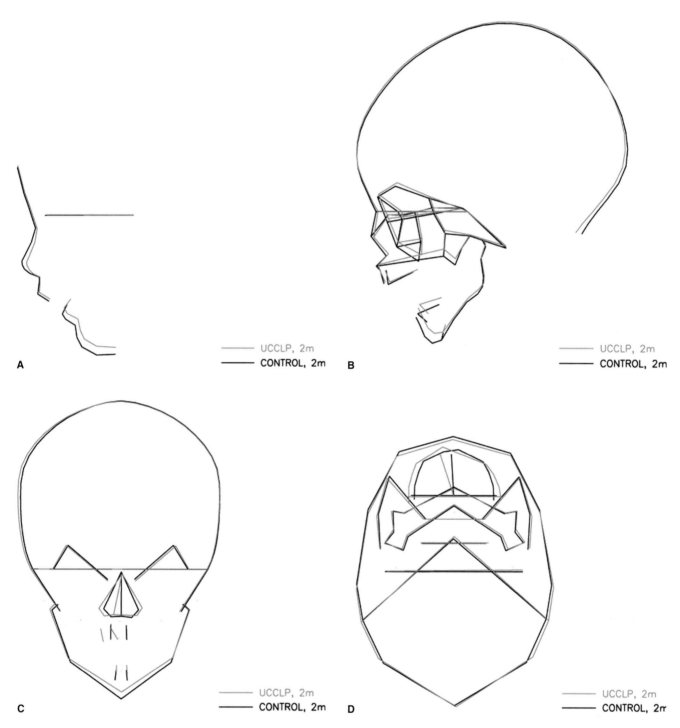

A

——— UCCLP, 2m
——— CONTROL, 2m

B

——— UCCLP, 2m
——— CONTROL, 2m

C

——— UCCLP, 2m
——— CONTROL, 2m

D

——— UCCLP, 2m
——— CONTROL, 2m

Figure 48–3.   A: Mean plot of the soft tissue profile and the skeletal craniofacial structures (**B:** lateral view, **C:** frontal view, and **D:** axial view) in 2-month-old infants with UCCLP ($N = 48$) superimposed on mean plots of an age-matched control group ($N = 45$). (*Modified from Hermann NV, Jensen BL, Dahl E, Bolund S, Kreiborg S. A comparison of the craniofacial morphology in 2-month-old unoperated infants with unilateral complete cleft lip and palate, and unilateral incomplete cleft lip. J Craniofac Genet Dev Biol 19:80–93, 1999.*)

the mandible is short (Fig. 48–5); and there is bimaxillary retrognathia and reduced pharyngeal depth and height. As seen in Fig. 48–6, superimposing the mean plot for the lateral projection the UCCLP-group on the mean plot for the ICP-groups gives a much closer "fit" than when superimpos-

ing the mean plot for the UCCLP-group on the mean plot for the normal controls (see Fig. 48–2). The major difference between the UCCLP-group and the ICP-group being the relative protrusion of the premaxilla and the upper lip in the UCCLP-group. This difference can be explained by the

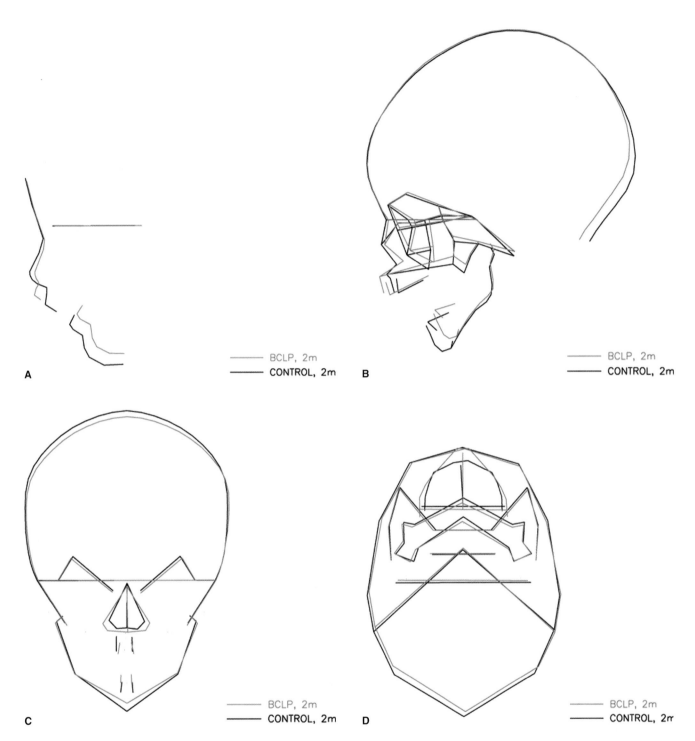

Figure 48–4. A: Mean plots of the soft tissue profile and the skeletal craniofacial structures (**B:** lateral view, **C:** frontal view, and **D:** axial view) in 2-month-old infants with BCCLP (*N* = 19) superimposed on mean plots of an age-matched control group (*N* = 45). (*Modified from Hermann NV, Kreiborg S, Darvann TA, Jensen BL, Dahl E, Bolund S. Early craniofacial morphology and growth in children with bilateral complete cleft lip and palate. Cleft Palate Craniofac J 41:424–438, 2004.*)

complete cleft of the lip and alveolous in this group. We suggest that cleft of the secondary palate, with or without cleft lip, is associated with the facial type described above.[3,7–9,12] Therefore, when analyzing the outcome following closure of the lip and palate in children with combined clefts (e.g.

UCCLP and BCCLP), comparison should, in our opinion, not be made to a normal control group or normative data, but rather to a group of children with nonsyndromic ICP. Such comparisons are employed in a later section of this chapter.

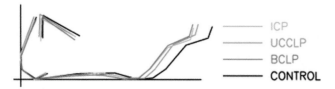

Figure 48–5. Superimposed mean plots of the mandible in 2-month-old infants with unoperated ICP (*N* = 53), UCCLP (*N* = 48) and BCCLP (*N* = 19), respectively, and an age matched control group (*N* = 45). (*Modified from Eriksen J, Hermann NV, Darvann TA, Kreiborg S. Early postnatal development of the mandible in children with isolated cleft palate and children with nonsyndromic Robin sequence. Cleft Palate Craniofac J 43: 160–167, 2006.*)

Early Facial Growth in Unoperated Children with ICP

The average craniofacial growth patterns from 2–22 months of age in the unoperated ICP-group and in the control group, are illustrated in Fig. 48–7A, B, C, and D. The growth pattern was very similar in the two groups except for a somewhat more vertical facial growth pattern in the ICP-group (Fig. 48–8). It is noteworthy that at 22 months of age the mean differences between the ICP-group and the control group were of the same nature as observed at 2 months of age, described above (Figs. 48–2 and 48–9); most notably, the soft tissue profile was still receding, the maxilla was short and retrognathic; the mandible was short and retrognathic; and the size of the pharyngeal airway was reduced.

Discussion and Conclusion

These findings support the hypothesis that subjects with non-syndromic clefts of the secondary palate, as a group, have a craniofacial morphology and a facial growth pattern that is within the limits of the normal variation, but their mean facial type is skewed within the normal distribution toward bimaxillary retrognathia, short mandible, and a more vertical facial growth pattern.[3,7,8,10–21] It has even been hypothesized that reduced mandibular length is a risk factor in the development of cleft palate.[22,23]

THE EFFECT OF LIP SURGERY ON EARLY FACIAL GROWTH

In the present context, this description will be limited to the group of children with UCCLP.

Unilateral Incomplete Cleft Lip

The effect of surgical closure of the cleft lip by a Tennison procedure at about 2 months of age on the soft tissue profile and the craniofacial growth pattern was analyzed by three-projection cephalometry and compared to the findings in the control group and in the ICP-group, respectively.

Fig. 48–10 illustrates the average craniofacial growth in the UCCLP-group from 2 to 22 months of age based on the lateral cephalometric projection. Lip surgery was performed just after the cephalometric examination at 2 months

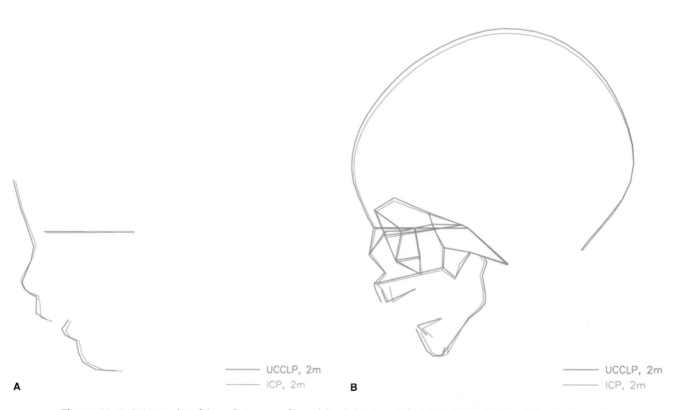

Figure 48–6. A: Mean plot of the soft tissue profile and the skeletal craniofacial structures (**B:** lateral view) in 2-month-old infants with UCCLP (*N* = 48) superimposed on mean plots of 2-month-old infants with ICP (*N* = 53).

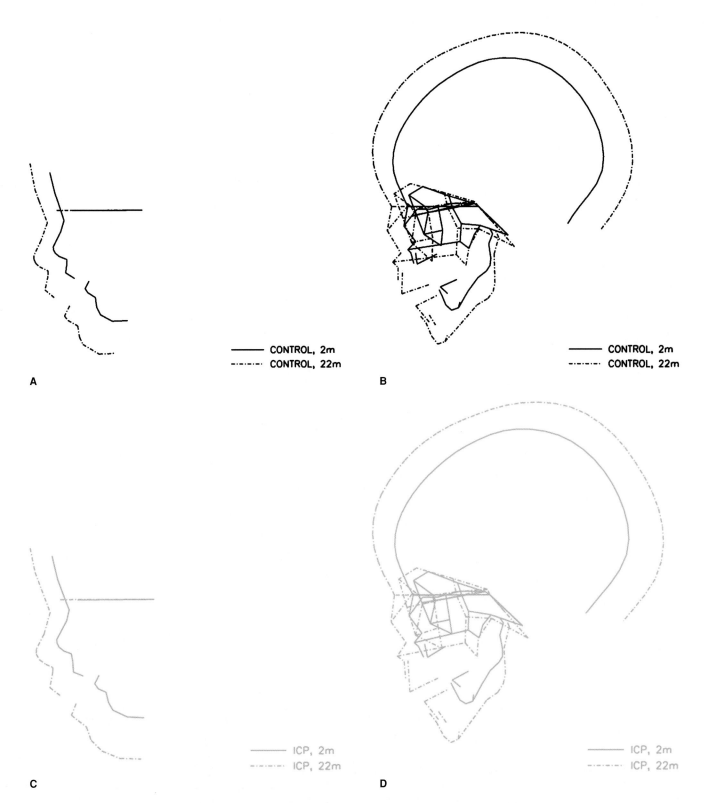

Figure 48–7. A: Superimposed mean plots of the soft tissue profile and the skeletal craniofacial structures (**B:** lateral view) of children with ICP (*N* = 53) from the ages 2 months and 22 months. **C:** Superimposed mean plots of the soft tissue profile and the skeletal craniofacial structures (**D:** lateral view) of control children without cleft palate (*N* = 45) from the ages 2 and 22 months. (*Modified from Hermann NV, Kreiborg S, Darvann TA, Jensen BL, Dahl E, Bolund S. Early craniofacial morphology and growth in children with unoperated isolated cleft palate. Cleft Palate Craniofac J. 39:604–622, 2002.*)

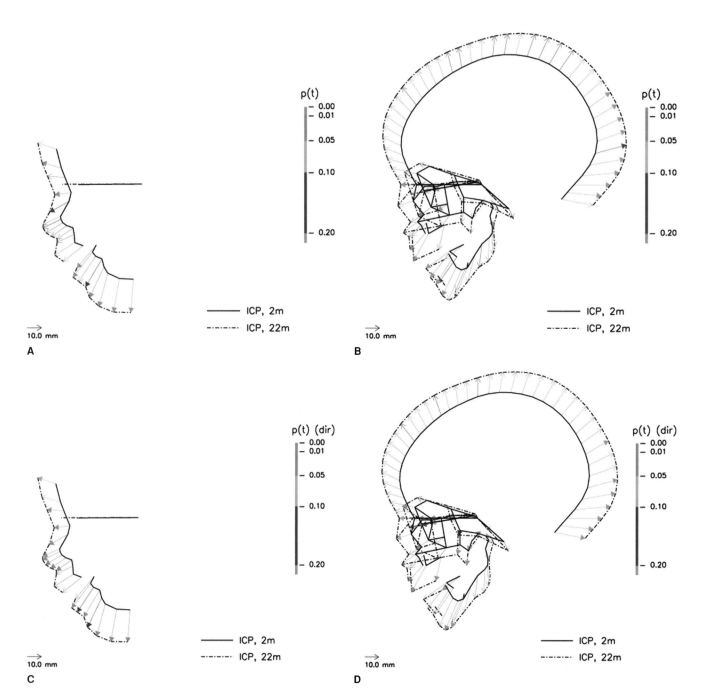

Figure 48–8. A: The average amount of growth of the soft tissue profile and the skeletal craniofacial structures (**B:** lateral view) of children with ICP (*N* = 53) from 2 months to 22 months of age. The significance of differences in the total length, *p(t)*, of the growth vectors when compared to the controls is indicated. Vectors with filled arrowheads indicate a larger growth in the ICP-group than in the control group, whereas vectors with unfilled arrowheads indicate a smaller growth in the ICP-group than in the control group. **C:** The average direction of the facial growth pattern in ICP-group. Vectors with filled arrowhead indicate a larger angle of the vector in relation to the NSL, meaning a more vertical growth direction in the ICP-group than in the control-group. **D:** Whereas vectors with unfilled arrowheads indicate a smaller angle of the vector in relation to the NSL, meaning less vertical growth in the ICP-group than in the control-group. (*Modified from Hermann NV, Kreiborg S, Darvann TA, Jensen BL, Dahl E, Bolund S. Early craniofacial morphology and growth in children with unoperated isolated cleft palate. Cleft Palate Craniofac J. 39:604–622, 2002.*)

of age. In general, the growth pattern seemed very harmonious, both for the soft tissue profile and for the skeletal structures. In fact, the growth pattern was somewhat similar to the growth pattern observed in the control group (Fig. 48–7B). The magnitude of growth was about the same in the

UCCLP-group and in the control group, except for the upper lip and the reference points related to the primary incisors, as shown in the vectorgram illustrated in Fig. 48–11A and B. In these regions, the growth vectors were significantly reduced in the UCCLP-group compared to the control group.

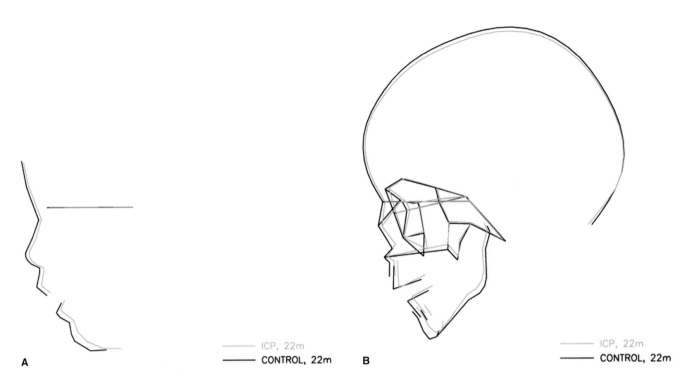

Figure 48–9. A: Mean plot of the soft tissue profile and the skeletal craniofacial structures (**B:** lateral view) in 22-month-old ICP-children (*N* = 53) superimposed on mean plots of age-matched controls (*N* = 45). (*Modified from Hermann NV, Kreiborg S, Darvann TA, Jensen BL, Dahl E, Bolund S. Early craniofacial morphology and growth in children with unoperated isolated cleft palate. Cleft Palate Craniofac J. 39:604–622, 2002.*)

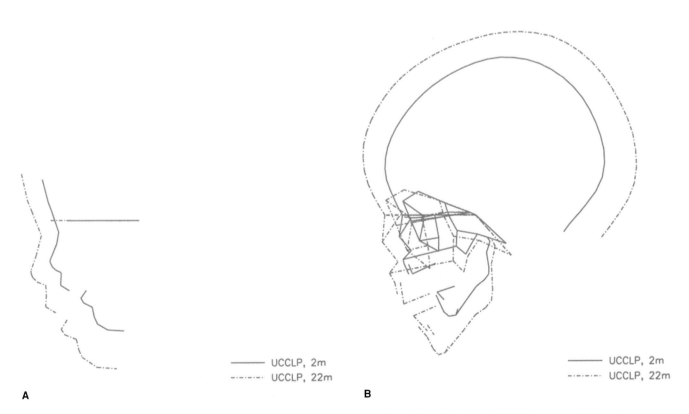

Figure 48–10. A: Superimposed mean plots of the soft tissue profile and the skeletal craniofacial structures (**B:** lateral view) in 22-month-old children with UCCLP (*N* = 48) and age-matched controls (*N* = 45). (*Modified from Hermann NV, Jensen BL, Dahl E, Bolund S, Kreiborg S. Craniofacial comparisons in 22 months old lip-operated children with unilateral complete cleft lip and palate, and unilateral incomplete cleft lip. Cleft Palate Craniofac J 37:303–317, 2000.*)

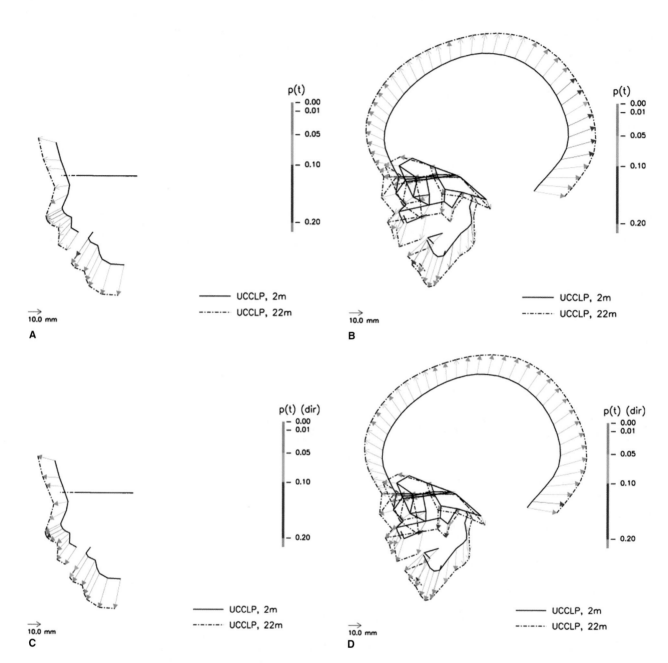

Figure 48–11. A: The average amount of growth of the soft tissue profile and the skeletal craniofacial structures (**B:** lateral view) of children with UCCLP (*N* = 48) from 2 months to 22 months of age. The significance of differences in the total length, *p(t)*, of the growth vectors when compared to the controls is indicated. Vectors with filled arrowheads indicate a larger growth in the UCCLP-group than in the control group, whereas vectors with unfilled arrowheads indicate a smaller growth in the UCCLP-group than in the control group. **C:** The average direction of the facial growth pattern in UCCLP-group. Vectors with filled arrowhead indicate a larger angle of the vector in relation to the NSL, meaning a more vertical growth direction in the UCCLP-group than in the control-group. **D:** Whereas vectors with unfilled arrowheads indicate a smaller angle of the vector in relation to the NSL, meaning less vertical growth in the UCCLP-group than in the control-group. (*Modified from Hermann NV, Jensen BL, Dahl E, Bolund S, Kreiborg S. Craniofacial comparisons in 22 months old lip-operated children with unilateral complete cleft lip and palate, and unilateral incomplete cleft lip. Cleft Palate Craniofac J 37:303–317, 2000.*)

In addition, the direction of facial growth was significantly more vertical in relation to the nasion-sella line (NSL) in the UCCLP-group (Fig. 48–11C and D). When the craniofacial morphology at 22 months of age in the UCCLP-group was compared to the controls (Fig. 48–12), it was observed that the UCCLP-group had a receding soft tissue facial profile, a short and retrognathic maxilla, a short and retrognathic mandible, and reduced size of the pharyngeal airway. These morphological characteristics were also described for unoperated 22 month-old ICP-children (see above); when

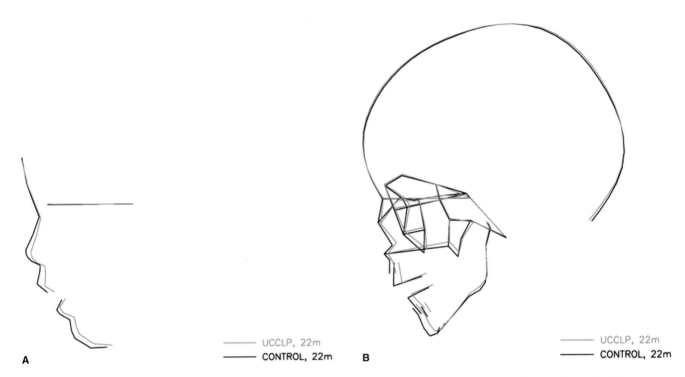

Figure 48–12. A: Mean plot of the soft tissue profile and the skeletal craniofacial structures (**B:** lateral view) in 22-month-old UCCLP-children ($N = 48$) superimposed on mean plots of the control group ($N = 45$) at 22 months of age. (*Modified from Hermann NV, Jensen BL, Dahl E, Bolund S, Kreiborg S. Craniofacial comparisons in 22 months old lip-operated children with unilateral complete cleft lip and palate, and unilateral incomplete cleft lip. Cleft Palate Craniofac J 37:303–317, 2000.*)

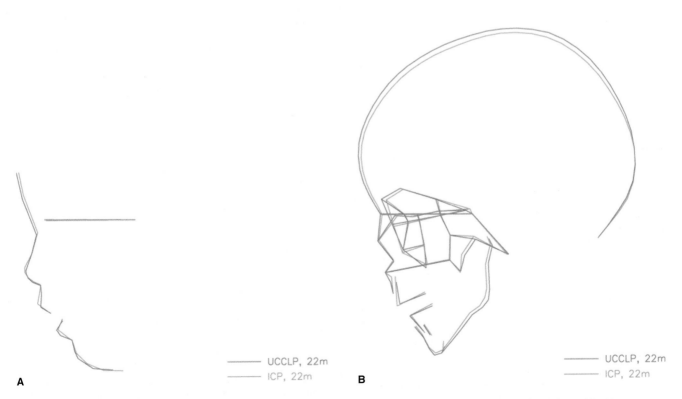

Figure 48–13. A: Mean plot of the soft tissue profile and the skeletal craniofacial structures (**B:** lateral view) in 22-month-old UCCLP-children ($N = 48$) superimposed on mean plots of ICP-children ($N = 53$) at 22 months of age.

the mean plots of the UCCLP-group at 22 months of age were superimposed on the mean plots of the ICP-children at the same age (Fig. 48–13), it was observed that the soft tissue profile and the skeletal morphology were nearly identical in the two groups. On an average, the upper lip was slightly less protruding in the UCCLP-group and the inclination of the maxillary primary incisors was also reduced in the UCCLP-group. Otherwise, the average differences in the soft tissue profile and facial skeleton were negligible.

Discussion and Conclusion

The effect of lip surgery at about 2 months of age, using a Tennison procedure, on the soft tissue profile and facial growth up to 22 months of age in children with UCCLP is, in general, favorable, leading to a harmonious soft tissue profile and a balanced jaw relationship. The resulting average morphology is, however, not identical to that of a control group but rather resembles the morphology observed in 22 month-old children with unoperated ICP.

CONCLUSION

This chapter has presented available knowledge concerning:

- facial morphology in newborns with ICP, UCCLP, and BCCLP
- early facial growth in unoperated children with ICP from 2–22 months of age
- the effect of lip surgery on facial growth in the first 2 years of life in UCCLP-children

It is suggested, based on comprehensive studies of a large consecutive sample of cleft individuals, using three-projection cephalometry, that newborns with clefts of the secondary palate, with or without cleft lip, have a characteristic *facial morphology* with a receding soft tissue profile, bimaxillay retrognathia, and a reduced size of the pharyngeal region.

In the individuals with combined clefts of the lip and palate, the maxillary retrognathia in the newborn is masked by relative (UCCLP-group) or true (BCCLP-group) protrusion of the premaxilla, caused by the lack of integrity of the maxilla and upper lip.

The early *facial growth* in the unoperated ICP-group from 2 to 22 months of age shows a harmonious growth pattern with the same magnitude of facial growth as observed in the control group but with a more vertical growth pattern, maintaining the morphology found at birth.

The effect of lip surgery (Tennison procedure) at 2 months of age on the subsequent facial growth up to 22 months of age in children with UCCLP has been shown to lead to a favorable molding of the premaxilla into place in the intrinsically retrognathic maxilla, thereby creating a facial morphology similar to that of 22 month-old children with unoperated ICP.

It is further suggested that future studies on the effect of lip surgery and palatal surgery on subsequent facial growth in individuals with nonsyndromic combined cleft lip and palate (CLP) should be made with comparison to individuals with ICP and not to normal controls or to normative data. Otherwise, it is to be expected that the importance of iatrogenic factors (surgery) and functional or adaptive factors will be overemphasized, since the intrinsic facial morphology in CLP-individuals is characterized by bimaxillary retrognathia and the intrinsic growth pattern is, on average, more vertical than in normal individuals without clefts of the secondary palate.

References

1. Broadbent H. A new X-ray technique and its application to orthodontia. *Angle Orthod* 1:45–66, 1931.
2. Semb G, Shaw WC. Facial growth in orofacial clefting disorders. In Turvey TA, Vig KWL, Fonseca RJ (eds). *Facial Clefts and Craniosynostosis. Principles and Management.* Philadelphia, PA, WB Saunders Company, 1996, pp. 28–56.
3. Kreiborg S, Hermann NV, Darvann TA. Characteristics of Facial Growth and development in children with clefts. In Berkowitz S (ed). *Cleft Lip and Palate. With an Introduction to other Craniofacial Anomalies. Perspectives in Management.* Berlin, Germany, Springer Verlag, 2005, pp. 225–235.
4. Jensen BL, Kreiborg S, Dahl E, Fogh-Andersen P. Cleft lip and palate in Denmark, 1976–1981: Epidemiology, variability, and early somatic development. *Cleft Palate J* 25:258–269, 1988.
5. Kreiborg S, Dahl E, Prydsø U. A unit for infant roentgencephalometry. *Dentomaxillofac Radiol* 6:29–33, 1977.
6. Heller A, Kreiborg S, Dahl E, Jensen BL. X-ray: Cephalometric analysis system for lateral, frontal, and axial projections. Presented at the *5th European Craniofacial Congress*, Copenhagen, Denmark, 1995, Abstract 61:33.
7. Hermann NV, Jensen BL, Dahl E, Bolund S, Darvann TA, Kreiborg S. A method for three projection infant cephalometry. *Cleft Palate Craniofac J* 38:299–316, 2001.
8. Hermann NV, Jensen BL, Dahl E, Bolund S, Kreiborg S. A comparison of the craniofacial morphology in 2-month-old unoperated infants with unilateral complete cleft lip and palate, and unilateral incomplete cleft lip. *J Craniofac Genet Dev Biol* 19:80–93, 1999.
9. Hermann NV, Kreiborg S, Darvann TA, Jensen BL, Dahl E, Bolund S. Early craniofacial morphology and growth in children with unoperated isolated cleft palate. *Cleft Palate Craniofac J* 39:604–622, 2002.
10. Hermann NV, Kreiborg S, Darvann TA, Jensen BL, Dahl E, Bolund S. Early craniofacial morphology and growth in children with bilateral complete cleft lip and palate. *Cleft Palate Craniofac J* 41:424–438, 2004.
11. Dahl E. Craniofacial morphology in congenital clefts of the lip and palate. *Acta Odontol Scand* 28(Suppl. 57):1–167, 1970.
12. Eriksen J, Hermann NV, Darvann TA, Kreiborg S. Early postnatal development of the mandible in children with isolated cleft palate and children with nonsyndromic Robin sequence. *Cleft Palate Craniofac J* 43:160–167, 2006.
13. Dahl E, Kreiborg S, Jensen BL, Fogh-Andersen P. Comparison of craniofacial morphology in infants with incomplete cleft lip and infants with isolated cleft palate. *Cleft Palate J* 19:258–266, 1982.
14. Dahl E, Kreiborg S, Jensen BL. Roentgencephalometric studies of infants with untreated cleft lip and palate. In Kriens O (ed). *What is a Cleft Lip and Palate? A Multidisciplinary Update.* Stuttgart, Germany, Georg Thieme Verlag, 1989, pp. 113–115.

15. Dahl E, Kreiborg S. Craniofacial malformations. In Thilander B, Rönning O (eds). *Introduction to Orthodontics*, 2nd ed. Gothia, Stockholm, 1995, pp. 239–254.

16. Hermann NV, Jensen BL, Dahl E, Bolund S, Darvann TA, Kreiborg S. Craniofacial growth in subjects with unilateral complete cleft lip and palate, and unilateral incomplete cleft lip, from 2 to 22 months of age. *J Craniofac Genet Dev Biol* 19:135–147, 1999.

17. Hermann NV, Jensen BL, Dahl E, Bolund S, Kreiborg S. Craniofacial comparisons in 22 months old lip-operated children with unilateral complete cleft lip and palate, and unilateral incomplete cleft lip. *Cleft Palate Craniofac J* 37:303–317, 2000.

18. Hermann NV, Kreiborg S, Darvann TA, Jensen BL, Dahl E, Bolund S. Early craniofacial morphology and growth in children with non-syndromic Robin sequence. *Cleft Palate Craniofac J* 40:131–143, 2003.

19. Hermann NV, Kreiborg S, Darvann TA, Jensen BL, Dahl E, Bolund S. Craniofacial morphology and growth comparisons in children with Robin sequence, isolated cleft palate, and unilateral complete cleft lip and palate. *Cleft Palate Craniofac J* 40:373–396, 2003.

20. Kreiborg S, Cohen MM, Jr. Syndrome delineation and growth in orofacial clefting and craniosynostosis. In Turvey TA, Vig KWL, Fonseca RJ (eds). *Facial Clefts and Craniosynostosis. Principles and Management*. Philadelphia, PA, WB Saunders Company, 1996, pp. 57–75.

21. Kreiborg S, Hermann NV. Craniofacial morphology and growth in infants and young children with cleft lip and palate. In Wyszynski DF (ed). *Cleft Lip and Palate: From Origin to Treatment*. Boston, Oxford University Press, 2002, pp. 87–98.

22. Hermann NV, Kreiborg S, Darvann TA, Jensen BL, Dahl E. Mandibular retrognathia in infants with cleft of the secondary palate. *Proceedings of the 9th International Congress on Cleft Palate and Related Craniofacial Anomalies*, Gothenburg, Sweden, 2001; pp.151–154.

23. Kreiborg S, Hermann NV, Darvann TA, Petersen I, Christensen K. Reduced mandibular length is a risk factor in development of cleft palate. *10th International Congress on Cleft Palate and Related Craniofacial Anomalies, Durban, South Africa*, 2005, Oral Presentation/Abstract.

49

Prosthetic Management of Patients with Clefts

Lawrence E. Brecht, DDS • Mohammad Maraheri, MDD, DDS

Restorative dentistry or prosthodontic care for the cleft palate patient is often not considered until the patient has reached adulthood or until all the surgical and orthodontic care has been completed. At this point, the patient is referred to the prosthodontist to replace any teeth that are missing or are in need of restorations. Little consideration may have been given to the prosthetic or restorative treatment planning required to provide the optimum overall care for the patient. In fact, the cleft palate patient is best served by having a prosthodontist or restorative dentist become involved as early as possible in the treatment planning process.

With the generally accepted principle that the *team approach* to management of the patient with cleft lip and/or palate provides the best results, it is recommended that the prosthodontist become involved in treatment planning at the onset of cleft care, even as early as in infancy. The prosthodon-

tist working with the orthodontist, pediatric dentist, and other members of the cleft palate team at the onset of treatment is the most effective model of care. The prosthodontist must not be considered the treatment provider of last resort, to simply manage the unrepaired cleft palate, the failed pharyngeal flap or to merely replace missing teeth.[1]

ORAL AND DENTAL CONDITIONS AND THE CLEFT ANOMALY

There are a number of dental conditions unique to the patient with the cleft palate anomaly. In the unilateral cleft condition, while the most common finding is the lack of the maxillary lateral incisor on the affected side. It is not uncommon, however, to find that the lateral incisor has been duplicated. Similarly, in the bilateral situation, there may be a second lateral incisor on one or both sides, located on the premaxillary segment or on the lateral alveolar segments. This duplication of dental units often poses esthetic challenges in the development of a natural appearance in the patient's smile. Teeth adjacent to the cleft are often hypoplastic, as well as dysmorphic in shape. Prosthetic intervention may be required to provide balance and symmetry in the development of an esthetic, as well as functional, final tooth arrangement. These teeth may be either larger or smaller than the tooth would normally be in a noncleft situation. Consideration should be given to the selective extraction of teeth that will not enhance the long-term functional or esthetic outcome. Therefore, it is particularly important that the orthodontist and prosthodontist work closely together in establishing a symmetrical and balanced tooth arrangement while orthodontics is underway, rather than waiting for the "final" tooth position determined by the orthodontist alone.

The dysmorphic shape and malposed position of teeth in the cleft patient, combined with the increased tendency for mouth breathing, greatly increases the potential for dental caries in this patient population.[2] The introduction of fixed or removable orthodontic appliances (or both) increases the potential for plaque accumulation and makes oral hygiene measures more challenging. Cleft patients have a higher incidence of dental caries. These patients in particular should be thoroughly instructed on the proper methods of daily oral hygiene. Professional dental prophylaxis and examinations should be increased from the usual regimen of a twice a year to a minimum of three times per year during the childhood and adolescent years, and perhaps even more frequently while they have fixed orthodontic appliances in place.

Early prosthodontic interventions, such as placement of a fixed dental prosthesis to restore badly decayed teeth, or to replace missing teeth, must take into consideration the presence of enlarged pulp chambers in the younger patient, thereby making either a carious or mechanical pulpal exposure more likely. Patients and their parents should be advised of the increased risk potential for the need for endodontic therapy for teeth that require extensive restorations. Every attempt should be made to keep tooth preparations for composite restorations, veneers, or crowns as conservative as possible. An adequate amount of tooth structure should be reduced to provide for physiologic tooth forms in the final restorations. These restorations should not increase the amount of plaque retention or compromise gingival health.

In addition to the unique dental conditions that exist in the cleft patient, there are other important oral factors that must be taken into consideration when providing prosthodontic care. There must be a meticulous examination of the hard and soft tissues of the oral cavity, with particular attention paid to the possible presence of small or pinpoint-sized fistulae (Fig. 49–1).

Dental impression material may be trapped in an unrecognized fistula or be pushed into the nasal cavity. The removal of this material may be difficult or impossible without nasal exploration. The presence of an unseen fistula may

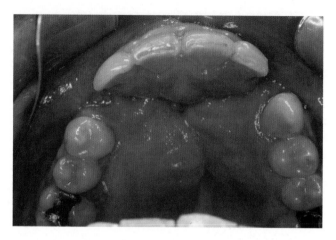

Figure 49–1. Oronasal fistula at the junction of the primary and secondary palate.

be discovered by pinching closed the patient's nostrils and directing the patient to attempt to blow air out through the nose. A high-pitched "hissing" sound may be heard or bubbling of mucous or saliva may be seen if a fistula is present.

The presence of postoperative palatal scarring tends to produce posterior arch width collapse and the recurrence of posterior crossbite if retainers are not fabricated and *used regularly* by the patient who has completed prosthodontic care to replace missing anterior teeth. While a fixed dental prosthesis may serve to maintain tooth position in the anterior maxilla, unless the prosthesis is large enough and encompasses enough teeth to extend to the maxillary molars, there will be the tendency for orthodontic relapse, arch-width collapse, and the development of a crossbite.

PROSTHODONTIC CONSIDERATIONS FOR THE INFANT AND CHILDHOOD CLEFT PATIENT

In cleft centers employing presurgical infant orthopedics, such as nasoalveolar molding, the management of early infant oral and nasal molding may be undertaken by the team's orthodontist, prosthodontist, or pediatric dentist on the team, if the practitioner has been trained in the technique.[3] The early use of presurgical infant orthopedics appliances was advocated by a prosthodontist.[4] In helping to manage the infant undergoing presurgical orthopedic care, the prosthodontist can become familiar with the development of the patient's oral structures from the earliest onset of care.

For the child who has had successful repair of their cleft, there are unique factors that should be taken into account as they grow and progress through orthodontics and eventually into prosthodontic care. Following a successful repair of the alveolar cleft, with or without a gingivoperiosteoplasty, the decision must be made prior to the eruption of the adult canine if autogenous alveolar bone graft surgery is indicated. This determination is often made by the orthodontist or surgeon alone, as is the decision to move the adult canine into

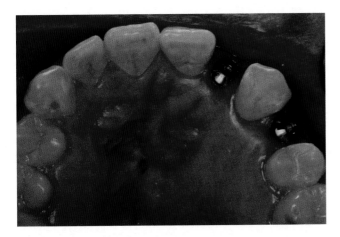

Figure 49–2. Osseointegrated maxillary alveolar implants.

the position of the missing lateral incisor. These decisions are ideally made in the setting of the cleft team, including the input of the prosthodontist who will ultimately be responsible for restoring, both functionally as well as esthetically, the teeth in that area. This requires early collaboration between the prosthodontist and the orthodontist in order to determine the treatment option best suiting each particular child as they progress through their dentofacial growth. There are often a variety of orthoprosthodontic pathways that might be pursued.

At the Institute of Reconstructive Plastic Surgery at New York University Medical Center, the orthodontic–prosthodontic evaluation usually begins at approximately age 8 years. The determination regarding what is needed to establish a solid and stable posterior occlusion is made while developing a maxillary dental midline that is as closely coincidental with the facial midline as is possible.

Consideration will then be given to establishing an intact maxillary alveolus if this has not already been accomplished through an early gingivoperiosteoplasty following nasoalveolar molding therapy. The position of the remaining

teeth, relative to the available space, are then worked out using a series of diagnostic waxups as the child ages and until early adulthood is achieved. Often, it is not finally determined until age 16 whether a missing lateral incisor(s) will best be restored with a transported canine or an osseointegrated implant (Fig. 49–2).

Spaces around the anterior teeth are developed if needed, allowing for properly proportioned teeth in the final restorations. These spaces may be maintained using direct composite restorations bonded to the proximal surfaces of the teeth or through the use of processed composite interim veneer restorations (Figs. 49–3A and B). These interim veneers serve to maintain spaces and provide for normal tooth function and esthetics, all with minimal to no tooth preparation. These interim restorations should not irreversibly alter the tooth or change it in such a manner precluding the placement of definitive restorations once the patient has fully grown and has reached adulthood. Larger, tooth-sized spaces are maintained using a removable Essix-type appliance, a conventional removable Hawley-type retainer, or an acrylic pontic bonded to fixed orthodontic appliances.

OSSEOINTEGRATED IMPLANTS AND THE CLEFT PALATE PATIENT

With sophisticated advances in surgical technique, along with our ability to orthodontically move teeth into fairly ideal positions, the replacement of the missing lateral incisor may be best achieved with a single osseointegrated implant placed once the patient has reached age 21 or even older.[5] A number of studies report greater than 90% success rates for implants placed into cleft sites adequately grafted or developed to receive an implant (Figure 49–4).[6] An osseointegrated implant should not be placed in the growing maxilla, and every attempt should be made to assure that growth has indeed been completed prior to implant placement. Although not reported specifically in the cleft patient population, the

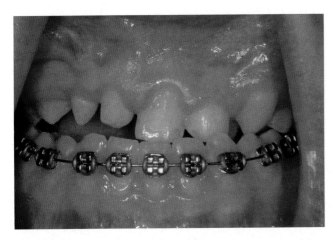

A

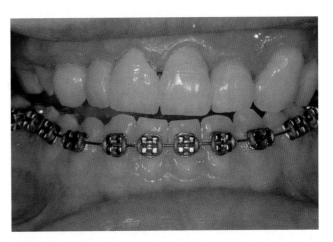

B

Figure 49–3. Processed composite interim veneer restorations (**A and B**).

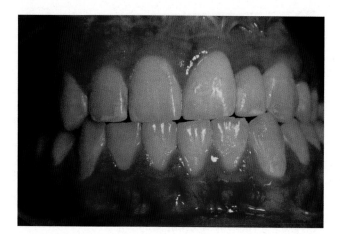

Figure 49–4. Osseointegrated dental implant in the cleft.

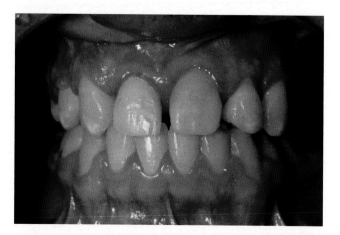

A

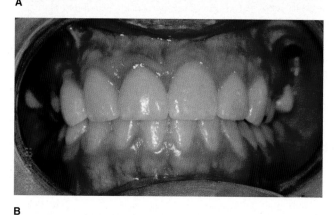

B

Figure 49–5. Adhesive-retained or "bonded" ceramic restorations, also referred to as "veneers" or "porcelain laminates" (**A and B**).

changes in anterior clinical crown height in younger patients having received single-tooth implant restorations have been well documented.[7] Over time, the position of the implant-supported single tooth restoration is at risk of developing an intruded vertical position relative to the natural teeth proximal to the implant.

Adequate bone quality and quantity in the region of the cleft is required to consider this conservative prosthetic intervention.[8] Often, additional bone grafting or implant site development is indicated even if there was sufficient bone present for the earlier eruption of the adult canine. Secondary or even tertiary bone grafting may be required to develop sufficient bone mass able to adequately support an endosseous implant and sustain a functional masticatory loading force.[9] We believe the ideal bone graft likely includes corticocancellous bone with marrow from the iliac crest region, and less preferably from the chin, tibia, or calvarium.[10] The placement of the endosseous implant should not be delayed beyond 4 months following the alveolar bone graft, or there is an increased risk that the volume of bone in the grafted site will begin to resorb. While it may be contended that the surgical placement of an osseointegrated implant is an aggressive approach to the management of the missing lateral incisor, an implant will serve to preserve the alveolar bone in the area, and will preserve tooth structure on the teeth proximal to the cleft site. In addition, an implant will reduce the potential for caries and endodontic complications that may accompany the early placement of a fixed dental prosthesis with the requisite tooth preparation and removal of natural tooth structure.

ANTERIOR BONDED CERAMIC RESTORATIONS

The replacement of missing anterior teeth or the development of an esthetic anterior tooth arrangement may, in select patients, be achieved through the use of adhesive-retained or "bonded" ceramic restorations.[11] These may be more commonly referred to as "veneers" or "porcelain laminates."

Again, the early and close collaboration between the orthodontist and the prosthodontist is imperative in order to provide the proper tooth arrangement where bonded ceramic restorations may be considered as an option for the young adult cleft patient. Ideally, as the orthodontic treatment is nearing completion, impressions of the teeth are obtained with the orthodontic wires off but the brackets left in place. The prosthodontist may then develop a diagnostic waxup and determine if additional tooth movement needs to be performed in order to consider "veneers" as an option (Figs. 49–5A and B). If veneers are deemed an acceptable treatment option, the orthodontics are completed, the patient is placed into orthodontic retention, gingival health is optimized if it is less than ideal, and the usual process of veneer fabrication is implemented. Once again, following the placement of the bonded ceramic restorations, a new orthodontic retainer must be fabricated for the patient.

Tooth preparation for bonded ceramic restorations should be as conservative as possible and remain in enamel whenever possible. The patient and/or the patient's parents must be informed that veneers require (1) the removal of tooth structure, (2) strict oral hygiene, and (3) at some point, replacement and perhaps the need for a full-coverage crown restoration if a "veneer" is no longer possible.

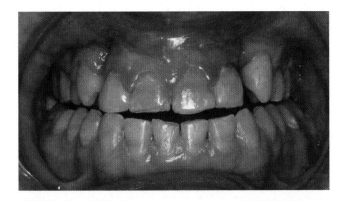

A

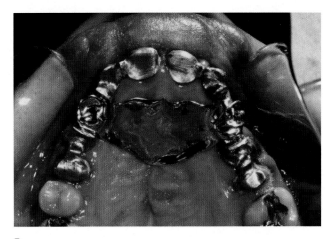

B

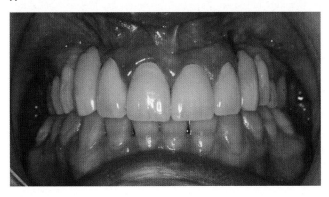

C

Figure 49–6. A combined "fixed–removable" maxillary prosthesis (**A, B, and C**).

PROSTHODONTIC CONSIDERATIONS FOR THE OLDER CLEFT PATIENT

As prosthodontic care progresses into the later years of life for the patient with a successfully repaired cleft, decisions must be made regarding the potential extraction of hopeless teeth with inadequate bone support or teeth that are severely malposed. Overdenture prostheses still have a place in the prosthodontic armamentarium for the appropriately selected cleft palate patient.

Consideration should be given to bone grafting the cleft alveolus before embarking upon any fixed dental prosthesis that spans the cleft gap and that is retained on abutment teeth located in mobile alveolar segments.[12] A fixed prosthesis placed across an unrepaired cleft will likely result in fracture of the restorative materials, loosening of the prosthesis or the abutment teeth, washout of the luting agent retaining the fixed prosthesis on the abutment teeth, and/or the subsequent development of dental caries. Encompassing additional teeth as abutments for a fixed dental prosthesis spanning an unrepaired cleft may still not prevent the movement of the alveolar segments when they are functionally loaded. It is axiomatic that a resin-bonded or "Maryland bridge"-type fixed prosthesis is *not* indicated in the situation where there are mobile alveolar segments, or when the proposed abutment teeth are mobile. In situations where the patient declines the recommendation for alveolar bone grafting, or has perhaps had a failed bone graft, some mechanism must be incorporated into the prosthesis design allowing for the

displacement of the mobile alveolar segments without transferring all loading forces to a rigid fixed prosthesis. This will often require the use of a removable prosthesis as well, in a combined "fixed–removable" prosthesis (Figs. 49–6A, B, and C).

SUMMARY

The prosthodontist is an integral person on the cleft palate interdisciplinary team and should become involved in the management of the patient's treatment planning at an early point in the patient's care. A prosthodontist engaged in treating patients with oral, facial, and speech deficits should be thoroughly familiar with the anatomic and physiologic deviations of the cleft defect, and involved with the basic principles involved in prosthetic dentistry. Prosthetic restorations for the older patient with a repaired cleft may include a fixed dental prosthesis, either tooth- or implant-supported. A removable appliance should be considered across a cleft defect where mobile alveolar segments remain. As long as sufficient alveolar bone is present, the placement of an osseointegrated implant in the repaired alveolus, replacing a missing lateral incisor is a predictable and conservative method of tooth replacement. Similarly, bonded porcelain restorations may conservatively address esthetic issues associated with anterior teeth in the cleft patient. The prosthodontist caring for cleft patients should always be willing to acquire further knowledge in this field.

References

1. Cooper HK, Long RE, Cooper JA, Mazaheri M, Millard RT. Psychological, orthodontic, and prosthetic approaches in rehabilitation of the cleft palate patient. *Dent Clin North AM* XX:381–393, 1960.

2. Stec-Slonicz M, Szczepanska J, Hirschfelder U. Comparison of caries prevalence in two populations of cleft patients. *Cleft Palate Craniofac J* 44(5):537, 2007.

3. Grayson BH, Santiago PE, Brecht LE, Cutting CB. Presurgical nasoalveolar molding in infants with cleft lip and palate. *Cleft Palate Craniofacial J* 36(6):486–498, 1999.

4. Winters JC, Hurwitz DJ. Presurgical orthopedics in the surgical management of unilateral cleft lip and palate. *Plast Reconstr Surg* 95:755–764, 1995.

5. Matsui Y, Ohno K, Nishimura A, Shirota T, Kim S, Miyashita H. Long-term study of dental implants placed into alveolar cleft sites. *Cleft Palate Craniofac J* 44(4):444–447, 2007.

6. Cune, MS, Meijer, GJ Koole. Anterior tooth replacement with implants in grafted alveolar cleft sites: A case series. *Clin Oral Implants Res* 15:616, 2004.

7. Jemt T, Ahlberg G, Henriksson K, Bondevik O. Changes of anterior clinical crown height in patients provided with single-implant restorations after more than 15 years of follow-up. *Int J Prosthodont* 19(5):455–461, 2006.

8. Kearns G, Perrott DH, Sharma A, Kaban LB, Vargerik K. Placement of endosseous implants in grafted alveolar clefts. *Cleft Palate Craniofac J* 34:520, 1997.

9. Murthy AS, Lehman JA. Evaluation of alveolar bone grafting: a survey of ACPA teams. *Cleft Palate Craniofac J* 42(1):99–101, 2005.

10. Ramstad T, Semb G. The effect of alveolar bone grafting on the prosthodontic/reconstructive treatment of patients with unilateral complete cleft lip and palate. *Int J Prosthodont* 10(2):156–163, 1997.

11. Moore D, McCord JF. Prosthetic dentistry and the unilateral cleft lip and palate patient. The last 30 years. A review of the prosthodontic literature in respect of treatment options. *Eur J Prosthodont Restor Dent* 12(2):70–74, 2004.

12. Murthy AS, Lehman JA. Evaluation of alveolar bone grafting: a survey of ACPA teams. *Cleft Palate Craniofac J* 42(1):99–101, 2005.

Otologic, Audiologic, and Airway Assessment and Management

50

Cleft Palate and Middle-Ear Disease

J. Brett Chafin, MD • Charles D. Bluestone, MD

EPIDEMIOLOGY

In the 1960s, Stool and Randall were among the first to report the high incidence of middle-ear disease (MED) in infants with cleft palate.[1] In 1969, Paradise and Bluestone noted the universality of the MED in unrepaired infants, with over 80% having persistent disease after repair.[2] This high rate of otitis media is attributed to abnormalities of Eustachian tube function (ETF).[1–3] Others corroborated these finding, with 90–100% having abnormal findings prior to repair, and a reported incidence of disease of 40–100% in the patient with a repaired cleft palate.[3,4] In this chapter, unless otherwise noted, the term "cleft" will relate specifically to clefting of the palate. Associated clefting of the lip will be included, only when associated with that of the palate as well as isolated cleft lip places the child at no higher risk for the development of Eustachian tube dysfunction (ETD) or MED, than children without clefts.

EUSTACHIAN TUBE ANATOMY AND PHYSIOLOGY

The otologic disease encountered by children with cleft palate is due to abnormalities associated with the Eustachian tube (ET). This structure consists of mucosa, cartilage, paratubal muscles (tensor veli palatini, tensor tympani, levator palatini, and salpingopharyngeaus), and bony support (sphenoid sulcus and medial pterygoid plate). The term middle ear refers to the ET, middle-ear space, and mastoid gas cells (Fig. 50–1).

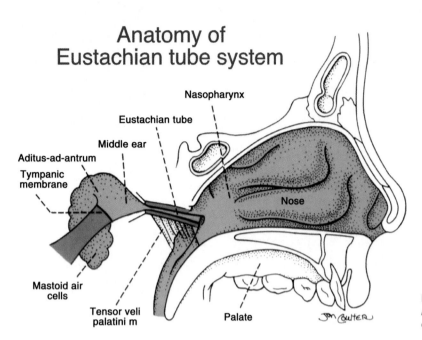

Anatomy of
Eustachian tube system

Figure 50–1. The middle ear. (*Reprinted with permission from B.C. Decker Inc., Hamilton, Ontario, Canada.*)

The ET connects the middle ear to the nasopharynx and has three main functions: ventilate, protect (from nasopharyngeal secretions), and drain the middle ear cavity.[5] The tensor veli palatini (TVP) muscle is composed of two muscle bundles that attach to the cartilaginous portion of the ET, and then wrap around the hamulus in the form of tendon. They then move on to insert on the palatine bone as the palatine tensor aponeurosis. This muscle is primarily responsible for tube dilation; and therefore, adequate middle-ear ventilation. (Fig. 50–2 and Fig. 50–3) represent the association of the TVP and ET.

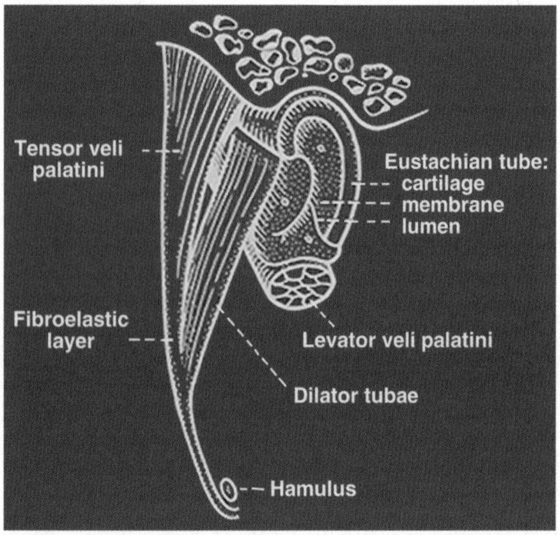

PATHOPHYSIOLOGY

Failure of the ET opening mechanism has been identified as the primary cause of dysfunction.[3,6,7] Histopathologic studies, noted further in the following section, demonstrate that the dysfunction is an obstructive process, which is not anatomic in nature, rather functional, i.e., failure of the opening mechanism as the underlying defect. In addition, craniofacial abnormalities may contribute to tubal dysfunction,

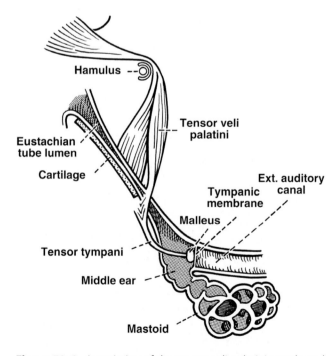

Figure 50–2. Association of the tensor veli palatini muscle and Eustachian tube. (*Reprinted with permission from B.C. Decker Inc., Hamilton, Ontario, Canada.*)

Figure 50–3. Association of the tensor veli palatini muscle and Eustachian tube. (*Reprinted with permission from B.C. Decker Inc., Hamilton, Ontario, Canada.*)

resulting in subsequent MED and hearing loss.[8,9] Interestingly, submucous cleft and congenital velopharyngeal insufficiency patients do suffer with a higher rate of MED, likely due to a similar mechanism found in their clefted colleagues.[10–12]

The underlying problem in cleft patients appears to be constriction of the ET during swallowing.[13,14] During the swallowing process, ET constriction impairs pressure regulation function, resulting in relatively asymptomatic middle-ear effusions in unrepaired infants. This form of otitis media is most commonly found in the cleft patients, as opposed to the recurrent acute condition found in their non-clefted counterparts.[2] Forced response function testing reveals that the ET of cleft patients have an elevated resistance to airflow, with evidence to suggest failure of tubal closing in these patients.[15]

An unrepaired palate prohibits velopharyngeal closure with swallow and speech. Children with intact palates are able to inflate their middle ears during crying, thus, attempting to regulate middle ear pressure; however, during this process, they are at risk of aspirating infected nasopharyngeal contents into the tube and middle-ear space. By contrast, the cleft child is unable to regulate in such a way, and therefore, has less of a chance of aspirating infected contents.[16] This may be a reason for recurrent acute ear disease in the nonclefted children and persistent asymptomatic fluid accumulation in the cleft group. The generally asymptomatic nature of this disease process was an important reason the diagnosis of "universality" of persistent otitis media with effusion was not accepted until the 1960s.[1,2] In fact, it is following cleft palate repair that one tends to see an increase in acute otitis media, especially if adequate velopharyngeal function has been achieved, as the child can develop positive nasopharyngeal pressure.

With regard to long-term sequelae of disease, persistent effusions are associated with inflammatory and infectious biochemicals that may initiate epithelial proliferation, keratinization, and subepithelial events, leading to hearing loss, chronic otitis media, and cholesteatoma.

Investigations of associated craniofacial measurements (other than ET placement) and their prognostic roles are emerging, with one recent report noting that a smaller sphenopalatine angle may be associated with a higher risk of developing hearing loss.[17] This angle is typically larger in the cleft patient, and the significance of these findings has not been fully elucidated. Chu and Bradley found a lower incidence of hearing loss in the Chinese cleft population when compared to Western nations.[18] Other studies, as well, have documented the relative hearing protection found in Asians with cleft palate.[19–21] As treatment strategies are similar, it was suggested that racial and associated craniofacial features may, again, play influential roles in disease development and outcome.

HISTOPATHOLOGY

Understanding the underlying structural and functional abnormalities that lead to MED in the child with a cleft palate will assist in establishing solutions to the development of otitis media in those patients with an intact palate. There is evidence to suggest that the tubal dysfunction in children with cleft palate is similar to those in their noncleft counterparts.[6,22,23] The ET is shaped like a shepherd's hook and possesses a medial and lateral lamella (both poorly developed in the cleft patient).[24] The levator veli palatini muscle's role in ET opening may be by isometric contraction, although others argue it has no role. The tensor's role is to open the tube directly by traction on its lateral portion, and indirectly by rotating the medial portion of the cartilage by this traction during swallowing.

Using extended temporal bone histopathologic specimens from infants with cleft palate, computer-aided three-dimensional reconstructions have shown anatomic differences between specimens with and without cleft palate. This aids in our understanding of the pathophysiology of MED in the cleft patient.

In comparison to their noncleft counterparts, patients with cleft palate have been found to have at least nine known abnormalities in the structure of the ET. These have been identified from studies of extended histopathologic cleft specimens. Table 50–1 summarizes these differences, which include: a shorter ET, insertion abnormalities of the TVP muscle, including a larger angle, onto the cartilaginous portion of the ET, poor dilatory function of the muscle, and smaller tube lumen with less pressure equalization ability. In addition, altered cartilaginous features such as increased cellular density, medial–lateral lamellar ratios, aberrant curvature, increased compliance with increased tube collapse, and less elastin content have been reported.[10,25–27] Finally, the ET lumen lies higher relative to the pharyngeal roof; and it is felt that the internal pterygoid muscles are more medial, therefore encroaching and compressing upon the ET.[6]

These findings are significant as they help explain the high incidence of otitis media in this special population. Reduced tubal length may enable aspiration and reflux of nasopharyngeal secretions into the middle ear.[28,29] Kitajiri et al. found that the severity of inflammation in this disease process was worse in the middle ear, and the bony middle-ear end of the ET, rather than in the cartilaginous portion. This indicates a functional obstruction being responsible for the disease process, rather than one due purely to inflammation.[30]

NATURAL HISTORY

As ETD with resulting middle-ear effusion are essentially inevitable in the cleft palate population, one's goal should focus on arresting the natural history of this process. This is important because persistent effusions can lead to hearing loss, speech and language impairment, tympanic membrane perforation, and cholesteatoma. Reports have noted, by diagnostic myringotomy, the near universal incidence of disease within the first few months of life; and, when the onset of disease is before 1 year, a trend toward worse hearing occurred.[1,2] One must be aware of the high incidence of MED,

Table 50–1.

Summary of the Differences in Structures of the Eustachian Tube in Extended Temporal Bone Specimens from Infants and Young Children with Cleft Palate Compared with Specimens without Cleft Palate

Abnormality Compared with Specimens without Cleft Palate	Reference
Length of tube shorter	Sadler-Kimes et al. [28]; Siegel et al. [29]
Angle between cartilage and TVP larger	Sadler-Kimes et al. [28]
Cartilage deformed	Shibahara and Sando [27]; Sando and Takahashi [9]
Cartilage cell density greater	Shibahara and Sando [27]
Ratio of lateral and medial laminae area of cartilage smaller	Takasaki et al. [24]; Matsune et al. [26]
Curvature of lumen less	Matsune et al. [26]
Elastin at hinge portion of cartilage less	Matsune et al. [26]
Insertion of TVP into tip of lateral lamina abnormal	Matsune et al. [26]
Insertion ration of TVP to cartilage less	Matsune et al. [26]

TVP = tensor veli palatini

and therefore, the associated risk of hearing loss, speech delay, and chronic ear disease in this patient population. Regardless of the subscribed mode of intervention, close observation must be mandated in order to monitor and intervene as necessary, in order to arrest and avoid sequelae.

Several studies indicate that between 6 years and late adolescence, approximately 70% of cleft palate patients will experience an improvement or even resolution of their ET dysfunction.[31–34] While the majority of scientific evidence indicates the presence of effusion in 100% of cleft patients, others have reported an incidence of 6–16%[31] of patients with no observed ear disease; athough, the methodology of diagnosis in these studies was often suboptimal. Most importantly, the reader should be reminded that all patients with clefts require the same level of monitoring.

Ramana et al. reported on the otologic and audiologic disease in a population of unrepaired cleft patients who were followed prospectively.[35] This population (15 patients) received no ear care and ranged in age from 8 to 18 years. Over 85% were "asymptomatic" for hearing loss and otologic complaints, and the most common otoscopic finding was mild retraction of the tympanic membrane (50%). In general, the audiologic profile revealed mild-to-moderate hearing impairment (76%), with less than one in six ears having a pure tone average at or below 20 dB. This population, unique to the literature, had a rate of cholesteatoma at 6.6%, and the same for tympanic membrane perforation. One of the more interesting aspects was the overall lack of symptoms. This was attributed to insidious onset, low socioeconomic conditions, illiteracy, social stigmatism, and perception that poor hear-

ing is incurable. Unfortunately, there was no assessment of language, speech, or cognitive skills in this population, making major inferences difficult. However, as previously noted, classic repair of the palate does not result in immediate improvement of ETF. In Ramana's population, receiving little to no ear care, one notes a very high incidence of abnormal ear findings, and low incidence of normal hearing, advocating an aggressive approach to ear disease.

The outcomes for children with repaired clefts, receiving little to no ear care, have been noted in several studies.[36–40] Between 20–40% of these patients demonstrated abnormal audiologic results, and at least one in three exhibited suboptimal language skills. While these authors failed to note a significant advantage of early tube insertion and advocate a watchful waiting policy, many would argue that the existence of otologic, hearing, and speech sequelae is simply too high without appropriate intervention. Another study has also associated the child with a cleft as having an increased risk of developing hearing loss in the extended high frequencies (levels above 9000 Hz). This is possibly due to the cleft sequelae, extended ear disease, surgical procedures for cleft repair, and the medication used during surgery.[41]

The long-term complications of untreated otitis media with effusion include hearing loss, middle-ear adhesions, tympanic membrane perforation, and cholesteatoma.[42,43] Incidences of conductive hearing loss have ranged from 0–90%, with an average of 50% reported in several studies.[44] The presence of MED is felt to negatively impact language aquisition, as well as cognitive and academic performance.[45] In addition, approximately 5% of cleft patients will have an additional sensorineural component to their hearing loss or a persistent conductive hearing loss associated with other syndromes.[46,47]

MANAGEMENT OVERVIEW

Management of MED is based on restoring ETF, and preventing the sequelae of disease. Until adequate tubal function is achieved, the problem is generally bypassed and aeration is generally restored to the middle ear via tympanostomy tubes. Children with clefts have MED that is characterized by persistent or recurrent high pressures, effusions, or both. They may also, subsequently, develop chronic suppurative otitis media, and are also prone to acute or chronic otorrhea.

This condition may be particularly troublesome prior to palatal repair, occurring through a tympanic membrane perforation, or via a patent tympanostomy tube. One must remember that chronic otorrhea fails to exist if acute otorrhea is successfully treated.[48] Cleft palate repair has been shown to reduce this problem significantly, possibly due to reduction of nasopharyngeal reflux, and muscle repositioning restoring the "muscular sling."[49,50] This, in turn, may improve muscular active opening of the tube.

Our general approach for patients with cleft lip and palate includes an evaluation at the time of lip repair. A myringotomy is performed, and a tube is placed, in the presence of fluid or inflammation, or if there is a history of MED. The ear is also evaluated at the time of palatal repair with similar guidelines for tube placement, or replacement if necessary. Following the surgical repair of the lip and palate, the ears are monitored closely as an outpatient, and at times of subsequent surgical procedures. Management is based on the status of the tube and evidence of ETF.

MIDDLE-EAR STATUS FOLLOWING PALATOPLASTY

The effect of palatal repair on otitis media with effusion has been reviewed in several studies. In one study, up to 30% of patients were noted to have improvement of middle-ear effusion on isolated otoscopy at 3 months after repair, resulting in the advocation to delay tube placement until after palatal repair.[51] However, several others, such as Robinson et al., have noted minimal improvement of disease after repair, persistent in 70% of 140 children at age 4 years.[52] They also noted that the age of repair, and type of cleft, had no significance on MED outcomes. Other studies have also noted that cleft palate type had no impact on degree, extent, or persistence of ear disease.[18,53]

Following palatoplasty, some infants experience a reduction in the rate of otitis media, while others do not.[1,2,52] This is felt to be related to the status of the ET, and/or possibly the type of palatoplasty. Doyle et al. found that in those patients with persistent ear disease, 70% had tubal constriction, as opposed to dilation, with swallowing.[6,54] Even after repair, the ET remains less able to open with swallow,

less able to equilibrate negative than positive applied pressure, and unable to equilibrate with Valsalva. These results confirm a retrograde (nasopharynx to middle ear) type of obstruction.[3,6,55] Studies with nonhuman primates indicate that associated ear disease may not lay solely in tubal function and abnormalities, but also abnormalities in nasopharyngeal structure.[56] It has been demonstrated that ETs with persistently low opening pressures, and inability to sustain lower middle-ear positive pressures, will be associated with a more prolonged course of MED, and require more frequent tympanostomy tube insertion.[17] Ultimately, it is the ET's ability to equilibrate positive and negative pressures, and maintain an elevated opening pressure that will lead to resolution of MED. Additional pharyngoplasty, to assist with velopharyngeal closure, has been noted to reduce otitis media. As previously mentioned, chronic ear drainage tends to resolve after palatal repair.

It has been hypothesized that closure of the palate would reorient the tensor and levator palatini muscles resulting in better ETF; however, this has never been definitively proven. Studies do show improved function occurring eventually, with the question not being "If," rather "When."[57,58] Studies clearly indicating improvement of ETF tend to have longer follow-up periods. In general, it is felt that while repair is a factor in the improvement of tube function, the benefits may take years; and other factors, such as growth and immunocompetence, may have a significant contribution as well. Smith et al. reviewed their long-term otologic findings, including 81 children; and determined that the average time to ET recovery after cleft palate repair was 6 years, with 94% of patients having normal ETF 10 years following palatoplasty.[59] The average number of sets of tubes was 3.1 (traditional Armstrong tubes and 0% perforations) and 1.1 long-term tubes (long-term Goode T-tubes with 6% perforations). While most failed their pretube hearing screen, over 90% had and maintained normal audiometric thresholds 2 years after tube placement. They concluded that the hearing loss before tube placement and palatoplasty resolves after aeration of the middle ear and did not result in any significant permanent hearing deficit. In addition, it has been shown that the improvement of conductive hearing loss following tube placement is often rapid, if not immediate.

Some have questioned whether early closure of the palate would lead to reduced MED. A previous study noted that palate closure before 18 months resulted in decreased permanent hearing loss, when compared with repair after 2 years of age.[60] Master et al. reviewed the hearing of those who had repaired palates to those children whose palates were left unrepaired.[61] He found a higher prevalence of permanent hearing loss in the latter group. Bluestone et al. reported the improvement of ETF was not likely due to increasing age alone; although, the contribution of age, including increased cartilaginous support and muscular vector change with growth, are felt to be important.[62] Nunn et al. reviewed the results of 19 infants receiving palatoplasty at 1 month of age (12 closed within first week of life). Seventy-two percent of these patients still required myringotomy with tubes within

30 months.[63] They concluded that there was no substantial benefit to very early closure with regard to ETF and MED. Unfortunately, one third of their study population had other associated craniofacial anomalies, making conclusions for the isolated cleft difficult to interpret.

Our position remains that while appropriate palatal closure is necessary to achieve adequate tube function and restoring normal middle-ear status, the benefits are not immediate. Therefore, timing of palatoplasty is left to the discretion of our colleagues, and ears are treated based on this knowledge of delayed improvement, as previously described.

INFLUENCE OF CLEFT TYPE AND METHOD OF VELOPLASTY ON MIDDLE-EAR DISEASE

It is generally felt that neither cleft type nor severity has a significant impact on MED severity or development of hearing loss.[36,64] There is also little information on the impact of cleft laterality and associated ipsilateral ear disease.

For the child with a cleft and functional tubal obstruction, surgical repair of the levator sling, achieving velopharyngeal competence, is possible. However, the most effective surgical procedure likely corrects the functional tube obstruction and reduce the rate of otitis media, awaits future investigation. A comparison of tube function in patients receiving the Veau-Wardill-Kilner repair to those who underwent Furlow repair failed to reveal any significant otologic difference.[65] Ideally, it is felt that reconstitution of the levator sling, while restraining from excessive dissection in the space of Ernst, results in better middle-ear outcomes. In addition, controversy regarding how to address the hamulus[66] and tensor tendon remains.[5] Some studies have found little difference with regard to hamulectomy, while others advocate greenstick fracture, or complete preservation, in order to achieve adequate ETF.[11]

Few studies speak to the role of cleft type or severity with regard to hearing and middle-ear outcomes. Handzic-Cuk et al. compared the hearing levels between bilateral cleft lip and palate (BCLP), unilateral cleft lip and palate (UCLP), and isolated cleft palate (ICP) groups receiving minimal otologic care.[67] Overall, most had a moderate conductive hearing loss by age 5 years; and, while all groups improved hearing scores with advancing age, the ICP group had the best scores, though few achieved completely normal hearing. Few ICP patients had moderate or severe hearing loss in early childhood. The BCLP group had the poorest hearing overall with time. Meanwhile, the UCLP population with established hearing loss, had the least chance of improvement or normalization of hearing. No group had significant improvement in hearing over the first 5 years; rather the significant change occurred between years 5 and 10. They surmised that the craniofacial dysmorphology burden was greater for the BCLP group; and greater structural malpositioning, more septal deviation and nasal airway obstruction, and hypoplasia of the tensor muscle, resulted in greater ETD.[68] They recommended early and aggressive tube placement for all patients, as this, they

felt, allowed for earlier normalization of hearing, and a better chance for normal long-term hearing.

In general, the severity or laterality of clefting and its effect on the ipsilateral/contralateral ear, have not been adequately elucidated, and remain a topic requiring further investigation.

TREATMENT OF MIDDLE-EAR DISEASE

Currently, for functional obstruction, we can only bypass the problem with myringotomy and tube insertion. In this regard, there are two general approaches to treatment. The first, based on the works of Paradise and Bluestone, advocates early and aggressive intervention with myringotomy tubes.[58] As the incidence and natural history of disease secondary to clefting is universal and persistent, early intervention may reduce the otologic complications, and the effects on speech and language development. In addition, there is good evidence to suggest that the development of proper speech is more dependent on the level of hearing rather than the severity of the cleft.[69]

However, the alternative approach to treatment, emerging over the last decade, advocates a more conservative stance, arguing that the added cost, risks associated with tubes, and need for repeated surgery, implore a more selective approach. Though these studies note more extensive evidence of chronic ear disease and a lack of "significant" improvement in speech, hearing, and articulation, they are largely retrospective, symptom-based, and nonvalidated.[70–72] These studies give very little evidence regarding long-term sequelae associated with this approach. Finally, they fail to account for the possibility that worsened outcomes occurring in the ears requiring repeated tube insertion, may not be due to the tubes, rather a reflection of more severe ETD.

Sheahan et al. retrospectively reviewed the sequelae of OME of 104 cleft palate children over an average of 7 years.[73] Ninety percent of these patients received at least one set of tubes, the average number of tubes was 2.1, with the first set placed on average at $3^1/_2$ years of age (late). Fifty percent had unilateral or bilateral hearing loss (>20 dB), less than 2% sensorineural loss. Twelve percent of the long-term tubes were associated with TM perforation, yet all but one patient had associated normal hearing. He found an incidence of overall chronic otitis media of 19% (including perforation of TM, fixed deep retraction pockets, and cholesteatoma); and specifically, 1.9% for cholesteatoma. Ears with these problems had a higher incidence of tubes, and had them placed "earlier," at 2.4 years (still later than U.S. standards). They surmised that in the long term, there existed a high correlation between abnormal TMs, decreased hearing, and repeated tube insertion. However, one must ask whether this is the natural history for these patients' advanced ear disease, or a complication from the tubes. They recommended tube placement not empirically, rather for monitored persistent effusion for more than 3 months and when there is associated hearing loss.

There are few studies directly comparing the outcomes of cleft palate patients whose MED is treated aggressively (i.e., myringotomy with tube placement with evidence of disease) to those more conservatively (i.e., watchful waiting). A report from 1990 compared hearing results from children treated conservatively before 1969 (as that was the standard of care) and those treated after with early tube placement.[21] Results indicated that the incidence of bilateral hearing loss was reduced in the later group. They also noted no influence based on gender or type of cleft palate, and did note a higher prevalence of hearing loss in the African American population; however, it was suggested that the latter may be more related to socioeconomic factors. In both groups, the incidence of hearing loss diminished with increasing age. Finally, it is challenging to draw major conclusions as the two groups differ in time periods, differ in racial/socioeconomic status, and level of access to health care. Despite the improvement, they still noted 25% of children with repaired clefts, below the age of 5 years, were found to have bilateral hearing level worse than 15 dB, and another 25% had similar loss unilaterally, and emphasized that this unacceptable level of hearing loss hinders proper language acquisition.

Many authors do promote an aggressive approach including Stool's paper advocating early microscopic evaluation,[1] to early tube placement recommended by Paradise and Bluestone,[58,74] Moore,[53] and Gordon.[32] These studies offer validated evidence of disease and generally superior study design. The fact remains that these children universally have ETD and resultant middle-ear effusions, with a high probability of associated sequelae. Hubbard et al. found impaired speech, articulation, and hearing more often in those receiving tubes only for overt problems (and then at an average age of 31 months) than in the children treated with early empiric tympanostomy (3 months).[37] They warned of the risk of such hearing loss as well as ensuing cognitive and language problems for ears left untreated, or treated for only overt problems. They further warned that these issues may manifest later in childhood, after key periods for developmental growth.

Based on the quality of evidence available, our opinion and approach follows a more aggressive protocol, including frequent office otoscopy, validated with intraoperative binocular microscopy and myringotomy, and a low threshold for myringotomy tube placement. Thereafter, we advocate close follow-up with regard to otoscopic findings, audiometric results, persistence of ETD, and the development of complications.

OUTCOMES

The ultimate questions involve the extent of ET dysfunction, its effect on MED, speech and language development, and the extent to which myringotomy tubes are effective in allowing proper development. The final hearing status of these patients is based on palatal correction, developmental factors, and appropriate treatment of MED. Though early intervention has been considered the standard of care, long-term hearing and language results have been deemed by some as "acceptable" in children receiving a more conservative approach. It is important to understand that in addition to one's approach to MED, improvement in hearing with advancing age is likely multifactorial.

In general, the degree of persistent MED, long-term effects on hearing and speech, and resultant complications vary from study to study. In a recent study from Greece, nearly two thirds of the repaired cleft patients over 5 years had mild hearing loss (20–40 dB), and this was significant enough to be associated with speech delay.[64] Palates were repaired between 18 and 24 months, and little information was given regarding the extent of infant and early childhood ear care.

A recent study from Finland investigated the development of MED in children with clefts, and their age-matched, noncleft peers with associated ear disease.[75] The groups were followed prospectively for 6 years after their first set of tubes, at which point audio results were compared. The group sizes were relatively small (39 cleft vs. 33 control), and assessed for audiometric, tympanometric, and otoscopic findings as well as radiologic evidence of mastoid air cell development. All cleft patients had early tube placement, and when compared to their noncleft persistent otitis media peers who had tubes as well, were found to have no differences in otoscopic exam, development of otologic complications, hearing, or mastoid development. The only obvious differences between the groups were (1) the greater number of children with clefts requiring more than one set of tubes (70% cleft vs. 40% controls), (2) a slightly higher perforation rate, and (3) a slower resolution of middle-ear disease (70% still had ETD 3 years after repair). Both groups demonstrated similar diminished mastoid air cell development when compared to children with no history of middle-ear disease. The pneumatization of the mastoid bone is dependent on regression of embryonic mesenchyme, starting at the end of the fetal period. In addition to genetic factors, amniotic fluid reflux into the middle ear and mastoid spaces may impair this regression secondary to a foreign body reaction, halting the mastoid air cell system development. Tube placement allows aeration of the system, allowing for improved development. They concluded that an aggressively treated child with a palatal cleft had the same prognosis as their chronic ear diseased noncleft counterpart both being, overall, favorable. The study by Robinson et al. supports the decisive effect of tympanostomy and tube placement in allowing the continued pneumatization of the mastoid.[52] In 22 patients with clefts, 1 ear was randomly selected for tube placement, and the other ear was left undisturbed. At 4 years of age, the mastoid air cell system size was found to be significantly larger on the tube side in 19 of the 22 patients. We concur that early onset of otitis media with effusion results in underaeration of the mastoid system, and that early resolution of this condition allows for more normal development.

When directly comparing otologic histories of aggressively treated children having palatal clefts with noncleft children, Broen et al. found that the cleft patients required earlier tube placement, more tubes, and still failed more hearing screens.[76] Their data indicated that the later the first of tubes were placed, the poorer the child's hearing. Those children with earlier intervention had better hearing and sound production when older, but no significant difference in cognitive, social, and emotional development were found. They did not find improvement in ear status after palatal repair, and argued no advantage to watchful waiting. They concluded that, without tubes, cleft children do not have normal middle-ear function; and without this function, hearing is depressed. Therefore, they advised placing tubes at the time of palatal repair.

Several studies address the influence of this ear disease and hearing loss on language, speech, and articulation. Schonweiler et al.[77] retrospectively reviewed the results of 370 children receiving veloplasty at 18–24 months and examined the effect of cleft extent, velopharyngeal competency, and hearing loss, on speech and language outcome. Results demonstrated that children with conductive hearing loss were more severely affected than the normal hearing children. They noted that patients' speech and language function were predominantly related to their hearing status, even in children with mild fluctuating hearing loss. Believing this loss results in a discontinuity of hearing and reduction of long-term hearing input and hearing quality, they recommended a very aggressive approach to tube placement. Fortunately, as with hearing, speech normalized in 95% of patients by 6–10 years of age. Other studies have echoed these findings.[78,79]

Overall, it remains challenging to compare the results, particularly long-term results, of many of these studies; for they vary in many respects including techniques of palatal repair, age of palatoplasty, indications for tube placement, means to assess, define, and confirm hearing loss, follow-up periods, and, most importantly, validation of the presence of otitis media.

COMPLICATIONS

As the majority of patients have received repeated placement of tympanostomy tubes, it has been somewhat difficult to identify which complications are directly due to these tubes, and which are due to the existing ear disease requiring tube placement. Complications include tympanic membrane perforation with a general risk of about 1%, and chronic ear drainage or otorrhea, with up to a 4% incidence. These are not significantly different from the incidence of complications found in noncleft counterparts. Patients with a history of long-term tubes (T-tubes), which we do not routinely advocate, have been noted to have perforation rates at 6–30%,[80–82] and even higher rates of chronic otorrhea.[48] In addition, tubes have been associated with focal atrophy of the TM, tympanosclerosis, and cholesteatoma.[38,56,71,83,84] One must also consider that children with more severe ear disease often require more tubes, and are at a higher risk of complications. It remains difficult to make major assumptions about the complications of tubes as they are, by definition, already associated with significant ear disease, effectively selecting out a cohort with poorer outcomes. Therefore, it is possible that some outcomes would likely have been even worse in these ears had they not received tube placement.

A common clinical finding in the repaired or unrepaired cleft palate patient is chronic middle-ear negative pressure. This often results in atelectasis of the tympanic membrane, which may lead to the development of a tympanic membrane retraction pocket, most frequently located in the posterior superior portion of the tympanic membrane. This, in turn, may ultimately result in the development of a cholesteatoma, which is a destructive mass of keratinizing epithelium. Prevention of complications remains key, and is accomplished by early and repeated efforts to maintain adequate middle-ear pressure, including palate repair and repeated insertion of tympanostomy tubes (which remain in place on average of 12–18 months).[85]

Cholesteatoma is a known complication in children with cleft palate. In his longitudinal study from Iowa, Severeid found the incidence to be 7.1% in the cleft palate population (160 patients, 70% between 10 and 16 years old).[31] The most common location for a cholesteatoma was the posterosuperior portion of the pars tensa of the tympanic membrane. A later report from the same institution found a rate above 9% (1 of 16 bilateral).[86] All had conductive hearing loss and a protracted history of otitis media with effusion. Most of these patients had disease leading to ossicular chain abnormalities. This complication was generally present by the mid-teen years. Not surprisingly, the cholesteatoma group had a greater number of tympanostomy tubes (6.8 sets vs. 5 sets in the noncholesteatoma group), reflective of more severe and persistent MED. Fortunately, only one recurrence was noted in this Iowa report. Other studies have noted a lower incidence of cholesteatoma in the general population, between 4 and 9 per 100,000.[87–89] The pathogenesis of this complication begins with atelectasis of the tympanic membrane, followed by a retraction pocket that leads to the development of cholesteatoma.[90] It is felt this course is similar in both the cleft and noncleft patient as there are no mesotympanic or epitympanic differences between these patient populations, and in addition, the clinical and surgical findings are similar. Both repaired cleft and nonclefted patients, who experience more severe and prolonged the ETD, are at higher risk for cholesteatoma formation. Interestingly, it has been proposed that with more frequent examinations due to elevated suspicion, earlier detection may be achieved in the cleft patient, resulting in more confined disease.[91] Finally, the goal is to arrest the disease process with early and frequent tubes as necessary to prevent the development of a retraction pocket. This, in turn, is associated with a reduced risk of cholesteatoma and associated hearing loss.

Outcomes of the management of these complications appear to be quite favorable. For tympanic membrane perforation, repair of the hole via tympanoplasty (fascia grafting) is the treatment of choice. In order to have a successful outcome, proper ETF must be present and persistent, and one must have a dry ear, without otorrhea or infection. When comparing the results of 26 cleft ears to 52 control ears, Gardener et al. found no difference in outcome, including graft survival, need for further tube placement, or postoperative hearing results.[92] Excellent results were achieved in both groups at an average follow-up of 2 years. It should be noted that the average age of tympanic membrane repair was 24 years. Many of these patients underwent concomitant mastoidectomy, and they often used cartilage for additional support in the grafting process.

CONCLUSION

In summary, infants with cleft palate universally suffer from ETD and MED. The vast majority experience a continuation of this problem through adolescence. The persistence of otitis media with effusion remains the primary cause of hearing loss; and contributes to other developmental sequelae. The associated ETD is the result of multiple anatomic pathologies associated with the clefting of the palate; and in general, persists for years after palatal repair. This obstruction is functional in nature and is not due to a fixed anatomic abnormality.

With appropriate care and treatment, the health of the middle ear, and prognosis for normal hearing and speech, for children with palatal clefts, is quite favorable. Although some debate exists on the most appropriate protocol to manage the MED, we feel that treatment should be based on validated evidence of disease (i.e., diagnostic myringotomy) generally at the time of lip and/or palate repair. The presence of disease mandates intervention with tube placement. Finally, these patients are recognized as a "high-risk population" for the development of hearing loss, speech and developmental delay as well as chronic ear disease; and therefore, require frequent and prolonged follow-up.

FUTURE DIRECTIONS

Evaluating the etiology of the tubal constrictive process in this population should be a specific aim of future research. Functional studies, which are more physiologic, would be helpful in determining the pathogenesis of ear disease in this high-risk group. Comparison of nasopharyngeal pressures generated during open and closed mouth swallowing in unrepaired, repaired, and control subjects should be undertaken. Assessment of tubal constriction, as a prognostic marker for persistent MED would assist practitioners in determining who might benefit from closer follow-up and more aggressive treatment. Radiologic-guided functional–anatomic evaluation of the ET may aid in the understanding of the mechanical interactions leading to dysfunction, and ultimately to their correction.

The impact of postoperative palatal fistulazation on hearing and ear disease has not been assessed, nor the significance of fistula size or location. In addition, it remains unclear if a particular form of veloplasty or associated operative ma-neuvers (i.e., management of the hamulus) are particularly beneficial with regard to MED and ETF.

Finally, a randomized, prospective, controlled investigation, comparing the short- and long-term outcomes of patients treated aggressively with tubes compared to those not treated under routine guidelines, has not been undertaken. The impact of palatoplasty technique, severity of the cleft, laterality of ear disease and cleft, hearing loss, chronic ear conditions, and influence on speech and language could potentially be determined for this unique population of children.

References

1. Stool S, Randall P. Unexpected ear disease in infants with cleft palate. *Cleft Palate J* 4:99–103, 1967.
2. Paradise J, Bluestone C, Felder H. The universality of otitis media in 50 infants with cleft palate. *Pediatrics* 44:35–42, 1969.
3. Bluestone C. Eustachian tube obstruction in the infant with cleft palate. *Ann Otol Rhinol Laryngol* 80:1–30, 1971.
4. Cole R, Cole J, Intaraprason S. Eustachian tube function in cleft lip and palate patients. *Arch Otolaryngol* 99:337–341, 1974.
5. Huang M, Lee S, Rajendran M. A fresh cadaveric study of the paratubal muscles: Implications for Eustachian tube function in cleft palate. *Plast Reconstr Surg* 100(4):833–842, 1997.
6. Doyle W, Cantekin E, Bluestone C. Eustachian tube function in cleft palate children. *Ann Otol Rhinol Laryngol* 89:34–40, 1980.
7. Bluestone C, Paradise J, Beery Q, et al. Certain effects of cleft palate repair on Eustachian tube function. *Cleft Palate J* 9:183–189, 1972.
8. Seigel M, Doyle W, Gest T, et al. A comparison of craniofacial growth in normal and cleft palate rhesus monkeys. *Cleft Palate J* 22:192–196, 1985.
9. Sando I, Takahashi H. Otitis media and various congenital diseases. Preliminary study. *Ann Otol Rhinol Laryngol Suppl* 148:13–16, 1990.
10. Kitajiri M, Sando I, Hashida Y, et al. Histopathology of otitis media in infants with cleft and high arched palates. In Lim D, Bluestone C, Klein J, Nelson J (eds). *Recent Advances in Otitis Media with Effusion—Proceedings to the Third International Symposium*. Hamilton, ON: BC Decker, 1984, pp. 195–198.
11. Odoi H, Proud G, Toledo P. Effects of pterygoid hamulotomy upon Eustachian tube function. *Laryngoscope* 81:1242–1244, 1971.
12. Sheahan P, Miller I, Earley M, et al. Middle ear disease in children with congenital velopharyngeal insufficiency. *Cleft Palate Craniofacial J* 41:364–367, 2004.
13. White B, Doyle W, Bluestone C. Eustachian tube function in infants and children with Down syndrome. In Lim D, Klein J, Nelson J, (eds). *Recent Advances in Otitis Media—proceedings of the Third International Symposium*. Hamilton, ON: BC Decker, 1984, pp. 62–66.
14. Casselbrant M, Doyle W, Cantekin E, et al. A. Eustachian tube function in the rhesus monkey model of cleft palate. *Cleft Palate J* 22:185–191, 1985.
15. Falk B, Magnuson B. Eustachian tube closing failure in children with persistent middle-ear effusion. *Int J Pediatr Otorhinolaryngol* 7:97–106, 1984.
16. Bluestone C. *Eustachian Tube: Structure, Function, Role in Otitis Media*. London: BC Decker, 2005, pp. 106–109.
17. Tasaka Y, Kawano M, Honjo I. Eustachian tube function in OME patients with cleft palate. *Acta Otolaryngol (Stockh)* 471:5–8, 1990.
18. Chu K, McPherson B. Audiological status of Chinese patients with cleft lip/palate. *Cleft Palate Craniofacial J* 42:280–285, 2005.
19. Lau C, Loh K, Kunaratnam N. Middle ear diseases in cleft palate patients in Singapore. *Ann Acad Med Singapore* 17:372–374, 1988.
20. Abdullah S. A study of the results of speech language and hearing assessment of three groups of repaired cleft palate children and adults. *Ann Acad Med Singapore* 17:388–391, 1988.

21. Gould H. Hearing loss and cleft palate: The perspective of time. *Cleft Palate J* 27:36–39, 1990.

22. Bluestone C, Paradise J, Beery Q, et al. Certain effects of cleft palate repair on Eustachian tube function. *Cleft Palate J* 9:183–193, 1972.

23. Cantekin E. Eustachian tube function in children with tympanostomy tubes. *Auris Nasus Larynx* 12(Suppl 1):S46–S48, 1985.

24. Takasaki K, Sando I, Balaban C, et al. Postnatal development of Eustachian tube cartilage. A study of normal and cleft palate cases. *Int J Pediatr Otorhinolaryngol* 52:31–36, 2000.

25. Sando I, Doyle W, Okuno H, et al. A method for the histopathological analysis of the temporal bone and the Eustachian tube and its accessory structures. *Ann Otol Rhinol Laryngol* 95:267–274, 1986.

26. Matsune S, Sando I, Takahashi H. Abnormalities of lateral cartilaginous lamina and lumen of Eustachian tube in cases of cleft palate. *Ann Otol Rhinol Laryngol* 100:909–913, 1991.

27. Shibahara Y, Sando I. Histopathologic study of Eustachian tube in cleft palate patients. *Ann Otol Rhinol Laryngol* 97:403–408, 1988.

28. Sadler-Kimes D, Siegel M, Todhunter J. Age-related morphological differences in the components of the Eustachian tube-middle-ear system. *Ann Otol Rhinol Laryngol* 98:854–858, 1989.

29. Siegel M, Cantekin E, Todhunter J, et al. Aspect ratio as a descriptor of Eustachian tube cartilage shape. *Ann Otol Rhinol Laryngol* 97(Suppl 133):16–17, 1988.

30. Kitajiri M, Sando I, Hashida Y, et al. Histopathology of otitis media in infants with cleft and high-arched palates. *Ann Otol Rhinol Laryngol* 94:44–50, 1985.

31. Severeid L. Development of cholesteatoma in children with cleft palate: A longitudinal study. In McCabe B, Sade J, Abramson M (eds). *Cholesteatoma: First International Conference.* Birmingham, AL: Aesculapius, 1977, pp. 287–292.

32. Gordon A, Jean-Louis F, Morton R. Late ear sequelae in cleft palate patients. *Int J Pediatr Otorhinolaryngol* 15:149–156, 1988.

33. Gopalakrishna A, Goleria K, Raje A. Middle ear function in cleft palate. *Brit J Plastic Surg* 37:558–565, 1984.

34. Moller P. Long-term otologic features of cleft palate patients. *Arch Otolaryngol* 101:605–607, 1975.

35. Ramana Y, Nanda V, Biswas G, et al. Audiological profile in older children and adolescents with unrepaired cleft palate. *Cleft Palate Craniofac J* 42:570–573, 2005.

36. Tuncbilek G, Ozgur F, Belgin E. Audiologic and tympanometric findings in children with cleft lip and palate. *Cleft Palate Craniofac J* 40:304–309, 2003.

37. Hubbard T, Paradise J, McWilliams B, et al. Consequences of unremitting middle-ear disease in early life: Otologic, audiologic, and developmental findings in children with cleft palate. *New Engl J Med* 312:1529–1534, 1985.

38. Maw R, Wilks J, Harvey I, et al. Early surgery compared with watchful waiting for glue ear and effect on language development in preschool children: A randomized trial. *Lancet* 353:960–963, 1999. [Erratum, *Lancet* 354:1392.]

39. Paradise J, Feldman H, Campbell T, et al. Effect of early or delayed insertion of tympanostomy tubes for persistent otitis media on developmental outcomes at the age of three years. *New Engl J Med* 344:1179–1188, 2001.

40. Wilks J, Maw R, Peters T, et al. Randomized controlled trial of early surgery versus watchful waiting for glue ear: The effect on behavioural problems in preschool children. *Clin Otolaryngol* 25:209–214, 2000.

41. Ahonen J, McDermott J. Extended high-frequency hearing loss in children with cleft palate. *Audiology* 23:467–476, 1984.

42. Bluestone C. Epidemiology and pathogenesis of chronic suppurative otitis media: Implications for prevention and treatment. *Int J Pediatr Otorhinolaryngol* 42:207–223, 1998.

43. Braganza R, Kearns D, Burton D, et al. Closure of the soft palate for persistent otorrhea after placement of pressure equalization tubes in cleft palate infants. *Cleft Palate Craniofac J* 28:305–307, 1991.

44. Butow K, Louw B, Hugo S, et al. Tensor veli palatine muscle tension sling for Eustachian tube function in cleft palate. *J Craniomaxillofac Surg* 19:71–76, 1991.

45. Bennett M. The older cleft palate patient. *Laryngoscope* 86:1217–1225, 1972.

46. Moller P. Long term otologic features of cleft palate patients. *Arch Otolaryngol* 101:605, 1975.

47. Rohrich J, Byrd H. Optimal timing of cleft palate closure. *Clin Plast Surg* 17:27–36, 1990.

48. Lewis N. Otitis media and linguistic incompetence. *Arch Otolaryngol* 102:387–390, 1976.

49. Yules R. Hearing in cleft palate patients. *Arch Otolaryngol* 91:319–323, 1970.

50. Bardach J, et al. Results of multidisciplinary management of bilateral cleft lip and palate at the Iowa cleft palate centre. *Plast Reconstr Surg* 89:419–432, 1992.

51. Crysdale W. Rational management of middle ear effusion in the cleft palate patient. *J Otolaryngol* 5:463–466, 1976.

52. Robinson P, Lodge B, Jones B, et al. The effect of palate repair on otitis media with effusion. *Plast Reconstr Surg* 89:640–645, 1992.

53. Moore I, Moore G, Yonkers A. Otitis media in the cleft palate patient. *Ear Nose Throat J* 65:291–295, 1986.

54. Doyle W. Eustachian tube function in special populations: Cleft palate children. *Ann Otol Rhinol Laryngol* 94:39–42, 1985.

55. Bluestone C, Wittel R, Paradise J. Roentgenographic evaluation of the Eustachian tube function in infants with cleft and normal palates. *Cleft Palate J* 9:93–100, 1972.

56. Doyle W, Cantekin E, Bluestone C, et al. A nonhuman primate model of cleft palate and its implications for middle-ear pathology. *Ann Otol Rhinol Laryngol* 89:41–46, 1980.

57. Frable M, Bandon G, Theograj S. Velar closure and ear tubings as a primary procedure in the repair of cleft palates. *Laryngoscope* 95:1044–1046, 1985.

58. Paradise J, Bluestone C. Early treatment of the universal otitis media of infants with cleft palate. *Pediatrics* 53:48–54, 1974.

59. Smith T, DiRuggiero D, Jones K. Recovery of Eustachian tube function and hearing outcome in patients with cleft palate. *Otolaryngol Head Neck Surg* 111:423–429, 1994.

60. Yules R. Hearing in cleft palate patients. *Arch Otolaryngol* 91:319–323, 1970.

61. Master F, Bingham H, Robinson D. The prevention of hearing loss in the cleft palate child. *Plast Reconstr Surg* 25:503–509, 1960.

62. Bluestone C, Beery Q, Cantekin E, et al. Eustachian tube ventilatory function in relation to cleft palate. *Ann Otol Rhino Laryngol* 84:333–338, 1975.

63. Nunn D, Derkay C, Darrow D, et al. The effect of very early cleft palate closure on the need for ventilation tubes in the first years of life. *Laryngoscope* 105:905–908, 1995.

64. Paliobei V, Psifidis A, Anagnostopoulos D. Hearing and speech assessment of cleft palate patients after palatal closure—Long-term results. *Int J Pediatr Otorhinol* 69:1373–1381, 2005.

65. Guneren E, Ozsoy Z, Ulay M, et al. A comparison of the effects of Veau-Wardill-Kilner palatoplasty and the Furlow double-opposing Z-plasty operations on Eustachian tube function. *Cleft Palate Craniofac J* 37:266–270, 2000.

66. Virtanen H, Palva T. Surgical treatment of patulous eustachian tube. *Arch Otolaryngol* 108:735, 1982.

67. Handzic-Cuk J, Cuk V, Risavi R, et al. Hearing levels and age in cleft palate patients. *Int J Pediatr Otorhinol* 37:227–242, 1996.

68. Fara M, Dvorak J. Abnormal anatomy of the muscles of palatopharyngeal closure in cleft palates. *Plast Reconstr Surg* 46:448–496, 1970.

69. Schonweiler R, Schonweiler B, Schmelzeisen R. Hearing capacity and speech production in 417 children with facial cleft abnormalities. *HNO* 42:691–696, 1994.

70. Shaw R, Richardson D, McMahon S. Conservative management of otitis media in cleft palate. *J Craniomaxillofac Surg* 31:316–320, 2003.

71. Robson A, Blanshard J, Jones K, et al. A conservative approach to the management of otitis media with effusion in cleft palate children. *J Laryngol Otol* 106:788–792, 1992.

72. Andrews P, Chrobachi R, Sirimanna T, et al. Evaluation of hearing thresholds in 3-month-old children with a cleft palate: The basis for a selective policy for ventilation tube insertion at time of palate repair. *Clin Otolaryngol* 29:10–17, 2004.

73. Sheahan P, Blayney A, Sheahan J, et al. Sequelae of otitis media with effusion among children with cleft lip and/or cleft palate. *Clin Otolaryngol* 27:494–500, 2002.

74. Cantekin E, Doyle W, Bluestone C. Effect of levator veli palatini muscle excision on Eustachian tube function. *Arch Otolaryngol* 109:281–284, 1983.

75. Valtonen H, Dietz A, Qvarnberg Y. Long-term clinical, audiologic, and radiologic outcomes in palate cleft children treated with early tympanostomy for otitis media with effusion: A controlled prospective study. *Laryngoscope* 115:1512–1516, 2005.

76. Broen P, Moller K, Carlstrom J, et al. Comparison of the hearing histories of children with and without cleft palate. *Cleft Palate Craniofac J* 33:127–133, 1996.

77. Schonweiler R, Lisson J, Schonweiler B, et al. A retrospective study of hearing, speech and language function in children with clefts following palatoplasty and veloplasty procedures at 18–24 months of age. *Int J Pediatr Otorhinolaryngol* 50:205–217, 1999.

78. Schonweiler R, Radu H, Ptok M. A cross-sectional study on speech and language outcome of children having normal hearing, mild fluctuating conductive hearing loss of bilateral profound hearing loss. *Int J Pediatr Otorhinolaryngol* 44:251–258, 1998.

79. Broen P, Devers M, Doyle S, et al. Acquisition of linguistic and cognitive skills by children with cleft palate. *J Speech Lang Hear Dis* 41:676–687, 1998.

80. Rosenfeld R, Bluestone C. *Evidence Based Otitis Media.* Ontario, Canada: BC Decker Publisher, 1999.

81. Brockbank M, Jonathan D, Grant H, et al. Goode T-tubes: do the benefits of their use outweigh their complications? *Clin Otolaryngol* 13:351–356, 1988.

82. Hawthorne M, Parker A. Perforations of the tympanic membrane following the use of Goode type long term tympanostomy tubes. *J Laryngol Otol* 102:997–999, 1988.

83. Golz A, Goldenberg D, Netzer A, et al. Cholesteatomas associated with ventilation tube insertion. *Arch Otolaryngol Head Neck Surg* 125:754–757, 1999.

84. Golz A, Netzer A, Joachims H, et al. Ventilation tubes and persistent tympanic membrane perforations. *Otolaryngol Head Neck Surg* 120:524–527, 1999.

85. Paradise J, Bluestone C. Early treatment of the universal otitis media in infants with cleft palate. *Pediatrics* 53:48–54, 1974.

86. Harker L, Severeid L. Cholesteatoma in the cleft palate patient. In Sade J (ed). *Cholesteatoma and Mastoid Surgery: Proceedings of the Second International Conference on Cholesteatoma and Mastoid Surgery.* Amsterdam: Kugler, 1982, pp. 32–40.

87. Harker L, Koontz F. The bacteriology of cholesteatoma. In McCabe B, Sade J, Abramson M (eds). *Cholesteatoma: First International Conference.* Birmingham, AL: Aesculapius, 1977, pp. 287–292.

88. Karma P, Perala M, Kuusela A. Morbidity of very young infants with and without acute otitis media. *Acta Otolaryngol (Stockh)* 107:460–466, 1989.

89. Tos M. Incidence, etiology and pathogenesis of cholesteatoma in children. *Adv Otorhinolaryngol* 40:110–117, 1988.

90. Bluestone C, Casselbrant M, Cantekin E. Functional obstruction of the Eustachian tube in the pathogenesis of aural cholesteatoma in children. In Sade J (ed). *Cholesteatoma and Mastoid Surgery: Proceedings of the Second International Conference on Cholesteatoma and Mastoid Surgery.* Amsterdam: Kugler, 1982, pp. 211–214.

91. Harker L, Severeid L. Cholesteatoma in the cleft palate patient. *Cholesteatoma and Mastoid Surgery Proceedings IInd Intl Confernce.* Amsterdam: Kugler, 1981, pp. 37–40.

92. Gardner E, Dornhoffer J. Tympanoplasty results in patients with cleft palate: An age- and procedure-matched comparison of preliminary results with patients without cleft palate. *Otolaryngol Head Neck Surg* 126:518–523, 2002.

93. Rynnel-Dagoo B, Lindberg K, Bagger-Sjoback D, et al. Middle ear disease in cleft palate children at three years of age. *Int J Pediatr Otorhinolaryngol* 23:201–209, 1992.

94. Cantekin E, Bluestone C, Saez C, et al. Normal and abnormal middle-ear ventilation. *Ann Otol Rhinol Laryngol* 86:1–15, 1977.

95. Cantekin E, Doyle W, Bluestone C. Comparison of normal Eustachian tube function in the rhesus monkey and man. *Ann Otol Rhinol Laryngol* 91:179–184, 1982.

96. Seagle M, Nackashi J, Kemker F, et al. Otologic and audiologic status of Russian children with cleft lip and palate. *Cleft Palate Craniofac J* 35:495–499, 1998.

97. Sheahan P, Miller I, Sheahan J, et al. Incidence and outcome of middle ear disease in cleft lip and/or cleft palate. *Int J Pediatr Otorhinolaryngol* 67:785–793, 2003.

51

Audiologic Assessment and Management of Children with Cleft Palate

Diane L. Sabo, PhD • Gretchen Probst, MAT

■ INTRODUCTION

One of the few populations who are offered coordinated health care by a multidisciplinary team is children with cleft palate. The reasons behind this are the multifaceted issues faced by those with orofacial clefting. This multidisciplinary care has not changed dramatically throughout the years. New advances in medicine and surgery have improved the outcomes for those with cleft palates, but the fact remains that coordinated, multidisciplinary care is still important for those with clefts.

In hearing health care, advances in the early detection of hearing loss have been made recently. There has been an emergence of newborn hearing screening into the routine care of newborns, thus reducing the age of identification of hearing loss that was not achievable prior to routine newborn

hearing screening. This improvement in the age of identification of hearing loss should not have significantly altered the care of children with cleft palates; because, for over 30 years, children with "defects of the ears, nose, or throat" have been considered to be at risk for hearing loss.[1] The recommendation made was that, even if hearing loss was not evident in the newborn period, these infants would continue to have regular assessments of their hearing.

Changes are being seen, not only in hearing screening, but also in better systems of care for those children who do not pass their hearing screen, or who are at risk for delayed onset of hearing loss. For example, better and more timely evaluation of hearing, better ability to assess middle-ear function more reliably for very young infants, and better amplification and other habilitation options are available. Consequently, as a result of newborn hearing screening, what has also emerged over the last decade is a refinement of techniques that are used to determine hearing levels in young infants, and a focus in recruiting and training of professionals to assess hearing in this young population. In addition to clinics routinely utilizing better techniques to evaluate hearing in young infants (e.g., more testing with both air and bone conduction, and more frequency specific testing conducted), there is also improved technology. What has not changed, though, is the continued need to monitor the hearing of those who are at risk for hearing loss, including infants and children with cleft palates. This chapter will review the audiologic tests in current use, commonly found results, and management of children with cleft palates.

CLEFT PALATE AND HEARING LOSS

Children with clefts need to be seen for audiologic testing as soon as possible to obtain a baseline of their hearing, because children with cleft palates are at increased risk of both conductive and sensorineural hearing loss. Conductive hearing losses may be transient, in association with fluctuating middle-ear fluid, or permanent due to structural anomalies of the ear, such as atresia of the ear canal, ossicular anomalies, and/or absence of the middle ear. Cleft palates can occur in isolation or as part of a syndrome that can have conductive, sensorineural, or mixed conductive and sensorineural loss associated with the syndrome. For example, atresia and cleft palate can be found in such syndromes as Treacher Collins and Nager syndromes. Other syndromes, associated with cleft palates, can have conductive losses due to middle-ear fluid and/or other structural anomalies. Examples of these syndromes include Oral-Facial-Digital, Brachio-Oculo-Facial, Oto-Palato-Digital, Dubowitz, Stickler's syndrome, and Robin sequence. Sensorineural hearing loss and cleft palate are found together in a number of syndromes involving the head and neck such as in Goldenhar's syndrome. Additionally, some syndromes, less often associated with cleft palates, can have both conductive and sensorineural hearing losses, such as CHARGE, de Lange, Crouzon syndrome, and Trisomy 13 and 18.

The literature is rich with studies that have shown an association between otitis media with effusion (OME) and hearing loss; and, OME has been found to be almost universal in infants with cleft palate.[2-4] The primary reason for the high prevalence of OME in children with cleft palates is abnormal Eustachian tube function, which may or may not resolve following palatal repair.[5-8] The main consequence of OME in the general population is conductive hearing loss.[9] However, there is variability found in the literature with regards to the amount of hearing loss associated with cleft palate. This variability can be attributed to various diagnostic definitions, particularly with regard to the definition of hearing loss in the pediatric population and ranges from 10 dB[10] to 15 dB[11] to 20 dB.[6,7,12] Although there is this variability in the literature, when taken together, there is consensus that (1) nearly all infants with cleft palate have OME, (2) OME declines with increasing age but can remain even into adulthood, and (3) hearing loss can be either transient or permanent.

Recently, Goudy et al.[13] reviewed the hearing in 101 cases of children who had cleft palate. The median age of the patients was 19 years, and the median age of palate repair was 16 months. Myringotomy and tubes were routine either at the time of lip repair or when middle-ear effusion persisted for greater than 3 months. They found that approximately one-half of the patients had conductive hearing losses less than 20 dB, approximately one-fourth had normal hearing, and approximately one-fourth had conductive loss greater than 20 dB. Of this latter group, 75% of the conductive hearing losses were mild, 21% moderate, and 4% severe losses. The average age of resolution of hearing loss was 5 years. These findings highlight the prevalence OME and associated hearing loss as well as the persistence of OME and hearing loss. Furthermore, these findings go along with reports of OME and hearing loss following surgical repair of the clefts.[14-16] However, the reports vary and range from 24% to 82% of the patients showing normal hearing after cleft palate repair. A confounding issue in many of these studies is the routine insertion and reinsertions of tympanostomy tubes in their treatment of otitis media.[6,7,11,12,17,18] The report by Goudy et al.,[13] regarding the age of resolution of hearing loss, is consistent with the literature showing resolution of Eustachian tube dysfunction by 5–6 years of age in 75–94% of the subjects studied. This agreement would be expected since Eustachian tube dysfunction is felt to be the primary reason for middle-ear effusion.[8,11,15] There are varying reports of longer persistence of hearing loss ranging from 2% to 24% of the hearing losses persisting beyond 5–6 years.[11,19] Persistent hearing loss in patients with repaired cleft palates has been attributed to postoperative scarring and poor palatal mobility.[20]

Tunçbilek et al.[16] conducted a retrospective evaluation of 50 children (100 ears) to evaluate the association of audiologic and otologic outcomes in relation to cleft type. The median age of the subjects in this study was 10 years, and only one had a history of ventilation tube insertions. When analyzed according to ears, normal hearing (≤ 15 dB HL) was found in 63% of the ears, 22% of the ears had minimal losses (16–25 dB HL), and 11% had mild loss. When analyzed according to subjects, 54% were found to have normal hearing, and 18% had unilateral hearing losses. They found no statistical difference between type of cleft and amount of hearing loss.

The management of this higher prevalence of OME is often tympanostomy tube insertion; although, there continues to be debate regarding the routine insertion of tympanostomy tubes. In one of the few prospective studies, Valtonen et al.[21] recently evaluated the long-term outcome of children with cleft palate who had tympanostomy tubes placed prior to 7 months for otitis media with effusion. They found no difference 6 years after tympanostomy tube insertion in the hearing levels between children with and without cleft palate, with average hearing levels of 10 dB in both groups. Their conclusion was that the tympanostomy tube insertion was beneficial as a treatment option to ensure normal hearing levels during the critical time of language development.

AUDIOLOGIC TESTS

Currently, there is no standard for conducting newborn hearing screening. The Joint Committee on Infant Hearing (JCIH) position statement of 2007[22] and prior publications, such as NIH 1993,[23] have recommended a two-stage or two-tier screening, utilizing both otoacoustic emissions (OAEs) and auditory brain stem response (ABR) screens. These tests are both objective measures, and for screening are often automated. The recommendation is to first screen with OAEs, followed by ABR, if the OAEs are not a pass result. The exception to this recommendation is for children who are in the neonatal intensive care nurseries, who may be neurologically compromised; wherein, ABR, with or with out OAEs, is the test of choice.

Newborn hearing screening is usually conducted while the newborn is in the hospital following birth. While it can be surmised that children with cleft palates will more often fail their newborn screening (due to higher prevalence of middle-ear involvement and sensorineural hearing loss), there is little evidence showing this to be true. Anteunis et al.[24] evaluated evoked OAEs in a feasibility study of infants with cleft palates. They studied infants from 1 to 11 weeks of age, using transient (click) evoked otoacoustic emissions. Of the 21 infants (42 ears) evaluated, 12 infants (24 ears) had emissions present and 9 infants (18 ears) had emissions absent; 3 infants (6 ears) of the 9 infants could not be tested due to high noise. All nine children with absent emissions were seen for follow-up testing using OAEs and ABRs. At follow-up, three children had emissions present and normal ABRs, four children had no emissions and normal ABRs, and two children had absent emission and sensorineural hearing loss. The authors concluded that it would be more appropriate to use ABR as a screening measure for children with cleft palates.

Regardless of newborn hearing screening outcome, diligent follow-up of all infants with cleft palates is indicated due to the high prevalence of middle-ear pathology present in this population. The same tests that are used for screening are used in the audiology follow-up for either those who fail their screening, or those who need continuous monitoring because of potential late onset or progressive hearing loss.

When evaluating the hearing of infants and young children, the use of any one test alone is insufficient. Rather, a comprehensive assessment, including behavioral and physiologic measures, is indicated to fully assess the auditory system, and determine the type, degree, and configuration of hearing loss for each ear. At very young ages, there needs to be a greater reliance on physiologic measures as the young child/infant is not capable of providing valid behavioral indications of hearing. This reliance on physiologic measures shifts to behavioral measures within the first developmental year of life. Furthermore, children who are at risk for fluctuating losses cannot be seen at a single point in time with the expectation that this is sufficient to characterize the child's hearing. Rather, continuous monitoring, in conjunction with otologic management, is warranted. The following is a review of the tests used for screening and evaluating infants for hearing loss.

PHYSIOLOGIC TESTS

Otoacoustic Emission Test

A test that has helped to propel newborn hearing screening into the standard of care for all newborns is an objective measure called the otoacoustic emission test. OAEs are sounds that originate from physiologic activity inside the cochlea and that can be recorded in the ear canal. There is much evidence that this activity is associated with normal to near normal hearing processes.[25,26] The sensory or outer hair cells within the organ of corti are thought to be responsible for the generation of otoacoustic emissions, specifically the electromotility of the outer hair cells.[27] Thus, the OAEs give us the ability to view the functioning of the cochlea, although not without contribution of the middle ear. That is, the sounds created in the cochlea are passed through the middle ear via the ossicular chain and eardrum (i.e., the middle-ear bones that are linked together and coupled to the eardrum). These sounds are then recorded by placing a microphone in the ear canal. Consequently, healthy middle ears—that can transmit sound to and from the cochlea effectively—are essential to being able to record the OAEs.

Recording OAEs allows measurement of cochlear function objectively and noninvasively. OAEs are generated exclusively by outer hair cells. Most hearing losses do not involve inner hair cell damage without outer hair cell damage because outer hair cells are generally more vulnerable to disease and damage than inner hair cells. Therefore, the presence of an emission provides us with reasonable assurance that hearing thresholds are 30–40 dB or better in the frequency range where the emission is present. OAEs may be absent, then, due to middle-ear dysfunction resulting in inability of the emission to be transmitted, or to sensory hearing loss affecting production of the emission. Prediction of hearing levels is not possible by measuring OAE. The absence of OAE can be associated with hearing levels of mild-to-moderate degree and greater, and their presence does not ensure normal hearing, When measuring OAEs in young children, their amplitude may be reduced in the low-frequency regions (1000 Hz and below) because of interference from the low-frequency physiologic and ambient noise in this region. Consequently, absent OAEs in low-frequency regions alone are insufficient for determining presence or absence of hearing loss. The OAEs, therefore, should constitute one test in a battery of tests for accurate interpretation.

Tympanometry

Other tests that are important to the test battery used for the audiologic assessment of infants and young children are acoustic immittance tests of tympanometry and acoustic reflex (AR) threshold monitoring. These tests are especially important when one considers the high incidence of OME in young children, and particularly in children with cleft palates. Tympanometry is an indication of tympanic membrane mobility, and middle-ear pressure used to infer middle-ear function. Tympanometry assesses the movement of the tympanic membrane in response to mechanically varied air pressure, and indirectly measures tympanic membrane mobility by measuring the amount of reflected sound, or inversely by the amount of sound passing through the tympanic membrane to the middle ear. Standard tympanometry uses a low-frequency probe tone of 220 or 226 Hz for measurement. However, the interpretation of the tympanogram and AR findings may be compromised when this probe tone is used with infants less than 4 months of age. Specifically, findings in the ears of infants with middle-ear fluid show normal-appearing tympanograms.[28] The reasons for this have not been definitively identified; although, it is known that the mass and stiffness contributions are different between adults and children, with children having a more mass dominated, compared to the adult stiffness dominated system at low probe tone frequencies. The use of a higher probe frequency (e.g., 1000 Hz) yields tympanograms that are a more valid indication of middle-ear function for infants aged 4 months or less.[29−38]

AR Threshold Monitoring

AR testing monitors a middle-ear muscle response to loud sound, which indicates middle ear and auditory brain stem activation. The AR can be a very useful part of the audiologic evaluation in infants. A present reflex is added support for normal middle-ear function as well as information about the integrity of a portion of the auditory brain stem pathway. It is important to use a high-frequency probe to measure the AR in infants under 6 months of age.[38] Tympanometry and AR testing are both objective measures, but abnormal acoustic immittance findings, and/or the presence of fluid, do not determine hearing levels. Furthermore, the tests used for assessment of hearing do not determine the presence of fluid. Therefore, acoustic immittance measures, in combination with hearing assessment measures, help to provide a complete picture of the status of the ear and hearing, and can help with ensuring proper recommendations.

Auditory Brain Stem Response (ABR)

For the very young child, physiologic assessment procedures, using auditory evoked potentials, such as ABR, are particularly important. The ABR can be used for both identification and assessment of hearing, and can provide accurate estimates of threshold sensitivity.[39] Under good recording conditions, and using frequency specific stimuli, the ABR can provide reliable estimates of sensitivity across the frequency range of hearing.[40] Using the ABR in infants as young as the newborn, reliable estimates of pure tone thresholds/hearing levels have been shown for both air- and bone-conduction stimulation.[41,42] The ABR has been used to evaluate infants' and children with cleft palate for some time. Fria et al.[43] evaluated 29 infants with cleft palates at the time of myringo-

tomy with tympanostomy tube placement. Testing was conducted under anesthesia either immediately before, after, or both before and after surgery. The ABR findings showed that 78% had bilateral mild or moderate conductive losses prior to surgery. After surgery, 75% showed normal hearing, and the remaining 25% showing a reduction in the amount of hearing loss. These results indicated that the ABR is a viable method of monitoring hearing in children with cleft palates who are too young to be tested by behavioral methods. More recently, Andrews et al.[44] evaluated 40 children at 3 months of age under natural sleep using both air- and bone-conducted click stimuli. Only 13 of the children could be successfully tested by bone conduction, while all remained asleep for air-conduction testing. The results estimated hearing threshold levels ranging from mild to severe. Bone-conduction scores, in general, were better than air-conduction scores, indicating a probable conductive component to the hearing loss. The authors point out that the responses to click stimuli are not frequency-specific, and that hearing could be poorer for the lower frequencies. Therefore, there is a need to use more frequency-specific stimuli for testing. The authors concluded, though, that the ABR was a viable means of evaluating the hearing in naturally sleeping young infants with cleft palate in order to make management decisions. Unfortunately, the results also indicated that bone-conduction testing was not always feasible, as the infants did not remain in a deep enough sleep. These results point out that, while bone-conduction testing is the standard of care in the presence of elevated air-conduction thresholds,[45,46] it can present feasibility problems in children who are not sedated or anesthetized for the ABR. An ideal time for testing infants or young children who could have both conductive and sensorineural hearing loss, is in association with other procedures that might be done under anesthesia or sedation.

AUDITORY STEADY–STATE RESPONSE TEST

The auditory steady-state response (ASSR)—an emerging physiologic-evoked potential test—holds promise for predicting frequency-specific thresholds in individuals who cannot provide reliable or valid behavioral thresholds.[47−50] The advantage of this measure is that it is truly an objective measure because the response presence or absence is based on statistical analysis and not on visual detection methods as with the ABR. The generation of the 80-Hz ASSR, like the ABR, is believed to be primarily in the brain stem.[51] ASSR uses relatively tonal stimuli (carriers), that are amplitude- and/or frequency-modulated, to evoke a response, and can provide accurate frequency-specific estimates of air- conduction hearing levels. For pediatric applications, the modulation occurs at a frequency appropriate for infants and children (about 80–100 Hz). Single or multiple stimuli presented simultaneously have been used to elicit the ASSR.[52] Furthermore, the 80-Hz ASSR can be obtained in infants and young children who are asleep.[53] The test has the ability to monitor both ears simultaneously, making it attractive for possible reduction in test time, compared to the ABR, although more research is needed in this area before conclusions can be drawn as to whether there is truly a time saving.

Threshold prediction, using the ASSR conducted on adults and children with hearing loss, has been shown to provide fairly accurate estimates of the behavioral audiogram.[49,54–59] Hearing thresholds have been estimated within about 10–15 dB in adults with normal hearing and hearing loss using the multifrequency ASSR.[48,60] Less data, however, exist regarding the use of the ASSR for measurement of hearing in infants and children. Perez-Abalo et al.[61] found that although they were able to determine hearing loss in the severe and profound range, in general, only fair agreement was found between ASSR thresholds and hearing levels in children with mild hearing loss or normal hearing. Recently though, concerns have arisen regarding artifact under certain stimuli conditions.[62,63] Little data exist regarding the use of ASSR employing bone-conduction stimulation. Small and Stapells[64] used multiple bone-conduction stimuli that were both frequency- and amplitude-modulated in a group of preterm infants (32–43 weeks) and a group of postterm infants (0–8 months). The results indicated that the findings in infants were different from those obtained in adults; and this suggests that for infants, the threshold estimates are better in the lower frequencies and poorer in the higher frequencies, when compared to adult data.

The influence of age on the ASSR suggests that maturation has some influence on threshold determination in very young infants. Rance and Rickards[65] found that in infants with hearing loss, the prediction of hearing thresholds was similar between young infants (1–8 months of age), and older subjects with hearing loss. However, results obtained from infants with normal hearing have suggested that maturational factors, which are sufficient to affect the differentiation between normal hearing and mild-to-moderate hearing loss, may influence the findings of ASSR assessments carried out in the first few weeks of life.[47,50,55,65–68] Recently, Rance and Tomlin[69] evaluated neonates and young infants with normal hearing and found that ASSR threshold levels are different from those observed in older subjects. They concluded that when used clinically, the ASSR will need to take into account developmental changes occurring in the first weeks of life. Furthermore, their findings indicated that ASSR thresholds in normal-hearing babies at 6 weeks of age were not yet mature. Clearly, this is a tool that has much promise as an assessment tool for infants and young children, but further research and refinement is needed on all aspects of the ASSR to determine if the ASSR will produce accurate audiogram predictions in all infants.

BEHAVIORAL ASSESSMENT

While it is possible to obtain unconditioned responses to sound in infants younger than the age of 6 months (e.g., changes in motor activity, sucking, eye movement, or startle response), this is not a valid means of determining hearing levels in young children. This technique of observing response changes to stimuli is known as behavioral observation audiometry (BOA). Since infants' responses will occur at levels above threshold and are quite variable, BOA cannot be used to assess threshold. For the very young infant, reliance on physiologic measures for threshold estimation is indicated. For children developmentally 5–6 months of age, it is possible to use a conditioned auditory response, called visual reinforcement audiometry or VRA, to measure hearing threshold levels. This is an operant-conditioning paradigm that reinforces a motor activity, usually a head turn, with an appealing visual display, usually a lighted, animated toy. The auditory signal or stimulus cues the infant that a response, i.e., head turn, will result in reinforcement. Studies have shown that frequency-specific thresholds can be obtained from infants at developmental levels of 5–6 months, producing accurate measures of hearing sensitivity.[70–77] VRA can be conducted using insert earphones (the transducer of choice), for ear-specific responses, and with a bone-conduction vibrator. If the child will not tolerate the use of earphones, results can be obtained using stimuli presented via sound field, such as presentation via speakers into the test booth or sound-isolating room.

As children get to be about 2 years of age, they can usually perform testing using a play task called play audiometry. The child is conditioned to respond to pure tones by playing a simple game using toys such as stacking rings, peg boards, or simple puzzles. Thresholds obtained using play audiometry, in a cooperative child, are assumed to be adult-like in accuracy.

MANAGEMENT OF HEARING LOSS

The management of children with cleft palate who have either transient or permanent hearing loss is a challenge due to the higher prevalence of otitis media and middle-ear effusion in this population, and often drainage from the ears. Tympanostomy tubes are often inserted to manage the middle-ear fluid, thereby reducing conductive hearing losses associated with middle-ear disease. It is possible that ventilation tubes can become blocked and/or fall out, requiring reinsertion. Aggressive otologic management is needed to minimize the amount of time that fluid, and possible associated conductive hearing loss, are present.

Children who have permanent sensorineural or conductive hearing losses are in need of amplification, usually in the form of personal hearing aids. As has been discussed, the child with cleft palate is at risk for recurrent middle-ear disease. If this child also has permanent hearing loss, hearing aid use can be especially challenging and its benefit compromised. Fluctuating conductive impairment, in a child with permanent hearing loss, will result in the child receiving inadequate gain from the hearing aid during times of ear disease, and possibly cause the child to reject the aid. Drainage from the ear can (1) block earmolds reducing the sound from the aid, (2) damage the hearing aid, or (3) cause a feedback whistle from the hearing aid by blocking the ear canal. Lack of air circulation in the ear, when the hearing aid is in place, can exacerbate external- or middle-ear infection, and result in inability to use the instrument consistently.

For children with permanent conductive losses and malformed outer ears that preclude the use of standard behind-the-ear (BTE) hearing aids, bone-conduction hearing aids are appropriate. Often, these children will receive an implantable hearing system, a bone-anchored implant (BAHA), when they are old enough. Until that time, the use of the bone vibrator, from the BAHA system, with a soft headband is a viable option, as it provides good, and a somewhat better, quality signal than a traditional bone-conduction hearing aid; and it is esthetically more appealing. This option of a bone-conduction hearing aid may also be appropriate for children who have chronic drainage from their ears, as it would allow better aeration of the middle ear.

BTE hearing aids are ideal for the child with a sensorineural loss, and should be fit as soon as the hearing loss is defined. However, diligent monitoring is needed because of the issues of otitis media and possible additional intermittent conductive hearing loss. Ideally, a hearing aid with multiple memories, or a volume control that is active, should be fit to ensure that there is an option to provide additional amplification during times when the ears are not clear of effusion.

The use of hearing aids, as a treatment option for otitis media, was studied by Mahashwar et al.[78] They conducted a retrospective evaluation of 70 children with cleft palate to evaluate the usages of tympanostomy tubes and/or hearing aids as a feasible way to manage the child's otologic care. Approximately 40% of the children had hearing aids alone (24%) or ventilation tubes and hearing aids (20%), while 17% had ventilation tubes only and the remaining 39% had neither. Otologic complications were evaluated between the two groups with a significant difference noted with the tympanostomy tube group having more complications than the group with hearing aids. However, speech and language outcomes were not evaluated formally, and aided hearing thresholds were not documented. While the use of hearing aids, for management of ongoing otologic problems in a population at risk for hearing loss due to otitis media, is appealing; given the fluctuating nature of the hearing losses and middle-ear condition, it would be difficult to ensure adequate amplification without regular, perhaps weekly, visits.

Recommended Protocol

Given the prevalence of both transient and permanent hearing loss associated with the presence of cleft palate, children with cleft palates are in need of a baseline hearing assessment, regardless of their newborn hearing screening outcome. Furthermore, routine hearing evaluations are needed at every visit with their cleft palate team. For children not involved in a center offering a multidisciplinary approach to care, referral to an audiology clinic for routine monitoring of their hearing is required. Audiologic monitoring should also occur in conjunction with otologic care for proper management of

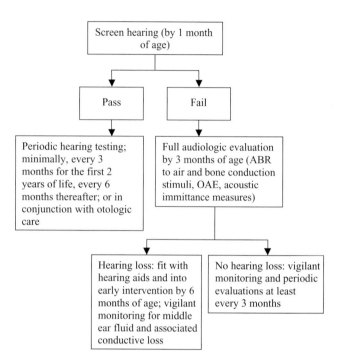

Figure 51–1. Flow chart depicting the time lines set forth nationally for early hearing detection and intervention programs and essential for the care and optimal outcome of infants with cleft palate.

any associated hearing loss. Figure 51–1 is meant to serve as a reminder of the time lines that are critical to maximize optimal outcome, particularly speech and language outcome, of children with hearing loss.

References

1. Joint Committee on Infant Hearing (JCIH). Supplementary statement on infants hearing screening. A Publication of the American Speech-Language Hearing Association 16:160, 1972.
2. Paradise JL, Bluestone CD, Felder H. The universality of otitis media in 50 infants with cleft palate. *Pediatrics* 53:48–54, 1969.
3. Grant HR, Quiney RE, Mercer DM, et al. Cleft palate and glue ear. *Arch Dis Child* 63:176–179, 1988.
4. Dhillon RS. The middle ear in cleft palate children pre and post closure. *J R Soc Med* 81:710–713, 1988.
5. Moller P. Long-term otologic features of cleft palate patients. *Arch Otolaryngol* 101:605–607, 1975.
6. Gordon ASD, Jean-Louis F, Morton RP. Late ear sequelae in cleft palate patients. *Int J Pediatr Otorhinolaryngol* 15:149–156, 1988.
7. Ovesen T, Blegvad-Anderson O. Alternations in tympanic membrane appearance and middle ear functions in 11-year-old children with complete unilateral cleft lip and palate compared with healthy age-matched subjects. *Clin Otolaryngol* 17:203–207, 1992.
8. Smith TL, DiRuggiero DC, Jones KR. Recovery of Eustachian tube function and hearing outcome in patients with cleft palate. *Otolaryngol Head Neck Surg* 111:423–429, 1994.
9. Fria TJ, Cantekin EI, Eichler JA. Hearing acuity of children with otitis media. *Arch Otolaryngol* 111:10–16, 1985.
10. Handžći-Ćuk, Ćuk V, Rišavi R, et al. Hearing levels and age in cleft palate patients. *Int J Pediatr Otorhinolaryngol* 37:227–242, 1996.
11. Gould HJ. Hearing loss and cleft palate: The perspective of time. *Cleft Palate J* 27:36–39, 1990.
12. Rynnel-Dagöö B, Lindberg K, Bagger-Sjöback D, et al. Middle ear disease in cleft palate children at three years of age. *Int J Pediatr Otorhinolaryngol* 23:201–209, 1992.

13. Goudy S, Lott D, Canady J, et al. Conductive hearing loss and otopathology in cleft palate patients. *Otolaryngol Head Neck Surg* 134: 946–948, 2006.

14. Nunn DR, Derkay CS, Darrow DH, et al. The effect of very early cleft palate closure on the need for ventilation tubes in the first years of life. *Laryngoscope* 105:905–908, 1995.

15. Moller P. Hearing, middle ear pressure and otopathology in a cleft palate population. *Acta Otolaryngol* 92:521–528, 1981.

16. Tunçbilek G, Özgür F, Belgin E. Audiologic and tympanometry findings in children with cleft lip and palate. *Cleft Palate Craniofac J* 40: 304–309, 2003.

17. Schönweiler R, Lisson JA, Schönweiler B, et al. A retrospective study of hearing, speech and language function in children with clefts following palatoplasty and veloplasty procedures at 18–24 months of age. *Int J Pediatr Otorhinolaryngol* 50:205–217, 1999.

18. Sheahan P, Blayney AW, Sheahan JN, et al. Sequelae of otitis media with effusion among children with cleft lip and/or cleft palate. *Clin Otolaryngol* 27:494–500, 2002.

19. Sheahan P, Miller I, Sheahan JN, et al. Incidence and outcome of middle ear disease in cleft lip and/or cleft palate. *Int J Pediatr Otorhinolaryngol* 67:785–793, 2003.

20. Bluestone CD. Eustachian tube obstruction in the infant with cleft palate. *Ann Otol Rhinol Laryngol* 80(Suppl 2):1–30, 1971.

21. Valtonen H, Dietz A, Qvarnberg Y. Long-term clinical, audiologic, and radiologic outcomes in palate cleft children treated with early tympanostomy for otitis media with effusion: Acontrolled prospective study. *Laryngoscope* 115:1512–1516, 2005.

22. Principles and guidelines for early hearing detection and intervention programs. Joint Committee on Infant Hearing. 2007 Position Statement. *Am J Audiol* 9:9–29, 2000.

23. National Institutes of Health Consensus Statement. Identification of hearing impairment in infants and young children. *Pediatrics* 120:898–921, 2007.

24. Anteunis LF, Brienesse P, Schrander JJ. Otoacoustic emissions in screening cleft lip and/or palate children for hearing loss—A feasibility study. *Int J Pediatr Otorhinolaryngol* 44:259–266, 1998.

25. Kemp DT. Stimulated acoustic emissions from within the human auditory system. *J Acoust Soc Am* 64:1386–1391, 1978.

26. Probst R, Lonsbury-Martin BL, Martin GK. A review of otoacoustic emissions. *J Acoust Soc Am* 89:2027–2067, 1991.

27. Schrott A, Puel JL, Rebillard G. Cochlear origin of $2 f_1 - f_2$ distortion products assessed by using 2 types of mutant mice. *Hear Res* 52: 245–254, 1991.

28. Paradise J, Smith C, Bluestone C. Tympanometric detection of middle ear effusion in infants and young children. *Pediatrics* 58:198–210, 1976.

29. American Speech-Language-hearing Association. Tutorial on tympanometry. ASHA Working Group on Aural Acoustic-Immittance Measurements Committee on Audiologic Evaluation. *J Speech Hear Disord* 53:354–377, 1988.

30. Bennett M, Weatherby L. Newborn acoustic reflexes to noise and pure tone signals. *J Speech Hear Res* 25:383–387, 1982.

31. Himelfarb M, Popelka G, Shannon E. Tympanometry in normal neonates. *J Speech Hear Res* 22:179–191, 1979.

32. Marchant CD, McMillan PM, Shurin PA, et al. Objective diagnosis of otitis media in early infancy by tympanometry and ipsilateral acoustic reflex thresholds. *J Pediatr* 109:590–595, 1986.

33. Margolis RH. Tympanometry in infants. State of the art. In Harford ER, Bess FH, Bluestone CD, Klein JO (eds). *Impedance Screening for Middle Ear Diseases in Children*. New York: Grune & Stratton, 1978, pp. 41–56.

34. Margolis RH, Bass-Ringdahl S, Hanks WD, et al. Tympanometry in newborns infants—1 kHz norms. *J Am Acad Audiol* 14:383–392, 2003.

35. Margolis RH, Hunter L. Tympanometry: Basic principles and clinical applications. In Musiek FE, Rintelmann WI (eds). *Contemporary Perspectives in Hearing Assessment*. Boston: Allyn & Bacon, 1999, pp. 89–130.

36. Margolis RH, Popelka GR. Static and dynamic acoustic impedance measurements in infants ears. *J Speech Hear Res* 18:435–443, 1975.

37. McKinley AM, Grose JH, Roush J. Multi-frequency tympanometry and evoked otoacoustic emissions in neonates during the first 24 hours of life. *J Am Acad Audiol* 8:218–223, 1997.

38. Weatherby L, Bennett M. The neonatal acoustic reflex. *Scand Audiol* 9:93–110, 1980.

39. Ballachanda B, Crawford M, Ferraro J, et al. Auditory Evoked Potentials. Audiologic Evaluation Working Group on Auditory Evoked Potential Measurements. Guidelines from the American Speech-Language-Hearing Association Rockville, MD, 2004.

40. Stapells DR, Gravel JS, Martin BA. Thresholds for auditory brainstem responses to tones in notched noise from infants and young children with normal hearing or sensorineural hearing loss. *Ear Hear* 16:361–371, 1995.

41. Cone-Wesson B, Ramirez GM. Hearing sensitivity in newborns estimated from ABRs to bone-conducted sounds. *J Am Acad Audiol* 8:299–307, 1997.

42. Sininger YS, Abdala C, Cone-Wesson B. Auditory threshold sensitivity of the human neonate as measured by the auditory brainstem response. *Hear Res* 104:27–38, 1997.

43. Fria TJ, Paradise JL, Sabo DL, et al. Conductive hearing loss in infants and young children with cleft palate. *J Pediatr* 111:84–87, 1987.

44. Andrews PJ, Chorbachi T, Sirimanna B, et al. Evaluation of hearing thresholds in 3-month-old children with a cleft palate: The basis for selective policy for ventilation tube insertion at time of palate repair. *Clin Otolaryngol* 29:10–17, 2004.

45. Stapells DR. Frequency specific evoked potential audiometry in infants. In Seewald RC (ed). *A Sound Foundation Through Early Amplification: Proceedings of an International Conference.* Chicago, IL: Phonak AG, 2000, pp. 13–31.

46. Stapells DR, Herdman A, Small SA, et al. Current status of the auditory steady-state responses for estimating an infant's audiogram. In Seewald RC (ed). *A Sound Foundation through Early Amplification: Proceedings of an International Conference.* Chicago, IL: Phonak AG, 2005, pp. 43–59.

47. Cone-Wesson B, Dowell RC, Tomlin D, et al. The auditory stead-state response: comparison with the auditory brainstem response. *J Am Acad Audiol* 13:173–187, 2002.

48. Dimitrijevic A, John MS, Van Roon P, et al. Estimating the audiogram using multiple auditory steady-state responses. *J Am Acad Audiol* 13:205–224, 2002

49. Vander Werff KR, Brown CJ, Gienapp B, et al. Comparison of auditory steady-state response and auditory brainstem response thresholds in children. *J Am Acad Audiol* 13:227–235, 2002.

50. Rance G, Roper R, Symonds L, et al. Hearing threshold estimation in infants using auditory steady-state responses. *J Am Acad Audiol* 16:293–302, 2005.

51. Herdman A, Lins O, Van Roon P, et al. Intracerebral sources of human auditory steady-state responses. *Brain Topogr* 15:69–86, 2002.

52. Picton TW, John MS, Dimitrijevic A, et al. Human auditory steady-state responses. *Int J Audiol* 42:177–219, 2003.

53. Cohen LT, Rickards FW, Clark GM. A comparison of steady-state evoked potentials to modulated tones in awake and sleeping humans. *J Acoust Soc Am* 90:2467–2479, 1991.

54. Aoyagi M, Suzuki Y, Yokota M, et al. Reliability of 80-Hz amplitude-modulation-following response detected by phase coherence. *Audiol Neurootol* 4:28–37, 1999.

55. Lins OG, Picton TW, Boucher BL, et al. Frequency-specific audiometry using steady-state responses. *Ear Hear* 2:81–96, 1996.

56. Rance G, Dowell RC, Beer DE, et al. Steady-state evoked potential and behavioral hearing thresholds in a group of children with absent click-evoked auditory brain stem response. *Ear Hear* 19:48–61, 1998.

57. Rance G, Rickards FW, Cohen LT, et al. The automated prediction of hearing thresholds in sleeping subjects using auditory steady-state evoked potentials. *Ear Hear* 16:499–507, 1995.

58. Stueve MP, O'Rourke C. Estimation of hearing loss in children: Comparison of auditory steady-state response, auditory brainstem

response, and behavioural test methods. *Am J Audiol* 12:125–136, 2003.

59. Swanepoel D, Hugo R, Roode R. Auditory steady-state response for children with severe to profound hearing loss. *Arch Otolaryngol Head Neck Surg* 130:531–535, 2004.

60. Kaf WA, Durrant JD, Sabo DL, et al. Validity and accuracy of electric response audiometry using the auditory steady-state response: Evaluation in an empirical design. *Int J Audiol* 45:211–223, 2006.

61. Perez-Abalo MC, Savio G, Torres A, et al. Steady state responses to multiple amplitude-modulated tones: An optimized method to test frequency-specific thresholds in hearing-impaired children and normal-hearing subjects. *Ear Hear* 22:200–211, 2001.

62. Gorga MP, Neely ST, Hoover BM, et al. Determining the upper limits of stimulation for auditory steady-state response measurements. *Ear Hear* 25:302–307, 2004.

63. Small SA, Stapells DR. Auditory steady-state responses: Stimulus artifact issues. Paper presented at the *2003 meeting of the American Auditory Society*, Scottsdale AZ, 2003.

64. Small SA, Stapells DR. Multiple auditory steady-state response thresholds to bone-conduction stimuli in young infants with normal hearing. *Ear Hear* 27:219–228, 2006.

65. Rance G, Rickards F. Prediction of hearing threshold in infants using auditory steady-state evoked potentials. *J Am Acad Audiol* 13:236–245, 2002.

66. Levi EC, Folsom RC, Dobie RA. Coherence analysis of envelope-following responses (EFRs) and frequency-following responses (FFRs) in infants and adults. *Hear Res* 89:21–27, 1995.

67. Rickards FW, Tan LE, Cohen LT, et al. Auditory steady-state evoked potentials in newborns. *Br J Audiol* 28:327–337, 1994.

68. Savio G, Cardenas J, Perez-Abalo M, et al. The low and high frequency auditory steady-state responses mature at different rates. *Audiol Neurootol* 6:279–287, 2001.

69. Rance G, Tomlin D. Maturation of auditory steady-state responses in normal babies. *Ear Hear* 27:20–29, 2006.

70. Bernstein R, Gravel J. A method for determining hearing sensitivity in infants: The interweaving staircase procedure (ISP). *J Am Acad Audiol* 1:138–145, 1990.

71. Diefendorf A. Pediatric audiology. In Lass J, McReynolds L, Northern J, Yoder D (eds). *Handbook of Speech-language Pathology and Audiology*. Toronto, Ontario, Canada: BC Decker, 1988, pp. 1315–1338.

72. Diefendorf A. Behavioral hearing assessment: Considerations for the young child with developmental disabilities. *Semin Hear* 24:189–200, 2003.

73. Gravel J. Behavioral assessment of auditory function. *Semin Hear* 10:216–228, 1989.

74. Gravel JS, Wallace IF. Otitis media and communication during pre-school years. Paper presented at *ICIS2000 Doctorial Consortium*, Brisbane, Australia, 1999.

75. Nozza R, Wilson WR. Masked and unmasked pure tone threshold in infants and adults: Development of auditory frequency selectivity and sensitivity. *J Speech Hear Res* 27:613–622, 1984.

76. Sabo DL, Paradise JL, Kurs-Lasky M, et al. Hearing levels in infants and young children in relation to testing technique, age group, and the presence or absence of middle-ear effusion. *Ear Hear* 24:38–47, 2003.

77. Widen JE, Folsom RC, Cone-Wesson B, et al. Identification of neonatal hearing impairment: Hearing status at 8–12 months corrected age using visual reinforcement audiometry protocol. *Ear Hear* 21:471S–487S, 2000.

78. Maheshwar AA, Milling MAP, Kumar M, et al. Use of hearing aids in the management of children with cleft palate. *Int J Pediatr Otorhinolaryngol* 66:55–62, 2002.

52

Pierre Robin Sequence

Richard E. Kirschner, MD, FAAP, FACS • Alison E. Kaye, MD

INTRODUCTION

The clinical triad of micrognathia, glossoptosis, and airway obstruction is known by many names, all of which highlight the contributions made by Pierre Robin. Now most commonly known as *Pierre Robin sequence* (PRS), this clinical association has been historically described as *Pierre Robin syndrome, complex, anomalad, malformation,* and *deformity,* to name a few. The large number of names serves as a testament to the still incomplete understanding of its biological origins. Decades of study and arguments over the developmental conditions that give rise to the manifestations of Pierre Robin sequence have still not been able to fully characterize this clinical entity. It is generally held that PRS does not constitute a distinct syndrome, but instead may occur in isolation or with other syndromes and with varying degrees of severity.[1–7]

The most fundamental understanding of PRS is that developmental disturbances in the fetal mandible and/or tongue (whatever the cause) may secondarily lead to growth disturbances in the upper airway and palate. Mandibular deficiency and growth abnormalities cause the tongue to remain displaced posteriorly, resulting in glossoptosis and postnatal airway obstruction.[1–5,8,9] Failure of the tongue to descend from between the developing palatal shelves due to malpositioning of the fetal head or to motor impairment during the early weeks of fetal development may also obstruct palatal fusion. The resulting cleft of the secondary palate is one of the most commonly associated findings occurring in children with PRS. Palatal clefting is so common, in fact, that many authors define PRS as an anomaly that includes micrognathia, glossoptosis, and cleft palate.[3–5,8,11–13] It should be noted, however, that palatal clefting is not a universal

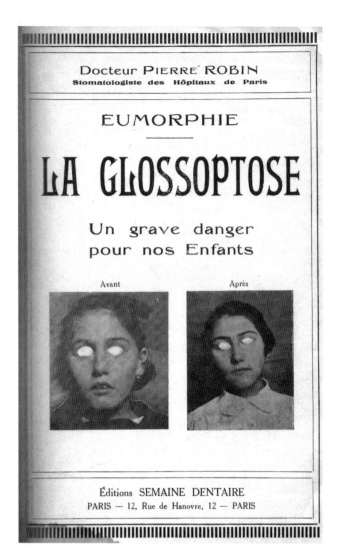

Figure 52–1. Title page of Pierre Robin's *La Glossoptose, un Grave Danger pour Nos Enfants.* Paris: Gaston Doin, 1929.

Nevertheless, Robin is credited with providing an early detailed understanding of some of the clinical findings in affected children and for dedicating much of his professional energies to the study of the malformation. Robin coined the term *glossoptosis* to describe the posterior displacement of the tongue that results in mechanical upper airway obstruction:

> "... This obstruction of the oral pharynx is due to the backward and downward fall of the base of the tongue which in diminishing the oral pharynx presses on the epiglottis and closes the superior opening of the larynx. This obstruction of the oral pharynx by the lowering of the tongue, let's call it glossoptosis, immediately disappears when the subject clips his mandible in a gaping position and holds his lips open..."[2]

In subsequent publications, Robin noted that treatment should aim to improve both respiration and feeding as "athrepsia [failure to thrive] and death are caused by respiratory and nutritional insufficiency following congenital glossoptosis due to mandibular hypotrophy."[17] Robin noted a high mortality rate in infants with severe mandibular hypoplasia. He recommended prone positioning as a treatment strategy for affected infants in order to counter the potential for hypoxia and death. Those infants who died were noted to suffer cachexia and pulmonary infection before 18 months of age. Robin even noted the common association of otitis, gastroesophageal reflux, and aspiration in these children.[2,17] Over time, Robin became perhaps overzealous in his characterization of the sequence, associating the "glossoptotic syndrome" with an extraordinary multitude of ailments (Fig. 52–2).[1,3]

feature of the sequence, whereas airway obstruction is always present to some degree in affected children. Moreover, it is the degree of airway compromise that is the primary determinant of morbidity and mortality suffered by infants with PRS.

HISTORY

Throughout the scientific literature of the last century, Pierre Robin (1867–1950), a French stomatologist, has been honored with the name for this congenital abnormality. Robin first published his article "A Fall of the Base of the Tongue Considered as a New Cause of Nasopharyngeal Respiratory Impairment" in the *Bulletin de l'Academie Nationale de Medicine, Paris* in 1923. As many authors have pointed out, several others, including St. Hilaire, Fairbairn, Shukowsky, and Lannelongue and Manard all predated Robin in describing the association of micrognathia and airway embarrassment.[2,3,5,14–16]

DEMOGRAPHICS

Because of the variety of diagnostic criteria and the widespread degree of clinical severity, the reported incidence of PRS varies widely between 1 in 5000 to 1 in 50,000 live births.[5,12,13,18–21] The apparent etiological heterogeneity of PRS further confounds attempts at descriptive statistics for this malformation. Differences in diagnostic inclusion criteria, such as whether cleft palate must be present, and attempts to limit case series to those with "isolated PRS" versus those with other malformations can exclude many affected patients and obscure the true descriptive picture. As a result, reports vary greatly as to the gender predilection of PRS, the rate of concomitant syndromology, the inheritance risk, and the predicted morbidity and mortality.[22,23]

ASSOCIATED SYNDROMES

It remains unclear what percentage of children with PRS can be correctly categorized as "isolated." Robin, himself, stated

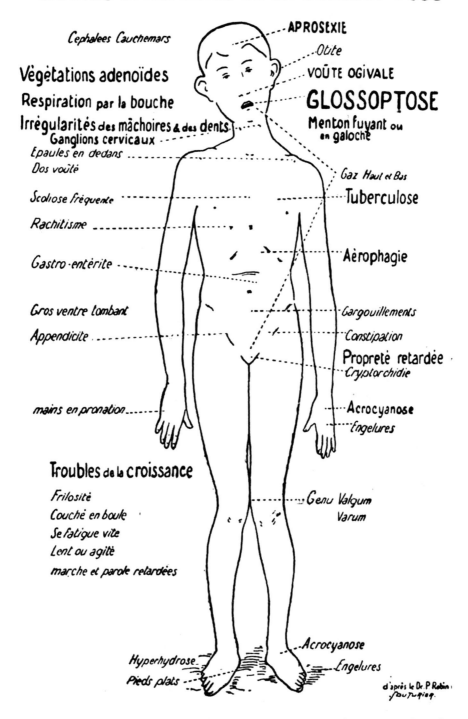

Figure 52–2. Robin's "grands syndromes de la glossoptose." (*From Robin P. La Glossoptose, un Grave Danger pour Nos Enfants. Paris: Gaston Doin, 1929.*)

that "'mandibular hypotrophy' was never idiopathic" and accurately pinpointed maternal alcoholism as one cause of these problems. He also named hereditary syphilis, tuberculosis, and "parental jaw disequilibrium" as causative factors, however, findings which others have not corroborated.[2,17] Since Robin's time, many studies have attempted to define the inci-

dence of "isolated" PRS but with little agreement. Reported rates vary from as low as 17% to as high as 63%.[4,11,13,22–24] For this reason, use of the name "Pierre Robin *sequence*" appropriately emphasizes the multitude of potential underlying etiologies that can contribute to the clinical findings. The vast number of syndromes that have been associated with PRS, as well as the large number of cases that are truly isolated occurrences, confirms that this is a multifactorial condition or, at the very least, the common clinical pathway of many possible derangements of development that can affect the mandible and upper airway.

The syndromes most frequently associated with PRS include Stickler syndrome, 22q11.2 deletion syndrome, fetal alcohol syndrome, and Treacher–Collins syndrome.[3,4,12,13,23,25] Stickler syndrome is by far the most common syndrome associated with PRS, occurring in one-third of affected patients. This connective tissue disorder is inherited in an autosomal dominant fashion and affects the developing eyes, ears, palate, joints, and heart. Affected children have a characteristic facial dysmorphology with a flattened midface, flat nasal bridge, long philtral columns, epicanthal folds, proptosis, and micrognathia. The degree of palatal clefting can range from a submucous cleft to a complete cleft of the secondary hard and soft palate. Stickler patients have normal mental development but typically have severe visual and hearing problems and early joint degeneration.[25,26]

PRS has been associated with a number of rare syndromes (see Chapter 8), each likely accounting for fewer than 1% of affected patients (Table 52–1). In fact, many of these associated syndromes include one or more of the clinical components of PRS as part of their defining features, making the overlap in diagnosis understandable. Knowledge of these common co-existing syndromes is important for ensuring proper referral for genetic testing and appropriate clinical examination for other expected congenital malformations. As the list of associated syndromes continues to grow, the potential for late findings and delayed diagnosis of a named syndrome in a PRS patient previously categorized as "non-syndromic" continues to grow as well.[4,5,13,20,23,25] As gene defects and developmental errors are identified for each of these syndromes, a more complete understanding of the etiologies of PRS will certainly emerge. There are many PRS infants who display congenital anomalies that are either not specific enough for a specific syndromic diagnosis that represent an as-yet unnamed syndrome. These co-existing findings most commonly include cardiac anomalies, such as ventricular septal and atrial septal defects, and central nervous system malformations, such as corpus callosum defects, microcephaly, and aplasia of the tractus corticospinalis.[4,13,22,23]

CLINICAL PRESENTATION

Recognition of the triad of micrognathia, glossoptosis, and airway obstruction does not begin to give the full picture of the medical challenges faced by infant with PRS. In Robin's era, these children suffered a high degree of morbidity and mortality from the associated airway obstruction and inability to feed. Early death rates were reported to range from 19 to 65%.[1,5,6,27,28] Those who survived infancy frequently suffered from psychomotor retardation due to chronic hypoxia and/or malnutrition.[17,22] To some extent, this remained true even into the 1980s, when algorithms for management were still being defined. The historically poor outcomes for affected children have led to the development of multidisciplinary management protocols for PRS. Team-based approaches to these patients have brought current mortality rates to between 5 and 30%, with nonsyndromic patients having better outcomes than those with associated syndromes.[11,12,20,23,29,30]

Table 52–1.		
Syndromes Reported with PRS as a Feature[3,4,12,13,23,25]		
Stickler Syndrome (34%)	Hemifacial Microsomia	Klinefelter Syndrome
22q11.2 Deletion syndrome (11–15%)	Cerebro-oculo-facial syndrome (Cockayne syndrome Type II)	OSMED (non-ocular Stickler's syndrome)
Fetal alcohol syndrome (10%)	Marshall syndrome	Miller-Dieker syndrome
Treacher-Collins syndrome (5%)	Cerebro-Costo-Mandibular syndrome	Spondyloepiphyseal dysplasia syndrome
Orofacialdigital syndrome	Kabuki syndrome	Moebius syndrome
Nager syndrome	Atelosteogenesis type III	Popliteal Pterygium syndrome
Silver-Russell syndrome	Beckwith-Wiedemann syndrome	Saethre-Chotzen syndrome
Trisomy 22	Distal arthrogryposis	ADAM sequence
Down syndrome	Bilateral femoral dysgenesis	Diastrophic dysplasia syndrome
Valproate teratogenicity	Catel-Manzke syndrome	Larsen syndrome

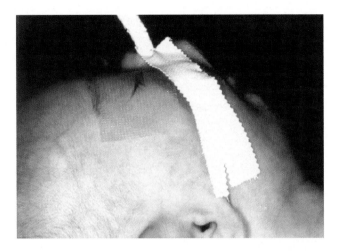

Figure 52–3. Infant with Pierre Robin sequence: The clinical triad of micrognathia, glossoptosis, and upper airway obstruction.

PRS is now widely recognized by pediatricians and neonatologists, and affected infants are typically identified within the first few days of life (Fig. 52–3).[23] Early recognition of PRS is important in order that affected infants can be adequately monitored for respiratory and feeding disturbances. Respiratory problems commonly appear with supine positioning or with feeding and include apnea, hypopnea, hypoxia, or frank respiratory distress. Reflux and aspiration of feeds is also common and can lead to devastating pneumonias, bronchial injuries, and septicemia. The combination of respiratory and feeding difficulties, if untreated, can ultimately result in an overall failure to thrive. Global oropharyngeal dysfunction and abnormal food bolus propagation can cause eustachian tube malfunction and obstruction, resulting in chronic middle ear effusions, conductive hearing loss, and speech impairment. An associated palatal cleft can also compound feeding difficulties. Infants with associated syndromes may have even more profound difficulties at birth related to associated congenital anomalies.[3,11,16,17,22,27,30,32]

MICROGNATHIA, GLOSSOPTOSIS, AND AIRWAY OBSTRUCTION

Because they are developmentally linked, it is difficult to separate the roles that micrognathia and retropositioning of the tongue play in the pathogenesis of airway distress in infants with PRS. Mandibular growth disturbance may prevent elongation and function of the genioglossus muscles, which normally serve to hold the tongue forward in the mouth. Alternatively, foreshortened genioglossus muscles may secondarily restrict mandibular development.[3,33] According to Robin, "glossoptosis is always the consequence of dysmorphic atresia of the mandible, and upon examination of the pharynx and the larynx, we never noticed any local lesion."[2] Regardless of the ultimate cause, this developmental combination sets the stage for airway compromise. Robin focused on glossoptosis

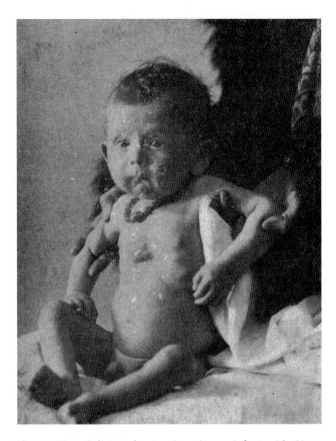

Figure 52–4. Substernal retractions in an infant with Pierre Robin sequence. (*From Robin P. La Glossoptose, un Grave Danger pour Nos Enfants. Paris: Gaston Doin, 1929.*)

as the key airway problem; namely, the tongue, the position and movement of which are restricted by a small mandible, is pushed backward and inferiorly in the airway. Douglas later used endoscopy to confirm that the tongue of affected infants falls posteriorly, pushing on the epliglottis to create a "ball-valve" obstruction of the airway. The negative pressure generated by inspiration sucks the tongue into the airway, preventing air from entering. When a newborn is placed in the supine position, the effect of gravity adds to the forces pulling the tongue base into the airway. Douglas pointed out that inspiration against this stopper-action results in the severe suprasternal, substernal, and intercostal retractions often manifested by PRS infants (Fig. 52–4).[2,9,17,27,30]

Natural resolution of glossoptosis and airway obstruction depends on the expansion of the oropharyngeal airway by forward and downward mandibular growth originating from the condylar growth centers. The concept of "mandibular catch-up growth" has been long debated. Cephalograms and computed tomographic data have allowed researchers to investigate mandibular growth in children with PRS. Early studies documented normal mandibular growth, with complete correction of micrognathia over 4–6 years.[6,27,30] More recently, it has been argued that such is almost never the case and that more than two-thirds of PRS children have persistent mandibular hypoplasia.[34,35] Most likely, both situations exist, depending upon the etiology of the sequence. Some children with PRS are thought to have suffered intrauterine mandibular constraint that, once relieved, yields to rapid correction of micrognathia. Patients with Stickler syndrome may have both maxillary and mandibular hypoplasia and, while they may appear to have resolution of their maxillo-mandibular discrepancy, they remain micrognathic.[4] Cephalometric studies comparing patients with isolated PRS to unaffected controls demonstrate approximation of growth in PRS children toward the normal pattern over the first 2 years of life. This pattern of partial catch-up growth is evidenced by data that the PRS mandible grows 10% more than the normal mandible, with a greater rate of monthly growth in PRS infants in the first 2 years. Although there is a significant increase in the area of the PRS airway during this time, there remains persistent Angle Class II occlusion.[3,36] The presence of associated syndromes with intrinsic craniofacial growth abnormalities, however, may affect the ability of the mandible to demonstrate catch-up growth.

SECONDARY AIRWAY ISSUES

In addition to primary airway obstruction in PRS, there are many secondary airway issues that can contribute to respiratory problems in affected infants. In large measure, this explains why the degree of micrognathia is not well correlated to the severity of symptoms seen in PRS. The most common secondary airway issues in PRS include central apnea, pharyngeal hypotonicity, laryngomalacia, and oroesophageal dysmotility. Other problems, such as ankyloglossia and lymphoid hyperplasia, may also negatively impact the ability to maintain airway patency.[9,16,37–39] Endoscopic views of the pharynx in PRS infants demonstrates not only the obstructive effects of glossoptosis during inspiration but also collapse of hypotonic pharyngeal walls.[40] Even after infants with PRS are placed in a prone position to relieve glossoptotic obstruction, many children may still suffer from the effects of chronic hypoxia. With the use of polysomnography, it has been shown that PRS children may have centrally mediated apnea that causes silent respiratory compromise and desaturation events during sleep. Relaxation of pharyngeal muscular support during sleep may prompt an infant who can successfully maintain airway patency while awake to decline into recurrent hypoxic events at rest.[9] Since centrally mediated apnea is not position-related, a PRS infant who appears comfortable when prone may still have significant respiratory compromise.[41–43] The presence of tracheomalacia or laryngomalacia can also cause position-independent airway obstruction and chronic hypoxia. Continued noisy and disrupted breathing, even in the prone position, may be a clue to the presence of secondary airway issues.[41]

PRS AND CLEFT PALATE

The cleft that is usually seen in PRS is a wide U-shaped or "horseshoe" cleft of the secondary palate rather than the V-

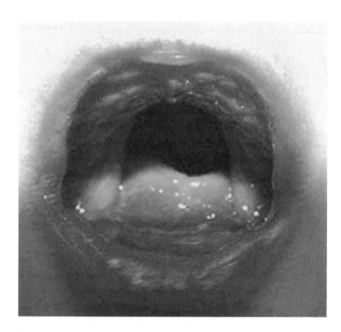

Figure 52–5. Characteristically wide U-shaped cleft palate in an infant with Pierre Robin sequence. (*Photo courtesy of Dr. Don LaRossa.*)

shaped cleft usually seen with other isolated clefts of the secondary palate (Fig. 52–5).[44] The absolute association of cleft palate and PRS has been debated ever since Robin failed to acknowledge palatal clefting in his original description. Several reports document a 58–90% incidence of cleft palate in PRS, with some infants having other palatal anomalies even when an overt cleft is absent.[5,7,19,22,45] Some authors assume palatal clefting to be a requirement for the diagnosis of PRS, although infants are certainly seen with the findings of glossoptosis, micrognathia, and airway obstruction without cleft palate.[7,41] These infants rely on the same diagnostic and therapeutic measures employed for PRS babies with cleft palate. The wide spectrum of severity in PRS suggests that there may be a significant number of cases that escape medical attention, and thus the true prevalence of PRS with or without cleft palate may never be known.

With the majority of PRS research focused on airway management, relatively little has been written specifically on PRS-associated cleft palate, despite its frequency. The U-shaped cleft palate is an interesting feature of PRS because it suggests a mechanism for abnormal development. Although the purported developmental sequence remains unproven, it has been suggested that the pattern of palatal clefting in PRS indicates that, in some children, fetal constraint prevents neck extension and subsequently impairs mandibular growth. The resultant micrognathia leads to palatal clefting as the fetal tongue fails to descend and blocks fusion of the advancing palatal shelves.[46] Cephalometric studies show the palate of the PRS infant with a U-shaped cleft to be more deficient in the antero-posterior dimension and in overall tissue than that of the non-PRS infant with an isolated cleft.[3,36] This is not to suggest that V-shaped clefts are never seen with PRS. Such clefts may themselves suggest an alternate intrinsic clefting pathway during development.

In 1956, Champion suggested the palatal cleft worsens airway obstruction in PRS children secondary to impaction of the tongue tip into the cleft. He proposed palatal closure in the first few days of life to improve respiratory insufficiency, based upon empiric evidence derived from his experience with two patients.[7,16,37] Others believe, however, that the cleft expands the oronasal airway to the child's advantage and should not be closed until airway maturation.[7] No randomized study to answer this question has ever been performed, and most authors now support traditional palatal closure at or around the same age as in non-PRS patients, assuming there is an adequately managed airway and no other medical contraindications. Post-palatoplasty speech data indicates similar outcomes for intelligibility and rates of secondary pharyngoplasty and fistula formation as non-PRS cleft children.[47]

An important concern is the increased difficulty in intubating PRS children at the time of cleft repair.[7,28,47,48] The anterior and inferior displacement of the PRS airway makes it difficult to view the vocal cords and epiglottis without fiberoptic assistance.[37,45] Intubation can exacerbate airway compromise in PRS due to local tissue trauma and edema formation. Because of acute airway changes induced by palatoplasty, a previously compromised airway in a PRS child may again become problematic postoperatively. These airway concerns have encouraged some to postpone palatoplasty until 18–36 months of age in order to allow further airway growth and maturity.[7,47] While most data indicate that cleft palate repair in PRS can be approached in the same fashion and time frame as in non-PRS clefts, the impact of concomitant congenital anomalies and significant potential for airway compromise must not be underestimated.

FEEDING ISSUES IN PRS

The negatively synergistic effects of respiratory distress, poor sucking, and disorganized swallowing provide a significant challenge for the feeding of PRS infants. Recurrent airway obstruction prevents normal sleep in affected infants. In turn, decreased sleep increases the metabolic demands and caloric needs. PRS infants are often slow to feed and can even develop an aversion to feeding secondary to the trauma of repeated gagging and aspiration of feeds. Prolonged feeding times may be a sign of airway obstruction, as affected infants struggle to coordinate breathing and eating. Inability to consume the necessary calories in a timely fashion leads to poor weight gain, and affected infants may be labeled as "failure to thrive." It is important to note that inadequate weight gain is itself a useful criterion for surgical intervention[8,49]

Recent examination of the feeding issues encountered with PRS has shed light on the particular problem of airway obstruction as related to motor dysfunction of the pharynx and esophagus. Typically, feeding difficulties in PRS are directly proportional to airway difficulties. An infant with an obstructed airway in the supine position will almost certainly have difficulty when trying to feed in a similar position. If gravity acts to pull the tongue into the pharynx, both inspiration and deglutition will be affected. Weak suction, direct tongue base stimulation of the gag reflex, and respiratory distress combine to create an uncoordinated breathing–feeding pattern that results in regurgitation of food. Gasping for breath also fills the stomach with air and may thus promote vomiting and aspiration. Aspiration, in turn, can cause caustic airway damage and pneumonia, leading to further respiratory compromise in affected infants.[9,12]

Although feeding difficulties in PRS infants typically occur in conjunction with respiratory insufficiency, poor feeding can be observed in the absence of clinically evident airway obstruction.[4,5] Cross-cut nipples and special bottles for cleft palate patients may be all that is required to allow affected infants to feed successfully. Infants with PRS associated with cleft palate may require upright or prone positioning during feeds and may need more frequent burping. Many affected infants, however, are still unable to sustain adequate nutrition. Manometry and pH measurements should be performed in order to determine the presence of gastroesophageal reflux, and if such is identified appropriate medical and/or surgical treatment is indicated. Several studies have shown that there may be synergy between gastroesophageal reflux and upper airway obstruction.[29,43,50] Once the reflux is adequately treated, airway insufficiency often improves. Conversely, successful airway management often results in improved feeding. For some patients, however, nasogastric or gastrostomy tube feedings are necessary in order to ensure adequate caloric intake. Often, infants may be successfully weaned off of tube feedings over several months. Infants with PRS associated with other syndromes, however, are more likely to require long-term tube feeds to optimize nutrition.[31,51]

Coordinated manometric, electromyelographic, cardiac monitor, and endoscopic studies have further delineated the airway-feeding problem in PRS. Most affected children exhibit a degree of uncoordinated sucking and swallowing to an extent greater than that observed in children with isolated cleft palate. Electromyelography of the genioglossus and thyrohyoid muscles demonstrates an abnormal synchronization or tonic activity in these tissues in place of the rhythmic alternating pattern seen in normal infants. Despite changes in the firing pattern, individual cranial nerve conduction is normal, and there is no evidence of denervation of the muscles of the palate, tongue, palate, or mandible.[42] Cardiac monitoring during reflux events demonstrates a high resting vagal tone that is not coordinated with obstructive events. Manometric studies demonstrate that these patients have a high rate of esophageal dysfunction related to hypertonic esophageal musculature. Abnormal upper esophageal sphincter relaxation, esophageal body dysmotility, and persistently elevated lower esophageal sphincter pressures combine to promote reflux and esophagitis in PRS infants. The high resting esophageal sphincter tone and high amplitude multi-peaked esophageal waves seen in PRS infants differ in the pattern seen in infants suffering from gastroesophageal reflux disorder (GERD) alone, suggesting a PRS-unique mechanism.[40,42,43,50]

EVALUATION AND MANAGEMENT OF THE PRS INFANT

A comprehensive approach to the PRS infant is essential to limiting morbidity and optimizing outcome in these patients. As prenatal ultrasound diagnosis has become more advanced, it has become possible to visualize cleft palate, mandibular deficiency, and glossoptosis in utero.[21] Thus, health care providers can now be prepared to care for affected infants at the time of delivery. At birth, Apgar scores may be diminished in these infants, particularly in those with associated syndromes.[23] It is important, however, to keep in mind that many PRS infants may do well initially after birth, only to suffer respiratory compromise a few weeks later. Infant evaluation and treatment is performed with the cooperation of a multidisciplinary team including nurse specialists, pediatricians, neonatologists, pediatric pulmonologists, geneticists, plastic surgeons, otorhinolaryngologists, anesthesiologists, speech/feeding therapists, and nutritionists.

Initial assessment of the PRS infant includes a methodical approach to the airway. In the supine position, infants may present with noisy and labored breathing, stridor, cyanosis, intercostal and substernal retractions, and evidence of accessory muscle use (Fig. 52–4). Switching the infant to a prone position may alleviate some or all of these findings as gravity allows for the obstructing tongue to fall forward in the mouth and out of the airway. Special prone positioning beds and neck-extension head caps designed to support the infant in this position have long been proposed and utilized by some.[5,22] Although prone positioning may be adequate for airway management in the majority of PRS infants, it is important to remember that silent obstruction can still occur in some infants, thus necessitating ongoing vigilance.

It is important to gather objective data in order to determine if the PRS airway is adequately treated by positioning alone. Although continuous pulse oximetry can document the adequacy of oxygenation, it may not detect brief, intermittent obstructive episodes during sleep. Polysomnography has been shown to provide a more complete picture of an infant's ability to maintain adequate oxygenation and ventilation, as it correlates O_2 and end-tidal CO_2 measurements with apnea, hypopnea, bradycardia, end EEG tracings. Polysomnography should be repeated as the infant grows and with the addition of intervention in order to objectively document airway improvement.[28,38,42]

When evaluating a child with PRS, polysomnographic data can help divide patients between those with desaturations associated with obstructive apnea and those without such. Those patients with persistent hypoxic obstructive events despite prone positioning must then be considered for airway intervention. There are several options for airway intervention. Nonsurgical airway choices include supplemental oxygen, intraoral prosthetic devices, oral airways, nasopharyngeal (NP) airways, and laryngeal mask airways.[3,5,12,23,52] Of these, NP airway placement is the most frequently used, and such may be combined with continuous positive airway pressure (CPAP). Successful use of an NP airway requires accurate placement of the tube in the pharynx. Incorrect position may stimulate gagging and/or aspiration or may obstruct the airway. Supportive attachments to the head or face can be made to limit motion of the NP airway, but the risks of malposition and dislodgement make NP airway therapy not ideal for home use in children who need prolonged airway intervention.[8,53]

If a nonsurgical airway does not provide relief of obstructive episodes, then the infant may require endotracheal intubation and/or surgical intervention. In this situation, close inspection of the entire airway is important in order to diagnose the true cause of airway obstruction. Flexible endoscopy allows for visualization of secondary airway abnormalities such as choanal atresia, laryngomalacia, tracheomalacia, vocal cord paralysis, and subglottic stenosis that may indicate a need for tracheostomy. Tracheo-esophageal fistula and severe CNS abnormalities may also require early tracheostomy for adequate airway management. Tracheostomy is also a suitable solution for airway obstruction due to glossoptosis alone, but surgical opinion is divided on the appropriateness of tracheostomy for primary airway management. Tracheostomy requires skilled care that can be more involved than some parents are capable of managing at home. Plugging and dislodgement of tracheostomy tubes represent major causes of morbidity and mortality in infants so treated. In addition, long-term tracheostomy use may be associated with subglottic stenosis.[12,53–55]

Historically, several techniques using surgical wires to help maintain airway patency in infants with PRS have been described.[16] Circum-mandibular Kirschner wire placement, with either direct pull on the wire or attachment to a pulley system to distract the jaw, is perhaps the oldest such intervention.[5,56] Use of a transmandibular Kirschner wire passed transversely through the posterior mandible to stabilize the base of the tongue in a forward position has also been described.[57–59] Hyomandibulopexy was first described by Bergoin et al. in 1971. Although this technique can successfully open the airway, its use may render endotracheal intubation difficult, thereby forcing tracheostomy in the setting of an airway emergency. Moreover, anchoring the mandible to the hyoid may ultimately impede forward mandibular growth.[53,57,60]

The earliest (and still frequently employed) surgical intervention for glossoptosis is glossopexy, or tongue–lip adhesion. Although first described by Shukowsky in 1911, tongue–lip adhesion was not widely utilized until Douglas described his technique in 1946.[3,27,28,30] Modifications to the Douglas procedure have since been proposed by several authors. In 1960, the Routledge modification of the Douglas glossopexy was the first major change in operative approach. Routledge altered the mucosal incision to form a transverse cut in the tip of the tongue and along the deep buccal groove to create a broad attachment when sutured together.[16] Randall proposed a further modification of the Routledge procedure that also used a horizontal incision but placed a retention suture through the posterior tongue, securing it over buttons

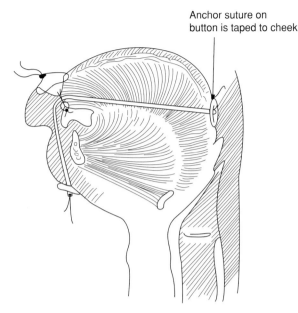

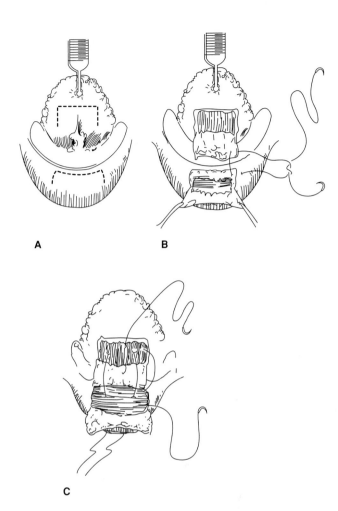

Figure 52–6. Randall modification of the Routledge glossopexy. (*From Randall P. The Robin sequence: Micrognathia and glossoptosis with airway obstruction. In McCarthy JG, May JW, Littler JW (eds). Plastic Surgery, Philadelphia: W.B. Saunders, 1990, p. 3132.*)

on the posterior tongue and beneath the chin (Fig. 52–6).[3] Further refinements of this technique include the placement of deep sutures between the muscularis propria of the tongue and the orbicularis oris of the lower lip to reinforce the attachment and decrease the rate of dehiscence (Figs 52–7 and 52–8).[31] Release of the genioglossus attachments to the mandible has been described to allow greater mobilization of the tongue. This floor-of-mouth release can be used alone or in combination with tongue–lip adhesion to relieve upper airway obstruction in PRS infants.[33,61]

Tongue–lip adhesion has been reported to relieve the specific tongue-to-posterior wall obstruction pattern of glossoptosis, but not other pharyngeal closure patterns such as lateral wall collapse, circular constriction or soft palate interposition.[9,62] Large series have shown, however, that when used with thorough preoperative assessment, glossopexy can be a reliable procedure for the treatment of airway compromise in PRS.[31,34,45,63] Perhaps the largest drawback of tongue–lip adhesion is the potential for dehiscence and need for repeat operation. Several authors point out, however, that dehiscence rates decrease with experience as well as with the use of intermuscular sutures. Failure of tongue–lip adhesion to successfully relieve upper airway obstruction has led some authors to favor primary tracheostomy or mandibular distraction in affected infants.[51,64,65] Failure of airway stabilization after tongue–lip adhesion occurs more commonly in children with associated syndromes than in those with isolated PRS. When preceded by thorough assessment with flexible endoscopy and/or polysomnography, however, tongue–lip adhesion successfully relieves airway obstruction in 80–100% of affected children.[31,45,63]

Figure 52–7. Authors' technique for tongue-lip adhesion. (A) Design of the mucosal flaps. (B) Inset of the tongue mucosal flap. (C) Suture of the muscularis propria of the tongue to the orbicularis oris prior to inset of labial mucosal flap. (*From Kirschner RE, Low DW, Randall P, et al. Surgical airway management in Pierre Robin sequence: Is there a role for tongue-lip adhesion? Cleft Palate Craniofac J 40:13–18, 2003.*)

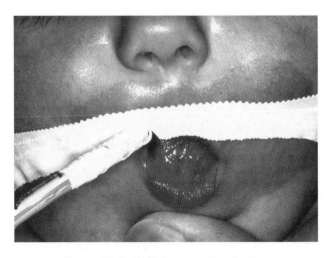

Figure 52–8. Healed tongue–lip adhesion.

There is conflicting evidence as to whether tongue–lip adhesion inhibits normal infant tongue movements used in feeding, thereby preventing normal bolus propagation.[8,34] Indeed, feeding is improved in most infants after glossopexy due to the associated improvement in airway obstruction. Some authors have expressed concern that speech development may be delayed in these children due to fixation of the tongue tip in a non-anatomic position. Studies of speech in patients after glossopexy demonstrate that there may be associated delays in babbling and first words, but such is only temporary, with rapid catch-up to normal after takedown of the adhesion.[67] It should be noted as well that children with prolonged tracheostomy have been found to demonstrate both receptive and expressive speech and language delays.[5,22,41,53,66]

There is lack of agreement on the most appropriate time to reverse the tongue–lip adhesion. Some practitioners favor combining the timing of release with cleft palate repair in order to limit the exposure of the patient to anesthesia. Others argue that releasing the adhesion before the palate repair can help to determine if the airway will remain patent once the palate is closed.[7,47] Preoperative polysomnogram and endoscopy may help predict if the infant airway will tolerate tongue–lip takedown. In addition, improvements in maxillo-mandibular discrepancy and neurological maturation, indicated by normalization of tongue and esophageal movements, may suggest readiness for adhesion takedown. Rarely, respiratory compromise after tongue–lip adhesion take-down requires tracheostomy or mandibular distraction.[31,34,51,63,67]

Distraction osteogenesis on the infant mandible has recently been described as an alternative for surgical airway management of infants with PRS (see Chapter 63). There is ample evidence that mandibular distraction may be successfully used to treat respiratory and feeding difficulties in PRS infants. Surgical intervention on the neonatal mandible, however, requires precise operative technique as the bone is very soft. Similar to glossopexy, distraction will not improve respiratory compromise in children with secondary airway problems such as laryngomalacia or subglottic stenosis. Distraction can, however, play a role in older children with PRS who have failed decannulation after tracheostomy.[57,59–61] Long-term follow-up of PRS patients treated by mandibular distraction is limited, and some have voiced concern over external scarring and the potential for long-term mandibular growth disturbance.

Other common surgical interventions in PRS patients outside of primary airway treatment include: cleft palate repair, myringotomy tube placement, gastrostomy tube placement, Nissen fundoplication, secondary palatal repair, and pharyngoplasty. The timing of these procedures must be selected with careful consideration status of the child's airway and overall medical condition. In all cases, safe airway management is of critical importance. Anesthesia for such patients should be entrusted only to a pediatric anesthesiologist experienced with PRS patients and with management of the difficult airway.

CONCLUSIONS

It is perhaps too simplistic to describe Pierre Robin sequence as merely a triad of clinical findings when its presentation and prognosis can be so varied. In its simplest form, PRS may call for only repositioning, close observation, and careful follow-up. When more severe, or when associated with multiple other congenital anomalies, PRS may require prolonged hospitalization, treatment of associated morbidities, and surgical airway management. Should surgery be required, several options are available, including tongue–lip adhesion, tracheostomy, and distraction osteogenesis. Selection among these is currently based both on rigorous assessment of the affected infant and on surgical preference and skill. The treating clinician must always consider that each PRS infant is unique, and only a thorough multidisciplinary approach to the child's care can assure optimal outcomes. Whether or not a PRS child will need surgical intervention is only one of many questions that arise during that child's care. The dangers of airway complications and the complex relationship between an infant's patterns of breathing and feeding make precision in diagnosis essential. When the available tools for clinical assessment are used appropriately, the information gained will help health care professionals responsible for the care of infants with PRS to make correct decisions regarding appropriate treatment. As children with PRS grow and develop, interval reassessment will ensure optimization of their care and long-term outcomes.

References

1. Robin, P. *La Glossoptose, un Grave Danger pour Nos Enfants*. Paris: Gaston Doin, 1929.
2. Paletta CE, Dehghan K, Hutchinson RL, et al. A fall of the base of the tongue considered as a new cause of nasopharyngeal respiratory impairment: Pierre Robin sequence, a translation. *Plast Reconstruct Surg* 93(6):1301–1303, 1994.
3. Randall P. The Robin sequence: Micrognathia and glossoptosis with airway obstruction. In McCarthy JG, May JW, Littler JW (eds). *Plastic Surgery*, 1st edn. Philadelphia, PA: W.B. Saunders, 1990.
4. Shprintzen RJ. The implications of the diagnosis of Robin sequence. *Cleft Palate Craniofac J* 29(3):205–209, 1992.
5. Sadewitz VL. Robin sequence: Changes in thinking leading to changes in patient care. *Cleft Palate Craniofac J* 29(3):246–253, 1992.
6. Kiskadden WS, Dietrich SR. Review of the treatment of micrognathia. *Plas Reconstruct Surg* 12:364–373, 1953.
7. Hoffman S, Kahn S, Seitchik M. Late problems in the management of the Pierre Robin syndrome. *Plast Reconstruct Surg* 35(5):504–511, 1965.
8. Singer L, Sidoti EJ. Pediatric management of Robin sequence. *Cleft Palate Craniofac J* 29(3):220–223, 1992.
9. Sher AE. Mechanisms of airway obstruction in Robin sequence: Implications for treatment. *Cleft Palate Craniofac J* 29(3):224–231, 1992.
10. Beers MD, Pruzansky S. The growth of the head of an infant with mandibular micrognathia, glossoptosis and cleft palate following the Beverly Douglas operation. *Plast Reconstruct Surg* 16:189–193, 1955.
11. Williams AJ, Williams MA, Walker CA, et al. The Robin anomalad (Pierre Robin syndrome) – follow up study. *Arch Dis Childhood* 56:663–668, 1981.

12. Tomaski SM, Zalzal GH, Saal HM. Airway obstruction in the Pierre Robin sequence. *Laryngoscope* 105:111–114, 1995.

13. Holder-Espinasse M, Abadie V, Cormier-Daire V, et al. Pierre Robin sequence: A series of 117 consecutive cases. *J Pediatr* 139(4):588–590, 2001.

14. Fairbairn P. Suffocation in an infant, from retraction of the base of the tongue, connected with defect of the frenum. *Mon J Med Sci* 6:280–282, 1846.

15. Shukowsky WB. Zur Atiologie des Stridor Inspiratorius Congenitus. *Jahrb Kinderheilk* 73:459, 1911.

16. Routledge RT. The Pierre-Robin syndrome: A surgical emergency in the neonatal period. *Br J Plast Surg* 13:204–218, 1960.

17. Robin P. Glossoptosis due to atresia and hypotrophy of the mandible. *Am J Dis Child* 48:541–547, 1934.

18. Bush PG, Williams AJ. Incidence of the Robin anomalad (Pierre Robin syndrome). *Br J Plast Surg* 36:434–437, 1983.

19. Dykes EH, Raine PAM, Arthur DS, et al. Pierre Robin syndrome and pulmonary hypertension. *J Pediatr Surg* 20:49–52, 1985.

20. Bartlett SP, Losee JE, Baker SB. Reconstruction: Craniofacial syndromes. In Mathes SJ (ed). *Plastic Surgery*, 2nd edn. Philadelphia, PA: Saunders Elsevier, 2006.

21. Bronshtein M, Blazer S, Zalel Y, et al. Ultrasonographic diagnosis of glossoptosis in fetuses with Pierre Robin sequence in early and mid pregnancy. *Am J Obstet Gynecol* 193:1561–1564, 2005.

22. Caouette-Laberge L, Bayet B, Larocque Y. The Pierre Robin sequence: Review of 125 cases and evolution of treatment modalities. *Plast Reconstr Surg* 93(5):934–942, 1994.

23. van den Elzen APM, Semmekrot BA, Bongers EM, et al. Diagnosis and treatment of the Pierre Robin sequence: Results of a retrospective clinical study and review of the literature. *Eur J Pediatr* 160:47–53, 2001.

24. Kirschner RE, McDonald-McGinn D, Baker SB, et al. *Airway Management in Pierre Robin Sequence: Etiology as a Predictive Factor.* Abstract.

25. Pierre Robin Network, Quincy, IL,

26. Nowak CB. Genetics and hearing loss: A review of Stickler syndrome. *J Commun Disord* 31(5):437–454, 1998.

27. Douglas BA. A further report on the treatment of micrognathia with obstruction by a plastic procedure: Results based on reports from twenty-one cities, 1948–1949. *Plast Reconstr Surg* 5:113–122, 1950.

28. Benavent WJ, Ramos-Oller A. Micrognathia: Report of twelve cases. *Plast Reconstr Surg* 22(5):486–490, 1958.

29. Bull MJ, Givan DC, Sadove M, et al. Improved outcome in Pierre Robin sequence: Effect of multidisciplinary evaluation and management. *Pediatrics* 86(2):294–301, 1990.

30. Douglas B. The treatment of micrognathia associated with obstruction by a plastic procedure. *Plast Reconstr Surg* 1:300–308, 1946.

31. Kirschner RE, Low DW, Randall P, et al. Surgical airway management in Pierre Robin sequence: Is there a role for tongue-lip adhesion? *Cleft Palate-Craniofac J* 40(1):13–18, 2003.

32. Handzic J, Bagatin M, Subotic R, et al. Hearing levels in Pierre Robin syndrome. *Cleft Palate-Craniofac J* 32(1):30–36, 1995.

33. Delorme RP, Larocque Y, Caouette-Laberge L. Innovative surgical approach for the Pierre Robin anomalad: subperiosteal release of the floor of the mouth musculature. *Plast Reconstr Surg* 83(6):960–966, 1989.

34. Argamaso RV. Glossopexy for upper airway obstruction in Robin sequence. *Cleft Palate-Craniofac J* 29(3):232–238. 1992.

35. Shprintzen RJ. Pierre Robin, micrognathia, and airway obstruction: the dependency of treatment on accurate diagnosis. *Int Anesthesiol Clin* 26(1):64–71, 1988.

36. Figueroa AA, Glupker TJ, Fitz MG, et al. Mandible, tongue, and airway in Pierre Robin sequence: A longitudinal cephalometric study. *Cleft Palate-Craniofac J* 28(4):425–434, 1991.

37. Champion R. Treatment of cleft palate associated with micrognathia. *Br J Plast Surg* 8:283–290, 1956.

38. Schaefer RB, Gosain AK. Airway management in patients with isolated Pierre Robin sequence during the first year of life. *J Craniofac Surg* 14(4):462–467, 2003.

39. Bravo G, Ysunza A, Arrieta J, et al. Videonasopharyngoscopy is useful for identifying children with Pierre Robin sequence and severe obstructive sleep apnea. *Int J Pediatr Otorhinolaryngol* 69(1):27–33, 2005.

40. Abadie V, Morisseau-Durand MP, Beyler C, et al. Brainstem dysfunction: A possible neuroembryological pathogenesis of isolated Pierre Robin sequence. *Eur J Pediatr* 161(5):275–280, 2002.

41. Cruz MJ, Kerschner JE, Beste DJ, et al. Pierre Robin sequence: Secondary respiratory difficulties and intrinsic feeding abnormalities. *Laryngoscope* 109(10):1632–1636, 1999.

42. Renault F, Flores-Guevara R, Soupre V, et al. Neurophysiological brainstem investigations in isolated Pierre Robin sequence. *Early Human Dev* 58(2):141–152, 2000.

43. Baudon JJ, Renault F, Goutet JM, et al. Motor dysfunction of the upper digestive tract in Pierre Robin sequence as assessed by sucking-swallowing electromyography and esophageal manometry. *J Pediatr* 140(6):719–723, 2002.

44. Hanson JW, Smith DW. U-shaped palatal defect in the Robin anomalad: Developmental and clinical relevance. *J Pediatr* 87(1):30–33, 1975.

45. Hoffman W. Outcome of tongue-lip plication in patients with severe Pierre Robin sequence. *J Craniofac Surg* 14(5):602–608, 2003.

46. Latham RA. The pathogenesis of cleft palate associated with the Pierre Robin syndrome. An analysis of a seventeen-week human foetus. *Br J Plast Surg* 19:205–213, 1966.

47. Lehman JA, Fishman JRA, Neiman GS. Treatment of cleft palate associated with Robin sequence: Appraisal of risk factors. *Cleft Palate Craniofac J* 32(1):25–29, 1995.

48. Benjamin B, Walker P. Management of airway obstruction in the Pierre Robin sequence. *Int J Pediatr Otorhinolaryngol* 22:29–37, 1991.

49. Parsons RW, Smith DJ. Rule of thumb criteria for tongue-lip adhesion in Pierre Robin anomalad. *Plast Reconstr Surg* 70(2):210–212, 1982.

50. Baujat G, Faure C, Zaouche A, et al. Oroesophageal motor disorders in Pierre Robin syndrome. *J Pediatr Gastroenterol Nutr* 32(3):297–302, 2001.

51. Denny AD, Amm CA, Schaefer RB. Outcomes of tongue-lip adhesion for neonatal respiratory distress caused by Pierre Robin sequence. *J Craniofac Surg* 15(5):819–823, 2004.

52. Yao CT, Wang JN, Tai YT, et al. Successful management of a neonate with Pierre-Robin syndrome and severe upper airway obstruction by long term placement of a laryngeal mask airway. *Resuscitation* 61(1):97–99, 2004.

53. Myer III, CM, Reed JM, Robin TC, et al. Airway management in Pierre Robin sequence. *Otolaryngol Head Neck Surg* 118(5):630–635, 1998.

54. Bath AP, Bull PD. Management of upper airway obstruction in Pierre Robin sequence. *J Laryngol Otol* 111:1155–1157, 1997.

55. Gianoli GJ, Miller RT, Guarisco JL, et al. Tracheotomy in the first year of life. *Ann Otol Rhinol Laryngol* 99:896–901, 1990.

56. Callister AC. Hypoplasia of the mandible (micrognathy) with cleft palate: Treatment in early infancy by skeletal traction. *Am J Dis Childhood* 53:1057–1059, 1937.

57. Lapidot A, Ben-Hur N. Fastening the base of the tongue forward to the hyoid for relief of respiratory distress in Pierre Robin syndrome. *Plast Reconstr Surg* 56(1):89–91, 1975.

58. Hadley RC, Johnson JB. Utilization of the Kirschner wire in Pierre Robin syndrome. *Plast Reconstr Surg* 31(6):587–596, 1963.

59. Rawashdeh MA. Transmandibular K-wire in the management of airway obstruction in Pierre Robin sequence. *J Craniofac Surg* 15(3):447–450, 2004.

60. Bergoin M, Giraud JP, Chaix C. L'hyomandibulopexie dans le traitement de formes graves du syndrome de Pierre Robin. *Ann Chirur Infant* 12(1):85–90, 1971.

61. Parsons RW, Smith DJ. A modified tongue-lip adhesion for Pierre Robin anomalad. *Cleft Palate J* 17(2):144–147, 1980.

62. Wetmore RF, Thompson M, Marsh RR, et al. Use of polsomnography in the management of Pierre-Robin sequence and its variants. Presented at the 7th International Congress on Cleft Palate and Related Craniofacial Anomalies. Broadbeach, Queensland, Australia, Nov 1993.

63. Schaefer RB, Stadler III JA, Gosain AK. To distract or not to distract: An algorithm for airway management in isolated Pierre Robin sequence. *Plast Reconstr Surg* 113(4):1113–1125, 2004.

64. Monasterio FO, Drucker M, Molina F, et al. Distraction osteogenesis in Pierre Robin sequence and related respiratory problems in children. *J Craniofac Surg* 13(1):79–83, 2002.

65. Denny A, Amm C. New technique for airway correction in neonates with severe Pierre Robin sequence. *J Pediatr* 147(1):97–101, 2005.

66. LeBlanc SM, Golding-Kushner KJ. Effect of glossopexy on speech sound production in Robin sequence. *Cleft Palate Craniofac J* 29(3): 239–245, 1992.

67. Freed G, Pearlman MA, Brown AS, et al. Polysomnographic indications for surgical intervention in Pierre Robin sequence: Acute airway management and follow-up studies after repair and takedown of tongue-lip adhesion. *Cleft Palate Craniofac J* 25(2):151–155, 1988.

Nasal Airway Considerations

Gale Norman Coston, EdD • Harold Friedman, MD, PhD • Michael James VanLue, PhD

INTRODUCTION

Esthetic surgery of the cleft lip nose has received a great deal of attention over the years and has been greatly improved. The airway function of the nose, however, has received much less attention and often, even after the "definitive" repair, the patient may be left with ineffective nasal breathing. The goals of this chapter are to briefly review the anatomical defects of the cleft lip nose and to describe surgical correction for these disorders. The residual problems that may follow the initial repair are described with recommendations for their resolution. A major portion of this chapter is devoted to state-of-the-art diagnostic techniques related to the nasal airway that may be utilized in the clinical setting. It may not be necessary to carry out all of the techniques presented on every

patient. The key is to make certain that the nasal airway is patent and functioning properly.

As was noted in the first chapter, development of the nasal placode is clearly visible by the fifth week of gestation, and by 6 weeks the medial and lateral nasal processes are identifiable surrounding the nasal pit. During continued development of the embryonic facial features, there is eventual fusion of the medial nasal swellings with the maxillary swellings to give rise to the upper lip.[1] Thus, it is no great surprise that clefting of the lip is intimately associated with developmental nasal deformities. Given the prominent position of the nose in the center of the face and the importance of nasal esthetics to self-esteem, cleft patients are greatly concerned about their nasal appearance.[2] While this concern has caused an emphasis on esthetic results, increasing attention has been devoted to nasal airway competence.

ANATOMICAL DEFECTS OF THE CLEFT LIP/NOSE

Harold McComb[3] has contributed careful dissections that focus on the anatomic deformities of the unilateral and bilateral cleft nasal defects. With regard to the supporting framework of the nose, the cleft premaxilla tilts in a forward direction toward the cleft, causing the anterior portion of the nasal septum to bow into the noncleft nasal passage. In fact, the caudal septum may be displaced into the vestibule on the noncleft side. More posteriorly, the septum bulges outward into the cleft side. The lower lateral cartilage on the cleft side appears stretched over the nostril opening from its origin medially at the base of the columella to the lateral attachment near the pyriform aperture at the alar base. The caudal border of the lower lateral cartilage forms a curtain-like edge displaced downward (caudally) over the nostril opening. This position causes the alar domes to also be depressed downward, backward, and laterally. The cephalic border of the lower lateral cartilage is pulled inferiorly so that it no longer overlaps the lower border of the upper lateral cartilage. The stretching of the caudal border of the alar cartilage contributes to a shortening of the columella on the cleft side as the medial crus is drawn into the cleft.

The external appearance of the nose reflects the disorders seen in the underlying structural framework (Fig. 53–1). The cleft-side nostril opening lies in a horizontal plane compared with the noncleft side. When measured from the nasion to the margin of the alar rim, the nasal soft tissue is longer on the cleft side. The flattened alar dome on the cleft side causes broadening of the nasal tip with concomitant loss of prominence. The columella tilts to the noncleft side at its origin from the lip, paralleling the displaced septum. The alar base joins the cheek at an oblique angle. Salyer[4] lists 21 separate deformities of the unilateral cleft nose. In addition to those already noted, he includes: missing nasal floor, lower nasal floor on the cleft side, and hypertrophy of the inferior turbinate on the cleft side. Bardach and Cutting[5] also describe the anatomy of the unilateral and bilateral cleft lip and nose.

SURGICAL CORRECTION OF THE CLEFT LIP/NOSE

In an unrepaired cleft, there is little or no obstruction to nasal airflow. However, once the lip is repaired and certain portions of the anatomy, such as the nasal floor, are restored, cleft deformities may limit nasal airflow (Fig. 53–2). Modern techniques of unilateral cleft lip repair generally incorporate some variation of either a Millard[6] or Tennison[7] type of flap design while at the same time making an effort to reposition portions of the displaced and altered lower lateral cartilages.[5,8,9] Repositioning of the alar cartilages at the time of lip repair can reduce some of the secondary nasal tip and alar rim asymmetries observed when these techniques are not incorporated. However, even under the best of circumstances, residual deformities will still exist, requiring additional operative procedures as the child matures.[10–14] These techniques deal with the esthetic deformities of the cleft nose as well as nasal airway obstruction.[15–17]

The primary anatomical structures that contribute to airway problems are the nasal vestibule, the septum, and the turbinates. Once the position of the alar rim is corrected, the rim itself does not cause narrowing of the ostium. Rather, there is often a curtain of mucosa and skin on the lateral aspect of the vestibule that reduces the flow of air. If these tissues are not supported, they may collapse on inspiration, further impeding airflow. This problem can be remedied with Z-plasties and/or cartilage grafts to support the vestibular skin and soft tissues. Additionally, there may be scar contracture or stenosis of the nostril opening. It is rare, however, for these defects alone to impede airflow. Rather, a combination of nasal septal deformities, vestibular narrowing, and hypertrophied turbinates most often restrict airflow and contribute to mouth breathing.

Hogan and Converse[18] have described the cleft septal deformity, comparing the nasal complex to a tilted tripod. The more severe the bony abnormality, the more the central strut (septum) deviates in both the vertical and horizontal planes. Thus, the nasal septum buckles into the noncleft side

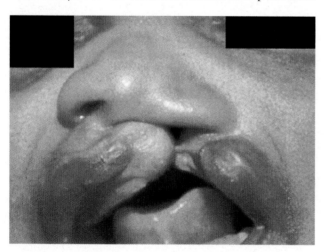

Figure 53–1. Disorders seen in the structural framework of the cleft nose.

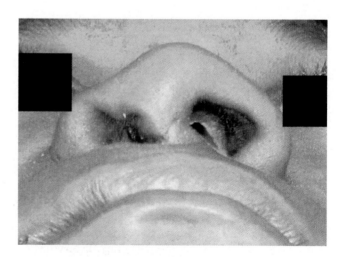

Figure 53–2. Post-surgical deformities of the cleft nose.

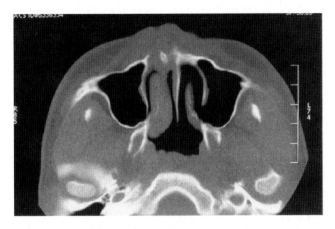

Figure 53–3. Axial CT scan demonstrating deviation of the nasal septum and hypertrophy of the inferior turbinate.

anteriorly and into the cleft side posteriorly. The most caudal portion of the septum is often dislocated from the nasal spine into the nostril opening on the noncleft side. In addition, there may be inferior turbinate hypertrophy on the cleft side that may lead to near total occlusion of the nasal passage[19] (Figs. 53–3 and 53–4).

Nasal airway obstruction presents with various sequelae: obligate oral breathing, recurrent sinus problems, hyponasal speech resonance, snoring and other symptoms of sleep apnea, and dental occlusal problems. In order to improve nasal airway patency, all of these abnormalities must be addressed. Correction of septal deviation may require a submucous resection along with repositioning and fixation of the caudal border in the midline. The hypertrophied turbinate may be either resected or in-fractured. Most surgeons opt to correct these problems at the same time that rhinoplasty is performed when the skeletal framework and nasal soft tissues are fully matured. Ideally, however, such intervention should be accomplished at an earlier age. The goal of the cleft palate/craniofacial team is to routinely assess the nasal function and to provide nasal airway patency as early as possible.

Cephalometric assessment of the posterior nasopharyngeal airway space has been shown to be of value.[20] Our team uses this technique routinely in evaluating adenoidal size and structure. We also use computed tomography and magnetic resonance imaging in the evaluation of our patients (Figs. 53–3 and 53–4). This chapter, however, focuses on the techniques used in our diagnostic laboratory.

ASSESSMENT OF NASAL AIRWAY FUNCTION

Case History

Assessment of nasal airway function should begin with a review of the clinical history,[21] including the list of the patient's current medications. It is important to determine if the patient has experienced chronic mouth breathing, snoring, hyponasality, chronic rhinitis, or nasal allergies. Any one or combination of these symptoms should trigger further evaluation. Questionnaires have been shown to be important tools in identifying the presence of symptoms.[22]

Hyponasal Speech Resonance

Hyponasalality is not often discerned by the patient or parents but can be an important clue to nasal airway interference. A clinician who is accustomed to listening to the resonance of speakers in an evaluative manner is essential. The clinician should have an evaluative tool to be used as a part of the diagnostic protocol. We have found the rating scales depicted in Fig. 53–5 to be helpful in judging hyponasality and/or hypernasality. Peterson-Falzone et al.[23] present a review of rating scales for resonance.

Examination of Nasalance

There are three techniques available for measuring nasalance: the Nasometer, NasalView, and the OroNasal System. Bressmann[24] presents a review of these techniques.

The KayPENTAX Nasometer 6200 and the more recent Nasometer II 6400 are the most frequently used of these tools.

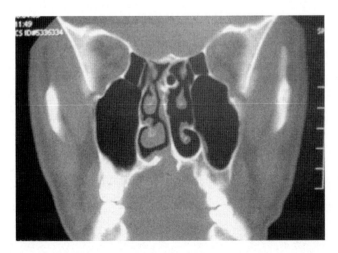

Figure 53–4. Coronal CT scan demonstrating deviation of the nasal septum and hypertrophy of the inferior turbinate.

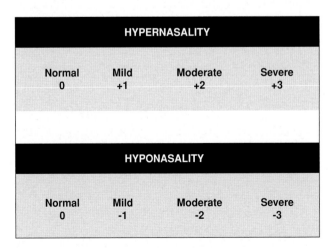

HYPERNASALITY			
Normal	Mild	Moderate	Severe
0	+1	+2	+3

HYPONASALITY			
Normal	Mild	Moderate	Severe
0	-1	-2	-3

Figure 53–5. Rating scales for speech resonance.

The MacKay–Kummer SNAP Test is a very useful companion in using the Nasometer and may be found in the Nasometer II manual. Kummer has provided a 2005 revision of the SNAP Test which has been re-normed for the Nasometer 6400.[25] As described in Chapter 37, the Nasometer is a computer-based instrument that measures the relative amount of nasal acoustic energy in a patient's speech and provides the results in the form of a mean score and a nasogram. Studies utilizing the Nasometer include the evaluation of velopharyngeal (VP) competence, upper airway obstruction, and normal speaker characteristics. The Nasometer results may be compared with the listener judgment of resonance discussed earlier.

As first presented by Awan[26] in 1996, the NasalView is a nasalance acquisition system. While the NasalView setup is very similar to that of the Nasometer, Lewis and Watterson[27] found the nasalance scores of the NasalView to be different from the Nasometer both qualitatively and quantitatively.

The OroNasal System differs from the Nasometer and NasalView techniques in that it uses a handheld facial mask that is placed against the patient's face. The mask has a sound separation plate. Similar to the Nasometer and NasalView equipment, the OroNasal system also has two microphones for nasal and oral components. The software, which is similar to the Nasometer and NasalView, calculates a nasalance score and a nasalance ratio. Bressmann[24] reports that, at present, there are no normative or clinical data for this system. It is important to note that the results from any one of these systems are interchangeable with those from another.

Rhinomanometry

Rhinomanometry is an evaluative procedure that measures the resistance to airflow through the nasopharyngeal airway.[28] Examples of the clinical uses of rhinomanometry include the documentation of nasopharyngeal airway resistance after adenoidectomy or turbinectomy in sleep apnea, in nasal provocation testing, in pre- and postoperative nasal surgery assessment, and in the evaluation of nasopharyngeal airway patency.[29] This technique shows the relationships of pressure, airflow, and time, resulting in an objective evaluation of air conduction through the nasopharyngeal airway.[30] Resistance to airflow is measured by the pressure difference (transnasal pressure) between the anterior and the posterior nasal airway. Rhinomanometry protocols differ in the location of the pressure sensing tube and in which areas of the nasopharyngeal airway are evaluated. Topical decongestants have been shown to reduce nasal airway resistance owing to the mucosal (soft) tissue vs. skeletal (hard) tissue; however, patients with severe rhinitis show less decongestion effect than patients without severe rhinitis.[31]

Rhinomanometry procedures can be classified as (1) anterior, (2) posterior, and (3) postnasal or pernasal.[32]. Within these classifications, an active or passive approach may be utilized. Passive methods require patients to hold their breath while air is introduced into the nose at a known flow rate. Active methods use the patient's own respiratory efforts as the source of pressure and flow offering a better represen-

tation of the actual physiology of the nose. This is the method more commonly used for clinical evaluation.[30]

Active anterior rhinomanometry is defined as the measurement of nasal airflow and pressure at the nostrils during respiration, and is the most commonly used method of rhinomanometry.[33] While the patient is actively breathing through one side of the nose, the narinochoanal pressure difference is measured in the contralateral side of the nose at the nares. Unilateral measurements for each side of the nasal cavity can be documented by reversing the procedure.

Active posterior rhinomanometry utilizes a pressure sensing tube placed in the posterior oropharynx while airflow is measured for both nasal cavities simultaneously at the nares.[33] This method allows for the measurement of the transnasal pressure difference from the nares through the nasopharynx to the oropharynx resulting in the documentation (when compared with active anterior resistance values) of the contribution of the tongue, palate, and pharyngeal walls to nasopharyngeal airway resistance.[34]

For pernasal rhinomanometry, the tube is placed in the posterior nasal cavity through one of the nares.[30]

Perci–SARS

In 1964, Warren and Dubois[35] introduced a method for measuring VP function based on the airflow and pressure to calculate VP area. This method, more commonly known as the pressure-flow technique, uses a modified hydrokinetic formula and was initially used for VP area estimates during speech production and also used to estimate nasal pathway resistance.[36] Many of the studies using the pressure-flow method provided the first descriptions of nasal patency status in patients with cleft lip and/or palate. Results from nasal airflow/pressure studies utilizing pressure-flow documented nasal airway impairment of patients with cleft lip and palate such as: (1) increased nasal airway resistances[36,37]; (2) increased nasal airway resistance secondary to restorative procedures on the nasopharyngeal airway in patients with cleft palate[38]; and (3) characteristic nasal airway profiles by type of cleft with documentation of oral vs. nasal breathing mode.[39] These studies emphasize key clinical sequelae that are important for clinicians to be aware of: individuals with cleft lip and palate have higher nasal resistances as compared to noncleft subjects; secondary surgical procedures such as a pharyngeal flap can add significant nasopharyngeal airway resistance and influence mode of breathing (nasal vs. oral); and patients with UCLP typically have smaller nasal cross-sectional areas as well as having the highest rate of oral breathing among the differing types of clefting.

The pressure-flow method has also been used in combination with standard rhinomanometry. Smith and Guyette,[40] using a combination of anterior rhinomanometry and VP resistance,[35] partitioned total nasal airway resistance into nasal cavity and VP components to assess the contribution of a pharyngeal flap to total nasal airway resistance. The two patients evaluated by this study demonstrated a 70–90% increase in the VP contribution to total nasopharyngeal airway resistance, measured at 7 months postoperative. At 10 months postoperative, one patient's VP contribution to total nasopharyngeal airway resistance was reduced to 33% and the other's VP contribution decreased only slightly from 90 to 80%. These outcomes demonstrate the utility of partitioning the total nasopharyngeal airway to evaluate the outcome of the pharyngeal flap procedure on nasopharyngeal airway resistance. Cohen et al.[41] emphasized this component approach technique as an essential part of a comprehensive evaluation for use in planning the correction of cleft nasal deformities and measuring esthetic and functional outcomes. The authors reported summary results for their first 30 patients: 22 (73.3%) of this cohort had functional and esthetic improvement, 5 patients (16.6%) demonstrated significant esthetic but only a modest functional improvement, and 3 patients (10%) had no esthetic or functional improvement and required additional surgery. Fukushiro and Trindade[42] used a combination of anterior and posterior pressure-flow (modified rhinomanometry) methods to document differences by cleft type in nasal airway dimensions. Fifty-three participants age 18–35 (17 BCLP, 16 UCLP, 20 CP, and 20 N) were evaluated using the pressure-flow procedure[37] to determine the smallest cross-sectional area to estimate nasal patency. Results of anterior and posterior methods indicated that participants with BCLP had a smaller nasal area than those with UCLP, and isolated CP did not compromise nasal area.

Acoustic Rhinometry

Hilberg et al.[43] introduced the technique of measuring the nasal cross-sectional area and its relationship to distance into the nasal cavity from the nares utilizing acoustic reflection. The acoustic rhinometer is a computer-assisted device with an analog-to-digital converter for data acquisition and processing. The instrument produces an acoustic pulse through a wave tube, an electric microphone, a 20 dB amplifier, and a 10 kHz low-pass filter. Two electrodes in the wave tube create an acoustic pulse which travels down the wave tube and enters the nasal cavity through a nosepiece inserted a few millimeters into the nostril. The size of the nose piece can be varied according to the size of the nostril. The analog signal from the microphone is amplified, low-pass filtered, and digitized at a sampling rate of 40 kHz. The data are converted to an area–distance function by the software with area plotted on either logarithmic or linear scale. The cross-sectional areas are determined for a distance of up to 20 cm with a spatial resolution of –0.4 cm. The measurement lasts 8 ms. The authors found a coefficient of variation of the areas of <2% by the acoustic rhinometry method as compared with 15% for the rhinomanometric measurements. Acoustic rhinometry areas correlated highly to similar areas obtained by computerized tomography (CT) scans ($r = 0.94$).

This technique is not dependent on nasal airflow, and due to its rapid, noninvasive nature, has a high compliance rate for patients of all ages. It may be used for infants and children.[44]

Acoustic rhinometry produces an area/distance curve, indicating the cross-sectional area of the nasal cavity as a function of proximal distance from the nares. The reported accuracy and reproducibility is in the 5–10% range.[45] Authors Hilberg and Pederson stress, however, that the clinician should be properly trained and should follow a standard procedure. Temperature and noise should be controlled, and the coupling between the equipment and nose should provide a sufficient seal without disturbing the anatomy. Calibration procedures, hygiene, and safety standards should be maintained.

When used properly, acoustic rhinometry provides a valid measure of anterior nasal cross-sectional area for at least the first 5–6 cm from the nares with the posterior portion susceptible to influence from the paranasal sinuses. When compared with magnetic resonance imaging in 10 subjects and CT measurements in a cadaver, acoustic rhinometry showed good correlation for the first 6 cm of the nasal cavity.[46]

Corey[47] presents an excellent review article related to the clinical applications of acoustic rhinometry. The importance of using a topical nasal decongestant pretest/posttest protocol (as in airflow measures) provides the added advantage of characterizing the actual locations of where mucosal vs. skeletal tissue is affecting nasal patency. Clinically relevant studies of acoustic rhinometry include those of allergic rhinitis, vasomotor rhinitis, nasal challenge studies, septoplasty, turbinoplasty, sinus surgery, facial/cosmetic surgery, cleft lip and/or palate, cleft nose, antrochoanal atresia, maxillofacial expansion procedures, adenoidectomy, sleep disorders, mechanical nasal dilation, air pollution, and drugs.

Video Recorded Fiberoptic Nasendoscopy

Use of fiberoptic nasendoscopy for assessment of VP function has been described in Chapter 36. The technique is also useful for capturing the landscape of the nasal chambers and nasopharynx. In addition to evaluating problems that may be related to VP valving, nasendoscopy can also document hypertrophy of the adenoids, nasal webbing, enlarged turbinates, septal deviations, nasal polyps, and scar tissue. Whether stored digitally or on videotape, it is important to preserve each examination for comparison over time. Because of the need for use of a nasal decongestant and topical anesthesia in preparing the patient for endoscopy, it is scheduled as the final procedure in our evaluation protocol.

▌ SUMMARY

As emphasized at the beginning of this chapter, children with cleft lip and/or palate experience significant deviations in nasal anatomy with concomitant sequelae that decrease normal nasal function. It has been our experience that the majority of children with cleft lip and/or palate do not receive objective nasopharyngeal airflow, interior nasal geometry, and speech resonance measures together in a comprehensive assessment of overall nasal patency and function. This is not surprising, since it is reported that experienced rhinologists and rhinosurgeons tend not to use objective assessments of nasal patency to determine the indications for nasal surgery, relying instead on clinical experience derived from trial and error.[48]

Specific, comprehensive evaluation protocols containing a diversification of measurements are necessary to assess the cleft nasal deformity. An example[41] includes esthetic, patient questionnaire, intranasal, rhinomanometric, and pressure-flow studies used specifically for providing comprehensive evaluation and planning for correction of the cleft nasal deformity. Many centers achieve good surgical results, but evaluation protocols remain unstandardized and do not use topical nasal decongestion. Topical nasal decongestion has been used extensively in rhinomanometric studies and acoustic rhinometry studies. It has been shown to significantly improve the coefficient of variation of estimating total nasal airway resistance (from unilateral rhinomanometry measures) using Ohm's law as compared to using a head-out body plethysmograph.[49] Yet many of the airflow studies of children who have cleft nasal deformity have not incorporated topical nasal decongestion. VanLue[50] proposed preliminary data using a pre-post topical nasal decongestion protocol with nasometry, acoustic rhinometry, and rhinomanometry studies for assessing the cleft nasal deformity. Pegoraro-Krook, Dutka-Souza et al.[51] further developed and replicated the results for using topical nasal decongestion with nasometry and concluded that nasometry, before and after decongestion, may assist in screening for the presence of nasal cavity congestion as part of addressing patient complaints of nasal airway obstruction. Protocols involving pre-test and then post-test topical nasal decongestion should be considered for inclusion into cleft nasal deformity functional assessment protocols involving acoustic (nasometry), airflow, and interior nasal geometry measures.

References

1. Langman J. Face, nose and palate. In *Medical Embryology Human Development-Normal and Abnormal*, 3rd edn. Baltimore: William and Wilkins, 1975, Chapter 18.
2. Randall P. History of cleft lip nasal repair. *Cleft Palate-Craniofac J* 29:527–530, 1992.
3. McComb H. Anatomy of the unilateral and bilateral cleft lip nose. In Bardach J, Morris HL (eds). *Multidisciplinary Management of Cleft Lip and Palate*. Philadelphia: W.B. Saunders Co., 1990, Chapter 18.
4. Salyer KE. Early and late treatment of unilateral cleft nasal deformity. *Cleft Palate-Craniofac J* 29:556–569, 1992.
5. Bardach J, Cutting C. Anatomy of the unilateral and bilateral cleft lip and nose. In Bardach J, Morris HL (eds). *Multidisciplinary Management of Cleft Lip and Palate*. Philadelphia: W.B. Saunders Co., 1990, Chapter 19.
6. Millard DR. How to rotate and advance in a complete cleft. In *Cleft Craft. The Evolution of It's Surgery. I. The Unilateral Deformity*. Boston: Little, Brown and Co, 1976, Chapter 37.
7. Tennison CW. The repair of the unilateral cleft lip by the stencil method. *Plast Reconstr Surg* 9:115–120, 1952.
8. De La Torre JI. Repairing the cleft lip nasal deformity. *Cleft Palate-Craniofac J* 37:234–242, 2000.
9. Verwoerd CDA, Mladina R, Trenite GJN, et al. The nose in children

10. Friedman HI, Stonerock C, Brill A. Composite earlobe grafts to reconstruct the lateral nasal ala and sill. *Ann Plast Surg* 50:275–281, 2003.
11. Millard DR. My own secondary correction of the unilateral cleft lip nose. In *Cleft Craft. The Evolution of It's Surgery. I. The Unilateral Deformity*. Boston: Little, Brown and Co, 1976, Chapter 53.
12. Bardach J. Secondary correction of the unilateral and bilateral cleft lip nasal deformity: Bardach technique. In Bardach J, Morris HL (eds). *Multidisciplinary Management of Cleft Lip and Palate*. Philadelphia: W.B. Saunders Co, 1990, Chapter 34.
13. Cutting CB. Secondary cleft lip nasal reconstruction: State of the art. *Cleft Palate-Craniofac J* 37:538–541, 2000.
14. Han S, Choi MS. Three-dimensional Z-plasty in the correction of the unilateral cleft lip nasal deformity. *Cleft Palate-Craniofac J* 38:264–267, 2001.
15. Warren DW, Odont D, Drake AF. Cleft nose. Form and function. *Clin Plast Surg* 20:769–779, 1993.
16. Drettner B. The nasal airway and hearing in patients with cleft palate. *Acta Oto-laryngol* 52:131–142, 1960.
17. Fukushiro AP, Trindade IEK. Nasal airway dimensions of adults with cleft lip and palate: Differences among cleft types. *Cleft Palate-Craniofac J* 42:396–402, 2005.
18. Hogan VM, Converse JM. Secondary deformities of unilateral cleft lip and nose. In Grabb WC, Rosenstein SC, Bzoch KR (eds). *Cleft Lip and Palate*. Boston: Little, Brown and Co, 1971.
19. Wolford LM. Effects of orthognathic surgery on nasal form and function in the cleft patient. *Cleft Palate Craniofac J* 29(6):546–555, 1992.
20. Rose E, Thissen V, Otten JE, et al. Cephalometric assessment of the posterior airway space in patients with cleft palate after palatoplasty. *Cleft Palate-Craniofac J* 40(5):498–503, 2003.
21. Grymer L, Hilberg O, Pederson O. Prediction of nasal obstruction based on clinical examination and acoustic rhinometry. *Rhinology* 35(2):53–57, 1997.
22. Grymer L. Clinical applications of acoustic rhinometry. *Rhinology* 16 (Supplement):35–43, 2000.
23. Peterson-Falzone S, Hardin-Jones M, Karnell M. *Cleft Palate Speech*, 3rd edn. Philadelphia: Mosby, 2001, pp. 226–227.
24. Bressmann T. Comparison of nasalance scores obtained with the nasometer, the nasal view, and the oronasal system. *Cleft Palate-Craniofac J* 42(4):423–433, 2005.
25. Kummer AW. Nasometry. In Kummer AW (ed). *Cleft Palate and Craniofacial Anomalies: The Effects on Speech and Resonance*. Clifton Park: Thomson Delmar Learning, 2001.
26. Awan S. Development of a low-cost nasalance acquisition system. In Powell T (ed). *Pathologies of Speech and Language: Contributions of Clinical Phonetics and Linguistics*. New Orleans: International Clinical Linguistics and Phonetics Association, 1996, pp. 211–217.
27. Lewis K, Watterson T. Comparison of nasalance scores obtained from the nasometer and the nasalview. *Cleft Palate-Craniofac J* 40(1): 40–45, 2003.
28. Sandham A, Solow B. Nasal respiratory resistance in cleft lip and palate. *Cleft Palate-Craniofac J* 24(4):278–285, 1987.
29. Gosepath J, Amedee RG, Mann WJ. Nasal provocation testing as an international standard for evaluation of allergic and nonallergic rhinitis. *Laryngoscope* 115:512–516, 2005.
30. Pallanch JF, McCaffrey TV, et al. Evaluation of nasal breathing function. In *General Face, Nose, Paranasal, Sinuses*. Vol. 1. St. Louis: Mosby Year Book, 1993, pp. 665–686.
31. Williams RG, Eccles R. Nasal airflow asymmetry and the effects of topical nasal decongestion. *Rhinology* 30:277–282, 1992.
32. Cole P. Rhinomanometry 1988: Practice and trends. *Laryngoscope* 99:311–315, 1989.
33. Clement PAR, Gordts F. Consensus report on acoustic rhinometry and rhinomanometry. *Rhinology* 43:169–179, 2005.

with unilateral cleft lip and palate. *Int J Ped Otolaryngol* 32:S45–S52, 1995.

34. Cole P, Aviomanimitis A, Ohki M. Anterior and posterior rhinomanometry. *Rhinology* 27(4):257–262, 1989.

35. Warren DW, Dubois AB. A pressure-flow technique for measuring velopharyngeal orifice area during continuous speech. *Cleft Palate-Craniofac J* 1:52–57, 1964.

36. Warren DW, Duany LF, Fischer ND. Nasal pathway resistance in normal and cleft lip and palate subjects. *Cleft Palate J* 6:134–140, 1969.

37. Warren DW. A quantitative technique for assessing nasal airway impairment. *Am J Orthodont* 86:306–314, 1984.

38. Warren DW, Trier WC, Bevin AG. Effect of restorative procedures on the nasopharyngeal airway in cleft palate. *Cleft Palate J* 11:367–373, 1974.

39. Warren DW, Hairfield M, Dalston ET, Sidman JD, Pillsbury HC. Effects of cleft lip and palate on the nasal airway in children. *Arch Otolaryngol Head Neck Surg* 114:987–992, 1988.

40. Smith BE, Guyette TW. Component approach for partitioning nasal airway resistance: Pharyngeal flap case studies. *Cleft Palate-Craniofac J* 30(1):78–81, 1993.

41. Cohen M, Smith BE, Daw JL. Secondary unilateral cleft lip and nasal deformity: Functional and esthetic reconstruction. *J Craniofac Surg* 14(4):584–593, 2003.

42. Fukushiro AP, Trindade IEK. Nasal airway dimensions of adults with cleft lip and palate: Differences among cleft types. *Cleft Palate-Craniofac J* 42(4):396–401, 2005.

43. Hilberg O, Jackson AC, Swift DL, Pedersen OF. Acoustic rhinometry: Evaluation of nasal cavity geometry by acoustic reflection. *J Appl Physiol* 66:295–303, 1989.

44. Djupesland P, Pedersen OF. Acoustic rhinometry in infants and children. *Rhinology* 16(Supplement):52–58, 2000.

45. Hilberg O, Pederson OF. Acoustic rhinometry: Recommendations for technical specifications and standard operating procedures. *Rhinology* 16(Supplement):3–17, 2000.

46. Hilberg O. Objective measurement of nasal airway dimensions using acoustic rhinometry: Methodological and clinical aspects. *Allergy* 57(Supplement 70):5–39, 2002.

47. Corey JP. Acoustic rhinometry: Should we be using it? *Curr Opin Otolaryngol Head Neck Surg* 14:29–34, 2006.

48. Grymer LF. Clinical applications of acoustic rhinometry. *Rhinology* 16(Supplement):35–43, 2000.

49. Cole P, Naito K, Chaban R, Aviomamitis A. Unilateral and bilateral nasal resistances. *Rhinology* 26:209–216, 1988.

50. VanLue M. *Nasometry, Acoustic Rhinometry, and Rhinomanometry in the Evaluation of Nasal Function.* Presented at the Annual Meeting of the American Cleft Palate-Craniofacial Association, Scottsdale, Arizona, 1999.

51. Pegoraro-Krook M, Dutka-Souza J, Williams WN, Teles Magalhães LC, Rossetto PC, Riski JE. Effect of nasal decongestion on nasalance measures. *Cleft Palate-Craniofac J* 43(3):289–294, 2006.

Management of Skeletal Deformities

The Functional Cleft Lip Repair, Maxillary Orthopedic Segment Alignment and Primary Osteoplasty: A Protocol for Complete Clefts

Diane Dado, MD • Sheldon Rosenstein, DDS, MSD

INTRODUCTION

The approach to the habilitation of complete unilateral and bilateral clefts of the lip, alveolus, and palate described herein begins at birth and utilizes both surgeon and orthodontist working together, in sequence, to optimize function, aesthetics, and growth. The newborn child with a cleft presents with intrinsic factors, such as hypoplasia of tissue, displacement of tissue, impaired growth potential, agenesis and ectopic eruption and placement of dental units, lack of a bony base within which to move teeth, and multicomponent maxillae that can compromise the ultimate aesthetic and functional result. It is the authors' belief that surgery is the single most important extrinsic factor affecting these treatment goals, and the surgeon, in conjunction with the orthodontist, can incorporate the principles of developmental genetics into a treatment plan that overcomes malocclusion and growth-related jaw discrepancies and that optimizes aesthetics and function of the lip and palate.

HISTORY

An awareness of a deficiency of tissue in complete clefts prompted the use of autogenous bone placement in the cleft area as early as the middle of the last century. By the mid-1960s, a myriad of techniques for early autogenesis bone placement were advocated, along with the use of palatal prostheses to move and manipulate maxillary segments and to aid in feeding. No attempts were made to define protocols; some utilized plates passively, and others used plates actively to move maxillary segments. Early autogenous grafts were markedly varied; some centers undermined extensively over large areas to place bone, and all continued to use lip and palate closures of their choice and sequence. The only common denominator was that these procedures were performed very early in life, and differences were many and varied. Koberg[1] reviewed over 175 published reports of treatment protocols and reached a similar conclusion. Fear of possible exacerbation of growth problems in an area already compromised by the cleft and its inherent growth deficiency eventually led many centers to use delayed autogenous bone grafts in the 1980s, and this approach continues to be extensively utilized.

RATIONALE AND PROTOCOL

The authors' rationale for treatment has always been predicated on two very important dictums: first, to do no further harm in the form of growth constraints through habilitative efforts and second, to attempt to create a functional and aesthetic facial environment that is better than if the early procedures had not been performed.

The authors' therapeutic approach has remained virtually unchanged since 1965 and is applied to almost all newborn infants with complete unilateral and bilateral clefts of the lip and palate. The timing and sequence of the protocol is specific and essential to its success (Table 54–1). When the newborn child is initially seen at the hospital or as an outpatient after a general pediatric evaluation, the orthodontist takes an impression of the maxilla, and the protocol is be-

Table 54–1.

Protocol for Early Alveolar Bone Grafting

Age	Intervention
First 2 weeks of life	Maxillary impression for construction and placement of passive self retaining appliance prior to lip closure
6–10 weeks of age	Functional cleft lip repair
10 weeks to 5 months	Appliance in place to control molding of segments by maintaining arch width posteriorly and allowing anterior segment approximation without collapse
5–8 months	Abutted segments stabilized with onlay, subperiosteal alveolar bone graft
8–12 months	Appliance in place in the mouth at least 6 weeks post graft or until palate repair
8–12 months	Complete palate repair

gun. Treatment includes fabrication and placement of the palatal prosthesis, a functional cleft lip repair at 6–8 weeks of age, and bone grafting at 3–5 months when the segments are aligned and have minimal or no gap between them. The palate is closed when the cleft is narrow enough for closure, but generally before the first birthday. This protocol has been extensively reported in the literature, along with modifications when indicated.[2,3]

Prior to the use of the infant prosthesis, the frequency of segmental collapse and mal-alignment was marked, even prior to the presence of the primary dentition. In the primary dentition, this presented as unilateral cleft side buccal cross-bite and often anterior cross-bite. The bilateral complete cleft would often present with bilateral buccal segment collapse and a mobile premaxilla. Use of the maxillary prosthesis allows for control of the local environment in an epigenetic fashion, so as to help create a more favorable arch and segment alignment. For unilateral clefts, the plate is constructed so that the anterior margin is terminated on the greater segment, where the fulcrum of rotation should be, and so that the anterior portion of this segment is directed back toward the midline. At the same time, the anterior border of the plate on the lesser segment can be relieved to allow the lesser segment to grow anteriorly in a controlled environment (Figure 54–1). The appliance is unique in that it gains retention from the undercut areas of the cleft, not from adaptation over the alveolar crest; it still maintains posterior width of the maxilla. Generally, only one appliance is sufficient, and, if desired, it can be used until palate closure. When the segments are in close approximation, graft placement can be executed. In the bilateral case, the anterior margin of the plate can be relieved bilaterally after lip closure, until growth brings the premaxilla into close approximation bilaterally, at which time the graft is placed. The appliance allows for continued growth in all planes of space. It does not act as an expansion appliance, but merely as a passive mechanism to allow molding in a controlled environment and to prevent medial movement of the buccal segments. The graft, in turn, creates a continuum to the maxilla, heretofore missing, so as to allow it to grow in a more normal fashion and relationship to the mandible.

Modifications to the sequence described above can occur. In the patient who initially presents with collapse of the lesser segment (in the unilateral cleft) or bilateral segment collapse (in the bilateral cleft), the appliance can be sectioned and a spring-loaded jackscrew placed for expansion prior to the placement of the passive appliance. Bone grafting is deferred until the segments are in optimum position with good arch alignment (Figure 54–2).

Short-term benefits of the prosthesis should not be overlooked. The appliance helps the infant to breathe primarily from the nose. Feeding is enhanced because the baby can build up better intraoral pressure and use the appliance and tongue to compress the nipple. Generally, 3–4 ounces of formula can be taken by the child within 15–30 minutes, with less air swallowed and less fatigue.

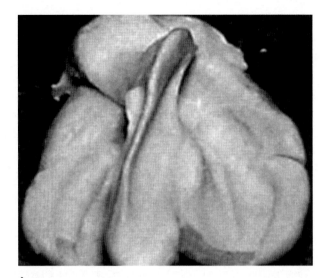

A

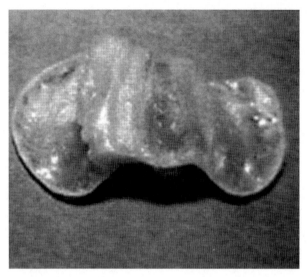

B

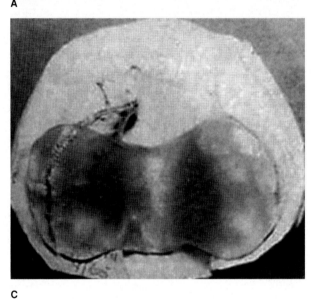

C

Figure 54–1. (A) Alginate impression of a complete unilateral cleft. (B) Superior view of an infant prosthesis for a unilateral cleft. Soft and hard acrylics have been bonded together. (C) Prosthesis on the cast. Note the position of the anterior margin of the prosthesis on the greater segment so that the action of the repaired lip will mold the segments to an end-to-end relationship. (*Reprinted with permission from Rosenstein SW. Early habilitation of the cleft lip and palate child. In: Johnston LE Jr., ed. New Vistas in Orthodontics. Philadelphia: Lea & Febiger, 1985, p. 325.*)

FUNCTIONAL CLEFT LIP REPAIR

In most cases, the lip is repaired at 6–10 weeks of age. By this time, the infant is gaining weight, and the palatal appliance has been placed. The infant is very accustomed to its presence and actually prefers to have it in the mouth. It is generally not removed for surgery.

The functional cleft lip repair with muscle realignment as designed by Kernahan is the procedure of choice in the protocol.[4,5] It is the first lip repair based upon an understanding of the abnormal anatomy of the orbicularis oris muscle and the principle of dissecting this muscle free and realigning it to reconstruct the sphincter. This lip repair addresses the lip as three separate layers to be closed: the mucosa, the muscle, and the skin. Generous dissection of the muscle as a separate layer lengthens the lip in both the horizontal and the vertical dimension by releasing the bunched up muscle of the lateral lip element and allowing it to lay flat.[6] Further

vertical lengthening of the lip is accomplished using the basic principles of Z-plasty closure, with one larger Z just below the floor of the nose and a second smaller Z just above the vermilion border, as necessary.

The specific step-by-step description of the lip repair is as follows (Figure 54–3):

A Keith needle dipped in methylene blue is used to tattoo key landmarks of the lip, namely, the columella, alar bases, high-point center and anticipated high point on the medial segment, and the point where the white roll disappears on the lateral segment of the lip. The medial and lateral edges of the cleft are paired so that a thin strip of skin and mucosa are removed. On the lateral segment, scalpel dissection frees up the muscle from the dermis, and the muscle is cut away from the alar attachment, the inferior lip border, and the mucosa. At this point the muscle lies flat and can be advanced as a separate layer to the medial side of the lip. On the medial side of the cleft, a few muscle fibers are freed up from the edge of

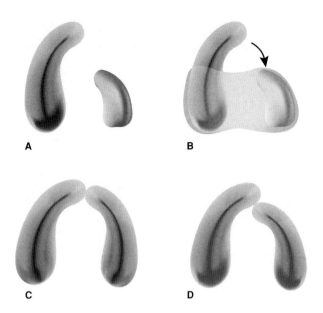

Figure 54–2. (A) Alveolar arch alignment before cleft is repaired. (B) Palatal appliance prevents alveolar arch collapse after lip repair. Arrow indicates direction of growth and molding of alveolus achieved with cleft lip closure. (C) Position of alveolar segments at a time of bone graft. There is a butt joint and good arch alignment. (D) Alveolar arch collapse when presurgical orthopedics not utilized. (*Reprinted with permission from Kernahan DA, Rosenstein SW, eds. Cleft Lip and Palate: A System of Management. Baltimore: Williams & Wilkins, 1990, p. 182.*)

the dermis, and scissor dissection creates a pocket near the nasal spine and at the inferior lip border. Further dissection of the mucosal flaps is done both medially and laterally. At this point of the operation, the nasal skin is dissected free from the alar cartilage on the cleft side of the nose. Access is gained through the lateral and medial cut borders of the lip; this allows redraping of the nasal skin and eliminates the buckling of the lateral ala when the lip is sutured closed.

The lip is closed in layers. The mucosal flaps are sutured together, first creating a buccal sulcus and eliminating a possible anterior alveolar fistula. The orbicularis oris muscle from the lateral lip element is advanced, and its superior corner is sutured to the tissue at the nasal spine. The muscle is split horizontally for several millimeters, dividing it into a lower one third and upper two thirds. The lower part of the muscle is sutured into the pocket created at the inferior lip border of the medial side of the cleft; there it will create some fullness to simulate a philtral tubercle. Further suturing to close the muscle layer results in a line of repair that lies under the skin on the medial side of the cleft and eliminates the gap between the medial and lateral skin edges; this will allow the skin to be sutured without tension.

The skin flaps in the floor of the nose are then sutured. A suture closes the lip segments at the white roll and is held on tension. Z-plasty flaps are then designed, cut, and interpolated at the upper segment of the lip without crossing the mid-line. Suturing of these flaps adjusts the width of the nasal floor and gives vertical length to the lip. Generally, additional length is needed to match the high point on the opposite side of the

lip, and a smaller Z-plasty closure is done just above the white roll of the lip. The rest of the skin is closed, and the mucosa of the inferior lip border is trimmed and closed as well.

This repair results in a lip with normal anatomic landmarks at rest and with normal function. There is no lateral muscle bulge when the lips are pursed. The functional cleft lip repair, as described here, is easy to learn and yields reproducible results. It follows the basic principles of adequate dissection and Z-plasty flap creation. It works well for incomplete cleft lips and for very wide cleft lips without using a preliminary lip adhesion. The zigzag appearance of the small flaps tends to disappear as the scars mature. Very little tissue is sacrificed, the alar crease is preserved, and there is no notching in the floor of the nose. Secondary revisions are generally minor and most commonly involve trimming labial mucosal fullness, correcting a notched vermilion, or placing a small Z-plasty above the white roll to further lengthen a short lip.

The principles of the functional cleft lip repair can also be applied to the complete bilateral cleft. If there is protrusion of the premaxilla and prolabium, external taping is done to reposition the premaxilla after the appliance is fitted. Since this may take several weeks, the bilateral cleft lip is often repaired at 8–12 weeks of age. The markings are made as for the unilateral cleft lip Figure (Figure 54–7). The lateral markings on the prolabium will determine the width between the created high points of the lip border and can usually be made about 4–5 mm apart. The medial and lateral borders of the cleft margins are pared and the cuts are continued to a V on the internal mucosa of the lip so that the prolabium can be elevated. On the lateral sides of the cleft, the mucosa is freed up and back cut as necessary so that the two edges can be approximated beneath the prolabium to create a buccal sulcus. The muscle on either side of the cleft is similarly freed up and sutured in the midline. If there is not too much tension, the muscle can be divided with about 1/3 the distance at the inferior pole sutured together to fill in the philtrum. The skin is approximated in a straight line with the suture lines lying where the philtral columns should be. The V-shaped mucosal flap is trimmed and sutured to fit into the mucosa from the lateral segments. No Z-plasties are used in the bilateral repair.

The palatal appliance is not removed until postoperative day 10. As discussed previously, the reconstructed orbicularis oris muscle sphincter exerts a force on the alveolar segments; with the fulcrum of the appliance and with growth and molding, the alveolar gap closes, generally within 6–12 weeks. The appliance maintains posterior palatal width and facilitates feeding.

EARLY ALVEOLAR BONE GRAFT PLACEMENT

Although the gap between the alveolar segments closes within weeks to a few months, a minimum of 2–3 months is needed before planning the bone graft in order to allow mucosal scar softening so that the small flaps can be more easily dissected.

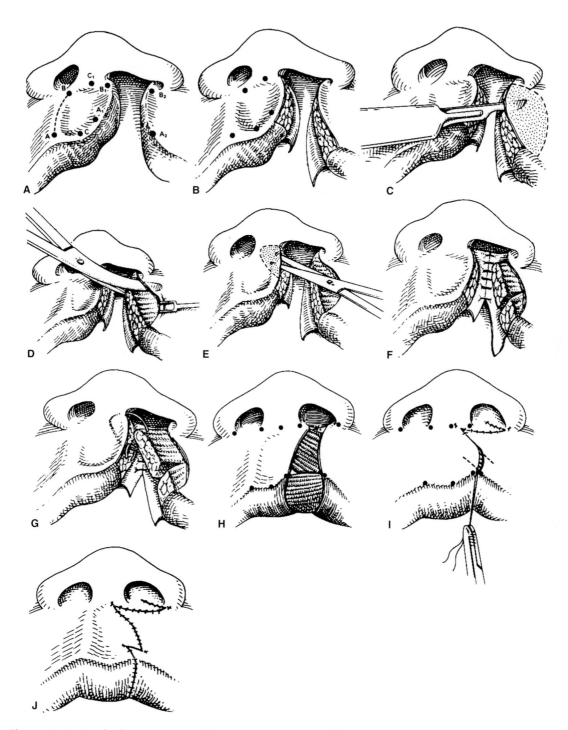

Figure 54–3. Muscle alignment repair. (A) Preoperative markings. (B) Mucosal flaps reflected. (C) Orbicularis muscle divided from dermal attachments. (D) Lateral muscle bundle divided from alar attachments. (E) Dissection of medial pocket to receive muscle flap. (F) Mucosal repair of buccal sulcus and nasal floor. Muscle flap divided. (G) Muscle flap drawn medially. (H) Muscle flap buried in medial pocket. (I) Z-plasty executed, lower planned. (J) Closure complete. (*Reprinted with permission from Kernahan DA. The functional cleft lip repair with muscle alignment. In: Kernahan DA, Rosenstein SW, eds. Cleft Lip and Palate: A System of Management. Baltimore: Williams & Wilkins, 1990, p. 149.*)

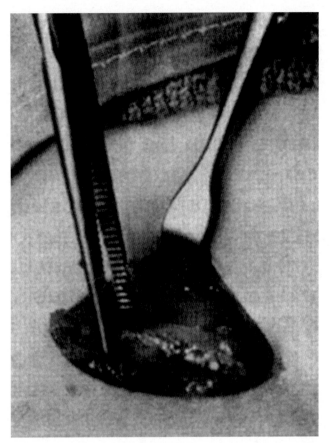

A

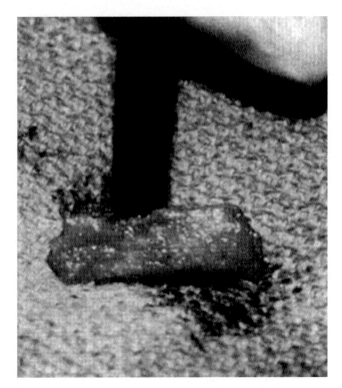

B

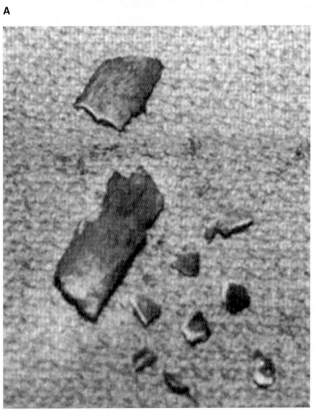

C

Figure 54–4. (A) After incision is made, dissection is done over sixth rib, and periosteum is dissected free from the rib, especially posteriorly, allowing traction to disarticulate rib at costocartilage junction. (B) Rib graft is split with an osteotome. (C) Anterior half of rib is kept intact; posterior half is cut into bone cips. (*Reprinted with permission from Kernahan DA, Rosenstein SW, eds. Cleft Lip and Palate: A System of Management. Baltimore: Williams & Wilkins, 1990, p. 182.*)

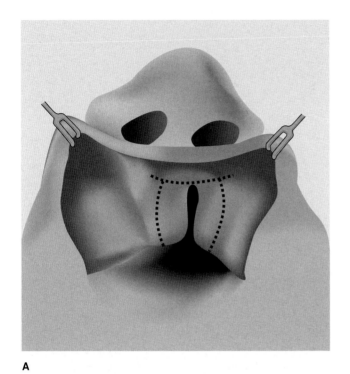

A

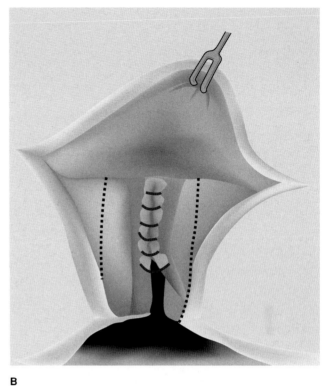

B

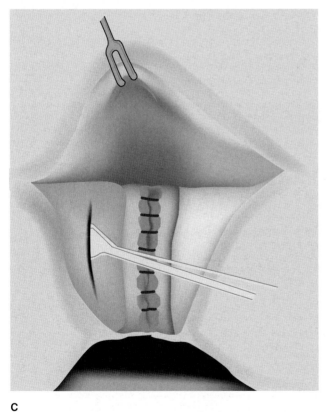

C

Figure 54–5. (A) Mucoperiosteal flaps are incised along cleft margins, and upper flag is incised along buccal sulcus. (B) Artist's representation of mucoperiosteal flaps sutured to create posterior wall of pocket (usually three sutures are sufficient). (C) Remaining periosteum is stripped off margins of cleft alveolus and anterior maxilla. (D) Anterior strut of rib is placed in pocket with smaller bone chips packed behind and around it. (E) Buccal flap is brought down to achieve closure of anterior wall of pocket. Again, fewer structures are usually required than demonstrated in this artist's representation. In addition, a notch at the inferior cleft margin still remains. (*Reprinted with permission from Kernahan DA, Rosenstein SW, eds. Cleft Lip and Palate: A System of Management. Baltimore: Williams & Wilkins, 1990, p. 182.*)

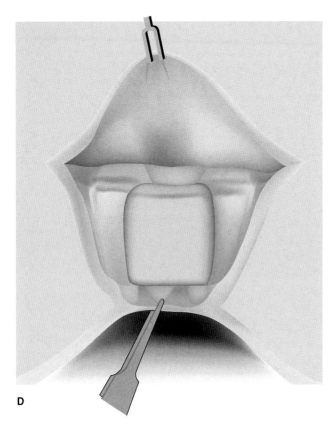

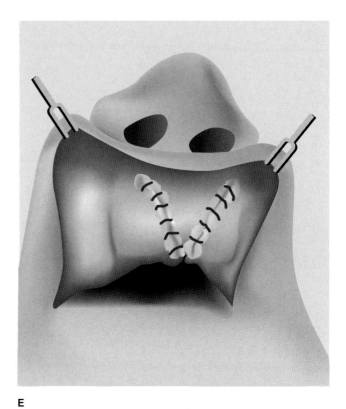

D

E

Figure 54–5. (*Continued*)

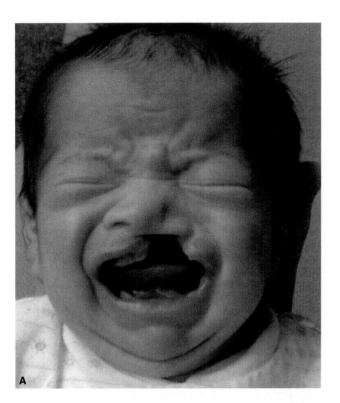

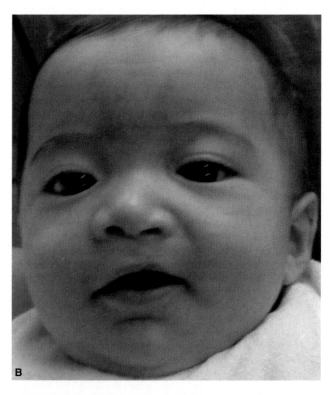

A

B

Figure 54–6. (A) Newborn (November 20, 2005) Caucasian male with unilateral complete cleft of the lip, alveolus, and palate; maxillary plate placed before lip closure (December 16, 2005). (B) lip closed (February 3, 2006) and frontal facial view (May 4, 2006).

The bone graft is placed when the gap at the alveolar cleft is small (1–3 mm) and the edges are almost touching. At this time, the graft is simply an onlay and is not required to bridge a gap.[7,8]

The bone is harvested through a 2–3 cm incision over the fifth rib (Figure 54–4). The resultant scar will fall into the inframammary fold in females and does not interfere with growth of the breast bud. The incision is deepened through the subcutaneous tissue and muscle fascia, and the muscle fibers over the rib are split. Near the costochondral junction, an H-type incision is made in the periosteum (one limb of the H lies on the junction), and the periosteum is freed circumferentially from the entire surface of the rib. At this age, the rib can be easily disarticulated at the costochondral junction, and a 1–2 cm length of rib is cut and removed. This segment of bone is then split; the anterior half becomes a strut of cortical and cancellous bone, and the posterior half is cut into small pieces (Figure 54–4). The periosteum is closed as a separate layer, allowing the rib to regenerate beneath it within 6–8 weeks. The remainder of the incision is closed in layers.

At the recipient site of the cleft alveolus, two flaps are incised, dissected free, and turned back on the medial and lateral alveolar segments (Figure 54–5). They are sutured together to create a posterior mucosal lining. A horizontal incision is made for a short distance in the buccal sulcus, and a mucosal flap is elevated. Periosteum is stripped off the maxilla above both sides of the alveolus for 4–5 mm. Thus, the anterior strut of rib, generally less than 1 cm, will fit nicely as an onlay graft just above the alveolus on the maxilla after a small amount of soft tissue dissection is done. The smaller bone chips are placed behind the strut to fill the created pocket, and the buccal mucosa is brought downward and sutured to the cut edges of the mucosa at the inferior margin of the alveolar segments. Thus, the bone graft is an onlay graft in the small created pocket and is completely covered by mucosa. There is no nasal buccal fistula, and the graft elevates the flattened floor of the nose on the cleft side.

BONE GRAFT INCORPORATION AND TIMING OF PALATE CLOSURE

As with the lip repair, the intraoral appliance remains in place during the bone graft placement and is not removed for 10 postoperative days. At that time, the mucosa is healed and the appliance can be safely removed for cleaning and replacement. It is necessary to use the plate for an additional 6–8 weeks until the bone graft is incorporated and the alveolar arch is stable. At that time, use of the appliance can be discontinued, although most parents prefer to keep using it in order to facilitate feeding until the palate is closed. The palate is repaired when the surgeon decides that the cleft is narrow enough and the palatal shelves are large enough to allow a complete closure of the hard and soft palate in one stage. Generally, at least 2–3 months should pass in order to allow

softening of the mucosa. In the majority of cases, the palate is repaired at 9–12 months of age. Occasionally, in very wide clefts, an additional few months may be necessary in order to assure that closure can be accomplished without tension and the associated risk fistula development. The author prefers using two unipedicle flaps based on the greater palatine arteries with an intravelar veloplasty.[9] At the time of palate repair, the buccal and lingual sides of the alveolus have already been closed, eliminating the presence of a buccal fistula or a fistula in the primary palate just behind the alveolus (Figure 54–6).

PROTOCOL ASSESSMENT AND DISCUSSION

This protocol has been followed without change or alteration for approximately 42 years. The protocol is unique and is distinct from other protocols of primary or early alveolar bone grafting. It results in successful management of the skeletal deformities associated with the inherent growth deficiency associated with cleft lip and palate. The methods of assessment have included cephalometric radiography, computer assisted tomography, plaster cast analysis, and intraoral and extraoral photography. Outcomes of patients who have been treated under this protocol have been compared to those of other teams and protocols[10–15] (Figures 54–8 through 54–14).

Long-term assessment of facial growth, incidence of orthognathic surgery, need for secondary grafting, height of the alveolar ridge, incidence of residual nasal fistulae and status of the lateral incisors adjacent to the cleft sites in 82 patients treated under this protocol was published in 2003.[16] Without exception, studies to date have shown that there is no growth attenuation caused by early grafting in this protocol, likely due to the very minimal undermining of the periosteum on the labial surfaces of the alveoli of the well aligned segments of the maxilla. After bone grafting, the maxilla can grow as a single unit, not as two or three segmental components. Thus, if need for orthognathic surgery can be considered a soft indicator of possible growth problems in complete clefts, because of an inherent lack of tissue initially, a less than ideal anterior–posterior, maxillary–mandibular relationship could be reasonably anticipated. It is essential, however, that one keeps in mind other previously mentioned extrinsic variables that influence growth, most notably lip surgery. If, in a wide cleft, lip closure necessitates excessive undermining, this too can create adhesion and scar tissue that will adversely affect growth and the anterior–posterior maxillary–mandibular relationship. Reports in the literature have shown that in complete clefts, the incidence of orthognathic surgery is in the vicinity of 25% or more.[17,18] The incidence in the authors' aforementioned report was 18.3%.[16]

The survivability and status of lateral incisor teeth has also been observed and found to be very good due to graft survival and tooth root formation and movement through the graft. This aids in cosmetic and functional dental reconstruction and reduces the need for secondary grafting.

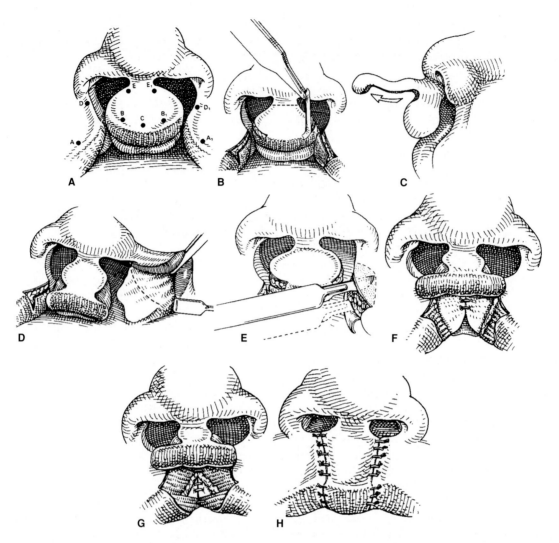

Figure 54–7. (A) Preliminary skin markings for bilateral lip repair. (B) Paring of a strip of tissue along the skin mucosal junction on either side of the prolabium and along the lateral margins of the cleft. (C) The prolabial skin and mucosa freed from the premaxilla and rotated forward. (D) Incision in the buccal sulcus to allow raising of an advancement flap of mucosa to form a deep buccal sulcus. (E) Primary realignment of muscle is possible, the muscle is freed from the skin and mucosa. (F) Closure of the lateral mucosal advancement flaps, leaving a V-shaped defect below to accept the prolabial mucosa. (G) Repair of the orbicularis which has been split to form larger superior and smaller inferior flaps. (H) The prolabial skin and mucosa are draped over the repaired muscle and sutured. The prolabial skin should be trimmed to have a philtrum of appropriate width. (*Reprinted with permission from Kernahan DA, Rosenstein SW, eds. Cleft Lip and palate: A System of Management. Baltimore: Williams & Wilkins, 1990, p. 157.*)

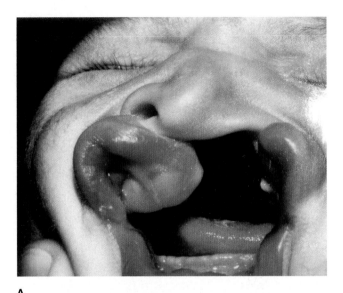

A

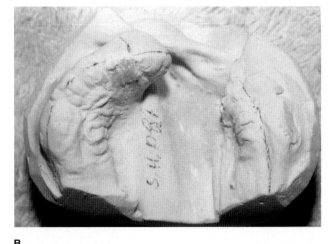

B

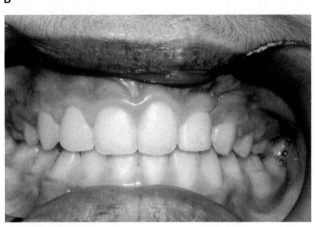

D

C

Figure 54–8. Case 1. (A) Frontal facial view of patient at birth with left complete cleft of the lip, alveolus, and palate. (B) Occlusal view of maxillary arch at birth. Maxillary void between segments was approximately 18 mm. (C) Frontal facial view (age 12) at finish of orthodontic treatment. (D) Frontal intraoral view of occlusion. (*Reprinted with permission from Rosenstein SW. Two unilateral complete cleft lip and palate orthodontic cases treated from birth to adolescence. Am J Ortho Dentofacial Orthop 1999;115:67.*)

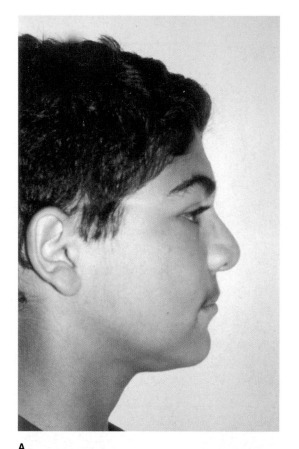

A

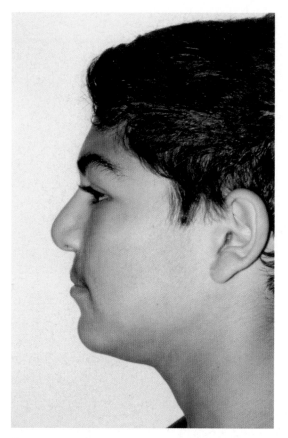

B

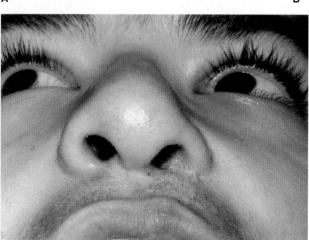

C

Figure 54–9. Case 1. (A) Right (noncleft) facial profile view (age 15). (B) Left (cleft side) facial profile view demonstrating lip and nasal symmetry. (C) Frontal caudal facial view demonstrating lip and nasal symmetry. (*Reprinted with permission from Rosenstein SW. Two unilateral complete cleft lip and palate orthodontic cases treated from birth to adolescence. Am. J Ortho Dentofacial Orthop 1999;115:70.*)

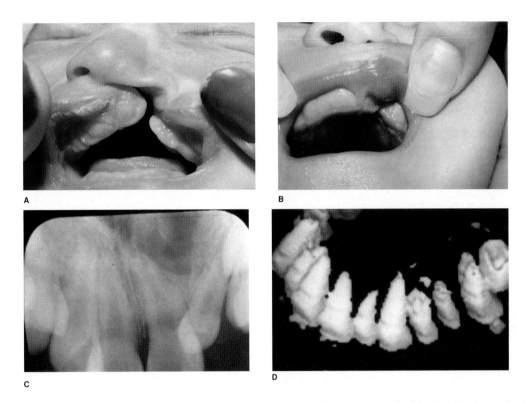

Figure 54–10. Case 2. (A) Frontal facial view of patient at birth with left complete cleft of the lip, alveolus and palate. (B) intraoral view of maxillary segment alignment after lip closure demonstrating segment approximation with palatal plate in place and before segment stabilization via bone graft. (C) Periapical X-ray view of cleft area before orthodontic treatment demonstrating tooth movement into area previously cleft. (D) Thee-dimensional CT scan demonstrating dental alignment and axial inclination of teeth in cleft area immediately before orthodontic appliance removal. (*Reprinted with permission from Rosenstein SW. Two unilateral complete cleft lip and palate orthodontic cases treated from birth to adolescence. Am. J Ortho Dentofacial Orthop 1999;115:62–63.*)

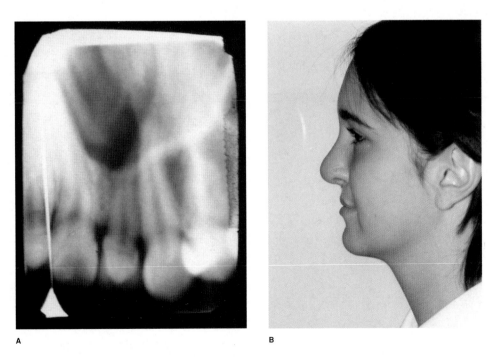

Figure 54–11. Case 2. (A) Periapical radiographic view of lateral incisor in area originally cleft, 4 years after orthodontic appliance removal; note root length, tooth position and alveolar bone integrity. (B) Cleft side profile view 4 years postorthodontic treatment. (*Reprinted with permission from Rosenstein SW. Two unilateral complete cleft lip and palate orthodontic cases treated from birth to adolescence. Am J Ortho Dentofacial Orthop 1999;115:65–66.*)

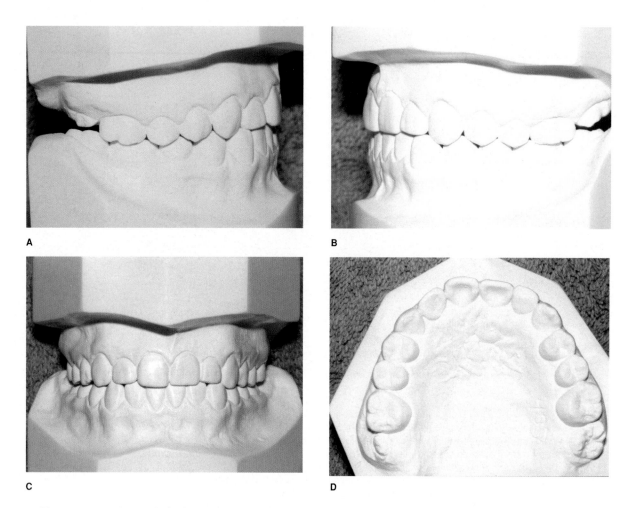

A   B

C   D

Figure 54–12. Case 2. Orthodontic diagnostic study models 4 years posttreatment (A–D). (*Reprinted with permission from Rosenstein SW, Two unilateral complete clefts lip and palate orthodontic cases treated from birth to adolescence. Am J Ortho Dentofacial rthop 1999;115:64.*)

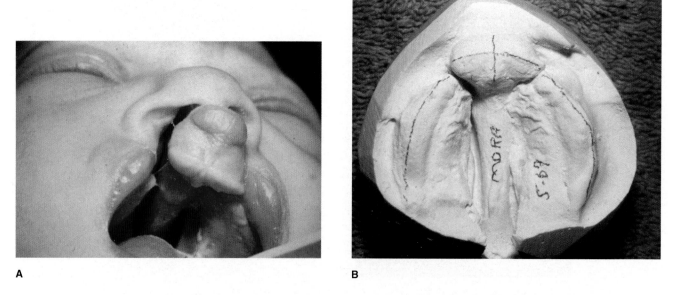

A   B

Figure 54–13. Case 3. (A) Female patient with a bilateral cleft born in November of 1968; frontal facial view. (B) Cast of maxillary arch alignment after maxillary plate placement and lip closure; note segment alignment prior to bone graft. (*Reprinted with permission from Rosenstein SW, Grasseschi M, Dado DV. A long-term retrospective outcome assessment of facial growth, secondary surgical need, and maxillary lateral incisor status in a surgical-orthodontic protocol for complete clefts. Plast Reconstr Surg 2003;111:8.*)

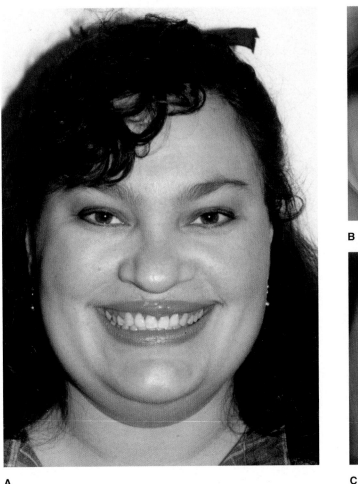

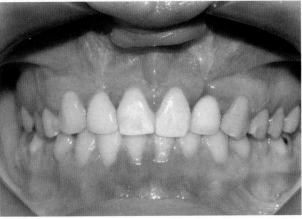

Figure 54–14. Case 3 (A) Frontal facial view smiling, age 35. (B) Frontal intraoral view of occlusion; all four maxillary incisors are present and in occlusion. (C) Frontal caudal facial view demonstrating lip and nasal symmetry.

CONCLUSIONS

The functional cleft lip repair, maxillary orthopedic segment alignment, primary osteoplasty, and early complete palate closure as described here is a straightforward, uncomplicated protocol that does not require numerous modifications and patient interventions. It is successful in managing the skeletal deformities of cleft lip and palate only when it is followed exactly. If the lip is repaired at the time of graft placement, if the graft is wedged into a large gap, if large periosteal flaps are elevated, or if an appliance is not used or does not maintain posterior palatal width, then the protocol is not the same and will probably not be successful. However, following this protocol will reduce the need for palatal expansion and maxillary osteotomies because fewer severe anterior crossbites occur. Periodontal health is good, and fewer teeth are lost because the early presence of bone allows eruption and better use of teeth that are present. The nasal buccal fistula is eliminated when the graft is placed. Secondary surgical procedures on the lip, nose, and palate are generally minor revisions. Good maxillary growth and/or compensation of the mandibular vector results in a balanced maxillary–mandibular relationship.

References

1. Koberg WR. Present view on bone grafting in cleft palate. (A review of the literature). *J Maxillofac Surg* 1:183–193, 1973.
2. Kernahan DA. Sequence of procedures and timing. In: Kernahan DA, Rosenstein SW, eds. *Cleft Lip and Palate: A System of Management.* Baltimore: Williams & Wilkins, 1990, pp. 115–119.
3. Rosenstein SW. Early maxillary orthopedics and appliance fabrication. In: Kernahan DA, Rosenstein SW, eds. *Cleft Lip and Palate: A System of Management.* Baltimore: Williams & Wilkins, 1990, pp. 120–127.
4. Kernahan DA, Dado DV, Bauer BS. The anatomy of the orbicularis oris muscle in unilateral cleft lip based on three-dimensional histologic reconstruction. *Plast Reconsrt Surg* 73:875–879, 1984.
5. Dado DV. Analysis of the lengthening effect of the muscle repair in functional cleft lip Repair. *Plast Reconstr Surg* 82:594–601, 1988.
6. Kernahan DA. The functional cleft lip repair with muscle alignment. In: Kernahan DA, Rosenstein SW, eds. *Cleft Lip and Palate: A System of Management.* Baltimore: Williams & Wilkins, 1990, pp. 149–156.
7. Dado DV. Early primary bone grafting. In: Kernahan DA, Rosenstein SW, eds. *Cleft Lip Palate: A System of Management.* Williams & Wilkins, 1990, pp. 182–166.
8. Rosenstein SW, Dado DV. Early bone grafting with the functional lip repair, *Semin Plast Surg* 19:306–307, 2005.
9. Dado DV. Early cleft palate repair with intravelar veloplasty. In: Kernahan DA, Rosenstein SW, eds. *Cleft Lip and Palate: A System of Management.* Baltimore: Williams & Wilkins, 1990, pp. 189–198.

10. Rosesntein SW, Long RE, Dado DV, et al. Comparison of 2-D calculations from periapical and occlusal radiographs versus 3-D calculations from CAT scans in determining bone support for cleft-adjacent teeth following early alveolar bone grafts. *Cleft Palate Craniofac J* 1997;34:199–205.

11. Dado DV, Rosenstein SW, Adler ME, et al. Long term assessment of early alveolar bone grafts using three-dimensional computer assisted tomography: a pilot study. *Plast Reconstr Surg* 99:1840–1845, 1997.

12. Trotman CA, Long RE, Rosenstein SW, Murphy C, Johnston, LE Jr. Comparison of facial form in primary alveolar bone-grafted and non grafted Unilateral cleft lip and palate patients: intercenter retrospective study. *Cleft Palate Craniofac J* 33:38–41, 1996.

13. Ross RB. Treatment variables affecting facial growth in complete unilateral cleft lip and palate. *Cleft Palate Craniofac J* 24:5–23, 1987.

14. Helms JA, Speidel TM, Denis KL. Effect of timing on long-term clinical success of alveolar bone grafts. *Am J Orthod Dentofacial Orthop* 92:232–240, 1987.

15. Whitney E, Tommasome DW, Enlow DH. Analysis of the craniofacial complex in cleft in cleft palate children. Case Western University School of Dentistry, Research Bulletin, 1964 p. 16.

16. Rosenstein SW, Grasseschi M, Dado DV. A long-term retrospective outcome assessment of facial growth, secondary surgical need and maxillary lateral incisor status in a surgical-orthodontic protocol for complete clefts. *Plast Reconstr Surg* 111:1–3, 2003.

17. Deluke DM, Marchard A, Robles C, et al. Facial growth and the need for orthognathic Surgery after left palate repair: Literature review and report of 28 cases. *J Oral Maxillofac Surg* 55:694–697, 1997.

18. Ross RB, Treatment variables affecting facial growth in complete unilateral cleft lip and palate. *Cleft Palate J* 24:5–7, 1987.

Gingivoperiosteoplasty

Richard A. Hopper, MD, MS • Craig B. Birgfeld, MD

INTRODUCTION

The primary goal of cleft care is to optimize function, appearance, and self-image with a minimum of surgical intervention. Although there is a consensus on this goal among cleft centers, the international cleft community continues to debate how best to attain it. One of the most controversial topics of debate in current cleft care is management of the alveolar cleft, specifically the indications for primary gingivoperiosteoplasty (GPP).

The theory of GPP is consistent with the goal of minimizing the number of secondary surgeries by optimizing results of primary surgery. Advocates of GPP report the primary benefit, obtained at the time of initial cleft lip repair, being the elimination of secondary alveolar bone grafting at the time of mixed dentition. The patient can therefore be spared the potential morbidity and cost of an additional surgery. Critics of GPP, in contrast, are concerned over the risk of iatrogenic

restriction of facial growth and malocclusion, secondary to early closure of the alveolar arch. If this occurs, the patient could be subjected to deteriorating facial projection with age, extensive orthodontics, and an increased risk of additional orthognathic surgeries at skeletal maturity. The debate over a GPP in an infant with a cleft therefore centers on weighing the chance of avoiding secondary bone grafting against the risk of the iatrogenic increase in treatment required by restricting facial growth.

GUIDED TISSUE REGENERATION

Initially described as, "boneless bone grafting," the basic principle of GPP is to surgically remove the soft tissue barrier within the alveolar cleft and replace it with a gingivoperiosteal tunnel that facilitates bone healing through guided tissue regeneration (GTR). In contrast to more traditional surgical reconstructive techniques, which repair defects by replacement with similar tissues from other parts of the body, GPP is a form of inductive surgery, similar to distraction osteogenesis, which creates a favorable environment for augmented local healing and tissue generation. The attraction of inductive surgery is the lack of donor morbidity.

The importance of the periosteum in bony healing has been well documented by a number of authors,[1,2] but Ollier is most often credited with first emphasizing the osteogenic potential of the periosteum.[3] The application of GTR in the healing of mandibular bony defects was first reported by Dahlin.[4] He demonstrated bony union of critical mandibular defects by creating a Teflon tunnel to guide bone regeneration, while impairing soft tissue in-growth and fibrous nonunion. More recent research on GTR in calvarial defect healing indicates that not only is an intact tunnel important for bony bridging to occur, but the nature of the guiding tissue, i.e., periosteum versus dura versus alloplast, is equally important.[5] Age also appears to have a major impact, in that tissues have augmented guiding regeneration capacity in immature compared to mature animals.[6] Based on these principles, the potential of GTR following a GPP is therefore dependent on the integrity of the guiding tunnel to restrict fibrous in-growth, the presence of viable periosteum in the created flaps, and the age of the patient.

EVOLUTION AND HISTORIC EVALUTION

References to the osteogenic properties of mucoperiosteum in healing a cleft palate date back to Langenbeck's descriptions in the 1800s,[7] but it was not until Tord Skoog's descriptions of primary GPP in the 1960s that the technique became popularized in cleft care. Skoog credited a case of unexpected maxillary regeneration for his interest in alveolar periosteoplasty. He performed a subperiostial maxillectomy in a 4-month-old patient, following which the patient's maxilla spontaneously regenerated without bone grafting. This case led him, and others, to consider the possibility that bone grafts are primarily conductive frameworks for bony regrowth instead of the traditional concept that they brought bone healing cells to the area.

In 1967, Skoog published his experience, with what he termed boneless bone grafting, in a series of 83 patients aged 3–6 months.[8] In this paper, he described the creation of local mucoperiosteal flaps to bridge unmolded alveolar clefts in a similar fashion to the flaps used for secondary bone grafting. Rather than adding bone graft to the bony defect however, Skoog inserted oxidized regenerated cellulose and subsequently found bony bridge formation across the alveolar cleft. Though not every patient grew bone initially, with repeated periosteal flaps, all patients eventually formed a bony bridge.[9] The bone formation was assessed by radiograph and confirmed by histochemical analysis, but he did not provide any information on the amount of bone or subsequent need for secondary bone graft. Since the "Skoog method" of GPP was performed on unmolded wide alveolar clefts, it required extensive undermining of mucoperiosteal flaps across the face of the maxilla, and in many cases, repeated surgical procedures. Skoog recognized the potential that repeated, wide subperiosteal maxillary dissection could threaten the viability of facial growth centers in the developing infant. When he evaluated his patients' maxillary growth at age 5 years using dental models and comparing them to patients with clefts who did not undergo GPP, he detected no facial growth disturbance.[10] Continuing concern for iatrogenic growth disturbance during pubertal growth, and the viability of the large mucoperiosteal flaps, however, led others to analyze and question the Skoog technique.

In 1972, Ritsilä and Rintala reported the use of free tibial periosteal grafts, to achieve the formation of a bony bridge across an alveolar cleft.[11] Seventeen years later, in 1989, Rintala and Ranta compared long-term results of this free grafting technique to the previously reported Skoog technique.[12] Over a 6-year time period, they had treated 67 patients with Skoog's maxillary periosteal flap technique and 23 with free periosteal grafts. Analyzing both groups using occlusal X-rays taken between ages 12 and 17 years, they reported bony formation in 64% of the clefts treated with the Skoog technique, and 85% in those treated with the tibial periosteum graft technique. Secondary bone grafts, however, were required in 72% and 73% of each group, respectively. Using cephalometric analysis, they did not detect a deficiency in facial growth, but they did report a lateral crossbite in all patients. Their analysis led the surgeons to abandon the technique of early GPP using the Skoog technique. They concluded that, because secondary bone grafting was not avoided in almost three quarters of the patients, maxillary collapse still occurred, adolescent orthodontics was not facilitated, and maxillary growth was not improved. They were also concerned that any GPP technique would prolong the initial surgery and create more scar tissue and the potential for secondary problems. They concluded that "... the more conservative and less scar-producing the early primary repair is, the lesser is the secondary growth retardation." A similar finding with the Skoog technique was reported by Renkielska and Dobke.[13] They used the Goslon yardstick[14] to evaluate occlusion after GPP, and found that 50% of patients treated with Skoog's GPP technique had Goslon scores of four or five, which would indicate the need for orthognathic surgery.

Around the same time as Rintala and Ranta's criticism of the Skoog technique, the next evolution of the GPP was taking place with the popularization of presurgical orthopedics in cleft care.[12] By preoperatively aligning the alveolar segments, the width of the cleft could be reduced and the closure of the lip and alveolus could be facilitated. The major criticism of the previous Skoog technique had been that the degree of dissection, and size of mucoperiosteal flaps required to achieve closure of the unmolded alveolar cleft, were not optimal for bone formation, and unnecessarily increased the risk of growth restriction. With approximation of the alveolar edges using presurgical orthopedics, less subperiosteal dissection was needed to achieve closure of the cleft, implying increased viability of the mucoperiosteal flaps, and less risk to facial growth. In 1974, Georgiade and Latham introduced an intraoral appliance for preoperative alignment of alveolar segments.[15] Millard began to use this device as part of his treatment protocol in Miami for patients with clefts.[16] His "POPLA" (Presurgical Orthopedics, Periosteoplasty, and Lip Adhesion) approach involved presurgical orthopedics with the "Latham device" followed by lip adhesion and GPP at 3–4 months of age. The "Millard GPP" involved elevation of gingivoperiosteal flaps from the interior of the alveolar cleft, with no dissection over the face of the maxilla. In 1999,[17] Millard and Latham reported good bone formation on dental radiographs, but also found a higher rate of anterior–posterior crossbite in patients treated with this technique. They analyzed occlusal casts of 63 patients treated with the POPLA technique and compared them to 61 patients who had been treated with their previous, conservative, technique of lip adhesion alone. Facial growth did not seem to be affected, but the authors admitted that the repeat evaluation at skeletal maturity would be needed for definitive conclusions.[17]

Critics of the POPLA technique included Berkowitz, the original orthodontist who worked with Latham and Millard as well as others with access to the Miami records.[17] Henkel and Gundlach analyzed occlusal casts and lateral cephalograms of 146 patients treated by Millard with either the POPLA or a conservative technique.[18] They reported worse crossbite in patients treated with the Latham device and GPP. Moreover, they found vertical growth disturbance of the maxilla in 42% of patients with unilateral and 40% of patients with bilateral clefts treated with Millard's technique.[18] Berkowitz analyzed the occlusion of these patients in a subsequent paper and found anterior and lateral crossbites in 100% of patients treated with GPP. His prime concern was that the crossbites were more difficult to correct orthodontically in patients treated with Millard's POPLA technique. He felt that "In most cases, LeFort I surgery or maxillary advancement with distraction osteogenesis is necessary."[19]

The most recent evolution of the GPP has attempted to address the potential negative impact of the Latham device on dentofacial growth, and has been in use in combination with naso-alveolar molding (NAM) as described by Grayson, Cutting, and Brecht.[20] This is the technique currently used by the senior author of this chapter. Contrasted to the POPLA technique described by Millard, the NAM-GPP differs not in the technical surgical details of the GPP, but in the method of presurgical molding of the alveolar segments in preparation for the GPP, and the criteria for selection of which patients are appropriate candidates for a GPP. Unlike the Latham device that actively molds the alveolar segments, NAM is a passive process that directs the rapid growth of the alveolar segments during the initial months of an infant's life. Grayson describes this technique in detail in a separate chapter dedicated to the topic. From the perspective of GPP success—bony union without impaired facial growth—the passive molding process of NAM is felt by its advocates to be a more accurate means of molding the leading edges of the alveolar cleft to optimize flap design and osteogenesis, while being less invasive and compressive to the growth centers of the immature face.

The history and evolution of GPP, from Skoog, to Rintala, to Millard, teaches us that it can take 15–20 years before the risks and benefits of a surgical technique, performed on an infant with a cleft, can be fully appreciated. As the NAM-GPP technique is practiced by more centers outside of the originating institution, over the next decade it will undergo objective external critical evaluation to find its appropriate place in the arsenal of cleft surgical care.

PRESURGICAL PREPARATION AND PATIENT SELECTION

Prior to undergoing a GPP, the infant with a cleft must be evaluated by the practitioner coordinating the NAM as well as by the surgeon who will be performing the GPP. Prior to initiating NAM, the guardians of the infant should be introduced to the concept of a GPP, the risks and benefits reported in earlier GPP techniques, and the current data on NAM-GPP. It must be emphasized that not all infants will be candidates for NAM due to individual compliance, but also that not all infants will be candidates for GPP due to individual variations of anatomy. Some infants with particularly wide unilateral clefts can be "mesenchymal deficient." This subjective term denotes alveolar arch anatomy that would unnaturally constrict the arch form were the segments to be pre-surgically approximated. These mesenchymal deficient infants are best identified by the NAM team early in the process, so that the parents can be notified of the likelihood that a GPP will not be possible. Isolated clefts of the primary palate are also difficult to predict if a GPP is possible. Due to the bony fusion of the secondary palate, the alveolar segments of the primary palate are more resistant to presurgical molding; and in many cases, cannot be adequately aligned for a successful GPP. Finally, in bilateral complete clefts, it is not always possible to align both sides of the premaxilla with the lateral alveolar segments. In these cases, one alveolar cleft can undergo a GPP to convert the arch form to a lesser and greater segment similar to a complete unilateral cleft. Although the contralateral cleft will need to be secondarily grafted, the premaxilla will be stabilized by the GPP to facilitate incisor mastication during early childhood, and the increased morbidity and failure associated with bilateral secondary bone grafting may be avoided.

During the NAM process, the critical assessment of alveolar ridge alignment and parallel alveolar molding is subjective, and benefits from a team presurgical evaluation. It must be remembered that the optimum alignment of the alveolar segments is based on the underlying bone, not on the visible gingival mucosa (Fig. 55–1A and B). In some cases, the gingival tissue can be hypertrophied in the area of the cleft, mimicking close approximation and alignment of the cleft, but the underlying bone gap is in misalignment and wide. In other cases, the alveolar cleft is compressed, but the bony arch forms are not in alignment, with the lesser segment posterior to the greater (Fig. 55–2A, B, C, and D) or the premaxilla wedged anterior to collapsed lesser segments. If a GPP is performed in these situations, the mucoperiosteal tunnel

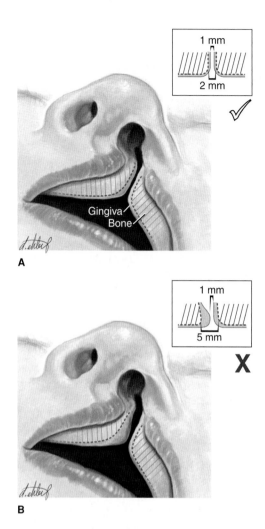

A

B

Figure 55–1. (A) An appropriately molded unilateral complete cleft for GPP. There is parallel alignment of the alveolar cleft edges with a 2-mm bone gap. **(B)** A molded unilateral complete cleft with gingival hypertrophy masking a deceptively wider cleft. The hypertrophy creates a nonparallel soft tissue gap of 1 mm, but the true bone gap is 5 mm. This cleft would not be an appropriate candidate for a GPP.

between the exposed bone edges will be "kinked" and create a soft tissue barrier instead of guided tissue regeneration.

Prerequisites for a GPP are therefore an informed consenting family, appropriate cleft anatomy to allow alveolar bony approximation, an optimally molded alveolar cleft, intact mucosa, and no dental eruption. Once these criteria are met, the GPP can be scheduled at the time of the primary lip repair.

SURGICAL TECHNIQUE

The GPP can be performed at any point during the primary cleft lip repair; however, it is technically easiest after all other dissection had been completed, and before repair of the lip elements. The "roof" of the GPP is the repair of the anterior palate, or the nasal floor, from the nasal sill back to the incisive foramen, which is typically done with most modern cleft

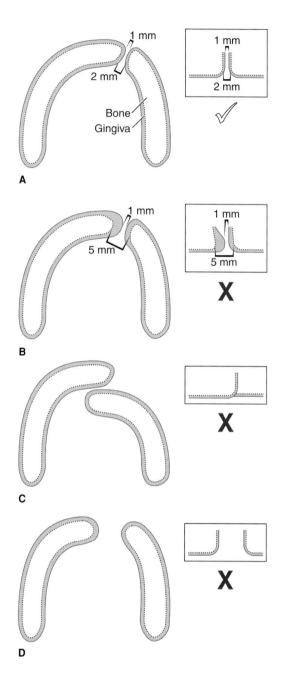

A

B

C

D

Figure 55–2. (A) An appropriately molded unilateral complete cleft for GPP. There is parallel alignment of the alveolar cleft edges with a smooth arch form. **(B)** Gingival hypertrophy in the alveolar cleft can mask a bone gap that is too wide for a GPP. **(C)** A collapsed arch form is not a candidate for GPP. Although the alveolar segments are touching, the edges of the cleft are not opposing, preventing the formation of a subperiosteal tunnel. **(D)** A mesenchymal deficient cleft arch form. If this cleft was approximated by preoperative molding, it would unnaturally constrict the projection of the alveolar arch due to a deficiency in either the lesser or greater segments.

lip repairs. In the Mohler modification of the Millard cleft lip repair technique used by the senior author, this is achieved by suturing the inferior edge of the reconstructed lateral nasal wall to a superiorly based mucoperiosteal vomer flap. The incision along the vomer to create the leading edge of the flap is at the level of the oral–nasal mucosa demarcation visible on the opposing lateral nasal wall. The vomer flap vertical dissection is kept to the bare minimum needed to achieve closure of the nasal floor, typically 1–2 mm at most, to avoid inadvertent damage to the premaxillary growth suture. After the mucosal incision, most of the vomer dissection can be achieved with an elevator, with the exception of the region of the suture, which will require sharp dissection with a small blade. This nasal floor closure with nasal flaps separates the nasal from the oral cavity back to the incisive foramen, and provides the superior barrier, or roof, of the GTR tunnel between the alveolar segments.

The "floor" of the GPP tunnel is created by elevating inferiorly based mucoperiosteal flaps from the oral edges of the alveolar cleft (oral flaps). These flaps are contained within the alveolar cleft itself, and extend from the labial surface of the alveolus back to the incisive foramen. They are typically 2–3 mm in vertical height, such that when they are inferiorly rotated, they meet across the oral boundary of the cleft, and can be sutured together with everting, resorbable 5–0 gut or vicryl sutures.

The attached mucoperiosteum that remains within the alveolar cleft, between the superior anterior–posterior (A–P) incision made to create the nasal roof closure flaps, and the inferior incision made to create the oral closure, or floor, is the tissue used to close the anterior border of the GPP. The alveolar cleft can be visualized as a pyramid, whose apex is at the incisive foramen, where the superior and inferior A–P vomer incisions converge (Fig. 55–3). Anteriorly, these two A–P incisions diverge, creating anteriorly based triangular flaps, on either side of the alveolar cleft, that are pedicled anteriorly and flipped across the cleft, closing the labial border of the GPP (labial flaps).

In designing the GPP flaps, the incisions on one side of the alveolar cleft are shifted slightly superiorly, so that one labial flap covers the upper half of the anterior labial border of the cleft, while on the contralateral side, the incisions are shifted inferiorly for the labial flap to cover the lower half. The superior edge of the upper labial flap is sutured to the lip mucosa, and the inferior edge of the lower labial flap is sutured to the anterior edge of the two oral flaps. In this fashion, a sealed GTR "chamber" is created. It is sealed nasally, orally, and labially by mucoperiosteal flaps, with two opposing bone surfaces on the mesial and distal walls. It is essential that this end goal is visualized throughout the GPP dissection to ensure that all soft tissue interference is removed from the alveolar cleft during creation of the flaps, and that the flaps are positioned correctly to direct bone growth across the cleft.

Technical pitfalls of the GPP include elevation of the flaps in a submucosal instead of subperiosteal plane, inaccurate planning of flaps such that viability of the anteriorly based labial flaps are compromised, and trauma to the flaps from compressive handling with forceps. Occasionally, a deciduous tooth follicle is encountered during the flap dissection. Careful sharp dissection between the follicle and the periosteum is required to prevent disruption of dental eruption. If the flaps appear too thin or nonviable during the follicle dissection, the GPP should be aborted and the mucosa replaced.

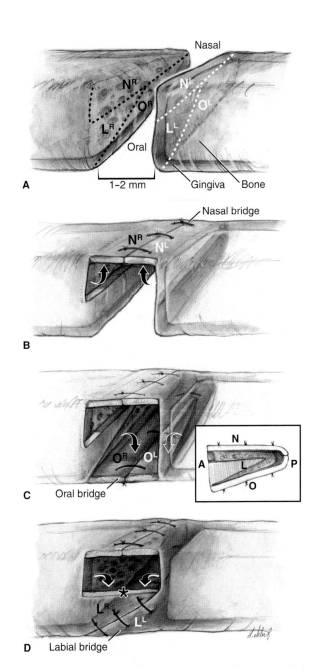

Figure 55–3. Gingivoperiosteal flap design and elevation for the Millard GPP. The dissection is limited to the tissues within the cleft. The flaps are named by the part of the periosteal tunnel they construct. See text for details. L^R: Right labial flap; O^L: Left oral flap; N^R: Right nasal flap; A: Anterior; P: Posterior.

EVALUATION OF NAM–GPP

The evaluation of the NAM-GPP must first include analysis of its success. Is bone formed? It has been known for over a century that the technique can form bone, but the results have been inconsistent. More importantly, is the bone formed of sufficient quality to allow normal tooth eruption and alveolar arch growth? Bone formation alone is not the sole measure of success; it is instead, the absence of the need for secondary bone grafting. Once the benefits of NAM-GPP are established,

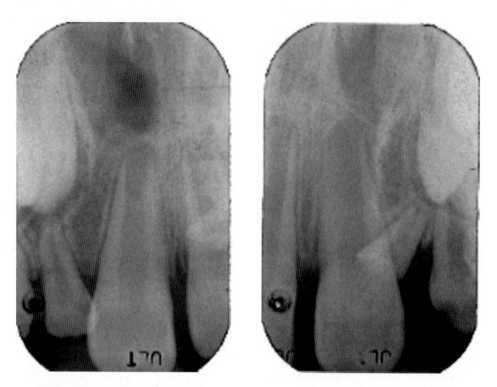

Figure 55–4. Periapical radiographs of a bilateral cleft lip and palate patient in mixed dentition with a successful previous bilateral GPP. There is adequate vertical bone height within the alveolar cleft to support tooth eruption. *(Courtesy of Dr. Barry Grayson.)*

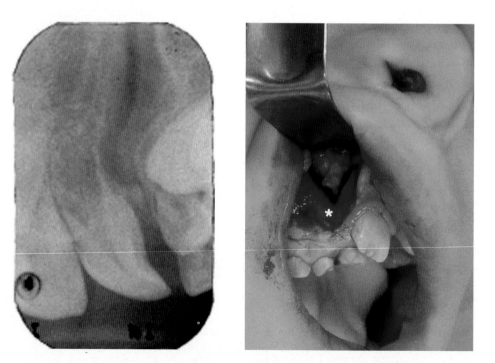

Figure 55–5. A right unilateral alveolar cleft following a "failed GPP." (A) A periapical radiograph at mixed dentition. There is formation of a bone bridge across the cleft, but insufficient vertical height to support tooth eruption. (B) At the time of secondary bone grafting, the bone bridge formation (asterisk) from the previous GPP provides a stable platform for the graft augmentation. *(Courtesy of Dr. Barry Grayson.)*

what are the opposing risks of this procedure? If the localized mucoperiosteal dissection and subsequent bone formation has the potential to impair facial growth, the impact of this must be weighed against the benefits of avoiding secondary bone grafting. Dental misalignment must also be distinguished from facial disproportion; the former can be corrected with orthodontics, the latter may require orthognathic surgery. Determination of this risk requires evaluation of a NAM-GPP cohort at skeletal maturity and comparing them with matched controls. Finally, in the age of cost-effective health care delivery, does a primary GPP save long-term expenses by decreasing the need of secondary bone grafting, or potentially increase them by resulting in more adolescent patients undergoing orthognathic surgery?

Answers to some of these pertinent questions have become available through the continued work of Grayson, Cutting, and Brecht—the developers of the NAM-GPP technique at New York University. In addition to their studies on the improved nasal morphology associated with the NAM technique, they have also evaluated their outcomes to date with the NAM-GPP. To date, the data is favorable compared to studies on earlier variations of GPP. They have reported bone formation in 80% of clefts treated with a primary NAM-GPP, with 40% requiring secondary bone grafting[21] (Fig. 55–4). In evaluating facial growth, they found no adverse effect on midfacial growth during mixed dentition,[22] or just prior to pubertal growth spurt,[23] when compared to an unmolded control group. Analysis of facial growth at skeletal maturity in this cohort, and the incidence of need for orthognathic surgery, should be available in the next 5 years; however, preliminary data on 14 of the original 20 patients did not reveal any attenuation of midfacial growth when compared to controls.[24] In a cost comparison between the nonmolded secondary bone graft control group and the GPP group, a savings of $2999 was seen when a primary GPP was performed.[25] The NYU group also has early data indicating that the 40% of NAM-GPP cases requiring secondary bone grafting ("failed GPP") have more favorable outcomes than non-GPP secondary grafting cases at time of mixed dentition. This is presumably due to a bone bridge formation in 80% of GPP cases (Fig. 55–5A and B).

Evaluation of outcomes of the NAM-GPP technique has been initially favorable. What remains to be seen is whether these results are maintained through skeletal maturity; and more importantly, whether they can be duplicated at other cleft centers using the published techniques.

CONCLUSION

In the quest for optimizing cleft care while minimizing surgical procedures, GPP plays a central and controversial role. It has the attraction of being one of the inductive surgical procedures that provides an opportunity for the patient's body to normalize form and function at an early age; however, it is set in a historical context of concern over iatrogenic restriction of dentofacial growth. The most recent evolution of the GPP technique is that associated with NAM. Compared to previous protocols, NAM-GPP uses passive guided presurgical molding of the alveolar cleft and strict criteria for patient selection. Comparison data available at this time is favorable for NAM-GPP, but further long-term outcome studies at other institutions are required before its final role in cleft care can be determined.

References

1. Sirola K. Regeneration of defects in the calvaria. *Ann Med Exp Biol Fenn* 38(Suppl 2):1–87, 1960.
2. Breitbart A, Grande D, Kessler R, Ryaby J, Fitzsimmons R, Grant R. Tissue engineered bone repair of calvarial defects using cultured periosteal cells. *Plast Recons Surg* 101:567–574; discussion 575–576, 1998.
3. Ollier L. *Traite Experimental et Clinique de la Regeneration des Os et de la Production Artificielle du Tissue Osseux.* Paris: V Masson et fils, 1867.
4. Dahlin C, Linde A, Gottlow J, Nyman S. Healing of bone defects by guided tissue regeneration. *Plast Reconstr Surg* 81:672–676, 1988.
5. Hopper R, Zhang J, Fournasier V, et al. Effect of isolation of periosteum and dura on the healing of rabbit calvarial inlay bone grafts. *Plast Recons Surg* 107:454–462, 2001.
6. Gosain A, Santoro T, Song L, Capel C, Sudhakar P, Matloub H. Osteogenesis in calvarial defects: Contribution of the dura, the pericranium, and the surrounding bone in adult versus infant animals. *Plast Recons Surg* 112:515–527, 2003.
7. Langenbeck von B: Die Uranoplastik mittelst Ablösung des mucösperiostalen Gaumenüberzuges. *Arch klin Chir* 2:205–287, 1861.
8. Skoog T. The use of periosteum and surgicel for bone restoration in congenital clefts of the maxilla. *Scand J Plast Reconstr Surg* 1:113–130, 1967.
9. Skoog T. Repair of unilateral cleft lip deformity: Maxilla, nose and lip. *Scand J Plast Reconstr Surg* 3:109–133, 1969.
10. Hellquist R, Skoog T. The influence of primary perioplasty on maxillary growth and deciduous occlusion in cases of complete unilateral cleft lip and palate. *Scand J Plast Reconstr Surg* 10:197–208, 1976.
11. Ritsilä V, Alhupuro S, Gylling U, Rintala A. The use of free periosteum for bone formation in congenital clefts of the maxilla. *Scand J Plast Reconstr Surg* 6:57–60, 1972.
12. Rintala A, Ranta D. Periosteal flaps and grafts in primary cleft repair: A follow-up study. *Plast Reconstr Surg* 83:17–22, 1989.
13. Renkielska A, Wojtaszek-Slominska A, Dobke M. Early cleft repair in children with unilateral complete cleft lip and palate: A case against primary alveolar repair. *Ann Plas Surg* 54:595–597; discussion 598–599, 2005.
14. Mars M, Plint D, Houston W, et al. The Goslon yardstick: A new system of assessing dental arch relationships in children with unilateral clefts of the lip and palate. *Cleft Palate J* 24:314–322, 1987.
15. Georgiade N, Latham R. Maxillary arch alignment in the bilateral cleft lip and palate infant, using the pinned coaxial screw appliance. *Plas Recon Surg* 56:52–60, 1975.
16. Millard D. Presurgical maxillary orthopedics. In Millard DR (ed). *Cleft Craft, Vol 3.* Boston: Little, Brown, 1980, p. 263.
17. Millard D, Latham R, Huifen X, Spiro S, Morovic C. Cleft lip and palate treated by presurgical orthopedics, gingivoperiosteoplasty, and lip adhesion (popla) compared with previous lip adhesion method: A preliminary study of serial dental casts. *Plast Reconstr Surg* 103:1630–1644, 1999.
18. Henkel K, Gundlach K. Analysis of primary gingivoperiosteoplasty in alveolar cleft repair. Part I: Facial growth. *J Craniomaxillofac Surg* 25:266–269, 1997.
19. Berkowitz S, Mejia M, Bystrik A. A comparison of the effects of the Latham Millard procedure with those of a conservative treatment

approach for dental occlusion and facial aesthetics in unilateral and bilateral cleft lip and palate. Part I: Dental occlusion. *Plast Reconstr Surg* 113:1–18, 2004.

20. Grayson B, Santiago P, Brecht L, Cutting C. Presurgical nasoalveolar molding in infants with cleft lip and palate. *Cleft Palate Craniofac J* 36:486–498, 1999.

21. Santiago P, Grayson B, Cutting C, Gianoutsos M, Brecht L, Kwon S. Reduced need for alveolar bone grafting by presurgical orthopedics and primary gingivoperiosteoplasty. *Cleft Palate Craniofac J* 35:77–80, 1998.

22. Wood R, Grayson B, Cutting C. Gingivoperiosteoplasty and midfacial growth. *Cleft Palate Craniofac J* 34:17–20, 1997.

23. Lee C, Grayson B, Cutting C, Brecht L, Lin W. Prepubertal midface growth in unilateral cleft lip and palate following alveolar molding and gingivoperiosteoplasty. *Cleft Palate Craniofac J* 41:375–380, 2004.

24. Garfinkle J, Grayson B, Brecht L, Cutting C. Long-term effects on midface growth of gingivoperiosteoplasty with presurgical infant orthopedics in unilateral cleft lip and palate. *2006 Annual Meeting of the American Cleft Palate-Craniofacial Association,* (Abstract #100), 2006.

25. Pfeifer TM, Grayson BH, Cutting CB. Nasoalveolar molding and gingivoperiosteoplasty versus alveolar bone graft: An outcome analysis of costs in the treatment of unilateral cleft alveolus. *Cleft Palate Craniofac J* 39(1):26–29, 2002.

Bone Graft Construction of the Cleft Maxilla and Palate

Timothy A. Turvey, DDS • Ramon L. Ruiz, DMD, MD • Paul S. Tiwana, DMD, MD

HISTORIC PERSPECTIVE

Historically, one of the most controversial issues in the comprehensive care of the patient with a cleft lip and palate has been the need for bone grafting the cleft maxilla and palate.

Although skeletal involvement with facial clefting conditions was recognized for centuries, little attention was directed to the importance of the skeleton prior to the last 30 years. The underemphasis of this is highlighted by a major textbook on cleft care, published 30 years ago, which dedicated less than 10% of its content to the importance of skeletal reconstruction.[1] The German literature documents that Lexar, Drachter, and von Eiselberg experimented with bone graft construction of the cleft maxilla and palate more than 100 years ago.[2–4] In the mid-twentieth century, Auxhausen summarized the problem of the skeletal deficiency in the cleft maxilla and palate, noting that the bone deficiency in cleft patients was the final problem to be solved in the repair of the clefts.[5] Schmid responded to Auxhausen's challenge in his 1955 contribution that introduced the concept of primary bone graft.[6] Following Schmid's report, there was a "bandwagon effect" around the world, with cleft palate teams embracing the concept of primary bone grafting.[7–14] As with most newly introduced surgical techniques, it required a decade to recognize the problems associated with the placement of bone grafts during infancy and early childhood. Reports of adverse growth following primary bone grafting appeared in the literature in 1968 and continued into the 1970s. It was the orthodontic community that documented growth disturbances of the maxilla; and the results were consistent, coming from multiple institutions in Europe, Scandinavia, the United States, Great Britain, etc.[15–17] For greater historic record, readers are referred to Koberg's article, which appeared in the inaugural issue of the *Journal of Maxillofacial Surgery* in 1973.[5] To date, a single center has reported favorable results with primary bone grafting.[18–20] It is significant that this work is representative of a center with a single surgeon and orthodontist whose patients were treated with the same protocol. This is unlike most other reports that involved multiple surgeons employing multiple techniques.

Following the reports of adverse facial growth, the enthusiasm for primary bone grafting rapidly faded; and the pendulum for bone grafting swung in the opposite direction. At the pinnacle of antibone grafting sentiment, Boyne introduced delayed bone grafting.[21,22] His rationale for placing the bone graft between the ages of 8 and 12 years was based on the preception that maxillary growth in the anterior and transverse direction was 80% completed by age 8 years. He demonstrated that the benefits of primary bone grafting could be achieved by placement of the bone graft nearing the end of the first decade with minimal effects on the growth of the maxilla. The concept was not readily embraced, principally because of the experience of primary bone grafting and the emotional outcry of some dissenters. This subject became the topic of heated discussions and correspondence. Consequently, it was several decades before cleft communities accepted that bone grafting, as proposed by Boyne, was soundly based and a significant contribution to cleft care. Today, bone graft construction of the cleft maxilla and palate is embraced by most and is considered a critical component of the habilitation of patients with cleft lip and palate when considering both the functional and esthetic concerns.

ANATOMIC CONSIDERATIONS

Clefts of the lip and palate almost always involve the maxilla and palate to at least some degree. Even in cases of incom-

plete clefts of the lip and palate, the anterior maxilla is commonly affected. Similarly, submucous clefts of the soft palate are almost always accompanied by skeletal involvement represented as a notch at the posterior edge of the hard palate. It is important to recognize that a cleft of the maxilla does not involve just the alveolar process. It also includes the nasal base and piriform rim. The defect is always greater along the nasal base than at the alveolus. In addition to the absence of bone in these areas, there is also hypoplasia of the lateral nasal structure causing distortion of the piriform rim on the affected side. It is impressive that the bone defect is always larger than the soft tissue defect. Of additional importance is the distortion of the anterior nasal spine and nasal crest of the maxilla, which is deviated away from the side of the cleft. The nasal septum, both bony and cartilaginous, is also affected with deviation toward the side of the cleft in the superior aspect of the nasal cavity and then deflection away from the cleft side toward the inferior part of the cavity (Fig. 56–1A, B, and C).

The soft tissues of the face and the nose depend upon skeletal support for projection and configuration. Without adequate skeletal support along the nasal base and anterior portion of the maxilla, the lip always lacks projection on the cleft side. The nasal cartilages, in addition to lacking structural integrity, are inadequately supported on the cleft side as well. Regardless of how well a cleft lip is repaired and its anatomic points matched, without appropriate skeletal support, there will always be distortion. The inadequate skeletal support in cleft lip and palate contributes significantly to the stigmata of cleft lip and palate, even when the soft tissues are closed with perfect alignment of all landmarks. The flat appearance of the lip, and the direct light reflection from the scar, are the distinguishing characteristics that can be improved by skeletal support.

The stigmata of cleft lip and palate can never be completely eliminated. Meticulous closure of the lip, by alignment of the cutaneous mucosal borders; construction of the orbicularis oris muscle; and appropriate placement of the alar base, may help alleviate asymmetry and distortion of the lip. The projection and support of the lip are derived from the underlying skeletal structures. Without this skeletal support, regardless of how well the lip is closed, the stigmata of cleft lip and palate remains. By appropriately supporting the lip and nasal base, the lip scar, configuration, and projection can be improved. The light reflection coming from the scar changes with improved lip support, even though the scar remains.

OBSERVATIONS OF NONBONE GRAFTED PATIENTS

A large number of patients, treated at a major cleft center with the state-of-the-art techniques not including bone grafting, were reviewed. It became obvious that although the lips and palates had been closed appropriately with anatomic elements aligned, most patients still possessed the stigmata of

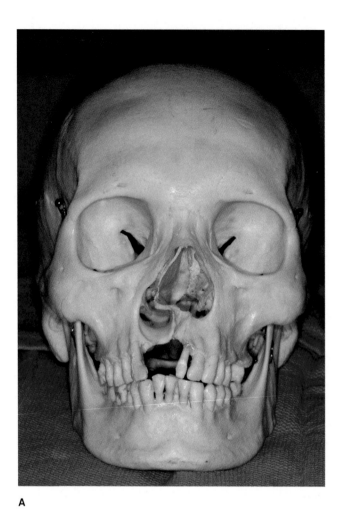

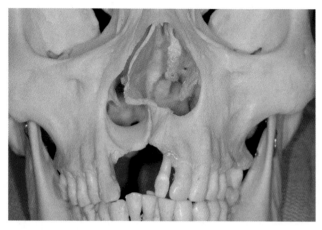

B

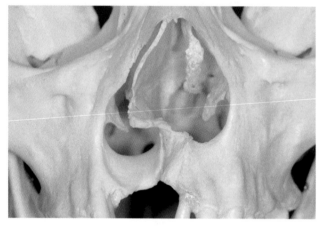

C

A

Figure 56–1. (A) An adult skull with a cleft of the maxilla demonstrating the extent of the skeletal involvement. Notice that the defect in the nasal base exceeds that of the alveolus. Also notice the hypoplasia of the margins of the cleft, the distortion of the lateral nasal alar region. (B) A close-up view demonstrating the deviation of the nasal crest of the maxilla and nasal spine away from the cleft. (C) A closer view demonstrating deflection of the septum toward the cleft in the superior part of the nasal cavity and then deviation away from the cleft inferiorly.

cleft lip and palate secondary to the flatness and asymmetric support of the lip. Most of the patients had residual oral nasal fistulas, in spite of multiple attempts to close these fistulas by soft tissue surgery alone. All of the patients lacked alveolar continuity, and they all required prosthetic rehabilitation with long, fixed bridges or large, removable prosthetic appliances. In most of the bilateral cases, the premaxilla remained mobile. In almost all cases, orthodontic treatment had been employed. At the completion of orthodontic care, prostheses were commonly placed. It was obvious that there was minimal bone support surrounding the teeth adjacent to the cleft and that often premolars were removed during orthodontic treatment. Many of the patients could not be treated satisfactorily with conventional orthodontics alone, and they would have benefited from skeletal surgery to assist with alignment of the facial bones. This was not available at the time, so many patients were left in anterior and/or posterior crossbite. After following this population for years, it became obvious that the prosthetic devices eventually failed and that periodontal

disease became rampant. This was especially true for the dentition adjacent to the cleft where the chronic inflammation from oral nasal reflux was greatest. Eventually, the teeth adjacent to the cleft were lost, and bridgework was redone as the patients continued to age. This occurred in spite of good oral hygiene.

TERMINOLOGY

When initially introduced, bone grafting the cleft maxilla and palate was named anatomically. As time passed, and as surgeons focused on the dental aspects of the procedure, the term "alveolar bone grafting" evolved. By contemporary standards, bone graft construction of the cleft maxilla and palate is well beyond construction of just the alveolus. The importance of the other benefits of the procedure have always been realized but were underemphasized, and the term alveolar bone grafting was adopted. Importantly, the nasal floor and lateral piriform rim are also constructed during the procedure as performed today. In consideration of this, the procedure described in this contribution is beyond alveolar bone grafting, and the name should accurately reflect the surgery. In contemporary settings, *bone graft construction of the cleft maxilla and palate* is the most appropriate terminology.

TIMING

Although Boyne introduced delayed bone grafting in the late 1960s, most centers were skeptical and shied away from bone grafting completely until the early 1980s. Cleft centers that had experience with the technique reported favorable results. After reviewing the experience of several centers who had adopted delayed bone grafting during the 1970s, it became obvious that the best results were achieved in patients where the bone graft was placed prior to the eruption of the secondary dentition and in particular the eruption of the cuspid.[23,24] There was better than 96% success compared to 75% success if the bone graft was placed after eruption of the permanent cuspid.[25] Further experience with bone grafting indicated that if the graft was placed prior to the eruption of the lateral incisor (if present), it could result in salvaging this tooth as well as the permanent incisor. Moving the age of grafting to 6 – 7 years has had no appreciable effect on the growth of the maxilla.

The potential benefits of placement of a graft during infancy or early childhood include early closure of all fistulas, providing adequate skeletal support for lip and nasal esthetics, preservation of the primary dentition, and fusing the premaxilla to the lateral segments in bilateral clefts. These are laudable reasons to consider early placement, but the practicality of achieving these goals early in life must be countered by the realities of limited amounts of cancellous bone available from the ilium in infancy and early childhood. Although rib grafts can be placed during infancy and early childhood, they do not permit teeth to migrate and/or to be moved through the graft as easily as cancellous iliac bone. The importance of early closure of all fistulas must also be questioned, since to date, no adverse health sequela has been ascribed to oral nasal fistulas persisting through early childhood. The changing periodontal pathogens with age set the stage for periodontal disease, especially around unrepaired oral nasal fistulas in adults, not children. Clearly, the persistence of oral nasal fistulas in adult years is detrimental to periodontal health, and the fistulas should be closed before adulthood. The wisdom of using these as arguments in favor of primary bone grafting is questioned.

The most appropriate time to place a bone graft is when the graft is needed to provide dental support to the permanent dentition. When originally introduced, delayed bone grafting focused on the preservation of the permanent cuspid. Today, the timing of bone graft placement is determined by the desire to preserve as much of the natural permanent dentition as possible. If a permanent lateral incisor is present and can be

salvaged, the graft is placed at a younger age. Supernumerary teeth, if large enough, can occasionally be used to substitute for a missing lateral incisor, and the root development should determine the timing of graft placement.

Root development of unerupted teeth in the cleft region is the key to bone graft placement. Ideally, the root of the salvageable tooth should be one half to two thirds developed when the graft is placed.

TEETH IN THE CLEFT AREA

If supernumerary teeth are present in the area of the cleft, and are not salvageable, they should be removed. Teeth in the cleft region are removed infrequently prior to bone grafting. For most young cleft patients, the administration of local anesthesia and even the manipulation of tissue in the cleft region is a traumatic episode. Unless the teeth are positioned so that soft tissue closure at the time of bone graft will be compromised, these supernumerary and/or ectopically positioned teeth are removed at the time of bone graft placement. If teeth are required to be removed before bone grafting, the removal is completed at least 6 weeks prior to surgery to assure adequate soft tissue healing.

PRESURGICAL ORTHODONTIC PREPARATION

Prior to bone grafting, it is desirable to have alignment of teeth initiated. When presurgical alignment is performed, care must be taken to avoid tooth movement into the cleft to prevent periodontal problems. Moving teeth away from the cleft may facilitate the surgery, making access to the cleft site easier.

Presurgical arch expansion is not always favorable or desirable. Widening the cleft before surgery necessitates more bone and soft tissues to close the defect. This makes success of the bone graft less predictable. Postgraft expansion is desirable for several reasons, including facilitating the maturation of the graft. This occurs by stressing the graft with the distraction forces required for expansion. Postgraft expansion should be delayed for about 6 weeks, while the revascularization of the bone occurs and the mucosal wounds are mature. Conventional orthodontic movement can commence after approximately 3 weeks.

Bone is a living tissue, which does best when stimulated. If bone is not stimulated, it will resorb, as seen when a tooth is removed and a bone defect occurs in the arch. If teeth are actively moved into the bone graft or erupt passively, the graft will survive and take on the characteristics of adjacent bone. Crestal resorption of the graft will always take place postsurgery. As the root matures and the tooth erupts, supporting bone will follow. Once the tooth is visible in the mouth, the orthodontist should position it adjacent to the central incisor so that the eruption of the permanent cuspid is not impeded.

TREATMENT OUTCOMES

The outcome of bone graft construction of the cleft maxilla and palate is determined by evaluating the success of each of the criteria for placement. Unfortunately, some have used only radiographs to determine the success or failure of the procedure. This judgment is based on evaluation of quantity and quality of bone as evidenced by a radiograph.[26,27] A well-designed study would include a weighted grading scale for each patient when determining success/failure of the graft. To date, no such study has been conducted.

It is the experience of the authors that the success of the procedure is primarily dependent upon the stage of dental development at the time of graft placement. Another factor determining success is the appropriate development of the graft bed. This requires complete exposure of the bone adjacent to the cleft closure, using fresh or autogenous bone, and developing a well-vascularized oral flap for coverage over the graft. Providing that the bone graft is placed prior to the onset of periodontal problems affecting teeth adjacent to the cleft, the degree of success is high.

The success of fistula closure is dependent upon adequate quality of soft tissue. Complete nasal and oral closure of mucosa is critical for the successful outcome. Another important factor is the patient's cooperation with eliminating habits of forcing fluids or mucus through the fistula during the healing phase. Improvement in lip projection and nasal symmetry can be assessed only by comparing standardized photographs, prior to, and at the completion of surgery.

The stabilization of the premaxilla will occur, providing that the premaxilla is appropriately prepared at the time of surgery. Adequate preparation includes subperiosteal dissection of the cleft margins, including the vomer. Adequate stabilization of the premaxilla requires elimination of traumatic occlusal forces. Any force that perpetuates movement of the premaxilla is detrimental to satisfactory healing. It is the surgeon's responsibility to be certain that adverse movement of the premaxilla is eliminated by orthodontic means prior to surgery, or it should eliminated at the time of surgery by repositioning the premaxilla.

Construction of an intact maxilla is almost always observed following bone graft habilitation. The height and width of the ridge is always determined by the presence or absence of teeth in the grafted bone. If teeth are not present in the grafted bone, the bone graft will act just as normal alveolar bone, and will resorb in height and width. This is not graft failure; it is predictable bone biology. Commonly, the grafted bone site will require additional bone grafting if endosseous implants are to be placed later in life.

The success of constructing an intact maxilla requires assessment of both the nasal base and piriform rim area as well as the alveolar ridge area. Factors that contribute to bone graft height and width at the alveolus include the presence of teeth in the graft and the quality of the soft tissue covering the graft. If roots of teeth are not in the bone graft, there is always resorption, as occurs at a normal extraction site. The graft site will resorb in all the three dimensions and an alveolar ridge defect will result. The degree of bone remodeling is always related to the tightness of the soft tissue flap covering the graft. Graft survival is more favorable with good quality loose soft tissue flaps, rather than tight and scarred tissue covering the graft. At the nasal base, the purpose of the graft is to support the nasal structure and the upper lip. After reviewing earlier cases of bone grafting, it became obvious that the dissections were not conducted to the level of the nasal floor. Consequently, the graft did not provide as much support for the lip and nose as desired. Today, an effort is made to complete the dissection to the nasal floor and piriform rim with dissection of the anterior nasal spine. The graft is always overpacked into the defect, realizing that resorption and remodeling occurs over time. In some patients, a cortical bone strut can be used to reconstruct the pyriform rim to the same height as the nonaffected side. A thin cortical strip can be used to bridge the defect from the anterior nasal spine to the lateral piriform rim.

THE SURGICAL MANAGEMENT OF THE CLEFT MAXILLA AND PALATE

Nasotracheal intubation is preferable through the nostril on the noncleft side, since it removes all obstructions from the surgical field. If nasotracheal intubation is not possible, the oral route can be used. If the oral route is used, the endotracheal tube can be sutured to the mandibular anterior teeth to remove it from the immediate surgical area and to secure its position. Occasionally, a mouth gag is helpful in positioning the endotracheal tube and gaining access to the palatal tissues, but it may also be cumbersome. The surgical field, including the buccal, palatal, and nasal tissue, is injected with local anesthesia and epinephrine (1:100,000). Sterile preparation of the surgical field is then performed.

Incision Design

The procedure begins by incision of the fixed gingival tissues from the cleft margin and around the adjacent teeth so that they are preserved. These tissues are reflected back on themselves and sutured to expose the crestal alveolar bone (Fig. 56–2). The tissues lining the cleft margin are then incised from the alveolus superiorly to the depth of the mucobuccal fold, where there is normally a buccal fistula. The incision continues around the margins of the fistula, but the depth of circumferential part of the incision is shallower than the marginal incision because there is no periosteum. This incision is made on both the sides of the cleft. A full-thickness flap is then developed, beginning from the alveolar crest superiorly to the height of the buccal fistula. Care is taken when the flap is elevated so that thin bone overlying the adjacent tooth root is not damaged. If bone is elevated and roots become exposed or damaged, periodontal defects will occur and/or external resorption will result. Secondarily, at the circumferential part of the buccal fistula, the tissues

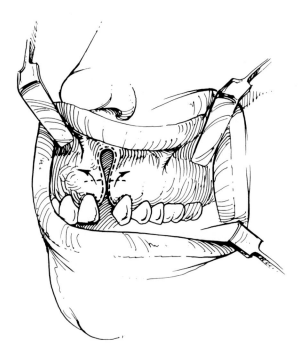

Figure 56–2. Outline of incision to prepare the cleft site for bone grafting. The fixed gingival tissues are preserved and sutured back.

are undermined sufficiently to permit the mucosal surface to be turned into the center of the fistula and elevated into the nasal cavity. The tissues lining the cleft must also be reflected from the palatal mucosa; this can be done by incising the tissue through the cleft from the buccal side. This flap is then elevated in the subperiosteal plane. The bone margins of the cleft are exposed to the level of the nasal cavity (Fig. 56–3A).

Closure of the tissues lining the cleft is accomplished with resorbable sutures on a small cutting needle. Mattress suture technique with the knots tied on the nasal side assists in establishing a watertight seal (Fig. 56–3B). Access to suturing in this confined area is facilitated by the use of a Castroviejo needle holder. If the fistula continues posteriorly on the palate, it is sometimes necessary to pass a traction suture through the nasal floor to the posterior palatal tissue to seal the posterior nasal floor. This is facilitated by bending a straight needle to the appropriate curved contour, passing it through the fistula and retrieving it on the palate (Fig. 56–4A, B, and C). Sometimes, it is necessary to mobilize the palatal tissue to achieve adequate palatal coverage. In such instances, an incision is made from the molar region approximately 5 mm from the gingival margin and parallel to the dental plane and can be extended to the cleft. The flap is then elevated in a subperiosteal plane and rotated medially and anteriorly to achieve coverage. An alternative is to elevate the palatal tissue from the first molar forward to the cleft area (Fig. 56–5A and B). A relaxing incision at the first molar area is then made to allow the flap to be advanced to cover the palatal defect. The relaxing incision should not extend to the greater palatine vessels. The vessels should be included in the flap (Fig. 56–6A and B).

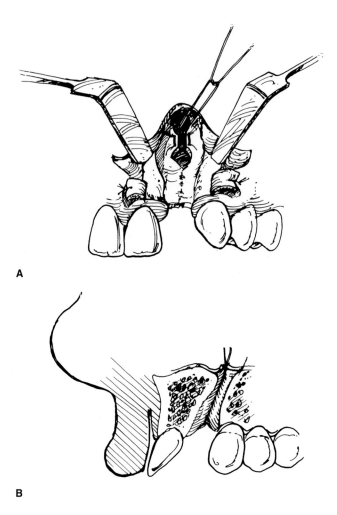

A

B

Figure 56–3. (A) The tissues lining the cleft are elevated to the nasal cavity to construct a floor (B) Closure of the nasal lining is accomplished with a horizontal mattress sutures to evert the edges toward the nasal side.

Placement of the Bone Graft

The anterior and posterior bone margins of the cleft should be completely stripped of all soft tissue. The lateral surface of the maxilla on either side of the cleft is exposed, and the hypoplasia of the bone margins is always apparent from the alveolus superiorly to the piriform rim. Autogenous particulate cancellous bone is densely packed into the entire cleft defect (Fig. 56–7). The success of this type of bone graft is enhanced by transferring osteogenic cells. This is facilitated by tightly condensing the graft. The bone must be extended from the piriform rim to at least the alveolar crest height in the region. Because bone margins of clefts are always hypoplastic, bone should be grafted over the margins. A strip of cortical bone can also be used at the piriform to bridge the lateral aspect of the defect from the anterior nasal spine to the lateral piriform rim. In older patients, this is normally secured with screws. In younger patients (< 10 years), it is normally placed into the defect and retained by the soft tissues (Fig. 56–8).

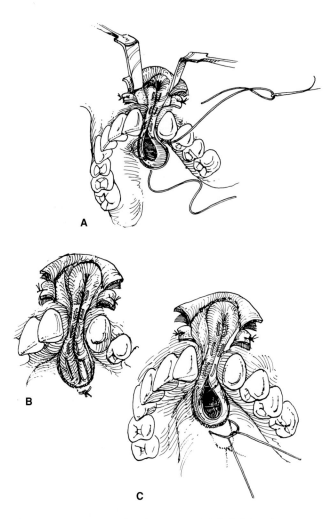

Figure 56–4. (A, B, and C) Sometimes it is helpful and necessary to pass a traction suture through the reconstructed nasal floor and the posterior palatal tissues in order to pull the reconstructed floor posteriorly to form a seal.

Choice of Bone Donor Source

Fresh autogenous bone is the graft material of choice for cleft construction. Although multiple sources for bone harvest are available, the ilium remains the donor site of choice for children and most adults. Cranial bone for adult cleft grafting is promising because of its density and the low morbidity with harvesting. Although the cranium is a good donor source for children, it requires more time to harvest than the ilium. When full-thickness cranial grafts are used in adults, harvesting requires the assistance of a neurosurgeon. The cranial defect is immediately reconstructed with split-thickness grafts harvested from the adjacent area.

Many bone substitute materials are also available, but none has proven to match the success of autogenous bone. Bone morphogenic proteins, delivered by a collagen sponge, is technology with promise but currently has limited availability; and the expense is considerable. As of this writing, autogenous iliac bone graft remains the source of choice for most patients. Tibia, rib, mandibular symphysis, and the cranium are other donor sites, but none has been as predictable as the ilium.[28–33]

Closure

Closure of the buccal side of the bone graft almost always requires the addition of more tissue to the area. A variety of flaps can be used for this purpose. Each has its own indications and potential pitfalls.

a. Buccal Mucosal Flaps
    Tissue can be rotated from the buccal mucosal or can be advanced from the buccal mucosa to cover the grafted bone. A rotational flap is the most predictable way of adding tissue to the cleft area with minimal tension. The flap is normally anteriorly based and incised to the level of the submucosa but above the periosteum. The base of the flap must be adequately undermined to permit the

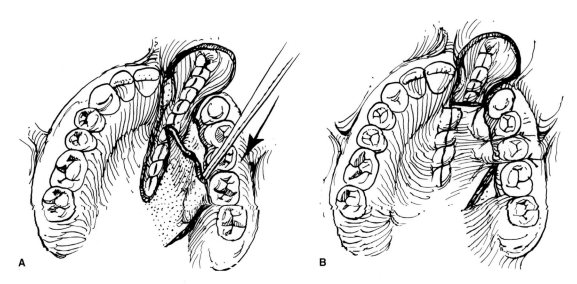

Figure 56–5. (A and B) A full-thickness palatal flap is elevated and rotated medially and anteriorly to provide palatal coverage.

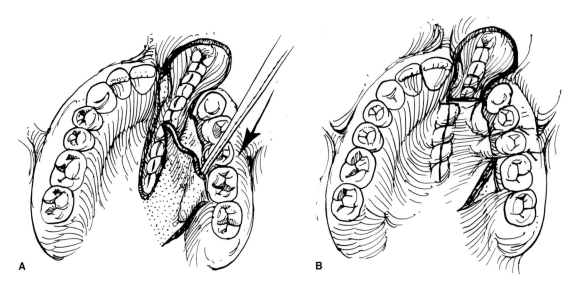

Figure 56–6. (A) A full-thickness flap is elevated from the teeth and a vertical relaxing incision is placed at the first molar region to allow the flap to advance. (B) The defect is left to granulate.

necessary 90° rotation (Fig. 56–9). As with all pedicle flaps, the base must be broad enough and thick enough to ensure perfusion of the tip. In general, the base should be at least /one third of the length of the flap. Once elevated and rotated, the tip of the flap is sutured to the palatal tissue with resorbable material. The base of the flap is also secured with sutures to the mucosa adjacent to the cleft. The fixed gingival tissues are preserved. Returning them to the original position is important for periodontal considerations. The mucosa of the flap in the area where the fixed gingival tissues have been elevated should be de-epithelialized. This is done with a #15 scalpel by shaving

this area of the flap (Fig. 56–10A). The fixed gingival flaps are released on either side and sutured together over the flap. They can also be further secured to the palatal tissues (Fig. 56–10B). Occasionally, the edges of the fixed gingival tissues cannot be stretched enough to allow primary closure. When this occurs, the adjacent fixed gingiva is not undermined further. Rather, the two edges are secured to the flap and the dehiscence is left. If necessary, a palatal graft can be placed later in life. The major advantage of rotational mucosal flaps is that they allow more soft tissue to be added to the region of the cleft. This is especially important because adequate volume of bone must be transferred to the cleft. Without more soft tissue, tension-free closure of the mucosa over the grafted bone is impossible. Another advantage is that

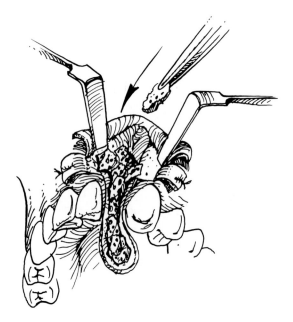

Figure 56–7. Cancellous bone particles packed into the defect must extend from the nasal rim to the alveolar crest.

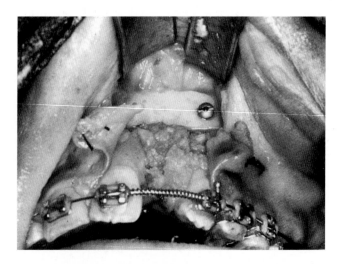

Figure 56–8. Cortical bone graft to construct a nasal rim is secured with a screw in older patients.

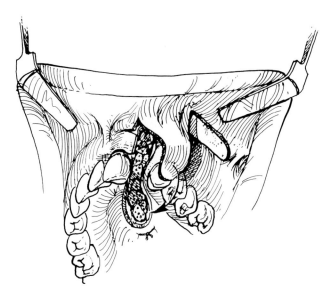

Figure 56–9. A buccal mucosal flap is elevated, maintaining a wide and thick anterior base. The flap is then rotated to cover the defect.

it does not require periosteal stripping. Such stripping is detrimental to further growth and is an important consideration in young children. The disadvantage of the rotational mucosal flap is that it transfers loose buccal mucosa to the dental supporting area of the alveolus. Some clinicians believe that this impedes the eruption of permanent teeth. Although this is possible, it has not been problematic in the author's experience, nor has the use of this flap increased the need to surgically uncover teeth in the area.

b. Advancement Buccal Mucosal Flap
This simple technique design can be employed to cover the bone graft site when there is minimal need for additional tissue to cover the cleft. It has a broad base in the lip, is undermined, and is advanced to cover the bone graft (Fig. 56–11). There is always tension on the closure when the flap design is used, and dehiscence is likely. In addition, it reduces the depth of the sulcus and may shorten the vermilion of the donor site area. Indications for the use of this flap are limited to situations in which the need for additional soft tissue over the bone graft is minimal.

c. Sliding Buccal Gingival Flap
This design is probably most commonly used to cover bone grafts of the cleft maxilla and palate. It requires elevation of a full-thickness flap, including the periosteum, from the lateral segment of the maxilla, sparing the fixed gingiva except at the cleft site. The flap is usually extended to at least the first molar, where a vertical release is placed. In addition, the periosteum along the flap's base often requires release, allowing for medial transposition. The lateral aspect of maxilla on this side of the cleft is stripped, and the full-thickness flap is advanced to cover the bone graft (Fig. 56–12). The major advantage of this flap is that it has a predictable blood supply and advances tissue into the cleft region. The fixed gingival tissues remain on the dental-bearing part of the maxilla. The major disadvantage of this is that it strips the lateral maxilla of its periosteum and leaves a defect posteriorly. The effect of the scarring on further growth is a consideration, especially when the flap is used in a young child.

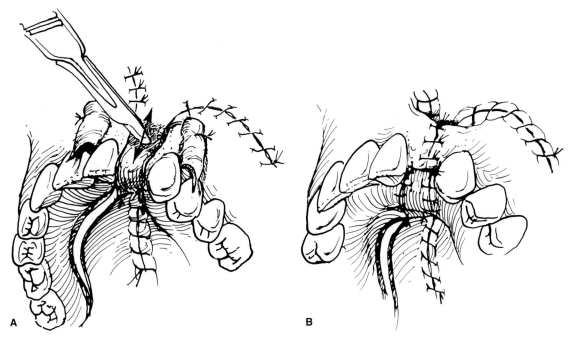

Figure 56–10. (A) The rotated flap is then de-epithelialized in the areas where the fixed gingival flaps will lie. (B) The fixed gingiva is then secured to the flap and around the margins of the teeth.

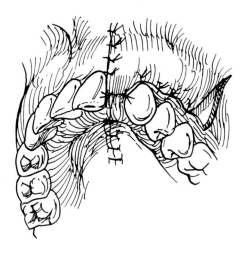

Figure 56–11. A broadly based mucosal flap can be advanced over the bone graft.

SPECIAL CONSIDERATIONS FOR BILATERAL CLEFTS

The principal steps involved in bone grafting bilateral clefts are identical to those in unilateral clefts. There is little reason to stage this procedure, because it can always be performed in one operation. Major differences in managing the bilateral condition include more operating time; and occasionally, the mucosa of the vomer must be elevated to facilitate nasal floor construction. When this is done, it is necessary to extend the bone graft to the vomer and then develop enough soft tissue to cover it. This often requires elevation and rotation

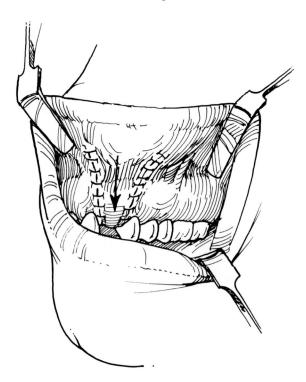

Figure 56–12. A sliding buccal gingival flap is elevated from around the teeth and advanced forward, leaving the posterior defect to granulate.

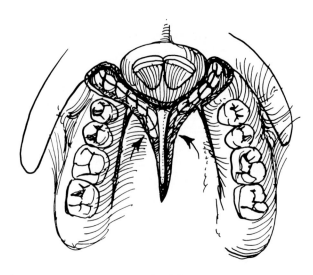

Figure 56–13. Sometimes palatal flaps must be elevated and mobilized toward the midline to close the palatal defects.

of palatal flaps toward the midline (Fig. 56–13). If this is done, the buccal flaps must be advanced into the alveolar cleft and attached to the palatal flaps (Fig. 56–14A and B). Sometimes, a bipedicle buccal mucosal flap can be developed and transposed over the entire buccal and palatal defect. The flap is less likely to dehisce and/or necrose at the midpalatal region where there are multiple flaps joining at the same place (Fig. 56–15A and B). The disadvantage of this flap is that it may shorten the buccal vestibule.

It is rarely necessary to reposition the premaxilla simultaneously with the bone grafting procedure. The need occasionally arises when the premaxilla is vertically overerupted. Under normal circumstances, orthodontic treatment can almost always resolve the situation in which the premaxilla is displaced forward or palatally inclined. Sometimes staging the osteotomy and the bone graft is necessary, especially if there are soft tissue deficiencies, which necessitate stripping.

When a premaxillary osteotomy and repositioning are undertaken, it is critical to design the flap so that the premaxilla remains perfused. In the bilateral cleft, the blood supply comes from the nasoseptal vessels, and adequate mucosa must be left attached to the premaxilla to ensure survival. If a bone graft is simultaneously performed, the nasal floor is constructed as usual. The premaxilla is either mobilized through a midline incision in the buccal mucosa to facilitate separation from the septum and vomer, or separated from the palatal side and fractured forward (Fig. 56–16). Large buccal pedicles must be detached, and occasionally a piece of the nasal and/or vomer must be resected to allow for adequate superior or posterior repositioning (Fig. 56–17).

COMPLICATIONS OF BONE GRAFTING THE CLEFT MAXILLA AND PALATE

Complications such as massive dehiscence, tissue necrosis, and infection are uncommon; and these are more likely

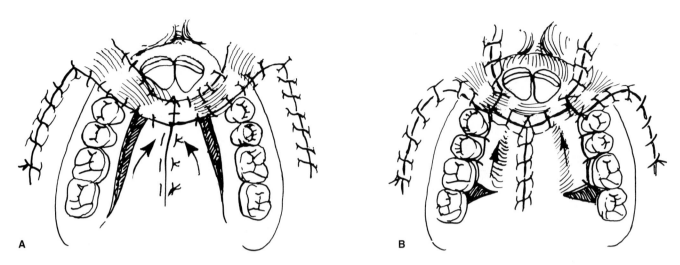

Figure 56–14. (A) Palatal flaps are elevated and rotated. (B) Palatal flaps are advanced, leaving he defect posteriorly.

age- and comorbidity associated. Minor complications such as small wound dehiscence and sequestration occur occasionally. When handled expeditiously and conservatively, they seldom compromise the result. Wound dehiscence and exposure of the graft is best treated conservatively with meticulous oral hygiene, a liquid or soft diet, the frequent use of medicated mouthwash (Peridex), and the administration of oral antibiotics. In an effort to prevent complications, all patients undergoing this procedure are administered prophylactic antibiotics (cephalosporin) to minimize the risks of infection, and some practitioners prescribe steroids to control swelling. The frequency of complications associated with bone grafting the cleft maxilla and palate appear age-related. Seldom do major complications occur in children, when the bone graft is placed prior to the eruption of the permanent dentition. In patients older than 25 years, the complication rate and failure of the bone graft procedure are considerable; a discussion regarding this can be found in the section on bone grafting in the adult that follows below.

When wound dehiscence occurs on the oral surface, it is usually identified within the postsurgical week. Minimal debridement with frequent irrigation and covering with petroleum jelly-impregnated gauze almost always resolves the condition with minimal loss of bone. When massive wound dehiscence and exposure of the graft occur, the wound is treated similarly; however, more extensive debridement of bone may be necessary. Attempting primary closure over the exposed bone is not indicated because the wound is contaminated. The exposed bone is almost always avascular.

When wound dehiscence occurs on the nasal surface, it is more difficult to detect initially because adequate visualization is not always possible, especially in children. In time, a distinct odor may become detectable. Any dead bone that has migrated to the surface can usually be removed with forceps.

Radical debridement is rarely indicated, as this usually means complete failure of the bone graft. Although some patients' parents may be inconvenienced by the conservative approach of irrigation and packing, this approach results in

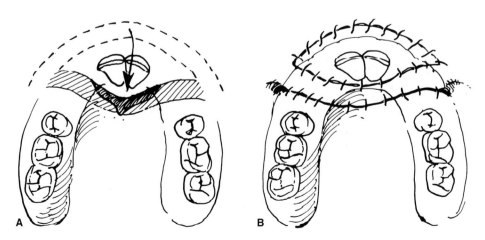

Figure 56–15. (A) Bipedicled or bucket-handle mucosal flap. (B) The flap is elevated and placed over the cleft defect.

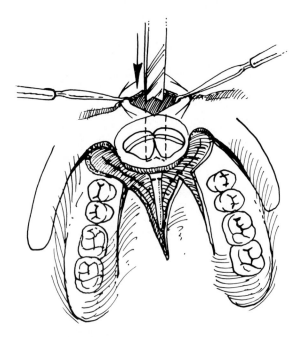

Figure 56–16. Separation of premaxilla with osteotome placed buccally to separate the nasal septum and the vomer.

better long-term graft survival than does the surgeon debriding the area.

BONE GRAFT CONSTRUCTION OF THE CLEFT MAXILLA AND PALATE IN ADULTS

Just as dental implants have revolutionized the practice of dentistry, they have similarly impacted cleft care.[34,35] Although the contemporary goals of cleft habilitation include the elimination of the prostheses care, this goal is not always possible. Additionally, there is a generation of adult cleft patients who have never had bone grafts and are in need of replacing failing prostheses. Whatever the circumstances, bone grafting the clefted maxilla in an adult for prosthetic reasons

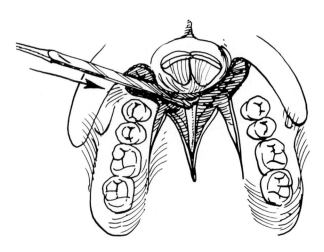

Figure 56–17. Osteotome placed through the cleft to separate the vomer.

requires a different technique than bone grafting the cleft of children.

When a bone graft is placed prior to the eruption of the secondary dentition, its special purpose is to provide periodontal support for teeth adjacent to the cleft, and to permit orthodontic movement of teeth into the graft. Once the permanent dentition has erupted, bone grafting cannot eliminate periodontal defects. Although moving periodontally involved teeth into the graft may be possible, it is not practical, since the periodontal defect around the tooth will always persist.

The success of bone graft placement prior to the eruption of the permanent dentition exceeds 96%. The success of bone grafting after the eruption of the permanent teeth drops precipitously with age.[23,25] Once the patient reaches 25 years of age, the success rate approaches 50% if the same technique of cancellous bone and a three-layered closure is used.

Children Versus Adults

Appreciating the difference between the functions of the bone graft in the adult and the child as well as the difference in healing between children and adults, are important to understanding the rationale for the different technique in the adult. The fundamental functional difference is that the bone graft placed in the adult is expected to support an implant for prosthetic rehabilitation. In the younger patient, its function is to support the natural dentition. The type of bone best suited for implant prosthetic rehabilitation is a corticocancellous block. In children, the cancellous bone graft is both osteogenic and osteoconductive. Revascularization occurs from both endosteal and soft tissue sources. In the adult, the bone graft is primarily osteoconductive, since live transference of osteogenic cells is markedly reduced. The bone graft in adults is much more dependent on vascularization from soft tissues and therefore a more robust soft tissue flap for coverage is required. In the child, a mucosal flap is usually all that is necessary. In the adult, a full-thickness mucoperiosteal flap is always used. In children, the clefts are usually smaller than in the adult. In the nonbone grafted adult, the teeth adjacent to the cleft usually are periodontally involved and are eventually lost. During aging, attrition of the dentition occurs, and the cleft on the oral side increases in size with the loss of teeth and bone.

In nonbone grafted adult cleft patients, periodontal loss of teeth adjacent to the cleft is common. It is likely that the chronic oral–nasal reflux, and the contamination of the nasal cavity with oral flora, contribute to this inflammatory response. Even in the presence of excellent hygiene, the chronic inflammation from the persistent fistulas takes its toll on the periodontal apparatus in adults. In children, the oral and nasal flora do not incite the same inflammatory response. The changing flora associated with age is responsible for the establishment of the periodontal pathogens. Given these significant differences, the principles of bone grafting the adult cleft patient differ significantly from the child.

Principles of Bone Grafting the Adult Cleft

1. Elimination of the inflammation and periodontally involved teeth adjacent to the cleft. This treatment should be done 6–8 weeks prior to bone graft placement to allow for adequate soft tissue response and healing.

2. Complete elimination of smoking and the use of other tobacco products at least 6–8 weeks prior to bone graft surgery. Drugs causing vasoconstriction of the nasal mucosa (recreational, prescription and/or non-prescription, including nose drops or sprays) should not be used for 6 weeks prior to surgery and for at least 4 weeks postoperatively.

3. Reduction of the size of bone defects. This goal should be accomplished by osteotomies and closure of the defects by advancing the posterior segments into the cleft.

4. Meticulous closure of the nasal floor. This is facilitated by principle #3. There is always adequate soft tissue lining the surface of the cleft to allow for closure and construction of a nasal seal, especially when the cleft is reduced in size. Care must be taken to assure the vascularity of the posterior segments, and therefore incision design is critical.

5. Corticocancellous block bone (usually harvested from the anterior ilium or cranium) is usually shaped, cut, and mortised into the cleft with the cortical crest facing the oral cavity. Small amounts of cancellous bone can be used to pack into the bone graft margins, but overpacking is not suggested, since this may contribute to wound dehiscence.

6. Stabilization of the bone graft with biodegradable plates and screws. Absolute immobilization of the graft will facilitate revascularization. Biodegradable plates and screws permit titanium implants to be placed without concern of the implant coming in contact with the screw or plate.

7. Soft tissue closure with full-thickness mucoperiosteal flaps. It is important to carefully design soft tissue flaps to assure perfusion of the segments that have been mobilized and yet provide robust perfusion into the flap resurfacing the bone graft. This often requires mobilization and advancement of full-thickness flaps from the noncleft side. In bilateral clefts, if the defects are large enough, staging the surgery may be necessary.

8. Dental implants must be placed into the grafts 4 months postsurgery. The patient and participating professionals must be willing and able to proceed with this, regardless of circumstances. Failure to place the implants in a timely fashion will jeopardize the result. If there is no assurance that this principle can be fulfilled, the procedure should not be undertaken.

CASE REPORT

T. I.

This 7-year-old girl (Fig. 56–18A and B) with a right unilateral cleft lip and palate was orthodontically prepared for a bone graft with minimal arch expansion (Fig. 56–18C and D). The bone graft was placed prior to the eruption of the permanent right lateral incisor with the expectation of preserving this tooth. The radiograph demonstrates the transposition of the cuspid and first premolar on the right side of the maxilla (Fig. 56–18E and F). The oral–nasal fistula was not symptomatic

A cancellous iliac bone graft was placed utilizing the three-layered closure, which included closure of the oral–nasal fistula. A mucosal rotational flap was used to cover the bone graft. Additionally, the fixed gingival tissues were preserved, as described in the text. As orthodontic treatment progressed, a decision was made to remove a left maxillary premolar and the right lateral incisor for occlusal concerns. The transposition remained, and the right first premolar was advanced adjacent to the incisor to substitute for the lateral incisor.

The patient was debanded at age 14 years with a satisfactory aesthetic and functional outcome. Improved lip and nasal symmetry can be appreciated (Fig. 56–18G and H). The first premolar was shaped, and a retainer was banded to the six anteriors (Fig. 56–18I and J). There was no need for a prosthesis. All fistulas are closed. The cephalometric radiograph confirms a favorable dental and skeletal relationship (Fig. 56–18K and L).

At age 34 years (27 years postoperatively), the patient continues to demonstrate a favorable result with good facial symmetry and preservation of natural dentition without the need for a prosthesis (Fig. 56–18M, N, O, P, and Q). Although the patient smokes, there is little adverse effect on the bone graft or periodontium adjacent to the cleft. The radiograph demonstrates good periodontal support in the cleft site (Fig. 56–18R).

CASE REPORT

E. C.

This 7-year-old boy with a left unilateral cleft lip and cleft palate (Fig. 56–19A and B) was bone grafted prior to the eruption of the permanent lateral incisor. Presurgical orthodontics was not initiated (Fig. 56–19C and D). The timing of surgery was determined by the root development of the lateral incisor (Fig. 56–19E and F). The intention was to preserve the natural dentition and close the remaining oral–nasal fistula.

An iliac cancellous graft was placed. A mucosal rotational flap was used to cover the graft and to close the oral–nasal fistula. The fixed gingival tissues were preserved. Orthodontic intervention occurred at age 11 years and he was debanded by age 14 years.

At age 16 years, the patient demonstrates symmetric support of the lip and nasal base (Fig. 56–19G and H). A complete natural dentition remains with the need for a prosthesis (Fig. 56–19I and J). Even though there is less than ideal bone support around the roots in the area of the cleft, the patient has excellent hygiene and it expected that these teeth will survive for his life (Fig. 56–19K and L). All fistulas remain closed.

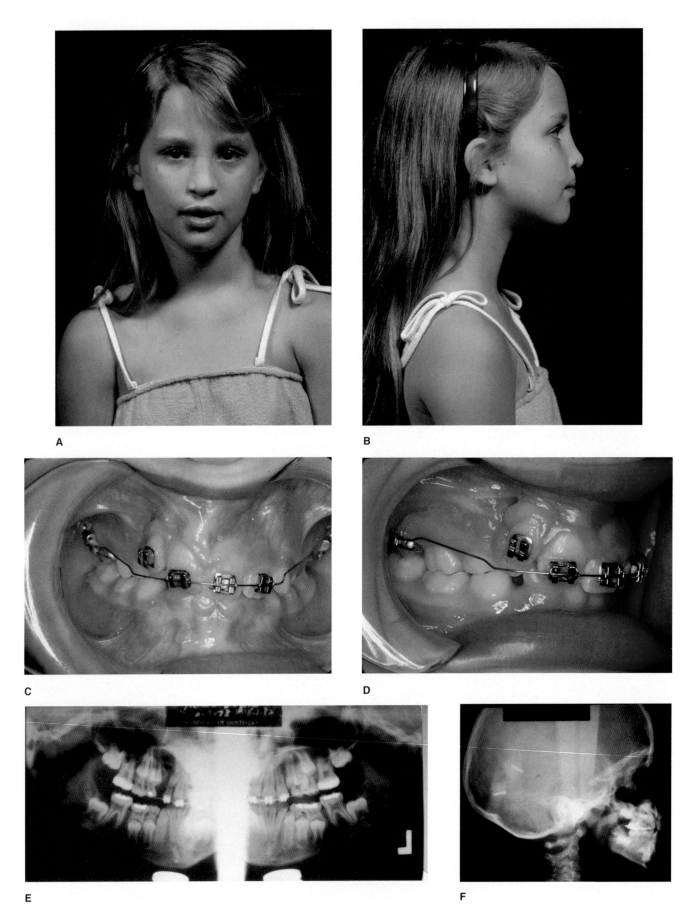

A

B

C

D

E

F

Figure 56–18. Figure 18–1 through 18–14 Case Report TI. (*contd.*)

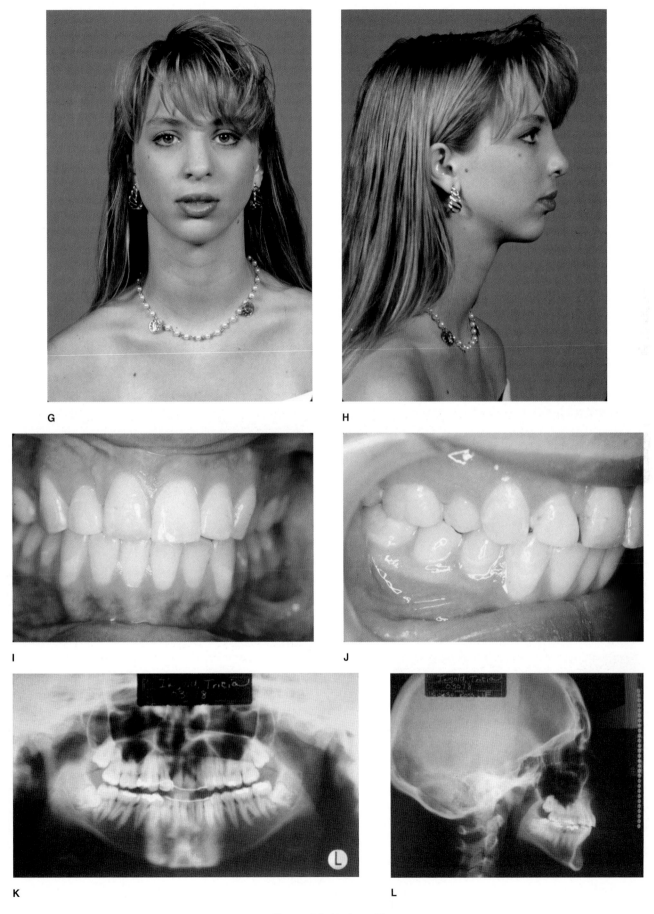

G

H

I

J

K

L

Figure 56–18. (*contd.*)

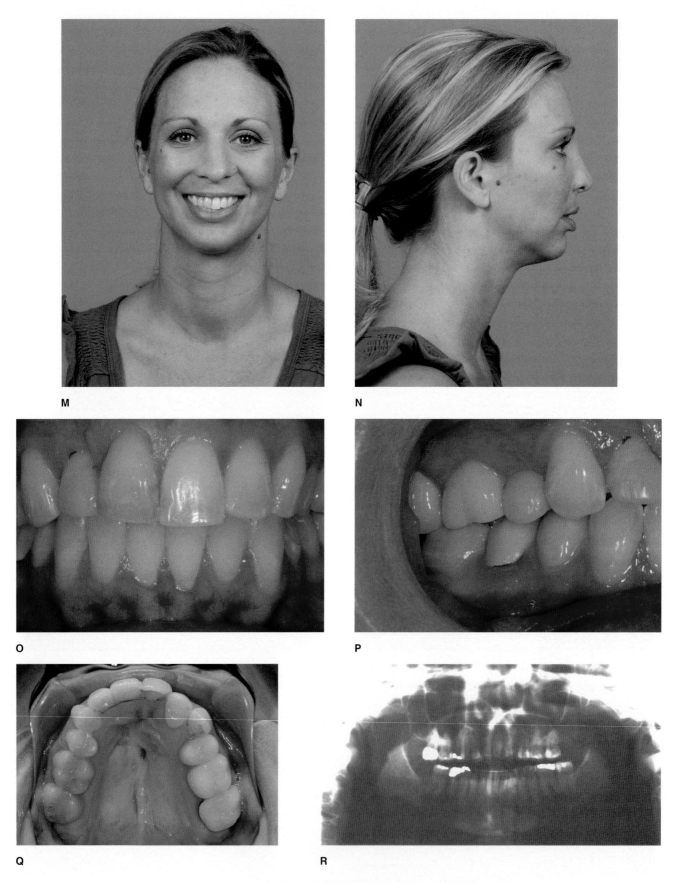

M

N

O

P

Q

R

Figure 56–18. (*Contd.*)

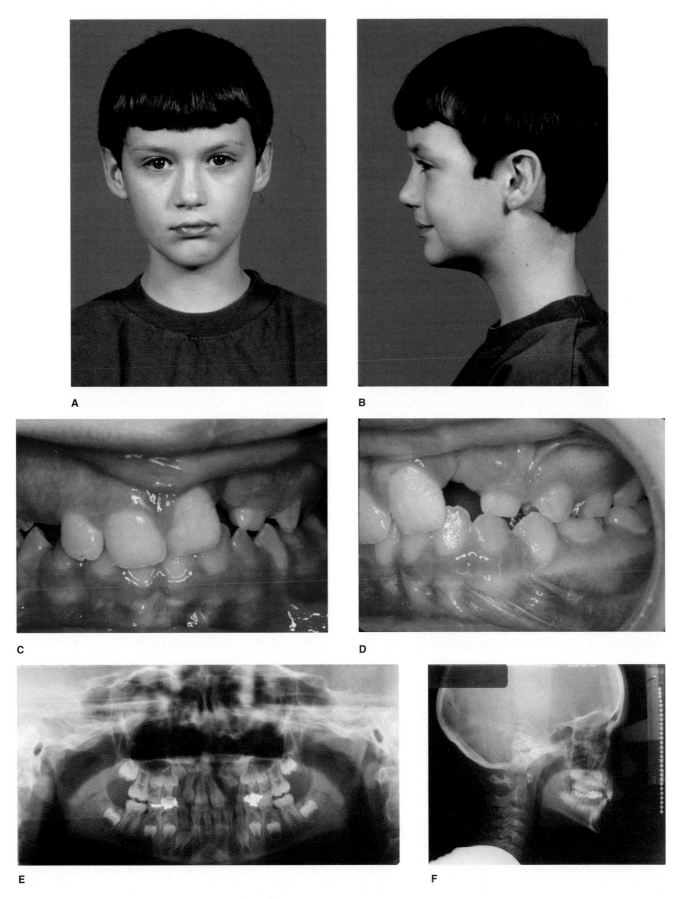

A

B

C

D

E

F

Figure 56–19. Figure 19–1 through 19–12 Case Report EC (*contd.*)

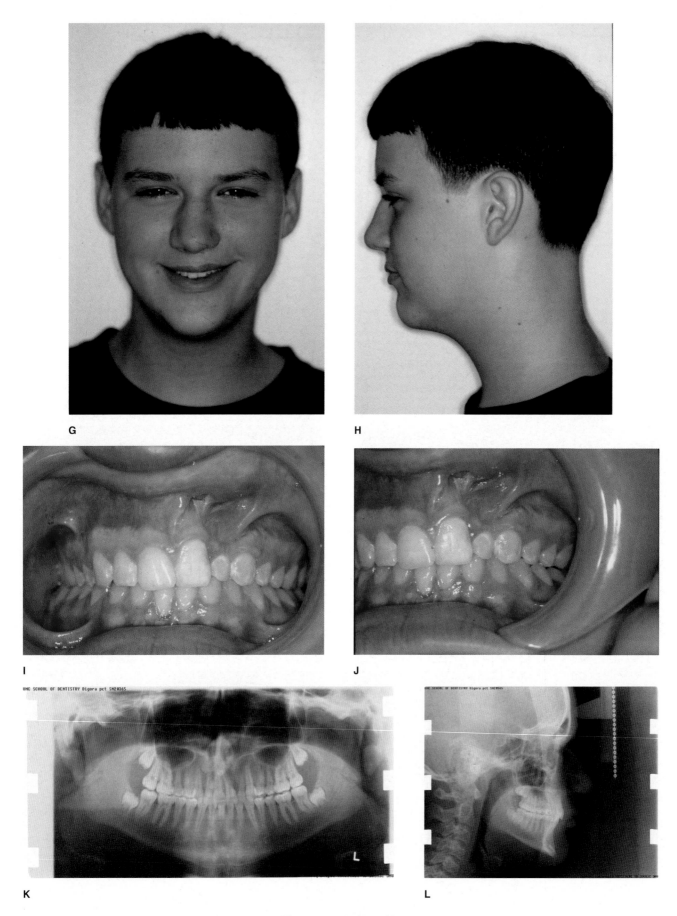

G

H

I

J

K

L

Figure 56–19. (*Contd.*)

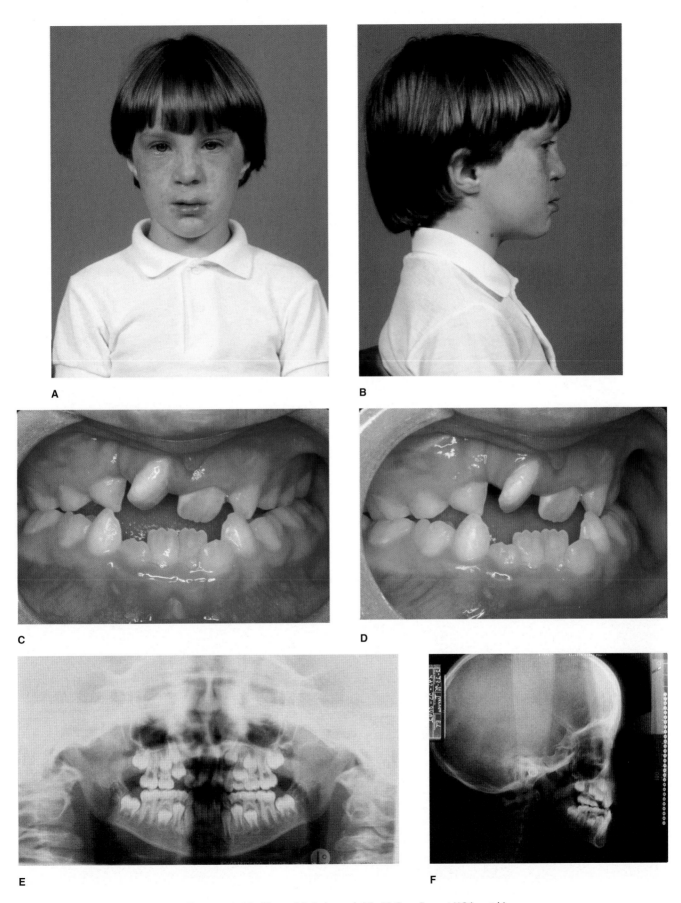

Figure 56–20. Figure 20–1 through 20–19 Case Report KC (*contd.*)

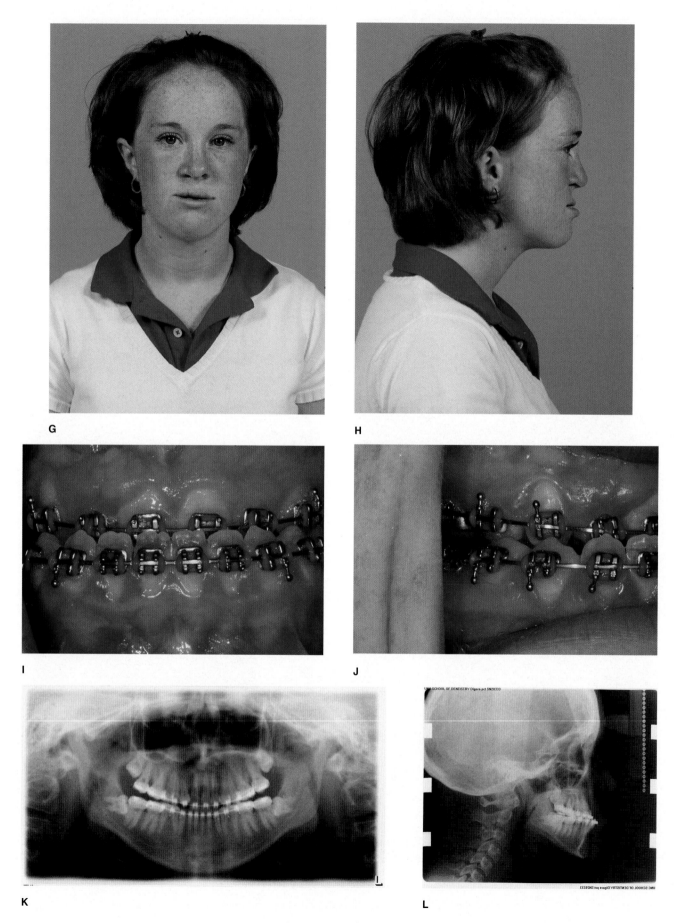

G   H

I   J

K   L

Figure 56–20. *(Contd.)*

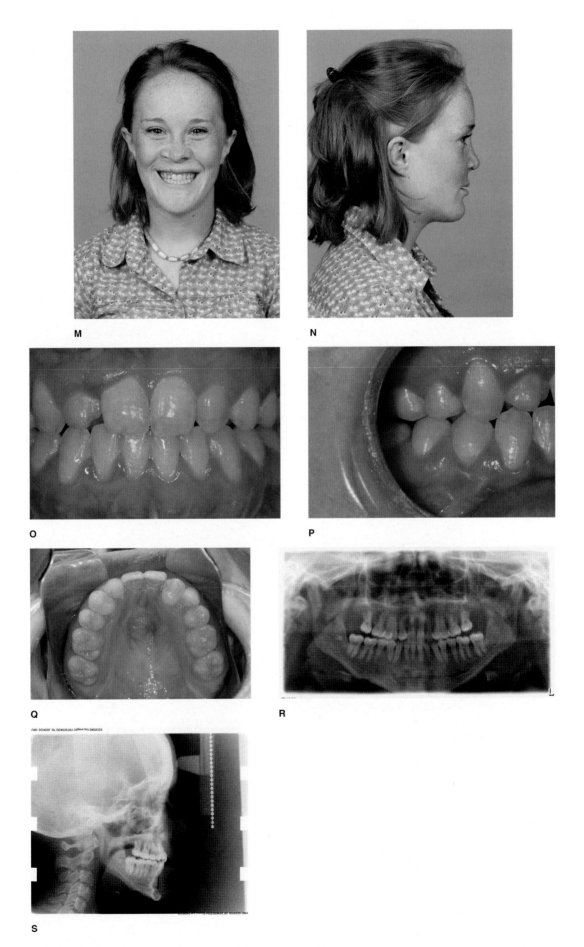

M

N

O

P

Q

R

S

Figure 56–20. (*Contd.*)

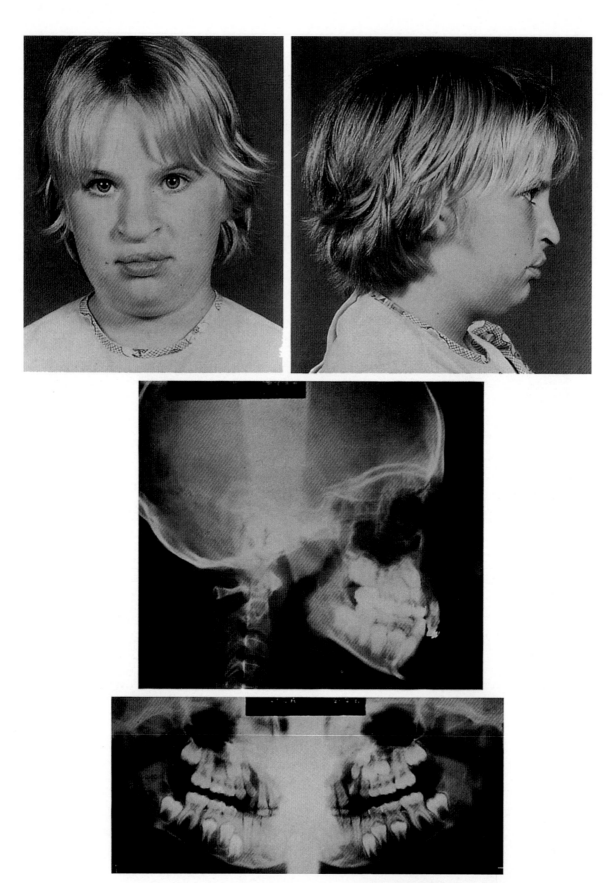

A

Figure 56–21. Figure 21–1 through 21–4 Case Report LS (*contd.*)

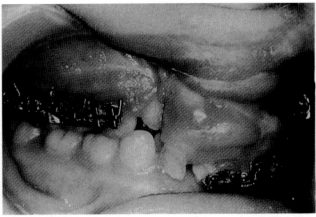

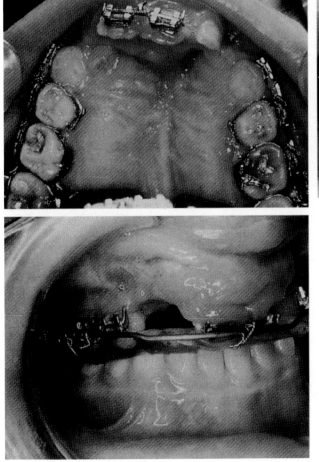

B

Figure 56–21. (*Contd.*)

CASE REPORT

K. C.

An 8-year-old girl with a right unilateral cleft lip and palate presented with maxillary deficiency and in need of a bone graft to the cleft maxilla and palate (Fig. 56–20A, B, C, and D). The incisor adjacent to the cleft was malrotated, and the cuspid and first premolar were transposed (Fig. 56–20E and F). Bone graft from the ilium was placed, and the oronasal fistula was closed at age 8 years.

The skeletal disproportion was ignored. Orthodontic preparation included maxillary and mandibular arch development independent of each other. The transposition was accepted. The first premolar was advanced adjacent to the central incisor on the right. By age 17 years, the patient was prepared to proceed with skeletal surgery to address the maxillary and mandibular disproportion. Midface deficiency involving the entire maxilla and infraorbital region and retrogenia were obvious, as was the class III malocclusion. Flatness of the upper lip and nasal asymmetry as well as fullness of the lower lip are visualized in the preoperative photos. The oronasal fistula remained closed, and adequate bone support for the natural dentition was available (Fig. 56–20G, H, I, J, K, and L).

Maxillary advancement, genioplasty, and cranial bone graft contouring to the cheeks and maxilla were performed at age 17 years. Biodegradable bone plates and screws were used to secure the position of the maxilla, chin, and cranial bone grafts placed in the midface and cheeks. Healing occurred uneventfully. Orthodontic treatment was completed without 6 months. One year after surgery, improved facial balance and symmetry are observed (Fig. 56–20M and N). No further lip or nasal revisions were performed, and none are anticipated. A positive overjet, lack of crossbite, sound periodontal health, and a natural dentition can be appreciated (Fig. 56–20O, P, and Q). Final contouring of the transposed premolar in the position of the right lateral incisor is awaiting. The postoperative radiographs demonstrated improved skeletal and dental harmony, excellent stability, and absence of biodegradable materials used at surgery (Fig. 56–20R and S).

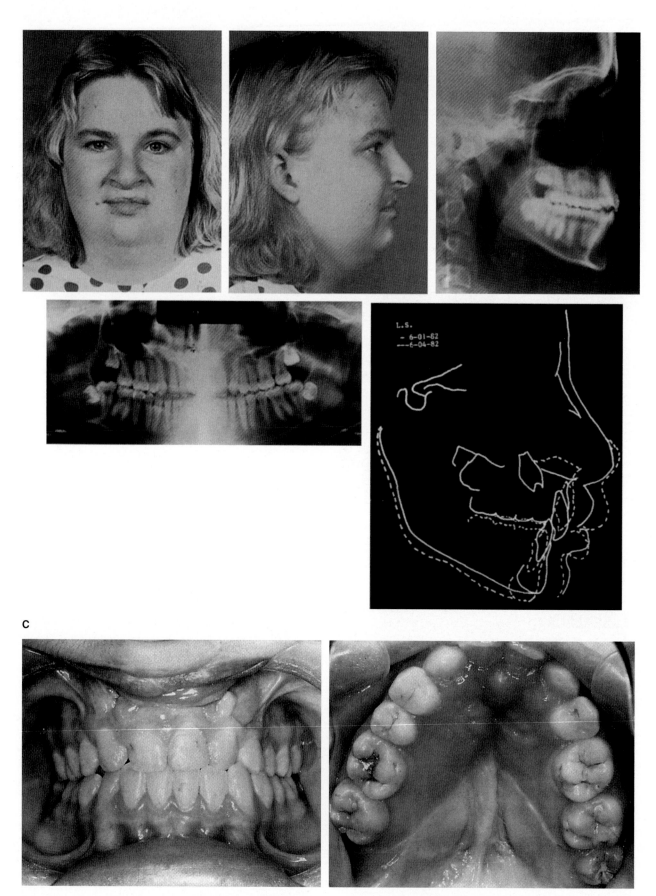

C

D

Figure 56–21. (*Contd.*)

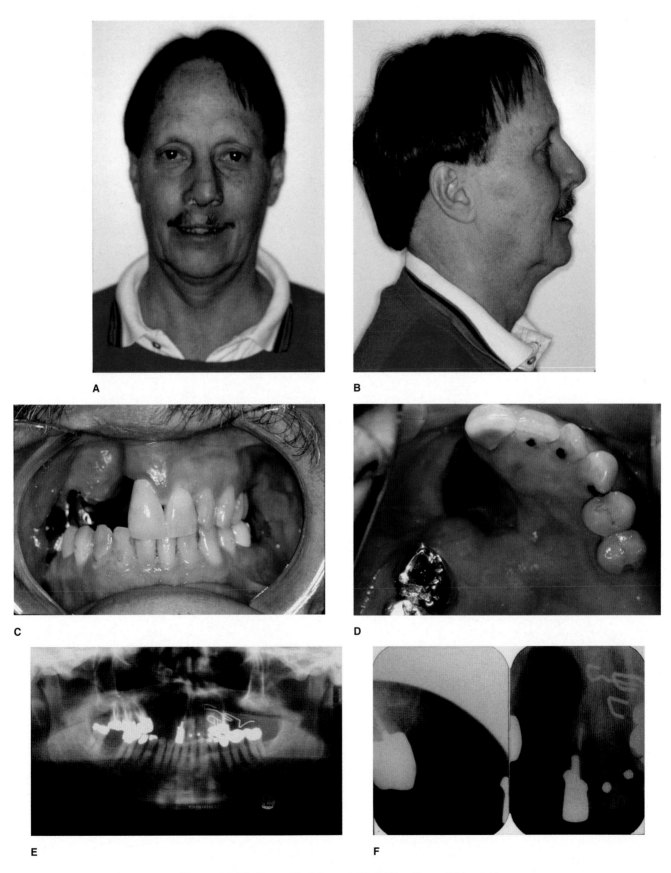

Figure 56–22. Figure 22–1 through 22–20 Case Report TJ (*contd.*)

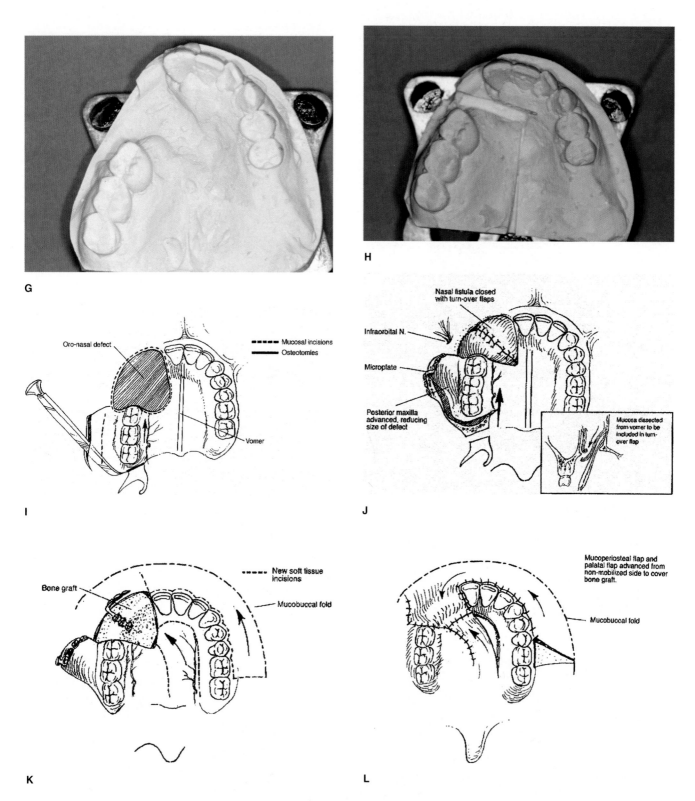

Figure 56–22. (*Contd.*)

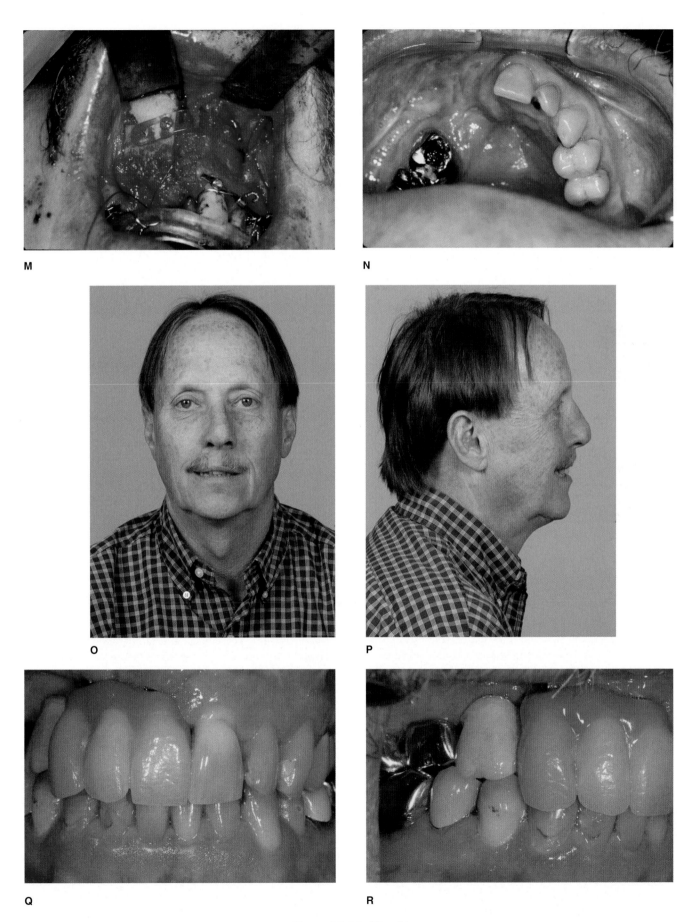

M

N

O

P

Q

R

Figure 56–22. (*Contd.*)

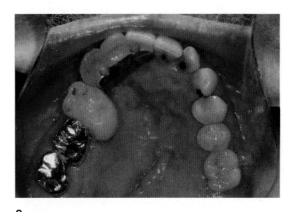

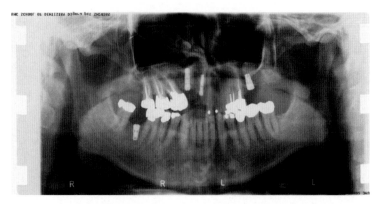

S   T

Figure 56–22. (*Contd.*)

CASE REPORT

L. S.

An 8-year-old girl with a repaired bilateral cleft lip and cleft palate was referred for treatment. She had undergone primary lip and palate closure and columella lengthening earlier in life (Fig. 56–21A). She initiated preliminary orthodontic treatment. Examination revealed overeruption of the premaxilla with the maxillary incisors contacting the mandibular alveolus when the posterior teeth were occluded. The molar relationship was class II. The arch width was adequate to accommodate the width of the premaxilla. Buccal and palatal fistulas were present, and the premaxilla was freely mobile. Multiple supernumerary teeth were identified in the cleft area, as were the developing permanent cuspids (Fig. 56–21B).

Previous experiences with similar conditions suggested that the condition of the maxilla was beyond orthodontic and/or orthopedic correction. Feasibility model surgery indicated that the premaxilla could be positioned superiorly and the incisors could be leveled with the posterior segments. There was adequate arch width so that orthodontic expansion before surgery was not necessary. Cuspid substitution for the lateral incisors was the anticipated plan, and so the unerupted lateral incisors and supernumerary teeth in the cleft were removed at the time of surgery.

Orthodontic appliances were placed with segmental arch wires on each of the three maxillary units. Molar bands with headgear tubes were used so that a 0.036 auxiliary wire could be placed during surgery to help stabilize the premaxillary segment with the two posterior maxillary segments. The surgery was executed as described in the text. Bone was harvested from the ilium and grafted to the defects. Mucosa was rotated from the cheek to cover the grafted bone. An occlusal index was also used during surgery to help maintain the position of the premaxilla.

After surgery, healing occurred uneventfully. Clinical and cephalometric examinations confirmed nasal tip elevation with the procedure as well as improved nasal base and upper lip support.

Continued alignment of the incisors after surgery was accomplished. At age 21 years, the premaxilla remains well positioned and in a stable relationship. The fistulas remain closed, and the occlusion has been detailed with cuspid substitution for the lateral incisors (Fig. 56–21C and D).

CASE REPORT

T. J.

A 54-year-old man with a repaired unilateral cleft lip and cleft palate presented with concerns of a failing prosthesis and a large oral–nasal fistula. He desired improvement of the condition, preferably with a fixed prosthesis and with closure of the fistula. The patient admitted to more than 14 previous surgeries. He wore a mustache for most of his adult life because it concealed the disfigurement of the lip.

The examination indicated a flat upper lip with asymmetry concealed by the facial hair (Fig. 56–22A and B). The oral exam revealed a large, removable prosthesis with full palatal coverage to obturate the nasal maxillary defect (Fig. 56–22C and D). The clinical and radiographic exams confirmed poor bone support for the central incisor adjacent to the cleft (Fig. 56–22E, F, G, and H).

Surgical and prosthetic options, including a bone graft and enosseous implants and a fixed prosthetic appliance, were discussed in addition to fixed and removable prostheses. Time and cost were not an issue. The patient opted for the surgical plan (Fig. 56–22I, J, K, and L).

The periodontally involved incisor adjacent to the cleft was removed. Feasibility model surgery indicated that a posterior maxillary osteotomy could be performed and the segment advanced approximately 1 cm to reduce the size of the nasal maxillary defect.

Turnover flaps from the tissues surrounding the nasal maxillary defect were used to close the nasal side. These flaps, combined with a vomer flap, facilitated the nasal closure.

The incision designed for the posterior maxillary osteotomy was a high, horizontal incision without a palatal incision on the cleft side. The blood supply was the mucosa of the posterior maxilla and palate. The segment was mobilized and advanced into an occlusal splint and stabilized with a biodegradable bone plate (Fig. 56–22M).

A block of corticocancellous bone from the ilium was carved, inserted into the nasal maxillary defect, and secured with a biodegradable bone plate. Oral–mucosal coverage was achieved by a rotational palatal flap on the left and a large mucoperiosteal flap from the left buccal side.

Healing occurred uneventfully. Six months later, a second bone graft was required to provide enough height and width to the ridge for endosseous implants. The implants were placed and restored so that no removable prosthesis was needed. Complete closure of the defect was achieved (Fig. 56–22N). Three years following prosthetic rehabilitation and 5 years postoperatively, the defect remains closed. The prosthetic and aesthetic results are satisfactory (Fig. 56–22O, P, Q, R, S, and T).

References

1. Millard DR. *Cleft Craft: The Evolution of Its Surgery.* Boston: Little, Brown and Co., 1976, 1977, 1980.
2. Lexer E. Die verwendung der freien knochenplastik nebst versucler uber gelenentransplantation. *Arch Klin Chir* 86:942, 1908.
3. Drachter R. Die gaumenpalate und cherenoperative berandlung. *Dtach Zachr Chir* 134:2, 1914.
4. Von Eiselsberg TW. Zur technik der uranoplastik. *Arch Klin Chir* 64:509, 1901.
5. Koberg WR. Present view on bone grafting in cleft palate: A review of the literature. *J Maxillofac Surg* 1:185, 1973.
6. Schmid E. Die Annaherung der Kieferstempfebei Lippen-Kiefer. Gaumensplaten: Ihre schadlichen Folgen und Vermeidung. *Forschr Keifer Gesichtschir* 1:168, 1955.
7. Schrudde J, Stellmach R. Primary osteoplasty of defects of the inferior maxillary arch in cleft palate and harelip in infants; preliminary report. *Zentralbl Chir* 12;83(15):849–859, 1958.
8. Schuchard K. Primary bone grafting in clefts of lip, alveolus and palate. In Gibson T (ed). *Modern Trends in Plastic Surgery, Vol 2.* London: Butterworths, 1966.
9. Brauer RO, Cronin, TD, Reaves EL. Early maxillary orthopedics, orthodontia, and alveolar bone grafting in complete clefts of the palate. *Plast Reconstr Surg* 29:625, 1962.
10. Georgiade HG, Pickrell LK, Quinn GW. Varying concepts in bone grafing of alveolar palate defects. *Cleft Palate J* 1:43, 1964.
11. Kriens O. Primary osteoplasty in patients with clefts of lip, alveolus and palate. *Acta Otorhinolaryngol Belg* 22:687, 1968.
12. Lonacre JJ. Diskussion zum Vortrag von R. Stellmach: Modern procedures in uni-and bilateral clefts of the lip, alveolus and hard palate with respect to primary osteoplasty. In Schuchardt K (ed). *Treatment of Patients with Clefts of Lip, Alveolus, and Palate: 2nd Hamburg International Symposium,* July 6–8, 1964. Stuttgart, Germany: Thieme, 1966.
13. Lynch JB, Lewis SR, Blocker RG, Jr. Maxillary bone grafts in cleft palate patients. *Plast Reconstru Surg* 37:91, 1966.
14. Pickrell KG, Quinn R, Massengill K. Primary bone grafting of the maxilla in clefts of the lip and palate: A four-year study. *Plast Reconstr Surg* 41:438, 1968.
15. Robertson NRE, Jolleys A. Effects of early bone grafting in complete clefts of the lip and palate. *Plast Reconstr Surg* 42:414, 1968.
16. Rohrmann AH, Koberg WR, Koch H. Long term postoperative results of primary and secondary bone grafting in complete clefts of the lip and palate. *Cleft Palate J* 7:206, 1970.
17. Jolleys A, Robertson NRE. A study of the effect of early bone grafting in complete clefts of the lip and palate: Five year study. *Brit J Plast Surg* 25: 229, 1972.
18. Rosenstein SW, Monroe CW, Kernaham DA, et al. The case for early bone grafting in cleft lip and cleft palate. *Plast Reconstr Surg* 70:297, 1983.
19. Rosenstein SW, Monroe CW, Kernahan DA, Jacobson BN, Griffith BH, Bauer BS. The case for early bone grafting in cleft lip and palate. *Plast Reconstr Surg* 70:297–309, 1982.
20. Rosenstein SW, Dada DV, Kernahan DA, Griffith BH, Grassechi J. The case for early bone grafting in cleft lip and palate. *Plast Reconstr Surg* 87:644–653, 1991.
21. Boyne PJ, Sands NE. 12 Secondary bone grafting of residual alveolar and palatal clefts. *J Oral Surg* 30:87, 1972.
22. Boyne PJ. Use of marrow-cancellous bone grafts in maxillary alveolar and palatal clefts. *J Dent Pros* 53:821, 1974.
23. Abyholm FE, Bergland O, Semb G. Secondary bone grafting of alveolar clefts. *Scand J Plastic Reconstr Surg* 15:127–140, 1981.
24. Turvey TA, Vig K, Moriarty J, Hoke J. Delayed bone grafting in the cleft maxilla and palate: A retrospective multidisciplinary analysis. *Am J Orthod* 86:244, 1984.
25. Semb G. *Analysis of the Oslo Cleft Lip and Palate Archive: Long term dentofacial development [Thesis].* Oslo, Norway: University of Oslo, 1991.
26. Rosenstein SW, Long JR, RE, Dado DV, Vinson B, Alder ME. Comparison of 2-D calculations from periapical and occlusal radiographs versus 3-D calculations from CAT scans in determining bone support for cleft-adjacent teeth following early alveolar bone grafts. *Cleft Palate Craniofac J* 34:195–198, 1997.
27. Kindelan JD, Nashed RR, Bromige MR. Radiographic assessment of secondary autogenous alveolar bone grafting in cleft lip and palate patients. *Cleft Palate Craniofac J* 34:195–198, 1997.
28. Wolfe SA, Berkowitz S. The use of cranial bone grafts in the closure of and anterior palatal clefts. *Plast Reconstr Surg* 72:659, 1983.
29. Harsha BC, Turvey TA, Powers SK. The use of autogenous cranial bone grafts in maxillary surgery: A preliminary report. *J Oral Maxillofac Surg* 44:11, 1986.
30. Sinder-Pedersen S, Enemark H. Reconstruction of alveolar clefts with mandibular or iliac crest bone grafts: A comparative study. *J Oral Maxillofac Surg* 48:554–558, 1990.
31. Tessier P, Kawamoto H, et al. Taking tibial grafts in the diaphysis and upper epiphysis–tools and techniques IV. *Plast Reconstr Surg* 116(Suppl): 47S–53S, 2005.
32. Maxon BB, Baxter SD, Vig KWL, et al. Allogeneic bone for secondary alveolar cleft osteoplasty. *J Oral Maxillofac Surg* 48:933–941, 1990.
33. Kraut RA. The use of allogeneic bone for alveolar cleft grafting. *Oral Surg Oral Med Oral Pathol* 64:278, 1987.
34. Verdi FJ. Use of Branemark implant in the cleft palate patient. *Cleft Palate Craniofacial J* 28:301, 1991.
35. Farmand M. Enossale implantate bei der kieferosteoplastik. In Schwamzer N (ed). *Fortscritt der Kiefer und Gesichts Chirurgie Band, Vol 38.* Stuttgart, Germany: Thieme, 1993, pp. 112–114.

57

Alveolar Transport Distraction Osteogenesis

Bruce B. Horswell, MD, DDS, MS, FACS • Nicholas J.V. Hogg, MD, DDS, MSc, FRCDS(c)

HISTORY OF ALVEOLAR CLEFT REPAIR

Management of the alveolar cleft defect has been a challenging and oft-experimented entity in the care of patients with orofacial clefts. The alveolar cleft defect (ACD) results from attempts at repair or partial repairs performed during cleft lip and/or palatal surgery. Typically, ACDs result in a collapsed, disunited arch with unsupported lip, nasal and dental elements. The concomitant oronasal fistula is a veritable depot of foul, inflammatory-provoking debris that contributes to sinonasal inflammation, drainage, and periodontitis. Therefore, closure and repair of the osseous defect is considered an important aspect of complete cleft management.

Repair of the ACD has a long history in cleft care. Goals for the ACD treatment are[1,2]

1. Continuous unified maxillary arch
2. Obturation of the oronasal fistula
3. Provide lip and nasal alar support
4. Provide dental and periodontal support

Attempts at closure by simply performing gingivoperiosteoplasty at lip repair has met with varying results, oftentimes necessitating future formal repair with bone grafts. Timing of ACD repair also has been controversial. Primary osteoplasty with placement of autogenous bone at or near

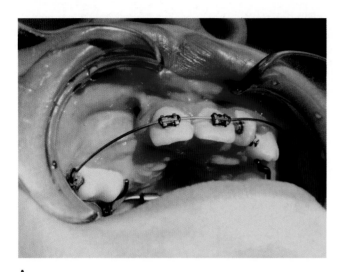

A

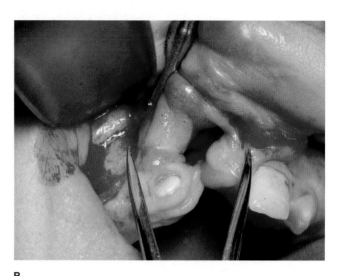

B

Figure 57–1. (A) Right unilateral cleft defect demonstrating wide, disparate alveolar segments. **(B)** Right unilateral cleft with deficient soft tissue and wide bone defect.

the time of initial lip repair has been both condemned and championed. Many results have been wanting, again with the need for further bony augmentation of the alveolar segment.[3–5]

Secondary osteoplasty of the ACD is considered the "gold standard" of many cleft teams principally because it is predictable and achievable, satisfying the goals of repair as stated above. Early secondary osteoplasty, as advanced by Boyne and Sands,[6–8] attempts to graft the ACD prior to eruption of the permanent incisors. Later secondary osteoplasty as reported by some[9,10] has been shown to be effective and predictable for most children when grafted prior to the complete root formation of the adult canine tooth or 10–12 years of age. Later secondary osteoplasty is usually performed in conjunction with preparatory orthodontics after some orthopedic manipulation to optimally position the cleft segment.

However, there still exists a significant number of patients who have failed bone graft attempts, have very wide defects or collapsed cleft segments with defects, or have significantly scarred ACDs with questionable soft tissue covering all of which make further attempts at bone grafting rather dubious and unsatisfying. This is an entity aptly termed the "recalcitrant" ACD (Fig. 57–1), which is a challenge due to the lack of healthy, unscarred mucogingiva covering the ACD; deficient alveolar bone height and width against which graft must be placed; older patients with decreased bony healing potential; or compromised dentition or prostheses with little bone support.[11]

Recently, distraction osteogenesis (DO) has been developed for application in the craniofacial region. Smaller regional areas of the facial skeleton have been distracted in order to optimize functional and aesthetic units for future orthopedic/orthodontic correction, grafting procedures, or prosthodontic rehabilitation. A summary of the history and application of DO follows.

HISTORY OF DISTRACTION OSTEOGENESIS

Principles of Distraction Osteogenesis

The concept of DO was initially described by Codivilla[12] in 1905. He used the technique to lengthen a femur to correct a limb length discrepancy. In the 1950s, this application was applied to orthopedic limb lengthening. The landmark research into this technique by IIizarov[13] looked at the development of distraction techniques, devices, and rates on bone formation. He developed the technique on canine long bones and then applied the protocol that he had developed to a human model. He pioneered many of the concepts of DO including recommendations on latency, distraction rate, and distraction rhythm.

Maxillofacial Application

McCarthy[14] was able to apply DO for unilateral mandibular deficiency found in hemifacial microsomia in which he lengthened the affected mandible in children. He used an external fixation device that allowed calibrated distraction between external pins holders. At the completion of the distraction phase, the mandibles were stabilized for a mean period of 9 weeks.

DO of the midfacial region has been accomplished by devices that can be categorized into internal and external devices. Various maxillary devices have been used for DO in the midfacial region to advance the maxilla through various osteotomies at LeFort levels or segmentation of the maxilla.[15] These procedures are more thoroughly presented in the chapter on Maxillary Distraction Osteogenesis by Polley et al. in this volume.

In terms of maxillary arch widening, a DO technique was applied via rapid palatal expansion by Bell and Epker,[16] who used a tooth-borne expander to increase the transverse dimension of the maxilla after osteotomies had been performed. These techniques were further developed by Guerrero and Bell.[17] These authors utilized incremental expansions of 1 mm every other day up to a total of 10 mm to obtain significant transverse expansion of the arch. This concept was applied to alveolar segment distraction by Chin and Toth,[18] who looked at regenerating alveolar bone after trauma using an internal device with a transmucosal activation screw. Block and Baughman[19] further applied DO to vertically deficient alveolar segments to increase bone height prior to implant placement. Simultaneous bone grafting was performed in many of these cases after final alveolar segment distraction. Use of alveolar distraction is now widespread for preprosthetic manipulation prior to rehabilitation.[20]

Cleft alveolar distraction has been performed and studied by Liou and coworkers.[21] Utilizing various osteotomies and appliances, they have been able to approximate cleft segments to narrow the defect and improve arch dimension. Others[22-25] also have applied DO to correct various cleft-related problems in the maxilla, narrow or collapsed arches, wide alveolar cleft, disproportionate and insufficient soft tissue, and a desire to avoid having to bone graft a defect. Distraction has become an important tool in the management of some difficult alveolar defects, as will be presented later in the chapter.

PREPARATION FOR ALVEOLAR DISTRACTION OSTEOGENESIS

Patient Selection

Alveolar distraction in those with a maxillary cleft defect requires careful patient selection. Most patients with sizeable ACDs will generally be in their mid-childhood years or older. This necessarily provides a large set of patients who may be eligible for consideration for distraction; however, several limiting factors reduce patient suitability. First and foremost, a very young or dentally immature person (less than 7-8 years of age) may be difficult to achieve a satisfactory result due to the presence of a mixed dentition or unerupted teeth, which may interfere with osteotomies or distractor placement. Young children will also have difficulty managing the aspect of intraoral distraction and the high demand for excellent oral hygiene practices. Also, those patients with handicapping conditions such as Attention Deficit Hyperactivity Disorder, neurodevelopmental delay or psychological issues probably will not be cooperative or be able to comply with postoperative distraction and care.

The optimal patient candidate for DO is established in team care, has a proven track record of compliance, can demonstrate basic oral hygiene practices, and has a supportive family or caregiver dynamic. Also, those patients and families who live a distance from the cleft team may have difficulty making many office or clinic visits for surveillance checks. These adjunctive resources may be utilized to give intermediate treatment or assistance should a need arise in the distraction and consolidation phases of treatment. All of these factors contribute to DO success on the smaller scale of intraoral alveolar transport.

Indications

There are several indications for alveolar transport DO. A very wide alveolar cleft defect may preclude a bone graft if there is deficient soft tissue and native alveolar bone (Fig. 57–1). A patient who has had a previous failed bone graft may be considered for transport DO to achieve the surgical and anatomical goals of alveolar cleft surgery (Fig. 57–2). Older patients who have not been treated for their alveolar cleft defect are less common, but these patients may be candidates for transport DO to narrow the defect and thus require minimal grafting and improve success for prosthetic rehabilitation.

Alveolar cleft defects that are by nature multidimensional may have different combinations of the defect in the anteroposterior, lateral, and vertical dimensions. Depending on the proportion between native tissues and the alveolar defect, transport DO may be considered for definitive treatment or to address the largest dimensional deficiency and thereby improve the quality and quantity of native alveolar bone to allow for an easier and minimal secondary bone graft procedure. This is particularly true in vertical alveolar deficiency. Vertical alveolar DO may also be considered to increase alveolar bone height after grafting for later prosthetic rehabilitation, most notably in planned placement of an implant.

Contraindications

There are several contraindications to alveolar cleft DO. If the patient, who is usually well known to the cleft surgeon by the time that the alveolar cleft defect needs to be addressed, has not been compliant in some aspects of their treatment, then the surgeon should be wary in initiating treatment. DO is a very labor-intensive process that requires a great deal of cooperation from the patient, the family, and their caregivers. If the patient has a poor compliance history, patient education is crucial before initiating treatment.

Patients with active dental issues should be addressed and consideration should be given to optimizing oral health prior to surgery. The presence of periapical disease should be investigated and eliminated to avoid infection during the distraction period. In patients who are younger than 10 years of age, potential exists for damage to developing teeth and impairing the eruption pattern in the area of distraction. This needs to be thoroughly discussed with the patient and family beforehand.

Indirectly associated with compliance is the patient's health and local tissue conditions. If there is a question about this issue, it may be prudent to avoid a very focused logistical and mechanical procedure than managing the problems of tissue breakdown and slough or loss of tissue and the device if plans were made to perform DO. Children who have poorly controlled asthma, diabetes, chronic allergies with nasal obstruction (mouth-breathing increases oral tissue inflammation), may be patients who are more prone to intraoral tissue problems and breakdown. For that reason, optimal tissue health will need to be documented and maintained through primary care and pediatric dental management. Once this has been satisfied then plans for distraction can be undertaken.

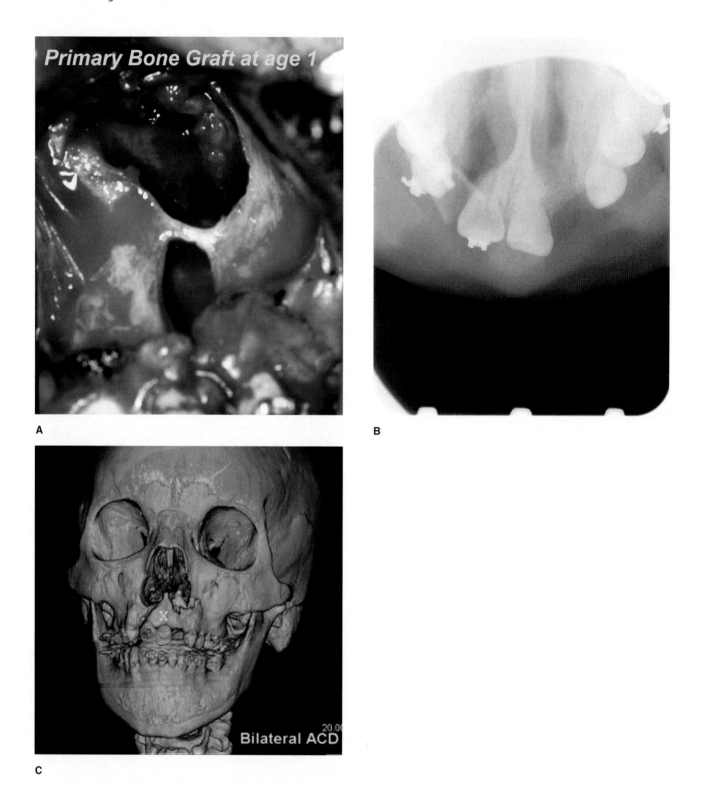

Figure 57–2. (**A**) Failed primary osteoplasty with persistent defect. Fistula and insufficient osseous support for dental structures. (Intraoperative photo). (**B**) Partial osteoplasty of a asymmetric cleft defect with failure of graft on the patient's right. (Radiograph). (**C**) Three-dimensional CT demonstrating partial osteoplasty on left and complete failure on the right side.

Patient Preparation

As with all aspects of cleft surgery, the management of the ACD is no different from other aspects of comprehensive cleft management and requires a team approach. Preparing the patient for the rigors that they will undergo is important

prior to the initiation of alveolar transport DO. There is a need for coordination of the team that will be involved in perioperative management.

Orthodontic consultation and management is important to address dental and arch discrepancies prior to the

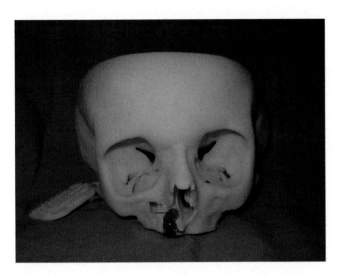

Figure 57–3. Acrylic model of right unilateral cleft defect (x) demonstrating planned distraction of the alveolar segment (arrow, →).

assessment of a patient for repair of the ACD whether by conventional bone grafting or by movement of the alveolar bone using distraction. The arch may require expansion prior to formal repair of the alveolar cleft. The orthodontist must be involved in the planning of and, possibly, management during distraction. Certainly, finishing dental and arch alignment is the orthodontist's responsibility.

Prosthodontic management of the patient may be required postoperatively for the replacement of missing teeth. This may involve the placement of crowns or bridges or the surgical placement of implants if there is satisfactory bone stock. The patient must understand that the bone must be completely mature prior to the placement of implants, a period of approximately 3 months.[26] Consultation with the prosthodontist is important to evaluate the arch space and bone height that will be needed for prosthetic rehabilitation.

The patient's pediatric dentist should be involved well before transport DO is started to optimize oral health at the time of surgery. Any carious lesions should be addressed and periodontal disease eradicated before the patient is assessed. Questionable or nonvital teeth should be addressed and treated before DO is begun to eliminate the possibility of infection jeopardizing the distraction process.

For reasons discussed before, the family members who will be involved in the day-to-day management of the distractor need to be prepared prior to the initiation of treatment. Three-dimensional acrylic models (Fig. 57–3) are a great help to the patient and caregivers who will perform the activation. Precise placement and activation of the device can be achieved and demonstrated, respectively. The caregivers need to be instructed in the cleansing and hygiene of the activation rod. Perioperative antibacterial mouthrinses (oral chlorhexidine) and indicated antibiotics should be carefully reviewed and dispensed. Pain medications and dietary instructions will need to be adjusted based on individual patient's needs. Most children will have adequate analgesia with ibuprofen, which

may be administered prior to and after each distraction event, as indicated.

Instructing the patient and caregivers in the objectives of DO and creating realistic expectations for what can be achieved is important. Instructions for care may need to be given in stages and over several appointments to create a thorough understanding before and during treatment. The patient and family need to know that DO may not be able to completely correct the anatomic deficits that preexisted prior to the initiation of treatment. Further, surgery as a second stage will be required to remove the distractor, and at this time, the defect can be simultaneously augmented with additional bone graft if necessary. As in many cleft defect reconstructions, final and acceptable soft tissue coverage may be needed to provide adequate attached gingiva around teeth and implants.

CASE EXAMPLES

Unilateral Cleft Defect

Unilateral ACDs are more common, obviously, and often have problems with significant asymmetry and excessive defect width. Although interceptive, skilled orthodontics can successfully align and position the lesser segment and narrow the defect width, there will remain some poorly positioned cleft segments or cleft defects, which will have suboptimal tissue conditions that compromise or prohibit orthodontic treatment.

A typical case is illustrated in Fig. 57–4. This patient had a long history of lip and nasal surgical procedures as well as two phases of orthodontics. The ACD is still poorly positioned, has extensively scarred soft tissue, and the radiographs verify significant bony defect width between the segments. This is a difficult condition to correct with conventional orthodontic preparation and bone grafting. Therefore, distraction of the cleft segment to prepare the defect by approximating the alveolar segments will increase the success of a smaller bone graft. A single vector alveolar distractor is placed on the buccal aspect of the lesser segment after vertical osteotomy between the bicuspids and transversely, approximately 7–8 mm above the level of the root apices, with the activating rod oriented in a favorable position under the lip for easy access. Pre- and postdistraction photos demonstrate a more favorably positioned ACD for bone grafting.

Many alveolar distractors offer various distracting lengths (10–20 mm) and multiple options for plate and screw placement (Fig. 57–5). This is necessary in order to position the device passively onto the bony contour surface such that activation will move the segment in the desired direction. Also, some distractors allow reorientation of the activation rod from 0° (coaxial to the distractor) to 30° in order to allow favorable rod positioning and access for daily activation. Minimal activation should be performed on table in order to avoid undue tension on the overlying soft tissue, which may tear and compromise vascularity if excessive activation

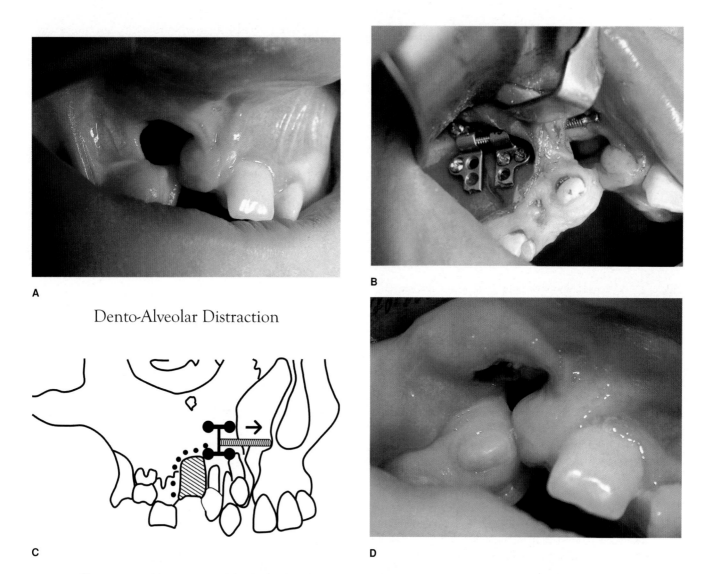

Figure 57–4. (**A**) Preoperative photo of wide unilateral cleft defect. (**B**) Intraoperative photo of alveolar distractor (15 mm) to move the dentoalveolar segment anteriorly 10 mm. (**C**) Illustration demonstrating dento-alveolar distraction of the cuspid-bicuspid segment. (**D**) Postoperative photo demonstrating firm docking of the alveolar segments and significant narrowing of the defect in preparation for final osteoplasty.

is performed. Two or three millimeters of activation to confirm mobility will suffice at the time of distractor placement.

There is no consensus on a latent period after distractor placement for maxillary alveolar cleft segments.[15] Since there is little intrabony interface and the soft tissue is often compromised, a latent period of 3–5 days is appropriate. Slow activation—0.5 mm/day to 1 mm every other day regimens will suffice to move the lesser segment into position. If orthodontic brackets are in place, "a light" elastic band can be applied to assist in segment orientation, particularly for vertical or lateral readjustments in orientation (see Fig. 57–5A). If elastics are utilized, vigilance to confirm and correct movement without soft tissue compromise is necessary.

After a period of active movement, the alveolar segments will firmly abut at the soft tissue interface. Blanching at the interface will confirm maximum distraction. At this time, the device can be left for a period of several weeks to

allow some osseous maturation. A second-stage procedure is then planned for removal of the device and simultaneous closure of the oronasal–palatal fistula with placement of a small bone graft.[22] The surgeon will note that simple gingivoperiosteoplasty is all that is necessary for a tension-free closure in many of these cases. Access to the nasal mucosa may be limited, thus nasal floor reconstruction is often performed via the nasal cavity. Additional access to this area can be gained through partial anterior turbinectomy, if hypertrophied, and endoscopic-assisted visualization may assist with nasal–mucosal elevation and effective nasal floor closure.

Bilateral Cleft Defects

Bilateral ACDs are less common but may be more problematic for treatment if considerable palatal collapse or premaxillary protrusion is present or if there is an amputated or stunted

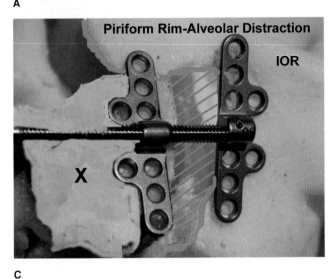

A

Dento-Alveolar-Piriform Distraction

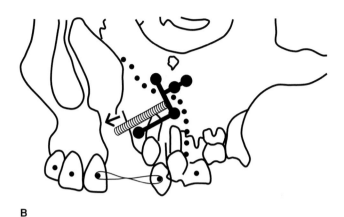

B

Piriform Rim-Alveolar Distraction

IOR

X

C

Figure 57–5. (A) Three-dimensional CT demonstrating a left alveolar defect and significant piriform rim and maxillary hypoplasia. **(B)** Illustration of left alveolar defect with piriform hypoplasia and planned dentoalveolar piriform distraction to narrow the defect and augment the piriform rim. **(C)** Acrylic model with left alveolar defect, planned alveolar piriform (x) distraction with device (20 mm) in place to determine vector, adaptation to the osseous surface, screw placement, and activation rod access. IOR: infraorbital rim, solid line: outline of osteotomy, dashed line: distractant distance.

premaxillary segment (Fig. 57–6). Orthodontic expansion through orthopedic devices, alone or surgical-assisted, will be the preferred method of alveolar positioning. Sometimes, the cleft defect dimensions are disparate or the cleft segments asymmetric, (Fig. 57–7) and if significant scarring is present, particularly on the palate, satisfactory orthodontic expansion may not be possible.[21] Surgical assistance, through tunneled buccal cortical osteotomy, and placement of an oblique palatal–tooth-borne expander as the first stage may be indicated. After adequate expansion has been achieved, then second-stage distraction can be planned. Generally, a latent period of several weeks after expansion will allow palatal mucosal maturation and safe reflection of the buccal mu-

coperiosteum for distractor placement (Fig. 57–8). During buccal segment exposure, vigilance is necessary to ensure adequate vascularity on the palate. If any ischemia of the palatal tissues is observed, the procedure should be deferred for 2 weeks, then plans made for a tunneling procedure and osteotomy without buccal soft tissue reflection. The lesser segment can then be digitally mobilized and slowly brought forward through a combination of orthodontics and elastics.

Simultaneous distraction of bilateral posterior segments can also be undertaken. A benefit of bilateral distraction is narrowing the defects to such a degree that minimal bone graft is required to finalize reconstruction i.e., less harvested bone from one site, or less alloplast necessary. A

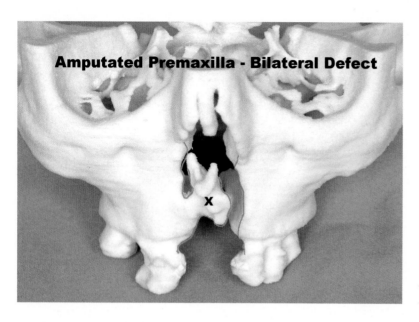

Figure 57–6. Amputated premaxilla in a patient with bilateral cleft demonstrating deficient and asymmetric bone stock on an acrylic model.

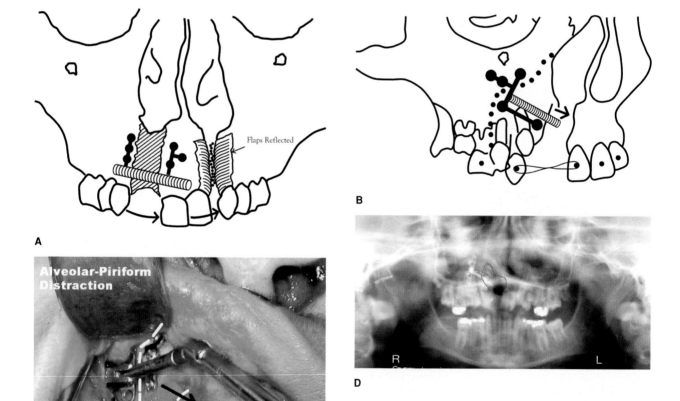

Figure 57–7. (A) Illustration demonstrating dentoalveolar distraction of asymmetric bilateral cleft defects due to failed osteoplasty with persistent defects. The figure demonstrates distraction of the premaxillary segment to the larger defect side in preparation for osteoplasty. Stippled: bone graft. Lines: distractant. **(B)** Illustration of asymmetric bilateral cleft defects after failed osteoplasty on the right. The figure demonstrates alveolar-piriform distraction to close or approximate the segment toward the premaxilla. **(C)** Intraoperative photo demonstrating distraction and vector of alveolar segment (arrow), the osteotomy (dashed line) and stable posterior maxilla (x). **(D)** Panoramic radiograph with distractor in place, the osteotomized alveolar segment (yellow dashed line) and large cleft defect (red line).

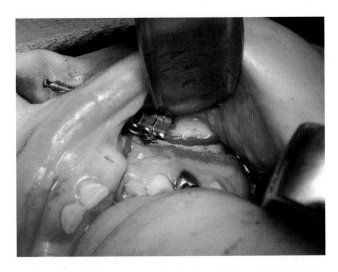

Figure 57–8. Intraoperative photo showing second-stage buccal corticotomy after palatal expansion of an asymmetric bilateral cleft.

disadvantage of simultaneous bilateral DO is the amount of oral hardware and consequent activation and hygiene required.

A patient with bilateral ACDs is illustrated in Fig. 57–9. This patient has undergone previous bone grafts with failure of the graft on the right side due to excessive width without adequate soft tissue coverage. The piriform rim is also more hypoplastic on the right side.

Therefore, unidirectional distraction is planned for anterior–inferior movement of the piriform alveolar cleft complex to narrow the left defect, move the piriform rim down and anteriorly, and finally, improve soft tissue coverage for a final bone graft. Three-dimensional CT reconstructions are helpful in evaluating the bone deficiencies as well as planning appropriate osteotomies and desirable movement of the distracted cleft segment. Simultaneous removal of the device and a small autogenous bone graft at a second stage will complete the alveolar cleft reconstruction. Postoperative finishing orthodontics can commence 3 months after grafting.

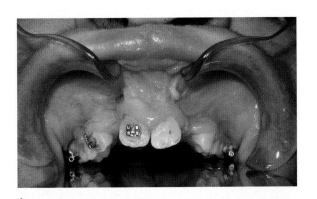

A

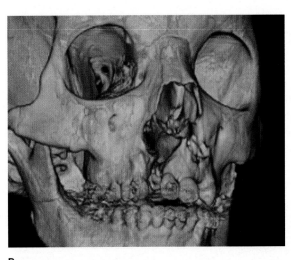

B

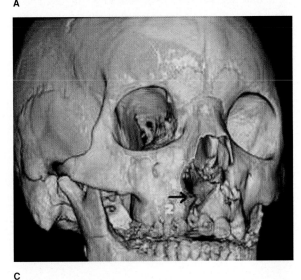

C

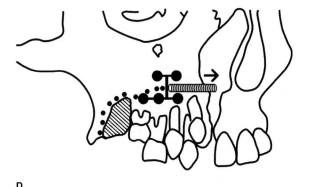

Dento-Alveolar-Piriform Distraction

D

Figure 57–9. (**A**) Patient with bilateral cleft postosteoplasty with failed graft on right. (**B**) Three-dimensional reconstruction of patient showing severe right alveolar defect and piriform hypoplasia. (**C**) Three-dimensional reconstruction demonstrating planned osteotomy for (1) dentoalveolar piriform or (2) dentoalveolar segment distraction to narrow the defect (red) and possibly augment the piriform rim, respectively. (**D**) Illustration of planned dentoalveolar piriform distraction.

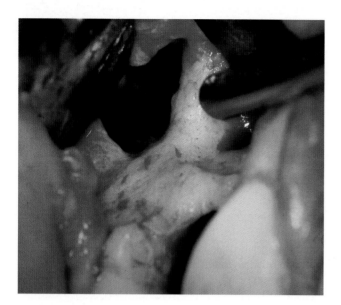

Figure 57–10. Intraoperative photo of a thin, hypoplastic alveolus after secondary osteoplasty.

Postgrafted Defect

Most well-planned and executed bone graft cases will heal with adequate bone stock to satisfy the objectives given earlier. However, some defects will heal with a small bone bridge or thin alveolar table and require further augmentation (Fig. 57–10). A very narrow bridge (less than 25% of the native alveolar height) probably is best augmented by retreatment as a full defect and/or distraction of the lesser segment to optimize subsequent regrafting.

A vertically deficient but sufficiently wide grafted defect can be distracted (Fig. 57–11) to augment the height of the

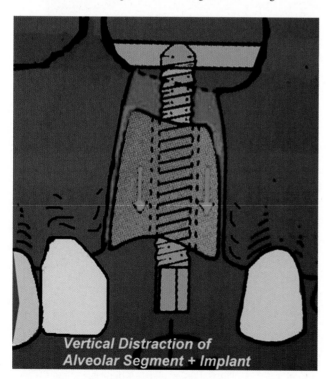

Figure 57–11. Illustration of vertical distraction of an alveolar segment to increase bony height.

alveolar bone.[19,20,26] Regenerated bone must mature before any implant placement or prosthetic rehabilitation is undertaken. Often further augmentation of the alveolar width with bone graft or substitute will be indicated, particularly on the facial aspect where implant threads may become exposed. If graft material is placed, then a barrier membrane or connective tissue graft should be placed to optimize bone healing and maintain sufficient bulk.[27]

HAZARDS AND COMPLICATIONS

Most of the complications with regard to distraction procedures have been observed and documented from the studies of mandibular and midfacial distraction. Smaller segmental distractions have been a more recent development and less is known about distraction problems and complications of the smaller and sometimes more challenging anatomical regions. As in the larger distraction cases, alveolar cleft distraction complications fall in three basic categories: poor patient compliance (and poor regional tissue); faulty surgical planning; and device (mechanical) failure.[28,29]

Poor patient compliance and health remain an area much outside of the surgeon's purview and control; however, every effort must be made to optimize this concern. As discussed previously, intraoral distraction requires tedious oral hygiene, careful and accurate activation, maintenance of periodic evaluation visits, and vigilance for any mechanical or tissue-related problems. Generally speaking, the surgeon will have some appreciation of a particular patient's compliance record and health history.

Poor surgical planning often results in a poorly vectored and positioned segment. If at all possible, having a three-dimensional acrylic model available with which to visualize, plan, and instruct is very valuable (Fig. 57–12). Placing surgical cuts and fashioning or molding the device on the model will help to determine the correct vector, distances necessary

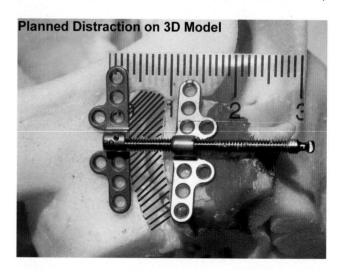

Figure 57–12. Planned distraction of cleft alveolar piriform process. Actual osteotomy, distractor placement, and distance necessary to achieve proper osseous bulk and contour can be accurately determined on an acrylic model. Red: defect, blue: distractant.

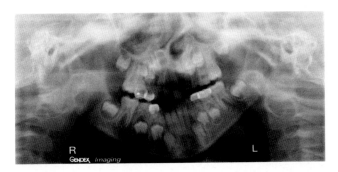

A

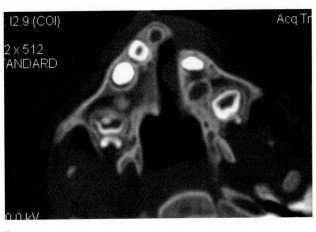

B

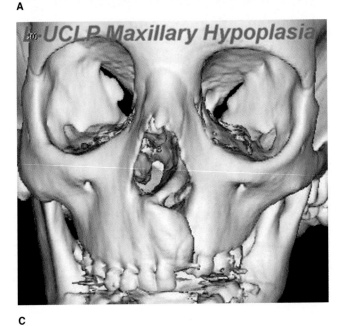

C

Figure 57–13. (**A**) Panoramic radiograph of left cleft defect. (**B**) CT (axial) scan demonstrating same defect with tooth roots visible for planned corticotomies. (**C**) Three-dimensional CT scan of left cleft defect.

for distraction (and appropriate length of device), and ideal placement of the activation rod. Actually, demonstrating the procedure on a model with device distraction will help the patient and family understand what is taking place, how to perform distraction, and the time involved until completion.

Obviously, precise narrow bony cuts, preservation of a vascular mucoperiosteum, and avoiding teeth roots are necessary to ensure a predictable and satisfactory result. Buccal corticotomies are planned for optimal placement between dental segments or the posterior alveolar segment in a modified LeFort I design. Precision corticotomy placement requires adequate radiographs (Fig. 57–13) to determine bone contour and bulk and root configuration. This may necessitate obtaining CT (axial and coronal sections) scans for accurate evaluation and confirmation of precise osteotomies.

Relapse of distracted segments has been reported.[15,29,30] Most reports are on maxillary or midfacial (LeFort I–III) distraction and the potential for relapse due to cleft-related scar retraction. There is one report of vertically distracted alveolar segments, which underwent "relapse" or significant remodeling after distraction and initial healing.[30] A 25% overcorrection was recommended to overcome this potential late problem.

Mechanical failure of a distractor device occurs as a result of two basic mechanisms: device fatigue from overapplied forces; and screw failure or pull out.[31] Device (metal) fatigue results from attempts at overdistraction of a rigid osseous segment, excessive torsional mechanics of the activation rod with thread stripping, and failure of coupling of rod to device, typically when disaxial forces are applied. Most of these problems will be eliminated if careful preoperative planning with acrylic skull models is carried out.[29] Also, care must be exercised to confirm that a nearly free alveolar (dentoalveolar) segment is achieved intraoperatively whilst preserving mucoperiosteal attachment and viability. On-table activation will confirm segment mobility.

Screw failure may result from inadequate fixation of either the stable or mobile segments. Usually, three screws are necessary to ensure alveolar device fixation. Also, placement of stable screws requires healthy cortical bone to hold and resist pressure and pull out forces placed across the screw–bone interface when activated. Finally, faulty screw manufacture may render a weak screw head–shank interface susceptible to shearing forces, which will ultimately give way under activation. Although unfortunate, planning for at least three screws will negate faulty screw placement or integrity.

Usually, all of the above problems will not result in loss of an alveolar segment, however, compromise of the vascular pedicle will. At all times, beginning from osteotomy and on-table activation to the distraction phase, if there is any suggestion of vascular compromise, i.e., prolonged cyanosis, ischemia, swelling, tissue slough, loosening of teeth, etc., then all activation should be halted, dental stabilization achieved, and consideration given to optimizing tissue health. This can be achieved through local hygiene measures and also the incorporation of hyperbaric oxygen management. Hyperbaric oxygen cannot reverse avascular necrosis and these segments will be ultimately lost; however, ischemic segments, as is typically seen in alveolar distraction, can be salvaged and go on to eventual healing.

CONCLUSIONS

DO is a valuable tool in the management of the alveolar cleft defect, especially wide defects with poor soft tissue. Approximating the alveolar segments is achievable through DO and helpful in preparation for final bone grafting and orthodontic/prosthodontic treatment.

Careful patient selection and preparation is paramount in DO technique and success. Preoperative (pre-DO) patient/family counseling, team coordination, planning with CT three-dimensional reconstruction and acrylic models, and perioperative vigilance during distraction for careful activation and hygiene, will ensure a successful outcome. With this in mind, the statement by Suhr and Kreusch[29] at the end of their treatise on distraction will serve well to remember in cleft management: "Clear advantages over conventional osteotomies and bone-grafting are still to be described... DO is a continuous and fluid process which requires careful planning and close observation ... "

References

1. Witsenburg B. The reconstruction of anterior residual bone defects in patients with cleft lip, alveolus and palate: A review. *J Maxillofac Surg* 13:197, 1985.
2. Horswell BB, Henderson JM. Secondary osteoplasty of the alveolar cleft defect. *J Oral Maxillofac Surg* 61:1082, 2003.
3. Ross RB. Treatment variables affecting facial growth in complete unilateral cleft lip and plate. Part 3: Alveolus repair and bone grafting. *Cleft Palate J* 24:33, 1987.
4. Enemark H, Sindet-Pedersen S, Bundgard M. Long-term results after secondary bone grafting of alveolar clefts. *J Oral Maxillofac Surg* 45: 913, 1987.
5. Keese E, Schmelzle R. New findings concerning early bone grafting procedures in patients with cleft lip and palate. *J Craniomaxillofac Surg* 23:296, 1995.
6. Boyne PJ, Sands NR. Secondary bone grafting of residual alveolar and palatal clefts. *J Oral Surg* 30:87, 1972.
7. Cohen M, Polley JW, Figueroa AA. Secondary (intermediate) alveolar bone grafting. *Clin Plast Surg* 20:691, 1993.
8. Lilja J, Kalaaji A, Friede H, et al. Combined bone grafting and delayed closure of the hard palate in patients with unilateral cleft lip and palate. *Cleft Palate Craniofac J* 37:98, 2000.
9. Long RE, Jr., Paterno M, Vinson B. Effect of cuspid positioning in the cleft at the time of secondary alveolar bone grafting on eventual success. *Cleft Palate Craniofac J* 33:225, 1996.
10. Tan A, Brogan W, McComb H, et al. Secondary alveolar bone grafting - five year periodontal and radiographic evaluation in 100 consecutive cases. *Cleft Palate J* 33:513, 1996.
11. Horswell BB. Current approaches to transport distraction of the alveolar cleft. *Preconference Symposium on Management of the Alveolar Cleft, 61st Annual Meeting, American Cleft Palate—Craniofacial Association*, Chicago, March 15, 2004.
12. Codivilla A. On the means of lengthening in the lower limbs, the muscles and tissues which are shortened through deformity. *Am J Orthop Surg* 2:353, 1905.
13. Ilizarov GA. The principles of the Ilizarov method. *Bull Hosp J Dis Orthop Inst* 48:1, 1988.
14. McCarthy JG. The role of distraction osteogenesis in the reconstruction of the mandible in unilateral craniofacial microsomia. *Clin Plast Surg* 21:625, 1994.
15. Swennen G, Schliephake H, Dempf R, et al. Craniofacial distraction osteogenesis: A review of the literature. Part 1: Clinical studies. *Int J Oral Maxillofac Surg* 30:89, 2001.
16. Bell WH, Epker BN. Surgical-orthodontic expansion of the maxilla. *Am J. Orthod* 70:517, 1976.
17. Guerrero CA, Bell WH, Intraoral distraction. In McCarthy JG (ed). *Distraction of the Craniofacial Skeleton.* New York: Springer, 1999, p. 230.
18. Chin M, Toth BA. Distraction osteogenesis in maxillofacial surgery using internal devices: Review of five cases. *J Oral Maxillofac Surg* 54:45, 1996.
19. Block MS, Baughman DG. Reconstruction of severe anterior maxillary defects using distraction osteogenesis, bone grafts, and implants. *J Oral Maxillofac Surg* 63:291, 2005.
20. Landers CA. Implant-borne prosthetic rehabilitation of bone-grafted cleft versus traumatic anterior maxillary defects. *J Oral Maxillofacial Surg* 64:297, 2006.
21. Lion EJW, Chen PKT, Huang CS, et al. Interdental distraction osteogenesis and rapid orthodontic tooth movement: A novel approach to approximate a wide alveolar cleft or bony defect. *Plast Reconstr Surg* 105:1262, 2000.
22. Binger T, Katsaros C, Rucker M, et al. Segment distraction to reduce a wide alveolar cleft before alveolar bone grafting. *Cleft Palate Craniofac J* 40(6):561, 2003.
23. Dolanmaz D, Karaman AI, Durmus E, et al. Management of alveolar clefts using dento-osseous transport distraction osteogenesis. *Angle Orthod* 73:723, 2003.
24. Mitsugi M, Ito O, Alcalde RE. Maxillary bone transportation in alveolar cleft-transport distraction osteogenesis for treatment of alveolar cleft repair. *Br J Plast Surg* 58:619, 2005.
25. Kuroe K, Iino S, Shomura K, et al. Unilateral advancement of the maxillary minor segment by distraction osteogenesis in patients with unrepaired unilateral cleft lip and palate. *Cleft Palate Craniofac J* 40(3):317, 2003.
26. Mazzonetto R, de Maurette MA. Radiographic evaluation of alveolar distraction osteogenesis: Analysis of 60 cases. *J Oral Maxillofac Surg* 63:1708, 2005.
27. Dempf R, Teltzrow T, Kramer FJ, et al. Alveolar bone grafting in patients with complete clefts: A comparative study between secondary and tertiary bone grafting. *Cleft Palate Craniofac J* 39:18, 2002.
28. Cheung LK, Chua HDP. A meta-analysis of cleft maxillary osteotomy and distraction osteogenesis. *Int J Oral Maxillofac Surg* 35:14–24, 2006.
29. Suhr MAA, Kreusch T. Technical considerations in distraction osteogenesis. *Int J Oral Maxillofac Surg* 33:89, 2004.
30. Saulacic N, Somoza-Martin M, Gandara-Vila P, et al. Relapse in alveolar distraction osteogenesis: An indication for overcorrection. *J Oral Maxillofac Surg* 63:978, 2005.
31. Mofid MM, Manson PN, Robertson BC, et al. Craniofacial distraction osteogenesis: A review of 3278 cases. *Plast Reconstr Surgery* 108: 1103, 2001.

58

Treatment Planning for Cleft Orthognathic Surgery

Alvaro A. Figueroa, DDS, MS • John W. Polley, MD

INTRODUCTION

The treatment of cleft patients with secondary maxillo-mandibular discrepancies requires a combined surgical-orthodontic approach. In addition, the nature of the skeletal discrepancy, which in these patients is in great part secondary to the cleft, requires special considerations regarding diagnosis. The thorough diagnostic evaluation will significantly impact the treatment plan and selection of surgical approaches to correct the cleft maxillomandibular discrepancy.

It is well established that the care of patients with maxillomandibular skeletal discrepancies requires a protocol that includes

1. A detailed medical and dental history.
2. A thorough clinical examination of the face, oral cavity, and temporomandibular joints.
3. A detailed photographic, radiographic, and cephalometric evaluation.
4. Evaluation of dental casts.

Based on the above, a treatment plan is formulated by the various specialists involved in the team management of the patient. These specialists include the maxillofacial surgeon, orthodontist, reconstructive dentist, and speech and language pathologist. On occasion, other team members are included, such as mental health professionals to emotionally support the patients and their families prior to and during the active phase of treatment.

Once the initial diagnostic data is evaluated and all involved professionals understand their role for the particular patient, the preparatory steps for care are initiated. This chapter will limit itself to treatment planning from the dental-orthodontic and surgical perspective.

After it is determined that the overall health and oral health of the patient is satisfactory, orthodontic treatment can be commenced. It is the role of the orthodontist to perform all necessary dental alignment procedures to facilitate surgery, and assure stability of the dentition and occlusion after surgery. The orthodontic appliances will also provide the surgeon with modes of fixation during the intraoperative and postoperative period of surgical care. In addition, the orthodontist must decide on the occlusal relations and specific dental positions required before surgery, and the desired postoperative dental occlusion and relations at the completion of treatment.

The stability of the dentition is achieved by positioning the teeth with the right inclination relative to their supporting bone bases. This applies to the anterior as well as the posterior dentition. The position of the anterior and posterior teeth, relative to their bases, is what orthodontists call "torque" of the crowns and roots. The orthodontist must place the posterior teeth in the correct vertical and transverse position relative to the supporting alveolar bone. The required movements are determined during the clinical examination, cast evaluation, and to a lesser extent, cephalometric evaluation. The use of a frontal cephalometric radiograph might be required to evaluate the inclination or torque of the posterior teeth.

Also critical to treatment planning is the sagittal position of the maxillary and mandibular incisors relative to their supporting bone. The position of the incisors is not only important for occlusion, but also have a significant impact on lip posture and aesthetics. To best assess incisor position, the cephalometric analysis is of significant value. During the cephalometric evaluation, the orthodontist can see the position of the tooth relative to the supporting bone, but also relative to the lips and the opposing incisors.

The correction of dental positions prior to surgery is commonly known as "removal of dental compensations." These are abnormal positions that the teeth have attained as a result of attempting to achieve contact despite the skeletal discrepancy.

Another critical element during treatment planning is to decide which position a tooth will be assigned at the end of treatment. Patients with orofacial clefts are commonly missing teeth, especially the maxillary lateral incisor and second bicuspids. These situations may force the orthodontist into making decisions such as shifting the position of a tooth to replace a missing one (i.e., maxillary canine replacing missing maxillary lateral incisor). At other times, the decision to extract teeth must be made in cases of moderate crowding in which a tooth may be missing; to achieve symmetry and adequate occlusal relationships, it becomes imperative to equalize the number of teeth. In cases with missing teeth but minimal crowding, the orthodontist may elect to maintain the space for the missing teeth for future prosthetic replacement. This is particularly important if the existing posterior occlusal relationships are satisfactory.

The surgeon must closely communicate with the orthodontist to decide on what is feasible surgically for the patient's situation. The orthodontist must rely on the surgeon's expertise to determine how far can segments be moved, and if the surgery will be done in stages or all in one procedure. The surgeon should also indicate if it is likely that the surgery will include one or two jaws, and whether segmentalization of the maxilla to close fistulas and eliminate dental gaps is expected. However, the orthodontist must be extremely vigilant of or-

thopedic changes such as overexpansion of the maxillary arch during the preparatory phase. If the arch is overexpanded before surgery, the surgeon may be forced to do a segmental procedure rather than a safer, single-piece osteotomy. Once the preparatory phase of orthodontic treatment is completed, and it is determined that the patient is ready for the proposed surgical intervention, the final treatment plan evaluation must be undertaken. The following steps need to be completed to properly and thoroughly evaluate a patient prior to surgery.

1. Clinical examination of the face, temporomandibular joints, and oral cavity including the velopharyngeal mechanism. The clinical examination is done in both functional and static situations. Various movements of the face are noted and special notations are made concerning asymmetric function of the lips, eyelids, etc. The aesthetic evaluation is done by means of standard anthropometric measurements.[1]

2. Diagnostic facial and intraoral photographs.

3. Two sets of dental casts with bite registrations in both centric occlusion and centric relation, a face bow transfer is also obtained, especially in cases in which both jaws will be operated.

4. Radiographic examination of dental structures and their supporting bone if necessary, as well as a panoramic radiograph, lateral and posterior/anterior cephalometric radiographs, hand/wrist (to assess growth stage), and on occasion screening TMJ tomographs. Depending on the severity of the maxillomandibular discrepancy and/or deformity, additional studies including CT scans and MRIs can be requested. CT scans are helpful when three-dimensional reconstructions are also obtained. In the last few years, the availability of cone beam tomography to obtain three-dimensional reconstructions has been used[2] as well as the use of stereo photography. Although the last two diagnostic tools are not routinely utilized, in the near future they will become more accessible to clinicians. This will allow for routine, accurate, three-dimensional analysis and evaluations of the face, skull, and dentition.

5. Cephalometric evaluation and surgical predictions.

6. Final discussion with the patient, by the surgeon and orthodontist, to discuss the proposed treatment plan, with the inherent risks, limitations, as well as potential benefits. In addition, a determination is made for the need of additional referrals such as evaluation by the speech and language pathologist, prosthodontist, psychologist, etc. The required presurgical information is not different from that required in patients with isolated dentofacial deformities.[3]

CLINICAL EXAMINATION

The most important part of the presurgical analysis of a patient is the actual clinical examination, when the clinician has the opportunity to directly interact with the patient and evaluate overall facial balance, activity of the lips during speech and smiling, head posture, quality and clarity of speech during communication, and overall attitude of the patient toward the upcoming surgery. The clinical examination is done with the aid of measuring calipers and rulers, using techniques previously published by Farkas.[1] The clinician can make enumerable measurements. Some of the measurements that, in our experience, are extremely helpful are illustrated in Table 58–1. These direct measurements are then used to evaluate the ratios of upper face and lower face, length and width of the nose, length of the upper lip, dental midlines, as well as the overall symmetry of the face, nose, upper lip, and chin. One of the key direct measurements, in patients undergoing correction for a maxillomandibular discrepancy, is the ex-

posure of the upper incisors below the upper lip at rest and during a forced smile. In conjunction with the measurement of lip height, these measurements are extremely valuable to determine vertical hypoplasia or hyperplasia of the maxilla, or a short or long lip. (Figs. 58–1A and B) In cleft patients, clinicians will encounter vertically asymmetric lips (short on cleft side); therefore, careful decisions must be made to either use the noncleft side as a guideline, or plan on postoperative lip revision to improve lip/tooth relations.

The position of the chin, and the horizontal position or cant of the occlusal plane, are additional critical

Table 58–1.

Clinical Form Utilized by the Authors to Record Key Direct Anthropometric Facial Measurements, Occlusal and TMJ Evaluation Findings

Patient's Name: _____   Birthdate: _____ Age: _____ Date: _____

ORTHOGNATHIC SURGERY: _____   CRANIOFACIAL SURGERY: _____

Doctor: _____

Midline-EN (endocanthion)_____ (Right-Side)   Midline-EN (endocanthion)_____ (Left-Side)

EX-EX (exocanthion- exocanthion)_____   Vertical Pupillary difference _____

RIGHT CORNEA/SUP.ORBITAL RIM: _____   LEFT CORNEA/SUP.ORBITAL RIM: _____

RIGHT CORNEA/LET.ORBITAL RIM: _____   LEFT CORNEA/LAT.ORBITAL RIM: _____

RIGHT CORNEA/INF.ORBITAL RIM: _____   LEFT CORNEA/INF.ORBITAL RIM: _____

UPPER FACE HEIGHT: _____ MM

LOWER FACE HEIGHT: _____ MM   OCCLUSION: _____ MM REST: _____ MM

TOTAL FACE HEIGHT: _____ MM   OCCLUSION: _____ MM REST: _____ MM

BIZYGOMATIC WIDTH: _____ MM   BIGONIAL WIDTH: _____ MM

NASAL LENGTH: _____ MM   NASAL TIP HEIGHT _____ MM   ALAR WIDTH: _____ MM

UPPER LIP LENGTH: _____ MM   INTERLABIAL GAP: Occlusion: _____ MM Rest: _____ MM

UPPER LIP-1 (Rest):   _____ MM

UPPER LIP-1 (Smile):   _____ MM   CROWN/GINGIVAL SHOW (Smile): _____ MM _____ %

UPPER MIDLINE: ON ( ) OFF ( )   RIGHT: _____ MM   LEFT: _____ MM

LOWER MIDLINE: ON ( ) OFF ( )   RIGHT: _____ MM   LEFT: _____ MM

CROSSBITE: ANTERIOR: YES ( )   NO ( )   RIGHT: YES ( ) NO ( )   LEFT: YES ( ) NO ( )

OVERBITE: _____ MM

OVERJET: _____ MM

MOLAR CLASS: RIGHT: _____ LEFT: _____

CANINE CLASS: RIGHT: _____ LEFT: _____

INTERCANTHAL LINE/OCCLUSAL PLANE: RIGHT: _____ MM   LEFT: _____ MM

CHIN POINT: ON ( )   RIGHT: _____ MM   LEFT: _____ MM

RIGHT TMJ: OK ( )   CLICK: EARLY ( ) INTERMEDIATE ( ) LATE ( ) OPENING ( ) CLOSING ( )

PAIN: YES ( ) NO ( )   WHERE:

LEFT TMJ: OK ( )   CLICK: EARLY ( ) INTERMEDIATE ( ) LATE ( ) OPENING ( ) CLOSING ( )

PAIN: YES ( ) NO ( )   WHERE:

OPENING DEVIATION: YES ( ) NO ( )   RIGHT: EARLY ( ) INTERMEDIATE ( ) LATE ( ) OPENING ( ) CLOSING ( )

PALATE SCARRING: MILD ( ) MODERATE ( )   LEFT: EARLY ( ) INTERMEDIATE ( ) LATE ( ) OPENING ( ) CLOSING ( )

   SEVERE ( )   PHARYNGEAL FLAP: YES ( ) NO ( )

   VPI: YES ( ) NO ( )

PLAN:

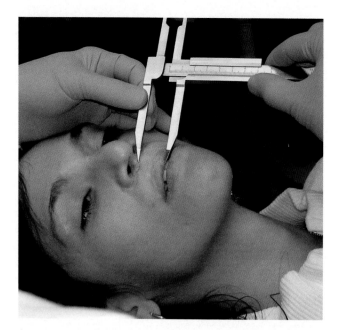

A

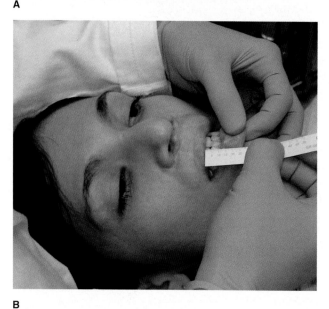

B

Figure 58–1. (A) Direct caliper and (B) ruler measurements of upper lip length and maxillary incisor to upper lip distance.

measurements to assess facial symmetry. When evaluating these findings, the clinician must also determine if the eyes, nose, and chin are symmetric. To assess symmetry, a string or piece of dental floss can be used, and in this way, easily visualize deviations relative to stable structures such as the eyes. (Fig. 58–2A) A critical aspect of symmetry is the occlusal plane as seen from the frontal view with the lips in repose and during forced smile. A tongue blade is used to determine deviation of the occlusal plane relative to the stable reference such as the bipupillary distance. (Fig. 58–2B) This should be recorded (Table 58–1), as these measurements will be critical during the execution of model surgery for preparation of splints, and also at the time of the actual surgical intervention.

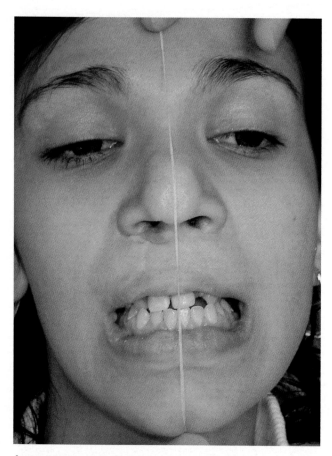

A

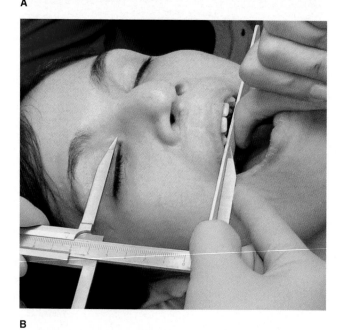

B

Figure 58–2. (A) Use of dental floss to assess position of the nose, maxillary dental midline, and chin. (B) Use of calipers and tongue blade to record cant of the occlusal plane relative to medial canthi.

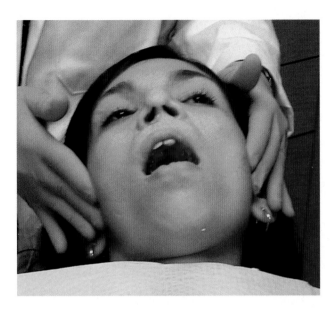

Figure 58–3. Palpation and evaluation of the temporomandibular joints required* to determine presence of abnormal sounds and condylar motion.

After evaluation of the face, the clinician evaluates the temporomandibular joints, and is done by assessing the ability of the patient to open and have lateral excursive movements, as well as determining the presence of joint signs or symptoms. Physical evaluation during opening movements is performed (Fig. 58–3). Deviations to the right or left, and also discrepancies between first occlusal contact (centric relation) and maximal occlusal intercuspation (centric occlusion) are noted. Presence joint sounds are important to record, as they may indicate internal derangement of the joint, and the clinician must determine if their presence needs special attention before, during, or after the surgical procedure. In many patients, joint sounds may be, in part, related to occlusal alterations related to the skeletal discrepancy.

At this point, the clinician directs their attention to the dentition. It is very likely that the patient's dental health is satisfactory, as the patient has been under the preparatory stages of orthodontic treatment. The clinician must note the presence or absence of crossbites, anterior or posterior openbites, molar and canine relationships, degree of overbite and overjet, any residual crowding, and the presence or absence of teeth and dental gaps. If it is noted that there are interdental spaces, planning segmentalization of the maxilla to consolidate these spaces, especially in the anterior region, is a common approach. The severity of scarring secondary to previous cleft surgeries, presence of residual alveolar or palatal fistulas, and existence of a pharyngeal flap or short soft palate should be noted.

Based on the clinical examination, the surgeon and orthodontist can perform a preliminary treatment plan, which will be eventually confirmed through other studies such as cephalometric evaluation, prediction tracings, study model analysis, and dental model surgery.

CEPHALOMETRIC EVALUATION AND PREDICTION TRACINGS

An important aspect of the presurgical evaluation and formulation of a surgical treatment plan includes cephalometric analysis of radiographs obtained within 2 months of surgery. With these radiographs, prediction tracings are obtained to evaluate the various desired skeletal movements and outcomes. There are many cephalometric analyses and measurements that have been used by orthodontists and surgeons for many years. Most analyses evaluate dental, skeletal, and soft tissue relations. The selection of a particular analysis is based, in great part, on the comfort level and experience of the clinician with that specific analysis. Most practitioners utilize a combination of measurements derived from various analyses, and they select what, in their experience, yields the most satisfactory overall evaluation for a particular situation.

Although cephalometric evaluation is helpful in all patients with dentofacial deformities, including cleft patients, the clinician has to be careful with the interpretation of results. This is especially true when prediction tracings are done, and the ratios of soft tissue to hard tissue movement are considered. Cleft patients have upper lips and noses, which are scarred and negatively affected by the deformity itself, as well as previous surgeries. Therefore, the response of these soft tissue structures to skeletal movements is not the same as that seen in noncleft individuals. However, the information obtained from the prediction, even when noncleft values are utilized for comparison, are still of value during treatment planning. Most predictions of facial changes with orthognathic surgery utilize the lateral cephalometric view. Although the frontal view can be utilized, especially in cases of asymmetry, its usefulness is limited because its limitations, as a two-dimensional analysis, do not provide accurate information of the expected facial changes. Future three-dimensional analyses, utilizing cone beam computed tomography with three-dimensional reconstructions, will be commonly utilized, and predictions will be done in all three planes of space.[2] At present, this technology is in its infancy, and the cost is still high. As with most technology, it is expected that, with time and further technical developments, it will be available in every orthodontist and surgeon's office that treats patients with dentofacial deformities.

Prediction tracings can be done from the cephalometric radiograph on acetate paper. The clinician will first draw all skeletal and soft tissue structures of interest, and subsequently will draw, on a separate piece of tracing paper, the structures that are planned for movement. In this way, the clinician can evaluate, over the original tracing, the skeletal and soft tissue changes based on the movement of the various skeletal parts.[4] Although accurate and inexpensive, these prediction tracings can be time consuming, and the visual effect for patient education may be limited.

For the past few years, most orthodontists and surgeons have available computerized programs that merge the cephalometric radiograph with a profile facial photograph. By means of proprietary software, these programs allow the

Digitized Landmarks

0   Sella
1   Porion
2   Basion
3   Hinge Axis
4   PT-point (Pterygoid)
5   Nasion
6   Orbitale
7   A-point
8   PM (superpogonion)
9   Pogonion
10 B-piont
11 PNS
12 ANS
13 R1
14 R3
15 Articulare
16 Ramus Down
17 Corpus Left
18 Menton
19 mx 1 crown
20 mx 1 root
21 md 1 crown
22 md 1 root
23 Occlusal Plane
24 mx 6 distal
25 mx 6 root
26 md 6 distal
27 md 6 root

A   B

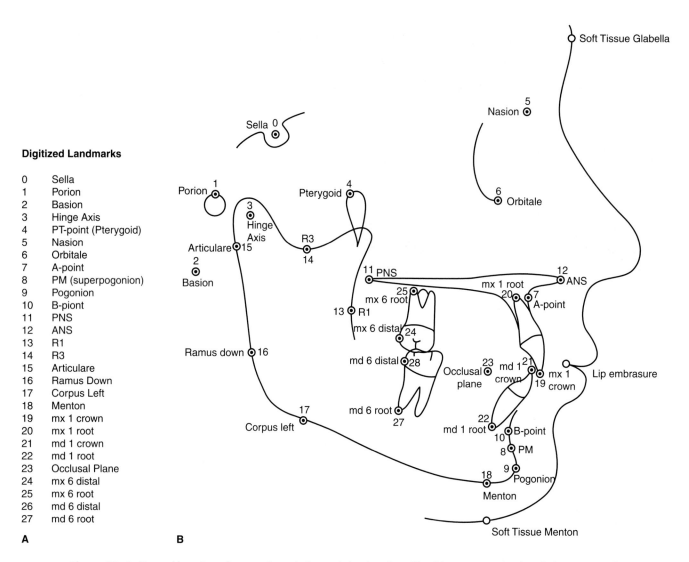

Figure 58–4. List and location of anatomic cephalometric landmarks utilized for computerized cephalometric analysis.
(*All cephalometric computerized tracings, predictions and measurements on the case reports illustrated in this chapter were done using Quick Ceph ® 2000 Version 3.5, October 19, 2005, Quick Ceph Systems, Inc., 9883 Pacific Heights Blvd., Suite J, San Diego, CA 92,121. (The authors do not have business or financial interests in Quick Ceph Systems, Inc.))*

clinician to make various skeletal manipulations, and see the predicted approximate soft tissue changes. These changes are based on published cephalometric studies that have determined, with a great degree of reliability, the changes that occur in the position of the nose and upper lip with advancement of the maxilla. In addition, one can see the concurrent changes affecting the lower lip and chin with anterior or posterior movement of the mandible, or by rotation of the mandibular body, hinged on the temporomandibular joint.

In Figs. 58–4A and B, commonly utilized skeletal anatomic landmarks required for developing a cephalometric analysis are shown, and the cephalometric measurements derived from them can be seen in the subsequent case reports. Most analyses available in literature provide race-, age-, and sex-specific normative standards.

With information obtained from the clinical examination of the patient, as well as the dental study model evaluation, the clinician will be able to make a preliminary plan. Once the clinician performs the cephalometric evaluation

and confirms which skeletal part is at fault, a problem list is developed, and the cephalometric digital or hand-traced prediction can be completed. During the prediction phase, the clinician aims to achieve: facial symmetry, adequate nasal tip projection, proper relationship of the nose to the upper lip (nasolabial angle), proper incisor exposure at rest and on smile, smile fullness, convexity to the face, bimaxillary lip projection and lip fullness, and adequate chin and neck definition.

In the cleft patient, it is not uncommon to find vertical and horizontal maxillary hypoplasia. In the majority of the patients, the mandible is either slightly small or of normal dimensions; however, an increased lower anterior facial height, secondary to a steep mandibular plane angle and short ramus height, is present.[5,6] The clinician must determine if the deformity can be corrected with surgery just to the maxilla, or if it will become necessary to also operate on the mandible. In order to determine the need for mandibular surgery, the first step of the prediction tracing is the counterclockwise autorotation of the mandible, hinged on the center of the mandibular condyle, until proper face height and upper and lower lip relationships are attained. If mandibular autorotation is able to place the mandible in the right position, and if the required maxillary movement to correct the overjet and overbite, as well as obtain adequate tooth exposure and lip and nose relations, is under 5–6 mm, only maxillary surgery is planned.

If the required advancement is less than 5–6 mm, conventional orthognathic LeFort I surgery can be performed. However, if the case has significant palatal scarring, a pharyngeal flap, and small segments with compromised vascular supply, the surgeon must consider distraction techniques, utilizing either an internal or external distraction device. If the maxillary advancement is over 8 mm and also requires changes in the infraorbital and paranasal areas, the surgeon must consider maxillary advancement with distraction utilizing an external device.[7–11]

If the mandibular autorotation produces excessive chin projection or excessive vertical contact with curling of the upper and lower lips, it is very likely that a mandibular osteotomy will be needed. In cases with a vertical facial pattern with an obtuse gonial angle, and a reduced posterior ramus height, the occlusal plane will be remain steep without a mandibular osteotomy. In these cases, even if the anteroposterior relationship is favorable, the occlusal plane needs to be adjusted, and a double jaw procedure, with counterclockwise rotation of the occlusal plane, is required. After the maxilla and mandible are in the proper position, relative to each other and to the face, a critical assessment of chin position is completed. A determination is made for the need of a genioplasty.

Cases in which the anterior/posterior position of the chin is satisfactory, but the lower lip and chin definition is deficient due to the mandibular incisor forward inclination, in place of a genioplasty, the clinician can consider a subapical mandibular osteotomy, done in conjunction with the maxillary advancement and mandibular autorotation.

DENTAL CAST ANALYSIS

Prior to surgery and after all necessary orthodontic tooth movements are completed, two sets of maxillary and mandibular dental alginate impressions are obtained in the patient. A wax "bite registration" is obtained. If there is a significant discrepancy noted in the bite between centric occlusion and centric relation, then separate bite registrations are obtained. The dental models obtained from the alginate impressions are used to assess arch coordination and occlusal relationships, as the casts are hand-articulated. The clinician determines if there is a need for maxillary segmentalization, with expansion or contraction of the arch, and the need for closure of dental gaps. If it is determined that a double jaw surgical procedure will be required, a face-bow transfer record needs to be obtained[11,12] (Fig. 58–5). The face-bow will then be utilized to mount the maxillary and mandibular dental casts in a semi-adjustable articulator (Fig. 58–6). If the patient will require only maxillary surgery, usually a face-bow

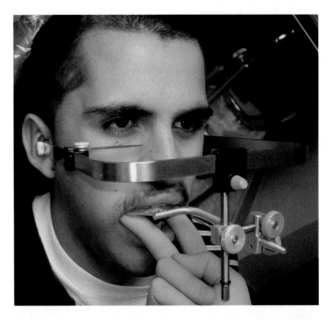

Figure 58–5. Face-bow transfer recording on a cleft patient requiring double-jaw surgery and need for intermediate and final occlusal splints.

mounting is not necessary, and the casts are mounted in a hinge articulator (Fig. 58–7). In situations where sub-apical maxillary or mandibular osteotomies will be performed, with or without changes in the posterior aspect of the maxillary and mandibular arches, it becomes imperative to mount these cases in a semi-adjustable articulator using the face-bow mounting as a guideline.

In cases requiring only maxillary surgery, the surgeon must base the surgical cuts on the cephalometric analysis and clinical evaluation, paying attention to the amount of

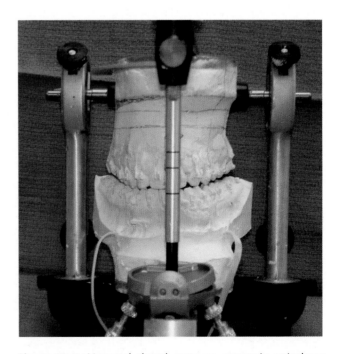

Figure 58–6. Mounted dental casts on anatomic articulator based on the face-bow mounting record and centric occlusion registration wax bite.

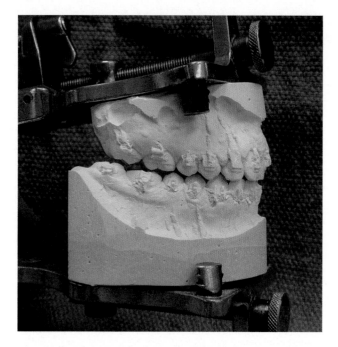

Figure 58–7. Dental casts used to prepare a final occlusal splint mounted on a hinge articulator with ideal occlusal relations.

maxillary posterior intrusion required to maintain or change the occlusal plane, and also achieving a close to ideal lip to tooth relation at rest and during function.

In cases requiring two-jaw surgery, an intermediate splint is prepared first, to guide the surgeon during maxillary repositioning, using the unoperated mandible as a reference. Based on the cephalometric and clinical evaluation, the surgery is performed on the mounted casts and exact values are obtained for moving the maxillary dentition in all planes of space. With the maxilla repositioned in the anatomic articulator, but with the mandibular cast unmoved, the intermediate splint is fabricated. Subsequently, the mandibular cast is repositioned to ideal occlusal relations with the pre-

viously moved maxillary cast, and the final occlusal splint is fabricated. The final occlusal splint can also be fabricated by simply taking the second set of casts and mount them on a hinge articulator with ideal occlusal relationships. The only time that this latter step is not recommended is when the surgeon needs to segmentalize the maxilla to achieve the desired treatment goals. In this situation, the mandibular cast should be moved in the anatomic articulator to avoid the replication of the desired maxillary movements in a different cast and further introduce error.

The fabrication and use of intermediate and final splints is extremely valuable, since many of the needed anatomic reference landmarks, are distorted or not accessible at the time of surgery. Based on the clinical, cephalometric, and cast analysis, as well as the model surgery, the surgeon expects to obtain: ideal occlusal relationships with correction of openbites or crossbites, correction of dental spaces due to missing teeth, and maxillary and mandibular midlines centered to each other and the face.

Preparation and evaluation of patients in a careful and methodical fashion assures obtaining ideal surgical and orthodontic outcomes after orthognathic surgery, even in patients with challenging cleft maxillary hypoplasia. The following examples illustrate various situations on which the preceding treatment planning approach has been successfully utilized.

CASE REPORTS

Patient 1 (Figs. 58–8 to 58–24): Bilateral cleft lip and palate with maxillary deficiency.

Patient 2 (Figs. 58–25 to 58–37). Unilateral cleft lip and palate with maxillary hypoplasia

Patient 3 (Fig. 58–38 to 58–51). Unilateral cleft lip and palate with maxillary hypoplasia and mild mandibular prognathism with mandibular dentoalveolar protrusion

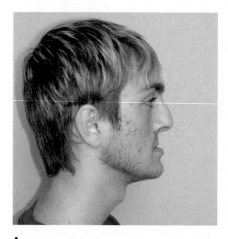

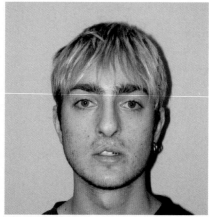

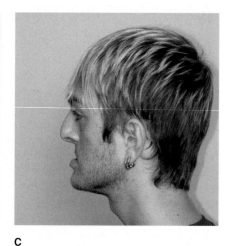

A **B** **C**

Figure 58–8. (A–C) Profile and frontal photographs of a 20-year-4-month-old male with a repaired bilateral cleft lip and palate and severe maxillary hypoplasia.

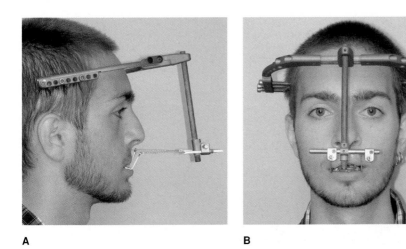
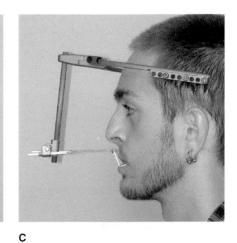

A   B   C

Figure 58–19. (A–C) Frontal and profile photographs of the patient undergoing maxillary advancement with a Rigid External Distraction Device. (*KLS Martin, Jacksonville, Fl*) Due to the extent of the maxillary advancement required for this patient, as well as the scarring from previous palatal surgery, a distraction approach was selected for the patient.

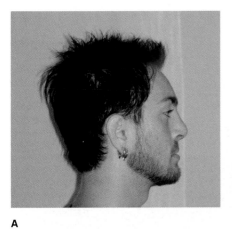
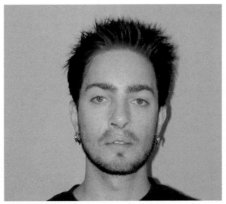
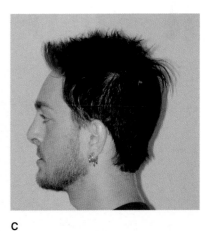

A   B   C

Figure 58–20. (A–C) Postoperative profile and frontal facial photographs after maxillary advancement utilizing a Rigid External Distraction Device. Note well-balanced nose and lip relations and overall facial improvement.

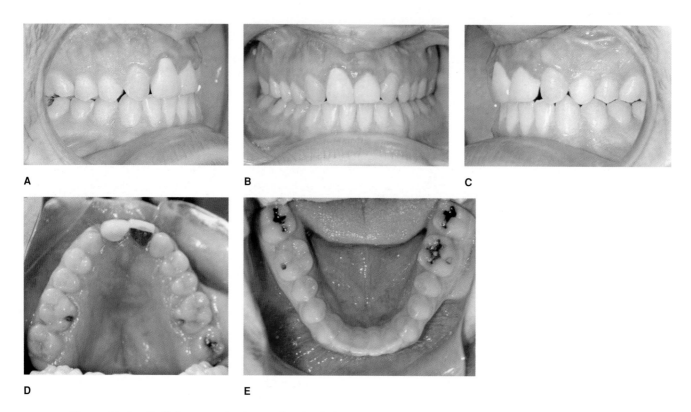

Figure 58–21. (A–E) Postoperative intraoral occlusal photographs. Note well-aligned arches, class II molar relationships (as a result of missing maxillary lateral incisors), and adequate position of the maxillary canines replacing the lateral incisors. Ideal transverse relations as well as overbite and overjet, with restoration of the maxillary midline, were also obtained.

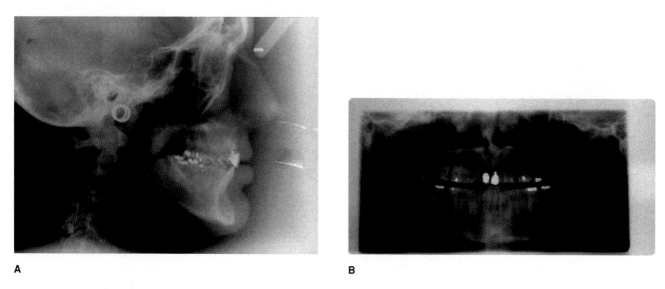

Figure 58–22. (A) Postoperative cephalometric and (B) panoramic radiographs demonstrating the maxillary advancement. Note absence of fixation hardware after surgery. Also note bone deposition posterior to the second molars by the distraction process.

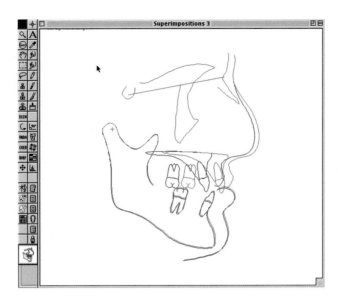

Figure 58–23. Pre- and postsurgical tracings demonstrating the degree of maxillary advancement as well as the upper and nose changes.

```
NAME:                                              Quick Ceph® 2000
BIRTH:    12/27/82    SEX:      M                  11/23/06
RECORD:   3/16/04     STATUS:   02                 Drs.Figueroa Polley
AGE:      21yr 2mo    CASE:
```

Analysis Figueroa		02	Norm	Clin.Dev.		Tr
SKELETAL RELATIONS						
SNA	(dg)	70.0	82.0	-4.0	***	78.7
SNB	(dg)	73.7	80.0	-2.1	**	72.8
A to N -| FH	(mm)	-12.5	-0.9	-4.7	***	-1.2
SNaOr	(dg)	52.3	60.0	-1.9	*	47.7
Facial Angle	(dg)	86.8	89.6	-0.8		86.9
Mandibular Plane	(dg)	23.0	22.9	0.0		22.6
Y - Axis	(dg)	60.9	59.4	0.4		60.4
Angle of Convexity	(dg)	-16.3	0.0	-3.2	***	4.5
Cant of Occl. Plane	(dg)	10.8	9.3	0.4		9.7
ANS-Menton	(mm)	71.7	65.4	1.0	*	70.7
Nasion-Menton	(mm)	130.8	119.3	1.9	*	129.9
ANS-Me./Nasion-Me.	(%)	54.8	55.0	-0.1		54.4
Mandibular Length	(mm)	121.2	121.8	-0.2		121.4
Midfacial Length	(mm)	84.8	93.6	-2.2	**	96.3
Maxillomand. Diff.		36.4	27.4	3.5	***	25.0
DENTAL RELATIONS						
Interincisal Angle	(dg)	139.6	130.0	1.7	*	137.6
Mx 1, to FH	(dg)	104.0	111.0	-1.2	*	105.4
Mx 1, to PPl.	(dg)	93.2	113.0	-5.0	***	98.0
Md 1, to APo	(mm)	2.4	1.0	0.6		-4.8
Md 1, to Md Plane	(dg)	3.4	1.4	0.5		4.5
Incisor Overjet	(mm)	-4.4	2.5	-2.8	**	3.7
Incisor Overbite	(mm)	-0.4	2.5	-1.5	*	1.0
ESTHETIC RELATIONS						
Lower Lip E-Plane	(mm)	-3.6	-2.0	-0.8		-5.0
Nasolabial Angle	(dg)	108.6	115.2	-1.1	*	107.6
G-Sn-Pg'	(dg)	-12.0	16.0	-5.6	***	-3.1
Ant. Cranial Base	(mm)	75.1	72.1	1.0		75.1

Figure 58–24. Cephalometric values before and after surgery demonstrating changes in the position of the maxilla (SNA, A-point to Nasion vertical, midfacial length) and mandible (SNB, facial plane, mandibular plane). The functional, structural, and aesthetic changes were dramatic and significant.

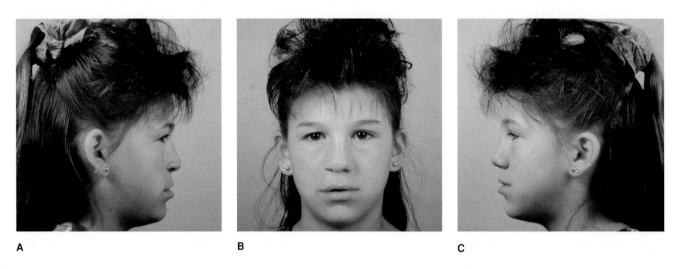

Figure 58–25. (A–C) Profile and frontal photographs of a 11-year-7-month-old female with a repaired complete right unilateral cleft lip and palate and maxillary hypoplasia.

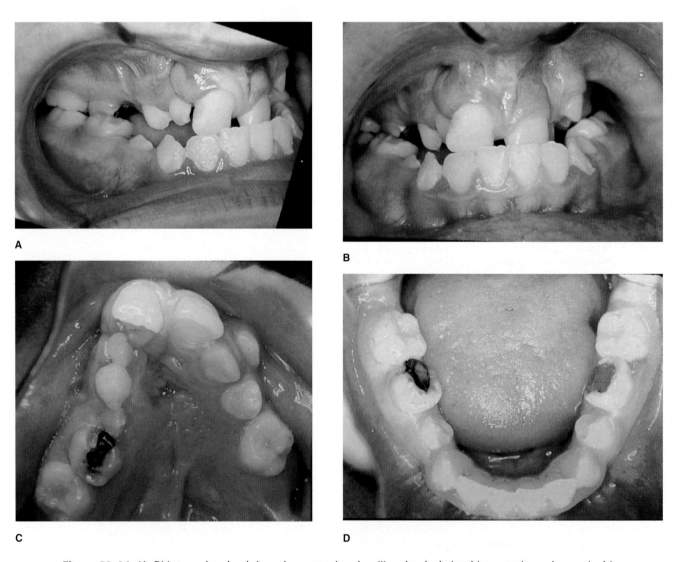

Figure 58–26. (A–D) Intraoral occlusal views demonstrating class III occlusal relationships, anterior and posterior bilateral crossbites, absence of maxillary right lateral incisor, deviation of the maxillary dental midline to the right, adequate hard palate and alveolar cleft reconstructions, and significant collapse of the maxillary arch due to scarring.

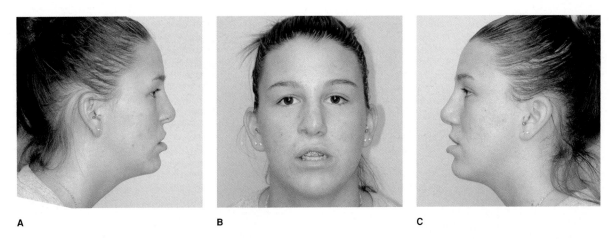

Figure 58–27. (A–C) Preoperative facial profile and frontal photographs of a 20-year-4-month-old female, with a repaired unilateral cleft lip and palate, and secondary maxillary hypoplasia. Note retruded upper lip position relative to lower lip; in the frontal view, the nasal asymmetry to the cleft side is obvious; a moderately short upper lip, increased interlabial gap and maxillary midline deviation to the cleft side are also noted.

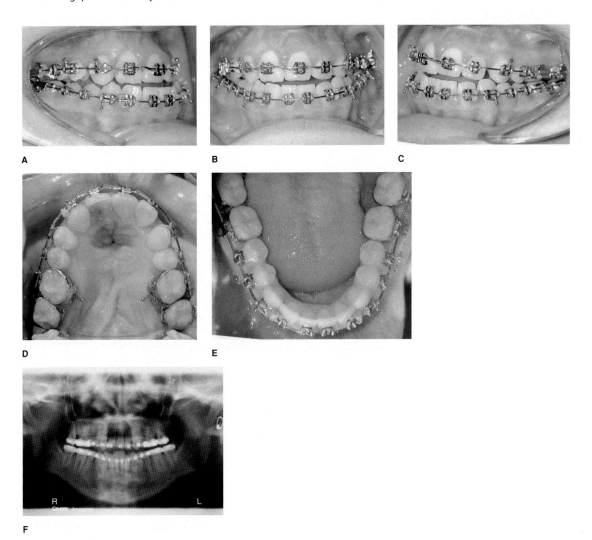

Figure 58–28. (A–E) Intraoral occlusal views. The patient underwent orthodontic preparation as well as previous secondary alveolar bone grafting to consolidate the maxillary arch. Note excellent gingival reconstruction but significant palatal scarring at the molar level. The patient was missing tooth #7, tooth #6 was moved into its position. Extraction of tooth #12 was performed to equalize the number of teeth in the maxillary arch. Note orthodontic appliances in all teeth in order to achieve a favorable arch form. In the mandibular arch no extractions were performed. (F) The panoramic radiograph demonstrates adequate supporting skeletal structures and a nicely reconstructed anterior maxillary region.

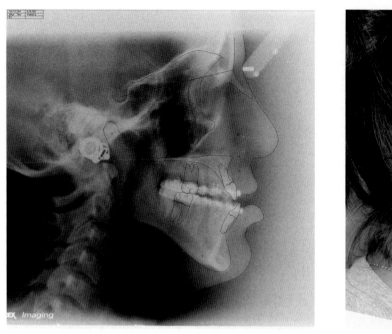

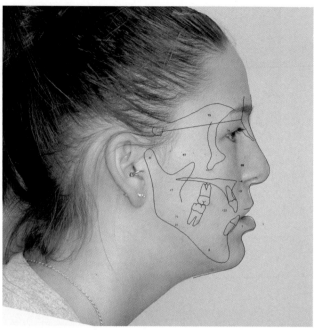

A

B

Figure 58–29. (A) Presurgical cephalometric radiograph with tracing as well as (B) superimposed tracing over the profile photograph. The cephalometric radiograph clearly demonstrates the degree of maxillary hypoplasia with an anterior crossbite and openbite. The mandible is relatively normal with slight proclination of the mandibular incisor.

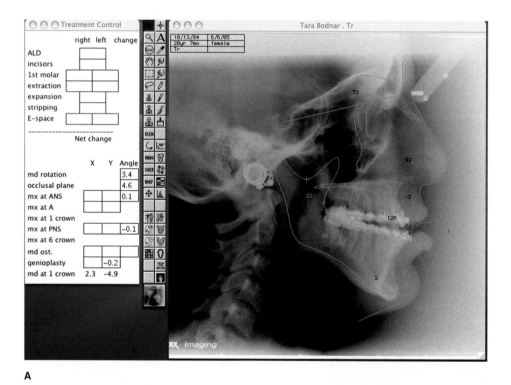

A

Figure 58–30. Digital cephalometric surgical predictions. The usual first step of a surgical cephalometric prediction is the autorotation of the mandible until the occlusal plane and anterior vertical lip relationships are normalized. Note the vertical and anterior posterior discrepancy between the mandibular outline and the tracing outline after the counterclockwise autorotation. (A) On the left side of the cephalometric image and software computer controls, note a table demonstrating the recorded changes after mandibular autorotation. The next step in the prediction process is to advance the maxilla until ideal occlusal and soft tissue relations are obtained. Note that ideal overbite and overjet have been achieved with improved lip relations. (*contd.*)

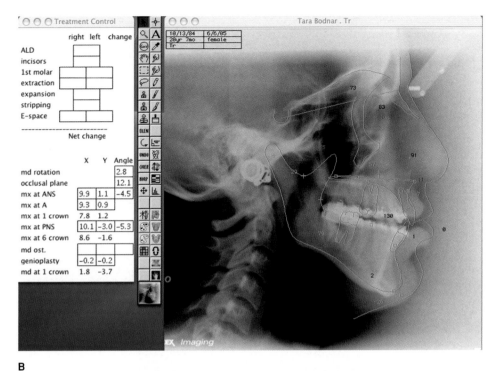

B

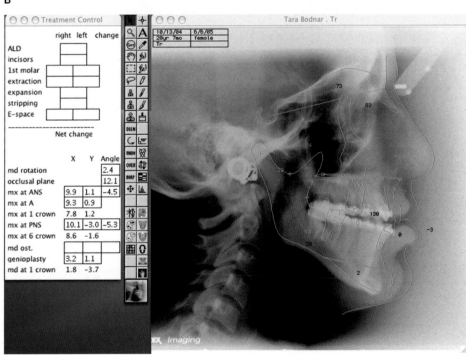

C

Figure 58–30. (*Contd.*) (B) On the left side, note the angular as well as the millimeter horizontal and vertical changes of the various structures that can be mobilized during the computerized prediction. (C) To improve facial balance, a genioplasty with advancement was planned and this is demonstrated on the prediction tracing.

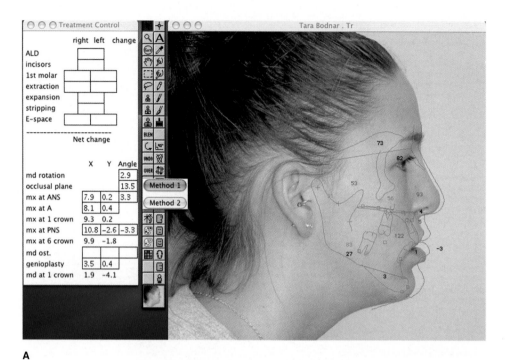

A

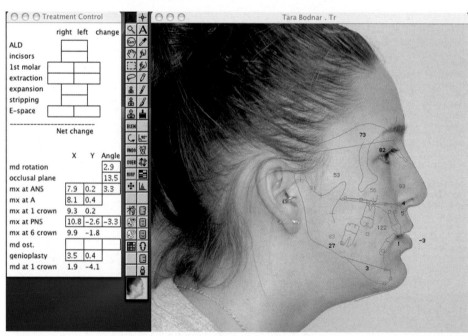

B

Figure 58–31. (A) The tracing is then superimposed on the digital facial image, and morphing of the soft tissues to the predicted tracing is performed. The software will fill in the existing distance between the soft tissue outline and the tracing lines of the nose, upper and lower lips, as well as chin. (B) After morphing, the anticipated changes after the maxillary advancement and genioplasty are noted. The software has now filled in color in the previous space between the soft tissue outline and the tracing lines.

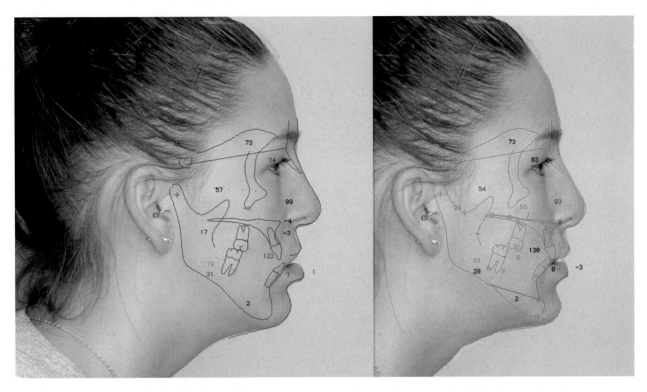

Figure 58–32. (A) Preoperative and (B) predicted soft tissue changes after maxillary advancement and genioplasty. Note improved relations between the upper lip and nose, upper and lower lips, and chin projection.

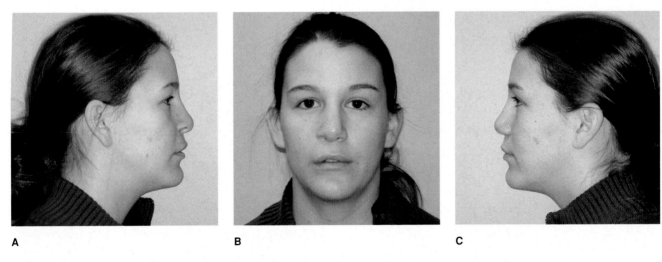

A   B   C

Figure 58–33. (A–C) Postoperative frontal and profile photographs. Note improvement on lip and nose relations as well as improved facial balance and lip posture.

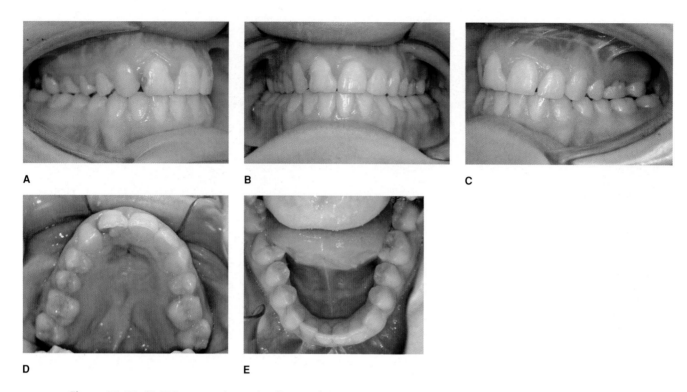

Figure 58–34. (A–E) Postoperative occlusal intraoral views. Note improved occlusal relationships with ideal overbite and overjet. The maxillary right canine has replaced the missing maxillary right lateral incisor. The patient occlusal relationships at the molar level are class II as she is missing two teeth in the upper arch and none in the lower arch.

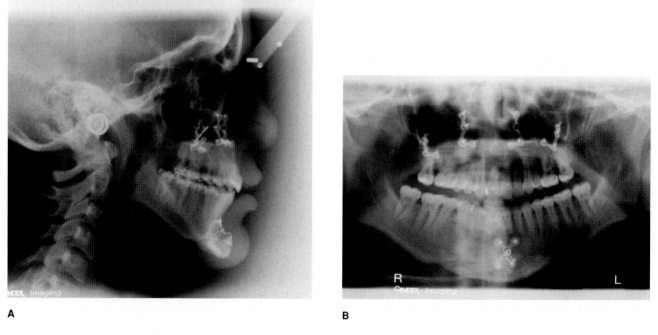

Figure 58–35. (A) Postoperative cephalometric and (B) panoramic radiographs. Note the presence of rigid fixation plates for stabilization of the conventionally advanced maxilla and genioplasty.

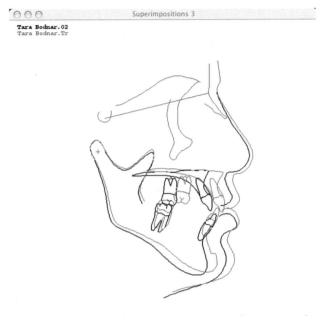

Figure 58–36. Pre- and postoperative tracings demonstrate the extent of the maxillary advancement, the mandibular autorotation, and the genioplasty as well as the nasal, lip, and chin changes.

NAME: Quick Ceph® 2000
BIRTH: 10/13/84   SEX: F   11/23/06
RECORD: 6/6/05   STATUS: 02   Drs.Figueroa Polley
AGE: 20yr 7mo   CASE:

Analysis Figueroa		02	Norm	Clin.Dev.		Tr
SKELETAL RELATIONS						
SNA	(dg)	74.1	82.0	-2.6	**	83.2
SNB	(dg)	74.6	80.0	-1.8	*	76.1
A to N -| FH	(mm)	-2.6	-1.7	-0.4		6.7
SNaOr	(dg)	56.9	60.0	-0.8		56.9
Facial Angle	(dg)	89.5	88.3	0.3		92.8
Mandibular Plane	(dg)	31.3	24.2	1.6	*	28.1
Y - Axis	(dg)	57.0	59.4	-0.7		53.8
Angle of Convexity	(dg)	-4.2	0.0	-0.8		7.6
Cant of Occl. Plane	(dg)	17.1	9.3	2.1	**	12.8
ANS-Menton	(mm)	69.2	62.1	1.2	*	65.7
Nasion-Menton	(mm)	121.5	112.4	1.5	*	119.2
ANS-Me./Nasion-Me.	(%)	57.0	55.0	0.7		55.1
Mandibular Length	(mm)	114.0	114.4	-0.1		117.2
Midfacial Length	(mm)	81.4	89.8	-2.1	**	90.7
Maxillomand. Diff.		32.6	24.1	3.3	***	26.5
DENTAL RELATIONS						
Interincisal Angle	(dg)	122.1	130.0	-1.4	*	129.7
Mx 1, to FH	(dg)	114.7	111.0	0.6		109.8
Mx 1, to PPl.	(dg)	99.1	113.0	-3.5	***	98.9
Md 1, to APo	(mm)	7.0	1.0	2.6	**	0.3
Md 1, to Md Plane	(dg)	1.9	1.4	0.1		2.4
Incisor Overjet	(mm)	-3.7	2.5	-2.5	**	3.4
Incisor Overbite	(mm)	-1.1	2.5	-1.8	*	2.1
ESTHETIC RELATIONS						
Lower Lip E-Plane	(mm)	1.0	-2.0	1.5	*	-2.8
Nasolabial Angle	(dg)	92.8	115.2	-3.7	***	93.1
G-Sn-Pg'	(dg)	6.8	15.8	-1.8	*	9.1
Ant. Cranial Base	(mm)	72.9	70.3	0.9		72.9

Figure 58–37. Pre- and postoperative cephalometric values. Note those changes related to the maxillary advancement (SNA, A-point to the Nasion vertical, midfacial length) and the mandibular autorotation and genioplasty (SNB, facial angle, mandibular plane, and Y-axis).

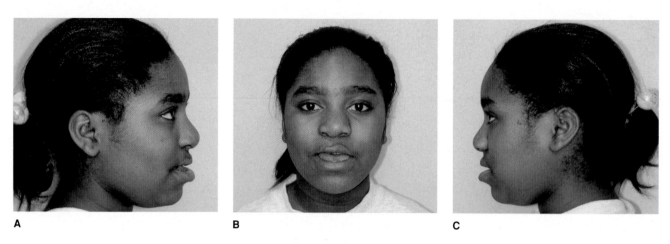

Figure 58–38. (A–C) Pretreatment frontal and profile facial photographs of a 13-year-old female with a repaired left unilateral cleft lip and palate. Note deficient upper lip and prominent lower lip as well as open mouth posture. Secondary cleft lip and nose deformities are also evident.

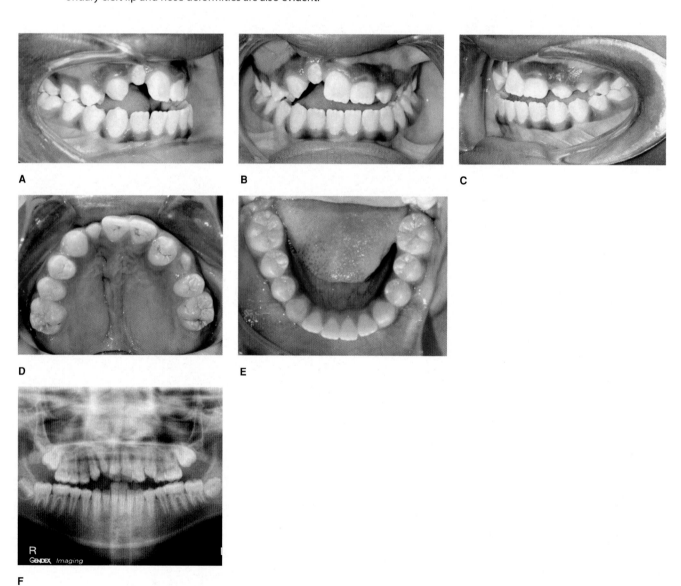

Figure 58–39. (A–E) Pretreatment intraoral occlusal photographs. Note left and anterior crossbites, anterior open-bite, diminutive tooth #7, absent tooth #10, and transposition between teeth #11 and #12. (F) The panoramic radiograph reveals a small size tooth #7 and absence of tooth #10. The transposition of teeth #11 and #12 is also evident. The alveolar cleft has been bone grafted.

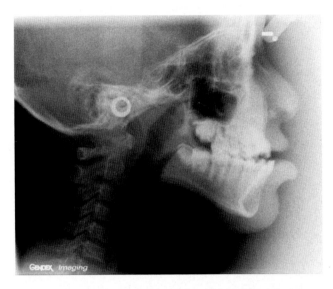

Figure 58–40. Pretreatment cephalometric radiograph demonstrating maxillary hypoplasia, moderate mandibular prognathism, and mandibular dental alveolar protrusion. The retruded upper lip position and prominent lower lip are also noted.

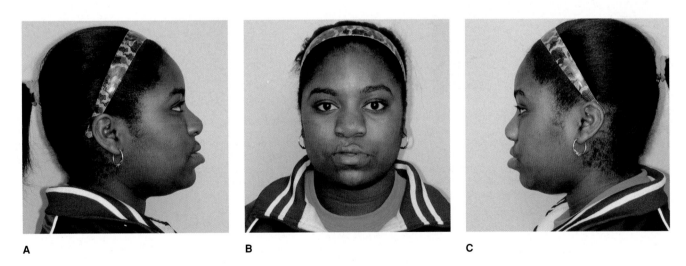

A   B   C

Figure 58–41. (A–C) Profile and frontal photographs after orthodontic alignment of the arches and before surgery.

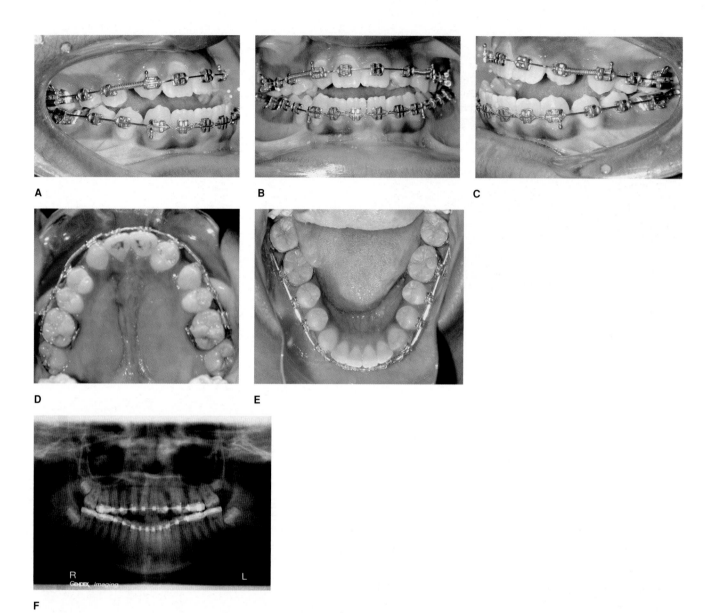

A B C

D E

F

Figure 58–42. (A–E) Intraoral occlusal views demonstrating alignment of the arches prior to surgery and an anterior openbite crossbite. Note that tooth #6 is in the position of the lateral incisor, as tooth #7 was extracted due to its small size. Also note that tooth #12 is in the position of tooth #10 due to the transposition between teeth #11 and #12. Both the maxillary and mandibular arches are aligned and coordinated. (F) The panoramic radiograph reveals adequate bone structure supporting the dentition. All third molars are present and unerupted.

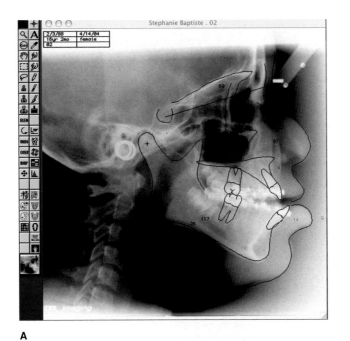

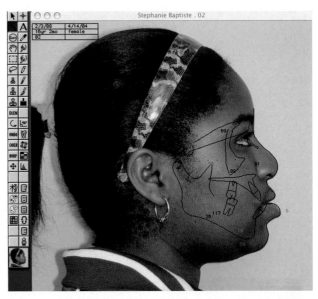

A

B

Figure 58–43. (A) Image from the computer screen demonstrating the lateral cephalometric radiograph with tracing overlaid. This radiograph reveals maxillary anteroposterior and vertical maxillary anterior deficiency. Both maxillary and mandibular incisors are proclined. The anterior crossbite and the retruded upper lip and prominent lower lip are evident. (B) Cephalometric tracings superimposed on the lateral facial photograph.

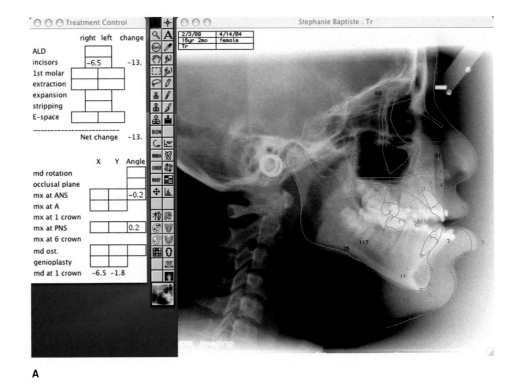

A

Figure 58–44. Digital cephalometric surgical prediction. The initial step of the prediction tracing in this case is the posterior movement of the mandibular incisor with correction of the extreme proclination. (A) The graph on the left of the software icons demonstrates the degree of the horizontal and vertical change of the lower incisor. (*contd.*)

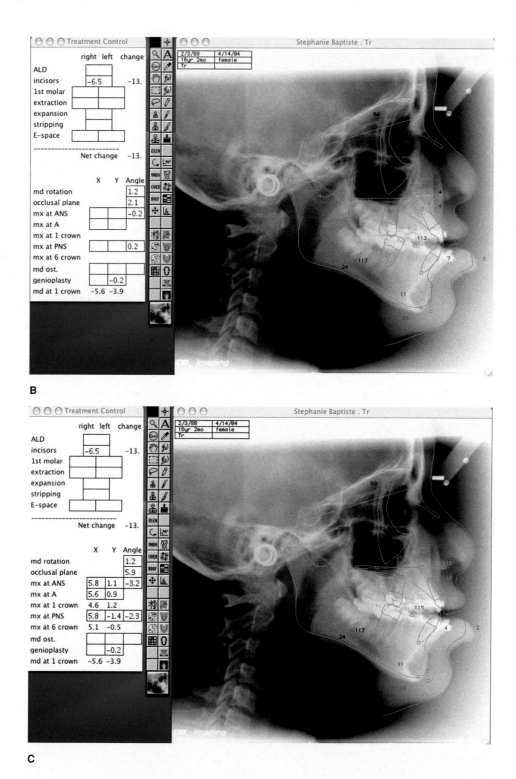

Figure 58–44. (*Contd.*) (B) The next step in the surgical prediction for this patient included the mandibular counter-clockwise autorotation until adequate vertical lip relations were obtained. The maxilla was advanced in one segment until ideal overbite and overjet were obtained as well as improvement in the lip relations. (C) The graph on the left side indicates the horizontal and vertical changes for the maxilla, maxillary and mandibular incisors, as well as maxillary first molars.

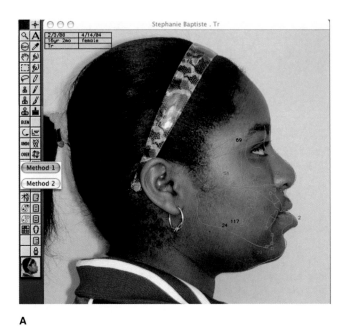
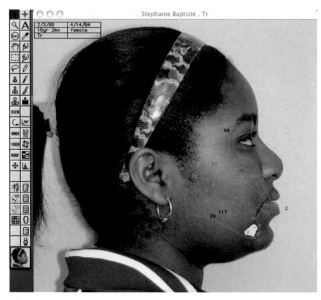

Figure 58–45. (A) The prediction tracing is superimposed on the facial profile photograph, and the predicted changes relative to the existing soft tissues are illustrated by the red line tracing of the nose, upper and lower lips. The software is prompting the clinician to morph the profile photograph into the new skeletal and soft tissue relations. (B) After morphing, the expected nose and soft tissue changes are seen.

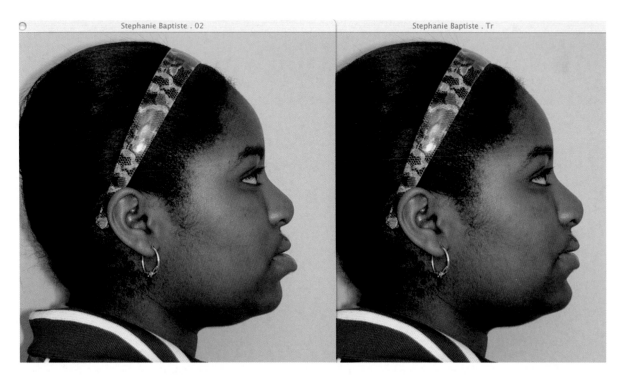

Figure 58–46. (A) Profile photograph on the left side is taken before morphing, (B) the image on the right side, is taken after morphing with the expected nose, lip, and chin changes after the planned maxillary advancement with mandibular subapical osteotomy with posterior repositioning of the lower six anterior teeth. Note improvement on the patient's facial balance and relations.

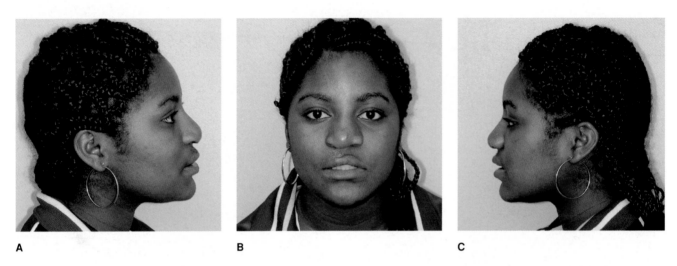

Figure 58–47. (A–C) Postoperative profile and frontal photographs. Note improvement on the facial balance, lip/nose and lip/chin relations, as well as significant aesthetic improvement. The patient will require finishing lip and nose revision at a future surgical procedure.

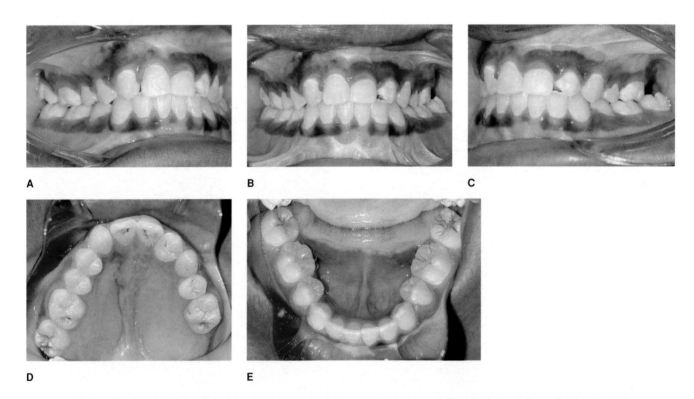

Figure 58–48. (A–E) Intraoral occlusal photographs demonstrating improved dental relations after orthodontics and orthognathic surgery. Note acceptable relationships of tooth #6 as well as tooth #12 and #13 with the opposing dentition. This patient will not require any additional prosthetic reconstruction and/or replacement. Both maxillary and mandibular arches are well coordinated and aligned. Note absence of teeth #21 and #28 in the lower arch with closure of the surgically created spaces.

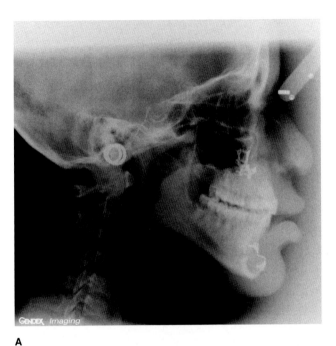

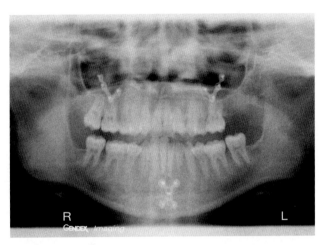

A

B

Figure 58–49. (A) Cephalometric (B) and panoramic radiographs after surgery, demonstrating the rigid fixation plates securing the maxilla, and the mandibular anterior segment. Note improvement in skeletal relations as well as nose, upper and lower lip, and chin relations.

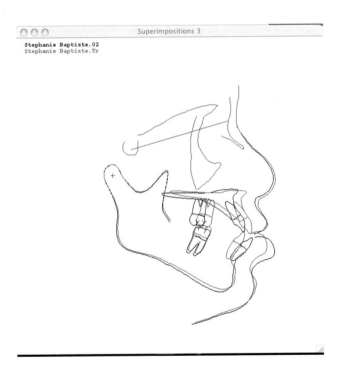

Figure 58–50. Before and after surgery, cephalometric tracings demonstrating the degree of maxillary advancement and posterior mandibular incisor repositioning. Note the modest change of the upper lip with the maxillary advancement but the significant change in the lower lip posture and chin definition.

```
NAME:                                          Quick Ceph® 2000
BIRTH:    2/3/88      SEX:      F              11/23/06
RECORD:   4/14/04     STATUS:   02             Drs.Figueroa Polley
AGE:      16yr 2mo    CASE:


Analysis Figueroa              02     Norm    Clin.Dev.      Tr       Tr

SKELETAL RELATIONS
SNA                    (dg)    78.5   82.0    -1.2   *       84.5     84.5
SNB                    (dg)    77.3   80.0    -0.9           75.8     75.8
A to N -| FH           (mm)     3.9   -1.7     2.2   **       9.5      9.5
SNaOr                  (dg)    62.4   60.0     0.6           62.4     62.4
Facial Angle           (dg)    91.3   88.3     0.8           92.2     92.2
Mandibular Plane       (dg)    25.8   24.2     0.4           24.5     24.5
Y - Axis               (dg)    55.1   59.4    -1.2   *       53.8     53.8
Angle of Convexity     (dg)     5.7    0.0     1.1   *       15.7     15.7
Cant of Occl. Plane    (dg)    18.0    9.3     2.3   **      23.9     16.4
ANS-Menton             (mm)    67.8   62.1     0.9           64.7     64.7
Nasion-Menton          (mm)   114.3  112.4     0.3          112.4    112.4
ANS-Me./Nasion-Me.     (%)     59.3   55.0     1.4   *       57.6     57.6
Mandibular Length      (mm)   116.8  114.4     0.6          116.8    116.8
Midfacial Length       (mm)    88.6   89.8    -0.3           94.5     94.5
Maxillomand. Diff.             28.2   24.1     1.6   *       22.3     22.3
DENTAL RELATIONS
Interincisal Angle     (dg)   102.5  130.0    -4.7   ***    115.3    115.3
     Mx 1, to FH       (dg)   122.2  111.0     1.9   *      119.6    119.6
     Mx 1, to PPl.     (dg)   110.9  113.0    -0.5          111.2    111.2
     Md 1, to APo      (mm)    13.9    1.0     5.6   ***      4.0      4.0
     Md 1, to Md Plane (dg)    19.5    1.4     4.8   ***     10.6     10.6
     Incisor Overjet   (mm)    -6.7    2.5    -3.7   ***      4.6      4.6
     Incisor Overbite  (mm)    -2.3    2.5    -2.4   **      -1.1     -0.5
ESTHETIC RELATIONS
Lower Lip E-Plane      (mm)     9.3   -2.0     5.6   ***      2.2      2.2
Nasolabial Angle       (dg)    93.1  115.2    -3.7   ***    103.7    103.7
G-Sn-Pg'               (dg)    11.0   15.8    -1.0           13.7     13.7
Ant. Cranial Base      (mm)    68.6   70.3    -0.6           68.6     68.6
```

Figure 58–51. Pre- and postsurgery cephalometric values, demonstrating the changes after maxillary advancement (SNA, A-point to Nasion vertical and midfacial length), and mandibular repositioning (SNB, inclination of the incisor relative to the A-point and mandibular planes, and occlusal plane). Note changes on soft tissue convexity (G-SN-PG' angle).

CONCLUSION

Care of cleft patients with cleft-related maxillary hypoplasia poses a significant challenge to the reconstructive team. However, if basic principles of diagnosis and treatment planning are carefully followed, satisfactory outcomes can be obtained. In addition, new technological and surgical advances allow clinicians to safely and predictably obtain the desired results for this difficult group of patients.

References

1. Farkas LG (ed). *Anthropometry of the Head and Face,* 2nd ed. New York: Raven Press, 1994, pp. 1–405.
2. Huang J, Bumann A, Mah J. Three dimensional radiographic analysis in orthodontics. *J Clin Orthod* 39:421–428, 2005.
3. Proffit WR, Sarver DM. Diagnosis: Gathering and organizing the appropriate information. In Proffit WR, White RP, Jr., Sarver DM (eds). *Contemporary Treatment of Dentofacial Deformity.* St. Louis, Mosby, Inc. 2003, pp. 127–171.
4. Epker BN, Fish LC. Essentials of treatment planning: Cephalometric prediction tracing. *Dentofacial Deformities: Integrated Orthodontic and SurgicalCcorrection, Vol 1.* St. Louis, MO: CV Mosby Co., 1986, pp. 73–93.
5. Semb G. A study of facial growth in patients with unilateral cleft lip and/or palate treated by the Oslo CLP team. *Cleft Palate Craniofac J* 28:1–21, 1991.
6. da Silva Filho OJ, Normando AD, Capelozza Filho L. Mandibular growth in patients with cleft lip and/or palate: The influence of cleft type. *Am J Orthod Dentofacial Orthop* 104:269–275, 1993.
7. Polley JW, Figueroa AA. Rigid external distraction (RED): Its application in cleft maxillary deformities. *Plast Reconstr Surg* 102:1360–1372, 1998.
8. Figueroa AA, Polley JW. Management of severe cleft maxillary deficiency with distraction osteogenesis: Procedure and results. *Am J Orthod Dentofacacial Orthop* 115:1–12, 1999.
9. Polley JW, Figueroa AA. Maxillary distraction osteogenesis with rigid external distraction. Atlas of oral Maxillofac. *Sur Clin North Am* 7:15–28, 1999.
10. Figueroa AA, Polley JW, Friede H, Ko EW. Long-term skeletal stability after maxillary advancement with distraction osteogenesis using a rigid external distraction device in cleft maxillary deformities. *Plast Reconstr Surg* 114:1382–1392, 2004.
11. Figueroa AA, Polley JW. Orthodontics in cleft lip and palate management. In Mathes SJM (ed). *Plastic Surgery, Pediatric Plastic Surgery, Vol 4,* 2nd ed. Philadelphia: Elsevier, 2006, pp. 271–310.
12. Tucker MR, White Jr., RP. Combining surgical procedures in the mandible and maxilla. In Proffit WR, White Jr., RP, Sarver DM (eds). *Contemporary Treatment of Dentofacial Deformity.* St. Louis, Mosby, Inc. 2003, pp. 345–356.

59

Surgical-Orthodontic Correction of Transverse Maxillary Deficiency

James A. Lehman, Jr., MD • Andrew J. Haas, DDS, MS

INTRODUCTION

With the increased interest in adult orthodontics, transverse maxillary width problems have been encountered, with greater frequency, by orthodontists in the nongrowing patient. The concept of widening the maxillary dental arch by means of opening the mid-palatal suture was first described by Angell[1] in 1860 and was reintroduced by Haas[2-4] in 1961. Rapid palatal expansion appliances have been used effectively in children and adolescents to correct real and relative maxillary transverse deficiency, skeletal Class II, Division I malocclusions with or without posterior crossbite, both surgical and nonsurgical Class III patients, and selected arch-length problems.[5-7] In adults, attempts at rapid palatal expansion are frequently associated with failure. Lateral tipping of the teeth, bending of alveolar bone, inability to open the mid-palatal suture, pressure necrosis of the mucosa from the expansion appliance, and relapse are all well-documented problems of this treatment.[8-11] In addition, the true unilateral crossbites cannot be as effectively treated by conventional rapid maxillary expansion, because the effects are bilateral.[5]

Historically, the difficulty with opening the mid-palatal suture in adults was attributed to fusion of this suture. Isaacson et al.[12,13] have shown that the facial skeleton increases its resistance to expansion with maturity and age; and, the major resistance to expansion of the maxilla is not the mid-palatal suture, but the remaining maxillary articulations. Various types of maxillary osteotomies have been described to facilitate lateral movement of the maxilla, either by palatal expansion appliances[8,14-16] or by repositioning the maxillary segments.[17-20] Kennedy et al.[17] have shown a statistically significant increase in the amount of lateral movement seen in animals who had a lateral osteotomy prior to the rapid palatal expansion. Lehman et al.[21] and others[22,23] have demonstrated in adults that the maxillary expansion can be achieved using a conservative approach, consisting of a lateral osteotomy of the zygomaticomaxillary buttress with or without osteotomy of the mid-palatal suture, combined with a rapid palatal expansion appliance.

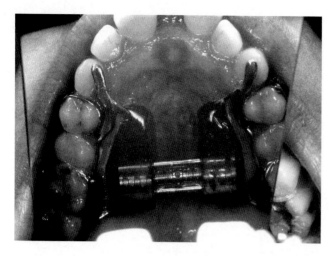

Figure 59–1. A rapid palatal expansion device cemented to the first premolar and first molar. This is a tooth-tissue-borne appliance.

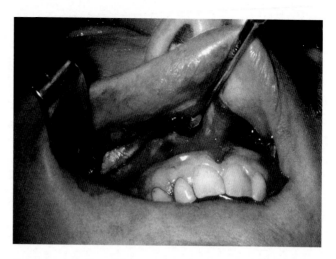

Figure 59–3. Elevation of the mucoperiosteum exposing the maxilla from the piriform aperture to the zygomatic maxillary buttress.

SURGICAL PROCEDURE

Before surgery, a rapid palatal expansion device is cemented to the maxillary first premolar and first molar teeth. This should be a tooth-tissue-borne appliance (Fig. 59–1). Under general anesthesia, an upper buccal sulcus incision is made through the mucoperiosteum from the first molar to the first molar (Fig. 59–2). The mucoperiosteum is elevated superiorly and laterally exposing the piriform aperture, anterior nasal floor, anterior lateral maxilla, and the zygomatic buttress (Fig. 59–3). The major areas to be osteotomized are the zygomaticomaxillary buttress and the anterior portion of the lateral nasal wall. A horizontal osteotomy is then made with a power saw (Fig. 59–4) through the lateral wall of the maxilla, approximately 4–5 mm above the apices of the teeth, from the inferior lateral aspect of the piriform aperture, to the

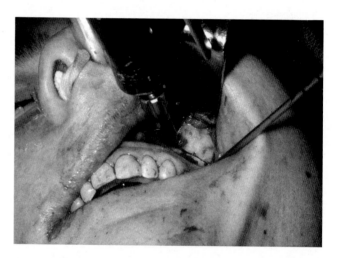

Figure 59–4. Horizontal osteotomy is made with a power saw.

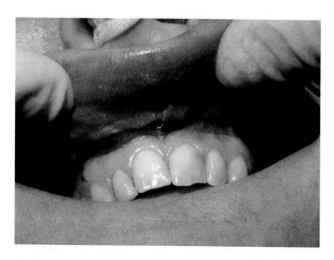

Figure 59–2. Incision line from first molar to first molar in maxillary sulcus.

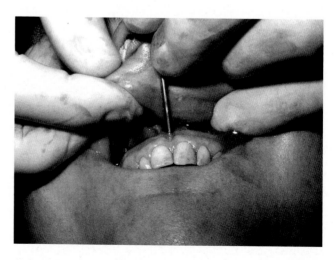

Figure 59–5. Start of expansion with a thin osteotome between central incisors.

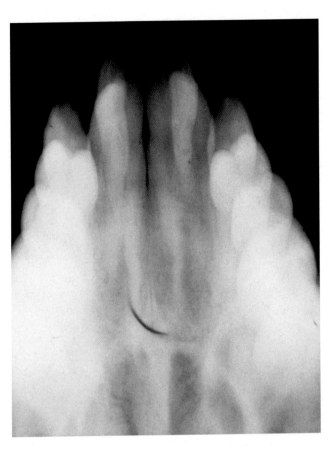

Figure 59–6. Palatal X-ray demonstrating ossification of mid-palatal suture.

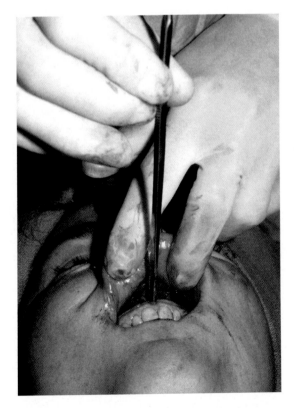

Figure 59–7. Mid-palatal osteotomy made with osteotome along the entire length of hard palate. Performed in patients with ossification of mid-palatal suture.

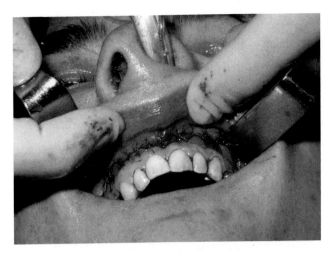

Figure 59–8. Closure of the incision.

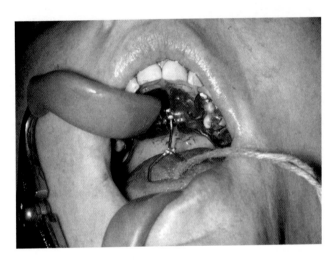

Figure 59–9. Activation of expansion appliance.

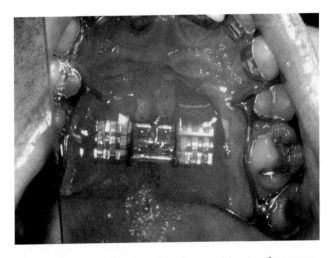

Figure 59–10. Stabilization of appliance with wire after expansion completed.

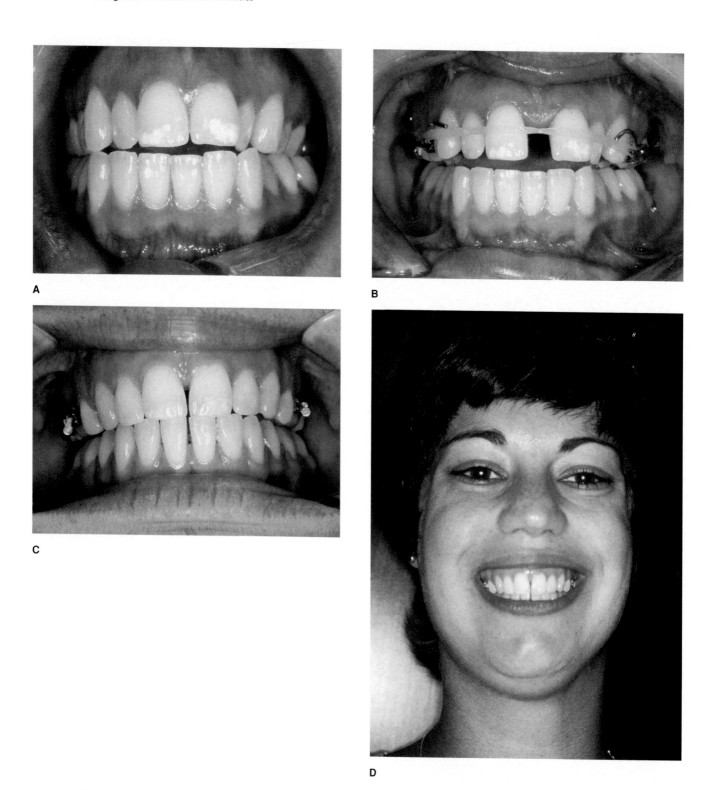

Figure 59–11. A: Bilateral maxillary crossbite in a Class I occlusion. **B:** Occlusion at completion of expansion. **C:** Final result 1 year after completion of orthodontia. **D:** Final facial photograph.

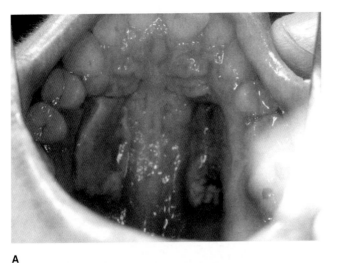

A

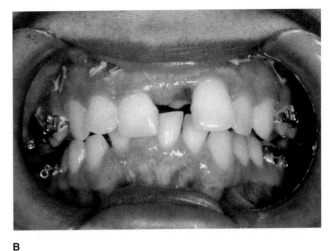

B

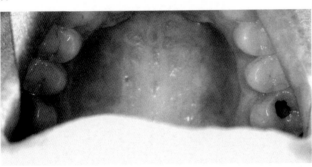

C

Figure 59–12. A: Severe mucosal ulceration after attempted expansion. **B:** Healed mucosa after 4 weeks. **C:** Expansion completed after mid-palatal osteotomy and repeat maxillary osteotomy.

inferior aspect of the junction of the maxillary tuberosity and the pterygoid plate. Certainly, the osteotomy through the thin anterior wall of the maxilla is not important, but it allows for rapid completion of the procedure. The anterior portion of the lateral nasal wall is included after elevation of the nasal mucosa. Sectioning of the pterygomaxillary suture is unnecessary. Expansion of the anterior portion of the maxilla can be started, by inserting a thin osteotome between the roots of the central incisors (Fig. 59–5), but this is not a necessary part of the procedure. Care must be taken not to cut too deeply, so as to sever the transeptal fibers linking the central incisors. Should the transeptal fibers be cut, the orthodontist may find it very difficult to bring the central incisors into approximation, and these teeth may be at risk for not exhibiting their usual physiological space closure.

In patients with ossification of the mid-palatal suture (Fig. 59–6), a mid-palatal osteotomy is performed in addition to the preceding procedure. After placing a thin osteotome between the roots of the central incisors, the osteotome is turned 90 degrees and malleted down the length of the hard palate staying in the submucosal plane (Fig. 59–7). A mid-palatal osteotomy was performed 30% of the time in the author's

reported series.[21] In the rare patient with a palatal exostosis, parasagittal osteotomies may be necessary to achieve expansion. In the patient with a true unilateral crossbite, only a unilateral maxillary osteotomy is required. However, most crossbites are bilateral with a unilateral manifestation, that is, mandibular shift to the crossbite side.

Following closure of the buccal mucosa (Fig. 59–8), the palatal expansion appliance is activated four one-quarter turns (Fig. 59–9). Each one-quarter turn is equivalent to a 0.25 mm movement of the screw. This is not translated into an equivalent movement in the bone. The operative procedure is performed on an outpatient basis and takes approximately 30 minutes. The patient is followed in the office. The palatal appliance is normally activated one one-quarter turn twice a day until the desired amount of expansion is achieved. The maxilla is always overexpanded, because there will be some relapse, owing to lateral tipping of the teeth. Expansion is usually completed in approximately 3 weeks; and, at this point, the appliance is stabilized with a wire or acrylic (Fig. 59–10). The expanded segments are retained for 3–4 months, but other orthodontic procedures can be initiated after the appliance is stabilized.

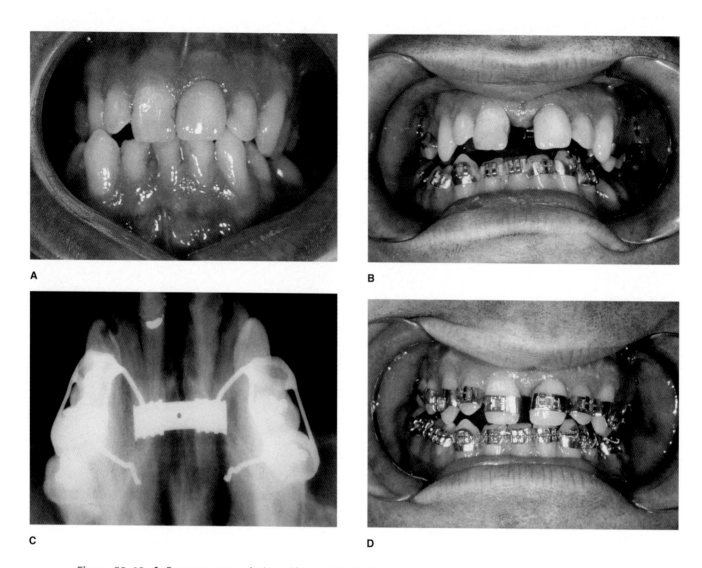

Figure 59–13. A: Pretreatment occlusion with crossbite. **B:** After expansion completed at three weeks. **C:** X-ray at three weeks showing wedge-shaped opening in palate. **D:** Orthodontic treatment under way. **E:** X-ray during orthodontic treatment. **F:** Final occlusion. **G:** Final X-ray after treatment completed with consolidation of the maxilla with new bone.

RESULTS

Since 1976, 92 patients with bilateral horizontal maxillary deficiency, and associated dentofacial disharmonies, have been treated by the conservative surgical-orthodontic approach herein described.[21] There were 54 females and 38 males, with age ranging from 19 to 47 years. There has been satisfactory expansion in all the patients, and the desired amount of maxillary expansion was accomplished in 12–28 days (Fig. 59–11). In two patients, palate expansion was discontinued prior to overcorrection because of pressure necrosis on the palate related to the appliance. There was enough expansion, however, treatment was subsequently completed after healing of the mucosa. Three other patients had some degree of mucosal ulceration, and expansion was stopped and then begun at a slower pace, which allowed treatment to be completed.

One patient was referred from another institution after expansion failed and there was severe mucosal ulceration (Fig. 59–12A). They failed to recognize an ossified mid-palatal suture. After the mucosa healed (Fig. 59–12B), a repeat transverse osteotomy, plus a mid-palatal osteotomy, allowed for successful expansion (Fig. 59–12C). Care must be taken with a tooth-tissue-borne appliance to generously bevel all line angles and corners of the acrylic appliance to avoid injury to the palatal mucosa. If some necrosis develops, it is best to stop expansion until the mucosa heals, and then proceed at a slower pace. As an alternative, you can remove the appliance, relieve the line angle or corner of the appliance causing the irritation, and immediately replace the appliance to full seating. With attention to these details, pressure necrosis of the mucosa has been avoided. In our reported series, there were no other complications.

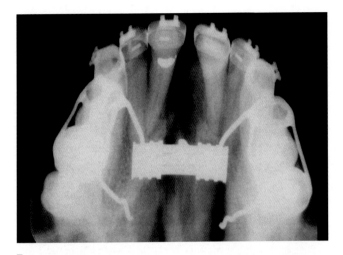

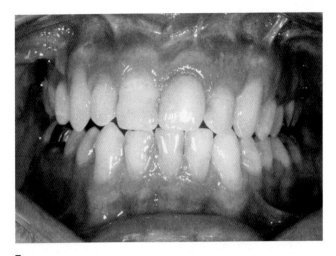

E

F

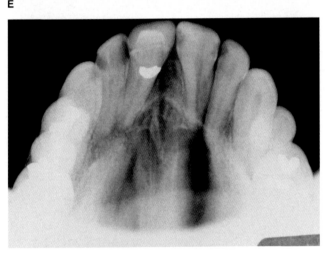

G

Figure 59–13. (*Continued*).

Occlusal X-ray films have demonstrated separation of the mid-palatal suture during the expansion (Fig. 59–13). The opening is slightly wider anteriorly. After completion of the expansion, there is gradual consolidation of the expanded maxilla with new bone; and, by 6 months, X-rays appeared normal. This is basically a form of distraction osteogenesis.

In the author's series,[21] twenty-eight patients had subsequent orthognathic surgery. Six patients had vertical and sagittal repositioning of the maxilla (Fig. 59–14). Fourteen patients had mandibular surgery (Fig. 59–15), and eight patients had combined maxillary and mandibular surgery to complete their dentofacial correction (Fig. 59–16). The cases illustrate how palatal expansion can be a complementary component in the overall treatment plan for patients with dentofacial deformities.

DISCUSSION

Transverse and anteroposterior maxillary deficiency can be seen with mandibular prognathism, mandibular deficiency,

and anterior openbite deformities. Once the diagnosis is made by cephalometric study, and by positioning the dental models into a Class I canine relationship, a decision must be made as to the method of expansion in the adult patient. Should expansion be accomplished by segmenting the maxilla at the time of vertical or sagittal repositioning, or should expansion be done with a horizontal osteotomy of the maxilla and rapid palatal expansion in a separate and prior procedure? The feasibility of each approach should be determined by an evaluation of the clinical problem, the dental models, and the cephalometric X-rays. In addition, all patients with maxillary constriction should have a palatal X-ray to see if the mid-palatal suture is ossified (see Fig. 59–6).

The major indication for surgery alone, without a staged preparatory palatal expansion, is the patient with a minimal transverse maxillary discrepancy, in which extraction of the first premolars is needed. In this situation, a three-piece segmental maxillary procedure will correct the problem. Patients who require maxillary advancement, vertical movement of the maxilla, or both can also be corrected using a three- or four-segment maxillary osteotomy.

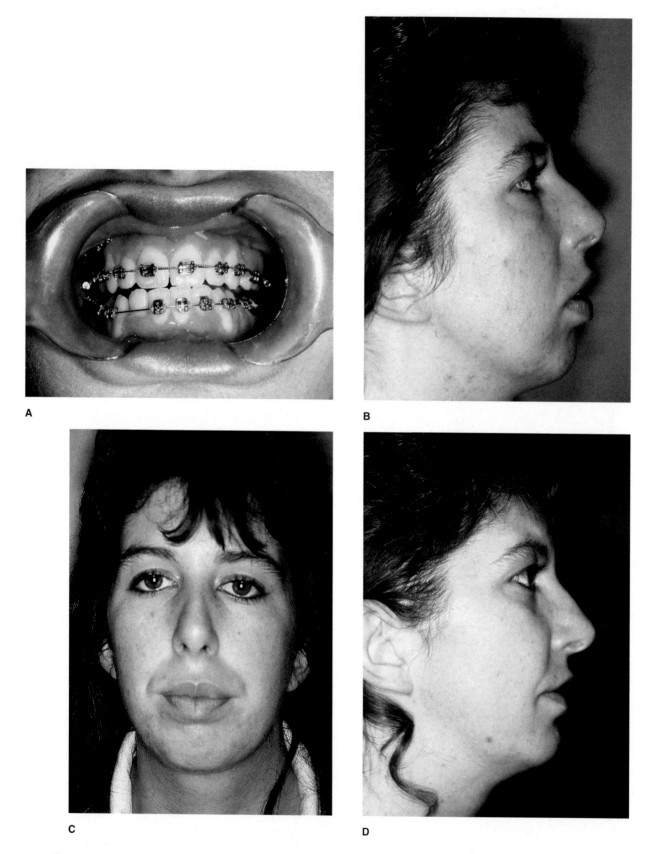

Figure 59–14. A: Occlusion after palatal expansion. **B:** Presurgical profile view. **C:** Presurgical frontal view. **D:** Appearance after LeFort osteotomy with superior repositioning and reduction genioplasty. **E:** Profile view. **F:** Final occlusion.

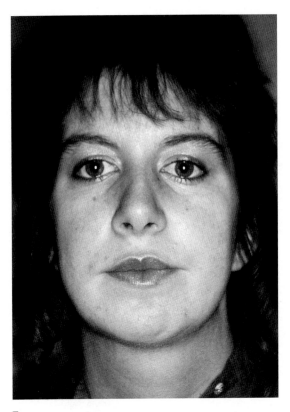

E

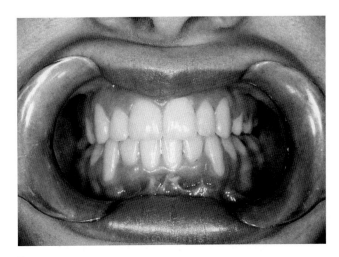

F

Figure 59–14. (*Continued*).

The primary indication for lateral maxillary osteotomy and rapid palatal expansion is the patient who does not require vertical or sagittal repositioning of the maxilla (Figs. 59–11 and 59–13). However, in patients with marked skeletal discrepancies, a preliminary rapid palatal expansion may eliminate the need for segmentation of the maxillae at the time of final orthognathic surgery and its accompanying risks.

While palatal expansion increases the width of the nasal cavity, without changing the position of the nasal septum,[24] its use for airway purposes alone is controversial. Warren et al.[25] feel that its use for airway improvement is not justified, but Haas[2] has shown significant clinical improvement in respiration if maximum anchorage appliances are used and the expansion is from 10 to 14 mm. Patients who have a significant anterior openbite, high mandibular plane angles, and convex profiles are generally not good candidates for rapid palatal expansion, because a secondary effect of palatal expansion may be molar extrusion, further opening the bite.[5] Haas[6,7] has noted that patients with mid-skeletal problems can be successfully treated if vertical control is started immediately after expansion is completed. In patients with marked skeletal problems, however, this treatment can be used to coordinate the arches prior to maxillary or mandibular surgery (Figs. 59–14, 59–15, and 59–16). Furthermore, it should be noted that segmentation of the maxilla increases the risk for skeletal, dental, and periodontal complications that do not exist when the maxilla is not segmented. This is another reason to consider rapid palatal expansion as a preliminary procedure, prior to orthognathic surgery, in patients with marked skeletal discrepancies.

Several other factors are also need to be considered, when deciding on the approach, for expansion. If the arch-length discrepancy is moderate, rapid palatal expansion will increase the arch circumference, and dental alignment can be accomplished without extractions. In the narrow tapered arch, rapid maxillary expansion is the preferred treatment to prevent a midline diastema. Finally, in patients in whom the transverse discrepancy is > 10 mm, the vascular limits of the three-piece maxillary osteotomy are exceeded, and rapid maxillary expansion is clearly the procedure of choice.

Virtually, all the maxillary articulations have been sectioned, in various combinations, to prevent the problems commonly seen when rapid palatal expansion is attempted in the nongrowing patient. Prior studies by Isaacson et al.[12,13] and Kennedy et al.[26] seem to indicate that the major resistance to expansion to the maxilla is zygomaticomaxillary buttress, and not the mid-palatal suture, or the pterygomaxillary articulation. The successful completion of rapid palatal expansion, in our series of 92 adult patients, and in other reports[22,23] using a conservative lateral maxillary osteotomy, supports this concept. It should be noted, however, that 30% of the cases (27 patients), needed an additional mid-palatal osteotomy

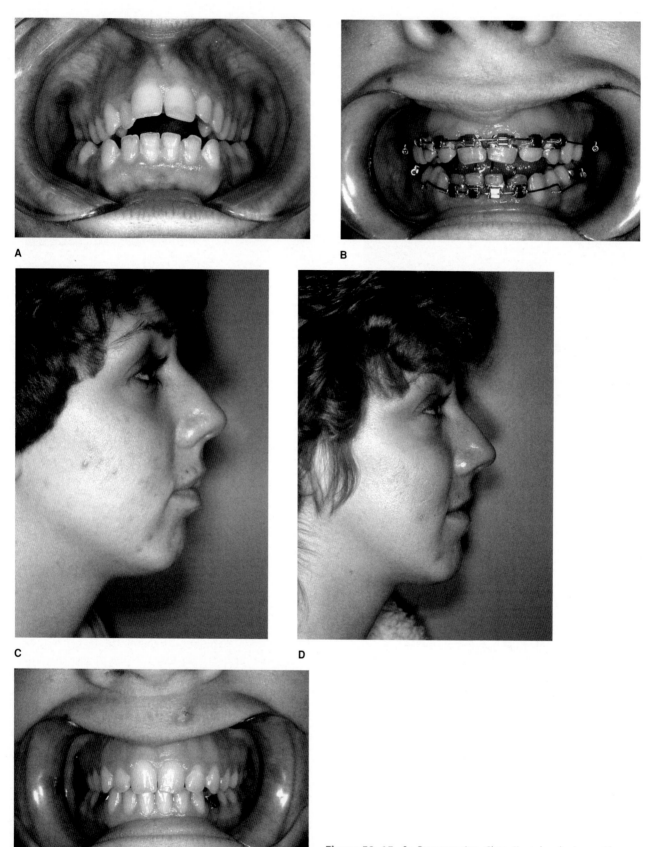

Figure 59–15. A: Preoperative Class II malocclusion with cross-bite and anterior openbite. **B:** Occlusion after palatal expansion. **C:** Presurgical profile of patient. **D:** Final profile after sagittal split osteotomy and advancement. **E:** Occlusion 1 year after completion of orthodontics.

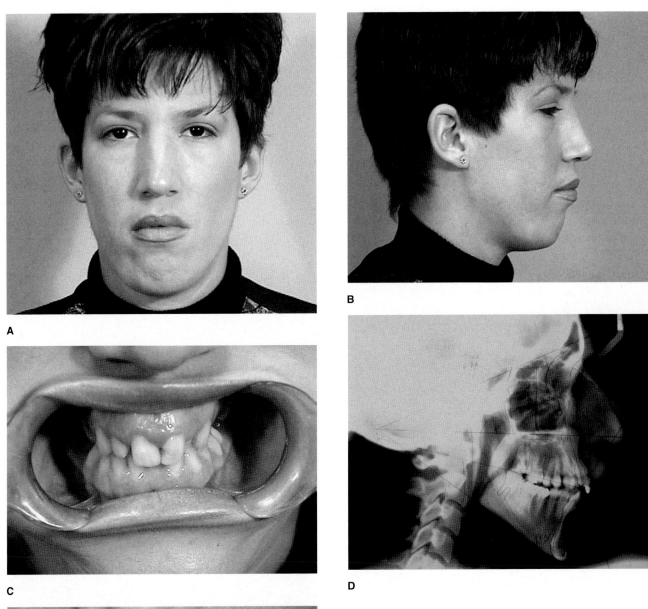

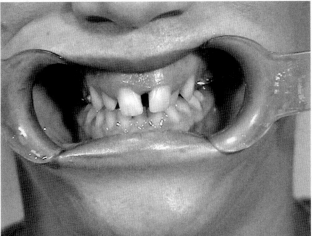

Figure 59–16. A: Presurgical frontal view of patient. **B:** Presurgical profile view. **C:** Presurgical occlusion demonstrating maxillary cross-bite. **D:** Presurgical cephalometric X-ray. **E:** Occlusion after palatal expansion. **F:** Appearance after LeFort I with superior repositioning, sagittal split and osteotomy with advancement and advancement genioplasty. **G:** Final frontal view. **H:** Final occlusion. **I:** Final cephalometric X-ray.

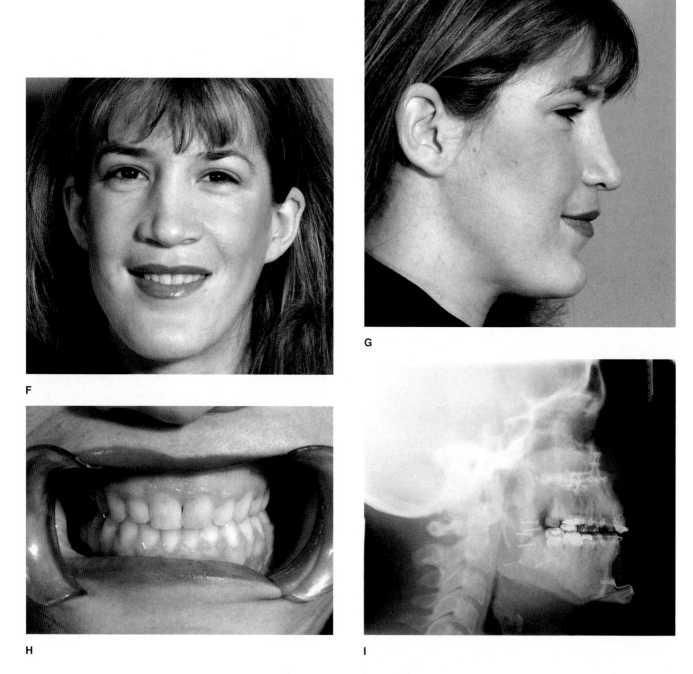

Figure 59–16. (*Continued*).

because of ossification of the mid-palatal suture. If the patient has a rare palatal exostosis, parasagittal osteotomies, as recommended by Bell and Epker,[14] are indicated.

Since the primary objective of palatal expansion is to coordinate the maxillary and mandibular arches, the appliance should be designed to enhance orthopaedic movement and curtail orthodontic response.[2,4] To obtain this, a fixed tooth-tissue-borne; acrylic palate expansion appliance is used. The acrylic portion is confined to the tissue between the first premolars and the first molars. Care is taken not to impinge on the rugae, the gingival tissue, or the tissue overlying the

posterior alveolar foramina, so that pressure necrosis of the mucosa does not occur.

SUMMARY

A conservative osteotomy of the zygomaticomaxillary buttress, in combination with a rapid palatal expansion appliance, is a dependable technique for the treatment of horizontal maxillary deficiency in adults. This procedure has been used successfully in 92 patients in our series, but 27 patients

(30%) required a mid-palatal osteotomy. In two patients, over-expansion was not achieved because of necrosis of the mucosa. In three other patients, expansion had to proceed at a slower pace because of mucosal ulceration. There have been no other complications. The procedure is indicated mainly for patients with a horizontal maxillary deficiency, that do not require subsequent surgery but for some patients with marked skeletal discrepencies, it may be the staged preliminary procedure. Twenty-eight patients (31%) had subsequent orthognathic surgery. Follow-up has been from 1 to 12 years, and there has been no relapse. In our opinion, the zygomaticomaxillary buttress is the primary area of resistance to lateral movement of the maxilla by rapid maxillary expansion appliances.

ACKNOWLEDGMENTS

We would like to thank the orthodontists David G. Haas, DDS; Roger Haas, DDS; Nicholas Mellion, DDS; Steve Misencik, DDS; Charles Schwarz, DDS; Michael Bernard, DDS; and Harry Osborne, DDS, who provided the treatment for some of the patients in this report.

References

1. Angell EH. Treatment of irregularities of the permanent or adult tooth. *Dent Cosmos* 1:540, 1860.
2. Haas AJ. Rapid expansion of the maxillary dental arch and nasal cavity by opening the midpalatal suture. *Angle Orthod* 31:73, 1961.
3. Haas AJ. The treatment of maxillary deficiency by opening the midpalatal suture. *Angle Orthod* 35:200, 1965.
4. Haas AJ. Palatal expansion: Just the beginning of dentofacial orthopaedics. *Am J Orthod* 57:219, 1970.
5. Bishara SE, Staley RN. Maxillary expansion: Clinical implications. *Am J Orthod Dentofac Orthop* 91:3, 1987.
6. Haas AJ. A biological approach to diagnosis, mechanics, and treatment of vertical dysplasia. *Angle Orthod* 50:279, 1980.
7. Haas AJ. Long-term post treatment evaluation of rapid palatal expansion. *Angle Orthod* 50:1819, 1980.
8. Lines PA. Adult rapid maxillary expansion with corticotomy. *Am J Orthod* 67:44, 1975.
9. Moss JP. Rapid expansion of the maxillary arch, Part I. *J Pract Orthod* 2:165, 1968.
10. Moss JP. Rapid expansion of the maxillary arch, Part II. *J Pract Orthod* 2:215, 1968.
11. Wertz, RA. Skeletal and dental changes accompanying rapid mid-palatal suture opening. *Am J Orthod* 58:41, 1970.
12. Isaacson RJ, Ingram AH. Forces produced by rapid maxillary expansion. II. Forces present during treatment. *Angle Orthod* 34:261, 1964.
13. Isaacson RJ, Wood JL, Ingram AH. Forces produced by rapid maxillary expansion. Design of force measuring system. *Angle Orthod* 34:256, 1964.
14. Bell WH, Epker BN. Surgical–orthodontic expansion of the maxilla. *Am J Orthod* 70:517, 1976.
15. Bell WH, Jacobs JD. Surgical–orthodontic correction of horizontal maxillary deficiency. *J Oral Surg* 37:897, 1979.
16. Kraut RA. Surgically assisted rapid maxillary expansion by opening the midpalatal suture. *J Oral Maxillofac Surg* 42:651, 1984.
17. Bell WH, Turvey TA. Surgical correction of posterior crossbite. *J Oral Surg* 32:811, 1974
18. Steinhauser EW. Midline splitting of the maxilla for correction of malocclusion. *J Oral Surg* 30:413, 1972.
19. Turvey TA. Maxillary expansion: A surgical technique based on surgical–orthodontic treatment objectives and anatomical considerations. *J Maxillofac Surg* 13:51, 1985.
20. Wolford, LM, Epker BN. The combined anterior and posterior maxillary osteotomy: A new technique. *J Oral Surg* 33:842, 1975.
21. Lehman, JA, Haas AJ, Haas DG. Surgical–orthodontic correction of transverse maxillary deficiency: A simplified approach. *J Plast Reconstr Surg* 73:62, 1984.
22. Alpern MC, Yorosko JJ. Rapid palatal expansion in adults with and without surgery. *Angle Orthod* 57:245, 1987.
23. Glassman AS, Nahigian SJ, Medway JM, et al. Conservative surgical orthodontic adult rapid palatal expansion: Sixteen cases. *Am J Orthod* 86:207, 1984.
24. Schwarz GM, Thrash WJ, Byrd DL, et al. Tomographic assessment of nasal septal changes following surgical-orthodontic rapid maxillary expansion. *Am J Orthod* 87:39, 1985.
25. Warren DW, Hershey HG, Turvey TA, et al. The nasal airway following maxillary expansion. *Am J Orthod Dentofac Orthop* 91:111, 1987.
26. Kennedy JW III, Bell WH, Kimbrough OL, et al. Osteotomy as an adjunct to rapid maxillary expansion. *Am J Orthod* 70:123, 1976.

Cleft Orthognathic Surgery

Stephen B. Baker, DDS, MD, FACS • Nathan Menon, MD

INTRODUCTION

Orthognathic surgery is the term used to describe surgical movement of the maxilla, mandible, or both jaws. The goal of orthognathic surgery is to establish ideal dental occlusion with the jaws in a position that optimizes facial form and function. It is common for patients who undergo surgical correction of cleft lip and palate in infancy to develop dentofacial deformities, and 25–30% will have severe enough midface retrusion to require orthognathic surgery. Maxillary

hypoplasia resulting in Class III malocclusion is the typical deformity seen in this patient population. The etiology behind maxillary hypoplasia remains unclear. There is evidence to support the fact that the inelasticity of scar tissue from surgical procedures restricts facial growth.[1,2] However, Weinzweig[3] has demonstrated midface retrusion in an unoperated caprine model of palatal clefting suggesting that an intrinsic mechanism may play a role in the midface deficiency associated with cleft palate. While mild Class III malocclusions may be camouflaged with orthodontic compensation alone, orthognathic surgery is needed to ideally correct the Class III dentofacial deformity.

The chance of a favorable surgical outcome is optimized if presurgical planning is performed with a cleft/craniofacial team. Speech and language pathologists play an integral role in the evaluation of the velopharyngeal mechanism and the potential effects that maxillary advancement may have on velopharyngeal competence, nasalance, nasality, and articulation. A preoperative perceptual speech evaluation may yield valuable information that can aid in predicting postoperative hypernasality.

The orthodontist's role in the preoperative evaluation and management of the orthognathic surgery candidate is critical. Prior to the surgery, the potential surgical candidate requires a comprehensive workup, including analysis of the occlusion and the age of the facial skeleton. If orthognathic surgery is attempted before the facial skeleton reaches maturity, the need for revision surgery will be increased because of unpredictable postoperative growth. Skeletal growth is usually complete between the ages of 14 and 16 in females and between the ages of 16 and 18 in males. One can assess the maturity of the facial skeleton and the cessation of growth by serial cephalometric radiographs or by looking for epiphyseal closure in hand radiographs.

It is important to obtain a thorough medical and dental history from every patient. Systemic diseases such as juvenile rheumatoid arthritis, diabetes, and scleroderma, may affect the treatment planning. Each patient should be questioned regarding symptoms of temporomandibular joint (TMJ) disease or myofascial pain syndrome. Motivation and realistic expectations are extremely important in ensuring an optimal final postoperative outcome. In cleft lip and palate patients, several factors are present that make this surgery more difficult. It is important for the patient to realize that some revision surgery and bone grafting may be needed to complete dental rehabilitation. Bone grafts are frequently necessary if edentulous spaces are to be restored with osseointegrated implants. Because implants cannot be moved orthodontically, they are placed after jaw surgery and postoperative orthodontics. It is important for the patient to have a clear understanding of the procedure, the recovery, and the anticipated result prior to the surgery. Orthognathic surgery is a major undertaking, and the patient should be appropriately motivated to undergo all necessary perioperative orthodontic treatment and rehabilitation in order to achieve the desired result.

PREPARATION FOR SURGERY

Physical Examination

A complete physical exam should be performed on the patient prior to the surgery. Intraorally, the patient must demonstrate evidence of good oral hygiene and periodontal health prior to the orthodontics and orthognathic surgery. The occlusal classification is determined, and the degree of incisor overlap and overjet is quantified. The surgeon should assess the transverse dimension of the maxilla. If a crossbite is present, models should be obtained to assess if it is a relative crossbite, based on maxillary retrusion, or a true crossbite when the models are articulated in a Class I position. An absolute crossbite is due to maxillary constriction and will require either orthopedic (orthodontic appliance) or surgical expansion to correct. In cleft patients, an absolute crossbite may be present despite a history of maxillary expansion prior to the alveolar bone grafting. In a severe Class III malocclusion, a degree of relative crossbite will also be present. To assess how much crossbite is truly present, the casts are articulated in a Class I position to determine if a two-piece osteotomy will be necessary to correct a transverse discrepancy. If the mandibular third molars are present, they will need to be extracted 6 months before performing a sagittal split osteotomy. Any missing teeth or abnormal periapical pathology should be noted and addressed prior to the surgery. Any signs or symptoms of TMJ dysfunction need to be evaluated before proceeding with the surgery.

The frontal facial evaluation consists of assessing the vertical facial thirds: Trichion to glabella, glabella to subnasale, and subnasale to menton. Each of these facial thirds should be about equal. If the lower third of the face is short, it can be increased by inferiorly positioning the maxilla. In the cleft patient, there is typically a degree of vertical shortening of the maxilla. Usually the patient benefits from both anterior and inferior positioning of the maxilla. The most important factor in determining the vertical height of the maxilla is the degree of incisor showing while the patient's lips are in repose. A man should show at least 2–3 mm while as much as 5–6 mm is considered attractive in a woman. If lip incompetence or mentalis strain is present, it is usually an indicator of vertical maxillary excess.

The alar base width should also be assessed prior to the surgery since orthognathic surgery may alter the intraalar width; and alar asymmetry is not uncommon in patients with a history of cleft lip. Asymmetries of the maxilla and mandible should be documented on physical examination, and the degree of deviation from the facial midline noted. When evaluating the chin, the clinician assesses the labiomental angle. An acute labiomental angle may indicate a short or prominent chin, while an obtuse angle with effacement of the crease typically indicates excessive vertical length or insufficient anterior projection.

The profile evaluation focuses on projection of the forehead, malar region, upper and lower jaws, nose, chin, and neck. An experienced clinician can usually determine whether the deformity is due to the maxilla, mandible, or both—simply by looking at the patient. This clinical assessment is verified at the time of the cephalometric analysis. The proper position of the nose relates to the upper lip, which is supported by the maxillary incisors, and the chin. Because both of these structures may be altered by orthognathic surgery, it is important to predict how the dimensions of the nose will fit into the new facial proportions. A rhinoplasty may be necessary to maintain proper facial proportions; and in cleft patients, a rhinoplasty is performed ideally after maxillary surgery.

Intraorally, the patient must demonstrate good oral hygiene and periodontal health. The maxillary and mandibular dental midlines are assessed to determine if they are congruent with each other and the facial midline. Any deviations are noted and quantified. The presence of mandibular third molars is noted; because, if a sagittal split osteotomy is planned, they will need to be removed 6 months before the surgery. The presence and degree of dental compensation is also recorded. The term 'dental compensation' is used to describe the tendency of teeth to tilt in a direction that minimizes the dental malocclusion. Often, the clinician can get a sense of the degree of dental compensation on physical exam, but radiographic analysis is necessary to quantify the degree of compensation. Typically, the cleft patient suffers from midface hypoplasia and a Class III malocclusion, so the lower incisors will be tilted lingually, and the maxillary incisors will be flared labially. Thus, dental compensation will mask the true degree of skeletal discrepancy. Precise analysis of the dental compensation is done on the lateral cephalometric radiograph.

Presurgical orthodontics will decompensate the occlusion, thereby reversing the compensation that has occurred. Decompensation has the effect of exaggerating the malocclusion but allows the surgeon to maximize skeletal movements. If the patient is ambivalent or not interested in surgery, mild cases of malocclusion may be treated by further dental compensation. Compensation may camouflage mild skeletal deformities and restore proper overjet and overlap. The importance of a commitment to surgery prior to orthodontics lies in the fact that the dental movements for decompensation and compensation are in opposite directions, so this decision needs to be made prior to the orthodontic therapy.[4]

Cephalometric Analysis and Models

A lateral cephalometric radiograph is performed under reproducible conditions so that serial images can be compared. It is important be certain the surgeon can visualize bony as well as soft tissue features on the image in order to facilitate tracing all the landmarks: sella, inferior orbital rim, nasion, frontal bone, nasal bones, maxilla, maxillary first molar and central incisor, external auditory meatus, condylar head and mandible, and the mandibular first molar and incisor. The soft tissue of the forehead, nose, lips, and chin are also traced. Once the normal structures are traced, several planes and angles are determined (Fig. 60–1).

The maxillary plane is a line drawn between the anterior nasal spine (ANS) and posterior nasal spine (PNS). The occlusal plane is drawn between the occlusal surfaces of the teeth. The mandibular plane is drawn between menton and gonion, and the Frankfort horizontal plane is delineated between the superior portion of the external auditory meatus (porion) and the inferior orbital rim (orbitale). Analysis of these planes, aids in establishing an accurate diagnosis.

The SNA and SNB are the two most important angles in determining the relative positions of the maxilla and mandible to each other as well as to the cranial base. These angles are determined by drawing lines from sella to nasion to

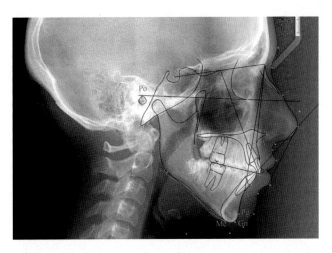

Figure 60–1. The cephalometric radiograph is used to identify skeletal landmarks used in determining the lines and angles that reflect facial development. These measurements aid in determining the extent to which each jaw contributes to the dentofacial deformity. S: sella turcica, the midpoint of the sella turcica; N: nasion, the anterior point of the intersection between the nasal and frontal bones; A: "A point," the innermost point in the depth of the concavity of the maxillary alveolar process; B: "B point," the innermost point on the contour of the mandible between the incisor tooth and the bony chin; Pg: pogonion, the most anterior point on the contour of the chin; Go: gonion, the most inferior and posterior point at the angle formed by the ramus and body of the mandible; Po: porion, the uppermost lateral point on the roof of the external auditory meatus; Or: orbitale, the lowest point on the inferior margin of the orbit; Gn: gnathion, the center of the inferior contour of the chin; Me: menton, the most inferior point on the mandibular symphysis.

A point or B point, respectively. By forming an angle with the sella and nasion, this position is related to the cranial base. The maxilla will be considered first. A point represents the anteroposterior position of the maxilla. If the SNA angle is excessive, the maxilla exhibits abnormal anterior position relative to the cranium. If SNA is less than normal, the maxilla is posteriorly positioned relative to the cranial base, typical in cleft patients requiring surgery. The same principle applies to the mandible; the only difference is that B point is used to relate mandibular position to the cranial base. The importance of the cranial base as a reference is that it allows the clinician to determine if one or both jaws contribute to the deformity. For example, a patient's Class III malocclusion (underbite) could develop from several different etiologies, including: a retrognathic maxilla and normal mandible, a normal maxilla and a prognathic mandible, a retrognathic mandible and a more severely retrognathic maxilla, or a prognathic maxilla and a more severely prognathic mandible. All of these conditions yield a Class III malocclusion, yet each requires a different treatment approach. The surgeon can delineate the true etiology of the deformity by the fact that the maxilla and mandible can be independently quantified to a stable reference point, the cranial base.

Plaster dental casts are also obtained during the treatment planning process. Casts are useful because they allow the surgeon to evaluate the occlusion when the casts are articulated into the proper position. Analysis of the new occlusion gives the clinician an idea of how intensive the presurgical orthodontic treatment plan will be. If a two-piece LeFort I osteotomy is planned to compress the segments and close an alveolar fistula, the casts can be cut and waxed into the anticipated position, determining if the new occlusion is acceptable. Casts also allow the clinician to distinguish between absolute and relative transverse maxillary deficiency. Absolute transverse maxillary deficiency presents as a posterior crossbite with the jaws in a Class I relationship. A relative maxillary transverse deficiency is commonly seen in a patient with a Class III malocclusion. A posterior crossbite is observed in this type of patient leading the surgeon to suspect inadequate maxillary width. However, as the maxilla is advanced, or the mandible retruded, the crossbite is eliminated. Articulation of the casts into a Class I occlusion allows the surgeon to easily distinguish between relative and absolute maxillary constriction.

Overview of Treatment up to Surgery

Prior to the surgery, the patient will have had multiple visits to the surgeon's office, and has undergone a thorough discussion of the surgical options. Having heard all the available options, to treat the problem, the patient is in agreement with the surgeon on the proposed plan. Good oral health has been achieved. The patient has had preoperative orthodontics to level, align, and decompensate the occlusion. Based on the physical and radiographic exams, a treatment plan has been developed that will achieve a Class I occlusion and optimize form and function. Cephalometric tracings have been used to determine the distances the jaws will have to move to achieve the desired result, and model surgery has been performed to fashion surgical splints that will intraoperatively position the jaws into the position determined by the cephalometric prediction tracing.[5] If a sagittal split osteotomy is to be performed, the lower third molars should be removed 6 months before the surgery, to reduce the chance of an unfavorable split. Similarly, if a segmental osteotomy is planned, the orthodontist will have diverged the root apices on either side of the proposed osteotomy to minimize the chance of damage to tooth roots. The surgeon should verify the splints fit, and that good surgical lugs have been applied to the arch wire. Soldered lugs work the best. If the lugs break during the surgery, the proper application of the splint can be compromised, making the ideal result much more difficult to obtain. In two-jaw surgery, auto-donation of packed red blood cells is useful.

The patient, presenting with a cleft lip and/or palatal anomaly, will have several anatomic differences, compared to an unaffected patient. The maxilla is typically deficient in both the anteroposterior and vertical dimensions. Because the midface retrusion can be significant, it frequently appears as if the mandible is prognathic, however, it is rare that the mandible demonstrates true prognathia. In the cleft patient, a relative prognathia secondary to the maxillary deficiency is the likely presentation. Finally, because of lesser maxillary

segment collapse, the dental midline is often deviated toward the cleft side.

Despite previous bone grafting of the alveolar cleft, many of these patients have deficient or missing bone in the region of the alveolus In addition, persistent palatal fistulas may be present as well. The lateral incisor is frequently missing in these patients, and closure of this space must be taken into consideration at the time of treatment planning. If a large fistula is present in the alveolus, modifications of the LeFort I procedure can be performed to facilitate a tension free alveolar closure. These modifications to the surgical procedure will be discussed in the following section.

■ SURGICAL TECHNIQUE

LeFort I Osteotomy

The preoperative vertical position of the maxilla is recorded by using a large caliper to measure the distance between the medial canthus of the right eye and the right central incisal edge. In a unilateral cleft lip patient, the standard incision can be made with little jeopardy to the premaxillary blood supply. If a labial-nasal fistula is present, an incision on either side of the cleft is made, similar to that of the alveolar bone graft incision, facilitating a two-layer closure of the palatal and nasal mucosa. If a bony defect exists and needs to be grafted, cancellous bone can be placed into the alveolar gap after fixation has been applied. If a wide fistula is present, the surgeon can compress the maxillary segments, reducing the size of the alveolar space. This maneuver will ensure the soft tissue closure is performed under minimal tension and the chance of fistula closure optimized (Fig. 60–2). The canine may now be adjacent to the central incisor, however, the restorative dentist can fabricate a prosthetic crown for the canine, making it look like a lateral incisor.

In the bilateral cleft patient, care must be taken not to make the vestibular incision across the premaxilla. The premaxillary blood supply will be from the vomer and the buccal mucosa. Since the mucosa of the vomer may be split, the majority of blood flow to the premaxilla will be from the premaxillary buccal mucosa. A complete buccal sulcus vestibular incision, violating the premaxillary buccal mucosa, will severely jeopardize the blood supply of the premaxillary segment. To minimize the risk of complications, the incision is made from lateral to medial, and stopped just distal to the alveolar cleft on either side of the premaxilla. In order to preserve blood supply, the surgeon minimizes dissection and reflection of the mucosa from the premaxilla. The osteotomy of the premaxillary segment is made from a posterior approach, just anterior to the incisive foramen. This allows mobilization of the segment without violation of the buccal mucosa. Similar to the unilateral cleft maxilla, residual fistulae and inadequate alveolar bone may be present. If either is identified, they can be corrected by a two-layer nasal and oral mucosal closure and bone grafting placed in the alveolar defect. If large gaps are present jeopardizing fistula closure, the segments can be compressed at the alveolar gaps to reduce tension on the

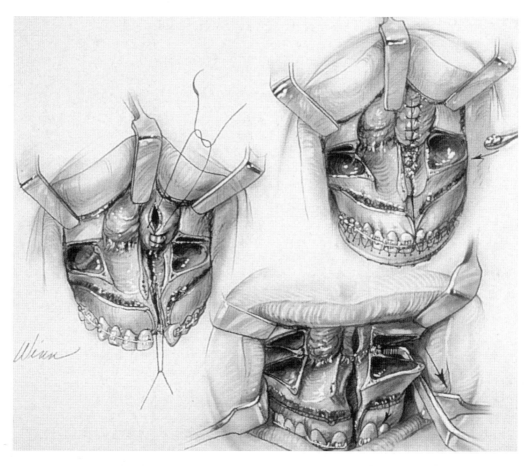

Figure 60–2. In the unilateral cleft deformity, the maxillary segments can be compressed to reduce the size of a persistent fistula. The proximity of the segments facilitates nasal closure. Bone grafting can be added to enhance the alveolar ridge and reduce the chance of wound breakdown.

repair (Fig. 60–3A and B). Postoperative orthodontics and prosthetic restorations of the teeth can correct almost any postoperative dental esthetic irregularities.

Once the incision is made, the mucosa is reflected in a subperiosteal plane to expose the piriform aperture, the zygomatio-maxillary buttress, and the posterolateral maxilla. A reciprocating saw is used to make a high LeFort I osteotomy in most cases. A high LeFort I osteotomy is cut horizontally in a direct line laterally from the piriform aperture to the zygomatico-maxillary buttress. One takes this line as high as possible, while staying at least 5 mm below the inferior orbital foramen. A vertical cut is now made from the lateral edge of the horizontal cut and taken to an area about 5 mm above the tooth root apices laterally. The lateral nasal walls are cut with a uniball osteotome and mallet. The vomer and septum can be reached through the lateral maxillary osteotomies so the buccal mucosa of the premaxilla remains preserved. The pterygomaxillary junction can be separated with a 10-mm curved osteotome, or the maxillary tuberosity can be cut posterior to the last molar in the arch. The latter choice makes downfracture easier and results in fewer complications (Fig. 60–4).

Downfracture of the maxilla is now completed with either digital pressure or application of the Rowe disimpaction

forceps. If a wide alveolar defect is present, the greater and lesser segments can be compressed at the alveolus. The occlusion resulting from segment compression would be anticipated from the preoperative model surgery on the dental casts. Any fistula is closed in layers, and deficiency of alveolar bone corrected with supplemental bone grafts, following application of fixation.

The surgical splint is then placed orienting the new position of the maxilla to the mandible. If a two-jaw procedure is to be performed, an intermediate splint is utilized at this time. Twenty-six gauge wire loops are used to place the patient in maxillomandibular fixation. It is extremely important to assure the condyles are seated in the fossa as the maxillo-mandibular complex is rotated to its new vertical dimension. Generally, cleft patients have vertical maxillary deficiency in addition to the sagittal deficiency. This requires the maxilla to be inferiorly positioned to its new position. If vertical lengthening greater than 5 mm is required, bone grafts are placed between the osteotomy segments to reduce relapse (Fig. 60–5). Rigid fixation is now used to secure the maxilla into its new position. If any instability remains across the maxillary segments, a small plate can be placed across the segments to reduce mobility and maintain the bone graft. Because the osteotomized cleft maxilla results in a multisegment maxilla,

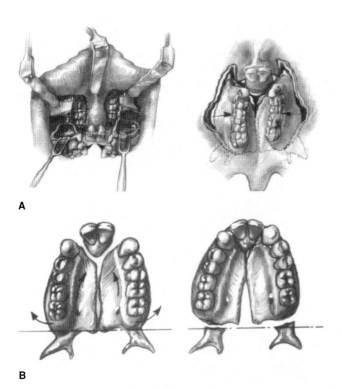

A

B

Figure 60–3. A and B: These pictures show compression of the segments in the bilateral cleft lip and palate patient. Anterior compression allows fistula closure. Note the posterior portion of the segments is expanded allowing correction of the posterior crossbite that is frequently seen in cleft patients.

the surgical splints are wired in place for 6–8 weeks in order to allow for bone healing.

Bilateral Sagittal Split Osteotomy (BSSO)

The Sweetheart retractor is placed to retract the tongue and tied with a sponge to the mouth prop. An incision is made from the point where the ramus meets the external oblique ridge anteriorly to the first molar. The tissue is dissected off the anterior ramus up to the top of the coronoid process. A

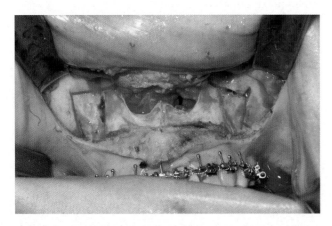

Figure 60–4. The maxillary osteotomy cuts have been made, and the maxilla is ready for down-fracture. Note the high LeFort I osteotomy cuts that will provide maximal cheek projection as the maxilla is advanced.

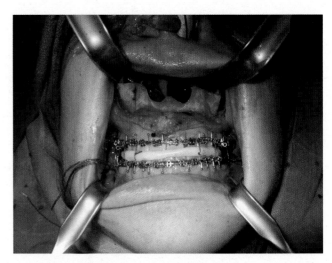

Figure 60–5. After down-fracture and maxillary advancement, the maxilla is secured to the mandible using a surgical splint to create the desired occlusion prior to the application of rigid fixation.

Kocher with a chain is clamped to the tip of the coronoid process. The chain is then clamped to pull the Kocher in a superior direction serving as a retractor for the intraoral mucosa (Fig. 60–6A and B).

The remaining mucosa and tissues are reflected from the medial ramus and external oblique ridge, and the Seldin retractor is placed medial to the ramus and turned clockwise exposing the medial ramus. As the Seldin is moved inferiorly it has a natural stop, the lingula, which is just above the point where the inferior alveolar nerve enters the mandibular foramen. The reciprocating saw is then placed above the Seldin retractor, about two-thirds to the posterior edge of the ramus, and a medial cut is made into cancellous bone of the lingual side of the ramus. Once the medial cut is complete, the osteotomy is extended anteriorly down the ramus just through the cortical bone. This cut follows the external oblique ridge to the inferior border of the mandible (Fig. 60–6B). Osteotomes are used along the osteotomy site, hugging the inner aspect of the outer cortex to minimize injury to the inferior alveolar nerve. The Smith spreader can also be used to free up any residual areas of cancellous bone (Fig. 60–7).

Once the osteotomy is complete, the distal segment is moved into the desired position, either with the final surgical splint or without a splint if the desired occlusion can be achieved by placing the jaws into maximal intercuspal position. Maxillomandibular fixation is again applied to secure the new position of the mandible to the new position of the maxilla. The distal portion of the proximal mandibular segment is grasped by a Kocher, that is used to seat the condyle and align the segments into the desired position. When the desired position is achieved, a second Kocher is positioned to hold the proximal and distal segments together, maintaining the new the position of the mandibular segments while fixation is secured.

The transbuccal trochar is used to allow percutaneous placement of the fixation screws. A mosquito hemostat is

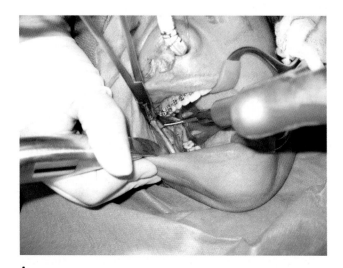

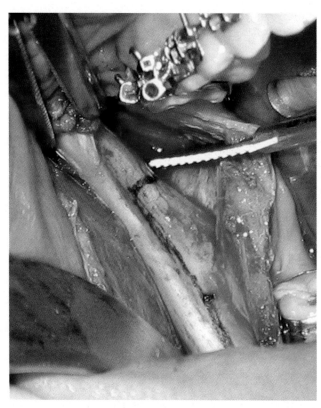

A   B

Figure 60–6. A: A Kocher with a chain is secured to the coronoid process and snapped to the head drape. The mandibular body retractor is placed lateral to the mandible and pulled laterally to give exposure. The reciprocating saw is then inserted medial to the mandible to initiate the osteotomy on the medial ramus. **B:** A close up of the osteotomy design.

placed inside the mouth near the area of desired screw placement. This is palpated on the cutaneous surface and a small stab incision is made through which the trocar is introduced into the oral cavity. The cheek retractor is attached to the trocar, and three screws are placed at the superior edge of the mandible in the region of overlapping bone. The surgeon should feel resistance as the outer cortex of the proximal segment is drilled, a loss of resistance as the cancellous bone is entered, and a second area of resistance as the inner cortex of the distal segment is encountered.

Once both sides are completed, the intermaxillary fixation is released and the final occlusion is verified. If the occlusion is not in the desired position, the screws are removed and the process is repeated. Typically, if the desired occlusion is not achieved, it occurs because the condyle was not properly seated during application of the fixation.

Two–Jaw Surgery

Moving the maxilla and the mandible in one procedure requires osteotomizing both jaws and precisely securing them into the position determined by the treatment plan. If proper treatment planning, model surgery, and splint fabrication are performed, each jaw should be able to be placed into its desired position with precision. The mandibular bony cuts

are made first, but the actual splitting of the bones is not performed. The open wounds are packed while attention is directed to the maxilla. The maxillary osteotomy is made, and the maxilla is placed into its new position using the intermediate splint. The splint is used to wire the teeth into intermaxillary fixation. The intermediate splint indexes the new position of the maxilla to the preoperative position of the mandible. With the condyles gently seated, the maxillomandibular complex is rotated so that the maxillary incisal edge is at the correct vertical height. The maxilla is plated into position, and the intermaxillary fixation is released. At this point, the mandibular osteotomies are completed, and the distal segment of the mandible is placed into the desired occlusion using the final splint. If the teeth are in good occlusion without the splint, the final splint may not be necessary to establish the desired occlusal relationship. Wire loops secure the occlusal relationship, and the rigid fixation is completed as previously described.

APPROACHES TO COMMONLY ENCOUNTERED PROBLEMS

Once the clinical and radiographic data are obtained, the surgeon can determine which abnormalities the patient exhibits

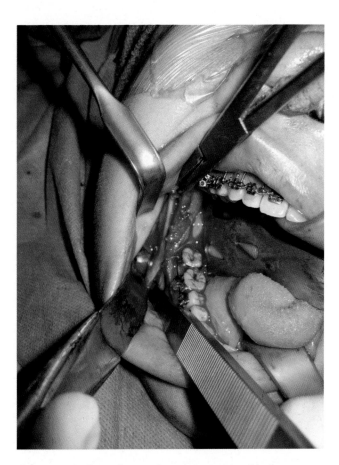

Figure 60–7. Once the cuts have been made with the saw, osteotomes are used to gently separate the proximal and distal segments. It is important to verify that the inferior alveolar nerve is within the distal segment.

and the extent to which these features deviate from the norm. However, the treatment plan is the application of these data, giving the patient the best functional and esthetic result while establishing a Class I occlusion. The following paragraphs outline basic treatment approaches to commonly encountered dentofacial deformities commonly seen in cleft patients.

Skeletal Class III Malocclusion

A Class III malocclusion may be treated by advancing the maxilla, posteriorly positioning the mandible, or by combining these procedures. It is important to consider the contributions of the mandible and the chin separately as each may require different treatments to achieve esthetic goals. Additionally, the patient may benefit from an advancement genioplasty, counteracting any skeletal contraction occurring from a mandibular setback. As in the Class II patient, a minor malocclusion with minimal dental compensation may be corrected with orthodontic treatment alone. In contrast, a minor malocclusion with dental compensation may become a significant malocclusion after dental decompensation, and the patient will be a good surgical candidate.

Maxillary Constriction

Cleft patients can present with a maxilla that is narrow in a transverse dimension. Maxillary constriction may occur as an isolated finding or as one of multiple abnormalities. Up to about 15 years of age, the orthodontist can expand the maxilla nonsurgically with a palatal expander. If orthopedic expansion cannot be done, a surgically-assisted rapid palatal expansion (SARP) can be performed.[6] If the maxilla requires movement in other dimensions, a two-piece (or multipiece) LeFort I osteotomy can be performed to place the maxilla in its new position while simultaneously achieving transverse expansion.

Apertognathia

An anterior open bite is usually caused by a premature contact of the posterior molars. The recommended treatment is a posterior impaction of the maxilla. By reducing the vertical height of the posterior maxilla, the mandible can come into occlusion with the remaining mandibular teeth. Posterior maxillary impaction does not necessarily result in incisor impaction; the posterior maxilla is simply rotated counterclockwise and upward using the incisal tip as the axis of rotation. Therefore, incisor show should not be affected. If a change in incisor show is also desired, the posterior impaction is performed, and then the whole maxilla can be inferiorly positioned or impacted to its new position.

Short Lower Face

A short lower face is marked by insufficient incisor show and/or a short distance between subnasale and pogonion. Treatment is aimed at establishing a proper degree of incisor show. The facial skeleton should be expanded to the degree that provides optimal soft tissue esthetics. As the maxilla is inferiorly positioned, resulting clockwise mandibular rotation leads to a posterior positioning of the chin. The surgeon needs to preoperatively assess the new chin position on the cephalometric prediction tracing to determine if an advancement genioplasty will be necessary to counter the effects of mandibular clockwise rotation.

GENERAL PRINCIPLES

It is useful for the surgeon to employ some basic perioperative principles in preparation for orthognathic surgery. Blood loss can be substantial in maxillofacial surgery. Standard techniques of head elevation, hypotensive anesthesia, blood donation, and the preoperative administration of erythropoietin are useful adjuncts to reduce blood loss and transfusion in orthognathic surgery. Before the incisions are made, an antimicrobial rinse is helpful to minimize the intraoral bacterial count. A topical steroid is applied to the lips to reduce pain and swelling associated with prolonged retraction. Intravenous steroids may also be useful to reduce the postoperative edema.

The postoperative desired occlusion may not be the same as the maximum intercuspal position. The splint is useful in maintaining the occlusion in the desired location when it does not correspond to maximal intercuspal position. It is easy for the orthodontist to close a minor postoperative posterior open bite, but very difficult to close an anterior open bite with orthodontics alone. At the end of the case it is important to have the anterior teeth and the canines in a Class I relationship without an open bite.

After the surgery, it is useful to use guiding elastics to control the bite. Class II elastics are placed in a vector to correct a Class II relationship (maxillary lug is anterior to mandibular lug). Class III elastics are applied to correct a Class III discrepancy. With rigid fixation, elastics will not correct malpositioned jaws, however, they serve only to help the patient adapt to their new occlusion. Many minor malocclusions can be corrected with postoperative orthodontics or occlusal equilibration.

Certain skeletal movements are inherently more stable than others. Stable movements include mandibular advancement and superior positioning of the maxilla. Movements with intermediate stability include maxillary impaction combined with mandibular advancement, maxillary advancement combined with mandibular setback, and correction of mandibular asymmetry. The unstable movements include posterior positioning of the mandible and inferior positioning of the maxilla. The least stable movement is transverse expansion of the maxilla. Long-term relapse with rigid fixation has not been demonstrated to be clearly superior to nonrigid fixation in single jaw surgery; however, in two-jaw surgery, rigid fixation results in less relapse.[7] The judgement of the surgeon will dictate the extent to which the facial skeleton can be expanded without resulting in unacceptable relapse.

COMPLICATIONS

Improper positioning of the jaws will result in malocclusion or an obvious unaesthetic result. If the complication results from improper condyle position during fixation or improper indexing of the splint, fixation must be removed and reapplied. It is wise to verify splint fit prior to the surgery. Meticulous treatment planning prior to the surgery minimizes splint-related problems.

Measures to reduce the chances of a bad mandibular split should always be employed. Removal of mandibular third molars, 6 months prior to the osteotomy, allows time for the sockets to heal, and this decreases the chance of a bad split. If the segments do not appear to be easily separating, the surgeon should verify that the osteotomies are complete. One does not want to use excessive force and increase the chance of an uncontrolled mandibular split. If a bad split occurs, the segments can be plated to reestablish normal anatomy, and the proximal and distal segments secured into the desired position with rigid fixation.

Bleeding may occur from any area but most commonly from the descending palatine artery in the maxilla. This can be stopped with packing or by placing a hemoclip on the artery. Bone wax is useful for bleeding bony edges.

Nerve damage is rare but may occur. The nerves associated with these procedures are the infraorbital, the inferior alveolar, and the mental nerves. If a transection is witnessed, coaptation with 7–0 suture is recommended if possible. Preoperatively, the patient should be informed that there is about a 25% chance of some paresthesia immediately after the surgery; however, permanent changes are seen only in 1–2% of patients.

The incidence of nonunion or malunion is rare after the surgery. If a malunion occurs, the jaw may need to be osteotomized again to move it into the proper position. A nonunion would require secondary bone grafting to establish osseous continuity.

SPEECH OUTCOMES

The primary goal of cleft palate surgery is to close the palate and create a properly functioning velopharyngeal mechanism allowing for the production of normal speech. Unfortunately, velopharyngeal incompetence may occur despite palatal repair because of a short, scarred, or immobile palate. Alveolar fistulas and a constricted arch can also contribute to resonance disorders or articulation defects.

Given the intricate attachment of the muscular apparatus of the velum to the maxilla, it follows that movement of the maxilla can change the preoperative velopharyngeal function. Because the soft tissues of the velum are attached to the posterior maxilla, maxillary advancement pulls the posterior edge of the soft palate away from the posterior pharyngeal wall. In many patients, a borderline or incompetent velopharyngeal mechanism is associated with midface deficiency; and, in these cases, a LeFort I advancement of the maxilla is necessary to restore a Class I occlusion. Patients undergoing maxillary advancement need to be counseled that there is a chance that their velopharyngeal function will deteriorate resulting in hypernasal speech. Patients who are at the highest risk for developing velopharyngeal incompetence after maxillary advancement are those who exhibit incompetence or borderline competence prior to the surgery. Janulewicz et al.[8] performed a retrospective study of the change in velopharyngeal function of 54 cleft lip and palate patients who underwent maxillary advancement with or without a mandibular set back procedure over a 21-year period. Their study demonstrated a decline in competent velopharyngeal function (42–18%), an increase in both borderline incompetence (9–22%) and complete velopharyngeal insufficiency (13–20%). The authors also noted that speech quality deteriorated when the patients were subjected to an overall speech score. Other published studies have shown similar results or no change in VPI function.[9] It is believed that those patients, who do not develop VPI after anterior maxillary positioning, do so as a result of adaptive changes such as velar stretching, and increased lateral wall movement.

Given that maxillary advancement leads to VPI, it would seem intuitive that the greater the degree of advancement, the higher the chance for developing hypernasality. However, multiple studies fail to show this correlation, and the majority of these studies are in agreement.[10,11] One study demonstrating a statistically significant correlation between maxillary advancement and speech intelligibility, reported that the average amount of maxillary advancement in the group with improved or no change in velopharyngeal function was 9.4 mm, while the average maxillary advancement in the group demonstrating decreased speech intelligibility was 12.2 mm.[12]

The potential for postoperative hypernasality following maxillary advancement justifies preoperative testing in order to determine the postoperative risk, and counsel the patient appropriately. Perceptual speech evaluations, video nasoendoscopy, nasometry, videofluoroscopy, and nasal airflow studies can all be used to evaluate velopharyngeal function for risk of speech deterioration. A perceptual speech evaluation appears to correlate well with the potential for speech deterioration. Recently, Phillips has questioned the necessity of routine video nasoendoscopy prior to the maxillary osteotomies. In a study of 26 cleft patients, Phillips et al.[11] showed that both perceptual speech evaluations and video nasoendoscopy are highly correlated with speech outcomes. However, it was statistically shown that video nasoendoscopy does not significantly ($p > 0.02$) contribute to the information obtained from a perceptual speech evaluation. Patients with normal resonance by speech evaluation are at much lower risk of postoperative hypernasality. Video nasoendoscopy may provide some additional information about the risk of postoperative hypernasality, but the additional information is not statistically significant.[11]

Some candidates for maxillary advancement have previously had posterior pharyngeal flaps (PPF). If these patients demonstrate hyponasality prior to the surgery, it can improve with maxillary advancement. Studies also show that patients with a PPF in place tend to have a lower risk of developing VPI after maxillary surgery.[8] Occasionally patients with a PPF in place requiring significant advancement may need to have the PPF taken down at the time of advancement to facilitate the movement. Many of these patients will subsequently require the replacement of their PPF in the future.

Patients have been shown to improve their velopharyngeal function and speech with time following maxillary advancement, it is recommended to wait at least 1 year after the surgery before performing a speech surgery. Posterior pharyngeal flaps (PPF) can be used to correct postoperative hypernasality following maxillary advancement with good results. Maegawa et al.[13] evaluated 13 patients who had a PPF after LeFort I advancement to correct postoperative hypernasality. Of the 13 patients, nine improved their hypernasality and 10 improved their intelligibility. Thus, it appears that a PPF may be a good strategy for the management of persistent hypernasality in this patient population.

Since the elements of speech are linked to hard and soft tissue relationships, advancing the maxilla could affect articulation. This appears to be the case, but the data from published studies appear to be inconsistent. Witzel et al.[14] showed that improving skeletal malocclusions with orthognathic surgery improved articulation, especially the production of sibilant sounds. Janulewicz noted that articulation defects improved, although the improvement did not achieve statistical significance. Preoperatively, 84% (46 patients) had at least one articulation defect as compared to 73% (40 patients) postoperatively.[8] In contrast, Dalston et al.[15] showed no improvement in articulation after the surgery.

In summary, it appears that while a positive effect on articulation might be achieved by orthognathic surgery, it might be at the expense of velopharyngeal function. Further prospective, controlled studies would be helpful in elucidating the relationships between maxillary advancement and speech.

STABILITY AND RELAPSE

The skeletal relapse associated with orthognathic surgery has been shown to be greater in patients with cleft lip and palate anomalies when compared to nonclefted patients. Scarring in the palatal and retromaxillary regions has been thought to be responsible for this observed relapse. The inelastic tissues attached to the posterior maxilla resist advancement and slowly pull the maxilla back to its original position. Aggressive mobilization of the skeletal maxilla from scarred soft tissues helps minimize theses forces. Relapse begins as soon as maxillomandibular fixation is removed and continues for approximately 1 year after the surgery, with most relapse occurring in the first 6 months. Rigid fixation and the use of bone grafts are recommended to reduce relapse; however, relapse remains an unavoidable and unpredictable aspect in the management of these patients.

It would seem intuitive that the degree of skeletal relapse following orthognathic surgery would correlate with the degree of maxillary advancement. However, several studies have found that this correlation does not exist. Posnick et al.[16] in a retrospective study evaluating relapse in cleft patients undergoing orthognathic surgery between 1987 and 1990, found that there was no significant correlation between the degree of horizontal or vertical movement and skeletal relapse. Furthermore, outcomes did not vary significantly with the type of autogenous bone graft used or the segmentalization of the osteotomy.[4]

In contrast to Posnick, Hirano[17] did observe a correlation between the amount of horizontal advancement and the degree of relapse. In the Hirano study, the mean advancement was the same as Posnick (6.9 mm), and the mean relapse was 1.5 mm (0.1 mm less than Posnick), however, Hirano did observe a correlation between the degree of advancement and relapse in both the horizontal and vertical dimensions. The vertical relapse was shown to be approximately 2 mm in most cases where the maxilla is inferiorly positioned; therefore, a

2-mm overcorrection is recommended when inferiorly repositioning the maxilla.[18,19] Finally, Hirano observed greater degrees of relapse in bilateral cleft patients when compared to the unilateral patients. An intact, stable alveolar arch was shown to be an important factor for the long-term stability of maxillary advancement.[17,20–22]

Surprisingly, Hirano's study failed to show a correlation between relapse and alveolar bone grafting. His un-grafted patients did not show greater relapse than those with stable alveolar bone grafts. Though relapse did not increase with ungrafted alveolar fistulae, other difficulties associated with grafting at the time of the surgery are possible. Changes can occur in the maxillary arch after mobilization of the LeFort I osteotomy, since downfracture results in two mobile segments. If the two segments are not synchronously moved during the downfracture and mucosal tears occur, recurrence of alveolar fistula is likely. In addition, the segments may collapse and orthodontic wires and brackets may break or fall off the teeth. The unanticipated mobility of maxillary segments may compromise the occlusion and the way the dentition fits into the surgical splints.

Because many studies have documented increasing skeletal relapse as the amount of horizontal advancement occurs, mandibular posterior positioning has been recommended in cases where more than 10–11 mm of maxillary advancement is required to create a Class I occlusion. By splitting the distance to be moved, it reduces the need for maxillary advancement to be the sole corrective procedure potentially leading to an instable result. Unfortunately, it potentially moves the mandible from a normal position to a retrognathic position compromising facial esthetics. Distraction osteogenesis offers a potential solution for patients with normal mandibles who require greater than 10 mm of maxillary advancement.

SURGICAL ALTERNATIVES: DISTRACTION OSTEOGENESIS

While patients with mild to moderate maxillary hypoplasia are good candidates for traditional orthognathic surgery, those with severe maxillary retrusion (>10 mm) are prone to a significant amount of relapse. Several previously cited studies have shown that patients with severe maxillary deficiency are prone to less predictable results and have a higher degree of relapse. Furthermore, the need for surgical revision and prolonged orthodontics is higher as well. This subset of patients might benefit from maxillary advancement by distraction osteogenesis.

Distraction osteogenesis at the LeFort I level has been recommended for early treatment of severe midface deficiency for the patient in the mixed dentition stage. Cho et al.[23] conducted a retrospective study to evaluate the long-term stability of maxillary distraction osteogenesis by use of a rigid external device, based on a 7-year experience.[23] In their study, the mean distraction length was 13.6 mm immediately after distraction was completed. However, at 6-month follow-up,

the mean distraction length was 10.8 mm and 10.4 mm at 1–6-year follow-up. Based on their results, the mean postoperative relapse rate was computed to be 23% at 1–6 years. The results demonstrate that most relapse occurs in the first 6 months after distraction, but was not statistically significant between 1 year and 6 years after distraction. They concluded that a 20–30% overcorrection is required in maxillary advancement in order to compensate for the relapse.

The results published by Polley[24] are in contrast to the results published by Cho et al.[23] In Polley's study, 16 patients underwent correction of maxillary hypoplasia using external distraction. The patients in their study, between 5 and 25 years of age, underwent distraction followed by a 2–3-month rigid retention phase. They achieved a mean advancement of 11.7 mm. The authors reported no relapse at 4-month and 12-month follow-up periods. In later reports, they attributed decreased facial convexity at 1-year follow-up to a combination of maxillary resorption, forward mandibular growth, and closed rotation of the mandible.

The benefits of the rigid external distraction device are the total versatility and flexibility in both the amount and the direction of the distraction process. With the skull anchored external head frame distractor attached to the orthodontic splint, one can achieve precise control of the maxillary segments, with the ability for accurate, consistent, and unlimited distraction. However, the only rigid aspect of this system is the halo attached to the head. The maxilla, therefore, is not held in strict rigid postoperative fixation after advancement, as the patients are allowed to function with an osteotomized maxilla. While studies have not shown a higher incidence of nonunion, this concept contradicts accepted principles of fracture management. It will be interesting to see if randomized, prospective, and controlled studies, comparing relapse and nonunion rates between distraction and classic orthognathic surgery patients, will prove external distraction to be superior. To date no such study, with a large sample size, has been reported.

Bradley et al.[25] compared the correction of severe maxillary retrusion by distraction to conventional orthognathic surgery. Fifty-one cleft lip/palate patients were divided into three groups based on the extent of maxillary retrusion and type of orthognathic treatment: (1) Group 1 (n = 20): mild to moderate deficiency (<10 mm) treated with conventional orthognathic procedure, (2) Group 2 (n = 11): severe deficiency (≥10 mm) treated with conventional orthognathic surgery, and (3) Group 3 (n = 20): severe deficiency (≥10 mm) treated with distraction osteogenesis. The results showed that Group 1 patients had a mean advancement of 7 mm. In this group, all patients finished with a Class I occlusion and had no complications, relapse, or revisions. Group 2 patients had a mean horizontal advancement of 11 mm. In this group of patients, one patient had a Class III malocclusion postoperatively, and 6 of 11 patients had Class III malocclusion at follow-up. Seven of 11 (64%) developed relapse, and five of 11 (45%) underwent re-operation. Group 3 patients had a mean advancement of 25 mm. In follow-up, a 15% relapse rate was noted (3 of 20 patients).

The authors suggest that the gradual skeletal advancement offered by distraction provides greater advancement with less relapse in patients with severe maxillary deficiency. They suggest that the cicatricial retraction in Group 2 patients most likely contributed to the high relapse rates seen in this group. Though Group 2 patients underwent less advancement than Group 3 patients, Group 2 patients had a higher relapse rate. The authors suggest that a gradual advancement with distraction osteogenesis allows the LeFort I segment to move a greater distance and remain stable in its new location because of slow adaptation of the scared tissues.

Effects on speech between distraction and orthognathic patients were evaluated. Patients who underwent distraction showed better speech scores and less velopharyngeal insufficiency, when compared with acutely advanced patients. Furthermore, nasal endoscopy in select patients showed that the patients who underwent distraction had fewer structural problems with oronasal closure than in the orthognathic group.

Bradley's study indicates that for patients with severe maxillary deficiency, LeFort I distraction may offer improved results when compared to traditional orthognathic surgery. It is the surgeon's choice to determine what will give the patient the best result given the surgeon's comfort with techniques in distraction osteogenesis and orthognathic surgery.

The best study to date comparing the effects of traditional LeFort I osteotomy and maxillary distraction on postoperative velopharyngeal function is by Chanchareonsook et al.[26] The study evaluated 22 cleft patients undergoing maxillary advancement in a blinded, prospective, randomized study. Any cleft palate patient (cleft lip and palate, or cleft palate alone), who had between 4–10 mm of maxillary retrusion and a grafted alveolus, was randomly placed into either a maxillary distraction group or a LeFort I orthognathic group. The mean planned advancement of the orthognathic group was 5.35 mm and 6.25 mm for the distraction group; this difference was not statistically significant. The mean advancement at 3 months, however, was statistically significant with the mean advancement of the orthognathic group being 3.28 mm and that of the distraction group being 7.39 mm. Although relapse was found to be less in the distraction group, the follow-up was only 3 months. This group plans to publish their results after longer follow-up, and it will be interesting to see if the stability of the distraction group remains after 1 year. Nasoendoscopy, by a blinded evaluator, was performed to evaluate velopharyngeal function. The nasendoscopy videos were given to a group of three surgeons who rated the results in a blinded fashion. A perceptual speech evaluation was performed in all patients, and nasality, nasalance, and velopharyngeal gap size were also evaluated. There was no statistically significant difference between the two groups on any of these four variables when evaluated at 3 months after the surgery. The authors plan to publish long-term results in an upcoming manuscript. Their early report concludes that factors influencing speech outcomes appear to be unrelated to the procedure performed, and that adaptation of the velopharyngeal mechanism after maxillary advancement is an individual response.

Orthognathic surgery is typically performed after skeletal growth is complete so that the patient's mandible does not outgrow the surgical correction achieved by the maxillary advancement. There is also the risk of injuring the tooth buds or roots of the permanent dentition if the teeth have not erupted beyond the site of the planned osteotomy. The benefit of the traditional orthognathic surgical procedure is precise control of the occlusion and application of rigid fixation to secure the maxilla's position.

In contrast to the one stage orthognathic procedure, advancement by distraction requires at least two operative procedures. The patient must also endure the appliance for 8–12 weeks. The LeFort I osteotomy for distraction is essentially the same as that performed in traditional orthognathic surgery, so the risk of injury to tooth buds, as well as the potential to outgrow the correction, is the same. Final control of the occlusion, when utilizing internal distraction, is not as precise, and mobility is present after external distraction. If the surgeon is to embark on a plan of distraction, this plan must have clear benefits to traditional orthognathic surgery. The indications that many see for maxillary distraction over traditional orthognathic surgery include reduced rates of relapse and possibly, velopharyngeal incompetence. In the extremely deficient maxilla when the surgeon is not comfortable with his/her ability to achieve adequate advancement with orthognathic techniques, distraction does allow a slow adaptation of the scarred palatal tissues, and possibly reduced relapse. Additionally, distraction has been shown to have a lower postoperative incidence of VPI in some studies.

Unless distraction achieves perfect occlusion without relapse or subsequent mandibular overgrowth, the patient will still require subsequent orthognathic surgery. If this situation arises, one must ask if the long process of distraction osteogenesis, followed by a second orthognathic procedure, is better than doing two LeFort I osteotomies in a staged fashion. It is the authors' opinion that while distraction osteogenesis is a valuable tool, its indications must be carefully weighed against those of traditional orthognathic techniques.

CONCLUSION

Orthognathic surgery is one of the effective treatment modalities available to the craniofacial surgeon to correct dentofacial deformities in the patient with a cleft anomaly. A review of the literature has shown that the operation can be performed safely. The benefits of the surgery, such as enhanced esthetics and optimal occlusion, have to be balanced by the functional outcomes such as a possible deterioration of speech patterns and a potential for other complications. Correction of maxillary hypoplasia by distraction osteogenesis, either internal or external, is an alternative to consider especially in the patient with severe maxillary hypoplasia. The most important aspect to the management of these patients is that each surgeon ultimately chooses the technique that produces the best result for the patient.

References

1. Mars M, James DR, Lamabadusuriya SP. The Sri Lankan cleft lip and palate project: The unoperated cleft lip and palate. *Cleft Palate J* 27:3, 1990.

2. Herber SC, Lehman JA, Jr. Orthognathic surgery in the cleft lip and palate patient. *Clin Plast Surg* 20:755, 1993.

3. Weinzweig J, Panter KE, Seki J, et al. The fetal cleft palate: IV. Midfacial growth and bony palatal development following in utero and neonatal repair of the congenital caprine model. *Plast Reconstr Surg* 118(1):81–93, 2006.

4. Tompach PC, Wheeler JJ, Fridrich KL, et al. Orthodontic considerations in orthognathic surgery. *Int J Orthod Orthognath Surg* 10(2):97–107, 1995.

5. Erickson K. An instructional manual for the model platform and model block. Great Lakes Orthodontics, Ltd., Tonawanda, New York, 1990.

6. Betts NJ, Vanarsdall RL, Barber HD, et al. Diagnosis and treatment of transverse maxillary deficiency. *Int J Orthod Orthognath Surg* 10:75–96, 1995.

7. Proffit WR, Turvey TA, Phillips C, et al. Orthognathic surgery: A hierarchy of stability. *Int J Adult Orthod Orthogn Surg* 11:191–204, 1996.

8. Janulewicz J, Costello B, Buckley M, Ford M, Close J, Gassner R. The effects of Le Fort I osteotomies on velopharyngeal and speech functions in cleft patients. *J Oral Maxillofac Surg* 62(3):308–314, 2004.

9. Kummer AW, Strife JL, Grau WH, et al. The effects of LeFort I osteotomy with maxillary movement on articulation, resonance, and velopharyngeal function. *Cletf Palate J* 26(3):193–199, 1989.

10. Watzke I, A. Turvey, D.W. Warren, et al. Alterations in velopharyngeal function after maxillary advancement in cleft palate patients. *J Oral Maxillofac Surg* 8:685, 1990.

11. Phillips JH, Klaiman PM, Delorey R, MacDonald DB. Predictors of Velopharyngeal insufficiency in cleft palate orthognathic surgery. *Plast Reconstr Surg* 115(3):681–686, 2005.

12. Maegawa J, Sells RK, David DJ. Speech changes after maxillary advancement in 40 cleft lip and palate patients. *J Craniofac Surg* 9(2):177–182, 1998.

13. Maegawa J, Sells RK, David DJ. Pharyngoplasty in patients with cleft lip and palate after maxillary advancement. *J Craniofac Surg* 9(4):330–335, 1998.

14. Witzel MA, Munro IR. Velopharyngeal insufficiency after maxillary advancement. *Cleft Palate J* 14:176–180, 1977.

15. Dalston RM, Vig PS. Effects of orthognathic surgery on speech: A prospective study. *Am J Orthod* 86:291, 1984.

16. Posnick JC. *Cleft –Orthognathic Surgery: The Unilateral Cleft Lip and Palate Deformity. Craniofacial and Maxillofacial Surgery in Children and Young Adults, Vol 2.* Philadelphia, WB Saunders Company, 2001.

17. Hirano A. Factors related to relapse after le fort I maxillary advancement osteotomy in patients with cleft lip and palate. *Cleft Palate Craniofac J* 38(1):1–10, 2001.

18. Bell WH, Scheidman GB. Correction of vertical maxillary deficiency: Stability and soft tissue changes. *J Oral Surg* 39;666–670, 1981.

19. Finn RA. Biomechanical considerations in the surgical correction of mandibular deficiency. *J Oral Surg* 38:257–264, 1980.

20. Luyk NH, Ward BR. The stability of LeFort I advancement osteotomies using bone paltes without bone grafts. *J Maxillofac Surg* 13:250–253, 1985.

21. Garrison BT, Lapp TH, Bussard DA. The stability of LeFort I maxillary osteotomies in patients with simultaneous alveolar bone grafts. *J Oral Maxillofac Surg* 45:761–766, 1987.

22. Eskenazi LB, Schendel SA. An analysis of LeFort I maxillary advancement in cleft lip and palate patients. *Plast Reconstr Surg* 90:779–786, 1992

23. Cho BC. Distraction osteogenesis of the hypoplastic midface using a rigid external distraction system: The results of a one- to six-year follow-Up. *Plast Reconstr Surg* 118:1201, 2006.

24. Polley JW. Rigid external distraction: Its application in cleft maxillary deformities. *Plast Reconstr Surg* 102:1360, 1998.

25. Kumar Anand, Gabbay Joubin S, Nikjoo Rabin. et al. Improved outcomes in cleft patients with severe maxillary deficiency after Le fort I internal distraction. *Plast Reconstruct Surg* 117(5):1499–1509, 2006.

26. Chanchareonsook N, Whitehill T, Samman N. Speech outcome and velopharyngeal function in cleft palate: Comparison of LeFort I maxillary osteotomy and distraction osteogenesis-early results. *Cleft Palate Craniofac J* 44:23–32, 2007.

Segmental Maxillary Osteotomies

Philip Kuo-Ting Chen, MD • Yu-Ray Chen, MD • Eric J.W. Liu, DDS, MS

INTRODUCTION

Even with present-day well-established multidisciplinary treatment approaches, most of the cleft patients continue to develop skeletal problems such as: (1) discrepancy between maxillary segments, (2) maxillary hypoplasia, (3) mandibular prognathism, (4) inappropriate facial proportions, and (5) wide alveolar gaps with complex alveolar oronasal fistulae. These may result in serious, long-lasting, functional and aesthetic problems such as malocclusion, poor dental hygiene, foul smell due to food impaction, nasal allergy from nasal regurgitation, and nasal deformity from an unbalanced nasal floor.[1-9]

Such skeletal problems can be addressed through well-designed single-stage orthognathic procedures after the patient has reached skeletal maturity.[10,11] The current approach for treating cleft skeletal deformity is typically a 1-piece maxillary advancement; this might be combined with mandibular setback or leveling, depending on mandibular sagittal position and canting of the occlusal plane, respectively. This results in a change of the positions of the maxillary and mandibular bones and alignment of the dental arches. The aforementioned complications related to skeletal problems, however, might arise long before a patient reaches skeletal maturity. This, combined with the inability of the traditional orthognathic approach to address certain anatomical deformities, provides the rationale for segmental maxillary osteotomies.

SEGMENTAL MAXILLARY OSTEOTOMY

The purpose of doing a segmental maxillary osteotomy in a cleft orthognathic procedure is to correct relative malposition within the maxilla. There are several clinical scenarios in which this is beneficial: (1) aligning the protruding or downwardly displaced premaxilla in a bilateral cleft, (2) differential repositioning of the greater and lesser segments during orthognathic surgery, (3) shortening the duration of orthodontic work in cases with significant anterior open bite, and (4) in very rare instances, reorienting severely proclined anterior teeth. For the patients who fall in any one of these first two scenarios (i.e., those who need either premaxilla repositioning or differential repositioning of the two segments), cleft orthognathic surgery (OGS) is a well-established approach for closing the dental gap and aligning the dental arches.[7-15] OGS for the above-mentioned third scenario is relatively controversial, as many orthodontists prefer to level the occlusal plane prior to proceeding with surgery. The final scenario rarely occurs in the cleft population, except occasionally in those patients who initially present with a cleft of the primary palate.

SEGMENTAL MAXILLARY OSTEOTOMY AND INTERDENTAL DISTRACTION OSTEOGENESIS

Another common deformity, that cannot be solved by the standard cleft OGS is, the severely-hypoplastic maxilla with dental crowding. The 1-piece Le Fort I maxillary osteotomy can only change the position of the entire maxilla. Since it does not change the length of the bone or relative tooth position within the bone, it cannot solve the problem of significant malocclusion from dental crowding.

Since a hypoplastic maxilla is usually identified at an early age in cleft patients, the technique of maxillary distraction osteogenesis provides the opportunity for early intervention, and thus serves as a solution to those primary and secondary problems related to cleft skeletal deformity.[16-20] Most of the maxillary distraction osteogenesis techniques described, involve a Le Fort I-type maxillary osteotomy and pterygomaxillary disjunction. Here, the maxilla is advanced in 1 piece, and new bone forms at the osteotomy sites, namely along the maxillary sinus walls and pterygomaxillary junction—the sites of the Le Fort I and pterygomaxillary separations, respectively. The drawbacks of this technique

are: (1) the maxillary bone remains similar to its previous size and without any anteroposterior lengthening of the alveolar process, (2) dental crowding is difficult to relieve, as it is difficult for orthodontist to move the molar teeth posteriorly into the regenerate in the pterygomaxillary region, and (3) there is a potential for deterioration of velopharyngeal closure when the maxilla is advanced significantly.

Combining the techniques of multiple segment osteotomies with rapid orthodontic tooth movement addresses several of these drawbacks. The technique of maxillary interdental distraction osteogenesis was developed in late 90s.[21] Here the maxilla or dental arch is lengthened through the formation of a new bony segment within the maxilla, between teeth, rather than along the maxillary sinus walls or pterygomaxillary region. This technique can expand the maxillary body and lengthen the alveolus in an anteroposterior dimension, helping the orthodontist to relieve dental crowding. It can close a wide dental gap, or bring together the bony walls associated with difficult oronasal fistulae, simplifying the surgical procedures used to close such fistulae (Fig. 61–1A and B).

ORIGIN OF THE TECHNIQUE

This technique combines two techniques previously published by the authors, *multiple segment osteotomies* and *rapid orthodontic tooth movement.*

Multiple Segment Osteotomies

This technique enables the surgeon to do fine osteotomies between the teeth safely, either with or without presurgical orthodontic separation of the teeth at the osteotomy site.[22,23] The only difference between the published technique, and the presently described technique, is that the previous technique was applied to OGS performed after skeletal maturity. This presently described technique is used for the early intervention of cleft skeletal problems at the time of late mixed or early permanent dentition. There are some modifications in the present technique to avoid injury to the tooth roots or developing dental follicles in the alveolar process.

Rapid Orthodontic Tooth Movement

The teeth adjacent to the regenerate can be orthodontically moved at a faster rate into the regenerate, soon after the distraction process.[24-26] This is because the regenerate is still soft. Furthermore, this may have a significant influence on the stability and long-term structural preservation of the bone created by distraction osteogenesis within the tooth-bearing segment of the maxilla.

ADVANTAGES AND INDICATIONS

The technique is best used in patients with a wide alveolar cleft, a difficult anterior palatal oronasal fistula, or a short

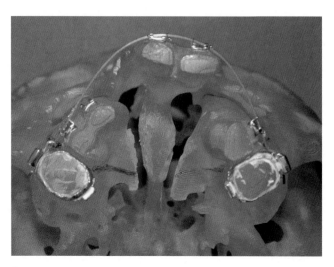

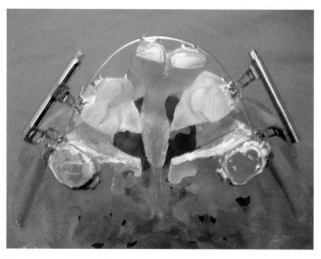

A

B

Figure 61–1. A: An acrylic model shows a case of bilateral cleft lip and palate with hypoplasia of both lateral segments and wide alveolar gap and difficult oronasal fistulae. The lines on the palatal shelf show the line of segmental osteotomy across the palatal shelf. **B:** After segmental maxillary osteotomy and interdental distraction osteogenesis with the bone-borne distractors, both anterior maxillary segments are moved forward. The alveolar gaps are approximated to facilitate surgical closure. The gaps in the osteotomy sites will be filled with new regenerate bone. The bony movement is controlled by the heavy arch wires. However, the vector of the distractors can further adjust the direction of bony movement, that is, forward movement or convergence.

maxillary segment with dental crowding. It will lengthen the maxillary bone and the attached gingiva. Through rapid orthodontic tooth movement, dental crowding is quickly solved as the malaligned teeth are rapidly moved into the regenerate. Once these teeth are aligned and occupying the regenerate, the risk of relapse is reduced. Theoretically, this approach should not affect the patient's speech since the posterior segment remains in situ; this should eliminate the need for speech therapy or velopharyngeal management that has sometimes resulted after traditional single-segment distraction. Gingivoperiosteoplasty, performed as a second stage after closure of the dental gap, followed by further approximation of the segments (compression osteogenesis in the alveolar cleft) will possibly achieve bony union across the cleft and thus eliminate a bone grafting procedure.

TECHNICAL ASPECTS

Timing of Surgery

The best timing for this procedure with the least surgical risk is, during late mixed or early permanent dentition, around the age of 11–12 years. The technique can also be performed during early mixed dentition, however, the risk of injury to the unerupted tooth buds is higher if performed at this stage.

Preoperative Orthodontic Preparation

The preoperative orthodontic approach includes tooth alignment, selective palatal expansion with a modified quadhelix, and opening a 2 mm space between the teeth at the distraction

site to facilitate the interdental osteotomy. The maxillary dentition must be well aligned, preoperatively, so that a stainless steel arch wire (0.016 × 0.022 or thicker) can be placed. The arch wire also serves as a track that helps guide the osteotomized anterior segments to be distracted in a curved and convergent pathway.

Surgical Procedures

The surgical procedure consists of two components: (1) a horizontal osteotomy, usually at the Le Fort I level and (2) a vertical interdental osteotomy, usually located between the second premolar and the first molar. The posterior segment remains in its original position, while the anterior segments are mobilized, and are distracted anteriorly to converge.

The procedure is performed under nasoendotracheal anesthesia. A horizontal intraoral incision is made along the buccal vestibule of the maxilla. Superior mucoperiosteal flaps are raised, exposing the site for the horizontal maxillary osteotomy on the buccal side. A vertical subgingival tunnel, extending superiorly from the interdental attached gingiva, to the horizontal incision is made, thus exposing the site of the vertical interdental osteotomy on the buccal side of the anterolateral maxillary wall. A second narrow and parallel tunnel is made on the palatal side of the maxilla, inside the gingival sulcus; this exposes the site of vertical interdental osteotomy along the palatal shelf. Care must be taken to avoid stripping all of the palatal mucosa, which would thereby devascularize the segment.

Preoperative radiographs are used to estimate the anatomic position of the dental roots, the location of permanent tooth buds, and the sites for interdental and horizontal

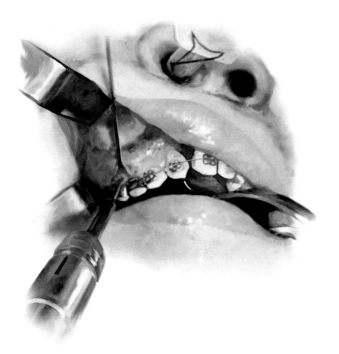

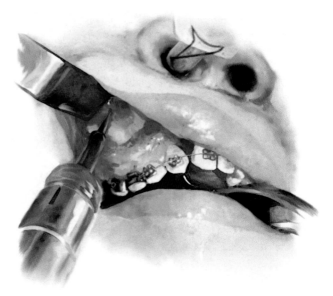

Figure 61–3. When the corticotomy reaches the anterior wall of maxillary sinus, it is deepened into a complete osteotomy using the rotary burr.

Figure 61–2. After exposure of maxilla through upper buccal sulcus incision, subperiosteal dissection and subgingival tunnel made by small Joseph elevator, vertical corticotomy is started in the subgingival tunnel with fine tipped (0.5 or 1 mm) rotary burr moving upward towards the anterior wall of maxillary sinus. A small retractor is used to elevate the gingiva for protection.

maxillary osteotomies. These positions are marked on the alveolar bone with surgical marking pencils. The vertical interdental osteotomy is started inferiorly in the subgingival tunnel with corticotomy using a 1-mm round bur (Fig. 61–2). It is deepened to become a complete osteotomy of the anterior maxillary wall (Fig. 61–3). This is followed by a similar procedure on the palatal shelf through the palatal tunnel (Fig. 61–4). A complete horizontal osteotomy is performed with a reciprocating saw through the anterior maxillary sinus wall, 3–5 mm superior to the dental root apex and tooth buds (Fig. 61–5). Next, a 4-mm-wide thin-blade osteotome is used from the vertical osteotomy line on the anterior maxillary sinus wall, passing medially through the medial maxillary sinus wall, to complete the cuts (Fig. 61–6). This thin-blade osteotome is also used to complete the cuts on the palatal shelf (Fig. 61–7). The last step, which is the most difficult part of the procedure, is the osteotomy of the teeth-bearing alveolar process. This is achieved by passing the thin-blade osteotome between the teeth and performing a green-stick fracture of the alveolar process by gently twisting the osteotome back and forth (Fig. 61–8). This avoids direct impact of the osteotome on the tooth root or tooth buds within the alveolar process. After the horizontal maxillary and interdental osteotomies are performed, the distal segment of the osteotomized dental arch should be completely mobile. The bone-borne distraction devices are mounted on the anterior maxillary sinus wall across the interdental osteotomies on both sides of the maxilla; this stabilizes the distal segments to the proximal segment

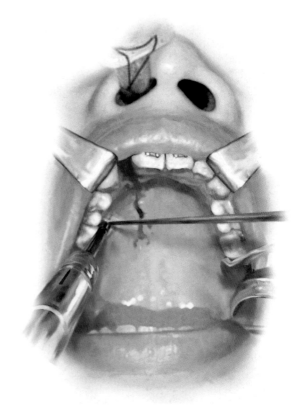

Figure 61–4. A similar corticotomy is performed with fine tipped rotary burr in subpalatal tunnel towards the palatal shelf with careful protection of the greater palatine vessels.

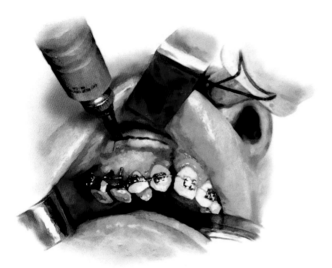

Figure 61–5. After finishing the initial vertical cuts, horizontal osteotomy is performed at the Le Fort I level using oscillating saw.

of the osteotomized dental arch of the maxilla (Fig. 61–9). A test turn must be performed to check for any hindrance of the bony movement during distraction. The incisions are irrigated and closed with absorbable sutures. The attached gingiva on the buccal and palatal sides of the interdental osteotomy sites must be sutured together to prevent any bony exposure of these regions during the distraction process.

Distraction Device

There are several devices that can be used for distraction. The authors initially designed a tooth-borne device, and subsequently changed to a bone-borne device (KLS-Martin, USA) (Fig. 61–10A). The tooth-borne device is designed to be anchored to the orthodontic brackets. With this device the

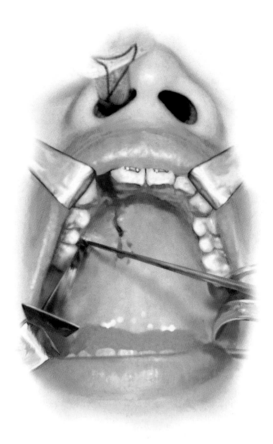

Figure 61–7. A similar procedure is performed on the palatal side using the same thin blade osteotome to penetrate the palatal shelf and finish the cuts on the floor of nasal cavity. Care must be taken for protection of nasal mucosa and the endotracheal tube.

distraction vector can be easily readjusted in the outpatient clinic, making it more flexible. Its major disadvantage, however, is lack of stability, and thus difficulty in performing postoperative rapid orthodontic tooth movement can be encountered. The bone-borne device, on the other hand, is rigidly fixed to the maxilla with screws. It allows better control of the maxillary segments during distraction. Its vertical connecting bars can be adjusted buccally and lingually, and the holes in the vertical connecting bars can be used as anchoring points for the subsequent rapid orthodontic tooth movement (Fig 61–10B). The RED device, designed by Polley and Figueroa, can also be used for this technique. It is relatively cheap and flexible, however, is bulky.

Distraction Protocol

A latency period of 5–7 days is observed before initiating the interdental distraction osteogenesis. The distraction device is activated daily until both ends of the alveolar cleft or oronasal fistula have been approximated. With the bone-borne device, the rhythmic distraction rate is 1 mm/day. During interdental distraction, the movement vector of the distracted segment can be adjusted by bending the vertical bars of the device with orthodontic pliers.

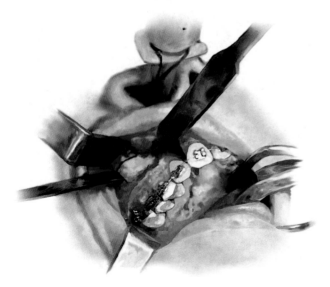

Figure 61–6. A thin blade osteotome is used passing from the vertical cut on the anterior wall of the maxillary sinus towards the medial wall of sinus with careful protection of the nasal mucosa.

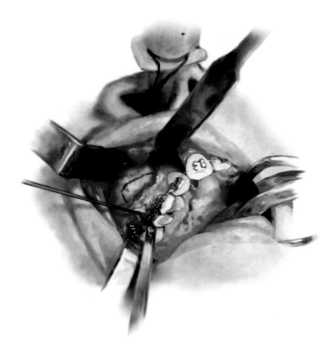

Figure 61–8. The last part of the osteotomy is to perform a greenstick fracture of the teeth bearing alveolar process by passing the thin blade osteotome in between the molar teeth and gently twisting the blade back and forth until the bony segment is completely mobile.

Gingivoperiosteoplasty

After approximating the alveolar segments, the patient is brought back to the operating room; and, a gingivope-

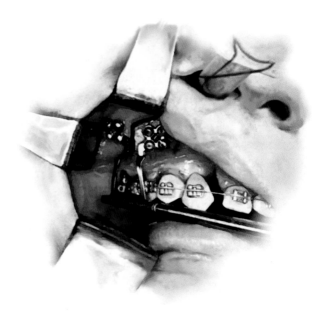

Figure 61–9. The bone-borne distractor is brought to the operating table. The connecting arms are bended into a suitable angle to avoid any pressure on the underlying gingiva. The device is then fixed to the maxilla by miniscrews. The device should be parallel to the occlusal plane with its long axis at the angle depending on the amount of advancement or convergence needed to correct the skeletal problem.

riosteoplasty is performed, by removing the interposing soft tissue from within the alveolar cleft or oronasal fistula. The buccal gingival and the palatal mucoperiostum are minimally raised and the cleft margins are freshened and closed without tension. The distraction is continued after the

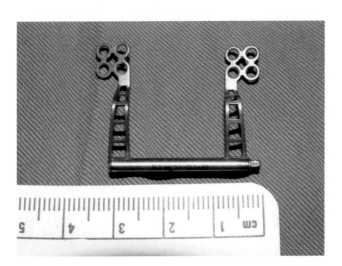

A

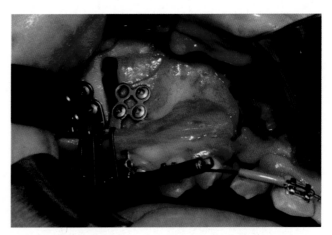

B

Figure 61–10. A: The bone-borne distractor. Its maximal distraction length is 25 mm. The distal end of the distractor is hidden inside the mouth thus the patient will not have any psychological embarrassment during the treatment period. The connecting bars are strong mesiodistally but malleable buccolingually. The holes for fixation miniscrews are arranged in a rectangular shape as the maxilla is usually hypoplastic in these cases thus has limited space for fixation. **B:** The device is fixed to the osteotomized maxilla. Three screws are used in the anterior segment due to space limitation. The bony movement must be tested on the table to avoid any possible bony hindrance during the distraction procedure. The vector of the distractor can still be adjusted buccolingually by the orthodontist in the outpatient clinic for more advancement or approximation.

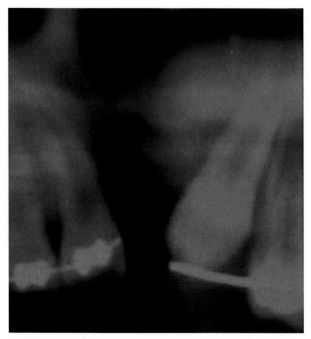

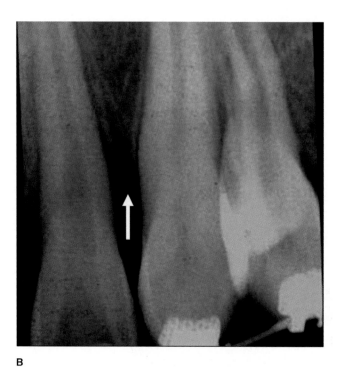

A   B

Figure 61–11. **A:** A 10-year-old unilateral cleft boy had a failed alveolar bone grafting procedure. The alveolar cleft was wide, with scarring surrounding the cleft, which made the secondary surgery quite difficult. An interdental distraction osteogenesis was planned for approximating of the cleft. This was the X-ray before operation. **B:** Bony union across the cleft was achieved after the distraction for gap approximation and compression osteogenesis across the cleft (Arrow).

gingivoperiosteoplasty until the alveolar segments are in firm contact with each other.

Postdistraction Maintenance and Rapid Orthodontic Tooth Movement through the Regenerate

After completion of distraction, the bone-borne distractor remains in place for an additional 3 months of consolidation and maintenance of position. Rapid orthodontic tooth movement is commenced during this period, usually 1-2 weeks after completion of the distraction. The tooth (or teeth) to be moved depends on the individual clinical situation of dental crowding. In using the bone-borne distraction device as the anchorage, an orthodontic elastic chain or nickel-titanium coil spring is attached between the distractor and the tooth (teeth) that is to be moved into the regenerate. Patients are evaluated on a monthly schedule until the entire edentulous space has been eliminated. This typically takes 3–5 months.

RESULTS

Since 1997, this technique has been applied to more than 50 cleft patients having a wide alveolar cleft, dental crowding, or a difficult fistula.[27] In most patients, the dental gap(s) have been approximated, and the fistulae have been successfully closed. The most difficult location for fistula closure has been at the premaxillary-vomerine junction, distant from the axis of bony movement. Some patients in recent years have achieved bony union across the cleft (Fig. 61–11A and B), In some earlier cases, where the technique was also used for maxillary advancement, the ANS point was easily advanced for more than 7 mm, and had no significant relapse at 6-year follow-up (Fig. 61–12A, B, C, D, E and F). No postoperative deterioration in velopharyngeal closure was observed, except for 1 patient who had a slight increase in hypernasality; no additional surgery was indicated.

Complications

Though performed with care, there were three tooth root injuries in our previous series. One patient had gingival recession at the vertical osteotomy site. One patient had postoperative nasal bleeding from a mucosa tear.

Long-term Results

In our long-term follow-up of over 6 years, this technique has resulted in stable facial profile and occlusion, without significant relapse. There was one case of delayed tooth eruption and one case of underdevelopment of the tooth root at the osteotomy site. Though the technique of interdental osteotomy can be performed in a relatively safe fashion, the authors currently are separating the teeth at the osteotomy site by

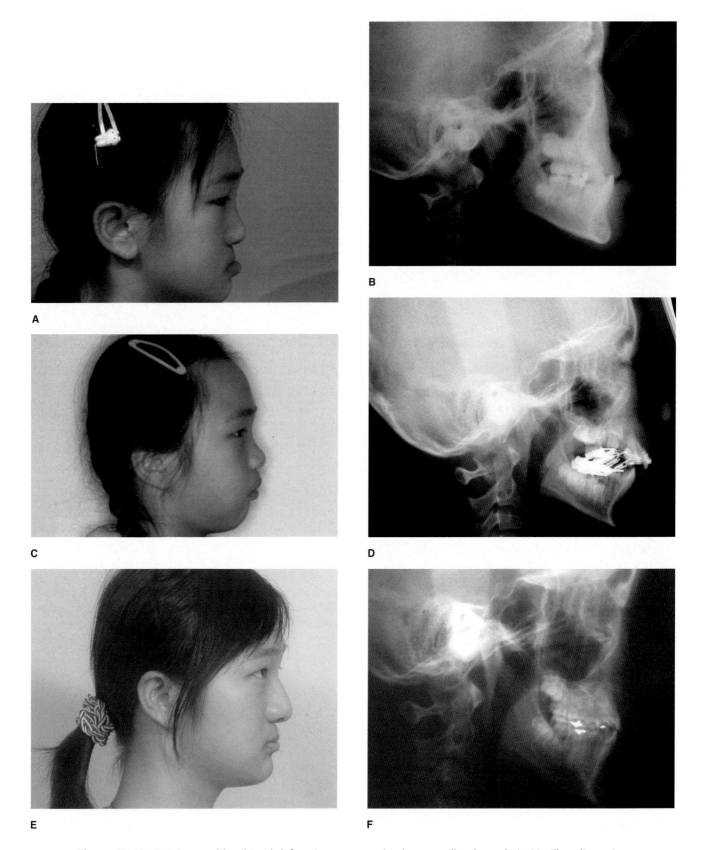

Figure 61–12. A: A 9-year-old unilateral cleft patient was noted to have maxillary hypoplasia. Maxillary distraction osteogenesis was planned to correct her midface retrusion and dental crowding. The lateral view before surgery. **B:** The lateral cephalometric X-ray before the distraction. **C:** The lateral view after the interdental distraction osteogenesis. The midface retrusion was corrected. **D:** The lateral cephalometric X-ray showed maxilla was over-corrected into a Class II occlusion after the distraction. **E:** The same patient 6 years after the distraction showed good maintenance of good facial profile. **F:** The lateral cephalometric X-ray showed good maxillary position with Class I occlusion.

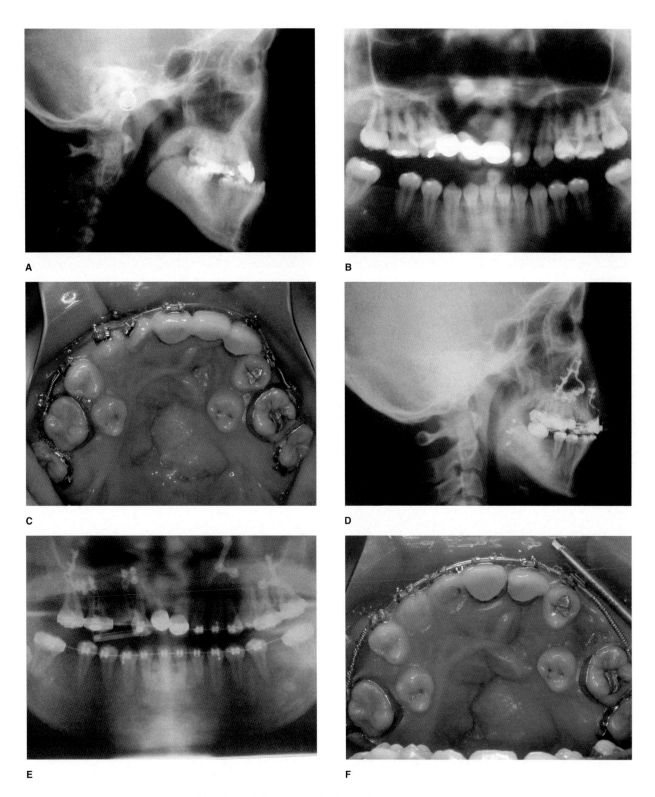

Figure 61–13. A: A 16-year-old unilateral cleft patient had maxillary retrusion, wide alveolar gap and dental crowding. She was planned to have an orthognathic surgery to correct her skeletal problem. **B:** Panoramic X-ray showed wide alveolar cleft (with a dental prosthesis) and dental crowding on her both greater and lesser segments. **C:** The intraoral photo showed the crowded teeth and wide alveolar cleft with prosthesis. **D:** She had an orthognathic surgery including a Le Fort I maxillary osteotomy with advancement and bilateral sagittal split mandibular ramus osteotomy with setback. **E:** An additional osteotomy was performed at her lesser segment for interdental distraction osteogenesis to lengthen her lesser segment, approximating the alveolar gap and relief of dental crowding. The panoramic X-ray clearly showed the distractor and interdental osteotomy site. The lesser segment was distracted forward with new bone regenerated in the osteotomy site. **F:** The intraoral photo during at the end of distraction. The lesser segment was lengthened and alveolar gap was approximated. There was new gingiva at the distracted site.

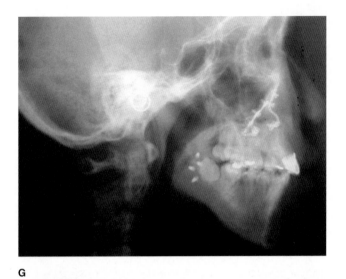

G

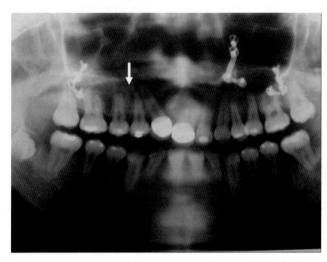

H

I

Figure 61–13. *(Continued)*. **G:** The lateral cephalometric X-ray at the end of the treatment showed good facial profile and Class I occlusion. **H:** The panoramic X-ray showed well-aligned teeth and approximation of the alveolar gap. The osteotomy site was hardly visible (Arrow). **I:** The intraoral photo after treatment showed relief of the dental crowding and approximation of the gap.

1–2 mm using preoperative orthodontics to prevent such dental complications.

USAGE IN COMBINATION WITH TRADITIONAL ORTHOGNATHIC SURGERY

The technique can be used in combination with traditional OGS to relieve dental crowding within a segment. The maxillary surgery is performed through a standard Le Fort I osteotomy combined with a vertical interdental osteotomy at the suitable location, usually the lesser segment. The greater and lesser segments are moved to the designed point with dental gap left open. A bone-borne device is fixed to the maxilla where the segmental osteotomy was performed and distraction is begun 5–7 days following the orthognathic surgery.

The dental gap can be closed and the lesser segment can be lengthened through distraction. Dental crowding within the lesser segment can easily be solved by distraction (Fig. 61–13A, B, C, D, E, F, G, H, and I).

CONCLUSION

The concept of performing segmental maxillary distraction osteogenesis through interdental osteotomy is more logical than traditional whole maxillary distraction osteogenesis for several reasons. It lengthens the short maxilla through the formation of new bone and gingiva within the maxilla, solving the problem of dental crowding, while not affecting the patient's speech. Relapse has been minimal, as the new regenerate is occupied by teeth. The technique can be performed

injury to the infraorbital neurovascular bundle and avoids all permanent tooth buds. Mobilization of the maxillary segments is achieved, including pterygomaxillary and septal disjunction. Aggressive down-fracturing is not necessary. No intraoperative repositioning of the maxillary segments is achieved, and no autogenous or alloplastic bone grafting or internal skeletal fixation hardware is utilized. The halo portion of the distraction device is placed immediately after closure of the intraoral incision. The halo device is illustrated in Fig. 62–2A, B, and C.

In our first clinical series, 18 consecutive patients were selected based on the above criteria, and were treated with maxillary distraction osteogenesis. There were 10 unilateral cleft lip and palate patients, 6 bilateral cleft lip and palate patients, and 2 patients with bilateral cleft lip and palate and severe congenital facial clefting. The patients' ages at the time of surgery ranged from 5.2 years to 25.2 years. Fourteen patients underwent rigid external maxillary distraction.[1] These patients had the rigid device placed at the time of surgery and had their distraction performed through mechanical

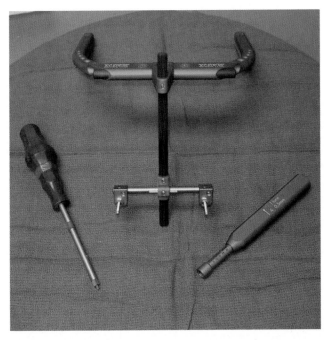

A

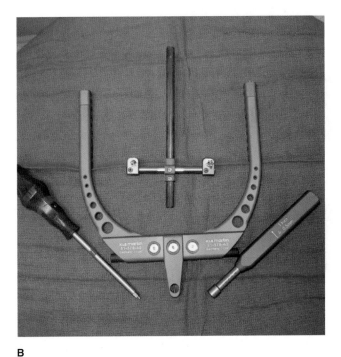

B

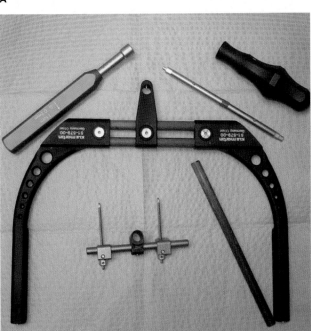

C

Figure 62–2. A, B, and C: The halo portion of the external distraction device.

activation of the distraction device. Four patients in this series underwent facemask elastic distraction osteogenesis, which was later abandoned because of poor results. All rigid external maxillary distraction patients underwent a latency period of 4–5 days following the osteotomy and then began distraction. The latency period is followed by the activation period, and this is the period of active distraction. The activation period typically lasts 12–15 days, but the duration is determined clinically by the severity of the midface deficiency and anterior crossbite. The patients are followed weekly during the activation period until satisfactory and stable skeletal and occlusal changes are achieved.

After the period of active distraction, a consolidation period of rigid retention of 3–4 weeks is undertaken. During consolidation, the distraction device is kept in place without any advancement. The purpose of this period is to allow the maxillary position to achieve clinical stability through bone mineralization. Following the consolidation period of rigid retention, the external distraction device is removed in an office setting for most patients. For very young patients, the distraction device is removed under mild sedation.

CEPHALOMETRIC EVALUATION

The preoperative and postretention lateral cephalometric radiographs were utilized for analysis of our case series. The radiographs were traced on 0.003-in acetate paper, and 12 anatomic landmarks were recorded (Fig. 62–3). Availability of serial radiographs in all patients permitted landmark verification. All X-rays were corrected to 0% magnification. Based on the recorded anatomic landmarks, 13 measurements were calculated, 6 angular and 7 linear (4 horizontal and 3 vertical). For the linear measurements, an *xy* coordinate system utilizing the sella-naison (SN) plane as the horizontal was employed. Linear horizontal changes were measured relative to a line perpendicular to the SN plane passing through the sella, and vertical changes were measured perpendicular to the SN plane. The preoperative and postoperative cephalometric values in the rigid external distraction group were statistically analyzed by means of a paired *t*-test. Changes in the soft tissue anthropomorphic measurements are evident after distraction as seen in Fig. 62–4A and B. The nasolabial angle has increased with concurrent raising of the pronasale. The changes in the soft tissue, as a result of the underlying bony framework alterations, have given this patient an impressive aesthetic improvement.

Angular Changes

In our series of patients who underwent rigid external distraction, the average predistraction SNA angle was 77.6°, and the postdistraction SNA angle was 85.3°, for an average increase in this group of 7.7° (Table 62–1). The average predistraction A-N-B was -1.2° and postdistraction 7.3° with an increase of 8.6°. For all patients who underwent rigid external distraction, the skeletal angle of convexity increased postdistraction by 17.2°. All of these three measurements were statistically significant.

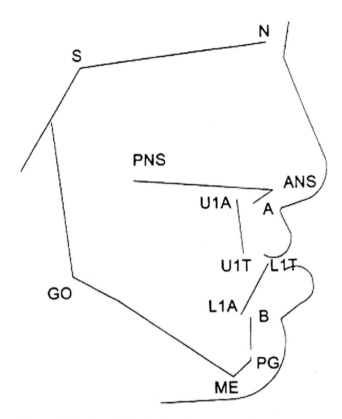

Figure 62–3. Anatomic landmarks and reference planes. Anatomic landmarks: S, sella, the center of sella turcica; N, naison, the most anterior point of the nasal frontal suture; A, "A point," the most anterior limit of the maxillary alveolar bone at the level of the incisor root apex; PNS, the posterior nasal spine, intersection between the nasal floor and the posterior contour of the maxilla; U1A, the apex of maxillary incisor root, uppermost point of the incisor root; U1T, the tip of maxillary incisor crown, maxillary incisor edge; L1T, the tip of mandibular incisor, mandibular incisor edge; L1A, the apex of manibular incisor root, lowermost point of the mandibular incisor root; B, "B point," the most anterior limit of the mandibular alveolar bone at the level of the incisor root apex; PG, pogonion, the most anterior limit of the mandibular symphysis; GO, gonion, the point at the greater convexity of the mandibular gonial region. Reference planes: sella-naison plane (SN), palatal plane (line passing through U1A and U1T): and mandibular plane (tangent to the lower border of the mandible through ME and GO).

Linear Changes

The A-N-S change between predistraction and postdistraction cephalometric radiographs in the rigid external distraction group was 7.1 mm. The average horizontal advancement of the "A point" following distraction was 8.3 mm. The horizontal advancement at the upper incisal edge averaged 11.6 mm and a positive correction of overjet by 12.7 mm postdistraction. All of the changes in the horizontal linear measurements in the rigid external group were highly significant between predistraction and postdistraction measurements at a *p* value of 0.001 (see Table 62–2).

Dental Changes

The dental changes in both groups between predistraction and postdistraction cephalograms are also given in Tables

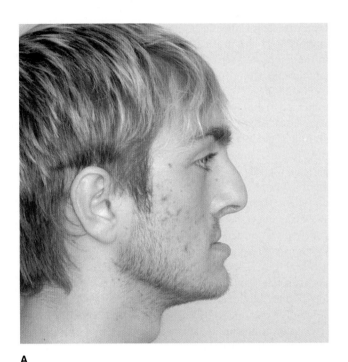

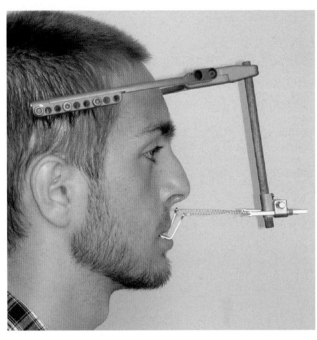

A

B

Figure 62–4. A and **B:** A 24-year-old male before and after midface advancement. Notice the 17° increase in the nasolabial angle and the raising of the pronasale.

62–1 and 62–2. In the rigid external distraction group, the change in the angle of the upper incisor edge of the palatal plane averaged 1.2° for all patients. This was not statistically significant. In none of the patients in this series, were spaces created posterior to the most distal point of anchorage of the intraoral splint.

DISCUSSION

Maxillary hypoplasia is a common finding in patients with orofacial clefting. It has been estimated that 25–50% of all patients born with complete unilateral cleft lip and palate will be potential candidates for maxillary advancement to correct the functional deformities and improve aesthetic facial proportions.[2] In addition, it is recognized that the majority of patients with facial clefts have morphologically normal or slightly smaller than normal mandibles.[3,4] Patients with severe cleft maxillary deficiency are difficult patients to treat with standard surgical/orthodontic approaches. These patients present with maxillary hypoplasia (vertical, horizontal, and transverse dimensions) characterized by thin or structurally weak bone. The maxillary hypoplasia in cleft patients is also compounded by residual palatal and alveolar fistulas, absent and aberrant dentition, and scarring of the palatal and pharyngeal soft tissues.

The physical deformities exhibited by patients with severe maxillary hypoplasia contribute to multiple functional

Table 62–1.

Predistraction and Postdistraction Angular Cephalometric Measurements for Rigid External Distraction Group

Distraction	Measurements (°)	Predistraction	Postdistraction (4 months)	Difference	Significance
Rigid external (n = 14)	SNA	77.6 ± 5.6	85.3 ± 5.6	7.7 ± 2.9	**
	SNB	78.8 ± 4.0	77.9 ± 4.1	−0.8 ± 1.8	NS
	ANB	−1.2 ± 3.5	7.3 ± 3.0	8.6 ± 3.6	**
	Convexity (NAPg)	−3.5 ± 7.5	13.7 ± 6.0	17.2 ± 7.3	**
	Mand. PL/SN angle	39.2 ± 6.7	41.4 ± 5.9	2.2 ± 2.4	*
	Ul-P.PL.angle	100.7 ± 15.7	98.8 ± 14.4	−1.2 ± 11.3	NS

* p <0.01
** p <0.001

Table 62–2.

Pre- and Postdistraction Linear Cephalometric Measurements for Rigid External Distraction Group

Landmark (Axis)	Pre- and Postdistraction Change Rigid External (mm)
ANS-x	7.1 ± 3.9*
ANS-y	−0.4 ± 3.0
A point-x	8.3 ± 3.3*
A point-y	−1.3 ± 3.4
Ul-x	11.6 ± 4.6*
Ul-y	−1.8 ± 3.5
Overjet	12.7 ± 3.0*

* $p < 0.01$

deficiencies as well. These include severe malocclusions, which result in compromised mastication, speech abnormalities, and nasal pharyngeal airway constriction.[5] The severe dish-face or concave facial profiles in these patients result in highly detrimental psychosocial ramifications as well.[6] Current protocols for the treatment of maxillary hypoplasia in cleft patients rely upon a surgical/orthodontic approach, including a Le Fort I maxillary advancement with concomitant fistula closure and maxillary and alveolar bone grafting. This surgery includes rigid internal fixation hardware for stabilization of the repositioned maxilla in the postoperative period. The long-term results of cleft patients with maxillary defi-

ciency treated in such fashion have been reported by several authors.[7–11] The mean horizontal maxillary advancement in these reported series has averaged between 5 and 7 mm, and the mean long-term horizontal relapse averages between 20 % and 25% (Table 62–3). Erbe et al.[7] presented a mean follow up of 59 months for 11 cleft patients who underwent segmental osteotomies, maxillary advancement with bone grafting, rigid internal fixation, and simultaneous fistula closure. On an average, the greater maxillary segment in these patients was advanced 3.9 mm and the lesser maxillary segment 5.3 mm. At nearly 5 years postoperatively, they found that the horizontal relapse of the maxilla was approximately 40%. Cheung et al.[8] reported a consecutive series of 46 cleft patients who underwent maxillary advancement with rigid internal fixation and simultaneous alveolar bone grafting with fistula closure. The mean horizontal maxillary advancement in this series was 4.5 mm. Relapse in the horizontal plane for the unilateral cleft patients in this series, at a mean of 28 months postoperatively, was 22%. Similar horizontal relapse rates, following maxillary advancement with rigid internal fixation in cleft patients, have been reported by others as well (Table 62–3).[9–11]

In this series, 14 consecutive patients underwent successful maxillary advancement at the Le Fort I level through maxillary distraction with rigid external distraction. Examples of our clinical experience with rigid external distraction are illustrated in Figs. 62–5 to 62–7. No rigid internal fixation hardware or autogenous bone grafting was utilized at the time of the osteotomy. The patients underwent distraction at the rate of 1 mm/day followed by a 3–4-week rigid retention period. In this group of 14 cleft patients, the mean effective maxillary advancement was 11.7 mm. The time of the postdistraction cephalometric radiographs analyzed in this group of patients averaged 4 months following completion of the distraction process. These data have been presented so that the immediate effects of the distraction process can be measured

Table 62–3.

Review of Long-term Results of Sagittal Maxillary Relapse in Cleft Patients Following Maxillary Advancement with Fistula Closure, Bone Grafting, and Rigid Internal Fixation

Author	N cleft Pt.	Mean Follow-up (months)	Mean Maximum Advancement	Mean Relapse (%)
Erbe et al.[7]	11	59	4.6	40
Cheung et al.[8]	46	28	4.5	22
Posnick et al.[9]	35	12	6.9	21
Hochban et al.[10]	14	12	8	25
Eskenazi and Schendel[11]	12	12	7.8	4
Polley and Figueroa[1]	14	4	11.6	—

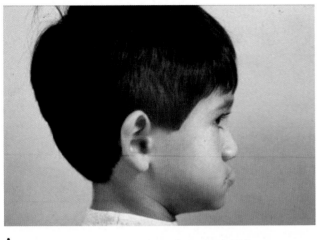

A

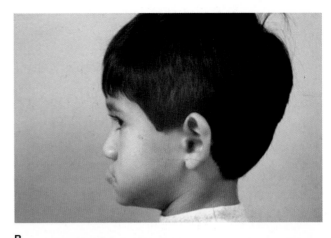

B

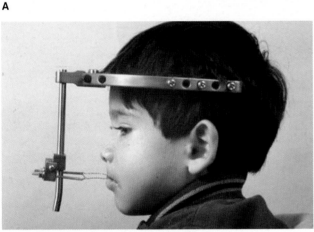

C

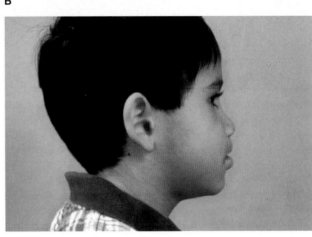

D

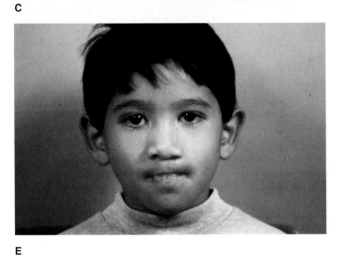

E

Figure 62–5. Clinical facial, cephalometric, and occlusal photographs of five year-old patient. **A**, **B**, **F**, and **H:** Before treatment with distraction, **C:** During distraction. **D**, **E**, **G**, and **I:** After distraction. These photographs illustrate maxillary advancement with good facial balance and occlusal relations.

accurately (Table 62–3). In the immature patients, maxillofacial growth will continue, and we are currently following the development of these patients.

Long-term skeletal stability after maxillary advancement with distraction osteogenesis has been documented in our series of 17 patients when comparing them at the completion of distraction and after two or more years of the follow-up[23] (Table 62–4 and Fig. 62–8). These patients demonstrated an increase in maxillary length of 1.9 mm (20%) when measured at the "A point" at two years of the follow-up. It is clear

from this data, and the corresponding average superimposition tracing, that the regression seen with traditional Le Fort I level advancements in the cleft population, is not a problem with distraction osteogenesis. The regression seen in the SNA in this series, is related to the forward growth at the nasion point over this period of follow-up, not a regression of point A. This is expected given the mean age of 12.6 years of the patients in the series. Other studies have demonstrated some relapse in the horizontal plane in the first 6–12 months after distraction with no regression after 12 months.[24–27] This

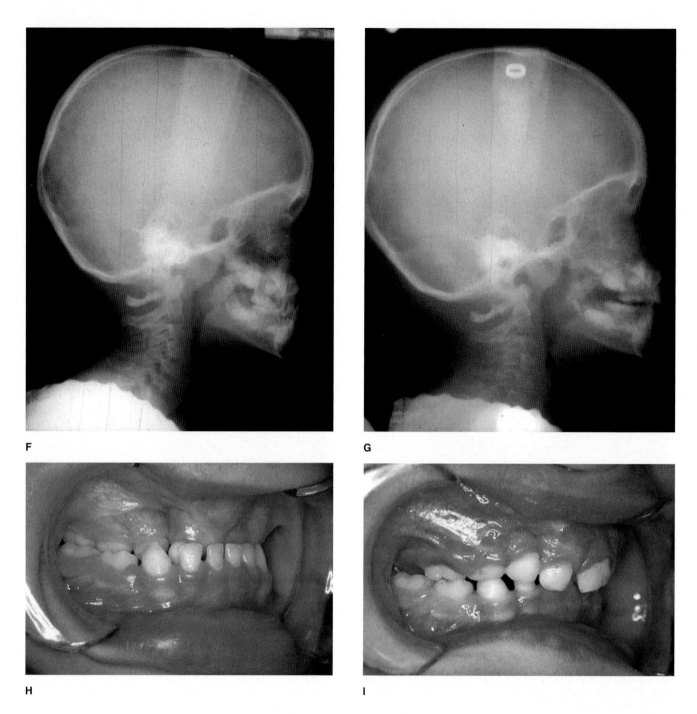

F

G

H

I

Figure 62–5. (*Continued*)

suggests that skeletal stability occurs at 12 months preventing relapse after that time.

In the past, it has been difficult to consistently and successfully treat patients with severe maxillary deficiency with maxillary advancement alone. Patients with large anteroposterior maxillomandibular discrepancies may require mandibular setback surgery in addition to maxillary advancement for correction of their severe horizontal deficiency. With the use of rigid external distraction, we can now gradually, and in a very stable fashion, reposition a severely hypoplastic maxilla to the exact horizontal and vertical position desired.

The patients create their own autogenous bone during this process, eliminating the need for a bone graft donor site, as well as eliminating the need for rigid internal fixation hardware (Fig. 62–9). The use of rigid external distraction has allowed rigid control over the distraction process, and has enabled us to follow our surgical and aesthetic guidelines for the reconstruction of these patients, by correcting the entire maxillary skeletal and soft-tissue discrepancy in the region of the hypoplasia only. The expansion of the soft tissue facial mask yields the most pleasing long-term aesthetic facial balance and harmony,[12,13] particularly in cleft patients.

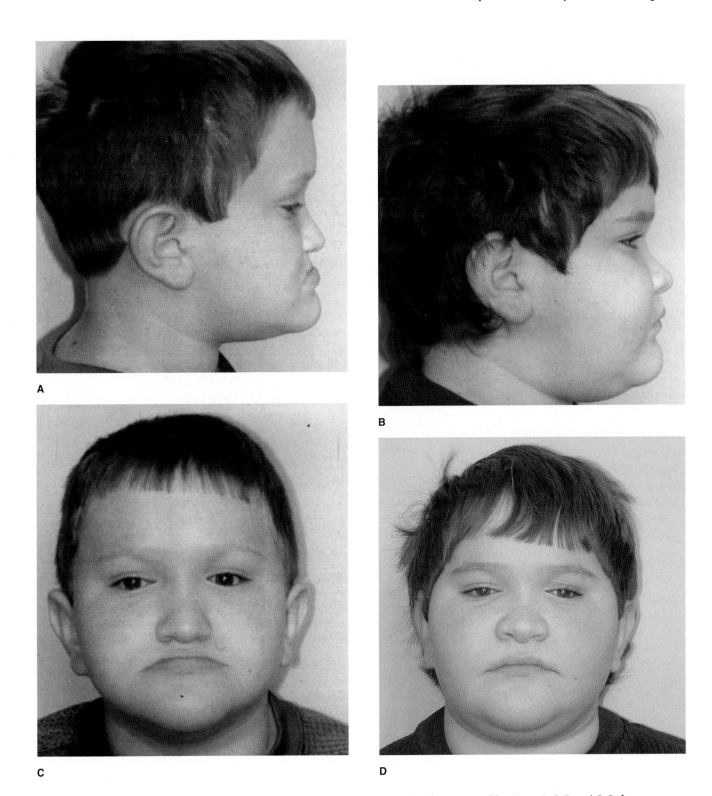

Figure 62–6. Clinical facial, cephalometric, and occlusal photographs of a 13-year-old patient. **A**, **C**, **E**, and **G:** Before treatment with distraction. **B**, **D**, **F**, and **H:** After distraction. These photographs illustrate maxillary advancement with good facial balance and occlusal relations.

In this initial consecutive series of patients, we utilized two different techniques for maxillary distraction. One group (facemask distraction) underwent maxillary distraction with the use of orthodontic facemask and elastic traction.[14] With the use of the elastic distraction, we were able to obtain only

partial correction of the horizontal maxillary deficiencies in these patients. We considered all of our facemask patients to have failed their surgical treatment. We therefore changed the design of the distraction technique to rigid external distraction, which utilizes the skeletally (cranial) fixed distraction

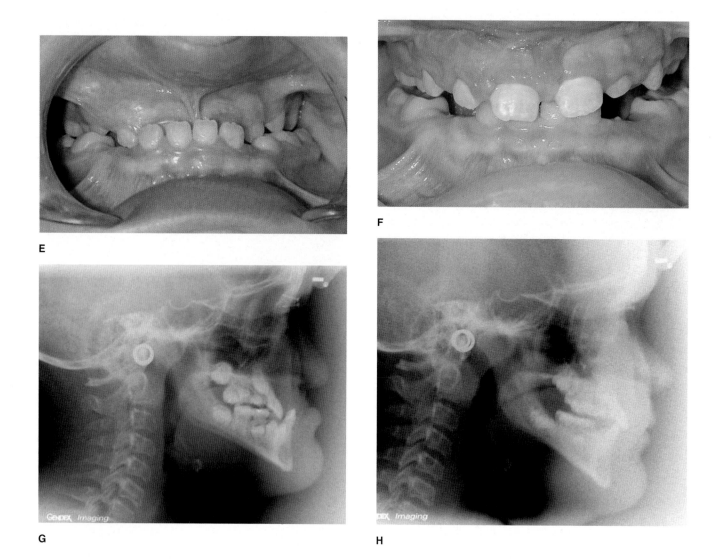

Figure 62–6. (*Continued*)

device, allowing for rigid and predictable control over the distraction process.

This halo device is readily adjustable, offering the ability to change the vertical and horizontal vector of distraction at any time during the distraction process. The tight control over the distraction process, afforded by rigid external distraction, is evidenced by the greater maxillary movements obtained with this device as compared with those patients who underwent facemask elastic distraction. For the patients who underwent rigid external distraction, the mean effective horizontal maxillary movement at the upper incisal edge averaged 11.7 mm. "A point" advancement in our series of patients with rigid external distraction averaged 8.3 mm. The change in the skeletal angle of convexity in the Rachmiel et al.[15] series with facemask traction averaged 5.0° compared with a change of 17.2° in our series of rigid external distraction. Diner et al.[16] obtained only 3 mm of horizontal maxillary advancement at "A point" in the series of patients who underwent maxillary distraction osteogenesis with the use of a facemask and elastic traction. The experience of Hung

et al.[17] was similar with the use of elastic forces for maxillary advancement in cleft patients. In their series, they found the mean horizontal maxillary advancement to be only 5.2 mm. Maxillary distraction at the Le Fort I level with the use of facemask and elastic traction is unpredictable and unreliable, allowing for horizontal advancement in the 4-6-mm range only. In our practice, patients who require only 4–6 mm of maxillary advancement are not routinely considered for treatment with distraction osteogenesis. In these patients, standard orthodontic surgical approaches at the appropriate age are generally performed.

Internal distraction devices have also been reported for use in midface advancement. Most of these reports have focused on advancements of the midface at the Le Fort III level or above.[18,19] Some, however, have advocated the use of an internal device for maxillary advancement at the Le Fort I level.[18] Internal devices may require multiple surgical approaches for their placement, a second operative procedure for their removal, and the necessity for an exit port for the activating arm of the device. The vectors of distraction with

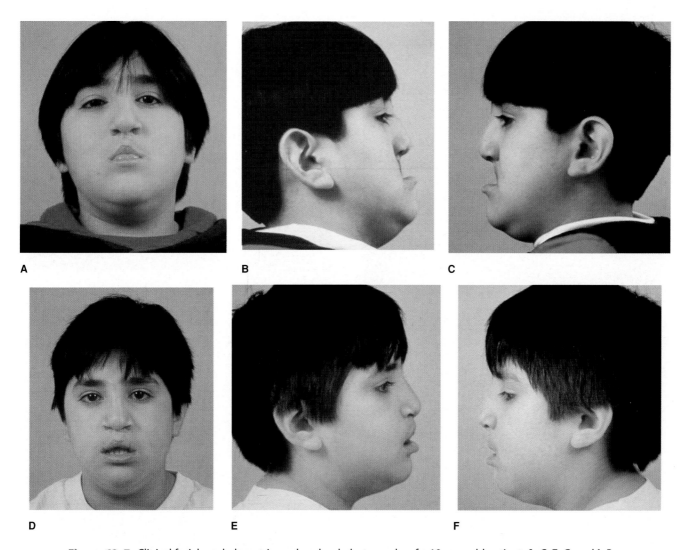

A   B   C

D   E   F

Figure 62–7. Clinical facial, cephalometric, and occlusal photographs of a 10-year-old patient. **A**, **C**, **E**, **G**, and **I:** Before treatment with distraction. **B**, **D**, **F**, **H**, and **J:** After distraction. The cephalogram shown demonstrates the clinical stability of maxillary advancement two years after distraction.

the use of internal devices will be limited by the placement of each device as well as its finite mechanics. Perhaps, the greatest disadvantage of internal devices is in the design of the transverse maxillary osteotomy. With internal distraction devices, the osteotomy must be designed so that there is enough stable bone above and below the osteotomy line to allow appropriate placement and fixation of the distraction hardware. This is not required with rigid external distraction. The osteotomy design with the external device is based upon the aesthetic requirements of each individual patient and not based upon the placement of internal hardware. This allows the transverse maxillary osteotomy to be carried as high as indicated along the pyriform aperture, as well as in the malar regions, allowing for maximal correction of the patient's preoperative facial concavity. Maxillary advancement with rigid external distraction allows total versatility and flexibility in both the amount and direction of the distraction process. The vectors of distraction can be, and frequently are, changed at any time during the distraction process. In addition, no additional sur-

gical procedure is required for removal of the rigid external device.

The use of the cranium as an anchorage point for the stabilization of maxillofacial surgery is not a new concept. Cranial stabilization devices for maxillofacial trauma reconstruction, as well as for elective maxillofacial surgery, have been reported with good success in the past.[20,21] In addition, our neurosurgical colleagues have used the cranium as a solid fixation point for the stabilization of cervical injuries and reconstructions for decades. The scalp pins (2–3 per side), which stabilize the halo component of the rigid external distraction device, are discomfort free. Not even the youngest patients have any complaints or problems with wearing of the device throughout the distraction process. No special scalp pin care is required, and the use of ointments and creams at the scalp pin interface is discouraged. The patients simply shampoo their hair in the shower with the device in place in a normal fashion. Currently, the device is readily removed without even local anesthesia in the clinic following the

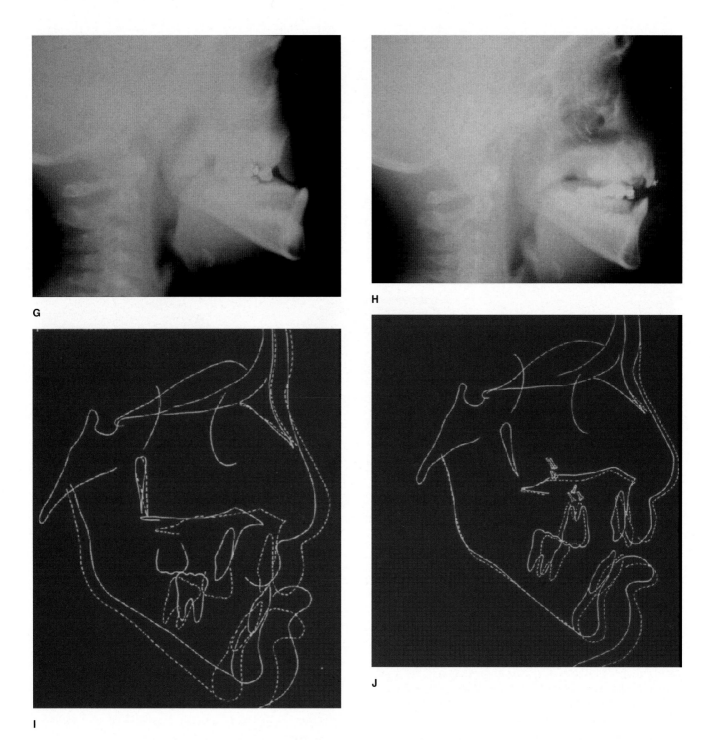

Figure 62–7. (*Continued*)

consolidation phase of rigid retention. In young apprehensive patients, the halo is removed with mild sedation. No secondary surgical procedure is required for removal of internal hardware.

One of the great advantages of distraction osteogenesis in the craniomaxillofacial skeleton is that, in theory, there is no limitation to the age at which patients can be treated. Contemporary surgical orthodontic approaches, for the treatment of maxillary deficiency in cleft patients, are dependent upon the patient having reached skeletal maturity before the

reconstructive surgery can be performed. Treating patients, in the transitional dentition stage, with the use of autogenous bone grafting and rigid internal fixation plates and screws, is technically difficult to perform without injury to the developing permanent tooth buds. The technique of rigid external distraction eliminates the negative technical factors associated with traditional orthognathic surgery in patients in transitional dental development. With maxillary rigid external distraction, only an osteotomy is performed. Repositioning skeletal segments, internal fixation hardware, and bone

Table 62–4.

Cephalometric Values Immediately After and 2 or More Years After Distraction

Variable	Mean	SD	Mean	SD	Difference	p
	Immediately after distraction ($n = 17$)		Two or more years after distraction ($n = 17$)			
SNA (°)	83.4	4.1	81	5.4	−2.4	0.01
SN/NL (°)	9.1	7.1	10	5.3	0.9	NS
SN/ML (°)	41.4	5.5	40.9	5	−0.5	NS
A-PM (mm)	52	5.3	53.9	5.2	1.9	0
ANS-PM (mm)	54	5.3	54	5	0	NS
ANS-S (H) (mm)	65.2	5.6	65.5	6	0.3	NS
ANS-S (V) (mm)	56	9	58.6	6.5	2.6	0.05

NS, nonsignificant

grafting are not required. The only limitations with rigid external distraction include adequate dentition, either primary or secondary, for fixation of the intraoral splint, as well as the ability of the patient to wear the device. Rigid external distraction now allows treatment of these patients from the age of 2 years and up. In special circumstances in patients with craniosynostosis (Crouzon and Apert syndromes), we have used the technique for monobloc advancement as early as 18 months of age. In these cases, the second or even the first primary maxillary molar has been used to support the intraoral splint. In addition, special plates have been developed to connect the edentulous maxilla to the rigid external distraction device.[22]

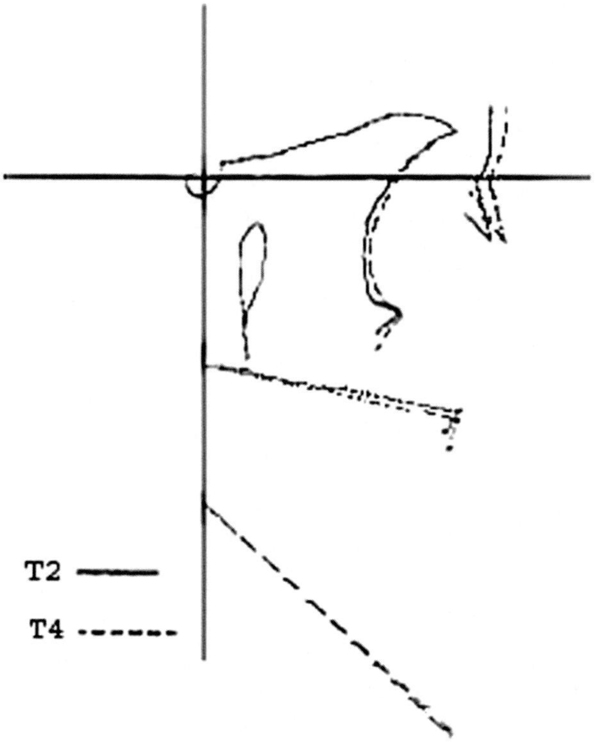

The three-year follow-up data, for this group of cleft patients after rigid external distraction, has demonstrated outstanding stability in maxillary position.[23] We believe that this stability is provided by substantial bone creation in the pterygomaxillary region with distraction as evidenced by Fig. 62–9.[23] However, we caution all young patients undergoing rigid external distraction that they may require a final "finishing" Le Fort I procedure at skeletal maturity for final arch alignment.

The advantages of maxillary rigid external distraction are numerous. This technique is an excellent modality for correcting, at any age, the severe midface concavities in patients with facial clefting and other hypoplastic anomalies (ectodermal dysplasia, Johansson Blizzard syndrome, etc.). Rigid

T2 ——

T4 ------

Figure 62–8. Average superimpositions illustrating changes occurring between soon after maxillary distraction (*T2, solid line*) and 2 or more years later (*T4, dashed line*). Note anterior growth, and anterior–posterior maxillary stability.

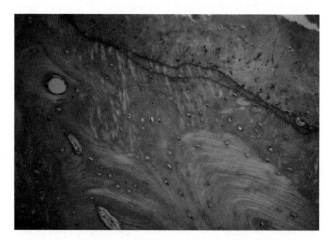

Figure 62–9. Histologic section of a bone biopsy specimen obtained from the pterygomaxillary region at the time of finishing Le Fort I surgery in a patient who underwent previous maxillary advancement with rigid external distraction. Note the well-ossified dense lamellar bone.

external distraction follows the important principles of aesthetic maxillofacial surgery by treating only the affected jaw, and offers the multiple benefits of distraction osteogenesis, including not only orthotopic bone creation with expansion of the facial skeleton, but soft tissue expansion as well. The technical advantages of rigid external distraction are numerous. The surgery is minor as compared with traditional orthognathic surgery. Only the osteotomy is performed, eliminating repositioning of skeletal segments, bone grafting, splints, intermaxillary fixation, and internal fixation hardware. Operative times are significantly decreased. Morbidity with rigid external distraction is very low (in our series zero). Blood transfusions are not required. Rigid external distraction can be performed on an outpatient or 23-hour admission basis. Patients begin a soft diet and normal oral hygiene the morning following surgery. The rigid external device is removed in the clinical setting, or with mild sedation for the young children. All of the above has resulted in a significantly decreased cost of care for these challenging patients.

In patients with severe cleft maxillary hypoplasia, distraction osteogenesis with rigid external distraction now offers the ability to fully restore facial convexity through a minimal procedure at almost any age. In our practice, this has dramatically changed our treatment philosophies and success for these patients who in the past have been extremely difficult to treat. The technique is currently applied with extreme success to those patients with severe maxillary nonsyndromal dentofacial deformities, as well as patients with severe syndromic conditions such as Apert's, Crouzon's, and Pfeiffer's syndrome.[24]

References

1. Polley JW, Figueroa AA. Management of severe maxillary deficiency in childhood and adolescence through distraction osteogenesis with an external, adjustable, rigid distraction device. *Craniofac Surg* 8(3):181–185, 1997.
2. Ross RB. Treatment variables affecting facial growth in complete unilateral cleft lip and palate: Part 7. An overview of treatment and facial growth. *Cleft Palate J* 24(1):5–77, 1987.
3. Da Silvia Filho OG, Correa Normando AD, Capelozza Filho L. Mandibular growth in patients with cleft lip and/or cleft palate-the influence of cleft type. *Am J Orthod Dentofacial Orthop* 104(3):269–275, 1993.
4. Semb G. A study of facial growth in patients with unilateral cleft lip and palate treated by the Oslo CLP team. *Cleft Palate Craniofac J* 28(1):1–21, 1991.
5. Witzel MA, Vallino LD. Speech problems in patients with dentofacial and craniofacial deformities. In Bell WH (ed). *Modern Practice in Orthognathic and Reconstructive Surgery, Vol 3*. Philadelphia, Saunders, 1992. pp. 1686.
6. Kapp-Simon K. *Psychological Adaptation of Patients with Craniofacial Malformations. Psychological Aspects of Facial Form*. Monograph No. 11, Craniofacial Growth Series, Ann Arbor, MI, Center for Human Growth and Development, University of Michigan, pp. 143–160.
7. Erbe M, Stoelinga PJW, Leenan RJ. Longterm results of segmental repositioning of the maxilla in cleft palate patients without previously

8. grafted alveolopalatal clefts. *J Craniomaxillofac Surg* 24(2):109–117, 1996.
8. Cheung LK, Sammam N, Hiu E, Tiderman H. The 3-dimensional stability of maxillary osteotomies in cleft patients with residual alveolar clefts. *Br J Oral Maxillofac Surg* 32(1):6–12, 1994.
9. Posnick JC, Dagys AP. Skeletal stability and relapse patterns after Le Fort I maxillary osteotomy fixed with miniplates: The unilateral cleft lip and palate deformity. *Plast Reconstr Surg* 94(7):924–932, 1994.
10. Hochban W, Gans C, Austermann KH. Longterm results after maxillary advancement in patients with clefts. *Cleft Palate Craniofac J* 30(2):237–243, 1993.
11. Eskenazi LB, Schendel SA. An analysis of Le Fort I maxillary advancement in cleft lip and palate patients. *Plast Reconstr Surg* 90(5):779–786, 1992.
12. Rosen HM. Facial skeletal expansion: Treatment strategies and rationale. *Plast Reconstr Surg* 89(5):798–808, 1992.
13. Rosen H. Aesthetics in facial skeletal surgery. *Perspect Plast Surgery* 6:1, 1992.
14. Molina F, Ortiz-Monasterio F. Maxillary distraction: Three years of clinical experience. In *Proceedings of the 65th Annual Meeting of the American Society of Plastic and Reconstructive Surgeons, Plastic Surgical Forum, Vol. XIX*. 1996. p. 54.
15. Rachmiel A, Laufer D, Aizenbud D. Surgically assisted orthopedic protraction of the maxilla in cleft palate patients by distraction osteogenesis (Abstract 198). *New Orleans: American Cleft Palate-Craniofacial Association 54th Annual Meeting;* 1997.
16. Diner PA, Martinez H, Tarbadar Y, et al. Experience with distraction in maxillary deficiency at Trousseau hospital *Paris: International Congress on Cranial and Facial Bone Distraction Processes;* 1997, Abstract 60.
17. Hung KF, Lin WY, Huang CS, Chen KT, Lo LJ. The maxillary movement distraction: Preliminary results. *Paris: International Congress on Cranial and Facial Bone Distraction Processes;* 1997, Abstract 55.
18. Cohen SR, Burstein FD. Maxillary-midface distraction in children with cleft lip and palate: A preliminary report. *Plast Reconstr Surg* 99(5):1421–1428, 1997.
19. Chin M, Toth BA. Le Fort III advancement with gradual distraction using internal devices. *Paris: International Congress on Cranial and Facial Bone Distraction Processes;* 1997, Abstract 76.
20. Stoelinga PJW, Van der Vijver HRM, Leenen RJ, et al. The prevention of relapse after maxillary osteotomies in cleft palate patients. *J Craniomaxillofac Surg* 15(6):326–331, 1987.
21. Houston WJ, James DR, Jones E, et al. Le Fort I Maxillary osteotomies in cleft palate cases. *J. Craniomaxillofac Surg* 17(1):9–15, 1989.
22. Hierl T, Hemprich A. Callus Distraction of the midface in the severely atrophied maxilla: A case report. *Cleft Palate Craniofac J* 36:457, 1999.
23. Figueroa AA, Polley JW, Friede H, et al. Long term skeletal stability after maxillary advancement with distraction osteogenesis using a rigid external distraction device in cleft maxillary deformities. *Plast Reconstr Surg* 114(6):1382–1392, 2004.
24. Figueroa AA, Polley JW, Ko E. Distraction osteogenesis for treatment of severe cleft maxillary deficiency with the RED technique. In Sanchukov ML (ed). *Craniofacial Distraction Osteogenesis, Chap. 55*. St. Louis, Mosby, 2001, pp. 485–493.
25. Suzuki EY, Motohashi N, Ohyama K. Longitudinal dento-skeletal changes in UCLP patients following maxillary distraction osteogenesis using RED system. *J Med Dent Sci* 51:27–33, 2004.
26. Ko EW, Figueroa AA, Polley JW. Soft tissue profile changes after maxillary advancement with distraction osteogenesis by use of a rigid external distraction device: A 1-year follow-up. *J Oral Maxillofac Surg* 58:959–969, 2000.
27. Krimmel M, Cornelius C, Bacher M, et al. Longitudinal cephalometric analysis after maxillary distraction osteogenesis. *J Craniofac Surg* 16(4):683–688, 2005.

Mandibular Distraction for Infants with Pierre Robin Sequence

Arlen D. Denny, MD, FACS, FAAP

INTRODUCTION

Pierre Robin sequence is a common congenital malformation. It appears in the general population with an incidence of approximately 1 out of 2000 live births. A French physician, Pierre Robin was the first to provide a detailed description of this malformation, and this was published in the Bulletin de l'Academy Nationale de Medecine Paris in 1923.[1] His description includes the triad of micrognathia, glossoptosis, and cleft palate.

Of greatest significance is his assertion that the triad of malformations will result in paroxysmal episodic airway obstruction in a small percentage of patients. From this episodic airway obstruction, a predictable pattern of other physiologic and developmental abnormalities follow. These include feeding disorders, gastroesophageal reflux disease, cachexia, pectus excavatum, and eventually cor pulmonale. Abnormalities of growth and development, progressing to death, will result when Pierre Robin sequence is untreated or inadequately treated. The symptoms of Pierre Robin malformation can be divided into two major classes: airway obstruction and feeding disorders. They are as intimately related as the anatomic structures which support these activities.

Pierre Robin states in his original description that airway obstruction, in approximately 90% of the patients, can be managed by positioning or other conservative measures.

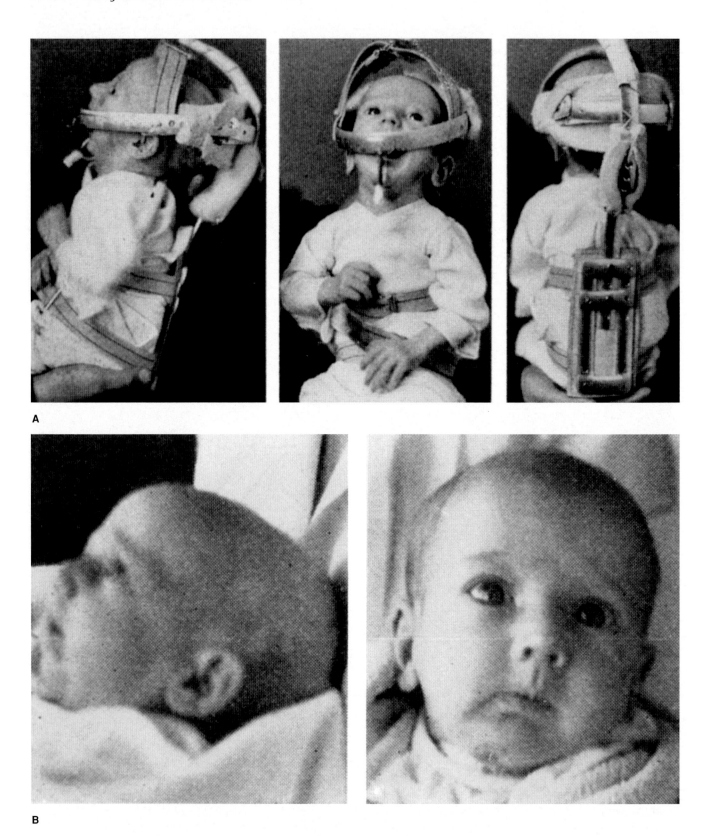

Figure 63–1. (**A**) Callister device, 1937. The lateral view shows the degree of maxillomandibular disharmony. (**B**) The patient, after 4 weeks of treatment in the Callister spring traction device.

However, the remaining 10% of patients are the most severely affected and will require more aggressive treatment.

HISTORY OF TREATMENT

Robin's description first appeared in English in 1934 in the *American Journal of Diseases of Children.*[2] In 1937, a report of successful treatment by Callister, of the University of Utah, was published, and described correction of micrognathia by applying traction to the mandible[3] (Fig. 63–1). A second published report of successful treatment, using traction on the mandible, appeared in 1949.[4] Longmeier and Sanford, of the University of California, Los Angeles, (Fig. 63–2) presented a technique utilizing orthopedic traction. Continuous traction, applied over a period of months, was required to achieve correction of micrognathia. Longmeier's unique contribution was the inclusion of radiographic documentation of the skeletal changes produced.

These early techniques were directed at correcting the skeletal abnormality, micrognathia. Correction of micrognathia resulted in resolution of airway obstruction and feeding difficulties. The principle of skeletal correction of micrognathia to eliminate airway obstruction was established by Callister in 1937 and reproduced by Longmeier in 1949. Eventually, techniques using traction on the mandible, to correct micrognathia and airway obstruction, were abandoned. A high incidence of temporomandibular joint ankylosis developed in patients following treatment. The application of traction forces to the mandible transmitted the applied force through the mandible, directly to the temporomandibular joint. Although micrognathia correction was achieved and airway obstruction relieved, the temporomandibular joints frequently ankylosed. No reliable correction for ankylosis of the temporomandibular joint was available at that time.

In 1946, an alternative technique of tongue advancement was described by Douglas.[5] It was strictly a soft tissue technique and was published in the first edition of the *Journal of Plastic and Reconstructive Surgery* (Fig. 63–3). Other soft tissue procedures have been proposed more recently.[6] The Douglas technique produced control of the tongue by suturing it over the mandibular alveolus into the labial sulcus, known as the tongue–lip adhesion. Although it did nothing to correct the skeletal malformation of micrognathia, it did provide some improvement in airway obstruction and gained wide acceptance.[7] Monitoring equipment, used routinely today to measure the effects of treatment, was not readily available at the time of these early studies, and would not emerge until nearly four decades later. These include pulse oximetry and neonatal polysomnography. Recently published reviews of single surgeon experiences with tongue–lip adhesion, up to 30 years, report complication rates up to 30%.[8,9] The tongue–lip adhesion procedure does not address the critical skeletal abnormality, micrognathia. It is the micrognathia that promotes glossoptosis, and the vertical tongue posture that produces episodic airway obstruction. In multiple studies based on serial cephalometry, it has been repeatedly shown that "catch-up" growth does not occur. Patients may survive their infancy without surgical correction

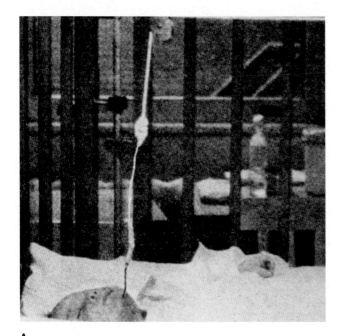

A

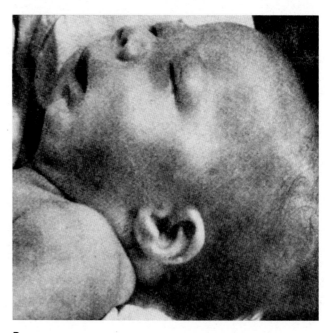

B

Figure 63–2. (**A**) The Longmeier traction apparatus. (**B**) The patient with micrognathia shown before treatment with the Longmeier device. (*continued*)

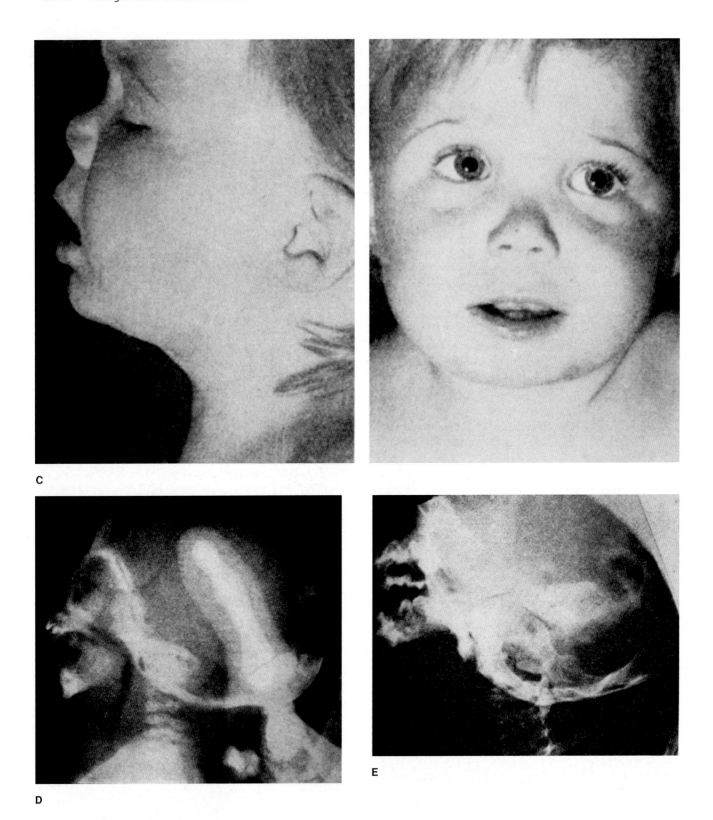

Figure 63–2. (*Continued*) (**C**) The same patient after 12 weeks in traction with the Longmeier device showing restoration of the proper maxillomandibular relationship. (**D**) Pre-traction, lateral view radiograph. (**E**) Post-traction, lateral view radiograph showing increased mandibular length.

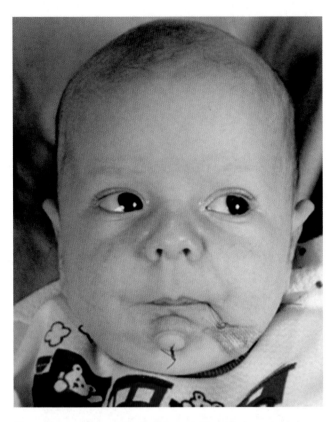

Figure 63–3. This patient is shown 32 days after repeat tongue–lip adhesion. He experienced recurrent airway symptoms after removal of the support button and went on to require mandibular distraction which relieved his airway obstruction.

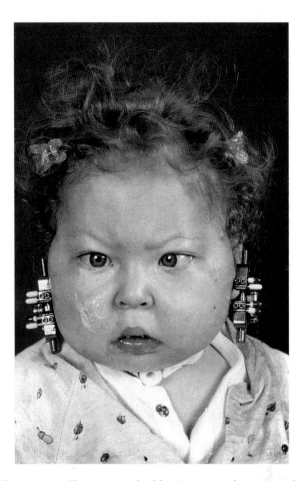

Figure 63–4. Thirteen-month-old patient treated as neonate by tracheostomy for airway obstruction. Shown under treatment by mandibular distraction to eliminate tracheostomy.

of micrognathia, but will achieve maturity with a persistent small jaw.[10–12]

Tracheostomy, although clearly a life-saving procedure, continues to produce high rates of mortality and morbidity, both in the hospital and home setting.[13–15] For decades, tracheostomy or tongue–lip adhesion has been the mainstay of surgical treatment for the most severely affected infants. These procedures do not provide skeletal correction of micrognathia. They can only be considered as temporizing measures as they do not provide definitive skeletal correction[16] (Fig. 63–4).

MANDIBULAR DISTRACTION OSTEOGENESIS

Mandibular distraction osteogenesis is significantly different from the traction only techniques previously used for the correction of micrognathia. With distraction osteogenesis, the mandible is surgically divided in preparation for distraction. The bone segments are controlled and separated incrementally by a mechanical device, and the distraction device functions as an adjustable force generator and bone segment stabilizer. Mandibular length is increased by activation. This is manipulation of the healing process, generating new bone formation. Traction only techniques, described in the past and performed without osteotomies, produced increased length by stimulating growth in response to applied force. These forces, applied by traction only techniques, were largely transmitted to the temporomandibular joint; while, distraction osteogenesis, as we understand it today, produces a minimal compressive force on the temporomandibular joint. These significant differences in force distribution may explain the rarity of temporomandibular joint ankylosis after contemporary mandibular distraction osteogenesis.

Published reports of initial experiences with mandibular distraction osteogenesis by Karp and McCarthy appeared in 1990.[17] Initially, only patients with hemifacial microsomia and Treacher Collins syndrome were treated by mandibular distraction to correct occlusal problems.[18,19] Experience with mandibular distraction increased over time; and, by 1999, reports from several centers described successful tracheostomy decannulation after mandibular distraction osteogenesis.[20–22] This concept of airway modification by mandibular distraction represented an important new application of the technique (Fig. 63–5). Improvements in airway dynamics, related to lengthening of the mandible, were independently confirmed by the adult obstructive sleep

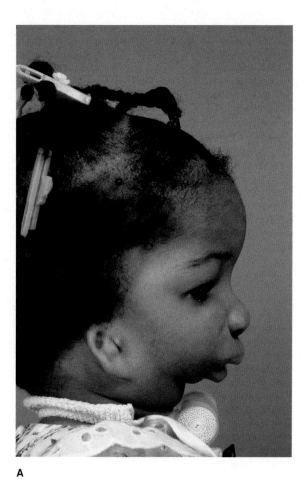

A

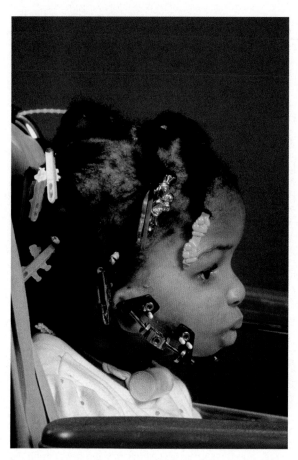

B

Figure 63–5. (**A**) Twenty-four month old patient with Nager's syndrome and severe micrognathia, treated in infancy by tracheostomy. (**B**) The patient in Fig. 63–5A after completion of active distraction of 22 mm.

apnea work of Riley et al. at Stanford University. Riley utilized the sagittal split osteotomy for mandibular lengthening, and clearly demonstrated the effective relief of airway obstruction.[23–26] Regardless of the surgical technique employed for mandibular lengthening, the attached soft tissues were advanced as a unit. The tongue was predictably pulled forward out of the airway, and it was this principle that allowed success using mandibular distraction to achieve tracheostomy removal.

A natural extension of the success experienced with tracheostomy decannulation following mandibular distraction was the consideration of utilizing mandibular distraction for tracheostomy avoidance. Published studies of airway cross-sectional area, before and after distraction, were followed by other reports demonstrating increases in the airway volume of the oropharynx following mandibular distraction. These studies documented a consistent and significant improvement[27] (Fig. 63–6). As clinical experience and objective data were collected, a more significant role for mandibular distraction has emerged. By this time, enough experience from several institutions has been gained to warrant application to the youngest and most fragile patients, the neonates. Reports of success, in single cases of neonatal distraction, lead us to initiate mandibular distraction for

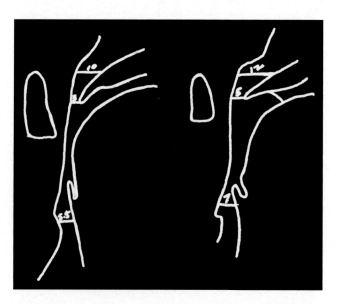

Figure 63–6. Lateral cephalometric x-ray tracing with measurements documenting key airway measurements. Left: Pre-distraction. Right: Post-distraction.

airway obstruction in a series of neonates.[28] These patients were selected because they were experiencing severe airway obstruction, and would otherwise have been treated by tracheostomy.[29]

CLINICAL INDICATIONS FOR TEAM EVALUATION

The diagnosis of Pierre Robin sequence, based on the triad of physical findings of small jaw, cleft palate, and glossoptosis, and resulting in paroxysmal airway obstruction, are followed closely for chest retractions on inspiration, intermittent oxygen desaturations, and persistent poor feeding. Feeding problems can present as a spectrum of dysfunction, from the inability to feed though interested, to refusal to accept the bottle. Persistent feeding problems in neonates with Pierre Robin sequence can be subtle but significant clinical indications requiring further evaluation. Our team experience indicates that, when obstructive airway problems are present, neonates will always preferentially breathe rather that eat. The neonate with Pierre Robin sequence may initially make a heroic attempt at feeding, while masking the seriousness of their airway obstruction. They may be discharged to the home setting only to deteriorate without benefit of medical observation.

The presence of intermittent airway obstruction in a neonate creates a very tenuous and dynamic situation. The newborn may manage adequately at first; however, the ability to self-rescue from airway obstruction may only be temporary. As time passes, nutritional stores present at birth are consumed and compensatory mechanisms are overwhelmed as the infant grows, and metabolic demand for nutrition and oxygen increase. Still today, deaths continue to occur in these patients who are not identified early after birth, appropriately evaluated, and aggressively treated. Most commonly, these deaths occur at home, during the night and outside the scrutiny of the medical community. They are commonly attributed to natural causes, and little useful information is returned to the medical caretakers. For these reasons, the clinical status of all Pierre Robin infants must be closely monitored.

TEAM EVALUATION

Our institution established an "Obstructed Airway Team" for the purpose of objectively evaluating and more effectively treating severely affected Pierre Robin patients. Our "Obstructed Airway Team" consists of specialists who are subspecialty fellowship trained in Pediatric Pulmonology, Intensive Care, Anesthesia, Otolaryngology, Craniofacial surgery, as well as Speech and Feeding. The Team evaluates all patients with Pierre Robin sequence who demonstrate episodic airway obstruction. Evaluations are assessed collectively, and treatment decisions are made by a consensus of team members. A neonatal intensive care environment is important. Intensive dedicated nursing, with continuous cardiac and O_2 saturation monitoring, is required. Daily weights, along with intake and output records, are also required. Feeding trials are attempted during the assessment period, and a detailed assessment by the feeding specialist is recorded. A thorough daily assessment, by the Pediatric Intensivist, considering all clinical parameters, is also provided. Since the Team was established, we have treated only 8% of all Pierre Robin patients diagnosed in this hospital using mandibular distraction. This corresponds well with Pierre Robin's early observation that approximately 10% of patients with the sequence experience severe airway obstruction and will require special care and treatment to survive.

ASSESSMENT PROTOCOL

The assessment protocol, which we have successfully utilized, requires flexible endoscopy of the entire upper and lower airway. This is the first step in the assessment protocol and is performed by the Pediatric Pulmonologist. Patients with Pierre Robin sequence, having micrognathia and cleft palate, frequently demonstrate glossoptosis, resulting in airway obstruction, when they relax in a supine position. This obstructive tongue posture is perpetuated by micrognathia. During the endoscopic airway examination, the patients are positioned supine and lightly sedated. A Pediatric Anesthesiologist is present for the exam to provide airway support if needed. The patient is purposefully placed in the "highest risk" position to assess the greatest potential for obstruction.

After performing a series of endoscopic examinations in these patients, the dynamics of glossoptosis are now well understood. As the tongue base falls posteriorly and inferiorly into the oropharynx, the tip of the tongue moves upward, passing through the cleft in the palate and obstructing the nasopharynx. The inferior movement of the tongue base obliterates the vallecular space, depressing the epiglottis and obstructing the airway. The posterior movement of the tongue base places it in contact with the posterior pharyngeal wall, obstructing the airway. This maneuver is regularly observed by oral inspection as a vertical tongue posture, and results in the simultaneous obstruction of the oral and nasal airway (Fig. 63–7). Negative pressures generated by inspiratory efforts by the patient perpetuate the obstruction. It is this glossoptosis, or vertical tongue posture, which can result in fatal airway obstruction. These obstructive components of glossoptosis are the only airway lesions that can predictably be corrected by using mandibular distraction to correct micrognathia.

Contraindications to distraction, identified by endoscopy, are flaccid ptosis of the epiglottis or arytenoids that collapse into the airway and obstruct airflow on inspiration. Circular collapse of the oropharynx (Sher Type III)[30] is also a contraindication to treatment by distraction. The same is true for obstructing degrees of laryngomalacia, tracheomalacia,

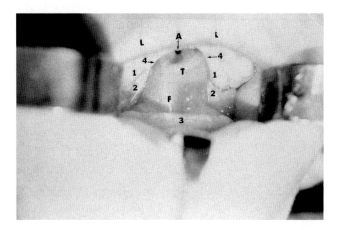

A

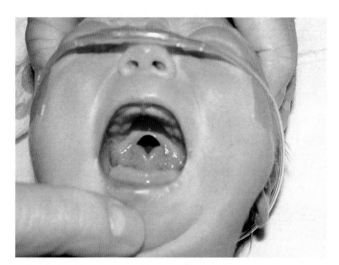

B

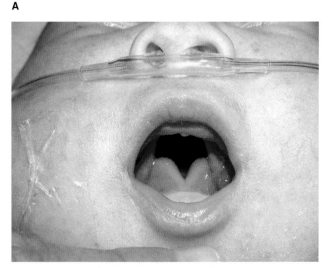

C

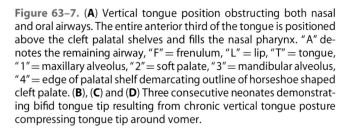

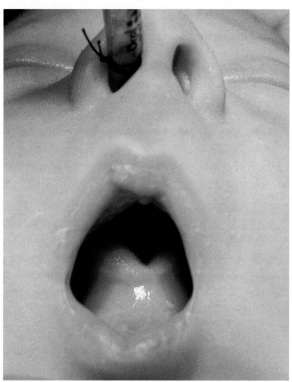

D

Figure 63–7. (A) Vertical tongue position obstructing both nasal and oral airways. The entire anterior third of the tongue is positioned above the cleft palatal shelves and fills the nasal pharynx. "A" denotes the remaining airway, "F" = frenulum, "L" = lip, "T" = tongue, "1" = maxillary alveolus, "2" = soft palate, "3" = mandibular alveolus, "4" = edge of palatal shelf demarcating outline of horseshoe shaped cleft palate. **(B)**, **(C)** and **(D)** Three consecutive neonates demonstrating bifid tongue tip resulting from chronic vertical tongue posture compressing tongue tip around vomer.

and bronchomalacia; these lower airway abnormalities will not be corrected by mandibular distraction.

The second objective parameter in assessing severity of airway obstruction is the infant polysomnogram. Repetitive obstructive desaturations during the study into the 80% p02 range or lower are strong indications of the need for treatment. These desaturations must be in the absence of central apneic events. A high frequency of central apnea, in addition to obstructive apnea, is a confounding variable. Although the obstructive apnea will be corrected by distraction, the central apnea will persist, is life threatening as well, and requires totally separate treatment. The ability to perform in-

fant polysomnograms in the intensive care setting, and their interpretation by an experienced Pediatric Pulmonologist is crucial.

Gastroesophageal reflux seen on polysomnogram studies is an indicator of strong inspiratory effort against an obstructed airway. This effort markedly increases negative intrathoracic pressure, pulling gastric contents into the esophagus. These symptoms can be expected to improve significantly after mandibular distraction.

The third modality in the evaluation protocol is a 3-dimensional CT scan. These images can provide visual impressions, as well as physical measurements, to assess

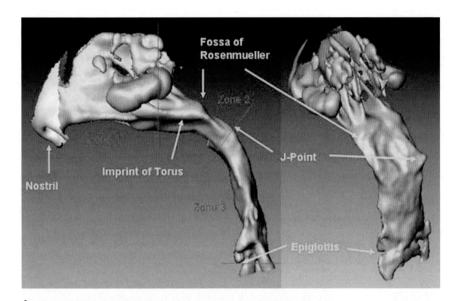

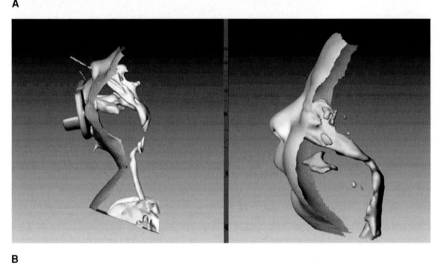

Figure 63–8. (**A**) Three-dimensional model of neonatal upper airway generated by Amira software. (**B**) Left: Pre-distraction. Right: Post-distraction. Three-dimensional model generated by Amira software from patient scan data.

the proportions of the mandible and maxillo-mandibular discrepancy. In addition, they provide a graphic tool for assessment of the entire craniofacial skeleton, and the temporomandibular joint. Mandibular distraction for airway obstruction requires a well-formed temporomandibular joint bilaterally to be successful. Using rapid CT scanning available today, in combination with various post-scan data processing programs, 3D images of the airway, and fly-through movies can also be generated. These are becoming increasingly useful in evaluating the internal airway configuration (Fig. 63–8).

The degree of maxillomandibular disharmony is a poor indicator of the need for distraction in the neonatal period. Several patients with as much as 14 mm difference have managed their airway without assistance, while others with only 8 mm discrepancy have demonstrated life-threatening airway obstruction. Measurements of maxillomandibular disharmony should be taken directly from a neonate placed briefly in a supine position using a small ruler. The ruler is placed

in the midline of the micrognathic mandible, and the measurement taken at the alveolar crest of the maxilla. These measurements can be safely taken at the bedside (Fig. 63–9). The combined analysis of these objective and clinical parameters by the team of specialists provides the basis for treatment recommendations.

SURGICAL TECHNIQUE

The procedure for application of mandibular distractors in neonates is truly technically challenging. One cannot overestimate the importance of surgical precision and correct application in the initial procedure. A neonatal airway case should never be the surgeon's first experience with mandibular distraction. It is necessary to develop a broad base of experience, beginning with older children successfully treated, and progressing to infants, prior to attempting distraction on neonates. As the patient age is progressively decreased, the

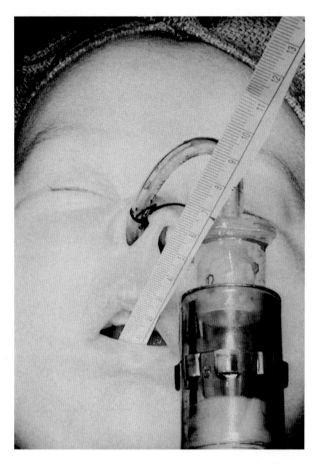

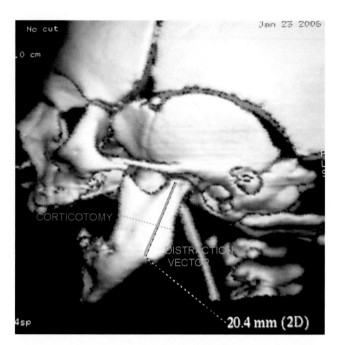

Figure 63–10. Three-dimensional CT scan showing ideal placement of corticotomy and distraction vector. Computer measurement from condylar neck to gonial notch. Indicates space limitation for distractor application along the ideal vector.

Figure 63–9. Ruler placed against the mandibular alveolus midline. Measurement taken at the maxillary midline alveolar crest showing a 12 mm disharmony.

size of the ramus and the density of bone are also reduced. The target area for pin placement is very small in neonates, with minimal margin for error. It is unwise to attempt placement on a neonate under 3 kg using the internal or external devices available today (Fig. 63–10). The physical size of

existing devices precludes application in neonates less than 3 kg in weight.

Internal distraction devices may be applied to neonates; however, they support their own set of problems.[31] With internal distractors, an open approach is essential; whereas, external devices can be applied, and the corticotomies performed, via the intraoral approach. Nonresorbable internal devices will require a second open procedure for removal, while an external device can be removed without incision. Internal devices remain strictly linear, while an external device allows the possibility of angular changes in the distraction vector.

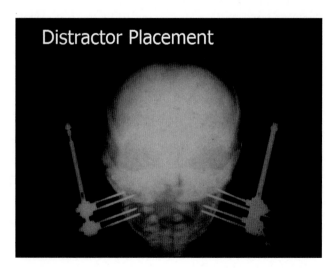

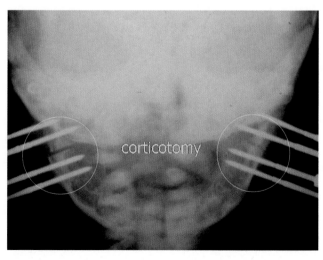

A

B

Figure 63–11. (A) Ideal distractor placement. **(B)** Bilateral ramus corticotomies highlighted.

Should an external distraction device fail, it can be replaced at the bedside. Failure of an internal device mandates a surgical procedure with general anesthesia and a very difficult airway.[32]

The author's preferred approach limits the surgical field to the area of the mandibular ramus posterior to the retromolar trigone. A four pin external device is used with bicortical pin placement. This prevents rotation of the mandibular segments on the pins, and allows the addition of controlled angulation if necessary (Fig. 63–11). Distraction vector selection is critical. Micrognathia is not a strictly horizontal deficiency. The most efficient vector for airway correction, and subsequent normal growth, is one perpendicular to the skull base. This vector is roughly parallel to the posterior border of the ramus in the neonate (Fig. 63–10). This provides both anterior projection and vertically increased intraoral volume. Some of the vertical lengthening will be translated into horizontal length increase by auto rotation and aid in restoring a normal skeletal relationship.[33] The vertical ramus osteotomy

combined with a horizontal distraction vector will be shown to cause significant growth and functional abnormalities, and should be avoided.

The recommended corticotomies are placed transversely across the ramus, above the mandibular angle, thus avoiding tooth buds and the entrance of the inferior alveolar nerve into the mandible. The corticotomies can be performed through an intraoral or extraoral route. Using an intraoral approach eliminates risk to the marginal mandibular nerve. However, procedures performed early in the surgeon's neonatal distraction experience are best done extraorally, through a small, modified Risdon incision, which provides the best visualization of the operative field. The marginal mandibular nerve must be protected. If an intraoral approach is selected, a sigmoid incision is made along the anterior ascending ramus, extending anteriorly in the mobile gingiva lateral to the alveolar ridge. After corticotomy and confirmation of complete separation, the distractor should be activated for several millimeters, then, returned to its original position. It is necessary

Table 63–1.

Patient Left Demonstrates Significant Deterioration in Oral Intake After Tongue–Lip Adhesion. Both Patients Demonstrate Substantial Improvement in Oral Intake and Weight Gain After Correction of Airway Obstruction by Mandibular Distraction

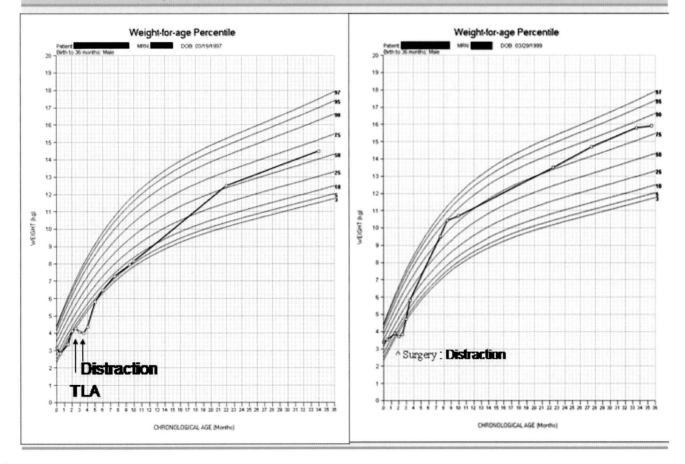

to confirm correct distractor function and bone separation under direct vision before closing the incision. This important maneuver will avoid many of the problems currently contributing to failure of distraction. Postoperative AP and lateral x-rays are obtained on the operating table to confirm pin placement and distractor alignment. Postoperatively, the patient should remain intubated and return to the neonatal intensive care unit.

PATIENT MANAGEMENT

During the evaluation and active distraction process, each of the team members provides specific services. The Pediatric Pulmonologist monitors lung physiology and interprets polysomnograms. The Pediatric Intensivist monitors clinical performance of the patient and performs endoscopy before, during, and after the distraction. The Pediatric Anesthesiologist monitors the progress of the patient, and assesses the airway by direct laryngoscopy and endoscopy. These services are necessary to assure safe airway management and anesthesia during the surgical procedures, before and after distraction is completed. The Pediatric Otolaryngologist also provides assessment of the airway, and identifies other airway pathology, which may contraindicate successful distraction. Most importantly, the otolaryngologist provides the "safety net" of tracheostomy, should distraction fail. This specialist must have a thorough knowledge of the patient's distraction progress and airway status at all times.

The Feeding Specialist provides expertise in assessing feeding skills, and provides training prior to distraction. Patients who have had even a short, monitored feeding experience prior to distraction, will be much more successful feeders once extubated. After the patient is extubated, feeding resumes under their guidance. A neonate will attempt feeding 8–12 times a day. Careful observation and recording of not only feeding volumes, but also time taken to feed, and characteristics of each feeding attempt, are critical. This will provide a much more rapid and accurate measure of the patient's growth characteristics than monitoring daily weights (Table 63–1). Cine studies of swallowing may also be necessary in some patients after distraction to document presence or absence of aspiration. A feeding plan, to guide the parents after discharge, is developed by the feeding specialist, and this plan must consider individual feeding skills and nutritional requirements.

The craniofacial surgeon is responsible for coordinating the team of pediatric specialists. The surgeon must integrate information produced by the team evaluation, and organize a timetable for treatment. This includes performing the distractor placement surgery, and managing all aspects of active distraction. The craniofacial surgeon should be involved in the evaluation for, and timing of, extubation. This is a critical point in the distraction process. Finally, the surgeon must determine the endpoint of distraction and timing of distractor removal.

DISTRACTION PROTOCOL

The distraction protocol is a very important part of patient management. The latency period, or time from corticotomy and distractor placement to the activation of the devices and start of distraction, is very short in the neonate because of the high rate of bone metabolism and healing. Activation of the devices and initiation of distraction is begun the next morning after distractor placement. Pain is managed with small amounts of IV morphine or oral oxycodone. When utilizing external pin-born devices, distraction proceeds at 2 mm/day for the first 3 days, with the distractors activated 1 mm every 12 hours. After 3 or 4 days, 6–8 mm of distraction will have been accomplished; and, the patient may be ready to be evaluated for extubation.

A good clinical indicator of readiness for extubation is tongue posture. As the distraction proceeds, the tongue will increasingly tend to lie on the floor of the mouth. The vertical tongue posture is no longer seen, and the resting position of the tongue tip will advance anterior to the apex of the cleft palate (Fig. 63–12). The advancement of the mandible prevents passage of the tongue tip through the cleft, avoiding nasal airway obstruction. These clinical indicators must be supported by improvements in the airway at the tongue base, confirmed by endoscopy. Endoscopy is performed with minimal sedation by the Pediatric Pulmonologist. To fulfill the

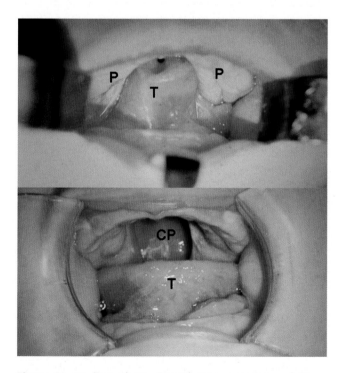

Figure 63–12. Top photo: Typical tongue posture of Pierre Robin neonate with airway obstruction. Tongue marked with "T", palate marked with "P". Lower photo: Same patient after 14 mm of distraction. Note both increased vertical and horizontal space intraorally. Tongue marked "T" now rests on the floor of the mouth with the tip of the tongue positioned anteriorly preventing passage of the tongue into the nasal cavity through the cleft palate (CP).

criteria for extubation, the tongue base must no longer be resting on, and partially collapsing the epiglottis. The vallecular space must be restored. When an airway is present constantly between the tongue base and the posterior pharyngeal wall, a trial of extubation may be warranted. The vigor and general health of the neonate must also be considered. If a team consensus is reached, extubation is performed. Close monitoring is required for the next 24 hours in an intensive care setting. If a correct decision has been made, an immediate and substantial improvement in the neonate's airway function will be apparent. If there is any question, the patient remains intubated for another 24 hours and active distraction continues for another 2 mm. The patient is then re-assessed by endoscopy. Swelling of the vocal cords and larynx may be treated by administration of a single dose of intravenous steroid. Continuous monitoring of cardiac activity and O_2 saturation after extubation is paramount. A polysomnogram should be repeated 1–2 days after extubation. Early interpretation of the results by the pulmonologist is necessary. A successful distraction will result in elimination of obstructive events and significant desaturations. It will also identify any persistent tendency for central apnea.

Once a safe and stable airway has been established for 24 hours, oral feeding trials should resume under the guidance of the feeding specialist. Since all of the oropharyngeal soft tissue relationships have been substantially re-arranged by the distraction, normal feeding of adequate volumes cannot be expected immediately. Nasogastric feeding support should be provided and weaned with progressively increased oral intake.

Distraction continues at 1 mm/day after extubation when using an external device. Continuing at a higher rate may result in shredding the skin around the percutaneous pins, breaking the distractors, or both. Internal devices may continue at distraction rates up to 2 mm/day. After extubation, pain is managed with oral oxycodone. The decision to terminate active distraction should be determined only by skeletal relationships between the mandible and maxilla. The airway obstruction issues should be resolved days before the skeletal endpoint of distraction is reached. The endpoint chosen should reflect a restoration of a normal relationship for age between upper and lower jaw. Overcorrection of the mandible in syndromic patients, with known high incidences of growth abnormality, is unlikely to avoid the need for repeat distraction in the future. Growth in syndromic patients cannot be predicted; and, not all patients with syndromes, such as Stickler syndrome, will require repeat distraction. Once overcorrection has occurred, it may become permanent, and extremely difficult to correct, requiring the patient to undergo mandibular setback via sagittal split osteotomy at skeletal maturity.

Once the normal maxillo-mandibular relationship has been established, active distraction is terminated, and a period of consolidation is begun. The consolidation phase, defined as the period of time between termination of active distraction and removal of the distractors when the bone regenerate has healed, will be 4 weeks in duration for the neonate less than 1 year of age.

FAILURE OF DISTRACTION

When employing external percutaneous pin-born devices, any loss of mechanical function of the distractors can be corrected at the bedside at any time. The device can be carefully removed from the pins to avoid dislodging them from the bone, and exchanged. Nonmechanical distraction problems are significant, based on the timing of their occurrence. Loss of distractor pin attachment to the bone, early in active distraction, may be uncorrectable, and the team should be notified immediately. If bone support is lost prior to achieving approximately 8 mm of distraction, replacement of the pins or screws under anesthesia should be attempted. If the attempt is unsuccessful, tracheostomy must be considered. If the distraction has proceeded effectively beyond 8 mm, and only one distractor is disrupted, the airway must be assessed (Fig. 63–13). If the airway is safe, active distraction should be terminated. The nonsupporting distractor should be removed, and the supporting distractor maintained until consolidation is complete. Asymmetric distraction can be performed months later if the patient redevelops symptoms. Some improvement in the airway will be maintained. Although ideal

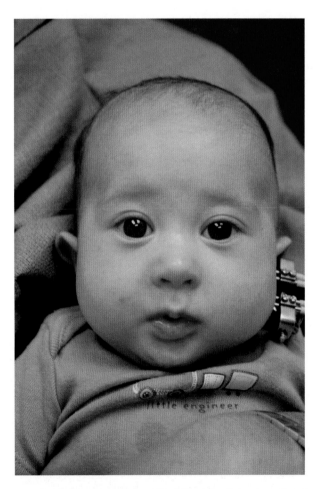

Figure 63–13. Neonate, 4 weeks following disruption of right distractor pins, after 8 mm of active distraction. Airway improvement allowed safe extubation. Note subtle rightward deviation of chin point.

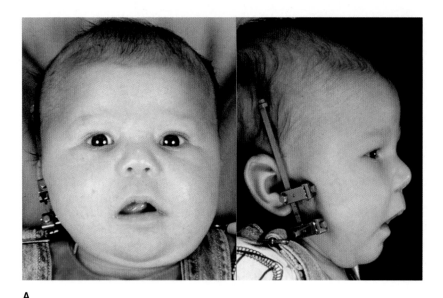

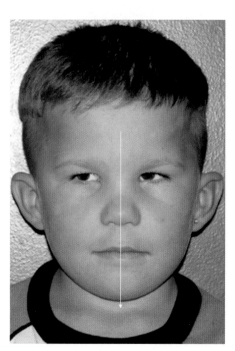

A

B

Figure 63–14. (**A**) Left mandibular distractor lost in neonate after 15 mm of active distraction and 2½ weeks of consolidation. (**B**) Patient 14a at 5 years of age with no mandibular deviation.

skeletal correction is lost, the advancement may be sufficient to prevent airway obstruction and avoid tracheostomy. If disruption occurs during the consolidation phase, minimal or no relapse may occur (Fig. 63–14). The airway should be carefully assessed, the nonsupporting distractor removed, the supporting distractor retained, and radiologic assessment of the mandible made. The supporting distractor can be safely removed at the end of the scheduled consolidation phase if protocol requirements are met. Redistraction may not be necessary. However, if the distraction process fails to provide an adequate airway after normal skeletal relationships have been established, tracheostomy must be considered. If the patient met all criteria for distraction initially, and distraction failed to establish a safe airway, temporizing solutions, such as nasopharyngeal intubation or tongue–lip adhesion, are unlikely to provide correction.

DISCHARGE PLANNING

After successful distraction, the neonate should be discharged to home on an apnea monitor, with thorough instruction to the parents. Endoscopy should be performed at three months postoperatively, and polysomnogram at 1 year after discharge. If no significant airway events are recorded after 90 days post-discharge, the apnea monitor is discontinued. Re-evaluation by the team is required at any time symptoms recur. Weight gains, and growth and feeding performance, should continue to be monitored by the feeding specialist and family pediatrician after discharge. Inadequate weight gain may be a subtle indicator of recurrent airway problems. Regular visits to the craniofacial surgeon should be made

to monitor subsequent mandibular growth, symmetry, scar maturation, and any airway symptoms. A post-distraction 3D CT should be obtained at 1 year to assess growth of the mandible and skeletal relationships. Regular visits to the pediatrician are required to monitor overall growth and development.

DISTRACTOR REMOVAL

The consolidation phase should be complete in infants under 1 year of age by 4 weeks. In the operating room, under general inhalational anesthesia, direct laryngoscopy is performed, and the findings are recorded by the anesthesiologist (Fig. 63–15). Endoscopy is performed by the otolaryngologist or pulmonologist to confirm a normal airway, and provide a reference for future evaluations. The external distractors are then removed from the pins carefully, leaving the pins in place. AP and lateral x-rays are taken to assess the quality and degree of calcification in the regenerate. While the films are being processed, the surgeon stresses the distraction site. No movement should be detected. The x-rays are then reviewed. Significant calcification should be readily apparent in the distraction gap. Complete reformation of medial and lateral cortices should be present on both rami. When union of the bone is present, the pins are removed (Fig. 63–16). If mobility or deficient calcification is present, the distractor should be replaced on the retained pins of the affected side, and be maintained for an additional 2 weeks, after which, a repeated evaluation is performed. When union is confirmed the pins are removed, and the process is complete.

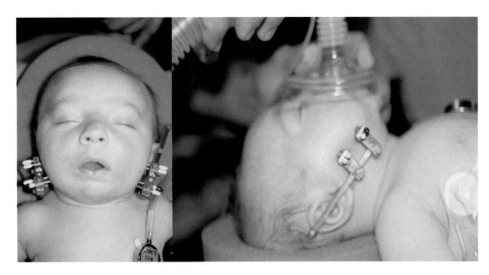

Figure 63–15. Patient after 14 mm of active distraction as neonate and 4 weeks consolidation with normal tongue posture restored and mask ventilation.

RE-DISTRACTION

Some syndromes associated with Pierre Robin sequence include a tendency for inadequate mandibular growth. These syndromic patients may re-develop obstructive airway symp-toms as early as 1 year or less after successful distraction. Repeat distraction can be readily performed with the same expectations and facility as the first procedure (Fig. 63–17); however, with the following caveat: Distraction repeated at 1 year or less can produce paresis in facial nerve branches,

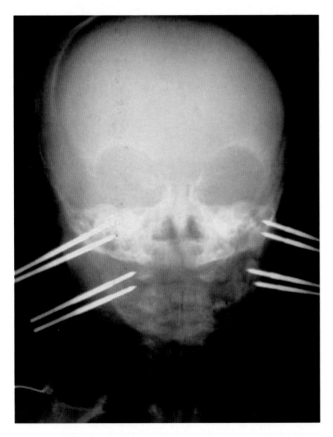

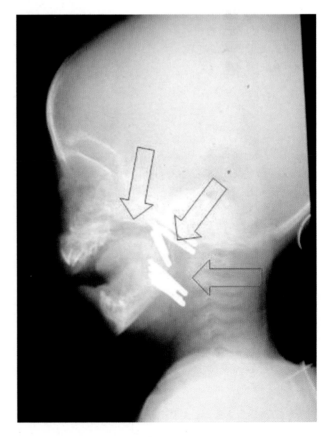

Figure 63–16. Left: Post-consolidation film with distractors removed. Consolidation sites are located between central pins. Right: Lateral view at time of distractor removal demonstrating restoration of nasal airway and horizontal tongue posture.

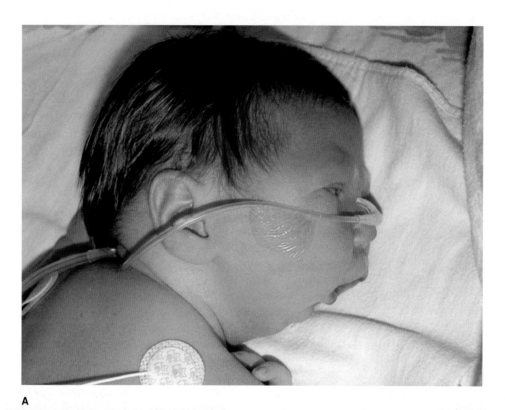

A

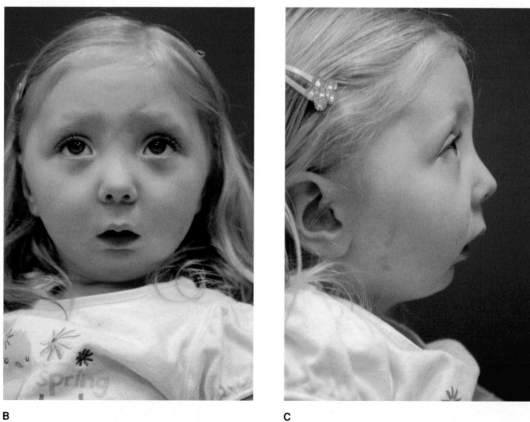

B

C

Figure 63–17. (**A**) Neonate with Pierre Robin sequence and severe micrognathia. Corrected by mandibular distraction. The patient redeveloped airway obstructive symptoms and required re-distraction at 1 year of age. (**B**) and (**C**) Patient 17a after repeat mandibular distraction at 1 year of age.

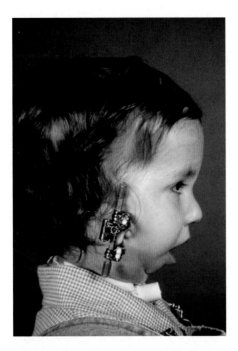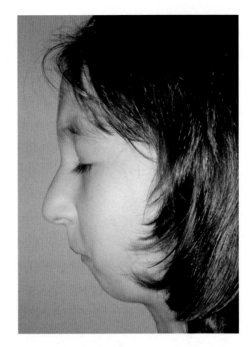

Figure 63–18. Left: Patient in infancy with severe Pierre Robin sequence and Goldenhar syndrome. Treated as neonate with tracheostomy. Undergoing bilateral mandibular distraction for tracheostomy removal in infancy. Right: 9 years of age after four successful mandibular distractions for recurrent airway obstructive symptoms related to inadequate mandibular growth.

and has been seen in the zygomatic and buccal branches. Paresis was noted only after 10 mm of distraction, performed at 1 mm/day. The paresis is temporary, and is thought to be a result of immature scar tissue in the region of the facial nerve, which has not completely softened. Traction forces generated by active distraction may be transmitted to the nerve branches causing the paresis. It has resolved completely in less than 1 year in all cases. This complication has not been observed in patients re-distracted 2 years after the original treatment. The earlier the distraction was repeated, the more scar tissue was present at surgery; however, the bone itself appeared completely normal in contour, density, and strength. Redistractions have been otherwise routine, with no increase in difficulty or complication rate, except as noted. Up to four successful distractions have been performed in the same syndromic patient over a 6-year period (Fig. 63–18).

LONG-TERM RESULTS

We have experience with mandibular distraction for airway obstruction in 15 neonates who have been followed for up to 7 years, and an additional 23 patients distracted before reaching 1 year of age (Fig. 63–19). All patients met the criteria for distraction with airway obstruction. No patients required more than 8 mm of distraction to achieve extubation. No reintubations or additional airway support was required.[34] In the neonatal group, three external distractors were lost. One distractor was disrupted on the day

of scheduled extubation, after 8 mm of active distraction. The contralateral distractor remained stable. An adequate airway was confirmed by endoscopy, and the patient was extubated on schedule, with a functionally normal airway. Eight months later, obstructive airway symptoms recurred, and elective re-distraction was repeated with resolution of symptoms, and without incident. In another patient, one distractor was disrupted at the completion of active distraction, and the contralateral distractor remained stable. The disrupted distal pins were replaced, and consolidation continued uneventfully. Ultimately, the patient has a normal airway, but mild skeletal asymmetry. Re-distraction, for symmetry, may be required in future. In the third patient, a distractor disruption occurred during consolidation, with no detectable midline shift 6 years later. Predicted complications, such as permanent nerve injury, dental disruption, and growth disturbance have not been experienced in our series.

CONCLUSION

Mandibular distraction is a useful technique in avoiding tracheostomy in selected newborns and infants with micrognathia and severe airway obstruction. It is a technically very demanding surgery, and experience with pediatric distraction is required. Because of the extremely young ages and fragility of the patients, strict adherence to suggested protocols is highly advisable to avoid catastrophic results.

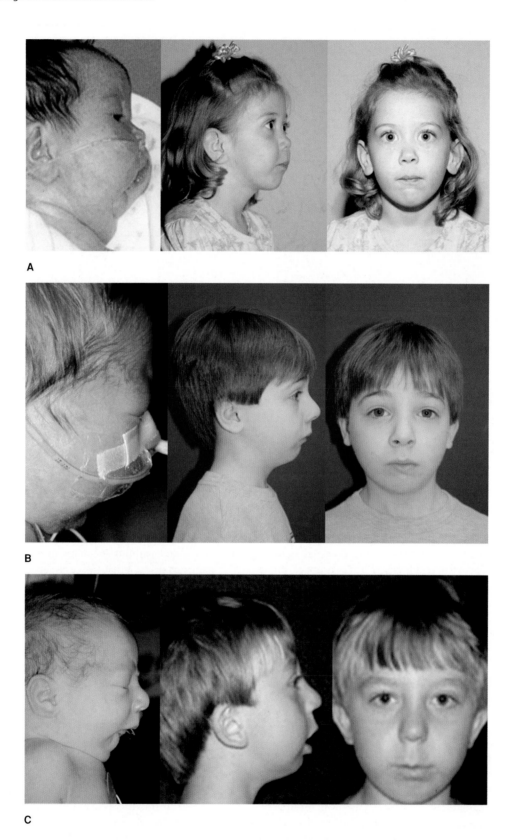

Figure 63–19. (A) Patient at birth and 7 year follow-up after neonatal mandibular distraction for airway obstruction. **(B)** Patient at birth and 7 year follow-up after neonatal mandibular distraction for airway obstruction. **(C)** Patient at birth and 7 year follow-up after neonatal mandibular distraction for airway obstruction.

References

1. Robin P. LaGlossoptose, son diagnostic, ses consequences, son traitment. *Bulletin de l'Academie National de Medecine*, Paris, 1923 and *J Med Paris*, 1923.

2. Robin P. Glossoptosis due to atresia and hypotrophy of the mandible. *Am J Dis Child* 48:541, 1934.

3. Callister AC. Hypoplasia of the mandible (micrognathia) with cleft palate: Treatment in early infancy by skeletal traction. *Am J Dis Child* 53:1057, 1937.

4. Longmire WP, Jr., Sanford MC. Stimulation of mandibular growth in congenital micrognathia by traction. *Am J Dis Child* 78:750, 1949.

5. Douglas B. The treatment of micrognathia associated with obstruction by a plastic procedure. *Plast Reconstr Surg* 3:300, 1946.

6. Delorme RP, Larocquie Y, Caouette-Laberge L. Innovative surgical approach for the Pierre Robin anomalad: Subperiosteal release of the floor of the mouth musculature. *Plast Reconstr Surg* 83:960, 1989.

7. Parsons RW, Smith DJ. Rule of thumb criteria for tongue-lip adhesion in Pierre Robin anomalad. *Plast Reconstr Surg* 70:210, 1982.

8. Hoffman W. Outcome of tongue-lip placation in patients with severe Pierre Robin sequence. *J Craniofac Surg* 14:602, 2003.

9. Kirschner RE, Low DW, Randall P, et al. Surgical airway management in Pierre Robin sequence: Is there a role for tongue-lip adhesion? *Cleft Palate Craniofac J* 40:13, 2003.

10. Figueroa AA, Glupker TJ, Fitz MG, BeGole EA. Mandible, tongue, and airway in Pierre Robin sequence: A longitudinal cephalometric study. *Cleft Palate Craniofac J* 28:425, 1991.

11. Daskalogiannakis J, Ross RB, Tompson BD. The mandibular catch-up growth controversy in Pierre Robin sequence. *Am J Orthod Dentofacial Orthop* 120:280, 2001.

12. Eriksen J, Hermann NV, Darvann TA, Kreiborg S. Early post-natal development of the mandible in children with isolated cleft palate and children with non-syndromic Robin sequence. *Cleft Palate Craniofac J* 43:155, 2006.

13. Zeitouni A, Manoukian J. Tracheostomy in the first year of life. *J Otolaryngol* 22:431, 1993.

14. Singer LT, Kercsmar C, Legris G, et al. Developmental sequelae of long-term infant tracheostomy. *Dev Med Child Neurol* 31:224, 1989.

15. Tomaski SM, Zalzal GH, Saal HM. Airway obstruction in the Pierre Robin sequence. *Laryngoscope* 105:111, 1995.

16. Denny AD, Amm CA, Schaefer RB. Outcomes of tongue-lip adhesion for neonatal respiratory distress caused by Pierre Robin sequence. *J Craniofac Surg* 15:819, 2004.

17. McCarthy JG, Schreiber J, Karp N, Thorne CH, Grayson BH. Lengthening the human mandible by gradual distraction. *Plast Reconstr Surg* 89:1, 1992.

18. Molina F, Ortiz-Monasterio F. Mandibular elongation and remodeling by distraction: A farewell to major osteotomies. *Plast Reconstr Surg* 96:825, 1995.

19. Moore MH, Guzman-Stein G, Proudman TW, Abbott AH, Netherway DJ, David DJ. Mandibular lengthening by distraction for airway obstruction in Treacher-Collins Syndrome. *J Craniofac Surg* 5:22, 1994.

20. Denny AD, Talisman R, Hanson PR, Recinos RF. Mandibular distraction osteogenesis in very young patients to correct airway obstruction. *Plast Reconstr Surg* 108:302, 2001.

21. Williams JK, Maull D, Grayson BH, Longaker MT, McCarthy JG. Early decannulation with bilateral mandibular distraction for tracheostomy-dependent patients. *Plast Reconstr Surg* 103:48, 1999.

22. Monasterio FO, Drucker M, Molina F, Ysunza A. Distraction osteogenesis in Pierre Robin sequence and related respiratory problems in children. *J Craniofac Surg* 13:79, 2002, discussion 84.

23. Bear SE, Priest JH. Sleep apnea syndrome: Correction with surgical advancement of the mandible. *J Oral Surg* 38:543, 1980.

24. Puckett CL, Pickens J, Reinisch JF. Sleep apnea in mandibular hypoplasia. *Plast Reconstr Surg* 70:213, 1982.

25. Riley RW, Powell, NB, Guilleminault C, Nino-Murcia G. Maxillary, mandibular, and hyoid advancement: An alternative to tracheostomy in obstructive sleep apnea syndrome. *Otolaryngol Head Neck Surg* 94:584, 1986.

26. Dierks E, Geller M, Roffwarg H, Johns D. Obstructive sleep apnea syndrome: Correction by mandibular advancement. *South Med J* 83:390, 1990.

27. Denny AD, Kalantarian B. Mandibular distraction in neonates: A strategy to avoid tracheostomy. *Plast Reconstr Surg* 109:896, 2002.

28. Judge B, Hamlar D, Rimell FL. Mandibular distraction osteogenesis in a neonate. *Arch Otolaryngol Head Neck Surg* 125:1029, 1999.

29. Denny AD. Distraction osteogenesis in Pierre Robin neonates with airway obstruction. *Clin Plast Surg* 31:221, 2004.

30. Sher AE, Shprintzen RJ, Thorpy MJ. Endoscopic observations of obstructive sleep apnea in children with anomalous airways: Predictive and therapeutic value. *Int J Pediatr Otorhinolaryngol* 11:135, 1986.

31. Burstein FD, Williams JK. Mandibular distraction osteogenesis in Pierre Robin sequence: Application of a new internal single-stage resorbable device. *Plast Reconstr Surg* 115:61, 2005.

32. Denny AD. Mandibular distraction osteogenesis in Pierre Robin sequence: Application of a new internal single stage resorbable device. Invited review. *Plast Reconstr Surg* 115:68, 2005.

33. Grayson B. Personal communication, May, 2006.

34. Denny AD, Amm CA. New technique for airway correction in neonates with Pierre Robin sequence. *J Pediat* 147:97, 2005.

Neuropsychosocial Aspects

Neuropsychological and Neuroimaging Aspects of Cleft Lip and Palate

Lynn C. Richman, PhD • Peg Nopoulos, MD

INTELLECTUAL ABILITY AND SCHOOL ACHIEVEMENT

Early studies suggested lower than average IQ in some groups of children with cleft; however, subsequent studies found that this finding was in part related to the inclusion of syndromic cases, as well as those with other conditions affecting IQ (e.g., seizure disorders). It was subsequently shown that the early findings of lower than average IQ were the result of uneven cognitive development with lower verbal intellectual development and higher nonverbal intellectual development in children with cleft. A review of these studies suggests that early reports were based on interview only, or on instruments which underestimated IQ due to high language load. With subse-quent control of samples using less biased instruments and excluding syndromes, most studies of children with cleft indicate average overall IQ with still some indication of slightly lower verbal IQ due to mild language deficits. This intellectual pattern has been associated with a high incidence of learning disabilities, primarily reading disabilities, memory deficits, and language disorders.

Intellectual Studies

Early Studies

Many early studies of IQ in children with cleft found lower IQ in these children than sibling controls, nonrelated controls, and the normative population.[1,2] When children with cleft were separated into those with and without other congenital anomalies, those with other congenital anomalies were found to have lower IQ than those with cleft alone.[3] Another contribution to the findings of lower overall IQ in children with cleft was related to specific verbal delay. When IQ tests were used which allowed specific verbal and nonverbal IQ scores it was found that these children were only lower on the verbal portion.[1,4]

There is increasing evidence that there may be a relationship between intellectual development and cleft type, age, sex, and specific language disorders.[5,6] Specifically, the findings indicate the possibility that there may be a cleft type by sex interaction with the least common occurrence (e.g., males with CPO) having the greater deficits in verbal intellectual skills. This is a complex interaction and further studies are needed to determine the validity of these findings. Nevertheless, there is increasing evidence that the intellectual skills of many children with cleft are within the average range with a higher frequency of mild cognitive deficits specific to language deficits or delay.[6–8] Furthermore, there is a suggestion that this language deficit in cleft may be age related with younger children showing a delay in language development, but tending to "catch up" by age 7. The relationship of verbal delay or deficit affecting intellectual and more specific cognitive skills is further examined in the subsequent section of this chapter on neuropsychological patterns.

Specific Patterns of Intelligence

There are only a few studies, which attempt to objectively examine unique patterns of the intellectual profiles of children with cleft. These studies have focused on the research already reviewed showing that there is often a lower verbal and higher nonverbal IQ in children with cleft. One study by Richman[6] demonstrated that there were two different types of language deficits in children with cleft, who had verbal intellectual deficits. This study examined cognitive patterns of 57 children with cleft, who had verbal IQs less than nonverbal. The children were identified as having verbal intellectual deficits and average or above nonverbal intellectual deficits with a standard intelligence test (Wechsler Intelligence Scale for Children). These children were then given an alternative intelligence test (Hiskey–Nebraska Test of Learning Aptitude), a test that requires no spoken language by either the examiner or child, pantomime and pictures are used. This test does, however, assess language mediation skills and short-term memory requiring manipulation of verbal labels even though it is nonvocal. One group showed average overall performance on this latter test showing that they had only expressive language deficits but not associative language deficits. The other group showed poor associative language (verbal mediation) reflecting a more global language disorder. Interestingly, this latter group comprised mostly males with cleft palate only (CPO). Also, this group of mostly males with CPO showed significantly greater school achievement problems.

Another study of the intellectual pattern of children with cleft by Richman and Eliason[7] compared 24 children with cleft lip and palate and 24 children with CPO on intellec-

tual test patterns. The groups were matched for age, sex, and IQ. A nonverbal intelligence test and other cognitive measures of associative language, memory, and visual–perceptual skills were also administered. The group with CL&P showed only verbal expression deficits, whereas the CPO group had more pervasive language deficits. These different patterns were also related to different patterns of reading deficits discussed in the next section on school achievement.

School Achievement

It has long been established that there is a higher than expected rate of educational problems for individuals with cleft. Early studies found significant educational attainment problems and subsequent studies have shown increased incidence of learning disabilities. Broder et al.[8] in a two-center comparison study found that there was a 30–40% incidence of learning disability in children with cleft. This is similar to the rate of reading disability (36%) in a large sample study of 172 children with cleft by Richman et al.[9] Learning disabilities in children with cleft have been related to verbal expressive problems and language problems.[6,8–11] There are an increasing number of studies suggesting that the learning problems manifested by children with cleft may be related to subtle neuropsychological deficits in memory, labeling, and speed of processing[12–14] which will be discussed more fully in the next section on neuropsychological patterns of children with cleft.

Although this chapter focuses on the intellectual and neurocognitive aspects of children with cleft and how this affects school achievement, there remains some controversy regarding whether school problems for these children relate more to biologic, cognitive factors or to environmental, social-emotional factors. Since this issue remains controversial, a brief review of both factors is provided. Several early studies surprisingly found visual–motor problems in samples of children with cleft[3,15] and related this to handwriting problems and written expression. However, several other careful studies of this possibility found no evidence of visual–motor deficits.[7,16] It was suggested that the visual tasks presented in some of these studies could have been contaminated by verbal mediation or naming factors more associated with language than with visual–motor skills. Similarly several early studies suggested that teacher and parent expectations may have an effect on school functioning,[17] and that teachers may underestimate the intelligence in children with more severe facial disfigurement.[18] Furthermore, both speech and facial appearance have been suggested to play a role in school underachievement.[19] In more recent studies, low self-esteem related to environmental effects of speech problems and facial differences have often been suggested as a source of low school achievement.[10,19–22] There are few studies, which examine the complex relationship of possible social-emotional aspects of speech problems and facial differences, along with cognitive variables, and how these relate to educational success.

One study by Millard and Richman[23] has attempted to examine the interacting effects of cleft type, speech, facial appearance, cognitive variables, and school success. In this study 65 children were placed in three groups CPO, CL&P

unilateral, and CL&P bilateral. Then speech, facial appearance, intellectual skills, and school achievement were examined. The CPO group showed more signs of anxiety and depression and school learning problems than the other groups. However, while this may suggest that the anxiety and depression could be causing school problems, it is important to note that this and several other studies have shown that children with CPO may also have more cognitive deficits suggesting more of a biologic basis for school learning problems, which might in turn create emotional problems. Furthermore, there was a relationship between facial appearance and school success in the CL&P groups. These findings show that the cognitive and emotional aspects of clefting are complex. It is most likely there are both biologic and environmental factors and their interactions, which point out the importance of objectively separating biologic and environmental factors. One recent development in the cleft literature has been the inclusion of neuroimaging studies, which should help to clarify some of the neurocognitive findings. These are discussed in the section on Neuroimaging.

NEUROPSYCHOLOGICAL ASPECTS OF CHILDREN WITH CLEFT

Neuropsychological studies of children with cleft indicate problems with expressive and associative language factors and delay in early verbal labeling skills. Children with cleft have been shown to have verbal labeling deficits similar to noncleft children with Dysnomia (word labeling problems), verbal fluency difficulties similar to noncleft children with Dysphasia (verbal expressive deficit) and lack of efficient verbal recall or short-term memory deficits. Children with cleft have also been shown to have neuropsychological and reading patterns similar to noncleft children with Developmental Dyslexia. Developmental Dyslexia is defined as a reading disability thought to be of neurological origin. All of these patterns indicate that clefting may be associated with atypical neuromaturation patterns. The documentation of specific neuropsychological patterns in children with cleft provides direction for studies related to direct brain measures through neuroimaging.

Language Development and Disorders in Cleft

Studies showing a significant lower verbal–higher nonverbal IQ have been reviewed earlier. These studies were the first to lead toward a language-based model for understanding the cognitive and learning deficits for children with cleft. Several previous studies[6,7] have indicated that there are at least two types of language disorders in children with cleft: (1) specific verbal expressive deficit without deficits in receptive language or verbal comprehensions and (2) general language disorder with deficits in both receptive and expressive language. The milder expressive language deficit was related more to children with CLP while the more severe general language deficit was associated more with children with CPO. The expressive language deficit has been associated with auditory memory and rapid labeling deficits[6,7]; whereas, the more general language deficit was related to more global verbal mediation deficits. These two language subtypes have also been directly related to specific reading patterns with the expressive type showing milder phonetic reading deficits and the general language type showing more severe global reading deficits in both word recognition and comprehension. Further discussion of these reading patterns is in the later section on Dyslexia.

One study by Eliason and Richman[24] has examined how early memory mediated verbal labeling may be delayed in children with cleft. This study examined 65 children with cleft (CPO & CL&P) at ages 4, 5, and 6. Children were excluded if there was mental retardation, unintelligible speech, significant hearing loss, neurological disorder, or syndrome. No cleft type or sex differences were found in vocabulary or verbal analogies. However, compared to norms, the children with cleft were deficient on tests which required the child to actively apply a verbal label to a visual stimulus in order to remember it. These findings indicate that while in noncleft children this verbal mediation skill (applying a verbal label to a visual stimulus) develops between ages 5 and 6, this skill does not develop for many children with cleft until approximately 1 year later. The authors suggest that this delay may be related to a delay of early organizational strategies or problem solving often associated with disruption of corpus collosum or prefrontal cortex. Whether these suggestions will be validated by neuroimaging studies remains to be seen.

Studies of language subtypes of children with cleft provide models of language-specific functions, which can then be associated with specific neurological locations and functions. In a series of studies,[6,7,9,12–14] Richman and colleagues developed a model of different language-specific functions of children with cleft. This model is based on subcomponents of language including auditory memory, expressive language, and associative language and differentiates these functions by cleft type. The studies will be summarized here. The overall findings indicate that children in both CPO and CL&P groups show some auditory memory deficits. However, the memory deficits of children with CL&P are sometimes so mild they do not show up in standard testing of auditory memory. In fact the problem appears to be primarily manifested when the child is asked to view a visual stimulus, which has a well-known verbal label (e.g., color, clock) and then remember a series of these visual stimuli and provide the verbal labels for them. This is a problem in rapid and efficient verbal labeling and is referred to as Dysnomia (verbal labeling deficit). Dysnomia is usually associated with dysfunction of the left prefrontal area of the brain. This area is referred to as Broca's area as in Broca's aphasia seen in adults, who sustain injury to this area, and have difficulty with word finding and labeling common objects. The more severe auditory memory deficit of children with CPO may be related to a more fundamental problem of associative language. Both groups, CPO and CL&P, show expressive language problems. This is a problem of word fluency and rapid naming. This problem is often referred to as expressive dysphasia in children. This problem is often associated with dysfunction of prefrontal motor strip, which controls oral-motor output, and also to Broca's area. Associative language refers to abilities in verbal comprehension and verbal reasoning. This problem is usually associated with dysfunction of the left temporal area and in adults who sustain damage to this area; it is called Wernicki's aphasia. This is a severe problem and may account for the greater language problems for some individuals with CPO.

Etiology of Language Subtypes

The different patterns and frequencies of these different language problems in children with cleft provide information which may help to guide neuropsychological and neuroimaging studies, as well as yield hypotheses related to neuromaturation, cell migration, and genetic aspects of clefting. Interestingly, children with nonsyndromic CL&P tend to fit a model of developmental expressive language problems which improve with age. Their developmental course is similar to children with specific language delay (SLD) who have dysnomia and/or dysphasia as well as to children with developmental dyslexia. Several studies by Richman and colleagues have shown how the patterns of reading and language development for children with CL&P are similar to these later mentioned groups.[6,10,12–14] These patterns are discussed further in the next section on Dyslexia.

The patterns and frequencies of language problems for children with CPO are more variable than those with CL&P. There appears to be a bimodal distribution of language functions in children with CPO, whereas the distribution of language problems for children with CL&P appears to be more linear. This suggests different models of neuromaturation and inheritance. The bimodal distribution seen in children with CPO suggests that some have quite severe and global language deficits and others show no apparent language deficits. This suggests that there may be at least two different modes of etiology and neuromaturation for these groups. In the early literature it was shown that there is a higher occurrence of other medical anomalies for children with CPO such as cardiac anomalies, seizure disorders, and other dysmorphologies. It may be that the children with CPO, who have more severe language impairment, are more likely to have mutations or as yet undiscovered syndromes. It may be that this global language impairment is a sign of neuromaturational factors related to CPO. It is also hypothesized that the children with CPO with good language and no other cognitive deficits may be a separate, independent group. The language models developed for CL&P and CPO provide us with direct hypotheses, which warrant further neuropsychological, neuromaturation, neuroimaging, and genetic investigation.

Memory and Naming Deficits in Children with Cleft

Children with nonsyndromic cleft show a high frequency of short-term memory and naming or verbal labeling deficits. At times these deficits are subtle and it is important to know how to detect these subtle deficits because they may be related to later reading problems. In a series of studies Richman and colleagues have shown that there is a developmental delay in

memory and naming skills in children with cleft.[6–8,24] These deficits can be identified through screening as early as age 5,[7] and they have been shown to be a strong predictor of reading disability even for children without cleft.[25] In fact these same deficits have been identified as important symptoms of later developmental dyslexia by the National Institutes of Child Health and Human Development.[26] Thus, it is important for Cleft teams to be aware of these subtle deficits and their high frequency in cleft children in order to better screen for these early signs and to institute earlier treatment of these symptoms and possibly prevention of reading disability.

There are three instruments, which have been shown to be useful in screening for early signs of memory, naming, and fluency in children with cleft.[7,12–14] These include the Rapid Automatized Naming Test (RAN),[26] the Word Fluency Test,[27] and the Color Span Test.[28] The RAN requires rapid naming of common objects, colors, letters, and numbers. The first two are particularly useful for younger children. This test differentiated children with cleft who had reading disability versus those who did not.[13] The child must rapidly name five pictures of common objects (e.g., shoe, clock) that appear repeatedly on a page. This only takes a few minutes to administer. It is a good test of labeling deficits (Dysnomia). The Word Fluency test assesses expressive language and is a good test for Dysphasia, expressive type. The child must say as many words as possible in one minute for three common letter sounds. This test also was shown to be related to reading disability in children with cleft.[12,13] The Color Span Test is a short-term memory test for colors, which varies the stimulus from visual to verbal, and the response from pointing to verbal. There are three cards with eight common colors on each placed in different positions on the card. The first two trials have the examiner point to the colors and then the child points to the colors on a different card (Trial 1) or says the name of the colors (Trial 2). Trials 3 and 4 have the examiner say the names of colors and on Trial 3 the child points to the same color on a card and on trial 4 the child says the name of the color. This allows assessment of intramodal and intermodal memory deficits often associated with reading disabilities. It has been shown that children with cleft are especially delayed on trials, which require them to verbally label a visual stimulus,[24] which is a sign of dysnomia and is related to reading disability.[14] Brief screening of children with these instruments or others like them is recommended due to their relationship to the prediction of reading disability which occurs quite frequently in the cleft population.

DYSLEXIA AND ADHD IN CHILDREN WITH CLEFT

Dyslexia Studies

Children with cleft have a high rate of reading disability, which is estimated to be 30–40% in several studies.[8,9] As reviewed in numerous studies, reading problems are thought to be related to verbal expressive deficits and language disorders.[6,8–10]

Reading disorder in children with cleft has also been related to subtle short-term memory deficits and word labeling problems as reviewed in the previous section. Recently, there has been accumulating evidence that some of the symptoms shown by children with cleft, who have reading disorders, are consistent with those shown by noncleft children with developmental dyslexia. This evidence is important because it leads to the hypothesis that cleft associated with reading disability and associated symptoms may be a sign of disruption or delay in the neuromaturation process similar to that seen in developmental dyslexia. This hypothesis by Nopoulos and colleagues suggests cell migration disruption in cleft. These studies will be described in the next section on Neuroimaging.

There are three important studies, which examine the reading symptoms of children with cleft which suggest some commonality to developmental dyslexia.[7,12,14] In the first study[7] Richman and colleagues examined reading disability symptoms by cleft type of 48 children with known language disorder identified by a lower verbal than nonverbal IQ but with overall IQ within the average range. This study controlled for connected speech ratings, which were not related to reading. The CPO group showed reading patterns of low word recognition, low reading comprehension, and many more sight word errors in reading. This pattern is similar to that seen in noncleft children with Dyslexia related to a receptive and expressive language deficit. This type of Dyslexia is thought to be related to disruption of both posterior and anterior left hemisphere function (e.g., left angular gyrus, temporal and frontal functions). The group with CL&P had a reading pattern marked by low word recognition level, only mild reading comprehension delay, and many more phonetic than sight word errors in reading. This reading pattern is similar to children with developmental dyslexia who have a primary difficulty with expressive language problem and memory deficits. This pattern is thought to be related to disruption or delay in development of left anterior prefrontal brain functions usually referred to as Broca's area. These different constellations of reading disability symptoms by cleft type are remarkably similar to that seen in two types of dyslexia.

A second study of dyslexic symptoms in children with cleft[12] examined three models of dyslexia in 92 children with nonsyndromic CL&P. This study did not include children with CPO since it was felt that the symptoms of CL&P groups more often fit common models of dyslexia than those children with CPO. The three models of dyslexia examined were: (1) Phonological awareness deficit model—difficulty blending individual letters or phonemes into words. The etiology of this type is a deficit in rapid auditory sequencing which does not allow the child to crack the code of words and be aware of individual sounds.[29] (2) Dysphasia (expressive type)—difficulty in fluent verbal expressive ability. The etiology of this type is a slowing of verbal expression due to neuromaturational deficits in motor planning and production causing a loss in word reading rate.[30] (3) The third type is the dysnomia model—a deficit in verbal label retrieval. This problem is related to a deficient short-term memory and the child cannot recall word labels in reading.[31] Tests of each

of these models were administered to 46 children with cleft, who had reading disability and 46 children with cleft, who had normal reading and were matched by age, sex, and grade. The findings indicated that the children with reading disability did not show symptoms consistent with the phonological awareness deficit model. However, the findings strongly support both the dysphasia model of dyslexia suggesting possible deficits in prefrontal and frontal brain areas related to motor planning and production as well as the dysnomia model suggesting deficits in Broca's area. These findings point out the importance of separating CL&P from CPO in studies of cognitive development and neuromaturation, and suggest the need for further research related to neuropsychological and neuroimaging studies of children with cleft on specific brain-based hypotheses.

A third study of dyslexia patterns in children with cleft[14] examined subcomponents of memory deficits. It is well documented that children with cleft often show short-term memory deficits and reading disability related to problems in slowed verbal expression (dysphasia) and retrieving verbal labels (dysnomia). However, it is also known that there are different neurological pathways related to different types of short-term memory problems. Baddeley[32] has mapped these pathways. He relates short-term auditory memory to left prefrontal brain pathways (Broca's area) and short-term visual memory to right prefrontal and parietal brain pathways. Since memory may be coded through either pathway, it is important to determine the type of short-term memory deficit in children with cleft, who have reading disabilities. In order to examine the memory deficits in children with cleft we examined[14] 48 consecutive children with cleft (CL&P and CPO) for visual and auditory memory skills and reading. All children had average intelligence. The findings indicated that for this group there were clear memory deficits for material presented visually (colors) than when the same colors were presented verbally. Children were then classified according to whether they showed deficits on the visually presented memory test ($n = 28$) or did not show such memory deficits ($n = 20$). The percentage of children with reading disability in each group was then examined. For those children with a memory deficit 61% showed a reading disability, and for those without a memory deficit only 30% showed a reading disability. The relationship of this memory deficit to reading was $r = .48$, $p < .01$. These results indicate that the memory skills of children with cleft were most deficient when they were required to spontaneously apply a verbal label to a visual stimulus. This finding is consistent with a dysnomia or inefficient verbal labeling often associated with deficient function of left prefrontal and frontal brain regions. This deficit was also related to reading disability consistent with the dysnomia model of developmental dyslexia. It has been shown in noncleft children that when this problem is recognized and remediation occurs with a reading teacher or speech clinician in applying verbal labels to visual stimuli, improvement in this memory capacity may be seen.[33] Also this finding suggests the need to avoid sight word approaches in reading and focus on auditory-based phonetic strategies.

Attention Deficit Study

Although there have been anecdotal reports of attention problems in children with cleft and a few reports of increased externalizing behavior in preschool[34,35] and school age children,[36] there is only one study directly examining attention deficit hyperactivity disorders (ADHD) in children with cleft.[13] This latter study examined 177 consecutive cases of children with nonsyndromic CL&P seen at a University-based Cleft Palate Center. There were 32 children from this sample, who had been diagnosed ADHD and were on medication for this. There were 18% of this group with cleft diagnosed with ADHD compared to 6%, the rate expected in the population at large. All children received comprehensive neuropsychological assessment as part of this study. The results indicate that only 10 of the 32 children (31%) previously diagnosed with ADHD actually had ADHD based on the more objective assessment. Most of the children actually had undiagnosed learning disorder rather than ADHD. The results suggest that many children with cleft may be misdiagnosed with ADHD when in fact they may have learning disorders that are not diagnosed. Most of the children misdiagnosed with ADHD showed memory deficits and dysnomia (word labeling problems) which are reviewed in the previous section.

These neuropsychological studies have helped to classify children with cleft according to different cleft types, different language types, and different reading disability categories. These categories have led to models of brain function and structure. These models in turn generate hypotheses of neuromaturation and function which can be verified via combined neuropsychological and neuroimaging studies. The next section reviews the neuroimaging studies on cleft.

NEUROIMAGING STUDIES

As outlined above, it has been known for decades that subjects with oral clefts have significant cognitive deficits. In syndromic clefting, the cognitive deficit is ubiquitous and severe with many patients suffering from mental retardation.[37] In isolated or nonsyndromic cleft lip/palate (CL&P), the cognitive deficit is less severe, but the impact on the lives of these patients should not be underestimated. What is the etiology of the cognitive deficits of individuals with oral clefting? Until recently, most hypotheses were focused on secondary factors such as hearing and/or speech deficits or even to the social effects of facial disfigurement.[38,39] More recently, it has been proposed that the cognitive dysfunction associated with oral clefting may be a primary manifestation of abnormal brain development.[40] First, some evidence to refute the hypothesis that the language deficits in subjects with cleft are secondary to hearing deficit is that although many studies have suggested that hearing deficit during childhood can have a substantial impact in language development, recent studies indicate that these deficits are transient with no long-term impact on language function.[41–43] Second, the study of embryology fully supports the notion that the face and the brain

grow together,[44,45] a phenomenon well-known enough that dysmorphologists have coined the phrase "the face reflects the brain." Therefore, since oral clefts are the result of abnormal development, it follows that there may well also be abnormal brain development.

This hypothesis—that the cognitive dysfunction in oral clefting is due to abnormal brain development—has driven our work in the neuroimaging of clefting. The field of neuroscience, and in particular, the study of the neurobiology of cognition and behavior, has been revolutionized in the past two decades by research techniques such as Magnetic Resonance Imaging (MRI) and Positron Emission Tomography (PET). Despite these advances, the systematic study of brain structure and function in oral clefting has been virtually absent until recent years. In the remainder of the chapter, a series of neuroimaging studies conducted at the University of Iowa in subjects with oral clefts will be reviewed (the only neuroimaging studies to date on subjects with oral clefts).

Evaluation of Brain Structure

The first series of studies were performed on a sample of adult males with CL&P.[40] Adult males were chosen to keep the study group homogenous and thereby eliminating the confound of development (age) and sex on brain structure. A total of 46 males, average age of 30 years old, were matched by gender and age to normal healthy controls recruited from the community. All subjects underwent an MRI scan and using state-of-the-art processing methods, quantitative measures of brain structure were obtained. The results showed that there was no difference in overall total brain size or cerebrum size compared to controls, however the volume of the cerebellum was substantially reduced in subjects with CL&P. Moreover, even though the total cerebral size was not different from controls, there was a substantial abnormality in the distribution of brain tissue types (gray matter and white matter). Specifically, the anterior portions of the cerebrum (frontal and parietal lobe) were abnormally *enlarged* compared to controls while the lateral and posterior regions of the cerebrum (temporal and occipital lobes) were substantially *reduced* in volume compared to controls (Fig. 64–1). Within the anterior cerebrum, gray matter or cortex volume accounted for the enlargement as white matter volume in the anterior cerebrum was not different in the two groups. In the temporal lobe (the most severely affected region), both white matter and gray matter were reduced in volume and the occipital lobe had normal volumes of gray matter, but reduced volume of white matter compared to controls.

Although no other studies have evaluated brain structure in CL&P, two studies have reported on brain structure in Velo-cardio-facial syndrome,[46,47] a genetic syndrome manifested by heart defects, cognitive impairment, and craniofacial abnormalities including cleft palate. Both these studies found a similar pattern of brain morphometry in which the frontal lobe or anterior portions of the cerebrum were proportionately *enlarged*.

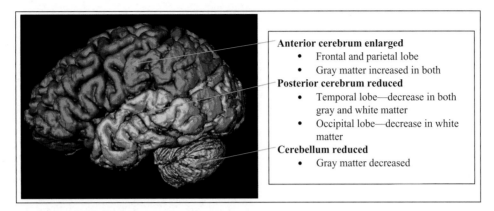

Anterior cerebrum enlarged
- Frontal and parietal lobe
- Gray matter increased in both

Posterior cerebrum reduced
- Temporal lobe—decrease in both gray and white matter
- Occipital lobe—decrease in white matter

Cerebellum reduced
- Gray matter decreased

Figure 64–1. An image of an MRI brain scan illustrating the abnormalities of regional brain volume in adult males with clefts of the lip and/or palate.

Are these structural abnormalities in subjects with CL&P related to their cognitive dysfunction? The finding of enlargement of the cortex in the anterior portion of the cerebrum was unexpected. One possibility is that this enlargement is not a primary abnormality, but an overgrowth, or compensation process. There is evidence to support the relationship between cerebral volume and cognitive function.[48] However, there is also evidence to suggest that larger than average cortical volume is actually "pathologic" and is associated with decreased cognitive function. This finding has been reported in both autism[49,50] and neurofibromatosis.[51,52] This pattern was also true for the CL&P subjects in that there was a significant *inverse* correlation between Full Scale IQ (FSIQ) and the volume of the anterior cerebrum—the larger the anterior cerebrum, the lower the IQ. Further the relationship for the posterior cerebrum was reversed with a significant positive correlation between volume and IQ, indicating that the smaller this region, the lower the FSIQ. These correlations were significant for FSIQ as well as for Verbal (IQ), but were nonsignificant for Performance IQ (PIQ—non-language based skills).

The finding of abnormal brain structure in subjects with CL&P, and the direct relationship between these abnormalities and cognitive function lend support to the notion that the etiology of the cognitive deficits in CL&P is indeed a primary problem with brain structure and function. A common concern about abnormal brain structure discovered in an adult population is that these abnormalities could potentially represent differential environmental factors between the groups, shaping brain morphology over time. There are indeed reports that show adverse childhood environments, such as abuse, result in smaller volumes of the cerebrum.[53] This is felt to be mediated by stress hormones. However, this report is far from supporting the theory that the abnormal brain changes in CL&P are due to environmental factors. First, these studies evaluated children who have endured extreme stress due to abuse, a situation much different than children with CL&P. Second, there are no studies to support environmental influences contributing to enlargement of the cortex, part of the pattern seen in CL&P. Third, although extreme environments may influence brain structure at some level, genetic/biologic factors determine the vast majority of gross cerebral structure (volume) as determined by previous studies.[54–56] Fourth, the sample of CL&P subjects described above were also qualitatively evaluated for the presence of brain anomalies. The subjects were found to have an increased incidence of a brain anomaly, an enlarged cavum septi pellucidi (CSP).[57] This anomaly is known to occur due to abnormal brain development, further supporting the idea that the structural abnormalities of the CL&P subject are developmental in nature.

Structure–Function Relationships

Social Function

Social inhibition or shyness has been demonstrated in high frequency in individuals with CL&P[58] along with fewer friends than noncleft controls.[59,60] Like cognitive dysfunction, this too has been attributed to secondary factors such as the development of poor self-concept as a psychological consequence of having a facial deformity. Yet, the literature on self-concept in CL&P has several studies that show normal or higher than normal levels of self-concept in subjects with CL&P relative to controls,[61–64] indicating the need for an alternative hypothesis.

A large body of literature has implicated the ventral portion of the frontal cortex as a critical region in the governance of social behavior in humans. This evidence comes from a long history of case studies as well as more recent neuroimaging studies.[65] Therefore, an alternative hypothesis to the etiology of social dysfunction in subjects with CL&P was posed, suggesting that the ventral frontal cortex is structurally abnormal and this manifested in the social dysfunction.[66] Using the same group of 46 adult males with CL&P and matched controls, the ventral frontal cortex was measured, subdivided into the orbitofrontal cortex and the straight gyrus. As discussed above, the volume of the total frontal lobe in the males with CL&P in this sample was enlarged compared to controls, therefore the subregions were measured as a proportion (volume of the region of interest divided by the volume of the frontal lobe). The findings showed that despite the overall enlargement of frontal cortex in males with CL&P, the orbitofrontal cortex was proportionately reduced in volume compared to controls. Further, the patients were measured on a scale of social dysfunction and these ratings were directly correlated with the morphology of the orbitofrontal cortex—the greater the social dysfunction, the greater the reduction in volume of this brain region. Once again, these findings support the notion that the social deficit seen in subjects with CL&P may not be due to secondary factors such as poor self-concept, but instead be due to a primary problem in brain structure due to abnormal development.

Functional Imaging

Positron Emission Tomography (PET) is a neuroimaging technique in which the activity of the brain can be visualized while it is engaged in a task. A radioactive label (e.g., O^{13} Water) is injected into the subject and they are instructed to engage in a cognitive task while the brain is then scanned. The labeled water appears as areas of increased or decreased blood flow (compared to a rest or baseline condition), a proxy to increased brain metabolism or activity. In order to better understand the functional neurocircuitry of speech and language function in subjects, we performed a PET scan on subjects while they were engaged in a series of language tasks with increasing complexity (reading a list of words, reading a list of sentences, reading a paragraph of a story). This study was done on a small subset ($n = 8$) of the males with CL&P described above and compared to a separate group of healthy male controls. During each of the reading conditions, CL&P subjects compared to healthy controls showed *increased* blood flow in areas previously reported to be involved in language processing and reading (inferior frontal lobe, cerebellum, and occipital lobe). This was not accounted for by increased volume of cortex as was reported above, as both the cerebellum and occipital lobe did NOT have enlarged cortex in the larger study. The increased blood flow suggests a possible neural inefficiency. In contrast, when analyzing the brain regions involved in more complex language functioning, control subjects showed an increase in blood flow in a distributed neural circuit whereas the subjects with CL&P had a decrease in flow in these regions (Fig. 64–2). Additionally, the subjects with CL&P had activation of several regions *not* activated by the healthy controls, suggesting a compensatory circuit used for this more complex reading task. These findings indicate that the function of the traditional circuits for speech and language are abnormal in subjects with the CL&P. In addition, subjects with CL&P are recruiting and using alternate neurocircuitry for these tasks that are not used by controls.

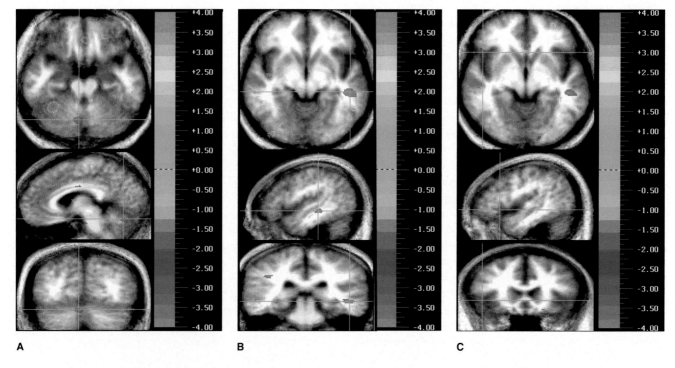

Figure 64–2. Three orthogonal views are shown, with transaxial at the top, sagittal in the middle, and coronal on the bottom. Green crosshairs are used to show the location of the slice. The statistical maps of the PET data, showing regions where the two groups differed significantly at a 0.005 level, are superimposed on a composite MR image. Regions in red/yellow tones indicate higher blood flow while regions in blue indicate lower blood flow. The "peak map" each image shows the small areas where all contiguous voxels exceed the predefined threshold for statistical significance. Selected brain regions showing clefting subjects having lower blood flow than controls in the complex language comparison. (**A**) Region in right cerebellum, (**B**) region in left temporal lobe, and (**C**) region right frontal lobe.

Brain Structure in Subjects with Van der Woude Syndrome

Van der Woude syndrome (VWS) is an autosomal dominant disorder manifested in cleft lip and/or palate and lip pits and is caused by mutations in the Interferon Regulatory Factor 6 (IRF) gene. In 12% of VWS cases, there is cleft lip/palate with no lip pits and these cases are phenotypically identical to subjects with CL&P. In addition, a recent report showed that DNA sequence variation in IRF6 confers risk for isolated cases of cleft lip and palate. Due to the substantial phenotype and genotype overlap between VWS and CL&P, it was hypothesized that subjects with VWS would have the same pattern of brain abnormalities as subjects with CL&P. The sample included 14 adult subjects with VWS (7 males and 7 females) compared to 14 age and sex matched healthy controls. Results indicate that the subjects with VWS show the same pattern of brain abnormalities as subjects with CL&P—enlarged cortical volume of the anterior cerebrum and reduced volume of the posterior cerebrum.[67] An important caveat is that the males had more severe abnormalities than the females, a phenomenon well documented in disorders that have their etiology in abnormal brain development.

Current Studies and Future Direction

We are currently in the process of a study of children, ages 7–18 with CL&P in order to further our study of the neurobiology of subjects with CL&P. Preliminary findings indicate that children with CL&P (average age 12 years), matched by age and gender to healthy normal controls are significantly smaller in stature (height), a fact reported by others, but seldom highlighted.[68] However, even after controlling for height, children with CL&P have substantially smaller total brain volumes compared to controls. Although both the cerebrum and the cerebellum are decreased, it is the reduction of the volume of the cerebellum that is most robust. In regard to distribution of tissue, boys, but not girls, with CL&P show proportionally larger volumes of gray matter, however in contrast to the adults where this increase in cortical volume is localized to the anterior regions, in the children, it is more evenly distributed, but particularly enlarged in the posterior cerebral regions.

Development of the human brain is a very long process with substantial changes in brain structure occurring during the adolescent years. Specifically, these changes are not in overall cerebral volume, but distribution of gray and white matter throughout the cerebrum with specific trajectories of volume changes throughout childhood and adolescence. These processes of change occur normally through the second decade of life. Therefore, the abnormalities that are seen in brain structure in children with CL&P are of a somewhat different pattern than that seen in adults, most likely due to the fact that there is a substantial period of brain development yet to happen. More importantly, it suggests that there is an abnormal developmental trajectory for not only brain size and brain tissue distribution, but for overall body growth (stature) in subjects with CL&P. Future studies will focus on evaluation growth and development of body and brain in subjects with CL&P from childhood through adulthood.

References

1. Estes R, Morris H. Relationship among intelligence, speech proficiency, and learning sensitivity in children with cleft palate. *Cleft Palate J* 7:763–773, 1970.
2. Lewis R. A survey of the intelligence of cleft palate children in Ontario. *Cleft Palate Bull* 11:83–85, 1961.
3. McWilliams BJ, Matthews H. A comparison of intelligence and social maturity in children with unilateral complete clefts and those with isolated cleft palates. *Cleft Palate J* 16:363–372, 1979.
4. Ruess A. A comparative study of cleft palate children and their siblings. *J Clin Psych* 21:354–360, 1965.
5. Lamb M, Wilson F, Leeper H. The intellectual function of cleft palate children compared on the basis of cleft type and sex. *Cleft Palate J* 10:367–377, 1973.
6. Richman LC. Cognitive patterns and learning disabilities in cleft palate children with verbal deficits. *J Speech Hear Res* 23:447–456, 1980.
7. Richman L, Eliason M. Type of reading disability related to cleft type and neuropsychological patterns. *Cleft Palate J* 21:1–6, 1984.
8. Broder H, Richman L, Matheson P. Learning disability, school achievement and grade retention among children with cleft: A two-center study. *Cleft Palate Craniofac J* 31:429–435, 1998.
9. Richman LC, Eliason M, Lindgren S. Reading disability in children with cleft lip and palate. *Cleft Palate J* 25:2125, 1988.
10. Kapp-Simon K. Self concept of primary school age children with cleft lip, cleft palate or both. *Cleft Palate J* 23:24–27, 1986.
11. Millard T, Richman L. Different cleft conditions, facial appearance and speech: Relationship to psychological variables. *Cleft Palate Craniofac J* 38:68–75, 2001.
12. Richman L, Ryan S. Do the reading disability of children with cleft fit into current models of developmental dyslexia? *Cleft Palate Craniofac J* 40:154–157, 2003.
13. Richman LC, Ryan S, Wilgenbusch T, et al. Overdiagnosis and medication for attention-deficit hyperactivity disorder in children with cleft: Diagnostic examination and follow-up. *Cleft Palate Craniofac J* 41:351–354, 2004.
14. Richman LC, Wilgenbusch T, Hall T. Spontaneous verbal labeling: Visual memory and reading ability in children with cleft. *Cleft Palate Craniofac J* 42:565–569, 2005.
15. Brennan D, Cullinan W. Object identification and naming in cleft palate children. *Cleft Palate J* 111:188–195, 1974.
16. Lamb M, Wilson F, Leeper H. The intellectual function of cleft palate children compared on the basis of cleft type and sex. *Cleft Palate J* 10:367–377, 1973.
17. Richman LC. Differing views of behavior of cleft palate children. *Cleft Palate J* 15:360–364, 1978.
18. Richman LC. The effects of facial disfigurement on teachers' perception of ability in cleft palate children. *Cleft Palate J* 15:155–160, 1978.
19. Richman LC. Self-reported social speech and facial concerns and personality adjustment of cleft lip and palate adolescents. *Cleft Palate J* 108–112, 1983.
20. Broder H, Strauss RP. Self-concept of early primary school children with visible and invisible defects. *Cleft Palate J* 6:114–117, 1989.
21. Broder H, Strauss RP. Effects of visible and nonvisible oral-facial defects on self-perception and adjustment across developmental eras and gender. *Cleft Palate J* 31:429–435, 1994.
22. Kapp-Simon K, Simon DJ, Kristovich S. Self-perception, social skills adjustment and inhibition in young children with craniofacial anomalies. *Cleft Palate Craniofac J* 29:352–356, 1992.
23. Millard T, Richman LC. Different cleft conditions, facial appearance and speech: Relationship to psychological variables. *Cleft Palate Craniofac J* 38:68–75, 2001.

24. Eliason M, Richman L. Language in preschoolers with cleft. *Dev Neuropsychol* 6:173–182, 1990.

25. Denkla M, Rudel R. Rapid automatized naming (RAN): Dyslexia differential from other learning disabilities. *Neuropsychologia* 14:471–479, 1976.

26. Lyon RG. *The NICHD Research Program in Reading Development, Reading Disorders and Reading Instruction.* Bethesda, MD: National Center for Learning Disabilities, Inc., 1999.

27. Benton AL, Hamsher K, Sivan AB. *Multilingual Aphasia Examination*, 3rd edn. Department of Neurology: University of Iowa, Iowa City, IA, 1994.

28. Richman LC, Lindgren SD. *Color Span Test.* Department of Pediatrics: University of Iowa, Iowa City, IA, 1988.

29. Tallal P. Temporal or phonetic processing deficit in dyslexia? *Appl Psycholinguist* 5:167–169, 1984.

30. Adams MJ. *Beginning to Read: Thinking and Learning about Print.* Cambridge, MA: MIT Press, 1996.

31. Vellutino FR, Scanlon DM, Tanzman MS. Components of reading ability. In Lyons GR (ed). *Frames of Reference for the Assessment of Learning Disabilities.* Baltimore, MD: Paul H. Brookes Pub, 1994, p. 279.

32. Baddeley AD. *Working Memory.* New York: Oxford University Press, 1986.

33. Brady HV, Richman LC. Visual versus verbal mnemonic training effects on memory-deficient subgroups of children with reading disability. *Dev Neuropsychol* 10:335–347, 1994.

34. Tobiasen JM, Hiebert JM. Parent's tolerance for conduct problems of the child with cleft lip and palate. *Cleft Palate J* 21:82–85, 1984.

35. Speltz ML, Morton K, Goodell EW, et al. Psychological functioning of children with craniofacial anomalies and their mothers. *Cleft Palate Craniofac J* 30:482–489, 1993.

36. Endriga MC, Kapp-Simon KA. Psychological issues in craniofacial care: State of the art. *Cleft Palate Craniofac J* 36:3–11, 1999.

37. Gorlin RJ, Cohen MM, Levin LS. *Syndromes of the Head and Neck*, 3rd edn. New York: Oxford Press, 1990.

38. Estes R, Morris H. Relationship among intelligence, speech proficiency, and hearing sensitivity in children with cleft palates. *Cleft Palate J* 7:763–773, 1970.

39. Sak RJ, Ruben RJ. Effects of recurrent middle ear effusion in preschool years on language and learning. *J Dev Behav Pediatr* 3:7–11, 1982.

40. Nopoulos P, Berg S, Canady J, et al. Structural brain abnormalities in adult males with clefts of the lip and/or palate. *Genet Med* 4:1–9, 2002.

41. Jocelyn L, Penko M, Rode H, et al. Cognition, communication, and hearing in young children with cleft lip and palate and in control children: A longitudinal study. *Pediatrics* 97:529, 1996.

42. Hubbard,TW, Paradise JL, McWilliams BJ, et al. Consequences of unremitting middle ear disease in early life. Otologic, audiologic, and developmental findings in children with cleft palate. *N Engl J Med* 3312:1529–1534, 1985.

43. Rovers MM, Straatman H, Ingels K, et al. The effect of ventilation tubes on language development in infants with otitis media with effusion: A randomized trial. *Pediatrics* 106:E42, 2000.

44. Sperber G. First year of life: Prenatal craniofacial development. *Cleft Palate Craniofac J* 29:109–111, 1992.

45. Kjaer I. Human prenatal craniofacial development related to brain development under normal and pathologic conditions (Review). *Acta Odontol Scand* 53:135–143, 1995.

46. Eliez S, Schmitt E, White C. Children and adolescents with Velocardiofacial Syndrome: A volumetric MRI study. *Am J Psychiatry* 157:409–415, 2000.

47. Kates WR, Burnett CP, Jabs EW, et al. Regional cortical white matter reductions in velocardiofacial syndrome: A volumetric MRI analysis. *Biol Psychiatry* 49:677–684, 2001.

48. Andreasen N, Flaum M, Swayze V. Intelligence and brain structure in normal individuals. *Am J Psychiatry* 150:130–134, 1993.

49. Piven J, Arndt S, Bailey S. An MRI study of brain size in autism. *Am J Psychiatry* 152:1145–1149, 1995.

50. Piven J, Arndt S, Bailey J. Regional brain enlargement in autism: An MRI study. *J Am Acad Child Adolesc Psychiatry* 35:530–536, 1996.

51. Said SM, Yeh TL, Greenwood RS. MRI morphometric analysis and neuropsychological function in patients with neurofibromatosis. *Neuroreport* 7:1941–1944, 1996.

52. Moore BD, Slopis JM, Jackson EF, et al. Brain volume in children with neurofibromatosis type 1: Relation to neuropsychological status. *Neurology* 54:914–920, 2000.

53. De Bellis MD, Keshavan MS, Clark DB, et al. A.E. Bennett Research Award. Developmental traumatology. Part II: Brain development. *Biol Psychiatry* 45:1271–1284, 1999.

54. Bartley AJ, Jones DW, Weinberger DR. Genetic variability of human brain size and cortical gyral patterns. *Brain* 120(Pt 2):257–269, 1997.

55. Pfefferbaum A, Sullivan EV, Swan GE, et al. Brain structure in men remains highly heritable in the seventh and eighth decades of life. *Neurobiol Aging* 21(1):63–74, 2000.

56. White T, Andreasen NC, Nopoulos P. Brain volumes and surface morphology in monozygotic twins. *Cereb Cortex* 2(5):486–493, 2002.

57. Nopoulos PS, Berg J, Canady J, et al. Increased incidence of a midline brain anomaly in adult males with nonsyndromic clefts of the lip and/or palate. *J Neuroimaging* 11:1–7, 2001.

58. Endriga MC, Kapp-Simon KA. Psychological issues in craniofacial care: State of the art. *Cleft Palate Craniofac J* 36(1):3–11, 1999.

59. Bressmann TR, Sader R, Ravens-Sieberer U, et al. Quality of life research in patients with cleft lip and palate: Preliminary results. *Mund Kiefer Gesichtschir* 3(3):134–139, 1999.

60. Noar JH. Questionnaire survey of attitudes and concerns of patients with cleft lip and palate and their parents. *Cleft Palate Craniofac J* 28(3):279–284, 1991.

61. Brantley H, Clifford E. Cognitive, self-concept, and body image measures of normal, cleft, and obese adolescents. *Cleft Palate J* 16:177–182, 1979.

62. Kapp K. Self-concept of the cleft lip and/or palate child. *Cleft Palate J* 16:171–176, 1979.

63. Leonard BJ, Brust HD, Abrahams G, et al. Self-concept of children and adolescents with cleft lip and/or palate. *Cleft Palate Craniofac J* 28:347–353, 1991.

64. Persson M, Aniansson G, Becker M, et al. Self-concept and introversion in adolescents with cleft lip and palate. *Scand J Plast Reconstr Surg Hand Surg* 36(1):24–27, 2002.

65. Adolphs R. The neurobiology of social cognition. *Curr Opin Neurobiol* 11(2):231–239, 2001.

66. Nopoulos P, Choe I, Berg S, et al. Ventral frontal cortex morphology in adult males with isolated orofacial clefts: Relationship to abnormalities in social function. *Cleft Palate Craniofac J* 42(2):138–144, 2005.

67. Nopoulos P, Richman L, Andreasen N. Brain structure and function in adults with Van der Woude syndrome. *Genes Brain Behav* (submitted).

68. Cunningham ML, Jerome JT. Linear growth characteristics of children with cleft lip and palate. *J Pediatr* 131(5):707–711, 1997.

Psychological and Behavioral Aspects of Clefting

Kathleen A. Kapp-Simon, PhD • Rebecca Gaither, PhD

Diagnosis of an orofacial cleft (OFC) sets in motion a variety of parental reactions that have significant consequences for the long-term emotional development of the child. Whether diagnosis occurs prenatally or at birth, the experience of becoming a parent is altered. Parents experience strong emotions, and there is a need for family reorganization and planning. Parents have an immediate need to learn about their child's diagnosis and the treatment that the child will require. In the midst of these stressful activities and emotions, parents must come to know and love their child. Most families cope well, despite the sometimes overwhelming feelings of anxiety and stress, and are ultimately successful in providing a healthy emotional environment for the child. This chapter will examine the psychological and medical factors that

ultimately influence both immediate and long-term adjustment for the child and family.

The chapter will be presented in two major sections: The initial section will provide a framework for thinking about psychological issues in OFC. Drawing from pediatric psychology literature, a multifactorial model will be described which identifies factors associated with risks for poor outcomes while also defining factors that have the potential to foster resiliency and thus serve as a counter to poor outcomes. The second section of this chapter will summarize what is known about risk and resistance factors within each developmental period in the life of an individual with OFC. Drawing on the extant scientific literature, this section will examine factors that hinder or promote adjustment during infancy/

preschool years, elementary school years, adolescence, and adulthood.

A MODEL OF RISK, RESILIENCE, AND ADAPTATION

Risk

Although it is not always conceptualized as such, cleft lip and palate (CLP) fits into a model of chronic childhood illness.[1] Children with CLP have a condition that can be treated but not cured or removed. They experience intermittent periods of intense medical care but also have extended periods of quiescence when no direct CLP-related treatment occurs. During these periods of quiescence, children may still need to manage secondary issues related to CLP, such as residual speech problems and facial scarring. They also have to be prepared to cope with required therapies, the inconvenience of extra medical appointments, and the likelihood of additional hospitalizations and operations during childhood and adolescence.

Wallander and Varni[2] proposed a model for studying chronic medical conditions and physical disabilities that used a paradigm of "risk, resistance, and coping." This model has been applied previously to CLP[3] and will be summarized briefly here.

Several categories of risk directly affect children with CLP. These include: (1) medical risks associated with having a birth defect, (2) the potential of both functional and cognitive problems, and (3) psychological stress. The impact of these risks may vary depending on the severity of the presenting condition, the parents' subjective impression of severity,[4] the degree to which the condition responds to treatment, the age of the child, and the quality of medical care available. For example, a severe bilateral cleft lip and palate may require more intensive initial treatment to address issues of cleft closure, feeding, and appearance. However, the support from early contact with a competent cleft team, guidance with feeding, and the dramatic changes in appearance during the early months of treatment may ameliorate some of the initial stress experienced by the family, resulting in a calmer home atmosphere.[5,6] In contrast, a child with an *undetected* submucous cleft palate may be subjected to several months of feeding problems, serious bouts of otitis media, hearing loss, and speech delays, resulting in considerable parental frustration and stress. Not knowing a cause can be a tremendous source of stress for parents and can cause strain in the relationship between the family and their primary care physician. Specific risks related to the child's medical condition, functional/ cognitive limitations, and psychosocial risks are described in greater detail in following paragraphs.

Medical Risks

For most children, specific medical risks associated with OFC include feeding problems with or without failure to thrive, chronic otitis media, the need for repeated operations to close clefts of the lip and/or palate, and the secondary sequelae of these conditions, including operations to improve appearance, dental concerns, and velopharyngeal dysfunction. Infants with OFC must also be screened for conditions associated with known syndromes or genetic mutations. Some of these conditions are associated with cardiac and metabolic problems (e.g., a 22q deletion), airway problems (as in Pierre Robin sequence), and hearing loss (as with mandibulofacial dysostosis). The presence of a secondary diagnosis increases the potential number and complexity of medical conditions with which a child must cope.

Functional Risks

The most common functional impairment associated with an OFC that includes cleft palate is speech and language impairment. Infants may experience delayed acquisition of early babbling skills depending upon the timing of cleft palate repair. Toddlers and preschoolers may experience difficulties with speech intelligibility, affecting language acquisition and communication skills. Continued speech problems into school age may result in the need for specialized therapies and potentially additional surgery to address velopharyngeal dysfunction. OFC is also associated with an increased risk of developmental problems. While the risk of mental retardation is slightly increased, occurring in approximately 6% of children with reportedly nonsyndromic cleft lip and palate (CLP),[7] the risk of specific learning disabilities is considerably higher, 30–40%, in isolated CLP.[8,9] Fluctuating hearing loss secondary to chronic otitis media may affect both speech and language acquisition and cognitive and academic functioning, adding yet another functional risk.

Psychosocial Risks

There are multiple stresses specifically associated with OFC that affect both parent and child. For a young family faced with obtaining care for a newly diagnosed infant, one of the first major stresses is sorting out treatment options and deciding which one is best for them. Many factors influence this decision, including parent sophistication, insurance options, and geographic location. When a child is newly diagnosed, parents will likely turn first for guidance to the medical providers they know: family doctor, pediatrician, and perhaps obstetrician. However, they also turn to the internet, family, friends, and colleagues. From this plethora of resources, they may find an abundance of contradictory information. Even if they are lucky enough to be referred to a multidisciplinary cleft treatment team, they may find that their local team does not provide the type of treatment that they have decided is best for their child, or they may find that their insurance will not cover treatment by the team with which they would most like to work.

Even desired medical interventions may cause stress. For example, nasoalveolar molding (NAM) may provide an excellent outcome for a child with a severe cleft lip and palate; however, its successful implementation may require weekly clinic visits over a 2–3 month period at great cost to the family in terms of time off work, transportation costs, and disruption of family routines. Parents may also be required to cope with "at home" procedures such as inserting the appliance or taping it in place. While some families may perceive their participation in the placement and maintenance of the appliance positively as their contribution to their child's treatment, others may see this participation as "hurting the child," thus increasing their stress. Similarly, parents differ in how they frame their child's need for adjunct treatments such as speech therapy. For some families, participation in early intervention is a positive experience as they learn how to support and teach their child; for others it is a source of embarrassment, tension, personal pressure, and possible financial strain. Finally, operations are stressful for both parent and child. Fear of hospitalization, worries about anesthesia, and disruption of routines create tension. Changing physical appearance may also pose a challenge. Parents frequently talk about "missing" the cleft after it is repaired, even though they very much want the child's appearance normalized.

Resilience

Synonyms for resilience include flexibility, buoyancy, spirit, hardiness, and toughness. All of these terms describe characteristics required by both child and family as they face the challenges of living with OFC.

Family Issues

A family's level of pre-pregnancy adaptation, cohesion, and general emotional health will influence its ability to cope with the birth of a child with an OFC and will continue to influence the child's adaptation throughout his/her life. Parents need to work out their own emotional reactions to the child's birth individually and they need to support each other. This process can be challenging because parents will move through stages of grieving and acceptance at their own pace. One parent may be feeling very sad or depressed while the other is angrily searching for someone or something to blame. The degree to which parents are able to validate each others' experiences and coping process will influence the family's long-term adaptation and their child's mental health.

Parental competence is enhanced when parents recognize their differing strengths. One parent may be better equipped to seek out information about available medical/therapeutic treatments while the other may do better supporting the young child through surgery.[3] Parents who believe that they can meet their child's needs, that feel satisfaction in their role as parents, and that realistically acknowledge the stresses of coping with the issues of raising a child with more complex medical needs enhance the parent–child relationship in important ways.

Family adaptation is also enhanced through social support. Often this support is provided by extended family. Other parents choose to reach out to families that have had similar experiences to their own. Parent to parent support can be an invaluable resource for parents who desire that type of contact. Organizations such as the Cleft Palate Foundation, http://www.cleftline.org/, AmeriFace (formerly AboutFace USA) http://www.ameriface.org/, The Children's Craniofacial Association, http://www.ccakids.org/, and Wide Smiles, http://www.widesmiles.org/ provide access to parent information and parent to parent support.

The financial resources available to a family have a tremendous influence on the family's ability to cope with some of the stresses related to caring for a child with CLP. Insurance coverage varies according to plan parameters. Even "good" insurance plans may exclude specific aspects of medically necessary care. The "working poor" often have the greatest difficulty coping with the financial demands of treatment. They often have limited or no insurance and time off of work may mean loss of pay. Consequently, social service support that helps families identify the financial resources available to them (e.g., Title V: Maternal Child Health funding which may support OFC services through Specialized Care for Children) is a critical component of CLP Team Care.

Child Factors

Child resilience can grow out of the interaction of child temperament and parenting skill. Child temperament has a strong biological basis. It can be defined in terms of three broad categories: emotionality, or how the child responds to distress, fear, or anger; activity level, as defined by attention span, response inhibition, and/or cognitive distractibility; and sociability, i.e., the tendency to withdraw in social situations and the ability to handle social stresses.[3]

Each of these characteristics occurs on a continuum for all children. At one end of the continuum are children who have an "easy temperament," those described as having the ability to easily moderate emotions, an intense interest in their environment, and an ability to remain focused. These children are often socially engaging. At the other end of the continuum are children with a more challenging temperament. These children may react strongly to new situations, experiences, or people; they will have difficulty moderating emotions—happy one moment and in tears the next—often leaving parents and professionals confused about what triggered the strong reaction. Finally, these children may have difficulty maintaining attention and focus.

The manner in which a child interacts with peers and adults is a critical determinant of social acceptance. Certainly, environment influences a child's ability to learn to modulate emotion, to use empathy, or to problem solve; however, children differ in their innate competence when encountering social situations, in part driven by the temperamental characteristics just discussed.

APPLICATIONS OF COPING MODEL ACROSS LIFESPAN

Infancy/Preschool Years

Longitudinal Research

The interrelationship between risk, resilience, and adaptation is best examined within the context of longitudinal research. However, controlled, prospective longitudinal studies of children with CLP that assess multifactorial predictors of psychological and social adjustment beginning in infancy are rare. A review of the literature reveals four recent multifactorial studies of children with craniofacial conditions that were begun during infancy/preschool years and that followed children with cleft and/or craniofacial conditions across time. Speltz and his colleagues[6,10–14] followed a group of infants with CLP, matched to a group of infants with sagittal synostosis and a group with no medical condition at multiple time points between early infancy until about 7 years of age. Hoeksma and Koomen[15] followed a group of infants with and without CLP at 3–6 month intervals from 3 months to 18 months of age. Kruekeberg and Kapp-Simon[16–18] evaluated a group of children with mixed craniofacial conditions including CLP and a control group during preschool and again when they entered elementary school. Finally, Pope et al.[19] assessed the relationship of parenting stress in infancy and preschool to child behavior and emotional adjustment.

Drawing on developmental psychology literature, a wide variety of variables were assessed in these four studies including (1) *maternal factors* such as parenting stress, social support, marital satisfaction, maternal sensitivity, emotional health, and child rearing styles; (2) *child factors* such as cognitive and motor development, child temperament, facial attractiveness, emotion self-regulation, reaction to medical procedures, vulnerability to stress, and behavior adjustment; and (3) *interactions between child and critical individuals* such as mother–child relationship during feeding, a measure of reciprocal sensitivity called interactional harmony, maternal teaching strategies, and mother–child attachment. Child interactions with peers provide measures of social skills and child problem-solving abilities.

A major strength of these studies is their longitudinal, multi-informant, multivariate nature and their use of comparison groups. Each study also includes more than one time point for measurement. A variety of assessment strategies are used, for example: (1) self-report based on standardized instruments assessing parenting stress or child self-concept and diary-type self-report where mothers kept track of behaviors such as length of feeding and who fed the baby; (2) multiple informant objective reports of child adjustment and social skills; (3) observational studies examining in-home natural behaviors, structured activities as in the Strange Situation or structured parent-teaching activities, and analogue situations such as a play interview in which children generated responses to hypothetical situations; and (4) objective ratings of appearance and of children's ability to produce recognizable facial emotions.

Maternal Support

This series of studies provides considerable support for the role of maternal stress in long-term adjustment of children with CFA. Similar findings have been reported for children with other chronic illnesses, e.g.[20,21] It is important to recognize that most mothers of children with CLP do not report mean levels of stress that are clinically abnormal; however, there is a group of mothers for whom stress is clinically elevated. Pope et al.[19] identified approximately 23% of mothers who demonstrated clinically elevated levels which persisted from infancy to toddlerhood. Mothers were more likely to report adjustment problems for their children when mothers' levels of stress remained significantly elevated during these early years.

Measures of parenting stress were associated with a variety of outcomes even when group means were not significantly elevated in relationship to norms. When their mothers were less stressed preschool children with CFCs displayed greater social competence.[16] Longitudinal follow-up of these children continued to show a relationship between early parenting stress and child behavior and social competence. Level of maternal stress at preschool age was associated with (1) parent, teacher, and self-report of social competence and (2) parent and teacher ratings of behavioral adjustment when children were in early elementary school.[18] Mothers who reported less stress related to their parenting role were more likely to have children who were socially competent and well-adjusted than mothers who reported high levels of stress. Endriga et al.[12] also found an association between maternal reports of parenting stress assessed when children with CLP were toddlers and levels of emotional regulation when the children were 5 years of age and internalizing and externalizing behaviors at age seven. Similar to the findings of Krueckeberg and Kapp-Simon,[16] Endriga and her colleagues[12] found that mothers reporting lower stress and less depression during infancy had children who displayed better emotional regulation and fewer behavior problems when they were 5 and 7 years of age.

Speltz et al.[10] reported that increased maternal stress during infancy was associated with mothers' perception that they were not competent to parent their children. Increased parenting stress was also associated with decreased feelings of well-being, increased marital conflict, and less social support.[10] Professionals treating infants with CLP should be on the alert for those mothers whose levels of stress are greater than typical. The Parenting Stress Index/Short Form[22] is a reasonable measure to use for screening.[23] Parental confidence can be enhanced by ensuring the parents of newborns have accurate information about their child's condition, treatment options, and information regarding important aspects of early care such as feeding. Both oral and written information is valuable. The Cleft Palate Foundation, http://www.cleftline.org/, is a good source of reliable information for parents. Contact with other mothers who have successfully negotiated early stages of CLP care may be particularly beneficial to some mothers experiencing high stress during the early stages of parenting. Support networks are available through AmeriFace's Cleft Advocate network, http://www.ameriface.org, as well as other local cleft support groups.

Mother–Child Interactions and Attachment

Mother–child interactions and mother–child attachment have also been the subject of some investigations. Early studies investigating mother–child pairs, where the child was affected with a CFA, reported disruptions to mother–child interactions.[24,25] Research findings suggested that these disruptions occurred because infants with CFA were less active and thus less likely to perform behaviors that signaled a desire for interaction, such as looking at the mother, touching mother, smiling, or cooing.[24,25] Field[26] noted that mothers whose high risk infants were less-responsive typically counter by becoming more active themselves, making greater efforts to elicit a reaction from the infant; however, mothers of infants with CFA in these two studies were passive. She hypothesized that mothers of infants with CFA were less active in response to their infants' lack of initiative due to depression. Endriga and her colleagues[14] did not replicate the findings of Field and Vega-Lahr[24] with a larger sample of 3-month-old infants with CP ($N = 30$), CLP ($N = 28$), and well-matched, unaffected controls ($N = 58$). Using a sequential lag analysis model, Endriga et al.[14] found that there were no differences between infants with CLP or CP and control infants in the frequency of infants positive affect, cooing, or fussiness. The one difference that did emerge among the groups was that infants with CP were *more* likely than the other two groups to engage in what the authors described as "social readiness" (gazing toward mother, neutral affect, without vocalization). There were no differences in social readiness between infants with CLP and controls. An unexpected finding was that *mothers* of the infants with isolated CP but not the mothers of infants with CLP or the controls were more likely to respond with *gaze aversion* in response to their infants' social alertness. In addition, low maternal involvement was associated with CP but *not* with CLP and with higher ratings by mothers of infant negative reactivity during routine home activities (feeding, sleeping, and play). The authors hypothesized that mothers of infants with CP may receive less emotional support from family and friends due to the invisibility of the defect. In addition they had less contact with the cleft team because no active intervention was planned until the child was near a year of age. Although they received less support, these new mothers were still coping with the fact that their infants had a CP and were difficult to feed.

The literature on maternal–child attachment describes the face-to-face interactions between parent and child in terms of harmony or reciprocity. Hoeksma and Koomen[27] summarize the scientific theory of harmonious interaction. A critical dimension relates to the responsivity of both infant and mother to each other's cues. A mother–child dyad is described as harmonious if mother–child behavioral states match. Thus in the Endriga et al.[14] study described above, the relationship between mother and child with CP was disharmonious on only one of several measures. When infants with CP cued a readiness for social interaction, mothers were more likely to avert their gaze rather than match their child's

initiation. On the other hand, harmonious interaction was coded for all five sequences involving mothers and children with CLP (positive vocal exchange, protest, calm disengagement, social play, and social readiness) and for four of the five interactions involving mothers and children with CP. Hoeksma and Koomen's[27] longitudinal study also investigated the harmony of interactions between mothers and children with CLP and control children at ages 3, 6, 9, 12, 15, and 18 months. Children with CP only were not included in this study. Hoeksma and Koomen[27] reported that harmony between mothers and infants in both groups increased between ages 3 and 12 months and decreased after 12 months due to the increased independence of the child. There were no significant differences in the frequency of harmonious interactions between the two groups. However, the behavior of mothers of children with CLP contributed less to the harmony equation. Hoeksma and Koomen[27] theorized that the mothers of children with CLP in their study were more initiating than control mothers, perhaps out of a perceived need to stimulate their children's development.

The different findings in the studies examining mother–child interaction are likely due to different methodologies utilized as well as to differences in the subjects assessed both in terms of diagnosis and age. In total, these studies provide some evidence that mothers of infants with OFC work harder to stimulate their infants and engage in more directive interactions, while being less responsive to the infants' initiations than mothers of children not affected with a cleft. There may be important behavioral consequences of the altered parenting style.[28] Speltz et al.[11] stated that a more directive, intrusive style of interaction between mother and child at 2 years of age, even during play, was associated with more behavior problems when the child was 6. Conversely, higher self-concept at age 6 was associated with a less critical, more child-directed style of interaction during toddler years. The findings of Speltz et al.[11] create some tension for mothers who are frequently counseled by clinic staff or therapists to elicit more speech from their child, to correct articulation patterns, or to stimulate other aspects of development. It is critical that research continue to examine the interaction between mother and child to identify the most advantageous ways of promoting optimal developmental outcomes while preserving a positive, warm relationship between mother and child.

Attachment Classifications

A central tenet of the attachment literature is that the quality of parent–child attachment is a significant force influencing the behavioral development of the child.[29] Attachment is a measure of caregiver–child relations, particularly in situations considered stressful. Aspects measured include the child's search for propinquity to mother during times that the child feels threatened, the extent to which the child uses a primary caregiver as a secure base from which to explore, and the manner in which a child responds to the caregiver after a separation. Formal assessment of infant attachment has generally been accomplished using the Strange Situation as described by Ainsworth et al.[30] The Strange Situation is a laboratory procedure that classifies a child into one of four attachment categories based upon the child's response to mildly stressful separation experiences. In current usage, the classifications include (a) avoidant attachment, when the child displays little distress during separation and avoidance of mother during reunion; (b) secure attachment, when the child displays moderate separation distress but a clear approach response to mother during reunion; (c) ambivalent or resistant attachment, when the child displays extreme distress during separation and when proximity seeking upon reunion is mixed with continued anger and rejection; and (d) disorganized attachment, when the child does not demonstrate any clear strategy during separation/reunion or displays contradictory behaviors. Insecure attachments (avoidant and ambivalent) have been associated with behavior problems[29,31] and social skills deficits at older ages in typically developing children,[32] as well as in medically compromised children.[33] While the Strange Situation has been the most commonly used strategy for systematic investigation of mother–child attachment in young children, there is considerable criticism of this methodology particularly as it relates to ecological validity (see Koomen and Hoeksma[28] and O'Connor and Zeanah[34] for further discussion of issues related to validity and reliability of the assessment of attachment). Despite the criticisms, the literature on attachment has been a dominant force in research examining mother–child relationships in typically developing and in chronically ill children but one that had been largely neglected in research on children with OFC.[35]

Two groups have recently completed longitudinal research that included Ainsworth's Strange Situation[30] to classify attachment in infants with CLP only[15] and with both CLP and CP.[6,36] These studies each included a comparison of classifications with control infants. Hoeksma and Koomen[15] investigated both maternal sensitivity and attachment behavior in a group of infants with CLP compared to controls when infants were 12 and 18 months of age. They observed that mothers of young infants with CLP were less sensitive and responsive to the signals of their infants even though they recognized and interpreted those signals appropriately. There were no differences in the distribution of attachment classification for infants with CLP compared to control infants; however, infants were more likely to display avoidant behaviors (little distress when separated and avoidance of mother during reunion) rather than proximity seeking in the period immediately after surgery for palate repair. Length of hospitalization was considerably longer (6–7 days on average) than in the United States, so this finding does not easily generalize to current United States practice.

In the studies by Speltz[6,36] infants with CLP, CP, and infants without OFC were assessed using the Strange Situation at 12 and 24 months. As in the studies by Hoeksma and Koomen,[15] the distribution of attachment classifications did not differ significantly among diagnostic groups at 12 or 24 months of age. A higher percentage of children with isolated CP than with CLP were rated insecurely attached at 12 months

of age in the subsample of children included in the longitudinal study; however, by 24 months of age these differences were no longer apparent.[36] At 12 months of age, girls in the cleft group were at greater risk of insecure attachment than boys, a finding not seen in the comparison group. Maternal characteristics associated with insecure attachment for the cleft group included being a young or first time mother, reporting depression (particularly in relationship to parenting competence), and reporting overly optimistic feelings about global well-being.

Risk and Resistance During the Elementary School Years

As children progress to school age, their developmental tasks shift to attaining academic achievement, gaining peer acceptance, and developing prosocial conduct.[37] Any child has the potential to hit stumbling blocks as they navigate these tasks and these stumbling blocks have the potential to impact the psychological well-being of the child. Children with clefts navigate these tasks with the added impact of a visible CLP or isolated CP, which, while not visible, often has associated speech difficulties.

Risks Related to Cognitive Factors

Whereas the majority of children with nonsyndromic cleft lip and palate have general intellectual functioning that falls within the average range, there is a 4–6% risk of mental retardation in children with nonsyndromic clefts, compared to 2% in the general population.[38] The risk of mental retardation is higher in those with syndromic clefts. A number of studies have revealed that, even in the presence of normal intelligence, children with clefts have a 30–40% risk of learning disabilities, particularly in the areas of reading, language, and memory.[8,9,39–41]

Children with learning disabilities without cleft lip and palate often have trouble developing positive, mutual friendships with their same age peers and have a higher incidence of behavioral and emotional problems than the general population.[42] Whereas the majority of children with clefts do not develop behavioral, emotional, or social difficulties, there is a significant subgroup that does so.[43] Given the relatively high incidence of learning disability amongst children with cleft lip and palate, such may be one risk factor for development of behavioral, social, or emotional difficulties in this population. A number of studies have found that children with CLP have difficulty in peer relationships, including social withdrawal, behavioral inhibition, and increased peer teasing.[37,44–46] In a study of facial and speech relationships to behavior of children with clefts, Richman[44] found that at age 9, children with fewer speech problems tended to have greater behavioral inhibition. Further exploration of that relationship revealed that higher IQ was also associated with greater behavioral inhibition. For the 12-year-old children in the study, greater facial disfigurement was associated with greater internalizing behavior and, as in the 9-year-olds, higher IQ was also associated with greater internalizing behavior. At age 6, no relationship was found between either speech or facial ratings and behavior. It appears that the impact of speech or facial differences may vary across the age span, and prospective longitudinal studies are needed to explore this possibility. There is evidence, however, that inhibited children without OFC are likely to make fewer attempts at social contact. Schneider[47] found that withdrawn children without CLP tended to make fewer verbalizations when interacting with their friends and tended to be less competitive with their friends. However, this lack of verbal communication did not necessarily compromise the quality of their friendships.

Self-concept, or the way one feels about oneself, plays a critical role in successful psychological adjustment.[48] Self-concept includes a number of different constructs including self-assessment of appearance, behavior, social acceptance, cognitive functioning, self-worth, and general life satisfaction. Low self-perception has been associated with peer rejection and victimization in 11–13-year-old children in a general school population.[49] Among children with clefts, 54–73% of early elementary aged children have been found to have self-concept scores on standardized self-report measures that fall within the "at risk" range.[48,50] Kapp-Simon's[48] study compared 50 five- to nine-year-old children with clefts with 172 controls and found that, compared to their nonaffected peers, children with clefts perceived themselves as less socially adept and more frequently sad and angry than their peers. Broder and Strauss[50] found similar results in their replication of the Kapp-Simon[48] study.

Slifer, Beck, Amari, et al.[51] examined self-concept and satisfaction with physical appearance in 8–15-year-old children with and without oral clefts. They found that these two groups varied very little on children's self-perception, social support, satisfaction, and discomfort measures. Interestingly, they did not find significant differences in child satisfaction with facial appearance between the groups. In fact, both groups indicated moderate dissatisfaction with their appearance, suggesting that this may be a normal developmental process. However, parent rated satisfaction with their child's facial appearance was significantly different between the groups. Parents of children with oral clefts indicated greater dissatisfaction overall than parents of noncleft children. Further examination revealed that when the parents of children with clefts were more dissatisfied than the child himself or herself, the child indicated higher degrees of satisfaction with quality of his or her life. The authors suggest that parents of children with clefts may respond in ways that serve to promote their child's quality of life when they have greater dissatisfaction with their child's appearance. For example, parents may be more proactive in seeking timely medical treatment for correction of their child's facial differences and may pursue more social activities for their child to provide positive social outlets. Parents of children without clefts tended to disagree with their child's dissatisfaction with their appearance and may tend to reassure their child of their physical attractiveness. These differences in parental response to what may be a normative developmental behavior (dissatisfaction with

facial appearance) provide a clue to a potential area of resilience. When parents are realistic and honest with children about their appearance and not dismissing of their child's dissatisfaction, the child may have a greater overall quality of life.

Protective Factors

Much of the research examining psychological adjustment in children with CLP and other CFCs has focused on the associated risks to psychological adjustment. In spite of the increased risks described herein, the majority of affected children studied have been found to have normal psychological adjustment. Strauss[52] has proposed taking a different approach to evaluating psychological adjustment in the craniofacial population, one that focuses our attention on factors that account for health, life success, and resiliency among individuals with CLP and other craniofacial conditions.

As noted previously, resistance factors include intrapersonal characteristics, social-ecological characteristics, and the way in which stress is processed by the child and his or her family members. Intrapersonal characteristics are those characteristics that are intrinsic to the individual, such as temperament, as well as learned characteristics, such as social skills and evaluation of personal competence and self-esteem/self-concept. As we have described, children with CLP demonstrate a tendency toward social withdrawal and behavioral inhibition.[44,53] When provided with appropriate support from parents and other adults, these children can successfully navigate their interactions with peers and adults and the various medical challenges they must face in the course of their treatment. Inhibited children may need more time to warm-up in the presence of strangers. This need may not match the needs of a fast-paced medical environment, but if parents can support their child by coaching him or her ahead of time about what to expect, such may allow the child time to "rehearse" in preparation for coping with the various aspects of their medical care. Parents may also be able to advocate for their child by cueing the medical staff as to their child's needs for a slower approach to implementation of procedures and even discussion of potential upcoming operations.

Social skills are those behaviors that enhance social interaction. Children with CLP who are rated by teachers or parents to have better social skills have fewer behavioral or emotional problems and are less likely to be socially inhibited or withdrawn.[16,18] Social skills, such as making eye contact, maintaining appropriate social distance, entering and maintaining conversations, managing social anxiety, and expressing empathy are all skills that can be taught.[54] One study of the effectiveness of social skills training in a group of children with CLP found that children who participated in the training significantly increased the frequency with which they initiated contact with their peers and the frequency with which these contacts progressed to full conversations. A control group of children with CLP who did not participate in the training group did not show any change in the frequency of their contact initiation.[55]

Social-ecological factors include family adaptation, financial resources, medical care, and school environment. A number of these factors were discussed in the above section on resilience. The degree to which families are able to adjust to the stress of having a child with CLP is an important factor in determining their child's ability to cope and to develop a positive self-concept.

Adolescence

Adolescence marks a time of change during which children become more aware of and sensitive to their appearance and attractiveness. It is also a time of separation and individuation during which they begin to achieve greater independence from their parents and during which their peer group has increasing influence on their interests and activities. Physical maturity is also achieved during this phase of development, bringing about the next stage of decision-making regarding treatment.

As in the younger age groups, global self-concept for adolescents with CLP and other craniofacial anomalies has generally been within the normal range with the exception of adolescent girls who have been shown to report more feelings of being unpopular, anxious, unhappy, and dissatisfied with their appearance (see Endriga and Kapp-Simon).[38] With regard to overall quality of life, adolescents with visible differences have been shown to be similar to other youth with chronic medical conditions and to have lower overall quality of life scores than their peers without chronic conditions.[56] However, in the area of overall relationship quality, youth with visible differences were similar to their peers without chronic conditions. The caveat here is that the youth with visible differences reported lower relationship scores in areas related to peer interactions but higher relationship scores in areas related to family interactions. Individuals with facial differences often have difficulties in the areas of peer interactions and have been shown to initiate fewer social contacts, to receive fewer positive responses, and to engage in shorter conversations than their nonaffected peers.[57] Owing to these difficulties, youth may turn more to their families than to their peers for support, and, to the extent that their families are able to provide that support, they find higher levels of satisfaction in their family relationships.

Risk and Resistance in Adulthood

Areas of Risk

The current literature on psychological adjustment of individuals with OFC is quite limited. The most frequently cited US studies are from the 1970s and early 1980s and could be thought to have little relevance to individuals coming into adulthood during the 21st century due to the many changes that have occurred in medical, educational, and psychological care as well as changes in how society views individuals with differences. The primary findings of these older studies were that individuals with OFC tend to marry later and less frequently than their unaffected siblings, that they participate less often in social activities, and that employment status and income are lower than expected.[58–61]

Most research on adults with OFC is currently being conducted in Europe and Asia. Similar to the results of the US research cited above, these studies have found that there are group differences between adults with CLP and unaffected individuals in educational attainment,[62,63] employment and/or income,[62–64] and marital status.[63,65] Psychological issues include increased rates of anxiety, depression, palpitations,[66] social concerns,[65,67,68] and appearance issues, particularly, but not exclusively, for females.[65,66,68–70]

Quality of Life

Differences in group means as identified in the above research provide some information about issues that may be of concern to individuals with an OFC. The concept of quality of life, however, examines the impact of a medical condition on specific aspects of functioning for the individual. Patient-reported quality of life is considered an important indicator of positive outcome in evidence-based medicine.[71] An important issue for CLP teams and individuals with OFC seeking treatment is that the degree of difference in facial appearance, dental status, or speech makes a difference in overall quality of life.

There are a few studies that have examined quality of life for adults with OFC.[62,69,70] Marcusson et al.[62] evaluated Swedish adults with CLP compared to a group of unaffected adults matched by age and gender. While overall quality of life was similar between groups, adults with CLP continued to view the CLP as impacting their quality of life, particularly in terms of global life satisfaction, overall well-being, social contacts, and family life. Adults who were more satisfied with their facial appearance reported significantly higher global quality of life, better health-related quality of life, fewer somatic complaints, and less depression. Positive valuation of facial appearance was also associated with positive global quality of life and less depression for unaffected adults.[69] Sinko et al.[70] reported that adults in Vienna with OFC reported lower scores than normative data on two aspects of quality of life, social functioning, and emotional concerns that affect role performance. They also reported that personal evaluation of facial esthetics was strongly related to quality of life. Adults with OFC who remained dissatisfied with treatment outcome (in this case, 44.3% of study participants) reported poorer quality of life related to physical role, bodily pain, social functioning, and general mental health.

Stress Processing

An important psychological coping skill identified in the research on risk, resilience, and coping in chronic illness relates to stress processing.[2] An important aspect of stress processing concerns an individual's cognitive appraisal of a situation.[72] Strauss has argued that having a CFC may have positive as well as negative sequelae,[52,73] depending on how one frames his or her condition with respect to oneself. Strauss and Fenton[73] drew on writings of individuals affected with facial differences to identify strategies that can be used to deflect negative social attention, foster resilience, and develop more intimate relationships with peers. Several themes emerged: (1) taking personal responsibility for educating others about facial differences; (2) embracing one's facial difference as a gift that has enhanced personal strengths; (3) placing one's energies in aspects of life that are unrelated to facial difference; (4) use of humor to deflect discomfort of self or others regarding facial differences (laughing at oneself); (5) drawing on faith or an internal belief system that allows one to value all experiences. Cochrane and Slade[68] provide some empirical support for the theories raised by Strauss and his colleagues. Cochrane and Slade reported that individuals who were able to identify positive gains from having an OFC reported more positive ratings of well-being. More adaptive coping strategies were also associated with emotional adjustment. Thus, there is some evidence to support the theory that psychological adjustment and emotional health is enhanced by positive attitudes toward the experience of having an OFC, including an acceptance of appearance differences that may persist after treatment is complete.

SUMMARY

Individuals born with an OFC face many challenges along the journey of reconstruction. Whereas these challenges may pose certain risks to psychosocial adjustment, the majority of individuals with an OFC lead happy and productive lives. An important role of the craniofacial team is to monitor the psychological functioning of the patient and family as medical treatment is planned and implemented. Members of the cleft team should keep in mind the areas of potential risk including parenting stress, parent–child interaction, cognitive functioning and learning, social interaction, and self-concept. Early identification and amelioration of emerging problems through referral to appropriate services such as early intervention, special education, social skills training, and parent/peer support networks will provide patients and families with tools needed to foster resilience and develop coping strategies that promote long-term psychological adjustment.

References

1. Eiser C. Psychological effects of chronic disease. *J Child Psychol Psychiatry* 31:85–98, 1990.
2. Wallander JL, Varni J. Adjustment in children with chronic physical disorders; programmatic research on a disability-stress-coping model. In La Greca AM, Siegel LJ, Wallander JL, Walker CE (eds). *Stress and Coping with Pediatric Conditions.* New York: Guilford Press, 1992, pp. 279–298.
3. Kapp-Simon KA. Psychological care of children with cleft lip and palate in the family. In Wyszynski DF (ed). *Cleft Lip and Palate: From Origin to Treatment.* New York: Oxford University Press, 2002, pp. 412–423.
4. Kazak AE, Kassam-Adams N, Schneider S, et al. An integrative model of pediatric medical traumatic stress. *J Pediatr Psychol* 31:343–355, 2006.
5. Nicholson J. Parents' perspective on cleft lip and palate. In Wyszynski DF (ed). *Cleft Lip and Palate: From Origin to Treatment.* New York: Oxford, 2002, pp. 474–480.
6. Speltz ML, Endriga MC, Fisher PA, et al. Early predictors of attachment in infants with cleft lip and/or palate. *Child Dev* 68:12–25, 1997.
7. Strauss RP, Broder H. Children with cleft lip/palate and mental retardation: A subpopulation of cleft-craniofacial team patients. *Cleft Palate Craniofac J* 30:548–556, 1993.
8. Richman LC. Cognitive patterns and learning disabilities in cleft palate children with verbal deficits. *J Speech Hear Res* 23:447–456, 1980.
9. Broder H, Richman LC, Matheson PB. Learning disabilities, school achievement, and grade retention among children with cleft: A two-center study. *Cleft Palate Craniofac J* 35:127–131, 1998.
10. Speltz ML, Armsden GC, Clarren SS. Effects of craniofacial birth defects on maternal functioning post infancy. *J Pediatr Psychol* 15:177–195, 1990.
11. Speltz ML, Morton K, Goodell EW, et al. Psychological functioning of children with craniofacial anomalies and their mothers: Follow-up from late infancy to school entry. *Cleft Palate Craniofac J* 30:482–489, 1993.
12. Endriga MC, Jordan JR, Speltz ML. Emotion self-regulation in preschool aged children with and without orofacial clefts. *Dev Behav Pediatr* 24:336–344, 2003.
13. Speltz ML, Goodell EW, Endriga MC, et al. Feeding interactions of infants with unrepaired cleft lip and/or palate. *Infant Behav Dev* 17:131–139, 1994.
14. Endriga MC, Speltz ML. Face-to-face interaction between infants with orofacial clefts and their mothers. *J Pediatr Psychol* 22:439–453, 1997.
15. Hoeksma JB, Koomen H. *Development of Early Mother-Child Interaction and Attachment.* Amsterdam: Pro Lingua, 1991.
16. Krueckeberg S, Kapp-Simon KA. Effect of parental factors on social skills of preschool children with craniofacial anomalies. *Cleft Palate Craniofac J* 30:490–496, 1993.
17. Krueckeberg S, Kapp-Simon KA, Ribordy SC. Social skills of preschoolers with and without craniofacial anomalies. *Cleft Palate Craniofac J* 30:475–481, 1993.
18. Krueckeberg S, Kapp-Simon KA. *Longitudinal Follow-up of Social Skills in Children with and without Craniofacial Anomalies.* American Cleft Palate-Craniofacial Association Annual Meeting, 1997.
19. Pope AW, Tillman K, Snyder HT. Parenting stress in infancy and psychological adjustment: A longitudinal study of children with craniofacial anomalies. *Cleft Palate Craniofac J* 42:556–559, 2005.
20. Kazak AE, Marvin RS. Differences, difficulties and adaptation: Stress and social networks in families with a handicapped child. *Fam Relat* 33:67–77, 1984.
21. Wanamaker CE, Glenwick DS. Stress, coping and perceptions of child behavior in parents of preschoolers with cerebral palsy. *Rehab Psychol* 43:297–312, 1998.
22. Abidin RR. *Parenting Stress Index (PSI) Manual*, 3rd edn. Charlottesville, VA: Pediatric Psychology Press, 1995.
23. Haskett ME, Ahern LS, Ward CS, et al. Factor structure and validity of the parenting stress index-short form. *J Clin Child Adolesc Psychol* 35:302–312, 2006.
24. Field TM, Vega-Lahr N. Early interactions between infants with cranio-facial anomalies and their mothers. *Infant Behav Dev* 7:527–530, 1984.
25. Barden RC, Ford ME, Jensen AG, et al. Effects of craniofacial deformity in infancy on the quality of mother-infant interactions. *Child Dev* 60:819–824, 1989.
26. Field TM. Early interaction of infants with craniofacial anomalies. In Eder RA (ed). *Craniofacial Anomalies: Psychological Perspective.* New York: Springer-Verlag, 1995, pp. 99–110.
27. Hoeksma JB, Koomen HMY. The development of harmony in interaction: A longitudinal comparison between children born with and

without cleft lip and palate. In Hoeksma JB, Koomen HMY (eds). *Development of Early Mother-Child Interaction and Attachment.* Amsterdam: Pro Lingua, 1991, pp. 75–90.

28. Koomen HMY, Hoeksma JB. Cleft lip and palate and the early mother-child relation. In Hoeksma JB, Koomen HMY (eds). *Development of Early Mother-Child Interaction and Attachment.* Amsterdam: Pro Lingua, 1991, pp. 21–45.

29. Burgess KB, Marshall PJ, Rubin KH, et al. Infant attachment and temperament as predictors of subsequent externalizing problems and cardiac physiology. *J Child Psychol Psychiatry* 44:819–831, 2003.

30. Ainsworth MS, Blehar MC, Waters E, et al. *Patterns of Attachment: A Psychological Study of the Strange Situation.* Oxford, England: Lawrence Erlbaum, 1978.

31. Warren SL, Huston L, Egeland B, et al. Child and adolescent anxiety disorders and early attachment. *Child Adolesc Psychiatry* 36:637–644, 1997.

32. Rubin KH, Dwyer KM, Booth-LaForce C, et al. Attachment, friendship, and psychosocial functioning in early adolescence. *J Early Adolesc* 24:326–356, 2004.

33. Goldberg S, Gotowiec A, Simmons RJ. Infant-mother attachment and behavior problems in healthy and chronically ill preschoolers. *Dev Psychopathol* 7:267–282, 1995.

34. O'Connor TG, Zeanah CH. Attachment disorders: Assessment strategies and treatment approaches. *Attach Human Dev* 5:223–244, 2003.

35. Speltz ML, Greenberg MT, Galbreath H, et al. Developmental approach to the psychology of craniofacial anomalies. *Cleft Palate Craniofac J* 31:61–67, 1994.

36. Maris CL, Endriga MC, Speltz ML, et al. Are infants with orofacial clefts at risk for insecure mother-child attachments? *Cleft Palate Craniofac J* 37:257–265, 2000.

37. Broder HL. Using psychological assessment and therapeutic strategies to enhance well-being. *Cleft Palate Craniofac J* 38:248–254, 2001.

38. Endriga MC, Kapp-Simon KA. Psychological issues in craniofacial care: State of the art. *Cleft Palate Craniofac J* 36:3–11, 1999.

39. Richman LC. The effects of facial disfigurement on teachers' perception of ability in cleft palate children. *Cleft Palate J* 15:155–160, 1978.

40. Richman LC, Eliason MJ. Type of reading disability related to cleft type and neuropsychological patterns. *Cleft Palate J* 19:249–258, 1984.

41. Richman LC, Michele J, Lindgren S. Reading disability in children with clefts. *Cleft Palate J* 25:21–25, 1988.

42. . Wiener J, Schneider B. A multisource exploration of the friendship patterns of children with and without learning disabilities. *J Abnorm Child Psychol* 30:127–141, 2002.

43. Slifer KJ, Amari A, Diver T, et al. Social interaction patterns of children and adolescents with and without oral clefts during a videotaped analogue social encounter. *Cleft Palate Craniofac J* 41:175–184, 2004.

44. Richman LC, Millard TL. Brief report: Cleft lip and palate: Longitudinal behavior and relationships of cleft conditions to behavior and achievement. *J Pediatr Psychol* 22:487–494, 1997.

45. Kapp-Simon KA. Psychological adaptation of patients with craniofacial malformations. In Lucker GW, Ribbens KA, McNamara JA (eds). *Psychological Aspects of Facial Form.* Ann Arbor, MI: Center for Growth and Development, 1981, pp. 143–160.

46. Pope AW, Ward J. Factors associated with peer social competence in preadolescents with craniofacial anomalies. *Pediatr* 22:455–469, 1997.

47. Schneider BH. A multimethod exploration of the friendships of children considered socially withdrawn by their school peers. *J Abnorm Child Psychol* 27:115–123, 1999.

48. Kapp-Simon KA. Self-concept of primary school-age children with cleft lip, cleft palate or both. *Cleft Palate J* 23:24–27, 1986.

49. Salmivalli C, Isaacs J. Prospective relations among victimization, rejection, friendlessness, and children's self- and peer-perceptions. *Child Dev* 76:1161–1171, 2005.

50. Broder H, Strauss RP. Self-concept of early primary school age children with visible or invisible defects. *Cleft Palate J* 26:114–117, 1989.

51. Slifer KJ, Beck M, Amari A, et al. Self-concept and satisfaction with physical appearance in youth with and without oral clefts. *Child Health Care* 32:81–101, 2003.

52. Strauss RP. "Only skin deep": Health, resilience, and craniofacial care. *Cleft Palate Craniofac J* 38:226–230, 2001.

53. Richman LC, Eliason MJ. Psychological characteristics associated with cleft palate. In Moller KT, Starr CD (eds). *Cleft Palate: Interdisciplinary Issues and Treatment.* Austin, TX: Pro-Ed, Inc., 1993.

54. Kapp-Simon KA, Simon DJ. *Meeting the Challenge: A Social Skills Program for Adolescents with Special Needs.* Chicago: Kapp-Simon & Simon, 1991.

55. Kapp-Simon KA, McGuire DE, Long BC, et al. Addressing quality of life issues in adolescent: Social skills interventions. *Cleft Palate Craniofac J* 42:45–50, 2005.

56. Topolski TD, Edwards TC, Patrick DL. Quality of life: How do adolescents with facial differences compare with other adolescents? *Cleft Palate Craniofac J* 42:25–32, 2005.

57. Kapp-Simon KA, McGuire DE. Observed social interaction patterns in adolescents with and without craniofacial conditions. *Cleft Palate Craniofac J* 34:380–384, 1997.

58. Peter JP, Chinsky RR. Sociological aspects of cleft palate adults: Education. *Cleft Palate J* 11:443–449, 1974.

59. Peter JP, Chinsky RR. Sociological aspects of cleft palate adults, I: Marriage. *Cleft Palate J* 11:295–301, 1974.

60. Peter JP, Chinsky RR, Fisher MJ. Sociological aspects of cleft palate adults, IV: Social integration. *Cleft Palate J* 12:304–310, 1975.

61. Heller A, Tidmarsh W, Pless IB. The psychological functioning of young adults born with cleft lip or palate. *Clin Pediatr* 20:459–465, 1981.

62. Marcusson A, Akerlind I, Paulin G. Quality of life in adults with repaired complete cleft lip and palate. *Cleft Palate Craniofac J* 38:379–385, 2001.

63. Danino A, Gradell J, Malka G, et al. Social adjustment in French adults from who had undergone standardised treatment of complete unilateral cleft lip and palate. *Ann Chir Plast Esthet* 50:202–205, 2005.

64. Ramstad T, Ottem E, Shaw WC. Psychosocial adjustment in Norwegian adults who had undergone standardised treatment of complete cleft lip and palate. I. Education, employment and marriage. *Scand J Plast Reconstr Surg Hand Surg* 29:251–257, 1995.

65. Bjornsson A, Agustsdottir S. A psychosocial study of Icelandic individuals with cleft lip or cleft lip and palate. *Cleft Palate J* 24:152–157, 1987.

66. Ramstad T, Ottem E, Shaw WC. Psychosocial adjustment in Norwegian adults who had undergone standardized treatment of complete cleft lip and palate. II Self-reported problems and concerns with appearance. *Scand J Plast Reconst Surg Hand Surg* 29:329–336, 1995.

67. Beck NW, Cooper ME, Lui Ye, et al. Social anxiety in Chinese adults with oral-facial clefts. *Cleft Palate Craniofac J* 38:126–132, 2001.

68. Cochrane VM, Slade P. Appraisal and coping in adults with cleft lip: Associations with well-being and social anxiety. *Br J Med Psychol* 72: 485–503, 1999.

69. Marcusson A, Paulin G, Ostrup L. Facial appearance in adults who had cleft lip and palate treated in childhood. *Scan J Plast Reconstr Surg Hand Surg* 36:16–23, 2002.

70. Sinko K, Jagsch R, Prechtl V, et al. Evaluation of esthetical, functional, and quality of life outcome in adult cleft lip and palate patients. *Cleft Palate Craniofac J* 42:355–361, 2005.

71. Wyrwich KW, Tierney WM, Babu AN, et al. A comparison of clinically important differences in health-related quality of life for patients with chronic lung disease, asthma, or heart disease. *HSR: Health Serv Research* 40:577–591, 2005.

72. Lazarus RS, Folkman S. *Stress, Appraisal and Coping.* New York: Springer, 1984.

73. Strauss RP, Fenson C. Experiencing the "good life": Literary views of craniofacial conditions and quality of life. *Cleft Palate Craniofac J* 42:14–18, 2005.

Sociocultural and Ethical Aspects of Prenatal Diagnosis and Care of Congenital Facial Differences

Ronald P. Strauss, DMD, PhD • Joshua S. Zukerman, BA • Barry L. Ramsey, BS

INTRODUCTION

How a society responds to people who have unusual or different physical attributes is an important indicator of the value they place on conformity and social control. Facial and speech differences are immediately apparent human features that elicit social responses from others. Indeed, people with facial differences may manage their first impressions by letting others see them from a distance or in a public setting at a first meeting in order to allow for accommodation and to reduce the element of surprise. Beyond first impressions, facial differences may call forward a societal effort to reduce the deformity and to make it visually acceptable. Societies have also sought to minimize the occurrence and presence of deformity in their midst.

Differences in appearance may result in stigmatization, teasing, or bullying, all of which are often deeply damaging.[1-13] Social and media norms (i.e., film, magazine, television, and advertising) frame self and peer expectations and reinforce the norm that one's face should be attractive and all efforts should be exerted to aesthetically correct appearance.

Appearance and facial difference have been shown to affect quality of life, social experience, school performance, dating, and employment. Persons who have birth conditions that result in altered appearance or speech disabilities often have altered social experiences.[14-21] Research also demonstrates that appearance is a powerful determinant of success and educational/work attainment.[22-30] However, many people with facial differences thrive in spite of their stigmatizing experiences.

Goffman's[25] classic work *Stigma* provides a theory of stigmatization useful in understanding the social responses to human difference and health conditions. Goffman describes how first impressions on meeting strangers are based on observations of attributes that are "transformed into normative expectations" and then into firmly held roles and responsibilities. Being visibly different is associated with being perceived by others as less than complete, as limited, or as otherwise reduced. The bodily signs of being different, known as stigma, are seen to carry a moral evaluation, usually a negative one. Stigma theory has been a powerful social science tool for over 40 years and continues to guide research today, especially that relating to HIV/AIDS and to mental health issues. Social researchers have sought to operationalize the concept of stigma by developing measures, including some in the realm of craniofacial research.[31,32]

The appearance of the face, head, and oral area are immediately observable by others.[33-35] Facial differences are quickly perceived in social discourse. The face is the initial focus of the gaze—it is the principal target of attention in interpersonal interaction—and there is much research to indicate that facial attractiveness has an important effect on psychological development and social relationships even when no deformity is present.[36-43]

Stigma has been described as "enacted" when the individual directly experiences damaging effects, such as discrimination, rejection, or physical abuse. Family members and persons working with those affected may also experience such enacted stigma. "Perceived" or "felt" stigma entails reduced self-perception; it is the internalization of enacted stigma.

This chapter explores how social and cultural norms about appearance translate into an impetus to sanitize facial difference, or even to reduce the chance that a child with a facial difference will be born. In societies in which the social ethic is to accept disability and difference, efforts to reduce stigmatization will occur in the context of socially integrating the person with a facial difference. However, in societies where a high value is placed on reducing deviance or difference, efforts will be extended to eliminate disability and difference as much as possible. Taken to the extreme, eugenic practice or even infanticide has been employed to control human facial difference.

The introduction of early cleft and craniofacial diagnosis and treatment raises many social and ethical questions about how families, craniofacial teams, and society respond when a prenatal craniofacial diagnosis is made and whether that knowledge leads to an overall enhancement of the child's and family's quality of life. The advancing sophistication and availability of prenatal diagnostic technologies, such as transvaginal or real-time ultrasound, have increased the medical capacity to visualize and detect congenital craniofacial conditions during pregnancy.

This chapter examines the ethical and social issues associated with counseling, managing information, and making treatment decisions that relate to the prenatally diagnosed facial birth defect. Families and health professionals often face ambiguity, uncertainty, and complex decision-making in dealing with a diagnosis and treatment plan. Embedded in parental and clinical decisions are values about children with

birth defects. Families are making decisions about whether to bear, or how to treat, an affected child based upon their perceptions of the craniofacial impairment and on their expectation of the social, emotional, and economic burdens involved for the family and the child.

On a broader societal level, pressures to conform and to minimize human differences are apparent in early biomedical and surgical interventions, in the Human Genome Project, in advertising and media images, and in social expectations to normalize disabilities. Social values, moral, legal, and ethical perspectives, and health policy factors influence how society and families deal with a craniofacial diagnosis. This chapter considers the societal impact of early craniofacial treatment and prenatal diagnosis in terms of tolerance for human difference and examines the issues that are likely to arise for parents, professionals, and craniofacial centers.

ISSUES ASSOCIATED WITH PRENATAL CRANIOFACIAL DIAGNOSIS

The increasing clarity and availability of prenatal diagnostic technologies in developed nations, such as transvaginal ultrasound, chorionic villus sampling, amniocentesis, and alpha feto-protein testing, have advanced the medical capacity to detect genetic and congenital conditions during pregnancy. The availability of this technology has made it possible for parents to learn a great deal about the health and physical status of a fetus while in-utero. Such information is clearly desired by parents who seek to screen the unborn fetus for birth defects and for other health conditions that can be identified by prenatal testing. Geneticists, ultrasonographers, and fetal medicine specialists have collaborated to provide information to expectant parents during pregnancy. Many prenatal diagnoses occur as inadvertent findings on a routine exam to find out about fetal position or to estimate the progress of the pregnancy and calculate an expected delivery date.

When faced with concerning prenatal diagnostic findings, parents may choose either to continue the pregnancy with a new awareness and seek prenatal therapy or to terminate the pregnancy. Prenatal diagnostic technology implies a high degree of parental choice regarding the fetus. However, little is known about how families and professionals deal with prenatally diagnosed conditions. How do they manage the inevitable ambiguity, uncertainty, and difficult decision-making that accompany a prenatal diagnosis?

Aside from the parental issues, there are societal implications of prenatal diagnosis.[44-46] One might seriously consider the societal impact of prenatal diagnosis in terms of tolerance for human difference. Issues relating to prenatal diagnosis affect parents and the extended family, but also have major impacts upon medical practice and on craniofacial centers.

The parental decision about whether to continue or terminate a pregnancy in the face of a birth defect is a personal and spiritual matter.[47] However, embedded in these parental decisions are values about the social and familial worth of children with birth defects. Some families will perceive a prenatally diagnosed birth defect to be acceptable and will plan to provide care and treatment to the child in the post-partum period. Some families will perceive a child with a known birth defect as a burden, or they may fear the child will ultimately not have a high quality of life. Some families weigh the risks and costs of treatment against the chance they could "try again" to have an unaffected pregnancy. Some families plan to place a child for adoption after delivery if they feel incapable of providing parenting and care to the affected child. Families also make decisions about what defects are so serious as to make the birth of an affected fetus undesirable.[48]

At the same time prenatal diagnosis occurs more commonly, the US and other developed nations are also investing ever more costly and scarce health care resources in the care of newborns with craniofacial and other birth defects. The neonatal intensive care unit and its remarkable capacity for helping seriously impaired infants survive represents a major societal and fiscal investment in the preservation and future health of disabled newborns. In developed nations, the capacity to survive and thrive with a birth defect has never been greater. However, some affected fetuses that are prenatally diagnosed are never born. Prenatal diagnosis and visualization has become a routine part of medical care for pregnant women and increasingly noninvasive tests allow for fetal screening without the risk of premature labor. While these various medical care trends might at first seem like contradictions or polarities, they represent a single position, one that all biomedical efforts must be exerted to reduce and repair disfigurations and disabilities in newborns.

Prior to the advent of prenatal diagnosis, most parents had little choice but to accept the birth of a child with a birth defect. The ever increasing ability to "know" in advance about a future child's special needs now allows parents to anticipate social pressures from the family or community regarding the integration and social roles for the child. If parents perceive that they or the child will be greeted with tolerance and that efforts will be made to accept the child, they will feel supported. If the parents perceive they or the child will face a high level of stigmatization and prejudice, the family may feel isolated and marginalized. The pressures for conformity to a common societal standard of appearance or function are overt, and some families report that family members and medical professionals pressure them to seek quick or early repairs of facial differences in the post-partum period.

The impetus to genetic conformity is also evident in other biomedical interventions, such as in the Human Genome Project. The describing of the "normative" genome creates a pressure to define other than normative genetic patterns as different and possibly as less acceptable. The drive for visual conformity is seen widely in advertising and media images and in social pressures placed on persons with disabilities to normalize by surgical and other treatment means. Even individuals without facial deformity undergo plastic surgery in response to media images and social expectations.

A variety of social and ethical questions must be posed about prenatal diagnosis. Is prenatal diagnosis a vehicle to normalize human difference and reduce variability in the human genome? Is there inherent, but unappreciated, value in the variation expressed in the human genome? Will the Human Genome Project and genetic research be used to define what is normatively human? Or, will such research show that all humans have diversity in their phenotypic manifestations and all people possess genes that are suboptimal and which encode their future illnesses? Are we as a society able to identify genetic differences between people and also to accept people with non-life-threatening genetic imperfections?[49] Are we ready to manage genetic knowledge?

Prenatal visualization and diagnosis are changing the emotional landscape of pregnancy. For families, the ability to visualize the fetus or determine its developmental stage, its health, or its sex, has changed the perception of pregnancy. Parents are bonding to and identifying with fetuses as children at a much earlier time. At one point, the "quickening" or movement of a fetus was a landmark for parents. Now, quickening is often preceded by hearing the heartbeat and getting a clear sonogram photograph of the unborn baby. Parents "bond" to their first baby picture months before the birth actually occurs. The use of prenatal visualization, even in 3-D, encourages families to personalize the fetus and to invest in what has essentially become a new member of the family.[50] When the family has received a photograph of the fetus, knows its gender, and selects a name on the basis of prenatal diagnostic information, does the meaning of birth change?

Craniofacial centers report that parents often seek prenatal consultation and referral in anticipation of their baby's needs or to collect advance information. Activist parents are arriving at craniofacial centers with extensive internet printouts about their future child's possible condition, making it clear there is a high level of parental concern and often anxiety. Families are sometimes feeling as though they need to have a clear treatment plan, and they seek to understand the extent of their treatment choices, in advance of their child's birth. The ease and access to prenatal diagnostic technologies raises other important emotional and psychological questions. Is prior knowledge of a craniofacial defect an advantage to families? What are the implications of aborting fetuses that have non-life-threatening conditions and that are largely repairable? Who should have access to prenatal diagnostic information?[51] Should prenatal testing be limited to the detection of conditions apparent in infancy, or should diagnosis seek to predict adult health status? Should fetuses be tested for a predisposition to develop breast cancer, cardiovascular disease, or diabetes as adults? As prenatal diagnosis becomes more accurate and available at ever-earlier times in pregnancy, other psychological and societal issues will arise.

Craniofacial centers have reported ethical issues related to prenatal diagnosis and nonlethal birth defects. Several authors[52–54] have discussed an Israeli center's experience with prenatal diagnosis. In 1996, Bronshtein et al. conducted a study in Haifa, Israel, analyzing the effects of prenatal transvaginal sonographic diagnosis of cleft lip for expecting parents.[55] Of the 15 detected cases with cleft lip, the pregnancy was terminated in all but one case. Parents of the 14 cases in which the fetus was voluntarily terminated were informed it was difficult to determine the size of the cleft lip. Interestingly, the decision for termination was made after the couples had consulted other parents of children who had been born with cleft lip and who had undergone surgical repair. The Israeli center's use of early prenatal diagnosis and the parents' subsequent decisions to terminate their pregnancies in response to prenatal diagnosis raised concerns. Some have concluded the Israeli parents and clinicians in that study were weighing the value of living a life against the impact of having a cleft lip. Fundamental questions about the rationale for prenatal diagnosis are raised if a repairable condition such as cleft lip can be widely seen as the basis for the termination of pregnancy. Is prenatal diagnosis meant to detect seriously impairing or life-threatening conditions, or is it meant to identify genetic or congenital traits that are compatible with a high quality life span? And, who should make that determination?

Anecdotal reports from Western Europe assert that craniofacial centers may be seeing declining numbers of children with cleft lip. Some European center clinicians have concluded that prenatal diagnosis may have led to aborted fetuses, resulting in a declining incidence of live-born cleft lip. If this hypothesis proves correct, craniofacial centers may see reduced calls for their services in the future. This is precisely what has occurred for teams that care for people with Down syndrome. A recent report[56] found that, as earlier Down syndrome screenings have become more available, women have been able to make "private" abortion decisions before other people perceive them to be pregnant. In a recent paper, Down syndrome prenatal diagnosis (using a combination of tests) has been shown to be correct about 85% of the time at gestational age of 12 weeks.[57] In a 1998 Brigham and Women's Hospital study in Boston, 86% of couples chose abortion when their unborn children were detected with Down syndrome.[58] The combination of readily available prenatal testing and abortion services in the US means that the incidence of Down syndrome will be in decline. Should we expect a similar outcome for the incidence of craniofacial conditions that can be prenatally diagnosed?

Blumenfeld et al. studied more than 30,000 transvaginal sonograms performed at 14–16 weeks' gestation.[52] Twenty-four cases of cleft lip were detected in the 30,000 sonogram images. Of these 24 cases, 23 underwent termination of pregnancy, and on post-abortion examination, 22 of the 24 cases only had cleft lip (with or without cleft palate). Most of these cases were in low risk parents without any medical history of fetal malformations.

In evaluating the social and ethical impacts of prenatal diagnosis it is important to carefully differentiate between fetuses with life-threatening and seriously impairing conditions and those with conditions that are compatible with a high quality of life. Where the line lies between these two groups is likely culturally and socially determined.[59] What criteria do people use to judge a future child's quality of life?

Who in the family or health professional community should participate in determinations of the quality of life for fetuses with prenatally diagnosed conditions?

For craniofacial health professionals who classically focus on the giving of care to individuals with cleft lip and other craniofacial conditions, other ethical quandaries arise. Advocates for persons with disabilities have asked whether a craniofacial team clinician has any reason to participate in efforts that might result in selectively preventing the birth of individuals who will become their patients when born. One may ask how craniofacial health professionals can treat patients with oral clefts one minute, then turn around the next minute and have a conversation in which a fetus with a cleft lip or palate is not seen as having the potential for a "good life." Can parents trust in a doctor who might not fully believe their child's life to be worthy?

Should the prenatal diagnostic advisor be entirely separate from the treatment team? How many centers have a geneticist who actively is involved with parents who have had a prenatal diagnosis? Does an overlap of treatment and prenatal diagnostic functions imply a conflict of interest? Some hold that craniofacial team professionals should focus on promoting the quality of life for all their patients and not become engaged in advising parents about prenatal diagnosis and about the possible termination of pregnancy. Others would assert that craniofacial team clinicians have unique knowledge and information that parents need to guide their decisions about whether to bear the affected child.

The establishment of optimism and hope around a craniofacial diagnosis may be a critical step in starting the process of professional treatment and care, even during the prenatal period. It is their special vantage-point that permits craniofacial health professionals to help families and individuals affected by cleft lip/palate to see their lives as rich with possibilities. They can help families envision good outcomes through treatment and prepare them for the course of therapy. They can help families to see that the unique and often difficult experiences faced by persons with cleft lip/palate may also afford them with special and worthwhile perspectives. To succeed in this role, craniofacial professionals must deeply believe in and value the lives of persons with cleft and craniofacial conditions.

For the affected individual, even the discussion about the value of a life lived with a cleft raises the fear that somehow their life was not worth it, that somehow they placed a burden upon their parents that was just too heavy. As Eiserman and Strauss suggest, "perhaps, some affected persons wonder 'what would my family's life have been like if they had been spared all the expense and heartache that I brought with me?"[54]

How professionals present information regarding a prenatal diagnosis may determine how much parents will respond. If the professionals present a gloomy prognosis and describe every possible complication, every frightening ramification, no matter how rare, then it becomes more likely that the parents will become deeply alarmed and possibly decide to terminate the pregnancy. What should be included in the professional's discussion with the parents about prenatal diagnosis? Where and with whom present should this discussion occur?

It is well accepted that professionals should not serve as opinionated advocates for or against the termination of pregnancy in the wake of a prenatal diagnosis.[60] Professionals must always respect the family's right to autonomously make such critical decisions without having a position about what the family "should" do. The decision about how to respond to a prenatal diagnosis is never easy for parents, and perhaps it should always entail a difficult, personal, and weighty consideration for the family. Prenatal diagnosis must be seen as a process that includes the professional provision of information and caring support after a finding occurs. It is critical to evaluate how prenatal counseling occurs and in what manner the professional provides the family with needed information. Parents must be offered support during this period and must be given the full spectrum of decisions and choices. It is possible that termination of pregnancy should only be offered or discussed if the family raises the question. All parents should be provided information about the treatment and support available for their unborn child.

The prenatal diagnosis of a congenital defect marks the beginning of a period of high stress and uncertainty for many parents. When people receive bad news, they experience a loss of control and are in crisis. This may be a time when parents are vulnerable and are easily swayed by the opinions of professionals or other parents. Prospective parents should be carefully informed of all of their possible options and afforded time to make their decision. In the prenatal period prospective parents should receive nonjudgmental and unbiased information, support, and advice from health professionals who are specifically trained to counsel and support their decisions. Family physicians and other professionals with a longstanding relationship with the family are ideal counselors at this time of considerable parental stress. The presentation of information to families[53] should be done in a positive and supportive manner.

The realm of early care does pose legal and ethical issues that have troubled health professionals. Issues of privacy and of the sharing of prenatal diagnostic information become apparent.[61] Insurance policies often do not cover persons who have pre-existing conditions. Will prenatal diagnostic information result in exclusions of such conditions as pre-existing? Might insurers avoid women known to be carrying an affected fetus, or might they selectively exclude those who choose to bear a child with a predictable health problem? Could insurers require mandatory prenatal diagnostic evaluations and demand to know the results? Could these studies be part of pre-employment physicals? Could prenatal ultrasound or genetic screening become mandatory, as has phenylketonuria screening? Other issues exist relative to the distribution of costly and scarce resources, such as prenatal diagnostic equipment. Will affluent societies commonly abort fetuses with genetic disorders, leaving those in impoverished nations with a greater relative burden of disease and disability than already exists?

ATTITUDES ABOUT CRANIOFACIAL PRENATAL DIAGNOSIS: INTERVIEWS WITH PROFESSIONALS AND AFFECTED PERSONS

In an effort to learn about the ethical and social issues surrounding craniofacial prenatal diagnosis, open-ended in-depth qualitative interviews were conducted in North Carolina with three craniofacial health professionals (craniofacial surgeon, medical social worker, and medical social scientist) and three affected persons (people living with a craniofacial condition). This qualitative pilot study was approved by the Human Subjects Committee and was conducted in 2005–2006. Audio-taped interviews were transcribed in-part, and the findings from this study are used in this chapter to explore perceptions of craniofacial prenatal diagnosis.

All interviews examined the implications of prenatal diagnosis. We asked health professionals:

(a) Do you think ultrasounds have become routine in pregnancy?

(b) Are craniofacial diagnoses based on prenatal screening accurate? How often is there a false diagnosis?

(c) How do you manage the situation of a prenatal diagnosis for cleft lip/palate? Do you have a specific role in prenatal counseling and if so, what do you do?

(d) Who informs the family of the diagnosis and how does one do that? Generally, how does the family react?

(e) Do you think it benefits the family to have access to this information?

(f) How often have people terminated the pregnancy?

(g) How do you manage discussion of termination or continuation of pregnancy? Should parents ever consider termination of pregnancy? What is your thinking about that as a possibility?

(h) How do you feel about prenatal diagnosis of craniofacial conditions?

(i) How do you think one's life quality is impacted by a craniofacial prenatal diagnosis?

(j) What, if any ethical questions exist in your mind about craniofacial prenatal diagnosis?

(k) How do you think society should deal with the termination of pregnancy in non-life-threatening fetal conditions?

We also asked adults with craniofacial conditions:

(a) How do you feel about prenatal diagnosis of craniofacial conditions? How would you respond if as an expectant parent, a prenatal craniofacial diagnosis was made of the fetus you or your spouse were carrying?

(b) How do you think one's life quality is impacted by prenatal diagnosis?

(c) What should be done to improve the life quality for parents from the time of prenatal diagnosis until the birth of the child?

(d) What, if any ethical questions exist in your mind about craniofacial prenatal diagnosis?

(e) Should parents ever consider termination of pregnancy? What is your thinking about that as a possibility?

(f) How do you think society should deal with the termination of pregnancy in non-life-threatening fetal conditions?

(g) From the vantage-point of having a craniofacial condition, are there issues or concerns you have about prenatal diagnosis of such conditions?

Critics and members of the disability rights community have raised concerns that prenatal diagnosis heightens preconceived notions that disability entails a low quality of life and that prenatal diagnosis will be utilized as means to produce a normalized and conformist society. In this pilot project, affected individuals voiced interesting perspectives relating to the social and ethical issues associated with the use of prenatal diagnostic technology to detect craniofacial conditions. Because some of these affected persons had spent a considerable amount of time adjusting to their condition, they provided personal examples of how people with facial differences are stereotyped and negatively perceived. Also, many of the affected individuals shared personal accounts of their interactions with family and clinicians and offered advice as to how the quality of life of a child with a craniofacial condition could be improved. They also provided recommendations about how clinicians could better interact with these future parents as well as with affected persons in general.

The most intense and controversial subject explored by affected persons was the issue of termination of pregnancy as a result of a prenatal diagnosis of a craniofacial condition. The social stigma attached to a prenatally diagnosed fetus can instill a fear of the unknown in anxious future parents. Affected adults wondered about how parents and clinicians should respond to the detection of a prenatal diagnosis of a craniofacial condition. What actions should be taken after the diagnosis is made? They considered how they as affected individuals would respond if presented with a positive prenatal diagnosis of an anomaly similar to their own. They pondered whether they would terminate the pregnancy and considered if their ability to cope with their own condition might empower them with a special empathy for an affected child.

In the interviews, all affected persons stressed that future parents should be entitled to all of the information revealed in an ultrasound. Some interviewees explained that care centers should implement educational programs to help future parents and families deal with prenatal diagnoses.

Both the health professionals and affected persons were opinionated about how they felt physicians and the health team should approach and treat discussion of the results of a craniofacial prenatal diagnostic study with parents.

From the vantage point of both the health professionals and the affected persons, the discussion of the prenatal diagnosis between the doctor and the parents is essential to the parents' course of action with regard to the pregnancy. The respondents asked if clinicians, like genetic counselors, take a nondirective approach in the way they approach their interactions and exchange of information with future parents

who have undergone prenatal diagnosis. In response to the criticism that medicine favors the prevention of unnecessary suffering of impaired children whose births could have been prevented by a positive prenatal diagnosis, they asked if clinicians urge future parents to "try again" in the hopes of giving birth to a healthy child? Do clinicians embody their role as healers and actively dissuade prospective parents from the decision to terminate a pregnancy and explain to these future parents that their child, despite an anomaly, can lead a rich life?

An affected adult interviewed expressed the idea that future parents and families should undergo a sonogram education program before they proceed with an ultrasound. This person felt that a clinician or social worker should explain to future parents and families "... some of the wonderful things a sonogram can show us and some of the anomalies a sonogram can reveal ... you can work parents through a bunch of hypothetical situations." This person felt that the "pre-sonogram training" would reduce the "knee-jerk reaction" to terminate a pregnancy in response to a craniofacial diagnosis.

A craniofacial plastic surgeon who interacts with numerous families who have received craniofacial prenatal diagnoses strongly asserted that all future parents and families should have complete access to the results of their ultrasound. This surgeon holds that, as a clinician, one must protect one's patients: "If I tell the patient everything I know, then I don't have to wonder what I said ... I cannot make a decision to protect a patient based on how much information a person can handle." The parents, this surgeon believes, must have full access to the findings of an ultrasound study because they may actually make a decision to abort based on incomplete information. This surgeon asserted that a cleft lip diagnosis by ultrasound is almost always valid and certain, whereas cleft palate is much more difficult to diagnose by this mechanism. As a result, the surgeon tells parents that have had a prenatal diagnosis of cleft lip that there is a chance that the child may also have an undetected cleft palate. This surgeon stressed that a clinician must always be completely honest and thorough in explaining all the information revealed by ultrasound to future parents.

In another interview, a medical social scientist affirmed that "the bottom line is that up until the third trimester, it is their [the future parent's] decision, and you may have pause about how people are going to act on that information. But once you start withholding information based on your assessment of what a person is going to decide, short of incompetence, you are going to run into a lot of trouble. You might think 'this is a non-lethal anomaly ... and termination would be an action of insidious eugenics, but you either have reproductive freedom or you don't, and you have to weigh these very tough principles." This respondent went on to assert that a health professional cannot withhold information or access to the results of a prenatal diagnosis simply because of a personal judgment or fear that a future parent or family will terminate a pregnancy for a non-life-threatening condition. This respondent provided a hypothetical vignette: A couple decides to divorce 6 weeks into their pregnancy, and, in response, the future mother feels that she must terminate the pregnancy. "Are you [the physician] going to restrict her right to do that?" By asking that question, this respondent made the point that termination based on a prenatal diagnosis for a non-life-threatening birth condition is not anymore indicative of an unethical act than in the case of a nonmedically complicated abortion. This respondent stated "...that does not mean you and I cannot have moral qualms about having created choices that can have untoward outcomes ...I think it's more important to ask these questions, but the answers are sometimes scarier than the questions." A clinician or medical establishment cannot threaten future parents and families who wish to terminate a future child prenatally diagnosed for a cleft lip, nor can they force future parents and families to terminate a pregnancy based on a prenatal diagnosis for a serious impairment. This respondent stated a concern that the "reproductive freedoms" not be "stripped of women who wish to terminate based on minor impairments," any more than they should be restricted for any other women.

In our interviews, we questioned whether younger or older future parents tended to terminate a pregnancy as a result of a positive prenatal diagnosis. In response, an experienced social worker who works in maternal and fetal medicine explained that "...the older families are the one's who usually terminate pregnancies ...they are able to realistically take into account the future ...while the younger future parents think about the here and now..." Although this social worker did not condone termination of pregnancy, the respondent held that the biomedical community does not do a thorough job of walking young future parents through the possible aftermath and long-term implications for themselves and their future child in continuing a pregnancy for a child that has been prenatally diagnosed with a condition. This respondent asserted that proper care is available to treat a majority of prenatally diagnosed conditions, but the long-term needs, actions, responsibilities, and abilities of young future parents rarely seem to emerge as a theme for discussion in their interactions with clinicians. Older future parents were portrayed as having a broader grasp of what is demanded from them in raising an affected child.

Through the advent and implementation of prenatal diagnostic technologies, the parental pregnancy experience was portrayed as changed over previous generations. The craniofacial surgeon interviewed felt that the craniofacial diagnosis is now often being shared with the parents 3–6 months earlier than it was when visualization was not possible. This surgeon stated that at some point in time parents are going to find out about the condition of their child, "so in a sense it [the prenatally diagnosed condition] is an earlier piece of information that they are going to find out about anyway." The surgeon stated that future parents and families struggle with their child's condition at some point, regardless if it is in the prenatal or the postnatal period. A prenatal diagnosis was portrayed as giving expectant parents extra time to prepare and to take action for their future child's health.

An affected adult with a surgically repaired cleft lip and palate confided his/her mother's personal experience with

pregnancy in the era before ultrasound diagnosis and how this mother reacted to the birth of an affected child. The respondent stated, "it's startling to give birth to a child who is different ... a good mother will not care that her child will appear different." This person's mother had a complicated pregnancy, and the respondent reflected that "she called the midwife, and they sat down and talked—the midwife told my mother she needed to decide if she really wanted to have the baby—'you need to decide right now because it is up in the air'—and of course my mother made her decision and from there everything was fine and she was ready. So it was not shocking for her to have a child who was different. What was shocking for her was how other people responded to me and she just pushed them all away." This respondent strongly urged clinicians to connect future parents with a stable person who has lived their life with a condition similar to that which was prenatally diagnosed. This person stated that it may also be helpful to talk with "other parents and learn what their life experience has been like." However, this person was aware the information provided by other parents is neither uniform nor predictable. This respondent stated that one parent may tell another parent, "you can do it" and "everything will be ok," whereas others may be less encouraging. Overall, the input from other parents and affected adults was seen as helpful.

In the interviews, we explored the issue of whether parents may feel the need or the desire to utilize advancing technology to screen, test, and ultimately terminate a pregnancy for any prenatally detectable condition, regardless of its severity, simply in hopes of producing the most perfect child? One respondent proposed that ethical quandaries with prenatal diagnosis may place those involved on a "slippery slope." This person posed a hypothetical situation: "Let's say we have a way of determining that this child is not going to be taller than 5'4" ...you can agree that [height] presents lesser justification for termination than cleft lip or palate. And then you can say that cleft lip or palate presents less justification for termination than missing limbs or heart defects. We go up the slope again—who decides?"

Some respondents found this slippery slope argument in relation to prenatal diagnosis to be a most frustrating issue. They perceived that a clinician and hospital cannot make a woman carry a fetus to term with a prenatally diagnosed minor non-life-threatening condition, nor can they force a woman to terminate a fetus diagnosed with a severe life-threatening condition. This perspective led respondents to wonder if there can be any regulation of the implementation of advancing biomedical technologies. The medical social scientist suggested that, since we have a "for profit" health care system, restricting the "use of this technology would not only involve fighting the technological imperative, but also the capitalist imperative." This respondent defined the technological imperative as the progressive and inherent driving force to advance technological development and said, "once you create something useful, then it's inevitable that the technology will be improved upon and that the technology will impact multiple facets of our life ...it has its own force." This respondent also asserted, "if I can make money doing this, then

I am going to do it," concluding that "...the American medical system reflects us and our values, and you cannot stop these large forces...but it is helpful to manage discussion of this issue by talking about all of the processes before a crisis occurs."

The most controversial issue raised in the interviews was that of termination of pregnancy. Responses were varied, often reflecting physician uncertainty and the sober worries of clinicians. The surgeon questioned, "Am I going to be including a kid [for abortion] that we are not assessing correctly?" He reflected on some of the information exchanged at perinatal conferences that enhanced the ambiguity, and said "It is amazing sometimes to see how well kids do, that were expecting to do very poorly. You know the opposite is true as well...based on the information we had from a prenatal diagnosis, a child who was expected to do well, may, in fact, not be doing so well." The surgeon related his experience in working with a family which elected to terminate a pregnancy based on a prenatal diagnosis of fronto-nasal dysplasia, saying: "On some level I cannot be responsible for any final decision that the family makes...it really is up to them...If they were to ask me 'what should I do?' I would say 'let this child be born' and we will take care of it. But, often, they are not asking that question directly...they are trying to arm themselves with as much information as possible...and sometimes the problem is that there is only so much that can be said...it's all indirect evidence."

In this situation, after three long conversations with the family, the surgeon sensed that the parents were hanging on to the "unknowns." The surgeon reflected that "the defect was potentially mild, and I really tried emphasizing this with the family. Despite the fact the ultrasound showed the brain appeared normal, they could not handle a child with a potentially mild defect with the unknown possibility of a considerably bigger defect. This family was very concerned that their child would have neurological abnormalities and at some point when a physician is pushed to a wall, he or she cannot be one-hundred percent...so if a family makes a termination decision on this uncertainty there is really not much that can be done." In this case, the surgeon reported information from the ultrasonographer, indicated the family had decided to terminate the pregnancy, and "felt beaten because clearly this child could have had a very productive life and...they chose to terminate." The surgeon asserted that the clinician's responsibility is to the entire family, regardless of what future parents and families decide with respect to the course of their pregnancy. Despite personal opposition to pregnancy termination, this surgeon was "always willing to serve as an educator and supplier of information to the family." Although the surgeon felt that it was unfortunate this family decided to terminate based on the unknown extent of the anomaly, he still felt that he had fulfilled the obligations and responsibilities of a physician.

The experience of this family is illustrative of how the "unknowns" associated with a prenatal diagnosis can instill fear in anxious future parents. This family was clinging to the unknowns of their child's prognosis because the physician could not completely guarantee that this child would have no neurological abnormalities. In responding to the "unknowns" in prenatal diagnosis, some future parents prepare for the worst. They often are anxious and desire as much information as possible about the health of their child. Future parents may fear the idea that their child may be born with impairment and that they may not be able to control the outcome of their pregnancy.

Prenatal diagnosis apparently serves as a vehicle to potentially address some of the worries future parents and families may have. A woman can undergo a noninvasive three-dimensional ultrasound providing her with numerous details with respect to the health of the fetus. As the surgeon respondent said, "If you look at all ultrasounds, a minimal percentage detect anomalies...truthfully the value of ultrasound is not the small detection of anomalies that it detects; rather, its value lies in the majority of cases in which anomaly is not detected—it alleviates fear and shows nothing is wrong." Parents may not be at ease until they discover that their ultrasound results deem that nothing is problematic with the fetus.

As part of this pilot project, we asked affected persons about what they would do if they were an expectant parent whose unborn child was diagnosed with a craniofacial condition. One participant, an affected adult, revealed that he/she would have terminated his/her own pregnancy if he/she had had access to the results of his/her own sonogram prior to birth. Though a successful adult, this person stated, "The extent to which the stigma is deeply engrained...you know that the function of the group is to maintain its identity and exclude anything—the *other*. That is the core of the problem...the stigma is real, it's not as my mother would have me believe that it was a figment of my imagination. The resistance that you are up against through a part of your life is real. It is not psychosomatic. Whatever one can do to be within the norm can make life easier. In an ideal world, you would live in this society where the aesthetic was not so narrow. You would ideally live in a world where there is room for more differences, but we do not and apparently we never have."

Several affected persons voiced a critique of the goals of prenatal diagnostic technology and highlighted the impacts prenatal diagnosis and abortion may have on the lives of currently affected persons. Affected persons considered how prenatal diagnosis may affect the stigma associated with their own facial difference. They noted that while American society prides itself on the acceptance of individual difference, facial abnormality is something that, as a culture, we have not substantially come to accept. The idea that a person, after years of life experience, would retract his/her own life prior to birth (had the option been feasible), speaks of society's intolerance for the anomalous. Similarly, one affected person described experiences in the numerous schools attended while growing up: "I went to many different schools of different sizes, and no matter where I was there was always someone I knew who had a cleft lip or palate or some sort of facial anomaly. And I can guarantee that these kids did not hang out with one another. You can always observe kids of the same ethnicity and those with similar interests hanging out with one another. The kids with a facial deformity do not hang out with one another because they do not want to draw any more attention to themselves than they have to."

This participant related that the social stigma associated with a craniofacial condition makes the anomaly much worse than it actually is, but this person did observe some of the potential benefits of having a craniofacial condition. Although this person explained he/she would rather not possess the anomaly, he/she saw the condition as a positive challenge. With admirable self-confidence and reassurance, this adult stated the anomaly allowed many life-advantages. The respondent felt those with a facial disfigurement tend to be much more compassionate toward others and are able to read others extremely well. This aspect of resilience has been explored with themes in poetry and prose.[62] However, the reality of stigmatization and the social expectations around facial differences create a context within which prenatal diagnosis of a craniofacial condition may be followed by termination of pregnancy.

LEGAL ISSUES

Legal issues have on rare occasion arisen as a result of elevated expectations regarding the precision and conduct of prenatal medical professional practice. Childbearing is increasingly perceived by the public as a process with controllable risks in which health professionals are expected to assure the birth of healthy offspring. When physicians have not informed parents of the availability of a prenatal test, performed the test improperly, failed to refer, failed to act upon a positive finding, or neglected to inform the parents about the risk to the child, the courts have sometimes intervened.[63] Such legal actions, called "wrongful birth suits," are based upon the claim that parents have been deprived of the right to make an informed decision about the pregnancy. "Wrongful birth" judgments have concluded that the physician may be at fault for effectively depriving parents of their right to make an informed decision about maintaining or terminating the pregnancy.[64] The "wrongful birth" suits have sometimes resulted in large financial awards to cover the expenses of health care, personal supervision, and maintenance for handicapped persons, sometimes through their lifespan (Phillips vs. US, 1981).[65] The parents of the child generally receive such settlements, often with few guidelines for how the funds are to be spent.

The "wrongful life" suit differs from the "wrongful birth" suit. The "wrongful life" suit is the claim on the behalf of the child it might have been better not to have been born than to have been born disabled. This provides an affected child with the possibility of receiving compensation for the health and special care he/she will require in life. These settlements are recognition that the child is a person with rights, including rights to have been aborted or never conceived. The courts have had to weigh whether there are children who would be better off having never been born. They have considered if it is ever parent negligence to permit a fetus's birth given the life risks that the newborn would face (i.e., fetal cocaine or alcohol exposure). This is an area of debate, and the legal awards that attempt to compensate for a specific condition are very controversial.

As of July 1, 2006, Brody's Law in Alabama enables prosecutors to file charges against anyone who attacks a pregnant woman and thus harms her fetus. In Utah, a woman is serving 18 months probation after she refused a Caesarian section to save one of her twins who died in childbirth. In Wisconsin and South Dakota, pregnant women can be arrested for abusing alcohol or drugs that might injure her fetus. In Arkansas, legislators are considering legislation that would make it a crime for a pregnant woman to smoke cigarettes. In South Carolina, a woman is serving a 12-year prison term for killing her unborn child by smoking crack cocaine. The growth of fetal rights legislation has been notable (Rick Montgomery, McClatchy Newspapers, 7-10-06),[66] and some have felt that these laws are difficult to enforce, if enacted.

The ultimate issue raised by fetal life lawsuits concerns the determination of who is responsible for the costs of the care of children with special needs. If the medical professional might have taken action to prevent the child from being born, should he or she have done so? Is it a parental right to have information available upon which to base a decision about a child's birth? Should parents who do not choose to abort or protect an impaired fetus be liable to later be sued by the child? The development of genetic screening methods implies not only their use, but also the availability of accurate results and nonjudgmental follow-up counseling. When prenatal or genetic tests were unavailable, congenital anomaly risk was generally unknown, and there was less possibility of disagreement over professional responsibility. With the advent of readily available genetic and prenatal diagnostic testing, the expectations for professional skill and follow-up have become high. Litigation is now seen as a means to create accountability; however, legal action does not often resolve moral quandaries or ethical dilemmas.

When prenatal diagnosis is performed, the impaired fetus comes to be thought of as a "patient," even though unborn. It raises basic questions about the rights and responsibilities of the mother, the physician, and the fetus. Do fetuses have rights? Do the mother's interests override the interests of the fetus up to the point of viability? Do fetuses that are going to be carried to term have rights that protect them from injury? Is it possible for a parent or other person to knowingly injure a fetus, by neglect or substance abuse, and be liable for such injury? Can parental liability be broadened to presume that a fetus has the right to demand consistent and caring maternal behavior? Should an alcoholic mother be subject to suit from her child with fetal alcohol syndrome? One wonders whether physicians or parents who chose not to pursue prenatal diagnosis might eventually be subject to future liability.

What rights does the mother have to freedom and autonomy over herself? Does her right to self-determination override the rights of the fetus or the physician? Currently, it is widely held that mothers have the right to refuse prenatal diagnosis. This right may become problematic as prenatal diagnostic testing becomes routine medical practice and it is assumed that parents will desire such information and screening. The potential for maternal-fetal rights conflicts is embedded in how the law has responded to decision-making around prenatal diagnosis.

IMPLICATIONS FOR CRANIOFACIAL CENTERS AND SOCIETY

Craniofacial centers can be places to assist families in understanding and responding to early diagnostic and prenatal information. The centers can help parents of yet unborn children evaluate the condition of their fetus, and they can help to project the range of possibilities that might occur in their child's life. They can help lighten the load of parents bearing internet printouts about their baby's condition by guiding their search, by assuring that their data is accurate, and by interpreting information. The centers can help the many families for whom prenatal diagnostic data may just be too much information to handle on their own. They can be constantly aware their medical advice in the delicate aftermath of prenatal diagnosis may easily sway a family's perspectives about a pregnancy. They must be careful to be neutral, nonjudgmental, and accurate. They can help a family assess whether a child with a less than perfect body or face could thrive in their home. They can help a family that has decided to bear an affected child to see the future in hopeful terms. The craniofacial team's ability to manage prenatal diagnostic and future genome technologies will depend upon their insight, their wisdom, and their vision of what constitutes a good life.

Only a limited number of craniofacial centers or teams includes the active and routine involvement of geneticists, genetic counselors, or specialists in fetal medicine. As unborn fetuses with clefts are detected, parents will seek the advice of the craniofacial team. It will be important that genetic counseling be accessible and that the genetic advisors be well informed about treatment options for the condition that has been detected. Furthermore, parents may seek input from other families that have managed similar prenatal diagnoses or from affected adults. The craniofacial center is in a position to offer parent-to-parent referrals and to assure that the family can locate effective advisors.

Research is needed to clarify the issues surrounding early starts about the prenatal cleft and craniofacial diagnosis from the vantage point of the diagnosticians, parents, affected persons, and craniofacial treatment teams. Prenatal diagnosis affords teams an opportunity to set priorities in early cleft care by choosing to look at the prenatal diagnostic encounter as the earliest possible moment to provide care and to establish positive ideas about the birth and future life of a child with a cleft. Centers have the opportunity to build strength and resilience in families choosing to bear a child with a cleft, and they can also make a statement that we, as a society, value human diversity. Centers can demonstrate that they respect people with differences and realize prejudice and stigma are ways to reduce human potential. For the sake of our culture and our society, craniofacial centers working with new parents carry the responsibility of conveying the rightness of human variation and human difference. If professionals can find the beauty and meaning in human difference, they can provide people who possess such difference with the acceptance and sense of rightness which will arm them for the difficult moments of growing up. It is a gift for craniofacial centers to provide support early, even before birth, and to set their goals as being supportive, kind, and positive from the very first family encounter.

On a societal and cultural level, supporting parents who have had a prenatal diagnosis of a cleft lip or palate has great merit. Helping families to see the value in having a child with a facial difference is an enormous statement of the faith health professionals have that they can help to provide a high quality of life for the child as he or she grows up. Having powerful surgical and other therapeutic approaches that produce outstanding clinical results is essential. Coordinated clinical team care reduces the number of interventions required for a child and generally results in improved clinical outcomes and cost savings. The concept of team care requires professionals to perceive the child with a facial difference as fundamentally of value and worthy of investment by a group of well-prepared and eager health professionals who project realistic goals and who can guide the family through the process of care.

A caveat is worth noting: Not all parents will decide to bear a child with a facial difference. Some will be fearful that the condition is more serious than has been estimated or will find the ambiguity unmanageable. Other parents will firmly believe that "trying again for an unaffected child" is their best course of action. Some parents will face much more dire diagnoses than cleft lip/palate and may feel compelled, sometimes even against personal moral values, to seek termination of the pregnancy. Craniofacial centers and society-at-large must be aware of how difficult such prenatal parental decisions are and must accept parental judgment as valid and appropriate. Support for parents who are making difficult determinations is essential.

On a broader societal level, questions will arise regarding the basic worth of children and adults with facial differences. If we find the live birth rates and incidence of cleft lip declining, we can ask whether increasing numbers of affected fetuses are being aborted. If that becomes the case, then we may find ourselves questioning the eugenic implications of prenatal diagnosis. We will also see a declining need for craniofacial teams or centers. Will prenatal diagnosis of clefts contribute to the notion that birth is predicable and children are perfectible? Will prenatal diagnosis diminish or inflate the stigmatization directed at affected children and adults? Will affected individuals perceive themselves as accepted or merely tolerated by their peers and society? How we respond to congenital human difference makes a fundamental statement about our moral, spiritual, and cultural foundations and beliefs.

References

1. Canady JW. Emotional effects of plastic surgery on the adolescent with a cleft. *Cleft Palate Craniofac J* 32:120, 1995.

2. Edwards TC, Huebner CE, Connell FA, et al. Adolescent quality of life, part I: Conceptual and measurement model. *J Adolesc* 25:275, 2002.

3. Heller A, Tidmarsh W, Pless IB. The psychosocial functioning of young adults born with cleft lip or palate: A follow-up study. *Clin Pediatr (Phila)* 20:459, 1981.

4. Kapp-Simon KA, McGuire DE. Observed social interaction patterns in adolescents with and without craniofacial conditions. *Cleft Palate Craniofac J* 34:380, 1997.

5. Kapp-Simon KA, Simon DJ, Kristovich S. Self-perception, social skills, adjustment, and inhibition in young adolescents with craniofacial anomalies. *Cleft Palate Craniofac J* 29:352, 1992.

6. McQuaid D, Barton J, Campbell EA. Body image issues for children and adolescents with burns. *J Burn Care Rehabil* 21:194, 2000.

7. Patrick DL, Edwards TC, Topolski TD. Adolescent quality of life, part II: Initial validation of a new instrument. *J Adolesc* 25:287, 2002.

8. Pope AW, Ward J. Factors associated with peer social competence in preadolescents with craniofacial anomalies. *J Pediatr Psychol* 22:455, 1997.

9. Richman LC. Self-reported social, speech, and facial concerns and personality adjustment of adolescents with cleft lip and palate. *Cleft Palate J* 20:108, 1983.

10. Richman LC, Holmes CS, Eliason MJ. Adolescents with cleft lip and palate: Self-perceptions of appearance and behavior related to personality adjustment. *Cleft Palate J* 22:93, 1985.

11. Strauss, RP, Broder H, Helms RW. Perceptions of appearance and speech in adolescent patients with cleft lip and palate and by their parents. *Cleft Palate J* 25:335, 1988.

12. Topolski TD, Patrick DL, Edwards TC, et al. Quality of life and health-risk behaviors among adolescents. *J Adolesc Health* 29:426, 2001.

13. Verhulst FC, van der Ende J. Agreement between parents' reports and adolescents' self-reports of problem behavior. *J Child Psychol Psychiatry* 33:1011, 1992.

14. Berk NW, Cooper ME, Liu Y, et al. Social anxiety in Chinese adults with oral-facial clefts. *Cleft Palate Craniofac J* 38:126, 2001.

15. Endriga MC, Kapp-Simon KA. Psychological issues in craniofacial care: State of the art. *Cleft Palate Craniofac J* 36:3, 1999.

16. Lansdown R, Rumsey N, Bradbury E, et al. *Visibly Different: Coping with Disfigurement.* Oxford, UK: Butterworth-Heinemann, 1997.

17. Leonard BJ, Boust JD, Abrahams G, et al. Self-concept of children with cleft lip and/or palate. *Cleft Palate Craniofac J* 28:347, 1991.

18. Marcusson A, Akerlind I, Paulin G. Quality of life in adults with repaired complete cleft lip and palate. *Cleft Palate Craniofac J* 38:379, 2001.

19. Pope AW, Snyder HT. Psychosocial adjustment in children and adolescents with a craniofacial anomaly: Age and sex patterns. *Cleft Palate Craniofac J* 42:349, 2005.

20. Slifer KJ, Amari A, Diver T, et al. Social interaction patterns of children and adolescents with and without oral clefts during a video-taped analogue social encounter. *Cleft Palate Craniofac J* 441:175, 2004.

21. Turner SR, Thomas PW, Dowell T, et al. Psychological outcomes amongst cleft patients and their families. *Br J Plast Surg* 50:1, 1997.

22. Blakeney P. School reintegration. In Tarnowski KJ (ed). *Behavioral Aspects of Pediatric Burns.* New York: Plenum Press, 1994.

23. Broder HL, Richman LC, Matheson PB. Learning disability, school achievement, and grade retention among children with cleft: A two-center study. *Cleft Palate Craniofac J* 35:127, 1998.

24. Bull R, Rumsey N. *The Social Psychology of Facial Appearance.* New York: Springer-Verlag, 1988.

25. Goffman E. *Stigma-Notes on the Management of Spoiled Identity.* New Jersey: Prentice-Hall, Inc., 1963.

26. Kelton RW. Facing up to stigma: Workplace and personal strategies. *Cleft Palate Craniofac J* 38:245, 2001.

27. Richman LC, Millard T. Brief report: Cleft lip and palate: Longitudinal behavior and relationships of cleft conditions to behavior and achievement. *J Pediatr Psychol* 22:487, 1997.

28. Richman LC, Harper DC. School adjustment of children with observable disabilities. *J Abnorm Child Psychol* 6:11, 1978.

29. Speltz ML, Morton K, Goodell EW, et al. Psychological functioning of children with craniofacial anomalies and their mothers: Follow-up from late infancy to school entry. *Cleft Palate Craniofac J* 30:482, 1993.

30. Tobiasen JM, Levy J, Carpenter MA, et al. Type of facial cleft, associated congenital malformations, and parents' ratings of school and conduct problems. *Cleft Palate J* 24:209, 1987.

31. Topolski TD, Edwards TC, Patrick DL. Quality of life: How do adolescents with facial differences compare with other adolescents? *Cleft Palate Craniofac J* 42:25, 2005.

32. Edwards TC, Patrick DL, Topolski TD, et al. Approaches to craniofacial-specific quality of life assessment in adolescents. *Cleft Palate Craniofac J* 42:19, 2005.

33. Harper DC. Children's attitudes to physical differences among youth from western and non-western cultures. *Cleft Palate Craniofac J* 32:114, 1995.

34. Okkerse JM, Beemer FA, Cordia-de Haan M, et al. Facial attractiveness and facial impairment ratings in children with craniofacial malformations. *Cleft Palate Craniofac J* 38:386, 2001.

35. Reed J, Robathan M, Hockenhull A, et al. Children's attitudes toward interacting with peers with different craniofacial anomalies. *Cleft Palate Craniofac J* 36:441, 1999.

36. Broder HL. Psychological research of children with craniofacial anomalies: Review, critique, and implications for the future. *Cleft Palate Craniofac J* 34:402, 1997.

37. Eiserman W. Unique outcomes and positive contributions associated with facial difference: Expanding research and practice. *Cleft Palate Craniofac J* 38:236, 2001.

38. Millard T, Richman LC. Different cleft conditions, facial appearance, and speech: Relationship to psychological variables. *Cleft Palate Craniofac J* 38:68, 2001.

39. Langlois JH, Kalakanis L, Rubenstein AJ, et al. Maxims or myths of beauty? A meta-analytic and theoretical review. *Psychol Bull* 126:390, 2000.

40. Partridge J. *Changing Faces: The Challenge of Facial Disfigurement,* 3rd edn. London: Changing faces, 1997.

41. Patterson DR, Everett JJ, Bombardier CH, et al. Psychological effects of severe burn injuries. *Psychol Bull* 113:362, 1993.

42. Sarimski K. Social adjustment of children with a severe craniofacial anomaly (Apert syndrome). *Child Care Health Dev* 27:583, 2001.

43. Thomas PT, Turner SR, Rumsey N, et al. Satisfaction with facial appearance among subjects affected by a cleft. *Cleft Palate Craniofac J* 34:226, 1997.

44. Bosk CL. *All God's Mistakes: Genetic Counseling in a Pediatric Hospital.* Chicago: University of Chicago Press, 1992.

45. Taylor JS. The public life of the fetal sonogram and the work of the sonographer. *J Diagnostic Med Sonography* 18:367, 2002.

46. Taylor JS. Image of contradiction: Obstetrical ultrasound in American Culture. In Franklin S, Ragone H (eds). *Reproducing Reproduction: Kinship, Power and Technological Innovation.* Philadelphia: University of Pennsylvania Press, 1998, pp. 15–45.

47. Eng C, Schechter C, Rabinowitz T, et al. Prenatal genetic carrier testing using triple disease screening. *JAMA* 278:1268, 1997.

48. Wexler A. *Mapping Fate: A Memoir if Family, Risk, and Genetic Research.* New York: Random House, 1995.

49. Strauss RP. Ethical and social concerns in facial surgical decision making. *Plast Reconstr Surg* 72:727, 1983.

50. Rothman BK. *The Tentative Pregnancy: Prenatal Diagnosis and the Future of Motherhood.* New York: Viking, 1986.

51. Murray TH, Botkin JR. Genetic testing and screening: Ethical issues. In Reich WT (ed). *Encyclopedia of Bioethics.* Revised. New York: Simon & Schuster, 1995, p. 174.

52. Blumenfeld Z, Blumenfeld I, Bronshtein M. The early prenatal diagnosis of cleft lip and the decision-making process. *Cleft Palate Craniofac J* 36:105, 1999.

53. Jones MC. Prenatal diagnosis of cleft lip and palate: Experiences in southern California. *Cleft Palate Craniofac J* 36:107, 1999.

54. Eiserman W, Strauss RP. The early prenatal diagnosis of cleft lip and the decision-making process. *Cleft Palate Craniofac J* 36:542, 1999.

55. Bronshtein M, Blumenfeld I, Blumenfeld Z. Early prenatal diagnosis of cleft lip and its potential impact on the number ob babies with cleft lip. *Br J Oral Maxillofac Surg* 34:486, 1996.

56. Malone FD, Canick JA, Ball RH, et al. First-trimester or second-trimester screening or both, for Down's syndrome. *N Engl J Med* 353:2001, 2005.

57. Wapner R, Thom E, Simpson JL, et al. First-trimester screening for Trisomies 21 and 18. *N Engl J Med* 349:1405, 2003.

58. Caruso TM, Westgate MN, Holmes LB. Impact of prenatal screening on the birth status of fetuses with Down syndrome at an urban hospital, 1972–1994. *Genet Med* 1:22, 1998.

59. Wertz DC, Fletcher JC (eds). *Ethics and Human Genetics: A Cross Cultural Perspective.* Berlin: Springer-Verlag, 1989.

60. Marteau T. Revealed identity: A study of the process of genetic counseling. *Soc Sci Med* 47:1653, 1998.

61. Weaver KD. Genetic screening and the right not to know. *Issues Law Med* 13:243, 1997.

62. Strauss RP, Fenson C. Experiencing the "good life": Literary views of craniofacial conditions and quality of life. *Cleft Palate Craniofac J* 42:14, 2005.

63. Lambert T. Tort liability for inadequate genetic counseling. *ATLA Law Reporter* 26:106, 1983.

64. Annas GJ, Elias S. Perspectives on fetal surgery. On the road from experimentation to therapy (and what to do when we arrive). In Milunsky A, Annas GJ (eds). *Genetics and the Law, III.* New York: Plenum Press, 1985, pp. 347–363.

65. Phillips v US, 508 F. Supp. 544 (S.C.), 1981.

66. Montgomery R, McClatchy Newspapers, printed in the Raleigh News and Observer, Jul 10, 2006.

Outcomes, Research, and Team Care

Fundamentals of Team Care

Marilyn A. Cohen, BA

INTRODUCTION

Advances in technology and refinements in surgery, dentistry, and speech pathology, together with a better understanding of the psychological and educational needs of a child born with a cleft, have allowed affected individuals a chance at a normal life. The care of such individuals has been further advanced through the establishment of multidisciplinary teams for evaluation and management throughout the world. Although the American Cleft Palate-Craniofacial Association (ACPA) established basic standards for cleft and craniofacial teams in the mid-1990s, interdisciplinary teams continue to be as diverse as the populations they serve.[1–3]

Until the dawn of the twentieth century, habilitation of an individual with a cleft was largely the responsibility of the surgeon. Although the need for other specialists to address several of the associated sequelae of clefts is noted in the literature, the true need for collaborative efforts in the management of affected individuals was not documented until the late 1930s.[4,5]

The availability of materials such as steel and rubber in the late 1800s and a more widespread use of x-rays in the early 1900s led to the development of additional nonsurgical management techniques for cleft lip and palate.[6] It was, perhaps, the availability of these relatively new materials and methods, together with the emergence of orthodontics as a dental specialty that led to the eventual emergence of cleft teams in the middle of the twentieth century. Although early textbooks on surgical management alluded to some of the sequelae of cleft lip and palate, it was not until the establishment of the first cleft palate team in the United States by Dr. Herbert Cooper of Lancaster that the need to manage these sequelae in a systematic and coordinated fashion was recognized. Cooper recognized that a cleft of the lip and/or palate could essentially become a crippling problem unless the associated complications were adequately managed. The need for a team approach was further recognized by Dr. Cloyd Harkins, a dentist, and Dr. Koepp-Baker, a speech pathologist. In the early 1940s, Harkins and Koepp-Baker offered practitioners the first interdisciplinary course dealing with nonsurgical management of cleft lip and palate. The course was one of the pivotal events leading to the establishment of the ACPA in 1943 as an educational society. These two practitioners recognized the need for various unrelated specialties to understand a similar nomenclature and to work in a collaborative fashion.[7,8]

Currently, over two hundred teams established to care for individuals with clefts and craniofacial anomalies are listed in the ACPA directory. Few of these teams would exist today without the pioneers in the field and the recognition that interdisciplinary collaboration and understanding is essential to cleft care. As teams evolved, so did an understanding and recognition of the sequelae associated with these birth defects. The acknowledgment of these associated problems ultimately advanced and expanded the composition of the cleft palate teams of today.

TEAM COMPOSITION

Although the composition of a cleft team may vary from center to center, it is generally agreed that, at the very least, teams should comprise a surgeon, orthodontist, speech pathologist, and coordinator. Without these basic disciplines, the major problems associated with orofacial clefts cannot be evaluated or treated. It is also extremely important that these basic disciplines work in a coordinated fashion and understand a basic nomenclature. Although surgery, orthodontics, and speech pathology are disciplines fundamental to cleft care, it is now widely understood that a more holistic treatment for individuals with clefts is needed. The *Parameters for Evaluation and Treatment of Patients with Cleft Lip-Palate and Other Craniofacial Anomalies*, adopted by a consensus conference in the 1990s by ACPA, essentially states that the care of individuals with clefts should be coordinated, interdisciplinary, longitudinal, and family-centered and that it should address the developmental and psychological needs of the affected individuals.[9] As a result of such understanding, the ACPA membership currently reflects specialists from over twenty separate medical and basic science fields.

Recognition of the importance of team care has led to legislative reform in some states. The state of New Jersey, for example, reformed its methods of providing and paying for cleft care through its Division of Maternal Child Health Services in 1979. As a part of that reform, the state established that care should be provided in centers with cleft teams comprising the following specialties: speech pathology, audiology, otolaryngology, plastic surgery, dentistry, orthodontics, pediatrics, social work, and psychology. New Jersey further established that consulting services from craniofacial surgery, oral-maxillofacial surgery, radiology, anesthesiology, cardiology, genetics, psychiatry, prosthetics, nursing, neurology, neurosurgery, and ophthalmology be available to children in the event that further diagnostic testing is needed as a part of their care. Recognizing the need to coordinate or orchestrate the services required by children with clefts, the state requires each team to have a designated coordinator and a medical di-

rector. The results of evaluations and recommendations provided by the team must be communicated to families using an individual plan of care that includes long- and short-term goals for each patient evaluated. It is also recommended that these long- and short-term goals be revised on a longitudinal basis. Although the basic standards for the composition of a cleft team have been established by ACPA and governmental agencies dealing with maternal and child health issues, the specialties represented on a team and the functioning of that team are dependent on its practitioners, the number of patients evaluated and treated, and the availability of appropriate funding.[10]

FUNDAMENTALS OF TEAM CARE

The actual fundamentals of team care are primarily dictated by the needs of children with clefts of the lip and/or palate and of their families. Early parental education about this birth defect and its expected outcome over the developmental continuum is, perhaps, one of the most fundamental roles of the team. Since many clefts are now diagnosed prenatally, a mechanism for counseling and reassurance by at least one member of the cleft team is indicated. Once a child is born, the team should establish a mechanism for early outreach and feeding education, especially for families of infants born in community-based hospitals without cleft teams. In addition to direct patient care, a primary function of the team is to serve as a resource for community-based practitioners treating patients with clefts. Essential to team care is effective communication between specialists from multiple disciplines, patients, and their families. It is therefore essential that services be provided in a culturally competent setting where differences in language and culture are taken in to consideration together with the medical needs of the patient. The psychological and social needs of the patient throughout the developmental continuum must always remain in the forefront of team services.

Teams should be organized to include specialists and allied health professionals, especially a designated patient care coordinator who helps to facilitate patient care and team interaction. This individual also ensures the provision of coordinated care for patients and families, assisting them in understanding, coordinating, and implementing treatment plans. The team members should be qualified by virtue of their education, experience, and credentials to provide appropriate care and to maintain current practice standards. The team should include (or have the ability to refer patients to) other healthcare professionals as required to meet their individual needs. These professionals must include individuals who provide services in mental health, psychology, audiology, genetics, general and pediatric dentistry, otolaryngology, pediatrics, and/or primary care.

Ideally, teams should meet on a regular face-to-face basis in order to provide interdisciplinary collaboration in the evaluation and treatment of each patient. A mechanism to provide communication with professionals treating patients outside the team setting should also be in place. In addition, a mechanism for referring patients to and receiving information from community-based providers, such as local speech-language pathologists, orthodontists, and mental health professionals, is essential. The proper sequencing of evaluations and treatments should be coordinated within a framework of the patient's overall developmental, medical, and psychological needs. Each patient followed by the team should have a comprehensive and shared record that includes findings and recommendations from each comprehensive evaluation as well as specific specialty records. The basic patient record should include a general medical history, social and psychological history, medical diagnosis, written treatment plans, dental and orthodontic findings, patient photographs, and radiographic findings. The team should also have a mechanism or process to share treatment plans (with the consent of patient and/or family) with other medical professionals outside the team, such as school nurses, counselors, and community-based speech pathologists. Moreover, teams should have resources and mechanisms that ensure delivery of care with sensitivity to the linguistic, cultural, ethnic, psychological, economic, and physical factors that may affect the dynamic relationships between the team, the patient, and the patient's family.

Fundamental to team care is a critical assessment of outcomes both for the types and extent of procedures employed to treat individuals and for the team practices in general. Therefore, a mechanism should be in place to monitor the short- and long-term outcomes for individual patients, including their psychosocial well-being in the context of their family and school. In addition to monitoring the outcomes of patient care, teams should have a performance improvement plan in place that includes periodic peer review of their clinical outcome data.[11]

PERFORMANCE IMPROVEMENT AND DATA COLLECTION

Since many teams are based in hospital settings and most institutions require performance monitoring, the systematic collection of data pertinent to cleft treatment is an essential part of the team's function. It is therefore recommended that patient data, at a minimum, include patient demographic and operative summaries. The use of a database that will enable the team to query this specific information about its cohort of patients is essential for both performance improvement and the monitoring of treatment outcomes. There are numerous software systems commercially available for this; however, it is suggested that the best system available be discussed with institutional information technology departments. It is also suggested (and, in fact, required by some governmental funding agencies for teams in the United States) that a system be put into place for consumer comment. In the author's institution, questionnaires are given to patients and their families on an annual basis at the time of their team evaluation. This information is then summarized and shared with team members and governmental funding agencies. The results of these evaluations can lead to modifications in the manner in which team care is provided and to an overall improvement of service provision.

CONCLUSION

The last seventy years have demonstrated that cleft care is best accomplished in a team setting. The availability of team care since the late 1930s has greatly contributed to a better understanding of the overall needs of individuals with clefts over the developmental continuum. This is particularly well demonstrated when one reviews the literature about clefts over the past several decades. The literature prior to 1950s primarily[12] described modifications related to techniques of surgical repair. Literature after the 1950s reflects the expansion of the cleft team and an understanding of the need for a holistic approach. This more recent literature, which reflects the expansion of the cleft team, includes papers that address the psychological and educational needs of individuals, recognition of middle ear disease and its effects on hearing, the effects of cleft surgery on facial growth, speech, and dental alignment. The goal of team care is a streamlined delivery system that ensures coordinated interdisciplinary care and that addresses the psychosocial, medical, dental, speech, hearing, and developmental needs of an individual born with an orofacial cleft.

The future of team care and its holistic approach to the habilitation of individuals born with clefts may well be dependent on our ability to prove its efficacy. The ability of diverse specialties to understand a similar nomenclature and to work in a collaborative fashion may well provide the framework for the documentation of the outcome evaluations needed to prove that team care is indeed the best practice. Current medical economics, especially in the United States, dictates the need for evidenced-based practice. The interdisciplinary structure of the cleft team is perhaps the best place to begin the evaluation process across disciplines. The fundamentals of team care have thus far been built on a strong hypothesis that interdisciplinary care is the best practice. The future of team care will be dependent on our ability to prove this hypothesis through both retrospective and prospective interdisciplinary studies.

References

1. American Cleft Palate Association. The cleft and craniofacial team. *ACPA Publication* 1996.
2. Strauss RP. Cleft and craniofacial teams in the United States and Canada. *Cleft Palate J* 35(6):473–480, 1998.
3. Strauss RP. The organization and delivery of craniofacial health services: The state of the art. *Cleft Palate J* 36(3):189–195, 1999.
4. Cooper H, Harding R, Krogman W, et al. *Cleft Lip and Cleft Palate: A Team Approach to Clinical Management and Rehabilitation of the Patient.* Philadelphia: W.B. Saunders Co., 1979.
5. Brophy T. *Harelip Cleft Palate: Oral Surgery.* Philadelphia: P. Blakistons Son & Co., 1915, pp. 506–736.
6. Case C. *Dental Orthopedia and Prosthetic Correction of Cleft Palate.* Chicago: CS Case Company, 1921.

7. Wells C. The American Cleft Palate Association: Its first 36 years. *Cleft Palate J* 16(1):86–123, 1979.

8. Richman L. Presidents' perceptions: A historic review of fifty years of the American Cleft Palate-Craniofacial Association. *Cleft Palate J* 30(6):521–527, 1993.

9. American Cleft Palate Association. Parameters for evaluation and treatment of patients with cleft lip/palate or other craniofacial anomalies. *ACPA Publication* 2000.

10. State of New Jersey. New Jersey special child and adult health services criteria for funding for centers providing evaluation and treatment services of cleft lip and-or palate and craniofacial anomalies. *New Jersey Publication* 2000.

11. American Cleft Palate-Craniofacial Association Draft Standards, 2007.

12. McDowell F. *Plastic Surgery*. Austin: Silvergirl, Inc. 1977, pp. 114–206.

International Missions—Cleft Care

Randy Sherman, MD, FACS • Bill Magee, MD, DDS

INTRODUCTION

Cleft care has evolved in such a way as to reflect the best that medicine has to offer. Through a highly coordinated team approach; populated by skilled professionals bringing very different competencies, listening, and adjusting their therapies as each patient's condition changes with growth and various comorbidities, the cleft team becomes truly transformative to a patient, his family and their community. A modern plastic surgeon, fully trained and newly minted by his or her national board, is deemed competent to accurately evaluate and perform appropriate corrective surgery for cleft lip and palate deformities as well as other various congenital and acquired maladies. Of course, even in the best of circumstances, the practitioner would never be able to achieve that goal without

the numerous medical, nursing and therapy personnel, instruments, facilities, funding, and follow up which make up the modern healthcare practice environment. Take away the above, as well as political stability, personal security, and reliable social service infrastructure, and the task of performing surgery becomes nearly impossible. It would be like asking a pilot to deliver passengers safely to a distant location without plane, fuel, runways, and control towers. Skilled professional attributes cannot take a plastic surgeon far at all without the aid and assistance of the entire delivery system. Such is the plight of the itinerant, well-intentioned cleft surgeon without a comparable mission team and structure.

Success in the execution of international cleft missions can be graded on many scales. Clearly, the most declarative claim of victory occurs at the moment a cleft lip repair is completed safely and precisely. To those children operated upon and their families, this event is no less than a magical gate which they pass through. To those fortunate physicians privileged to provide the gift, there is no greater professional reward. As plastic surgeons, our specialty has relied on pre and postoperative photographs of children with clefts to symbolize all that the pursuit of plastic surgery represents. How many young medical students have been drawn to this discipline after observing this procedure firsthand or seeing the results in a textbook? How many individuals of a philanthropic mind and heart have opened their purses towards the support of this work after witnessing these compelling pictures? Of course, our professional community judges success on a much more graduated scale. Current outcome measures for patients treated with this spectrum of deformities include, but are not limited to, multiple measures of lip and nasal aesthetics, dynamic perioral function, palatal closure complication rates, dental and alveolar abnormalities, speech and velopharyngeal sphincter function, subsequent midfacial growth, etc.

Peer critiques regarding the effectiveness of surgical missions have rightfully focussed on: (1) the quality of personnel involved in mission care delivery, (2) the lack of effective follow up care and absence of measurable outcomes, and (3) the paucity of local sustainability in the form of appropriately trained medical and other healthcare personnel. Given the adversarial circumstances, which engender the need for surgical mission programs in the first place, progress towards meeting such benchmarks of success can be agonizingly slow. Many organizations have significantly de-emphasized surgical mission work or abandoned it all together because of the many logistical obstacles inherent in trying to provide comprehensive cleft care in such hostile environments. Those that vilify international voluntary cleft surgical programs, on the basis of a suboptimal compliance with comprehensive cleft care paradigms practiced in well funded, stable western referral centers, should instead invest their energies in finding solutions to attack this entirely treatable but seemingly intractable global endemic disease.

HISTORY

Scholars have long argued as to the origins of planned excursions by missionaries in order to bring medical care and alleviate suffering to foreign populations in need. Most would agree that those who ventured forth early in the history of medical missions did so in the context of a religious Ministry.[1] Dr. David Livingstone, a native of Glasgow, representing the Presbyterian Church of Scotland, became synonymous with the modern medical missionary, bringing his skills, sense of adventure, and western view of the world to several locations in central and southern Africa. He fought endemic diseases, taught hygiene techniques, and tried to change attitudes towards disease and healing. While he persevered many privations working in the remote region now known as Malawi, and fell far short of his goals in many respects, prematurely succumbing to endemic malaria, he became iconic in this endeavor, and eventually symbolized the missionary doctor well through the modern age.[2]

Formally-organized units followed shortly with the establishment of the Edinburgh Medical Missionary Society in 1841 with a transcribed record of 40 physicians in the field by 1849. The Lutheran medical missions, because of their focus on providing medical care to whatever extent it could be delivered, were able to penetrate Zululand in present day South Africa where other ministries failed. A world missionary conference convened in Edinburgh in 1910, drew so much attention to the concerns of those physicians dedicating themselves to healthcare delivery, that a separate session was held to exclusively address their concerns. By 1925, the Protestant missions' organization recorded 1157 doctors and 1007 nurses in the field widely distributed over Africa and Asia.[3]

Massive displacement of populations during the great wars of the nineteenth and twentieth century led to establishment of several aid organizations which took it upon themselves to provide rudimentary healthcare to these otherwise hopeless refugees. The Red Cross Movement—best known among all—was begun in the mid-1800, by Henry Dunant after witnessing the carnage of battle outside the Italian town of Solferino. The Geneva Convention of 1864 chartered the International Committee of the Red Cross, providing tangible evidence worn by all aid workers of their special and protected status. In the United States, Clara Barton founded the American Red Cross in 1881. The American Red Cross has grown over succeeding decades; and now, well over a century old, has become our premiere healthcare support provider in times of natural or manmade disaster.[4]

While stories of harrowing individual efforts to treat both medical and surgical disease by volunteers around the world abound, the advent of modern international surgical missions did not evolve until well into the last half of the twentieth century. Throughout the majority of the last century, attempts to provide surgical relief internationally were limited by several factors. The evolution of medical knowledge, as well as surgical procedural safety and effectiveness, did not begin its remarkably rapid acceleration until the late 50s and early 60s. Safe and reliable anesthetic administration emerged early as a significant limiting factor on the success of any such endeavor. Other challenges included the ability to travel rapidly to remote locations, the capacity to move precious supplies without cargo being pilfered or stolen, and the recognition that some basic, sustainable social infrastructure on the receiving end would have to be built and maintained to allow these efforts to have any lasting effect.

One of the first organizations to successfully piece together all of the components needed to deliver medical care to the bush was the Flying Doctors of East Africa, otherwise known as the African Medical and Research Foundation (AMREF). Established in 1957 by Drs. Michael Wood of Nairobi, Thomas Rees of New York, and Sir Archibald McIndoe of Britain, this pioneering group of plastic surgeons built a flexible and responsive system of medical volunteers, support personnel, aircraft capabilities, supply delivery, and development expertise. What started out as a group of highly motivated volunteers traveling to remote areas to deliver otherwise unobtainable medical care, has now grown into a sophisticated, mostly African run healthcare delivery organization concentrating on endemic disease treatment and prevention, including but not limited to HIV/AIDS, malaria, and cholera. The Flying Doctors Service, currently serving as a medical evacuation platform, has a proud history if transporting medical teams into the bush to perform lifesaving surgery. Many notable plastic surgeons participated in these most valiant efforts. Cleft lip and palate surgeries were one of several procedures offered by those who were appropriately trained. Operating rooms and hospital facilities were constructed by local missionary groups and were rudimentary at best. Despite their valiant efforts, occasional perianesthetic morbidity and mortality presaged the problems that would be faced by similar minded organizations even to the present day. Significant obstacles were not only confined to building a safe and effective perioperative environment but, just as importantly, in getting teams into the field. Recounting the development of AMREF in his autobiography, Dr. Thomas Rees included a letter sent from his administrator to a prospective site at the mission in Shirati on the southern shore of Lake Victoria. It read:

AFRICAN MEDICAL AND RESEARCH FOUNDATION
On Feb. 6, 1960, Drs. Michael Wood and Thomas Rees will visit your hospital.

We would be grateful if you could confirm these dates and let us have an operation list at least a week before the projected visits with these details:

(I) Amount of low clouds, if any

(II) Thunderstorms in the vicinity or any rain

(III) Visibility: Smoke haze from bush fires, etc.

Please check the airstrip as follows:

1) Length of grass. If it is long or tufted, please cut it and remove hard tufts.

2) Inspect for and remove ant hills. Fill any holes.

3) Mark all trees and sisal poles, particularly on the approaches.

4) Windsock. If none available, light a small fire.

5) If your strip is murram or earth with little or no grass cover, overnight or recent rain will cause difficulty in bringing the aircraft to a stop. Drive your Land Rover or car up the whole length of the strip and apply the brakes fully; if the wheels lock and the vehicle skids or leaves deep tracks, the strip is probably unserviceable.

6) If for any reason the airstrip is unserviceable, place white crosses in the middle and at either end – cloth or pieces of wood, iron, etc., will do so long as they can be easily seen.

7) Keep all cattle and local inhabitants completely away from the strip when the aircraft is due to arrive. It is most important that all school children should be kept well back from the path of the aircraft: if a tyre should burst, the aircraft might go out of control and run into spectators causing loss of life and/or serious injury.[5]

While most transportation issues in today's international surgical mission work have evolved considerably from AMREF's early efforts as described above, logistical challenges continue to constitute the largest and most intractable obsta-

cles. Unfortunately, those difficulties are mostly man-made with limitations in technology playing an ever-diminishing role.

In 1969, under the leadership of Donald Laub at Stanford University, Interplast was born. This organization ushered in the modern era of mission-based, comprehensive cleft care, with focused, fully manned and equipped surgical teams delivering a recurring care package to a targeted locality and population. Interplast developed sites in Latin America, Africa, and Asia with the specific intention of delivering safe and effective cleft care, concentrating on providing the highest quality of surgical repair possible.

Over time, they realized the increasing importance of surgical education in sustaining these programs. Because of his leadership role in plastic surgical training at Stanford, Laub was able to both introduce his trainees to international surgical volunteer efforts, as well as provide a forum for education for visiting surgeons from underserved countries. Out of these efforts grew the Webster fellowship and the Visiting Educator Programs. More recent refinements have included a greater focus on support of regional Surgical Outreach Centers, where Interplast resources augment host countries' rudimentary infrastructure. Along with cleft care delivery, Interplast has made a special effort to offer both perioperative and rehabilitative care to burn victims in many of their host countries.

Other like-minded organizations began building similar mission oriented cleft care teams throughout the 1970s and 1980s. Some were locally or regionally oriented (Austin Smiles, Interface—UCSD), some aligned with religious denominations (Catholic Medical Missions, Esperanca), and some associated with more global nongovernmental organizations (Rotoplast International). Some were started as small, independent efforts (i.e., Philplast/Operation Rainbow—William Riley, Operation Smile—Bill and Kathy Magee, Physicians for Peace—Charles Horton, Reconstructive Surgery Foundation—Edward Falces.)

All of these, and many more, shared the belief that mobilization of concerned and competent professionals, along with sufficient supplies placed in underserved areas, would result in the partial alleviation of suffering borne by untold numbers of hopelessly deformed children in regions where local access to care was unthinkable. This may have been the golden age in the relatively young enterprise of international surgical charity work. While the concept of tight controls on measurable quality and outcome standards had not yet taken center stage, Albert Shweitzer's memorable aphorism "it is better to light a single candle than to curse the darkness" held sway. The number of dedicated professionals and voluntary organizations focused on this work dramatically increased.

Several notable surgeons took it upon themselves to invest in a different and more radical model of medical mission work, one that would require constant involvement over a prolonged period of time in one location. Legendary figures in this regard were the likes of Paul Brand in Velor, India, Jerome Webster in Bejing, China, and Sam Nordhoff in Taipei,

Taiwan. Each moved their families, made a radical commitment, and concentrated all their efforts on a chosen place, totally immersing themselves in patient care, teaching, mentoring, and institution building, all for the sake of transforming medical care and access to modern plastic and reconstructive surgery. Their efforts paid off handsomely, as we now see great centers of plastic surgery developed in no small part because of their deep personal investments in places like Beijing Union Medical College, Chang Gung Memorial Hospital, and Velor Medical College. These programs have each gone on to become world class centers of plastic surgery, caring for hundreds of thousands, teaching and graduating enormous numbers of well trained plastic surgeons, and dedicating themselves to surgical innovation and better healthcare delivery.

As these organizations grew in number and diversity of approach, the American Society of Plastic and Reconstructive Surgeons (ASPRS) acknowledged the importance of these activities to their membership by creating the Reconstructive Surgery Volunteer Program (RSVP), through the Plastic Surgery Educational Foundation. Membership was open to those programs whose leadership were members of the ASPRS, and who's operating bylaws subscribed to a basic set of guidelines agreed to by RSVP membership. Not attempting to dictate or drive policy or strategy, the RSVP became an annual forum for discussion of similarly encountered problems in carrying out these most challenging missions. Differences in organizational size, style, and approach would occasionally divert attention from the singular fact that hundreds of thousands of children throughout the world with cleft lips, palates, other facial and burn deformities were not receiving any recognizable care. The common bond amongst these groups recognizing the need, RSVP (later known as VIPS), the ASPRS (later known as ASPS), the American College of Surgeons, and all related humanitarian healthcare organizations, was the knowledge that solutions did indeed exist. The capacity and capability to attack the problems and the desire to overcome the obstacles were shared by all.

BUILDING QUALITY AND SUSTAINABILITY

While the nature of voluntary organizations is to provide maximum service with minimum expenditures, the evolution of cleft mission work has progressed to where organizations must be measured using objective criteria. Presently, our singular goal must be to assure the best possible quality of care delivery to all patients no matter where they reside. Areas of concentration should include:

- Identification of need
- Validation of host country partners
- Type and qualification of medical and other healthcare personnel
- Equipment
- Logistics
- Protocols
- Documentation
- Security
- Sustainability—Foundational Development
- Education—both onsite, distant learning, and exchange

Identification of Need and Host Country Partners

Given the fact that all populations carry some incidence of cleft lip and palate in their newborn populations, the need for cleft care is truly global. In most fully developed population centers, a combination of either government sponsored or private healthcare infrastructure provides this service to a greater or lesser extent. On the other extreme, highly remote, deeply impoverished countries with little healthcare delivery infrastructure may not offer any form of this service. Developing countries where some form of expertise resides and basic hospital services are maintained, tend to be the most productive locations for the provision of cleft care via the surgical mission model. A brief look at the country lists of most major organizations confirms this. To have any chance of executing a successful mission, let alone a sustainable presence for comprehensive cleft care, the host country, or significant constituencies therein, must be prepared to play a supportive, welcoming role. These groups may include, but are not limited to, the central or regional government usually through their ministries of health, established religious organizations, the military, the host medical community, or other established social welfare groups. Trying to push one's organization past hostile or adversarial hosts usually multiplies the obstacles and oftentimes may diminish any chance for long-term acceptance. Time taken to understand whatever healthcare system is in place is extremely valuable. Local champions usually emerge from within the medical community no matter how sparse. Oftentimes, it may be an individual who received their training abroad during their formative early years. Each country will have some set of customs and regulations designed to monitor, if not actively restrict, the practice of medicine by foreign nationals. These must be understood and respected, no matter how dire the healthcare needs appear to be. Early compliance will usually allow more long-term acceptance. Mission sites may be identified by local contacts on the basis of proximity of patients, relationships with a funding organization, affiliation with a religious group or other mutual benefit societies, or simply as a result of a personal, family, or community connection. Either way, due diligence should be given to "fact finding" in regards to those people who would sponsor the mission organization, as they will serve as the visiting group's initial access to patients, facilities, transportation, media, and play a critical role in country lay support (Fig. 68–1).

Type and Qualification of Medical and Other Healthcare Personnel

Given the complexity and life-threatening risk inherent in performing surgical procedures in unfamiliar circumstances far away from one's home, it is mandatory that all

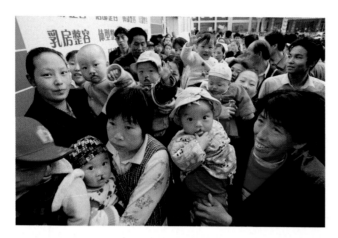

Figure 68–1. Patient candidates and their families facilitated by local health authorities.

participating professional volunteers be highly skilled, and well practiced in their respective fields. An international surgical mission is the last place where an unprepared surgeon, anesthesiologist, or nurse should go to learn the ropes or improve their self-image. Those taking primary responsibility for the perioperative care of children should be competent and qualified to provide similar duties in their country of origin. While it is a fact of life that many mission volunteers do not have a practice which mirrors their work on these trips, it is imperative that each individual participant be credentialed, qualified, and current in the general body of knowledge and experience as determined by their respective professional practice board, as well as trusted peers. It is not only a "best practice" for volunteer organizations to credential their members, but is more and more becoming a licensing requirement in many host countries. More recently, numerous volunteers have been prevented from participating in missions because of their inability to produce requested proof of licensure. It is incumbent upon the responsible aid organization to develop and maintain a sufficient screening process when choosing applicants for these positions. Common prerequisites should include a diploma, certificate of completion or board certification in their specialty, demonstration of clinical competency and currency, recommendation by well-known peers within the organization, and additional specialty training as required in their particular mission role. With anesthetic exposure posing the greatest perioperative risk, one example of this type of special preparation would include pediatric advanced life support (PALS), advanced cardiac life support (ACLS) or equivalent training for anesthesiologists, pediatricians, and recover room personnel. Volunteers should be encouraged to stay abreast of all current teaching in their respective fields, attending postgraduate courses, meetings, local or regional cleft team rounds, as well as reviewing videos or other teaching aids prior to deployment. Even though it increases the cost and logistical complexity of each mission, first time participants are best included as observers or assistants, partnered to a mentor so that they might completely experience all the inner workings of a typical mission, without

the pressure of taking primary responsibility for care. All of these investments in personnel selection pay off handsomely in overall margin of safety (Fig. 68–1). Teams can be as small as a plastic surgeon and anesthesiologist supported by familiar and trusted local healthcare providers with the plan of simply repairing presenting deformities, or as large as a fully articulated cleft care team designed to deliver an entire care package with the eventual plan of building sustainability and self-sufficiency over a multi-year interval. Such a team would include the following:

- Logistics coordinator
- Clinical coordinator
- Cleft surgeon(s)
- Anesthesiologist(s)
- Operating room nurses
- Pediatrician(s)
- Recovery room/PACU nurses
- Dentist
- Pediatric intensivist
- Medical records specialist
- Photo imaging technician
- Biomedical technician
- Speech therapist
- Child life specialist

As mentioned previously, organizations must continuously build volunteer team rosters with professional credentialing being just one component (Fig. 68–2). Availability for overseas travel is always problematic, as the voluntary nature of the work requires even the most dedicated professional to work around central commitments of their jobs and families. This leads to inevitable late cancellations, which then require others to be ready in reserve. Volunteer's health must be assessed and risks of injury or delay in treatment for sudden volunteer disabilities made known. Participants must be educated in team expectations, local customs and mores, and

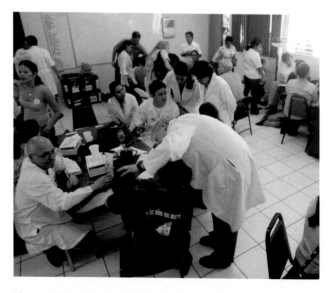

Figure 68–2. Credentialed volunteers manning various screening stations.

unacceptable behavior patterns. Many a mission has been confronted with the ugly after effects of isolated episodes of a team member's misconduct. These events can lead to a great deal of pain for both the mission organization and the host country, leading to a loss of continued association and the development of a hostile, mistrusting environment for other organizations who might offer aid in the future. It is best for each organization to thoroughly inculcate each volunteer with its core values, making them repeatedly aware of the mission *rules of the road*. This cannot be repeated too frequently and should be distributed in both print and spoken form before, during, and after the mission.

Equipment

Inevitably, surgically oriented endeavors are dependent on large amounts of instrumentation. It would be ideal if one could pack a change of clothes, a pair of clean scrubs, a set of loupes, and a good book before an all night flight, arriving at a mission site fully equipped with all of the necessary instruments, monitors, sutures, and pharmaceuticals to do one's job. Sadly, this rarely, if ever is the case. Acquisition, preparation, shipping, deployment, and maintenance of equipment *is* the air in which volunteer mission trips breathe. At a minimum, complete surgical trays, sutures and dressings, reliable and preferably state of the art anesthesia equipment, resuscitation packs, perioperative monitors, and sterility materials must be accounted for in one form or another. Long gone are the days when one could pilfer old, worn out supplies, outdated suture, and expired drugs to throw in one's backpack as a survival kit when doing surgery in the bush. Equivalency in material quality and safety is the order of the day. A partial list of recommended mission trip supplies follows (Fig. 68–3):

- Screening and Assessment
  - Vital sign monitors
  - Camera
  - Oto-ophthalmoscope
  - Lights, tongue blades, etc

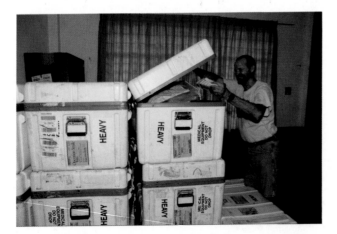

Figure 68–3. Equipment containers packed, inventoried, and cleared by the Customs.

- Medical Record
- Laboratory facilities for blood and electrolytes analysis
- Anesthesia
  - Anesthesia machine—with capabilities equivalent to those used in volunteer's home environments
  - Resuscitation boxes with current, unexpired drugs and pediatric dosage schedules
  - Airway equipment for pediatric patients including but not limited to masks, ET tubes, airways, laryngoscopes, positive pressure ventilation systems, non-invasive monitors, difficult airway management items, Sevoflurane anesthetic agent, and Dantrolene,
  - Blood matching and blood availability
  - Defibrillator and other appropriate emergency equipment
  - Intravenous fluids and fluid administration sets
- Surgery
  - Appropriately constructed surgical instrument trays for cleft lip, cleft palate, burn or hand care
  - Appropriate suture material
  - Sterilization materials with barrier devices, gowns and gloves
  - Electrocautery capability
  - Illumination
- Post Anesthesia Care
  - Full resuscitation packs
  - Oxygen and suction equipment at each bedside
  - Vital signs monitors with pulse oximetry
  - Documentation system
- Postoperative Intensive Care
  - Either built in capability in the host hospital or provisions made for the transport of critical patients
- Ward Nursing Units
  - Appropriate dressing and cleaning materials
  - Medications for pain, antisepsis, nausea, etc.
  - Vital sign monitoring equipment

Logistics

Personnel recruitment, equipment acquisition, movement, and security start long before a mission, and are never really complete. A weeklong endeavor where a dozen or so volunteers safely conduct 50–60 surgical procedures may take six months to plan and execute. Personnel schedules must be coordinated with the understanding that volunteers may want to team up with friends or other colleagues. Travel to and from sites can be very costly and must be planned well ahead of time for any hope of coordinated arrival and departure. Passports and visas must be prepared as should health alerts distributed. Local travel arrangements, housing, meals, social events, and security all play a crucial role in mission success and require meticulous planning with the expectation that many well-crafted plans will fail or change at the last minute. Equipment needed to execute the surgical program (as outlined above) should be acquired and tested to confirm normal operation well before shipping time. Drugs and expendables should be checked for expiration dates and any evidence of mishandling or breech in packing. All items to be shipped must be accurately inventoried and documented for there to be any chance of successful passage through customs. These issues continue to plague the most experienced of organizations, for political and economic exigencies are always the wildcard as to whether or not cargo passes through unconfiscated and undisturbed. Once again, this is where in-country partnerships play a crucial role in mission execution. Clearance to use local facilities must be sought out in advance and should be explicit and well documented. As well, advanced fact-finding trips, assuring adequate and acceptable facilities are critical. The mission's operational layout deserves focused attention early on, so that patient flow and the efficient use of human resources and materials are maximized. The operating room, recovery area, and intensive care region should be colocated to the maximum extent possible. This allows surgeons and anesthesiologists to monitor recently operated children in all perioperative phases. While not as crucial, postoperative nursing units should be in quick reach by surgical personnel. Cargo and supplies should be reinventoried using checklists, and those components, which are intended to be returned to the organization's home base, should be separated and differentiated from those that would remain behind. A clear explanation to the host medical leaders of the difference in equipment and supplies that stay versus return with the team will engender thankfulness; while, a confusing message may cause hard feelings. As in any medical care environment, drugs should be tightly controlled, and their access and distribution monitored.

Protocols

Competent surgeons, anesthesiologists, and nurses will each have their particular way of doing things. Often, times that keeps things interesting and lively. In most circumstances, however, protocols and priorities help focus the mission volunteers into a more coherent group. One example includes the priority-screening tool used while evaluating the patients which reads as follows:

1. Primary repair of cleft lip—6 months and older
2. Primary repair of cleft palate—1–6 years
3. Primary repair of cleft palate—6 years and older
4. Secondary repair of lips and palates—any age
5. Other conditions—including burn, scar, and hand problem

Operative protocols might recommend a certain procedure be used by all surgeons such as the Millard for cleft lip repair and the pushback palatoplasty for palatal defects Anesthesia might recommend limiting volatile anesthetics to one alternative, placement of tongue stitches, and the limited use of narcotics upon emergence. Nursing might recommend certain staffing ratios in the postoperative ward, and medical records may insist on a certain type of documentation. Clin-

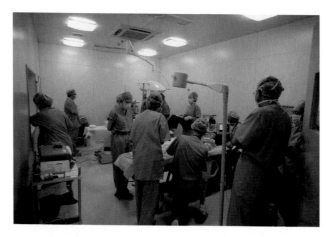

Figure 68–4. Personnel and procedure protocols are followed as closely as possible.

ical coordinators should mandate the use of translators in all phases of the operation. The more these protocols can be agreed upon and articulated to the group before the mission, the better. They insure a sense of consistency and decrease the margin of error in most circumstances (Fig. 68–4).

Documentation

As in all other endeavors, if it isn't written, it hasn't been done. This maxim is particularly important in three vital areas; the medical record, consents, and patient photographs. Medical record forms, whether written or electronic, should be identical throughout the organization. They should be explicit, simply and clearly designed, leaving no doubt as to what is being requested. The charts should be easily accessible and uniformly acceptable.

Histories should include familial background and other comorbidities. Physical examination data, pertaining to the congenital anomaly, should be collected diagrammatically and based on know classification schemes. Multiple copies of the document allow one to be left in the patient's chart in country, and another returned for tracking and statistical analysis. Preoperative and postoperative photographs should be taken of all patients in standard, well-lit poses, and labeled with the patient's name and ID number. Time spent educating the volunteer taking photographs, or recruiting a medical photographer is key to analyzing results. Consents for families to read and sign should be equivalent in content to those in the United States. They must be comprehensive and understood using a skilled interpreter. They must, at least, include the nature of the operation and its attendant risks, the use of anesthesia and potential blood transfusions, the taking of pictures, and HIV/Hepatitis testing in the case of a needle stick (Fig. 68–5).

Security

While we all long for days gone by when foreigners could roam free in distant countries without fear of threat, bodily harm, or abduction, it is unrealistic to disregard modern

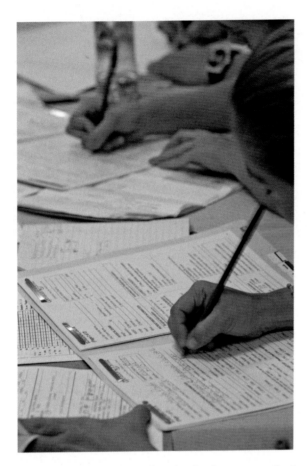

Figure 68–5. Medical records maintained on every patient.

security concerns. Several humanitarian healthcare organizations working in hostile environments have evolved very sophisticated methodologies for maximizing the protection of their volunteers. The International Medical Corps has developed a comprehensive protocol for security awareness and preparation with a booklet and mandatory questionnaire to be completed prior to the arrival on site of any volunteer. Caution must be practiced both at the mission work site and in all community environments. It is important that travel arrangements be scrutinized with respect to time and route of travel, as well as accompanying personnel. The overwhelming sentiment in virtually all of these programs is one of openness, sharing, trust, teamwork, and healing. The role of security in the modern mission world should be to insure an environment where these social paradigms can be maximized.

Sustainability

In all human endeavors, even the noblest, some form of payment is borne. One of the great misstatements made by many surgical charities is that a particular surgical procedure is done for free. In reality, this most likely means that someone besides the patient is paying for the service, as costs are shifted away from the recipient of the service. If this were not the case, then the need for charity would not exist. The very fact that children would otherwise grow to adulthood in their home-

land with unrepaired clefts is clear evidence that they do not have the financial means to obtain a repair on their own. This point should be understood and appreciated, as these endeavors consume resources and cost money. Participating medical personnel lose significant potential income and continue to pay expenses in their practices during their service time away. The volunteers' travel, food, and housing costs money. The equipment, supplies, and pharmaceuticals cost money. The organization's administrative expenses cost money. All of the cost shifting away from the patient, who would otherwise have no hope of cure, is the economic reality of international surgical charities. This reality comes at a price. To sustain and grow such an organization, fundraising, grant writing, and other development strategies must continually bring in money. These very efforts require the employment of several administrative staff to oversee these operations. To become sustainable, surgical charities with limited access to income must invest heavily in development efforts. For some organizations such as Rotaplast, or various religious based charities, there is a development arm already in place. For nonaligned organizations, development becomes a major source of effort and expenditure. Some organizations contribute to cleft care entirely as development and granting entities. In addition to traditional development strategies, Operation Smile, Interplast, and others have invested a great deal of effort in building foundations in host countries who then go on to build local development offices and infrastructure to share funding responsibilities. Many host countries not only mature to become financially self-sufficient, but are then able to contribute to the funding needs of much poorer hosts. Income is largely derived from grants, gala events, media campaigns, private donors, and annual fund drives.

Education

Providing educational opportunities and building sustainable capacity for care, is where surgical charity work, modern medical training, the communication revolution, and globalization coalesce. Through the last decade of the twentieth century, the ancient proverb, "Give a man a fish and you feed him for a day. Teach a man to fish and you feed him for a lifetime," became the rallying cry for those believing in the futility of surgical mission charities. Well run, effective organizations were continually criticized for failing to recognize their inability to effectively diminish the quantity of unrepaired lips and palates in the world using the mission model. However, like most proverbs, the cleverness of the phrasing masks the dramatic oversimplification of the meaning. The importance of education has never been lost on those who give of their time in these endeavors. Educational programming, no matter how rudimentary, became an integrated part of many organizational efforts. On-site education can be, and has been, very effective in transmitting small, focused, and discreet areas of knowledge and competencies like basic cardiac life support, ACLS, PALS, or sterilization techniques (Fig. 68–6). It also provides the opportunity for profoundly meaningful mentoring in the right circumstances. While enormously enriching

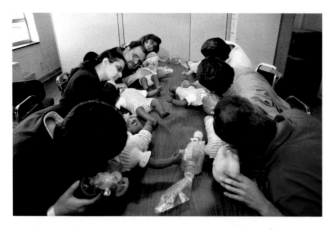

Figure 68–6. PALS/ACLS course delivered on site.

Educationally, the challenge has always been, and continues to be, matching resources with need. Just as most dependent host countries are impoverished in their healthcare delivery infrastructure, so are they deficient in professional educational programs. Plastic surgery residency training does not exist in many countries where international missions go. In others, the very few slots available train only a small fraction of surgeons needed to effectively service local populations. Many dedicated local doctors learn whatever they can by taking extended postgraduate preceptorships of 6 months to 1 year in mostly European and Asian centers. Unfortunately, the United States has made the least progress in offering non-traditional (less than full curriculum) subspecialty surgical training. This situation has only become worse with security concerns after 9/11. Slowly but steadily, University training programs in the United States and Canada are recognizing and responding to the ever-increasing needs of this type of focused study.

Medical Diplomacy and Beyond

When skilled professionals from foreign lands come together to overcome political and socioeconomic barriers, in order to deliver care to desperately needy children, medical diplomacy is the result. Barriers are broken, tensions are lowered, and interchange occurs at meaningful professional and personal levels. A classic example of this was the Vessey initiative to reengage Vietnam in 1988, authorized by President Reagan. After much discussion, it was concluded that the logical instrument in this effort should take the form of a humanitarian medical effort, more specifically, a voluntary surgical charity. Because of the non-threatening humanitarian nature of the work, the Vietnamese government allowed Operation Smile safe entry and the ability to care for their children. Barriers were broken; bridges were built (Fig. 68–8).

A handful of organizations have worked continuously to transcribe the language of volunteers, providing cleft care for desperately needy children, into the framework of medical diplomacy. As well, the use of humanitarian relief,

for both parties, it is wholly unrealistic to expect the pairing of an experienced volunteer cleft surgeon with a local host general surgeon, for merely a week, to result in anything more than the most rudimentary introduction to cleft surgery (Fig. 68–7). Surely, that brief association between teacher and resident in an American plastic surgical training program would not provide any measure of competency in cleft surgery. How are we to expect it then in much more hostile circumstances. Recognizing the need to go beyond on-site education, several organizations have dedicated themselves to long-term partnering in visiting educator programs, as well as visiting scholar programs. These are the efferent and afferent limbs of international education. Visiting educator programs take skilled western surgeons and allow them to stay with a host hospital and teach, both didactically and otherwise, for an extended length if they so choose. Visiting scholar programs bring a limited number of host country participants to educational program opportunities in various resource countries including Canada, the United States, Taipei, Singapore, and Europe. These programs last as little as three weeks or as long as 1–2 years. All of these efforts combined will be our only hope to truly address the entire problem.

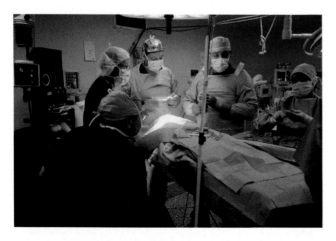

Figure 68–7. One-to-one mentoring at mission surgical site is only the beginning of the educational process.

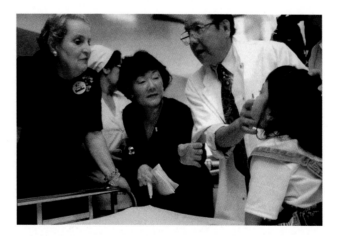

Figure 68–8. Former US Secretary of State acknowledging the importance of healthcare assistance as a diplomatic and humanitarian enterprise.

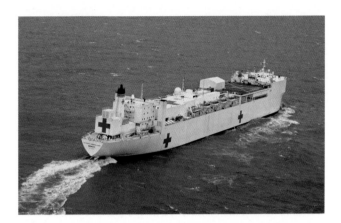

Figure 68–9. USNS Mercy Hospital ship on tour incorporating NGOs nongovernmental organizations performing cleft lip and palate surgery.

as a conversation starter towards greater interactivity, tolerance, and codependency between previously hostile nations, can become a reality. Currently, the United States Navy, after cooperative ventures with surgical charities, has realized the enormous effectiveness of these types of missions, and has included humanitarian assistance/disaster relief as an expected core naval competency in their global strategy update (Fig. 68–9).

CONCLUSION

The unique blend of skilled and dedicated medical professionals challenged with these complex surgical deformities in otherwise healthy children affords us the rare privilege to express ourselves in the most noble professional manner possible. Each child touched by a volunteer plastic surgeon and their colleagues during an international surgical mission, regains the opportunity to live a more normal life. There is no greater degree of satisfaction given to a conscientious healthcare provider. Obstacles to this delivery of care can be enormous; nefarious; and sometimes, overwhelming. The move away from itinerant surgery, and towards nurturing a host country's healthcare infrastructure and self-sufficiency, is universally supported. However, in so many environments, it remains no more than a faint hope on a distant horizon. Simultaneous efforts towards correcting facial deformities, building and equipping facilities, training competent local surgeons, developing comprehensive cleft care teams, and securing ongoing funding sources is what today's international voluntary surgical charity movement is all about. Whatever perspective one chooses to take, there can be no argument that this vital and fulfilling work will be there for years and years to come. Each and every child, whose life is changed for the better, is reason enough to proceed.

References

1. Porterfield A. Healing in the history of Christianity, Oxford: Oxford University Press, 2005.
2. Shepperson G. David Livingstone. 1813–1873. *Br Med J.* 2(5860):323–324, 1973.
3. McKay, A, Towards a History of Medical Missions. *Med Hist.* 51(4):547–551, 2007.
4. Buckingham, Clyde E. For humanity's sake: The story of the early development of the League of Red Cross Societies. Washington, DC: Public Affairs Press, 1964.
5. Rees T. *Daktari: A Surgeon's Adventures with the Flying Doctors of East Africa.* Santa Fe, NM: Sunstone Press, 2002.

Strategies for Improving Cleft Care

William C. Shaw, BDS, FDS, PhD, D Orth • Gunvor Semb, DDS, PhD • Pauline A. Nelson, BA (Hons)

In 2002, the World Health Organization published its first ever report focusing exclusively on craniofacial anomalies.[1] Together with reviews and recommendations for research concerning gene discovery, gene-environment interactions, and prevention, three interrelated priorities for improving the treatment of craniofacial anomalies (CFA) were set out:

- The identification and dissemination of optimal clinical interventions for the management of craniofacial anomalies (evidence-based care);
- The identification and dissemination of strategies to optimize the quality of services that deliver care (quality improvement); and
- The identification and dissemination of strategies to increase the availability of care to all affected citizens of the world (access and availability).

These will form the subsections of the present chapter.

EVIDENCE-BASED CARE

Evidence-based care is considered to be "the integration of best research evidence with clinical expertise and patient values." It is largely concerned with reducing clinical uncertainty by minimizing bias in the selection of optimal interventions.[2] The evidence considered should ideally allow choices to be made that also take account of the human burden and the financial costs of treatment.

Table 69–1.

Source of Bias when Comparing Groups of Patients

Source of Bias	Example
Case mix bias	Comparisons of facial growth data may be dubious where there are inherent differences in facial form between communities. Similarly, speech development may be less good in circumstances where the socioeconomic profile of the population served by a particular center is less favorable, or where the local spoken language requires different oropharyngeal skills.
Proficiency bias	The skill of a more gifted surgeon or clinical team can also inflate the apparent effectiveness of the technique. If operator A is 10% better than operator B and technique X is 5% better than technique Y, a false conclusion will be reached in a comparison of technique Y performed by A, versus technique X performed by B.
Follow-up bias	Without knowing about all the cases on whom a particular technique was tried, reliable conclusions cannot be drawn. Follow-up should be equally rigorous for cases that went badly.
Exclusion bias	Irregular application of grounds for retrospective exclusion e.g. "uncooperative" or "didn't really fit the criteria," can remove any equivalence that comparison groups may have had.
Analysis bias	When raters are not blinded to the treatment allocation of patients.
Reporting bias	When negative or disappointing findings remain unpublished.

There are some challenges ahead, however, for CFA care providers. Even for the longest established CFA intervention—the management of cleft lip and palate—the scientific basis of the discipline is weak. Virtually no elements of treatment have been subjected to the rigors of contemporary clinical trial design, and there is a bewildering diversity of practices, as Spriesterbach and others pointed out over 30 years ago.[3] A recent survey of European cleft services revealed that, in 201 teams, 194 different surgical protocols were followed for unilateral cleft lip and palate alone.[4]

Generally speaking, choices in surgical technique, timing, and sequencing, as well as choices in ancillary procedures such as orthopedics, orthodontics, and speech therapy, are arrived at after disappointment in the results of former practices, rather than after the establishment of firm evidence that the new protocol has succeeded elsewhere. As a consequence, the unsubstantiated testimony of enthusiasts for a particular treatment has done much to shape current practices. Typically, enthusiastic claims are made for a new type of therapy, the procedure is widely adopted, a flow of favorable anecdotal reports ensues, little or no positive evidence develops to support the desirability of the procedure, and, finally, there is a sharp drop in the number of clinical reports, again without evidence to support the change.[3]

Sources of Bias in Cleft Research

The general rules for making fair comparisons of alternative treatments are well established and conform to a widely accepted hierarchy, from anecdotal reports to systematic reviews of randomized trials. This hierarchy relates to the degree of effort made to minimize ever-present sources of research bias that readily lead to false conclusions. These are summarized in Table 69–1.

Not surprisingly, then, empirical research frequently demonstrates, in studies of healthcare interventions without randomization, an inflated view of effectiveness results.[5]

Minimizing Bias by Appropriate Designs for Comparison

While the general safety and potential effectiveness of novel methods of treatment may initially be assessed through accumulation of series of cases, direct comparisons with alternative treatments will be necessary to establish the true relative effectiveness of the method.

Nonrandomized comparison studies may provide insights of relative effectiveness, provided their limitations are recognized. Opportunities for nonexperimental retrospective comparisons of therapies or programs of care can arise in several ways: by the coexistence of different therapies at the same center, by the replacement of one therapy with another, or by collaboration of two or more centers. Prospective nonrandomized cohort studies in one or more centers may also be planned. Though all of these designs lack the reliability of randomized trials, efforts may still be made to reduce bias.

Comparison of Coexisting Therapies

When using retrospective material, such as case notes or clinical databases, checks can be made on the equivalence of the groups, commonly in terms of gender, age, or diagnostic subtype. Preferably, cases can be matched pair wise on these characteristics, or adjustment can be made in the analysis by stratification or the use of multivariate statistical methods. In either case, however, doubt will remain that important prognostic factors have been masked, for if two or more therapies were being used concurrently within a single center, selective allocation to treatment may have occurred. For example, decisions as to what age at which to perform surgery may be influenced by unrecorded aspects of the condition, the availability of personnel, the health of the child, or parental attitudes and characteristics. Should these factors influence outcome, confounding may distort the effect of age on surgical outcome.

Even if it is possible to match or adjust data to remove bias due to gender, age, or severity this gives no guarantee that some other prognostic factor that may affect outcome is not associated with choice of treatment. In addition, a critical factor in surgical outcome is the varying proficiency of different surgeons. Thus, a comparison of two techniques, one of which is preferred by one of the team's surgeons and the second of which by another, may essentially become a comparison of their relative surgical skill.

Comparison with Historical Controls

These studies may arise as natural experiments set up by changes in therapy within a treatment center. Such research is feasible when durable records (radiographs, study casts, speech recordings, photographs, etc.) are obtained in a standardized way for both those subjects treated by an earlier method (the historical controls) and those subjects treated by a subsequent one, allowing simultaneous evaluation. This design requires only half the number of patients to be gathered prospectively as in a randomized clinical trial and is clearly attractive where recruitment of cases is slow. Furthermore, it has been argued that, in circumstances of poor outcome, it may be unethical to withhold new treatment in order to create a control group.[6]

There are nevertheless several biases and possibilities for confounding that generally tend to favor the newly introduced procedure. In practice, changes in technique at a treatment center often come about as a result of changes in personnel who may have performed differently in respect of the previous method. This again leads to bias due to differences in skill of personnel associated with either treatment method. For example, a new method of treatment is often tested by an experienced and innovative surgeon who may be expected to achieve better results than the average surgeon. Even where there is stability of staff, bias reflecting gradual changes of ability and technique are highly likely, and definition or ascertainment of prognosis may change. New methods may also be initially applied with some selectivity to "suitable" cases as experience is gained. Other aspects of clinical management may have been altered with the intention of improving outcome, creating additional possibilities for bias in favor of the innovative procedure. Multivariate methods have been suggested as a way to adjust for these biases, but serial

changes in related aspects of treatment are likely to take place in parallel, resulting in a strong association between treatment variables.[7] This is one reason why historical control design is generally unsuited to evaluating primary cleft surgery, since other changes in the total program of care are likely to have occurred during the extensive recruitment period.

The bias favoring the innovative procedure is a major cause for concern with historical control studies, as they may either fail to resolve controversy or create ethical concerns that preclude further, more rigorous comparisons. Favorable outcomes suggested for a new procedure by historical control studies have often been disputed by subsequent randomized controlled trials.[8,9] The danger thus exists that historical control studies may set in motion an unwarranted cycle of change with no benefit to the patient and that such may consequently delay the process of development.

The reduction in recruitment time required for a historical control study is less important when extended follow-up is required. If, for example, the proposed follow-up of a trial of two methods of primary surgery is 10 years, and the recruitment time of patients sufficient for a randomized trial is 4 years, the total duration would be 14 years. The potential saving of time in such a partially prospective, historical control study would thus be only 2 years (14%).

Intercenter Comparison

The multicenter approach offers distinct advantages for cleft or CFA treatment centers, as the generation of adequate samples within specific subtypes treated by contrasting treatment modalities is hastened. Prospectively planned recall of patients at participating centers allows data on outcome to be collected in a standardized way, and rigorous planning and execution across centers can ensure consecutive case recruitment and consistent evaluation.[10,11]

Provided procedures for entry into the study are equivalent in all participating centers, this strategy is extremely valuable in assessing the outcome of surgery, together with other major components of the treatment program at respective centers. For primary cleft surgery, however, it is difficult, if not impossible, to establish the key beneficial or harmful features of the specific treatment due to the invariably complex and arbitrary mix of surgical technique, timing and sequence, ancillary procedures, and surgical personnel.[11] For example, if two centers differ in the use of presurgical orthopedics and type of primary lip and palate surgery, there is no way to determine which of these procedures might be responsible for any difference in outcome between centers, nor would a null result allow the conclusion that individual aspects of the treatment program are equivalent. The method is therefore better suited to comparative clinical audit and quality assurance than to definitive clinical research. The existence of significant disparities in outcome of the overall treatment process provides a basis for speculating as to the possible cause, and intercenter studies should, therefore, be highly motivating towards the generation of specific hypotheses for subsequent trials. This was certainly the case in the Eurocleft Cohort Study.

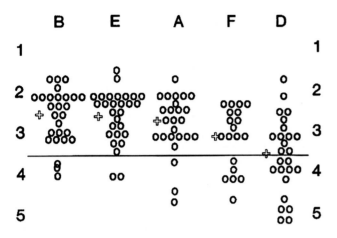

Figure 69–1. Goslon individual patient scores at age 9 years by center. A Goslon score of 1 represents excellent maxillary prominence and a score of 5 severe maxillary retrusion. One way to consider this outcome variable is the likely future need for subsequent maxillary osteotomy, cases falling below 3.5 at this age are likely candidates for osteotomy in the late teens.

The Eurocleft Cohort Study

The Eurocleft Cohort Study began in the late 1980s as an intercenter comparison of the records of 9-year-old children with complete unilateral cleft lip and palate. It sought to overcome, at least in part, some of the limitations and potential biases associated with the comparison of outcomes described in single center reports. A full account of the methodology and findings has been presented elsewhere.[10–16] Five of the original six teams agreed to continue follow-up of the cohort until age 17.

Outcomes at Age Nine

At 9 years of age, several differences between the centers were apparent, especially for dental arch relationship (Fig. 69–1).

Whereas only 7% of cases for center E were considered to have a likely future need for osteotomy, almost half (48%) did so for center D. It was not possible to ascribe success or failure to particular details of the surgical protocols, but poor outcomes appeared to be related to decentralized services without consistent protocols.

Follow-up

The aims of the follow-up were to quantify the burden of care imposed by respective protocols; to see whether the ranking of centers for different outcomes at age 9 was predictive for equivalent outcomes at age 17; to assess patient/parent satisfaction with care; and to explore interrelationships between outcome and burden.[17–20] A separate comparison of speech outcomes was carried out at ages 11–14.[21]

Survey of Treatment Experience

The amount of treatment provided by the five different teams between 1976 and 1979 was remarkably different (Table 69–2). Most notable was the lengthy hospital stay associated with presurgical orthopedics at that time in centers D and F. The subjects in center D also had more orthodontic visits for treatment and review and a greater overall number of operations compared to the other centers. The reason for the large differences in the intensity of treatment was not primarily related to clinical need but rather to differing beliefs and historical practices that shaped the clinical protocols of the period.

Consistency of Outcomes Over Time

The statistical analysis used to compare the five centers was a general linear mixed model applied to longitudinal data.[22] Variance terms were included in the model to account for between-subject variation in the intercept as well as fixed factor for assessment point (9, 12, 17 years) and center. Full details have been reported elsewhere.[23]

Table 69–2.

Amount of Treatment Provided by Five Different Teams from Birth to 17 Years of Age

		A	B	D	E	F
SURGERY						
Mean number of surgeries		4.8	3.3	6.0	4.4	3.5
Mean days in hospital		33	31	60	24	26
PRESURGICAL ORTHOPEDICS						
Months of treatment		13	0	15	0	5
Number of visits		11	0	8	0	17
Days in hospital		0	0	60	0	146
ORTHODONTIC TREATMENT						
Treatment length (years)		5.6	3.3	8.5	3.5	4.0
Number of visits	Treatment	52	41	54	33	47
	Follow-up	11	23	42	16	25
	Total	63	64	94	49	72

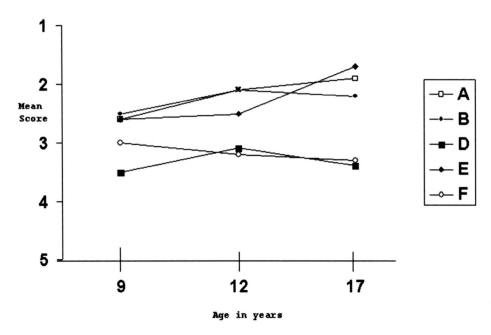

Figure 69–2. Mean dental arch relationship scores at ages 9, 12, and 17 years for participating centers.

As Figure 69–2 indicates, the scores for dental arch relationship tended to improve in centers A, B, and E, but not in D and F. There was a consistent relationship over time for most cephalometric variables (e.g., soft tissue profile; Fig. 69–3) and for nasolabial appearance.

Lack of Association between Outcome and the Amount of Treatment
Not surprisingly, follow-up of these five cohorts of patients from age 9 to age 17 confirmed the main finding of the first report, with some centers continuing to achieve considerably better outcome than others at all age points. Perhaps most sur-

prising is the lack of association between amount of treatment and final outcome (Tables 69–3 to 69–5). Especially ironic is the finding that the two centers with the highest intensity of early treatment (hospitalization in order to perform presurgical orthopedics), achieved the lowest rankings for eventual outcome (Figs. 69–2 and 69–3). The poorest ratings for nasal appearance were associated with the lengthy use of a presurgical device called T traction designed not only to reduce the alveolar gap but also to straighten the nasal septum.[24] Patients in the center with the least favorable dentofacial outcomes (center D) also experienced the longest orthodontic

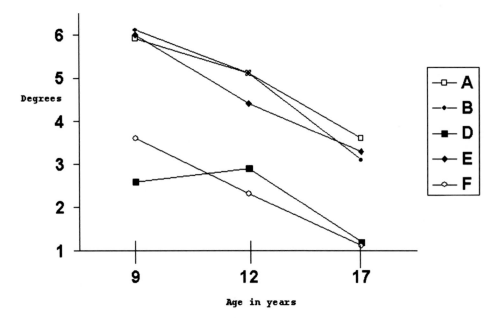

Figure 69–3. Mean soft tissue profile (angle SSS-NS-SMS) at ages 9, 12, and 17 years for participating centers.

Table 69–3.

The Relationship between Outcome Assessment (Dental Arch Relationship at 17 years) and Amount of Infant Orthopedic Treatment in the Different Centers

Objective Ranking	Center	Months of Treatment	No of Visits	Days in Hospital
Best	E	0	0	0
↑	A	13	11	0
↕	B	0	0	0
↓	F	5	17	146
Worst	D	15	8	60

treatment duration and the highest number of orthodontic visits. It appears that this was partly due to the complexity of center D's orthodontic treatment protocols, with almost continuous treatment from the eruption of the primary dentition, and partly to the unfavorable dentofacial outcomes of primary surgery.

The lack of association between treatment outcome and intensity may represent a key lesson for the development of future protocols. It justifies an emphasis on simplicity, economy, and minimized burden for the patient, rather than adherence to demanding protocols with unsubstantiated promise.

Lack of Association between Outcome and Satisfaction

Perhaps the most perplexing finding of the Eurocleft series is the inconsistency between objectively rated outcomes and patient/parent satisfaction. Investigators observed instances wherein the highest levels of dissatisfaction with treatment outcome were reported by subjects attending the centers with the best objective ratings (Table 69–6). The possible reasons for this disparity have been discussed elsewhere.[18] This finding underscores the need for concerted work on the understanding and measurement of patient satisfaction and the provision of more holistic models of cleft care.

Prospective Cohort Studies: A Preliminary Approach for Rare and/or Novel Interventions

During the introductory phase of a new therapy, it may be impossible to conduct a randomized trial if the intervention is undergoing constant modification and the population to which it is applied is heterogeneous and ill-defined. Such is currently the case with many CFA interventions. A case in point in the last decade is distraction osteogenesis in its increasing application to the craniofacial skeleton.

Pending the conduct of clinical trials, the establishment of prospective registration to enable critical appraisal of different kinds of CFA interventions will maximize collective experience and minimize the biases that inevitably occur with ad hoc reporting. Such studies would therefore play a similar role to Phase I trials of pharmaceutical interventions. One such registry has been set up for distraction osteogenesis in Europe as part of the EUROCRAN program, with centers submitting duplicate records prior to treatment as a step to minimize follow-up, analysis, and reporting bias (www.eurocran.org).

As records of all consecutive cases would be filed with the registry prior to the start of treatment as well as after it, justification for non-follow-up would be required. As in well-conducted clinical trials, analysis bias could be overcome by employing blinded independent raters, while

Table 69–4.

The Relationship between Outcome Assessment (Dental Arch Relationship at 17 years) and Amount of Orthodontic Treatment in the Different Centers

Objective Ranking	Center	Treatment Length (years)	No of Visits	
			Treatment	Check-up
Best	E	3.5	33	16
↑	A	5.6	52	11
↕	B	3.3	41	23
↓	F	4.0	47	25
Worst	D	8.5	54	42

Table 69–5.

The Relationship between Outcome Assessment (Dental Arch Relationship at 17 years) and the Mean Number of Surgeries Per Patient in the Different Centers

Objective Ranking	Center	Number of Surgeries
Best	E	4.4
↑	A	4.8
	B	3.8
↓	F	3.5
Worst	D	6.0

reporting bias could be overcome by the greater impartiality of the partnership and its predetermined conventions. Case mix bias and exclusion bias could not to be minimized with the assurance derived from random allocation, but some checks of equivalence might be possible. Clinical proficiency, however, would inevitably remain as a major bias. Thus, prospective cohort studies occupy an intermediate position between nonrandomized studies and randomized controlled trials.

Prospective registration also allows opportunities for preparatory work on outcome methodology: the early detection of extremely promising or unpromising clinical strategies, the definition of answerable questions amenable to clinical trials, and the building of interpersonal trust and institutional partnerships that will be necessary to mount such trials.

Randomized Controlled Trials

For the fairest comparison of therapies, there is little doubt that the randomized controlled trial is generally the method of choice, both scientifically and ethically. Prognostic factors, including clinical proficiency, whether known or unknown to the investigator, tend to be balanced between treatment groups. Since patients are registered prior to treatment and followed up prospectively according to a clearly defined pro-

tocol, missing data are less likely as the potential for loss to follow-up and late exclusion is reduced. Formalizing the protocol at the outset, as required by an ethical review board or funding agency, increases the likelihood of consistent record collection and impartial analysis. The likelihood of reporting the results is also increased by the conventions of trial registration and funding.

Randomized controlled trials can, of course, also be performed badly. If the randomization procedure is not strictly applied (i.e., if allocation is not fully concealed from the investigators), bias can enter. Inadequate concealment in clinical trials is associated with higher odds ratios, leading to an inflated view of effectiveness,[25] as in the case of nonrandomized studies. Trials with insufficient cases may also give misleading results.

Early Experience with Randomized Trials in Cleft Management
Over 30 years ago, Spriestersbach et al.[3] identified the need for prospective research to resolve central problems of cleft management, but in a review of 25 years of the Cleft Palate Journal reported in 1991, only five controlled clinical trials were identified, with only one involving follow-up of surgery for more than 4 years.[26] Since then, the situation has improved only slightly.

Robertson and Jolleys conducted two small randomized controlled trials of primary surgery in the 1960s. In the first study, a sample was randomized with respect of alveolar bone grafting at the time of primary surgery in infancy.[27] Follow-up revealed a detrimental effect on facial growth in the grafted group.[28] The second study involved two groups of 20 cases wherein one group's anterior palate closure was delayed until 5 years of age. No benefit for dentofacial growth was found when hard palate closure was delayed.[29] A follow-up study conducted when the children were 11 years of age reached the same conclusion.[30] In a quasi-randomized trial (patients entered on basis of birthdates), Wray et al.[31] found a difference in perioperative morbidity following three types of palate repair (V–Y pushback, von Langenbeck, or von Langenbeck with superiorly based pharyngeal flap) in 47 patients with a variety of cleft types. Speech outcomes were subsequently reported for 52 patients.[32] Morbidity was least with the von Langenbeck repair, and speech outcomes were

Table 69–6.

The Relationship between Objective Ranking of Nasolabial Outcome and Patient Dissatisfaction

Objective Ranking	Percentage of Respondents Dissatisfied with Nasal Appearance		Objective Ranking	Percentage of Respondents Dissatisfied with Lip Appearance	
Best	A	64	Best	B	14
↑	E	32	↑	A	41
	B	14		F	6
↓	D	45	↓	E	42
Worst	F	33	Worst	D	16

the same in all three groups. Chowdri et al.[33] compared rotation advancement and triangular flaps in unilateral cleft lip repair in 108 cases and found no differences in lip and nose appearance.

In another quasi-randomized controlled trial (patients alternated rather than randomized) on speech outcome, Marsh et al.[34] compared palate repair with or without intravelar veloplasty in 51 subjects with a broad range of palatal types. Speech evaluations were made at a 2 years follow-up. No difference in outcome was detected, but the use of intravelar veloplasty significantly prolonged operating time.

Another randomized controlled trial on speech outcome and maxillary growth in patients with unilateral complete cleft lip and palate operated on at 6 versus 12 months of age was undertaken in Mexico.[35] The study groups consisted of 41 subjects operated on at 12 months of age and 35 subjects operated on at 6 months. There was no statistically significant difference in velopharyngeal function, maxillary arch development, or soft-tissue profile as measured on cephalometric radiographs. However, phonologic development was significantly better in patients operated at 6 months, and none of the patients in this group developed compensatory articulation. The authors concluded that cleft palate repair performed at 6 months significantly enhances speech outcome and prevents compensatory articulation disorder. The same group compared minimal incision palatopharyngoplasty with and without individualized velopharyngeal surgery for velopharyngeal insufficiency in 72 patients with submucous cleft palate, finding no benefits to the more complex procedures[36]

For patients with velopharyngeal insufficiency, secondary surgery is often recommended. Whitaker et al.[37] found no difference in outcome in a randomized trial of 35 patients, comparing superiorly versus inferiorly based flaps. More recently, pharyngeal flap and sphincter pharyngoplasty were compared in a multisite randomized controlled trial of 97 patients. Patients were evaluated before surgery, then 3 and 12 months following surgery, by perceptual speech evaluation, video nasopharyngoscopy, nasometry, polysomnographic sleep study, audiometry, and tympanometry. Analysis revealed both techniques to be equally effective and equally safe.[38]

Most of the above trials have involved relatively small samples, but two recent surgical trials have adopted a more ambitious approach. The first of these, an NIDCR sponsored study "Velopharyngeal Function for Speech after Palatal Surgery" was coordinated by the University of Florida. All subjects were enrolled and treated at the University of São Paulo Hospital for Rehabilitation of Craniofacial Anomalies (USP-HRAC), Bauru, Brazil. A total of 475 subjects were included and preliminary results have been reported.[39]

Subjects were randomly assigned to receive either the Spina or Millard surgical procedure for lip repair and to receive either the Furlow double-opposing Z-palatoplasty or the von Langenbeck technique for palate repair. Subjects were also randomly assigned to one of two age groups for their palatal surgery (9–12 months of age or 15–18 months of age).

Therefore, the study design has eight subgroups of subjects: (1) those who received the Spina lip repair and the von Langenbeck palate repair at 9–12 months of age; (2) Spina lip repair and the von Langenbeck repair at 15–18 months of age; (3) Spina and Furlow at 9–12 months of age; (4) Spina and Furlow at 15–18 months of age; (5) Millard and von Langenbeck at 9–12 months; (6) Millard and von Langenbeck at 15–18 months of age; (7) Millard and Furlow at 9–12 months of age; and (8) Millard and Furlow at 15–18 months of age. Each subgroup had approximately 60 patients.

The preliminary results indicated that, although more favorable speech outcomes were achieved by the Furlow over the traditional von Langenbeck technique, there was a higher fistula rate with the former (21.5% vs. 14.1%, $p \leq 0.03$).

Since 1986, North European teams have been developing a concerted program of multidisciplinary intercenter research in cleft lip and palate. This includes a comparison of surgical outcome in four Scandinavian centers[40,41] and six European centers.[10–21,42] Following these collaborations, the limitations of intercenter studies became increasingly obvious to these teams, as it became clear that it would be impossible to separate and compare the single elements of the package of care provided in the different centers. This experience provided a compelling stimulus for starting randomized controlled trials in primary surgery of patients with unilateral cleft lip and palate. Ten centers are currently participating in a set of three parallel trials where groups of teams are testing their traditional local protocols against a common protocol.[43] The sample size requirements were 450 infants, 150 in each trial. The principle outcomes were speech and dentofacial relationship at age 5 years. Only 7% of the parents declined participation in the trials. At the time of this writing, entry into the trials is completed (456 infants), and 260 of these children have reached 5 years of age. The follow-up rate has so far been 100% in 8 of the centers and 94% and 90% in the other two centers.

Randomized trials of other interventions have also been completed. These include trials of artificial bone,[44] nasal floor augmentation,[45] anesthesia or analgesia,[46–49] perioperative steroid therapy,[50] perioperative antibiotics,[51] speech therapy following velopharyngeal surgery,[52] inclusion of the mother in speech therapy,[53] phonologic versus articulatory speech intervention,[52] use of presurgical orthopedics,[54–57] use of arm splints following surgery,[58] feeding after surgery,[59,60] feeding methods in infancy,[61,62] use of continuous airway pressure in the treatment of hypernasality,[63] and fluoride supplements for dental caries.[64]

Such efforts demonstrate the feasibility of randomized controlled trials in the CFA field and indicate the probable shape of future progress. Thus, trials of sufficient power are likely to be carried out through collaboration between funding agencies, clinical scientists, and high-volume centers (possibly in the developing world). Alternatively, they may be conducted as multicenter investigations within collaborative groups with strong geographical cultural links, as in the Scandcleft trials. Each will have a place.

Challenges in Performing Clinical Trials

Since interventions are often applied at an early stage of life and their full consequences only revealed some years later, achieving adequate length of follow-up represents a significant challenge in performing clinical trials concerned with cleft lip and palate include. Moreover, the impact of clefts calls for the quantification and balancing of diverse outcomes.

Above all, however, is the challenge of achieving sample size in light of the fact that the various subgroups of cleft lip and palate occur infrequently. Current estimates suggest that two groups of 75 cases or more of the same diagnostic subtype are required in trials of cleft surgery. Thus, more than one million births would have to occur in order to conduct a trial including 150 infants with complete, nonsyndromic, unilateral complete cleft lip and palate (assuming a rate of 1 per 7 of all cleft types, one cleft per 700 births, 75% compliance with all inclusion/exclusion criteria, and consent obtained in 90% of cases). On the basis of the actual rate of entry into the Scandcleft trial mentioned above, smaller countries, such as Denmark (population 5.4 million) and Norway (population 4.6 million) would take 8 and 11 years respectively to recruit 150 patients in a single-nation trial, despite a rate of one cleft per 500 births.

Ethical Issues in Randomized Trials

The ethical issues raised in randomized trials in CFA care are interesting,[65,66] in particular, the double standards that are applied in clinical experimentation. History indicates that not all surgical innovations are an enduring success. Discredited, though once fashionable, techniques include gastric freezing for bleeding peptic ulcer, carotid body denervation for bronchial asthma, portacaval shunt to prevent esophageal variceal bleeding, nephropexy for visceroptosis, removal of chronically inflamed appendix, and periarterial sympathectomy.[67,68] Indeed, numerous reports show that new treatments are as likely to be worse as they are to be better than existing alternatives.[69]

Where the doctor leads, however, most patients and parents will follow, raising an important ethical dilemma. If the surgical team wishes to test an innovative procedure in a randomized trial, it must obtain ethical approval from an appropriate authority and fully inform each patient (parent) of any uncertainty and/or risk prior to obtaining consent. Ironically, if the team wishes to try out the same innovation on its patients without a randomized trial, no such rules currently apply.[70] "Ethical codes that seek to protect patient . . . regulate the responsible investigator but not the irresponsible adventurer."[71] In the United States, the National Commission for the Protection of Human Subjects recommended that "medical committees should be responsible for ensuring that major innovations undergo proper scientific evaluation" and be charged with "determining which new treatments need to be evaluated, the proper method of evaluation, and how to limit the use . . . prior to the completion of that evaluation."[72] As yet no such body exists, either in the United States or elsewhere, yet it is manifestly clear to anyone attending a cleft conference that informal experimentation with patients is occurring all the time.

In the light of this, there exists a strong imperative to conduct clinical trials across a range of CFA where true uncertainty of effectiveness (equipoise) exists and to apply the customary rules for informed consent and ethical approval from appropriate authorities. When trials in a developing country are planned and funded by a developed country, it would offer reassurance if a cooperative or parallel trial were also to be undertaken in the developed country, unless, of course, the trial has relevance only for developing countries.

Systematic Review of Randomized Trials

Systematic review of all relevant randomized trials is the optimal method for establishing whether scientific findings are consistent and can be generalized across populations, settings, and treatment variations, or whether findings vary significantly by particular subsets. Explicit methods used in systematic reviews limit bias and improve reliability and accuracy of conclusions.[73] Meta-analysis—the use of statistical methods to summarize the results of independent trials—can provide more precise estimates of the effects of healthcare than those derived from individual studies. The Cochrane Collaboration is an international organization established to prepare, maintain, and promote the accessibility of systematic reviews of the effects of healthcare interventions, and as randomized trials in CFA are completed and reported, it will become a primary source of reviews and dissemination (www.cochrane.org).

The Cochrane Collaboration logo (Fig. 69–4) illustrates a systematic review of data from seven randomized control trials (RCTs), comparing one health care treatment with a

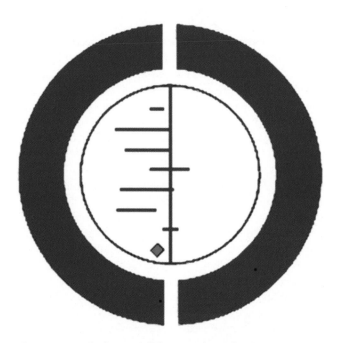

Figure 69–4. Cochrane Collaboration logo showing systematic review of data from seven randomized clinical trials.

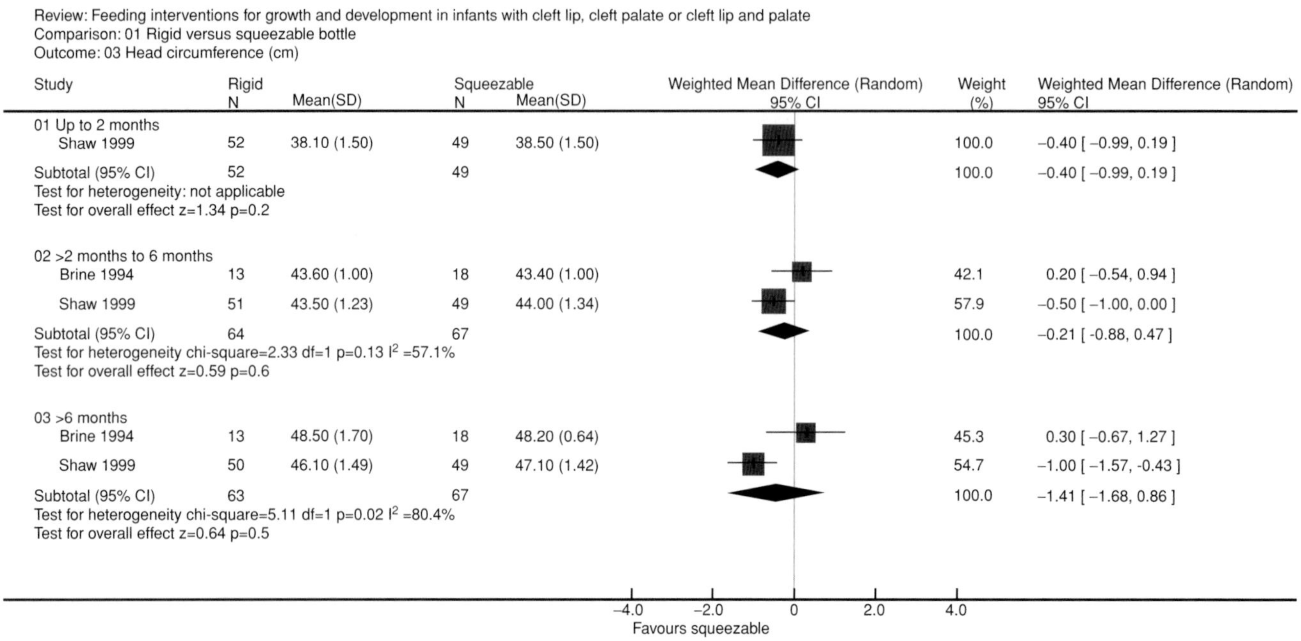

Review: Feeding interventions for growth and development in infants with cleft lip, cleft palate or cleft lip and palate
Comparison: 01 Rigid versus squeezable bottle
Outcome: 03 Head circumference (cm)

Study	Rigid N	Mean(SD)	Squeezable N	Mean(SD)	Weighted Mean Difference (Random) 95% CI	Weight (%)	Weighted Mean Difference (Random) 95% CI
01 Up to 2 months							
Shaw 1999	52	38.10 (1.50)	49	38.50 (1.50)		100.0	−0.40 [−0.99, 0.19]
Subtotal (95% CI)	52		49			100.0	−0.40 [−0.99, 0.19]
Test for heterogeneity: not applicable							
Test for overall effect z=1.34 p=0.2							
02 >2 months to 6 months							
Brine 1994	13	43.60 (1.00)	18	43.40 (1.00)		42.1	0.20 [−0.54, 0.94]
Shaw 1999	51	43.50 (1.23)	49	44.00 (1.34)		57.9	−0.50 [−1.00, 0.00]
Subtotal (95% CI)	64		67			100.0	−0.21 [−0.88, 0.47]
Test for heterogeneity chi-square=2.33 df=1 p=0.13 I²=57.1%							
Test for overall effect z=0.59 p=0.6							
03 >6 months							
Brine 1994	13	48.50 (1.70)	18	48.20 (0.64)		45.3	0.30 [−0.67, 1.27]
Shaw 1999	50	46.10 (1.49)	49	47.10 (1.42)		54.7	−1.00 [−1.57, −0.43]
Subtotal (95% CI)	63		67			100.0	−1.41 [−1.68, 0.86]
Test for heterogeneity chi-square=5.11 df=1 p=0.02 I²=80.4%							
Test for overall effect z=0.64 p=0.5							

```
        -4.0    -2.0    0    2.0    4.0
        Favours squeezable
```

Figure 69–5. Forest plot for the outcome head circumference.

placebo. Known as a forest plot, each horizontal line represents the results of one trial (the shorter the line the more certain the result), and the diamond represents their combined results. The vertical line indicates the position around which the horizontal lines would cluster if the two treatments compared in the trials had similar effects; if a horizontal line touches the vertical line, it means that the particular trial found no clear difference between the treatments. The position of the diamond on the left of the vertical line indicates that the treatment studied is beneficial. Horizontal lines or a diamond to the right of the line would show that the treatment did more harm than good.

This systematic review evaluated the effectiveness of a short, inexpensive course of a corticosteroid given to women at risk of giving birth too early. The first of these RCTs was reported in 1972. The diagram summarizes the evidence that would have been revealed had the available RCTs been reviewed systematically a decade later. It indicates strongly that corticosteroids reduce the risk of babies dying from the complications of immaturity. By 1991, seven more trials had been reported, and the picture had become still stronger. This treatment reduces the odds of the babies of these women dying from the complications of immaturity by 30–50%. Because no systematic review of these trials had been published until 1989, most obstetricians had not realized that the treatment was so effective. As a result, tens of thousands of premature babies have probably suffered and died unnecessarily (and needed more expensive treatment than was necessary).

So far, only one systematic review of trials concerning the care of children with clefts has been carried out.[74] The value of this review of feeding interventions for growth and development in infants with cleft lip, cleft palate, or cleft lip and palate, is, however, diminished by a lack of RCTs. Although a total of 290 articles with possible relevance were identified through electronic searching, only four reported RCTs. Two compared squeezable versus rigid bottles in various cleft types; one compared breast versus spoon feeding in cleft lip; and one compared passive palate obturation with a maxillary plate versus no obturation.

Figure 69–5 shows the forest plot for one of the outcomes (head circumference) from the meta-analysis carried out on the two trials that compared bottles in a total of 130 babies. The larger trial shows statistically significant benefit to head circumference after 6 months, but the pooled analysis shows no significant difference. This uncertainty can only be resolved by additional RCTs, as is almost certainly going to be the case in carrying out systematic reviews for the whole range of other interventions in the cleft field for the foreseeable future. There could not be a stronger imperative for the professionals in cleft care to form effective collaborative clinical trial partnerships.

Measuring Outcome

The ultimate goal of cleft care is restoration of the patient as far as possible to a "normal" life, unhindered by handicap or disability. However, the measurement of normalcy is a highly complex proposition and there is certainly no index at present that would allow sufficiently sensitive comparison between alternative treatment protocols. Clinical trials will focus more on "proximate" outcomes. These will mainly represent different aspects of anatomical form and function in the parts affected by the cleft, often reflecting the particular interest of individual provider groups. In essence, most measures will be an indication of the deficits that persist despite (or as a result of) treatment, such as shortcomings in appearance, speech, hearing, and dentofacial development. The general rules of reproducibility and validity apply, the latter being especially important when outcome is assessed before maturity. Longitudinal archives may be useful to determine the reliability of prediction for outcomes that are to be measured in the young.[75,76]

In relation to cleft surgery, experience with a number of outcome measures and scales has been obtained regarding speech, dentofacial outcomes, and patient satisfaction.[77–79] Further work is certainly needed to refine these and build consensus upon international standards. Reliable rating of appearance is still problematic, and for speech, linguistic differences represent a significant international challenge; however, efforts are underway to resolve these (www.eurocran.org;[80]). Outcomes should be patient centered, i.e., measuring things that matter to ordinary people, rather than sophisticated surrogate measurements that may have little relevance to everyday life.

Family Perspective in CFA Research: Qualitative Approaches

There is a need to integrate "patient values" with best clinical evidence if care is to be truly evidence-based in CFA. Methods of exploring such values must also aim to illuminate the health and social care issues that are of importance to parents and young people themselves, rather than valuing the development of outcome measures through the professional lens alone. Qualitative research methods used as a set of complementary tools can bring such issues to light and, in turn, encourage the self-evaluation of professional beliefs and behavior in relation to the provision of care. Uncovering evidence in qualitative ways to shed light on the questions "What do I do and believe that is different from what the patient I am treating does and believes?" and "What can I learn from this patient?"[81] will help ensure that important ideas about how CFA-affected families could be better supported in the future are not missed.

Qualitative research is concerned with interpreting and making sense of people's beliefs and behavior in complex social worlds, is based on data generation techniques that are flexible and sensitive to social context, and uses methods of analysis that seek to understand complexity through attention both to the detail and context of participants' lives.[82] Qualitative research is not a single method but rather a set of tools and approaches that can be selected on the basis of their suitability in relation to the nature of the particular research question.[83,84] Its methods have a long history in the social sciences, are underpinned by assumptions which differ from those of experimental or survey type research, and are now widely applied to questions in health and social care.[85–87] Rather than bringing value to questions such as the evaluation of the effectiveness of a medicine or treatment in a controlled setting, their worth is recognized for questions concerned with issues such as the appropriateness of care, or understanding lay/professional beliefs and behavior in the social setting.[88]

Despite its now widespread recognition in the health arena, qualitative research in the field of CFA has been rel-atively scarce. In spite of the call almost 20 years ago for an "interdisciplinary 'social science model'" to address questions related to patient values and experiences, including the use of both quantitative and qualitative methods,[89] only recently have qualitative methods made an appearance in the CFA literature. A search of the Cleft Palate Craniofacial Journal over the 43 years since its inception found only eight papers that had employed qualitative approaches, the majority in the last 5 years.[90–97] Additionally, only two published qualitative studies could be found elsewhere.[98,99] Such studies, using a range of qualitative techniques for data generation and analysis, have contributed unexpected insights about CFA from the lay perspective on a range of issues that can inform policy and practice: barriers to family–professional communication, cultural factors influencing beliefs, and behavior and self-perceived influences on quality of life, challenges, coping strategies and even positive aspects of living with CFA. Indeed, a call for research in CFA to be built upon the foundations of a "new craniofacial social science model" that seeks to understand the resourcefulness and health of affected families, rather than focusing only on deficits, has been made.[100] Such insights are unlikely to be brought to light through the use of traditional quantitative methods alone, but by means of the rich data that can be generated via qualitative techniques.[101]

Studies using qualitative approaches can facilitate the development of measurement tools that have been informed by the lay perspective. For example, it is known that measurements of aesthetic and functional outcomes in isolation are not good predictors of emotional (psychological) adjustment and well-being[102]; consequently, there is a pressing need to identify the self-perceived variables that contribute to the quality of life of affected individuals. The Eurocleft series highlighted the lack of association between outcome and satisfaction (Table 69–6). Meaningful ways to document the satisfaction of patients and families are essential, but present scales are rudimentary and may possess little validity. The development of techniques that have cross-cultural international validity has not begun and will be a significant challenge. Qualitative inquiry that incorporates the patient view could at least inform the theoretical basis for the development of such quantitative tools.

Old arguments about the superiority of either the quantitative or qualitative paradigms have now been superseded, and there is widespread acknowledgement complementary approaches are needed in order to adequately address questions of health and social care.[103] The Medical Research Council of the UK has recognized that the evaluation of complex interventions for health, i.e., interventions made up of multiple components, requires the use of a range of research tools in a phased approach, rather than those of the experimental model alone. The Council has established a framework for the design and evaluation of such interventions that integrates both quantitative and qualitative methods.[104] The value of an integrated approach to questions of health and social care is now a given in the wider health arena.

In order to enhance the evidence base for CFA, a range of tools from the qualitative repertoire must be used in an integrated approach so that patient values are able to appropriately influence policy and practice.

Measuring Treatment Burden

Since the consequences of cleft lip and/or palate may be apparent through every phase of childhood and adolescence, there is seldom a time when the disciplines involved in care cannot recommend one or another intervention. The powerful desire of patients and parents to reach the point where the stigma will be completely eradicated makes it likely that they will accept most proposals and willingly comply with protocols of care recommended by all members of the team no matter how demanding they may be. They have little choice.

So far, "burden of care" has received little attention in cleft studies, and yet the combined total of operations, other treatments, and follow-up appointments in the first 20 years of life can be enormous (Tables 69–3 and 69–4). Pain and suffering, disruption of family life, employment, and school attendance, and the dependent role into which the patient is placed may all have an adverse effect on his/her sense of self determination or locus of control.

A particular problem has arisen over the years with supplementary orthodontic interventions such as presurgical orthopedics, primary dentition orthodontics, and maxillary protraction. There is little evidence to suggest that the extra burden imposed on patients and the financial cost of these interventions is justified by any significant benefit.[105,106] Clearly it will be important in clinical trials to accurately record the total number of ancillary interventions and clinical visits in addition to surgical episodes.

Measuring Cost/Benefit

Economic pressures around the world have forced close examination of the true financial cost of treatment. With budget reductions, clinicians must either be involved in cost controls or have choices imposed upon them. Surgical procedures are invariably expensive treatment episodes, and successful primary operations that minimize the need for multiple secondary revisions are highly desirable. Furthermore, successful initial repairs are likely to reduce the duration and complexity of subsequent ancillary procedures.

Work has yet to begin in applying the techniques of health economics to the field of cleft care. Health status, the utility of care, and the associated quality of life may be estimated using the techniques of time tradeoff and conjoint analysis.[107–109] Economic prioritization models use decision analysis and simulation to assess the resource costs and patient benefits of current treatment patterns and the "cost effectiveness gap" or potential gain from alternative surgical procedures for cleft care.

Priorities for Research on Treatment

All of the above highlights an urgent need for the creation of collaborative groups in order to assemble a critical mass of expertise and to sufficiently access large samples of patients for adequately powered clinical trials. Given the current poor state of evidence for virtually all aspects of clinical management, there is an almost unlimited list of trials that could be initiated. However, the following were considered to be especially important in the recent WHO review:

- Trials of surgical methods for the repair of different orofacial cleft subtypes, not just unilateral cleft lip and palate
- Trials of surgical methods for the correction of velopharyngeal insufficiency
- Trials of the use of prophylactic ventilation tubes (grommets) for middle ear disease in patients with cleft palate
- Trials of adjunctive procedures in cleft care, especially those that place an increased burden on the patient, family, or medical services, such as presurgical orthopedics, primary dentition orthodontics, and maxillary protraction
- Trials of methods for management of perioperative pain, swelling and infection, and nursing
- Trials of methods to optimize feeding before and after surgery
- Trials addressing the special circumstances of care in the developing world in respect of surgical, anesthetic, and nursing care
- Trials of different modalities of speech therapy, orthodontic treatment and counseling.

Equally urgent is the need to create collaborative groups, or to improve the networking of existing groups, in order to develop and standardize outcome measures; there is an especially urgent need for work on patient-centered psychological and quality of life measures and economic outcomes. For rarer interventions, prospective registries should be established to hasten collaborative monitoring and critical appraisal, equivalent to Phase I trials. Relevant topics would be craniosynostosis surgery, ear reconstruction, distraction osteogenesis for hemifacial macrosomia and other skeletal variations, midface surgery in craniofacial dysostosis, and correction of hypertelorism.

QUALITY IMPROVEMENT

Previous research demonstrates that similar interventions achieve widely different outcomes dependent upon the manner and circumstances in which care is provided. For example, secondary complications have been found to occur up to 10 times more frequently when the care of children with unilateral cleft lip and palate is performed inexpertly or delivered in an uncoordinated manner.[110] It is evident too that simple care can achieve equivalent or superior outcomes to complex care at less human and economic cost.[11,105]

The exploration of methods to define attainable standards of care for CFA and to promote quality improvement protocols among the providers of care is considered by WHO to be an important priority.

Organization of Services

One program of quality improvement activity conducted under the auspices of the European Commission between 1996 and 2000[4] revealed great variability between countries in the provision of medical services for individuals with cleft lip and/or palate. While long-standing, high-volume centers of expertise prevailed in Scandinavia, countries such as Italy, Germany, Switzerland, and (until recently) the United Kingdom, provided cleft care via large numbers of local services with small caseloads. In other countries, such as Greece, Portugal, and Spain, the concept of comprehensive specialist team care was still undeveloped.

The challenge of improving services in a pan-European manner was addressed in part by the consensual development of clinical and organizational guidelines. The difficulties observed in configuring services into specialized units with sufficient caseloads to foster proficiency of care and secure adequate resources for comprehensive care were by no means solely economic. Instead, the obstacles were frequently reported to be

- personal egotism of individuals unwilling to discontinue the practice of treating a few children each year;
- competition between specialties for preeminence in the field;
- local pride, with every hospital, town, or region desiring its own small team;
- lack of clinical leadership; and
- lack of responsiveness of the health authorities at local and national level.

All the above problems have confronted the United Kingdom in the recent past and were not resolved until a national review was instigated by a government body.[111] The review included a national survey that revealed that Britain's fragmented, decentralized services were achieving a low standard of clinical success. As a result, the government instructed regions to provide care from a single regional center with a fully comprehensive specialist team, typically with two to three surgeons, each responsible for not less than 40–50 new personal cases requiring primary surgery per year. In this instance, government intervention was essential to the improvement of services when voluntary methods failed.[111]

Elsewhere in Europe, it was noted that the consensual guidelines on policies, practice guidelines, and record keeping had also been a powerful force in promoting reorganization of services for orofacial clefts, suggesting the influence of peer pressure at a national level. Thus, within months of the publication of the European guidelines, more than half the countries in Europe had to some extent reconfigured services, formed new multidisciplinary collaborative associations, and increased funding for clinical services.[4] These guidelines have since been endorsed by the WHO and are reproduced in the appendix of this chapter.

Monitoring Outcomes

It goes without saying that professionals entrusted with the provision of health care have an obligation to review the success of their practices and, where shortcomings are revealed, to take remedial action. Such efforts should constitute a continuous cycle, sometimes known as clinical audit. This has been defined as "the systematic critical analysis of the quality of care including procedures for diagnosis and treatment, the use of resources and the resulting outcome and quality of life for the patient."[112] Often, efforts in clinical audit are divided into evaluating the process of care (the way in which it is delivered) and the outcomes of care (what is achieved). Cycles of outcome audit are more easily established when the intervention is common and the consequences are clear-cut and quickly observable. Cleft audit therefore involves a considerable challenge because of the lengthy follow-up required, the complexity, subtlety and number of relevant outcomes, and above all, the relatively low number of cases.

Two general approaches are available for monitoring standards:

- **Intercenter comparisons**: These might take the form of a blinded comparison of records of consecutive patients from different centers, a number of which have been reported. Alternatively, one set of records may be compiled to serve as a standard reference archive against which any team could compare its outcomes. A "good practice" archive of this kind might include durable records such as study casts, radiographs, speech tapes, and so forth that would be representative of the ethnic population treated by well-established teams with consistent protocols. Other teams could measure their own outcome records against these. In time, a series of such archives for clefts and other CFA from different regions could become a web-based resource.
- **Registries**: There have been a number of attempts to establish a registry system that would allow ongoing self-monitoring. As yet, however, these have been difficult to fully establish. Under the auspices of the American Cleft Palate-Craniofacial Association, a web-based "Craniofacial Outcomes Registry" was recently piloted, enabling North American teams to anonymously enter diagnostic and outcome data. This intended that teams could rate their own outcomes and obtain an indication of their relative success compared with the Registry's aggregated data (www.cfregistry.org).

A national registry for Craniofacial Anomalies Network in the United Kingdom has also been established and is developing protocols for standardized outcome data collection (www.crane-database.org.uk/).

The Swedish Cleft Lip and Palate Association also has a web-based registry (Swedish National Quality Registry for Cleft Lip and Palate Treatment, http://natqa.uas.se/LKGreg/LKGreg.ihtml). It is intended that teams will display the actual records of consecutive cases, allowing peer review by each other.

ACCESS AND AVAILABILITY

The recent WHO review notes that by the early 1960s most industrialized countries had gained control of diseases caused by infection and/or malnutrition, so that genetic disorders and birth defects had attained public-health significance.[113] This situation is considered to occur when the infant mortality rate falls below 40–50/1000 live births, at which juncture countries tend to recognize the need for medical genetic services. Approximately 40 years later, a significant proportion of the world's developing nations has attained a similar situation: In 1997, 75 (53%) of the developing world countries, in which 60% of their population resided, had an infant mortality rate of less than 50 per 1000 live births.

Only a minority of CFA are lethal, and for the majority of affected individuals, there is a full life expectancy. Appearance, function, and social integration can, in nearly all cases, be improved by surgery and related multidisciplinary specialist care. The cost of treatment through infancy, childhood, and beyond can be considerable, however, and often unaffordable in the developing world, for example, in 1994 the medical costs for one individual with cleft lip/palate in the United States was estimated at $101,000.[114] In the United Kingdom, the estimated cost of one regional multidisciplinary cleft lip and palate service, receiving 140 new cases annually, was UK£ 6.4 million per year, excluding capital costs.[115] The social costs of unmet or partially met medical needs are also enormous. Affected individuals are liable to suffer stigmatization, social exclusion, and barriers to employment.

When malnutrition and communicable diseases represent more pressing priorities, cleft care provided by nongovernmental organizations (NGOs), through charitable missions of medical staff or the external sponsorship of local providers, may be the only chance of treatment that many individuals will have. Such efforts take place on a remarkably large scale and in a wide variety of ways. Because of the distinctive features of these services, WHO considered that particular research questions need to be addressed in order to maximize the benefit of NGO endeavors. In developing countries, for example, patients often present for surgery at later ages than in developed countries. Moreover, the services themselves may be of a rudimentary nature, and patients may be seen only once. Thus, a sound evidence base is needed in order to maximize effectiveness, safety, and capacity. Again, quality improvement strategies should be considered alongside this.

Main Approaches

Three main approaches to the provision of specialist care in the developing world have been noted. The first is the establishment of efficiently run, high-volume, indigenous centers of excellence, capable of serving large and widespread populations by a mixture of assisted traveling arrangements and outreach satellites. One such example of a center that had achieved considerable success, both in providing service and conducting research, has been developed in Brazil (www.centrinho.usp.br).

Secondly, some NGOs assist large numbers of individuals to receive surgery by providing financial support for indigenous clinical units to undertake operations that could not otherwise be afforded. Support for training indigenous specialists may also be provided (e.g., www.smiletrain.org).

Thirdly, a large number of NGOs provide care by forming surgical missions where teams of surgeons and ancillary staff make visits to selected sites where there is a shortage of resources or experienced personnel (e.g., www.operationsmile.org; www.rotaplast.org). In several instances, valuable research, especially of a genetic or epidemiological nature, has been conducted alongside these ventures.[116,117]

Ethical issues are a prominent concern in this work, and some programs have been criticized on grounds of safety, surgical competence and absence of follow-up. Although not a research issue per se, it was felt that WHO should attempt to encourage agencies involved in the charitable provision of treatment in the developing world to develop and adhere to a common international code of practice. Such an effort might build upon the survey undertaken by an earlier international task force on volunteer cleft missions[118] and consider:

- a survey of the charitable organizations involved and the scale of their work;
- an appraisal of the cost effectiveness and clinical effectiveness of the different models of aid;
- the promotion of dialogue between different NGOs to develop commonly agreed codes of practice and adoption of the most appropriate forms of aid for local circumstances, with an emphasis on support that favors indigenous long-term solutions;
- the initiation of clinical trials concerning the specifics of surgery in a developing country setting: one stage operations, optimal late primary surgery, anesthesia protocols (e.g., local anesthetic, inhalation, or sedation) antisepsis; and
- the development of common core protocols for genetic, epidemiological. and nutritional studies alongside surgery.

Regional Perspectives

WHO has published a partial review of international service provision and research capacity.

Africa

In sub-Saharan Africa clinical resources for CFA are scarce as a consequence of prevailing economic problems and the greater challenge of communicable diseases, particularly AIDS. In Namibia, for example, there are no cleft surgeons despite a high reported incidence of clefting. As the wealthiest sub-Saharan country, South Africa has approximately 12 centers that undertake cleft surgery, and these tend to work independently without common quality improvement protocols. There has been little formal study of CFA in the population of sub-Saharan Africa, and a regional "good practice" reference archive for this region would be valuable.

There are a number of centers in the cities of Northern Africa, but as elsewhere in Africa, a survey has yet to be undertaken to identify potential sites with capability for collaborative research.

Australia and New Zealand

There are well developed services in many cities, although in some instances, the caseload is quite low, limiting the potential for collaborative research. However, the establishment of the Australian and New Zealand Craniofacial Association makes coordination possible, and one center has a program of support and development for Indonesian and Malaysian centers.

China

In China there is reportedly a high level of unmet need for cleft and other CFA treatment. There is, however, a network of several large surgical centers that could form a potential research partnership.

Treatment, however, is not free, and follow-up is difficult. Speech therapists are especially scarce. Of those individuals receiving cleft surgery, only 30% are operated in the first year of life. Again, this points to a need for surgical trials to define preferred operative techniques in more mature patients. A survey of clinical services and potential collaborating sites would be valuable, as would development of a quality improvement strategy and "good practice" archive.

Europe

European clinical services have recently been surveyed.[3] In the main, Europe's problems arise from fragmentation of care over numerous small centers. The adoption of consensus recommendations, however, has begun to bring about some restructuring, at least for cleft services. Several international research collaborations are underway.

Indian Subcontinent

As yet, the subcontinent has not been surveyed regarding CFA or cleft services and research capability. However, an overview of India may be reasonably representative of adjoining countries. There are high levels of unmet need, and access is complicated because the majority of the population lives in rural communities. There are several hundred surgeons trained in cleft surgery and several large University hospitals, but no quality improvement protocols are yet in place. The subcontinent undoubtedly has numerous potential partners for clinical trials, although follow-up studies will be a challenge.

Latin America and the Caribbean

No survey has yet been done on clinical services and research capability across the continent. Mexico has at least one large center that has successfully completed clinical trials,[35,36,52] and is recognized as a center of excellence in the region. Brazil has a center of excellence at Bauru. Elsewhere in Latin America, there is undoubtedly a high level of unmet need.

South East Asia

Singapore has already embarked upon a surgical trial in collaboration with a large center of excellence in Taipei (www.nncf.org; www.cgmh.org.tw), and together they have a high research capability. In Indonesia, there are high levels of unmet need, but six cleft teams are established and would be potential sites for research collaboration. Both Indonesia and Malaysia are engaged in epidemiological, nutritional, and genetic research, with agencies in Australia, Europe, Singapore, and elsewhere. There are reportedly high local incidences of CFA, such as frontal encephalocele, that may be fruitful targets for multidisciplinary research.

Like Europe, Japan has a fragmentation of services in small centers; however the Japanese Cleft Palate Association has begun discussions on intercenter studies in clinical trials. In Korea, several high-volume centers are potential sites for collaborative research, and the Korean Cleft Palate Association has begun discussion on intercenter studies.

Middle East

A high level of unmet need has been reported with a few established CFA centers. A number of university hospitals in the region would be potential partners in research.

North America

North America also suffers from a fragmentation of cleft and craniofacial services, and there are difficulties in obtaining sufficient subjects for clinical trials because of the decentralized nature of services. The recent emergence of health management organizations is seen as a particular force for the fragmentation of services and dissipation of established cleft teams. Nonetheless, the Childhood Cancer Study Group has achieved a high level of coverage in the United States, and as a result, a high proportion of affected children are enrolled in trials.[119,120]

The American Cleft Palate-Craniofacial Association has promoted team care and has published several sets of guidelines.

References

1. World Health Organization: *Global Strategies Towards Reducing the Health-care Burden of Craniofacial Anomalies.* Report of WHO meetings on International Collaborative Research on Craniofacial Anomalies. WHO Human Genetics Programme, 2002.
2. Sackett DL, Straus SE, Richardson WS, et al. *Evidence-Based Medicine. How to Practice and Teach EBM.* Edinburgh: Churchill Livingstone, 2000.
3. Spriestersbach DC, Dickson DR, Fraser FC, et al. Clinical research in cleft lip and palate: The state of the art. *Cleft Palate J* 10:113–165, 1973.
4. Shaw WC, Semb G, Nelson P, et al. The Eurocleft Project 1996–2000: Overview. *J Craniomaxillofac Surg* 29:131–140, 2001.
5. Kunz R, Oxman AD. The unpredictability paradox: Review of empirical comparisons of randomised and non-randomised clinical trials. *Br Med J* 317:1185–1190, 1998.
6. Gehan AE. The evaluation of therapies: Historical control studies. *Stat Med* 3:315–324, 1984.

7. Semb G, Roberts CT, Shaw WC. Scope and limitations of single centre studies of cleft lip and palate. In: Vig PS, Dryland-Vig K (eds.). *Clinical research as the basis of clinical practice.* Monograph 25. Craniofacial Growth Series, Centre of Human Growth and Development. Ann Arbor: University of Michigan, 1991, pp. 109–123.

8. Pinsky CA. Experience with historical control studies in cancer immunotherapy. *Stat Med* 3:325–329, 1984.

9. Pollock AV. Historical evolution: Methods, attitudes, goals. In: Troidl H, Spitzer WO, Peak B, Mulder DS, McKneally MF, (eds). *Principle, practice of research: Strategies for surgical investigators.* New York: Springer Verlag, 1986, pp. 7–17.

10. Shaw WC, Asher-McDade C, Brattström V, et al. A six-center international study of treatment outcome in patients with clefts of the lip and palate: Part 1. Principles and study design. *Cleft Palate Craniofac J* 29:393–397, 1992a.

11. Shaw WC, Dahl E, Asher-McDade C, et al. A six-center international study of treatment outcome in patients with clefts of the lip and palate: Part 5. General discussion and conclusions. *Cleft Palate Craniofac J* 29:413–418, 1992b.

12. Mølsted K, Asher-McDade C, Brattström V, et al. A six-center international study of treatment outcome in patients with clefts of the lip and palate: Part 2. Craniofacial form and soft tissue profile. *Cleft Palate Craniofac J* 29:398–404, 1992.

13. Mars M, Asher-McDade C, Brattström V, et al. A six-center international study of treatment outcome in patients with clefts of the lip and palate: Part 3. Dental arch relationships. *Cleft Palate Craniofac J* 29:405–408, 1992.

14. Asher-McDade C, Brattström V, Dahl E, et al. A six-center international study of treatment outcome in patients with clefts of the lip and palate: Part 4. Assessment of nasolabial appearance. *Cleft Palate Craniofac J* 29:409–412, 1992.

15. Mølsted K, Dahl E, Skovgaard LT, et al. A multicenter comparison of treatment regimes for unilateral cleft lip and palate using a multiple regression model. *Scand J Plast Reconstr Surg Hand Surg* 27:277–284, 1993a.

16. Mølsted K, Dahl E, Brattström V, et al. A six-center international study of treatment outcome in patients with clefts of the lip and palate: Evaluation of maxillary asymmetry. *Cleft Palate Craniofac J* 30:22–28, 1993b.

17. Semb G, Brattström V, Mølsted K, et al. The Eurocleft Study: Intercenter study of treatment outcome in patients with complete cleft lip and palate. Part 1: Introduction and treatment experience. *Cleft Palate Craniofac J* 42:64–68, 2005a.

18. Semb G, Brattström V, Mølsted K, et al. The Eurocleft Study: Longitudinal follow-up of patients with complete cleft lip and palate. Part 4: Relationship between treatment outcome, patient/parent satisfaction and the burden of care. *Cleft Palate Craniofac J* 42:83–92, 2005b.

19. Brattström V, Mølsted K, Prahl-Andersen B, et al. The Eurocleft study: Longitudinal follow-up of patients with complete unilateral cleft lip and palate. Part 2: Craniofacial form and nasolabial appearance. *Cleft Palate Craniofac J* 42:69–77, 2005.

20. Mølsted K, Brattström V, Prahl-Andersen, et al. The Eurocleft study: Longitudinal follow-up of patients with complete unilateral cleft lip and palate. Part 3: Dental arch relationship. *Cleft Palate Craniofac J* 42:78–82, 2005.

21. Grunwell P, Brøndsted K, Henningsson G, et al. A six-center international study of the outcome of treatment in patients with clefts of the lip and palate: The results of a cross-linguistic investigation of cleft palate speech. *Scand J Plast Reconstr Surg Hand Surg* 34:219–229, 2000.

22. Diggle PJ, Liang KY, Zeger SL. *Analysis of Longitudinal Data.* Oxford: Oxford Scientific Publications, 1994.

23. Shaw WC, Brattström V, Mølsted K, et al. The Eurocleft Study: Longitudinal follow-up of patients with complete cleft lip and palate. Part 5: Discussion and conclusions. *Cleft Palate Craniofac J* 42:93–98, 2005.

24. Nordin K-E, Larson O, Nylén B, et al. Early bone grafting in complete cleft lip and palate cases following maxillofacial orthopedics. I. The method and the skeletal development from seven to 13 years of age. *Scand J Plast Reconstr Surg* 17:33–50, 1983.

25. Moher D, Jones A, Cook DJ. Does quality of reports of randomized trials affect estimates of intervention efficacy reported in meta-analyses? *Lancet* 352:609–613, 1998.

26. Roberts CT, Semb G, Shaw WC. Strategies for the advancement of surgical methods in cleft lip and palate. *Cleft Palate Craniofac J* 28:141–149, 1991.

27. Robertson NRE, Jolleys A. Effects of early bone grafting in complete clefts of lip and palate. *Plast Reconstr Surg* 42:414–421, 1968.

28. Robertson NRE, Jolleys A. An 11-year follow-up of the effects of early bone grafting in infants born with complete clefts of the lip and palate. *Br J Plast Surg* 36:438–443, 1983.

29. Robertson NRE, Jolleys A. The timing of hard palate repair. *Scand J Plast Reconstr Surg* 8:49–51, 1974.

30. Robertson NRE, Jolleys A. A further look at the effects of delaying repair of the hard palate, In: Huddart AG, Ferguson MWJ, (eds). *Cleft Lip and Palate. Long-term Results and Future Prospects.* Manchester University Press, 1990.

31. Wray C, Dann J, Holtmann B. A comparison of three techniques of palatorrhapy: In-hospital morbidity. *Cleft Palate J* 16:42–45, 1979.

32. Holtmann B, Wray RC, Weeks PM. A comparison of three techniques of palatorrhaphy: Early speech results. *Ann Plast Surg* 12:514–518, 1984.

33. Chowdri NA, Darzi MA, Ashraf MM. A comparative study of surgical results with rotation-advancement and triangular flap techniques in unilateral cleft lip. *Br J Plast Surg* 43:551–556, 1990.

34. Marsh JL, Grames LM, Holtman MD. Intravelar veloplasty: A prospective study. *Cleft Palate J* 26:46–50, 1989.

35. Ysunza A, Pamplona MC, Mendoza M, et al. Speech outcome and maxillary growth in patients with unilateral complete cleft lip/palate operated on at 6 versus 12 months of age. *Plast Reconstr Surg* 102:675–679, 1998.

36. Ysunza A, Pamplona MC, Mendoza M, et al. Surgical treatment of submucous cleft palate: A comparative trial of modalities for palatal closure. *Plast Reconstr Surg* 107:9–14, 2001.

37. Whitaker LA, Randall P, Graham WP III, et al. A prospective and randomized series comparing superiorly and inferiorly based posterior pharyngeal flaps. *Cleft Palate J* 9:304–311, 1972.

38. VPI Surgical Trial Group. A randomized trial of pharyngoplasty versus pharyngeal flap for individuals with velopharyngeal insufficiency following cleft palate repair. Paper presented at the 9th International Congress on Cleft Palate and Related Craniofacial Anomalies, Göteborg, Sweden, 25–29 June, 2001.

39. Williams W, Pegoraro-Krook MI, Dutka-Souza J, et al. The Furlow double z-palatalplasty vs the von Langenbeck surgical technique: A ten-year prospective randomized double-blind clinical trial comparing VP function for speech. *Proceedings of the 63rd Annual Meeting of the American Cleft Palate-Craniofacial Association*, Vancouver, Canada, 2006.

40. Friede H, Enemark H, Semb G, et al. Craniofacial and occlusal characteristics in unilateral cleft lip and palate patients from four Scandinavian centers. *Scand J Plast Reconstr Surg Hand Surg* 25:269–276, 1991.

41. Enemark H, Friede H, Paulin G, et al. Lip and nose morphology in patients with unilateral cleft lip and palate from four Scandinavian centers. *Scand J Plast Reconstr Surg Hand Surg* 27:41–47, 1993.

42. Morrant DG, Shaw WC. Use of standardized video recordings to assess cleft surgery outcome. *Cleft Palate Craniofac J* 33:134–142, 1996.

43. Semb G. *Scandcleft randomized trials of primary surgery for unilateral cleft lip and palate.* Working paper presented to WHO meeting, "International Collaborative Research on Craniofacial Anomalies", Geneva 5–8 November, 2001.

44. Ping F, Yan F, Chen J. A primary clinical analysis of artificial bone implantation of cleft palate. [Article in Chinese] *Zhonghua Zheng Xing Wai Ke Za Zhi* 17:353–355, 2001.

45. Chen PK, Yeow VK, Noordhoff MS, et al. Augmentation of the nasal floor with Surgicel in primary lip repair: A prospective study showing no efficacy. *Ann Plast Surg* 2:149–53, 1999.

46. Bremerich DH, Neidhart G, Heinmann K, et al. Prophylactically administered rectal acetaminophen does not reduce postoperative opioid requirements in infants and small children undergoing elective cleft palate repair. *Anesth Analg* 92:907–912, 2001.

47. Prabhu KP, Wig J, Grewal S. Bilateral infraorbital nerve block is superior to periincisional infiltration for analgesia after repair of cleft lip. *Scand J Plast Reconstr Surg Hand Surg* 33:83–87, 1999.

48. Ahuja S, Datta A, Krishna A, et al. Infra-orbital nerve block for relief of postoperative pain following cleft lip surgery in infants. *Anaesthesia* 49:441–444, 1994.

49. Nicodemus HF, Ferrer MJ, Cristobal VC, et al. Bilateral infraorbital block with 0.5% bupivacaine as post-operative analgesia following cheiloplasty in children. *Scand J Plast Reconstr Surg Hand Surg* 25:253–257, 1991.

50. Senders CW, Di Mauro SM, Brodie HA, et al. The efficacy of perioperative steroid therapy in pediatric primary palatoplaty. *Cleft Palate Craniofac J* 3:340–344, 1999.

51. Amland PF, Andenaes K, Samdal F, et al. A prospective, double-blind, placebo-controlled trial of a single dose of azithromycin on postoperative wound infections in plastic surgery. *Plast Reconstr Surg* 96:1378–1383, 1995.

52. Pamplona MC, Ysunza A, Espinosa J. A comparative trial of two modalities of speech intervention for compensatory articulation in cleft palate children, phonologic approach versus articulatory approach. *Int J Pediatr Otolaryngol* 49:21–26, 1999.

53. Pamplona MC, Ysunza A, Jimenez-Murat Y. Mothers of children with cleft palate undergoing speech intervention change communicative interaction. *Int J Pediatr Otolaryngol* 59:173–179, 2001.

54. Kuijpers-Jagtman AM, Prahl C. *A study into the effects of presurgical orthopaedic treatment in complete unilateral cleft lip and palate patients. A three-centre prospective clinical trial in Nijmegen, Amsterdam and Rotterdam.* Interim analysis. Nijmegen: University Press, 1996.

55. Kuijpers-Jagtman AM, Prahl-Andersen B. Value of presurgical infant orthopaedics: An intercentre randomised clinical trial. In: Lee ST, Huang M, (eds). *Transactions 8th International Congress on Cleft Palate and Craniofacial Related Anomalies.* Singapore: Stamford Press, 1997, pp. 1002.

56. Konst EM, Weersink-Braks H, Rietveld T, et al. An intelligibility assessment of toddlers with cleft lip and palate who received and did not receive presurgical infant orthopedic treatment. *J Commun Disord* 33:483–499, 2000.

57. Prahl C, Kuijpers-Jagtman AM, van't Hof MD, et al. A randomised prospective clinical trial into the effect of infant orthopaedics on maxillary arch dimensions in unilateral cleft lip and palate (Dutchcleft). *Eur J Oral Sci* 109:1–9, 2001.

58. Jigjinni V, Kangesku T, Sommerlad BC. Do babies require arm splints after cleft palate repair? *Br J Plast Surg* 46:680–685, 1993.

59. Darzi MA, Chowdri NA, Bhat AN. Breast feeding or spoon feeding after cleft lip repair: A prospective, randomized study. *Br J Plast Surg* 49:24–26, 1996.

60. Lee TK. Effect of unrestricted postoperative sucking following cleft repair on early postoperative course. *Proceedings of the 4th Asian Pacific Cleft Lip and Palate Conference* Japan: Fukuoka, 1999.

61. Brine EA, Rickard KA, Brady MS, et al. Effectiveness of two feeding methods in improving energy intake and growth of infants with cleft palate: A randomized study. *J Am Diet Assoc* 94:732–738, 1994.

62. Shaw GM, Todoroff K, Finnell RH, et al. Maternal vitamin use, infant C677T mutation in MTHFR, and isolated cleft palate risk [letter]. *Am J Med Genet* 85:84–85, 1999.

63. Kuehn DP, Imrey PB, Tomes L, et al. Efficacy of continuous positive airway pressure for treatment of hypernasality. *Cleft Palate Craniofac J* 39:267–276, 2002.

64. Lin YT, Tsai CL. Comparative anti-caries effects of tablet and liquid fluorides in cleft children. *J Clin Dent* 11:104–106, 2000.

65. Berkowitz S. Ethical issues in the case of surgical repair of cleft palate. *Cleft Palate Craniofac J* 32:271–276, 1995.

66. Shaw WC. Commentary to "Ethical Issues in the Case of Surgical Repair of Cleft Palate" by S. Berkowitz. *Cleft Palate Craniofac J* 32:277–280, 1995.

67. Baum M. Scientific empiricisms and clinical medicine: A discussion paper. *J R Soc Med* 74:504–509, 1981.

68. Salzman EW. Is surgery worthwhile? *Arch Surg* 120:771–776, 1985.

69. Chalmers I. What is the prior probability of a proposed new treatment being superior to established treatments? *Br Med J* 314:74–75, 1997.

70. Chalmers I, Lindley RI. Double standards on informed consent to treatment, In: Doyal L, Tobias JS (eds). *Informed consent in medical research.* London: British Medical Journal Publications, 2000.

71. Lantos J. Ethical issues. How can we distinguish clinical research from innovativebtherapy? *Am J Pediatr Hematol Oncol* 16:72–75, 1994.

72. Tonelli MD, Benditt JO, Albert RK. Lessons from lung volume reduction surgery. *Chest* 110:230–238, 1996.

73. Chalmers I, Altman DC. *Systematic Reviews.* London: British Medical Journal Publishing Group, 1995.

74. Glenny AM, Hooper L, Shaw WC, et al. Feeding interventions for growth and development for infants with cleft lip, cleft palate or cleft lip and palate. In: *The Cochrane Database of Systematic Reviews.* doi: 10.1002/14651858.

75. Shaw WC, Semb G. Facial growth in orofacial clefting disorders, In: Turvey TA, Vig KWL, Fonseca RJ (eds). *Principles and management of facial clefting disorders and craniosynostosis.* Philadelphia: WB Saunders Co., 1996, pp. 28–56.

76. Atack NE, Hathorn IS, Semb G, et al. A new index for assessing surgical outcome in unilateral cleft lip and palate subjects aged five: Reproducibility and validity. *Cleft Palate Craniofac J* 34:242–246, 1997.

77. Kuehn DP, Moller KT. Speech and language issues in the cleft palate population: The state-of-the-art. *Cleft Palate Craniofac J* 37:1–35, 2000.

78. Sell D, Grunwell P, Mildinhall S, et al. Cleft lip and palate care in the United Kingdom—The Clinical Standards Advisory Group (CSAG) Study: Part 3—Speech outcomes. *Cleft Palate Craniofac J* 38:30–37, 2001.

79. Williams AC, Bearn DR, Mildinhall S, et al. Cleft lip and palate care in the United Kingdom—The Clinical Standards Advisory Group (CSAG) Study: Part 2—Dentofacial outcomes, psychosocial status and patient satisfaction. *Cleft Palate Craniofac J* 38:24–29, 2001.

80. Henningsson G, Kuehn D, Sell D, et al. Universal Parameters for Reporting Speech Outcomes in Individuals with Cleft Palate. *Cleft Palate Craniofac J* (in press,).

81. Strauss R. Culture, health care and birth defects in the United States: An Introduction. *Cleft Palate Craniofac J* 27:275–278, 1990.

82. Mason J. *Qualitative researching,* 2nd ed. London: Sage, 2002.

83. Flick U. *An introduction to qualitative research,* 3r ed. London: Thousand Oaks, New Delhi: Sage, 2006.

84. Creswell J. *Qualitative Inquiry and Research Design. Choosing Among Five Approaches.* Thousand Oaks: London, New Delhi: Sage, 2007.

85. Green J, Thorogood N. *Qualitative methods for health research.* London: Sage, 2004.

86. Pope C, Mays N. *Qualitative research in health care.* BMJ Books: Blackwell, 2006.

87. Richards L, Morse JM. *Read Me First for a User's Guide to Qualitative Methods,* 2nd ed. London, Thousand Oaks, New Delhi: Sage, 2007.

88. Popay J, Rogers A, Williams G. Rationale and standards for the systematic review of qualitative literature in health services research. *Qual Health Res* 8:341–351, 1998.

89. Strauss R, Broder H. Directions and issues in psychosocial research and methods as applied to cleft lip and palate and craniofacial anomalies. *Cleft Palate Craniofac J* 28:150–156, 1991.

90. Tretsven V. Impressions concerning clefts in Montana Indians of the past. *Cleft Palate J* 2:229–236, 1965.

91. Eisermann W. Unique outcomes and positive contributions associated with facial difference: Expanding research and practice. *Cleft Palate Craniofac J* 38:236–244, 2001.

92. Meyerson M. Resiliency and success in adults with Moebius Syndrome. *Cleft Palate Craniofac J* 38:231–235, 2001.

93. Patel Z, Ross E. Reflections on the cleft experience by South African adults: Use of qualitative methodology. *Cleft Palate Craniofac J* 40:471–480, 2003.

94. Beaune L, Forrest CR, Keith T. Adolescents' perspectives on living and growing up with Treacher Collins Syndrome: A qualitative study. *Cleft Palate Craniofac J* 41:343–350, 2004.

95. Edwards T, Patrick DL, Topolski TD, et al. Approaches to craniofacial-specific quality of life assessment in adolescents. *Cleft Palate Craniofac J* 42:19–24, 2005.

96. Strauss R, Fenson C. Experiencing the "Good Life": Literary views of craniofacial conditions and quality of life. *Cleft Palate Craniofac J* 42:14–18, 2001.

97. Klein T, Pope A, Getahun E, et al. Mothers' reflections on raising a child with a craniofacial anomaly. *Cleft Palate Craniofac J* 43:231–235, 2006.

98. Silverman D. The clinical subject: Adolescents in a Cleft-Palate Clinic. *Sociol Health Illn* 5:253–274, 1983.

99. Johansson B, Ringsberg K. Parents' experiences of having a child with a cleft lip and palate. *J Adv Nurs* 47:165–173, 2004.

100. Strauss R: "Only Skin Deep": Health, resilience and craniofacial care. *Cleft Palate Craniofac J* 38:226–230, 2001.

101. Denzin NK, Lincoln YS. *Collecting and interpreting qualitative materials.* Thousand Oaks: Sage, 1998.

102. Robinson E. Psychological research on visible difference in adults (Chapter 16), In: Lansdown R, Rumsey N, Bradbury E, Carr T, Partridge J, (eds.). V*isibly Different: Coping with disfigurement.* Oxford: Butterworth Heinemann, 1997.

103. Morse JM, Field PA. *Nursing Research. The Application of Qualitative Approaches,* 2nd ed. Chapman and Hall, 1996.

104. Campbell M, Fitzpatrick R, Haines A, et al. Framework for design and evaluation of complex interventions to improve health. *Br Med J* 321:694–696, 2000.

105. Severens JL, Prahl C, Kuijpers-Jagtman AM, et al. Short-term cost-effectiveness analysis of presurgical orthopedic treatment in children with complete unilateral cleft lip and palate. *Cleft Palate Craniofac J* 35:222–226, 1998.

106. Kuijpers-Jagtman AM, Long RE. The influence of surgery and orthopedic treatment on maxillofacial growth and maxillary arch development in patients treated for orofacial clefts. *Cleft Palate Craniofac J* 37:527, 2000.

107. Torrance GW. Social preferences for health states: An empirical evaluation of three measurement techniques. *Socioecon Plann Sci* 10:129–136, 1976.

108. Ryan M, McIntosh E, Shackley P. Methodological issues in the application of conjoint analysis in health care. *Health Econ* 7:373–378, 1998.

109. Ryan M. Using conjoint analysis to take account of patient preferences and go beyond health outcomes: An application to in vitro fertilisation. *Soc Sci Med* 48:535–546, 1999.

110. Bearn D, Mildinhall S, Murphy T, et al. Cleft lip and palate care in the United Kingdom—the Clinical Standards Advisory Group (CSAG) Study. Part 4: Outcome comparisons, training, and conclusions. *Cleft Palate Craniofac J* 38:38–43, 2001.

111. Sandy JR, Williams AC, Bearn DR, et al. Cleft lip and palate care in the United Kingdom—The Clinical Standards Advisory Group (CSAG) Study: Part 1—Background and methodology. *Cleft Palate Craniofac J* 38:20–23, 2001.

112. Long AF. *Outcomes Within Audit: A Process and Outcome Perspective. Vol 7* Outcomes Briefing, UK: Clearing House on Health Outcomes, 1996, pp. 4–7.

113. Christianson A. Orofacial clefting in sub Saharan Africa. Working paper presented to WHO Meeting "International Collaborative Research on Craniofacial Anomalies", Geneva, 5–8 November, 2001.

114. Waitzman NJ, Romano PS, Scheffler RM. Estimates of the economic costs of births defects. *Inquiry* 31:188–205, 1994.

115. National Health Service: North West Regional Office, commissioning background paper. Warrington: United Kingdom, 2001.

116. Lidral AC, Murray JC, Buetow KH, et al. Studies of the candidate genes TGFB2, MSX1, TGFA and TGFB3 in the etiology of cleft lip and palate in the Philippines. *Cleft Palate Craniofac J* 34:1–6, 1997.

117. Murray JC, Daack-Hirsch S, Buetow KH, et al. Clinical and epidemiologic studies of cleft lip and palate in the Philippines. *Cleft Palate Craniofac J* 34:7–10, 1997.

118. Yeow VKL, Lee ST, Lambrecht TJ, et al. Recommendations of the international task force on volunteer cleft missions. In: Lee ST, Huang M (eds). *Transactions 8th International Congress on Cleft Palate and Related Craniofacial Anomalies.* Singapore: Stamford Press; xliii-li, 1997.

119. Ross JA, Severson RK, Pollock BH, et al. Childhood cancer in the US: A geographical analysis of cases from the pediatric cooperative clinical trials groups. *Cancer* 77:201–207, 1996.

120. Shochat SJ, Fremgen AM, Murphy SB, et al. Childhood cancer: Patterns of protocol participation in a national survey. *CA Cancer J Clin* 51:119–130, 2001.

APPENDIX: EUROCLEFT CONSENSUS RECOMMENDATIONS

Background

The Eurocleft Consensus Recommendations which follow take the form of four documents:

- *Policy Statements*
- *Practice Guidelines*
- *General Principles Governing Record Taking and Timing of Minimum Records*
- *Record Taking Methodology*

All but the last were agreed by a process of consultation amongst the national representatives of the Eurocleft Clinical Network, via a series of short personal interviews prior to consensus workshops held in Manchester during 1998 and 1999. Recommendations for *Record Taking Methodology* continue to be discussed, however the guidelines which appear below provide a suggestion that is currently being used widely in Europe.

Policy Statements

1. The professional involved in cleft care should provide basic information on cleft care and on the proposed treatment to any potential patient and/or patient's guardian. Basic information should contain at least:

   - a general explanation of the condition, the reasons for treatment, what may or may not be achieved, the stages of treatment including examination, record collection and general protocols. This may be supplemented by leaflets, booklets or other kinds of information.
   - an explanation of why a specific treatment is considered necessary for the individual patient, what specifically is involved:- method, timing, duration cost, what the specific goal is and possible side effects.

2. When a treatment is considered, the professional engaged in cleft care should take into consideration the desires and attitudes of the patient and/or those of the patient's guardian. The professional should also pay attention to and inform the patient/patient's guardian of the risks and benefits inherent in the potential alternative treatment options, including no treatment or no further treatment.

3. If requested, it is the professional's responsibility to provide a procedure for obtaining a second opinion for the patient. If requested, this procedure should be communicated to the patient before treatment starts.

4. After an episode of treatment, the professional engaged in cleft care should inform the patient and/or patient's guardian on:

   - outcome of treatment relative to the defined goal.
   - undesirable effects of treatment.
   - expected future development.

5. The professional engaged in cleft care should analyse and document any complaints or praise expressed by the patient and/or the patient's guardian.

6. The professional engaged in cleft care should give consideration to the burden of the treatment:

   - considerations should include financial as well as non-financial burden, such as treatment duration, effort from the patient and/or patient's guardian and discomfort as a result of treatment.

7. During the process of treatment, the professional involved in cleft care should continuously evaluate treatment progress against the planned treatment and act accordingly.

8. Organisations and institutes responsible for the provision of cleft care should:

   - encourage the cleft professional to follow the policies described above and to acknowledge the patient's rights.
   - recognise and encourage the professional's right to provide treatment that can be expected to improve the patient's condition whilst minimising adverse effects.
   - recognise and encourage that decisions on treatment priority should be based on criteria proposed by the cleft professionals in consultation with the patient and/or patient's guardian. This is especially so in a situation with insufficient treatment resources.
   - recognise and encourage that access to treatment should not depend on the patient's ability to pay.
   - recognise that co-operation of the patient with the advice and instructions of the cleft professional is necessary in order to achieve a successful result.

Practice Guidelines

Part I: Healthcare Needs

1. **Neonatal Emotional Support and Professional Advice**
   In the event of prenatal diagnosis and as soon as possible after the birth of a child with a cleft parents should be given emotional support and advice about the child's future management by a specialist in cleft care.

2. **Neonatal Nursing**
   Difficulties in feeding are common in the early days of life and specialist advice on feeding should be provided.

3. **Surgery**
   Primary surgery to close clefts of the lip and/or palate should be performed by an experienced and qualified surgeon according to a protocol agreed by the team. Further corrective procedures may be necessary for some patients in later years and should be performed by an experienced and qualified surgeon according to a protocol agreed by the team.

4. **Orthodontic/Orthopaedic Treatment**
   For children with cleft lip and palate orthodontic/orthopaedic treatment should be available when necessary and should be performed by an experienced orthodontist.

5. **Speech and Language Therapy**
   Early assessment of speech and language problems, advice to parents and the availability of corrective therapy by an experienced speech and language therapist should be provided.

6. **Ear, Nose and Throat (ENT)**
   ENT problems should be identified at an early stage and the necessary therapy should be provided.

7. **Clinical Genetics/Paediatric Developmental Medicine**
   As cleft lip and/or palate may be associated with other anomalies early assessment and diagnosis is necessary. Genetic counselling for patients and families should be available.

8. **Emotional Support and Professional Advice for the Growing Child and its Parents**
   Emotional support and professional advice for parents, patients and their environment is often necessary and should be available.

9. **Dental Care**
   Regular dental care should be available.

10. **National Register**
    A national register should be in place for accurate recording of children born with cleft lip and/or palate and related craniofacial anomalies.

Part II: Organisation of Services

1. Cleft care should be provided by a multidisciplinary team of specialists.
2. Members of the team should have special training in cleft care.
3. The team should agree on the stages of treatment including the examination, record collection and general protocols.
4. There should be one person responsible for quality improvement and communication within the team.
5. Co-ordination of the care of individual patients is important since numerous specialities are involved. This should be the responsibility of one member of the team.
6. The number of patients referred to the team should be sufficient to sustain the experience and specialist skills of all team members and to allow evaluation/audit of the team's performance within a reasonable period of time. It has been recommended that cleft surgeons, orthodontists and speech therapists should treat at least 40–50 new cases annually. However, it is recognised that individual member states have the right to provide care for their own population.

Part III: Finances

Resources should be available to cover the following care for children with cleft lip and palate:

1. Emotional support and professional advice during the neonatal period.
2. Neonatal nursing.
3. Surgery.
4. Orthodontic/orthopaedic treatment.
5. Speech and language assessment and therapy.
6. Ear, Nose and Throat treatment.
7. Clinical genetics/Paediatric developmental medicine.
8. Emotional support for the growing child and its parents.
9. Travel expenses.
10. General dental care including cleft related prosthodontics.

General Principles Governing Record Taking

1. **Records for Treatment Planning/Monitoring**
   - clinical records should be taken for individual patients to allow treatment planning, monitoring treatment progress and treatment evaluation.
   - the timing and nature of these records will depend on the clinical protocols followed by individual teams.
   - treatment and associated record taking protocols should be agreed and clearly set out by the cleft team.

2. **Records for Quality Improvement/Research**
   Additional records may be taken for a number of other reasons:
   - follow up of a series of patients to provide an overview of the outcome of care.
   - to allow retrospective comparisons of different protocols.

   - as part of a prospective clinical trial with ethical approval.
   - as part of an agreed protocol for intercentre quality improvement comparisons or comparison against known standards.
   - as part of an agreed research protocol.
   - other reasons such as medico-legal, second opinion.

3. **Safeguards**
   - exposure of patients to unnecessary radiation should be avoided.
   - research and quality improvement records should only be taken when there is an established written protocol on how they will be put to use.
   - research and quality improvement records should not be taken without the consent of the patient/parent/guardian.
   - research and quality improvement records should coincide as far as possible with the records for treatment planning/monitoring (statement 1).

Timing of Minimum Records

1. Complete Cleft Lip and Palate (UCLP & BCLP)

Timing	Models	Lateral skull radiograph	Photographs	Speech	Audiometry/ tympanometry	Patient/ parent satisfaction
Primary surgery	√		√			
3 Years				√*	√*	
5/6 Years	√		√	√	√	
10 Years	√	√	√	√	√	
18+ Years	√	√	√	√		√

* = *if hard palate is closed*

2. Cleft Palate Only

Timing	Models	Lateral skull radiograph	Photographs	Speech	Audiometry/ tympanometry	Patient/ parent satisfaction
Primary surgery	√		√			
3 Years				√	√	
5/6 Years	√			√	√	
15/16 Years	√	√	√	√	√	√

3. Cleft Lip Only

Timing	Models	Photographs	Patient/ parent satisfaction
Primary surgery	√*	√	
3 Years			
5/6 Years	√*	√	
10 Years			
18+ Years		√	√

* = only in cases with cleft of the alveolus as well as cleft lip

4. Alveolar Bone Grafting

Timing	Intra-oral X-ray	Photographs
Just before bone graft	√	√
6 months after graft	√	
After canine fully erupted	√	√

5. Pharyngoplasty

Timing	Speech sample
Just before operation	√
One year after operation	√

Record Taking Methodology

Discussion of the precise method of record taking is continuing. The following however, provide a suggestion that is currently being used widely in Europe.

6. Orthognathic surgery

Timing	Lateral cephalogram	Models
Just before operation	√	√
One year after operation	√	√

PHOTOGRAPHS

Background

The vast majority of surgeons and orthodontists use still photographs for documentation of clefts. Very few clinicians use video recording of clefts pre- or post-operatively. If photographs of clefts which appear in any publication are examined it is clear that there is no uniformity or standardisation of the way in which such photographs are taken. For comparative studies the following are recommended:

Basic views to be taken
- frontal, both laterals, inferior (columellar) view
- 3/4 facial (oblique) view

Dynamic views
- during smiling and whistling: in the co-operative older patient, these views will give an idea of function of the circumoral musculature
- video recording will be better for assessing circum-oral movement but this will also need to be standardised and cannot be used routinely at present

Lighting and Background
- lighting for the studio should be two fill-in lights and the main light synchronised with the camera. In the ward or operating theatre a single flash unit is appropriate
- the background should be blue

Framing of the Picture
- for frontal view, the camera should be set at a ratio of 1:8
- for lateral view, the camera should be set at a ratio of 1:8
- for inferior view, the camera should be set at a ratio of 1:4

Camera and Lens
- suggested camera is Nikon F3 with a 105 mm lens or equivalent
- film type and speed need not be standardised

Dental Casts

Background

Dental casts need to be made from well taken impressions which include all teeth, the palate and the buccal sulcus. For comparative studies the casts need to be prepared in a standard manner so that the source of the models cannot be identified.

Preparation
Models should be:

- cast in vacuum mixed white stone, for example Crystacal R
- hand trimmed using fine wheel to the standard heights and angles shown in Figures 69-Aa)., 69-Ab). and 69-Ac). below
- finished with wet and dry paper (not soaped)

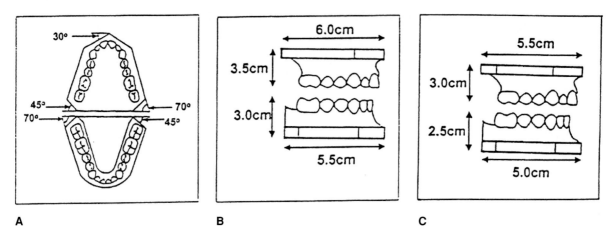

Figure 69-A. A. Dental casts' base angles. **B.** 10-year-olds' dental casts **C.** 5-year-olds' dental casts.

Speech

Background

A fundamental problem for speech and language pathology has been the lack of an acceptable framework for measuring speech. Various groups have proposed procedures for measuring, recording and reporting speech data cross-linguistically, but to date there is no one recognised method.

Proposals have come from Henningsson and Hutters 14, and also from Dalston, Marsh, Vig, Witzel and Bumstead 15. In Britain, Sell, Harding and Grunwell, developed GOS.SP.ASS 16. This is now a nationally agreed speech assessment tool for cleft palate and/or velopharyngeal incompetence in English. From GOS.SP.ASS was devised CAPS (Cleft Audit Protocol for Speech) by Razzell, Harding and Harland 17, a more succinct protocol specifically designed for audit purposes.

Ages
3–4 years
5–6 years
10 years
15–16 years (cleft palate only)
18+ years (UCLP and BCLP)
Equipment
A good quality audio recording using a high quality microphone.

Variables

Intelligibility: a rating should be made upon spontaneous speech. The CAPS scale can be used to judge how "understandable" a persons speech would be to familiar and unfamiliar listeners (there are however flaws with this method).

Nasality: the presence/absence and degree of hypernasality, hyponasality, audible nasal emission and nasal turbulence can be judged and rated on a five point scale (see CAPS). An agreed instrumental method for assessing nasality has yet to be recommended.

Assessing Articulation: set sentences and single words containing consonant sounds in different word positions (beginning, middle and end) should be repeated eg. "Bob is a baby boy" or equivalent in the native language, and recorded for CAPS. Targeted sounds are*: p, b, f, n, t, d, s, s, ʧ, ʤ, k, g. Errors made can be broadly categorised or grouped according to CAPS:

- front of mouth oral sound errors
- back of mouth oral sound errors
- non-oral sounds
- passive errors
- immaturities

---

* depending on the speech sound system in each language but should contain plosives, fricatives and a nasal consonant (p, b, t, d, k, g, f, s, n).

Assessment of Orthodontic Outcomes in Patients with Clefts

Ross E. Long, Jr, DMD, MS, PhD • Scott A. Deacon, BDS, MSc

INTRODUCTION

The role of the orthodontist has been pivotal for the effective functioning of the cleft lip/palate team and the assessment of the facial growth and development of the dentition and occlusion ever since Dr. Herbert K. Cooper, a Pennsylvania orthodontist, first championed the team concept.[1] The wide range of patient ages over which orthodontic involvement is possible and recommended is evident in the many chapters in this book describing such interventions. At each phase of intervention, the number of months of continuous orthodontic management required to produce the desired changes can be significant: 3–18 months for presurgical orthopedics, 6–12 months for primary dentition expansion, 12–24 months for mixed dentition management, and 18–30 months for end-stage treatment in the permanent dentition. Figure 70–1 is a graphical depiction of the very significant role played by the orthodontist relative to other team specialists in the longitudinal management of patients with clefts.

Figure 70–1 also highlights three additional points of importance to any discussion of outcomes either resulting from, or impacting upon, orthodontic treatments. First is the potential for orthodontic treatment to become an uninterrupted continuum of intervention, imposing an enormous burden of care on patients and their families and requiring careful assessment of the true benefits to be expected from each phase of intervention. Second is the obvious conclusion that, when dealing with outcomes related to orthodontic treatment for patients with clefts, those outcomes are not necessarily an assessment of orthodontic treatments in isolation, but rather reflect the sum total of all other treatments and interventions from many other disciplines that are carried out

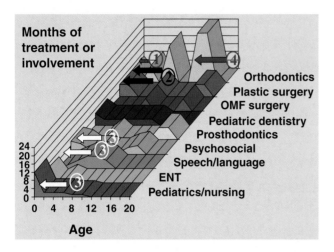

Figure 70–1. Graphic illustration of possible levels of involvement of several key specialties at various ages through the first 20 years of a patient's life. Numbers 1, 2, 3, and 4 are examples of the types of outcome measures. A *segregate* outcome of presurgical orthopedic treatment is shown at 1 where only the effect of the PSOT on infant arch form prior to surgery, might be measured. Similarly, a *segregate* outcome of end-stage orthodontic treatment using, for example, an occlusal index, is illustrated at 4. An *aggregate* outcome assessment at 2, in the context of orthodontics, would provide both a longer-term and multidisciplinary view of the results of the total infant management protocol used up to the point of the assessment, with obvious emphasis on surgery and PSOT (black arrows). An *ultimate* assessment of the multidisciplinary outcomes of an infant management protocol would involve consideration of the orthodontic outcomes (2) along with, among other things, *aggregate* outcomes of speech, psychosocial development, hearing, etc. (3 and white arrows) at a standardized referent time.

prior to or simultaneous with the orthodontic intervention. Likewise, the results of an orthodontic intervention can have effects on outcomes of other disciplines months and years later.

The most obvious examples of this lie in the inextricable relationship between surgical and orthodontic treatment strategies (primary repairs, management of the alveolar cleft, orthognathic surgery, etc.). For example, infant cast measurement following presurgical infant orthopedic treatment (PSOT) provides an assessment method *only* for the outcome of the PSOT procedure itself. An outcome measure of this short-term nature has been described by Tulloch and Antczak-Bouckoms[2] as a *proximate* outcome, but such might also be considered a *segregate* outcome due to its intent to isolate results of a specific intervention. While such a measure may define the effectiveness of an appliance to alter infant arch form, it provides no useful information about the effectiveness of PSOT in the context of the primary surgical treatment strategies for which it is most often used. Therefore, an orthodontic outcome assessment immediately after PSOT but before the surgery for which it was carried out (#1 in Fig. 70–1), provides less useful information for evidence-based multidisciplinary management than an orthodontic outcome as-

sessment that is carried out several years later and that therefore provides data on the total infant management protocol (#2 in Fig. 70–1).

Since few, if any, orthodontic treatment procedures on patients with clefts are carried out in isolation from the rest of the team, the need to realize the interactive nature of the outcomes being measured is critical. In this example, outcome measures of surgical results (facial esthetics, number of secondary revisions, etc.), orthodontic treatment impact (facial growth, arch form, etc.), and more global concerns (patient satisfaction, psychosocial adjustment, etc.) have been described as *ultimate* outcomes by Tulloch and Antczak-Bouckoms.[2] They might also be operationally defined as *aggregate* outcomes by moving the assessment into the context of total interactive, evidence-based *team* treatment, which is the core of comprehensive cleft care. In this chapter, we will use the operational descriptor of these types of outcomes as *segregate* outcomes for those measuring the immediate effect of an isolated intervention, versus *aggregate* outcomes to use discipline-specific measures to assess the longer-term, convergent and summative effects of earlier interventions. In this scheme, the term *ultimate* might best be reserved for a total, comprehensive outcome assessment that integrates outcomes from multiple disciplines in cleft care (i.e., considering collectively #2 and all #3s in Fig. 70–1).

The third lesson from Fig. 70–1 is that of the central responsibility of the orthodontist to develop longitudinal outcome measures related to the effects of orthodontic and surgical treatments on facial growth and development and dental occlusion and to oversee and manage the collection of longitudinal records necessary to assess such outcomes. Multiple phases of prolonged orthodontic treatment, preceded and concluded with standard records for treatment planning and documentations of results, enable the orthodontist to assume primary responsibility within the team for the appropriate recording of outcomes relative to growth, occlusion, and dental and facial esthetics.

This chapter addresses the progress, limitations, and failures of orthodontic assessments to date as well as highlights the obvious gains in our knowledge and understanding of the effects of our interventions when outcome assessments are designed and executed properly. The seemingly endless number of treatment strategies that include and require orthodontic input[3] demand that, for evidence-based decision making and treatment planning, orthodontic outcome assessments be rigidly applied to all phases of care.

STRENGTH OF EVIDENCE HIERARCHY AND ORTHODONTIC OUTCOMES

Numerous authors have emphasized the relative strengths of evidence obtained through various reporting methods and types of investigations.[4,5] Unequivocally, the randomized control trial (RCT) and the systematic review of multiple RCTs are the "gold standards" for establishing evidence upon which orthodontic and total team treatment regimens can be based. Unfortunately, in the field of cleft lip and palate treatment, such trials are difficult to execute due not only to the long time frame and huge costs involved, but more importantly due to the large sample sizes required. The incidence of cleft lip and palate is limited, and there are hundreds of cleft palate centers providing care for patients using protocols and methods unique to each particular center. Most centers and care providers have absolute faith and confidence in the particular methods they have chosen. Consensus agreement for participation in RCTs requiring multiple centers to randomly assign patients to different treatment groups is difficult to establish. Without such consensus, however, sample sizes from single centers are frequently inadequate.[6,7]

The cleft palate scientific literature has long depended on retrospective studies from individual centers, each often examining its own results using methods that are scientifically weak and unreliable due to the multiple sources of bias. As emphasized in the 2002 World Health Organization Report,[5] "differences arising from the biases…are likely to exceed actual differences attributable to the procedures." Furthermore, multi-center retrospective studies are often restricted due to a lack of standardization of recording and reporting treatment data.

As a case in point, reviews of the orthodontic and facial growth literature over the past 50 years[8,9] have highlighted the fact that the outcomes and benefits of presurgical orthopedic treatment (PSOT), which was introduced in 1950s and the subject of innumerable retrospective investigations since then, are still being debated. This is almost certainly due to the confusing array of findings of such studies, ranging from positive benefits to no effect to harmful consequences. Only recently has a randomized control trial been able to produce definitive data documenting the lack of any long-term measurable orthodontic benefit from the methods of PSOT examined in that trial.[10-13]

Fortunately, the effects of these methodological problems, confounding variables, and research biases can all be minimized by the study design. In the hierarchy of evidence, intercenter comparisons of outcomes are considered second strongest behind the RCT.[4,5] Therefore, the ultimate goal for the establishment and use of valid and reliable orthodontic outcome measures is to serve as the substance for the first line of comparative, rigorous scientific scrutiny of treatment interventions, following anecdotal case reports, case series, and retrospective studies using historical controls. Of interest in this regard, however, is that assessment of such outcomes is essentially another form of retrospective study. It is therefore of value to examine the characteristics of appropriate orthodontic outcomes and the planning sequence that allows for such assessments, strengthening the evidence they disclose and making them more valuable than other types of retrospective studies.

FROM ORTHODONTIC OUTCOMES TO CLINICALLY USEFUL EVIDENCE

The journey from conceptualization of a new orthodontic treatment intervention, or of one which would have orthodontic implications, through the process of scientific validation or refutation requires careful prospective planning. The four principal steps involved are (1) defining the outcome(s) of interest and value; (2) determining and/or developing records or reports which represent or allow evaluation of those outcomes; (3) utilizing objective methods of measurement or assessment which are reliable and valid; and (4) designing comparative intercenter studies which have recognized, controlled, or minimized bias and confounding variables. In practical common orthodontic terms, as an example: (1) facial growth or morphology following a particular intervention (outcome of interest/value); (2) could be evaluated using standardized lateral cephalometric radiographs (record); (3) and measured using computer digitization and Steiner, Downs, or McNamara analysis (reliable and valid assessment); and then (4) compared between centers using different interventions with equivalent data, and sufficient sample sizes of consecutively treated cases (control of bias, confounders).

Orthodontic Outcomes of Interest

The outcomes of interest to the orthodontist in the context of cleft lip and palate are no different from those in routine orthodontic treatment for the noncleft patient, with a few notable exceptions. These include, among other things, facial growth and morphology, dental alignment, maxillomandibular relations, dental occlusion, facial and dental esthetics, masticatory function, treatment stability, and patient satisfaction. Exceptions to this list, in the context of cleft care, are somewhat related to the degree to which the interest and/or value of the outcome may differ from the noncleft orthodontic realm. For instance, given the complexities of multidisciplinary cleft management and the severity of the problems encountered, concern over dental alignment issues such as marginal ridge and contact point relationships which are closely scrutinized in routine orthodontic assessment, would logically not be considered as outcomes of equal value to maxillomandibular relations, facial growth, etc. in the cleft population. There are also outcomes that are unique to cleft care and not found in noncleft orthodontics, such as the segregate outcome of infant arch form and segment relationships following PSOT.

Other important outcomes unique to orthodontics in the context of comprehensive cleft team care include, for example, aggregate outcomes which represent (1) future orthodontic treatment needs following various methods of primary infant management; (2) bone support for cleft-adjacent teeth following various protocols for alveolar repair and concomitant orthodontics; (3) the balance between perceived or measured benefits of an orthodontic or orthopedic intervention, and the total burden of care imposed on patient and family; and (4) the level of patient satisfaction and contribution of the treatment in eliminating the stigma of clefting.

Records and Reports for Evaluating Outcomes

The records used to evaluate outcomes relative to the orthodontic management of the patient with cleft lip and palate are typically the same records used by all orthodontists for treatment planning and documentation of results: cephalometric radiographs, panoramic radiographs, periapical radiographs, dental study casts, facial and intra-oral photographs, and clinical chart notes. More recently, the methods of three-dimensional radiographic and photographic imaging are becoming a routine part of this mix.

Use of these records for intercenter outcome comparisons, however, requires that the outcome records are standardized and comparable. The standardization of importance here includes both the methods of obtaining/preparing the records and the timing of when the records are taken. With regard to the former, most orthodontic records have been or can easily be standardized. For instance, lateral cephalometric radiographic methods have been standardized since the time of Broadbent.[14] Standard methods to obtain and prepare dental study casts are readily available. But for use in cleft orthodontic outcome assessment, it is the *timing* of obtaining the records which is most variable and most in need of standardization.

Historically, a limited number of cleft centers have either established standardized protocols for records or had research grant support for obtaining standard records. Unfortunately, support to obtain records (especially radiographs) for research purposes is now rare, and there is no uniformity between centers for the timing of record-taking for clinical purposes. The most successful attempt to date to establish a "standard" for orthodontic records useful for both treatment purposes and outcome assessment has been developed by the Eurocleft/Eurocran projects and adopted by a growing number of cleft centers in Europe and Asia.[3] These minimal standards include, among other things, infant presurgical study casts and photographs, 5-year-old dental study casts and photographs, 10-year-old dental study casts, photographs and lateral cephalometric radiographs, and the same following completion of all orthodontic and surgical treatment at age 18. Added to this are periapical radiographs before, 6 months after, and long-term after bone grafting. To date, similar standards have not been adopted or even attempted by centers in the United States, limiting the potential for intercenter outcome comparisons. Furthermore, it is likely that some modifications of the Eurocleft standards will evolve (e.g., panoramic radiographs, 3-D imaging, additional ages for records collection, etc.) as outcome studies in orthodontics improve and develop. Of primary importance is that the records chosen and the methods and timing of acquisition of these records be predicated on their value in both treatment planning and assessment of outcomes deemed important not only to the

orthodontist, but also to the entire team, thereby minimizing costs, risks, and burdens to the patient.

Methods of Measurement and Assessment

Once desired segregate and aggregate outcomes have been identified, objective methods for measuring and assessing those outcomes are essential to allow for statistical analysis. The characteristics of such methods have been well defined in the literature. *Reliability* is the degree to which a measure made by different investigators or by the same investigator at two different times would yield the same result. Statistical tests for inter- and intra-examiner reliability are well established.[15] *Validity* is the degree to which a measure actually represents the outcome it is meant to assess. These are foundation requirements for scientific research tools.

Cephalometric Analyses

The methods of cephalometric analysis available to the orthodontist for outcomes studies are nearly as numerous as the number of years standardized cephalometric radiography has been in use. A detailed description of these methods is beyond the scope of this chapter. Excellent summaries are available elsewhere.[16] There is also no consensus within the orthodontic community as to which method (e.g., Downs, Steiner, McNamara, Tweed, Wylie, Ricketts, etc.) is best suited for measuring growth and facial morphology in the cleft population. However, in general terms, several key points need to be considered in use of these methods.

The reliability of cephalometric analyses is well established and easily determined,[17,18] and often the variability of the method has more to do with landmark identification than the method of analysis used. In this regard, the error of the method in cleft cephalometric studies is especially important to determine due to the known difficulties in precisely determining anterior maxillary landmarks in these patients. The validity of the method also may be questionable inasmuch as the landmark points and quantitative data derived are two-dimensional representations of a three-dimensional object. Attempts to integrate lateral and frontal cephalometric data to simulate a three-dimensional analysis have generally not been successful. Current advances in three-dimensional imaging have not yet been associated with reliable and valid assessment methods. Finally, the existence of so many methods of cephalometric analysis, each with its own combination of linear, angular, and proportional measures, also suggests a lack of agreement on which measures are truly valid assessments of facial growth and morphology.

Another point to emphasize is that for outcomes assessed with cephalometric radiographic analysis to be amenable to intercenter comparative studies, those that utilize angular and proportional measures would be preferable. Since intercenter studies imply comparisons of results obtained using different cephalostats, on patient populations from different age groups, and different ethnic and racial mixes, variations in radiographic magnification and subject size can all be minimized if absolute linear measures are avoided.

In spite of these shortcomings, the cleft palate literature is filled with studies using various cephalometric radiographic analyses of facial growth and morphology outcomes after various treatment interventions.[8,9] Most of these have identified significant aberrations resulting from the original deformity and subsequent surgical interventions. None have yielded definitive evidence of specific favorable or unfavorable interventions, due mostly to methodological weaknesses endemic to most retrospective studies, rather than to shortcomings of the methods of cephalometric analysis used. While providing little strength of evidence regarding growth effects of primary surgical protocols, however, the volume of such studies has provided what might be called a cumulative weight of evidence, suggesting, for instance, the likely unfavorable growth consequences of primary bone grafting.[9] Such evidence may preclude the possibility of initiating an RCT since the ethical requirement of "equipoise" or "true uncertainty of effectiveness"[5] may not be possible. In this instance, well-designed intercenter orthodontic outcomes comparisons may remain the only option available to improve our strength of evidence.

Assessment of Dental, Occlusal and Arch Relations

Perhaps the most common and clinically useful orthodontic outcomes are those that assess treatment needs and treatment results in the context of dental, occlusal, and arch relations.

Maxillary Arch Dimensions

Starting in infancy, maxillary arch form, and cleft segment relations have been assessed using a number of methods. Two-dimensional measures on photocopies of maxillary casts have been used to show the changes occurring following lip and palate repair.[19] To address the problems of validity from two-dimensional evaluation of three-dimensional structures, others have used three-dimensional digitizing methods directly on maxillary casts to demonstrate the effectiveness of PSOT to realign cleft maxillary segments before surgery.[20] More detailed evaluation of entire maxillary arch morphology and palatal topography before and after primary surgical repair using three-dimensional stereophotogrammetry has been described by Berkowitz.[21,22]

Three-dimensional methods have also been used to measure the aggregate outcome of maxillary arch dimensions in the primary and mixed dentitions following various primary infant management protocols. For example, the reflex microscope has been used to digitize landmarks in three dimensions directly from dental casts by numerous investigators. Hathaway and colleagues[23] reported small but significant decreases in intercanine width and arch length using this method in a sample of patients treated with PSOT and primary bone grafting. In the Dutchcleft RCT,[13] a similar method was used to demonstrate the absence of any long-term effect of PSOT on maxillary arch dimensions.

Three-dimensional methods have also been developed using scanned images of dental study casts. Three-dimensional CT scans of dental study casts with computerized reconstruction were used to demonstrate the absence of any long-term effect of PSOT.[24] Other methods using three-dimensional scans of dental study casts have appeared in the literature with increasing frequency.[25,26] Many of these seem to show measurable and acceptable degrees of reliability. What remains to be established is the validity of the various forms of two- and three-dimensional measures of which we are now capable. While increasing sophistication of the method may appear to be an advance in the science of the outcome measure, it remains to be established whether they are in fact more reliable than other, simpler methods. It is also clear that the costs of equipment, trained personnel, and availability to clinical orthodontists of these advanced methods may limit their use on a regular basis for orthodontic outcome assessments. In this regard, it is of interest to note that the findings and conclusions reached in the CT scan study mentioned above[24] were identical to those reached in another study using 0.1 mm digital calipers to make simple two-dimensional linear measures on the same sample.[27] It is therefore important to bear in mind that while, in theory, increasing measurement sophistication may offer improvements over more traditional measures, the actual gains in reliability and validity may not necessarily outweigh the possible loss of practical utility.

Occlusal Indices

To increase the objectivity of assessment of orthodontic treatment outcomes, occlusal indices have been developed by the orthodontic community. These have included the Peer Assessment Rating (PAR)[28] and, more recently, the American Board of Orthodontics (ABO) Objective Grading System. The ABO Objective Grading System has not yet been evaluated as an orthodontic outcome measure that would have value for patients with clefts. This system could be useful as a proximate or segregate outcome measure for end-stage cleft orthodontic treatment in isolation. However, since the success or failure of orthodontic treatment by that age is so heavily influenced by the sum total of all convergent preceding interventions, its use as a more valuable measurement tool for aggregate outcome assessment may be questionable. The same may apply to the PAR index, although a number of investigators have attempted to apply it to the cleft population.

Several studies[29,30] have demonstrated the reliability and validity of the PAR index as an orthodontic outcome measure in a noncleft assessment. It is based upon weighted occlusal traits felt to describe malocclusion, as determined by a panel of 10 experienced orthodontists. The traits rated are (1) upper and lower anterior segment alignment; (2) right and left buccal occlusion in three-dimensions; (3) overjet; (4) overbite; and (5) centerline. Weightings varied in different validation studies indicating the subjectivity of the weighting.[29,30] Using a PAR Index ruler to measure dental casts, the occlusal traits are assigned scores based upon the degree of deviation from ideal. The scores are then added together to yield a cumulative score. Higher scores reflect worsening malocclusion, with scores over 40 reflecting a severe malocclusion.[31] Calculation of the difference between scores before and after orthodontic treatment allows for quantification of the efficacy of treatment.[30] Cases are then categorized as greatly improved, improved, or not improved/worse based upon the magnitude of the difference.

Originally the cohort of study casts used to develop the indices contained no cleft lip and/or palate patients. Subsequent research projects have addressed the need to adapt the index to reflect the differences in malocclusion that patients with complete clefts have compared to noncleft patients.[32–34] All of these studies use different weightings for the occlusal indices when applied to the cleft palate population, and suggest the need for modifications of the occlusal indices to address problems unique to clefts. For example, one of the traits for success for unilateral clefts is buccal occlusion. However, right and left sides have been weighted differently, reflecting the increased number of left-sided unilateral cleft cases.[33] This suggests that further work using cleft and noncleft side buccal segment weightings may increase the validity of the index in these cases. However, even without the adjusted weightings for cleft lip and palate, orthodontic outcomes of 128 patients with unilateral clefts were assessed using the PAR index to evaluate treatment provided by the UK National Health Service Consultants.[35] The mean reduction in PAR using UK noncleft weightings was 69% ± 22. This figure compared favorably with the noncleft cohort, also treated by the UK NHS Consultant Service,[31] although the mean severity ratings for the cleft sample were worse both before and after treatment.

In spite of such promising findings for using the PAR Index as an orthodontic outcome measure for clefts, it is well recognized that many factors make cases with clefts more difficult to treat and to compare using indices based on noncleft samples. The factors include poor oral hygiene and increased rates of dental caries,[36] missing teeth, and unfavorable growth.[8,9] For example, the prevalence of missing lateral incisors may affect dental symmetry and predispose to centerline discrepancies which can raise the score on the PAR index. Also, improving buccal segment relationships in the anteriorposterior dimension can be complicated due to missing teeth, microdontia, and poor growth and in the transverse dimension due to the relapse following the known instability of cleft arch expansion. Finally, although the PAR Index as a noncleft outcome measure has been shown to have excellent reliability, the intra- and inter-examiner reliability has been shown to fall to levels that may not be as acceptable when it is applied to cleft orthodontic outcomes.[32,34] In one study, the authors tested an indirect rating system based on severity and degree of improvement of the PAR occlusal traits. This seemed to improve the reliability.[34]

Perhaps the greatest shortcoming of the PAR index or other occlusal indices is that they use changes in characteristics of dental occlusion and alignment before and after orthodontic treatment to purportedly measure outcomes of that treatment. In that focus, they represent a segregate outcome measure of therapy that in the cleft patient is itself heavily influenced by the sum total of multiple other preceding or concurrent interventions in the context of comprehensive cleft care. Therefore, their use as an aggregate outcome mea-

sure suitable for use in intercenter comparisons may not be as suitable as their use in intracenter audits comparing end-stage orthodontic treatment outcome achieved by different orthodontists from the same center to treat patients who had similar prior treatment histories. Alternatively, the segregate outcomes of different end-stage orthodontic treatment approaches carried out by the same orthodontist at the same center would seem to be more suitably assessed using these occlusal indices. Clearly, further refinements and modifications of these outcome measures must be made to realize the potential for occlusal indices to be a valuable addition to the list of assessments of value to the cleft palate orthodontist.

Dental Arch Relationships

The concept with perhaps the greatest impact in the assessment of cleft orthodontic outcomes over the past 20 years was the use of simple assessment scales for the rating of maxillo/mandibular relations using dental study casts. Although the Angle classification system has been a standard in orthodontics since 1906, it lacks specificity for clefting and is too narrow in its focus for use as an aggregate cleft orthodontic outcome measure of dental arch relationship.

In 1987, Mars and colleagues published a landmark paper in which dental arch relationships were evaluated by ranking dental casts using a new arch relation analysis called the Goslon (named after the centers involved in the development of the rating system: Great Ormond Street, London, and Oslo) Yardstick.[37] All cases represented were in the late mixed or early permanent dentition. Using reference dental models ranked into five distinct groups based on arch relationships, the authors were able to compare treatment outcomes. These groups were differentiated primarily according to sagittal maxillo/mandibular relationship. Transverse and vertical occlusal relationships were assessed secondarily. The models were ordered from excellent to very poor: Goslon 1 – Excellent; Goslon 2 – Good; Goslon 3 – Fair; Goslon 4 – Poor; Goslon 5 – Very Poor.

Those ratings corresponded to the authors' estimation of a patient's future treatment needs in the permanent dentition. Those models that were rated in the first two groups were from those patients that were presumed to require routine orthodontic treatment or no treatment at all in their end-stage treatment. Group 3 models generally represented patients presumed to require complex orthodontic treatment due to the Class III malocclusion. Patients in group 4 were presumed very likely to require orthognathic surgical intervention. Patients categorized into group 5 clearly required orthognathic surgical treatment. Statistical analysis revealed that the Goslon Yardstick was a reliable method of evaluating and comparing treatment results from different centers.

In carrying out a Goslon Yardstick rating, dental casts to be studied are compared to these referent groups and assigned a score. Simpler means of arch assessment have been suggested such as crossbite evaluation[38–40] and incisal overjet measurement[41]; however, while these techniques correlate well with Goslon ratings, they do not explain all of the Goslon score variation and do not predict facial morphology outcomes as accurately as the Goslon Yardstick.

To evaluate the study models, the antero-posterior relationship is first scored. It is based on an anterior apical base relationship rather than a molar and incisal relationship, which have less impact on the score. Pre-existing dental compensation is not considered favorable, as it limits the effectiveness of future orthodontic treatment. A severe Class III relationship is least favorable, whereas a Class II division 1 relationship is considered most favorable. The former represents inhibited maxillary growth secondary to primary surgery, whereas the latter is felt to be most favorable in the 9-year-olds because of the potential for Class III growth through adolescence. The anterior vertical relationship is evaluated second. An overbite is considered more favorable than an open bite. The transverse relationship is evaluated last. Evaluation of the transverse relationship is based on the arch narrowness, rather than on dental crossbite. A referent set of models representative of each category has been established for use during the ratings. Ratings are generally done by a group of 3–6 unbiased raters, trained and calibrated in the use of the Yardstick, using dental casts that have been prepared identically to blind the examiners to the center of origin of the casts. The Goslon Yardstick standards are shown in Figs. 70–2 to 70–6.

The Goslon Yardstick is an outcome measure of current dental arch relationship in the context of future orthodontic treatment needs. It reflects the results of the sum total of all prior treatment interventions, especially infant management protocols. The Yardstick therefore represents an aggregate outcome measure (see #2 in Fig. 70–1) that impacts upon, but is not the sole result of, orthodontic treatment. With this understanding of its meaning, the Goslon Yardstick has been used extensively in a growing number of studies since 1987. Repeatedly, it has been shown to be a valid and reliable measure, with great utility, especially with regard to identifying favorable versus unfavorable outcomes of primary infant management protocols in the context of future orthodontic treatment needs.

The value of the Goslon Yardstick was convincingly demonstrated in the historic Eurocleft project.[42,43] This retrospective comparison of treatment outcomes in 8–10-year-olds utilized dental casts, cephalometric radiographs, and nasolabial photographs from six European cleft centers to evaluate craniofacial form,[44] arch relationships,[45] and nasolabial appearance.[46] All 151 subjects included in this study were born with complete unilateral clefts of the lip and palate. However, many differences in treatment regimens were evident both between centers and, in some cases, within the same center. The range of Goslon Yardstick scores for each center clearly demonstrated the value of this outcome assessment tool to discriminate between the results obtained following different infant management protocols. Although the use of such an aggregate outcome measure did not allow for identification of effects of specific features within an overall protocol, it was clear that better results, with better prognosis for end-stage orthodontic treatment, were obtained with higher volume operators, centralized and standardized care, and simple surgical management with no PSOT or alveolar repair.[43]

Since that time, the Goslon Yardstick has been used, tested, analyzed, and compared in a large number of studies. Of greatest interest are (1) studies that validated the assumption of predicting need or no need for orthognathic surgery in end-stage treatment[47]; (2) studies that consistently

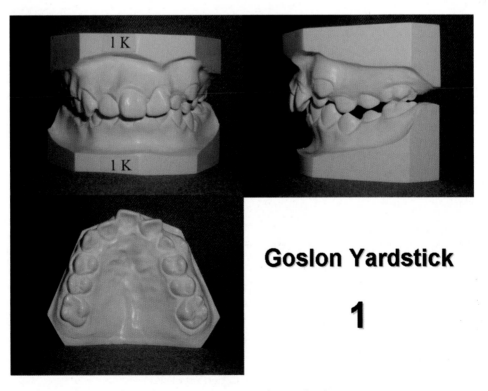

Goslon Yardstick

1

Figure 70–2. 9 Year Goslon Yardstick 1.

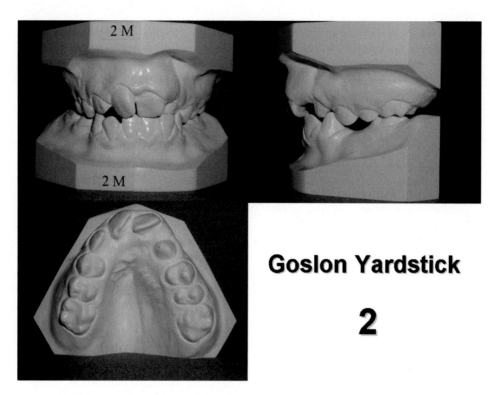

Goslon Yardstick

2

Figure 70–3. 9 Year Goslon Yardstick 2.

reconfirmed the findings mentioned above[48]; (3) studies that demonstrated the significant correlation between Goslon Yardstick scores and cephalometric variables of maxillo-mandibular relation,[44,49] and (4) studies that have proposed simpler, alternative methods of outcome assessment that at-

tempt to replicate or improve upon the reliability, validity, or sensitivity of the Goslon Yardstick. These include incisor overjet measurement,[41] use of photographic comparisons,[50] and scoring of anterior and posterior crossbite.[39,40] With regard to the latter, Mossey and colleagues modified the

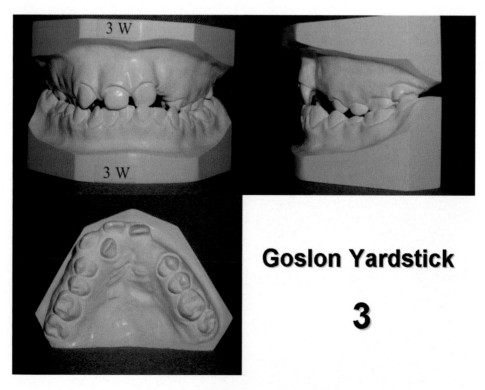

Goslon Yardstick

3

Figure 70–4. 9 Year Goslon Yardstick 3.

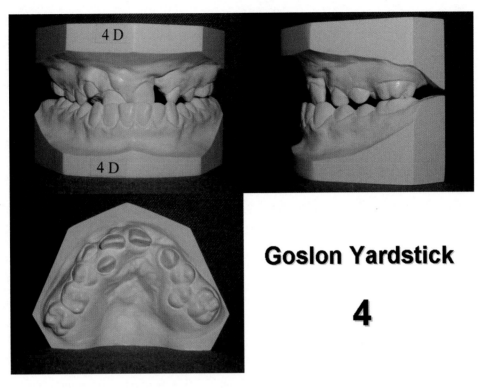

Goslon Yardstick

4

Figure 70–5. 9 Year Goslon Yardstick 4.

Huddart/Bodenheim system[38] to render it suitable for use at both the primary and mixed dentition stages. They applied a simple point system to grade presence, absence, and/or degree of crossbite in anterior and buccal segments of the dental arch as an outcome measure of arch relationship. The authors proposed that, by focusing the outcome on dental crossbite, the measure is a more valid representation of the outcomes of primary lip and palate surgery since inherent favorable or unfavorable growth patterns may not influence the score as much as they might in the Goslon Yardstick. When

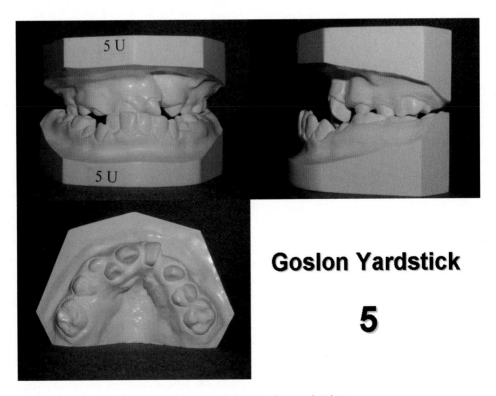

Goslon Yardstick

5

Figure 70–6. 9 Year Goslon Yardstick 5.

the method was applied to the referent models for both the Goslon Yardstick and the 5-Year Yardstick (see below), the result was appropriate rating of the models into the same Yardstick categories from which they came. When applied to a sample of 50 patients with unilateral clefts, there was also a high correlation between the Huddart/Bodenheim scores and the Yardstick categories. In addition, the assessment was found to have less subjectivity, greater sensitivity, greater utility, equal or greater reliability, and suitability for parametric statistics by use of a continuous variable scale (as compared to the categorical scale of the Yardsticks).

One additional outcome measure for dental arch relationships was an outgrowth of the Goslon Yardstick. When it became apparent that such a simple, noninvasive, utilitarian method for identifying favorable versus unfavorable early management protocols was available, the benefits of doing such assessments at younger ages were clear. A Goslon-type index for 5-year-olds was developed for this purpose, using the same assumptions, categories, and methods, including the creation of a reference set of dental casts.[51] When the dental casts of 27 UCLP patients were rated at the ages of five years and ten years in order to determine if any correlations existed, it was found that nearly all of the cases evaluated at age 5 either remained in the same category or deteriorated by the age of 10. A similar strong correlation between 5-Year Yardstick ratings and Goslon ratings was also reported by other investigators.[49,52] When used as an orthodontic outcome measure in a two-center study[53] and a three-center study,[54] the index revealed statistically significant differences between the centers that used differing primary protocols, suggesting that differences in surgical outcome may indeed be detectable by 5 years of age. Recently, others have attempted to compare the Goslon and 5-Year-Old Yardsticks for use in 5-year-old primary dentition assessments and have suggested the need to further refine and improve the reference models to reflect the normal differences in incisal relationship between primary and mixed dentitions.[55] Efforts to improve these dental arch outcome measures continue. It should be noted that the two Yardsticks apply only to unilateral cleft lip and palate. Efforts are currently underway to test a similar dental arch Yardstick rating scale for bilateral complete clefts, the Bauru Yardstick.[56] There is no rating method available or being developed for isolated clefts of the palate at the present time.

Assessment of Bone Support for Cleft-Adjacent Teeth

Another outcome measure of interest to the orthodontist is the assessment of bone fill-in and support of cleft-adjacent teeth following alveolar bone grafting protocols. Although such a measure would seem to be a segregate outcome of the surgery itself or surgical skill, it actually represents an aggregate outcome of orthodontic significance. Since most protocols for alveolar bone grafting involve a coordination of surgical and orthodontic interventions (expansion, incisor alignment, concomitant orthopedics, etc.),[8,57] an outcome measure of success of bone grafting provides data for

evidence-based decisions regarding favorable versus unfavorable orthodontic and surgical protocols and impacts upon future orthodontic treatment needs and capabilities.

There are two basic scales available for assessment of this outcome, categorical and continuous. The Bergland Scale[58] and Kindelan Scale[59] are examples of categorical scales. Both use a 4 point rating scale based on the height of the interalveolar septum achieved: With the Bergland scale 1 = normal height, 2 = 3/4 height, 3 < 3/4 height, 4 = failure with no bone in cleft. Using this method, authors were able to demonstrate a very high success rate (90% of their cases rated 1 or 2) using the Oslo, Norway protocol for grafting. The Kindelan scale offers the benefit of being able to score the interalveolar septum prior to the eruption of the permanent canine in the cleft site. While offering a simple and understandable method for assessment, the subjectivity of these categorical scales weakens their reliability, the two-dimensional representation of a three-dimensional object lessens the validity, and the use of categorical variables limits the strength of statistical testing. As a result, modifications have been made to address these issues, but using the same basic principles. In an attempt to improve on the interpretation of these radiographs, the Chelsea Scale was described by Witherow et al.[60] This method maps the bone in the interalveolar septum on an 8 point scale (1–8) and describes the position of any bony bridge with a 6-point categorical scale (A–F). Interobserver reliability was found to be lower around the root apices of the cleft-adjacent teeth. All other parts of the scales demonstrated good levels of agreement. In comparing the reliability of these three scales, all demonstrated similar levels of intra- and inter-observer reliability. Neither periapical nor occlusal films demonstrated improved reliability with these methods.[61]

From a research perspective, Long and colleagues developed a method of assessment using digitized landmarks on periapical and occlusal radiographs, with proportional measures of bone height compared to root length for cleft-adjacent teeth. The method has been shown to have excellent intra- and inter-examiner reliability.[62,63] Figure 70–7 illustrates the method where B/A and F/E represent support for the teeth mesial and distal to the cleft, respectively; C/A and G/E, the heights of the alveolar crests relative to root lengths; and D/E, the degree of alveolar ridge notching. In this manner, there is also added specificity to the outcome measure, since it takes into account bone grafts that may result in a bone bridge and acceptable location of the alveolar crest, but that have residual defects at the apical end of the tooth. Using this method, the confounders of foreshortening and elongation on these radiographs are eliminated, and averages and standard deviations of bone support for the entire sample can be calculated. In this particular sample of secondary grafted patients, differences in bone support were found between the mesial and distal tooth (72% vs. 86%).

A subsequent study[64] on a sample of primary grafted patients has supported the validity of the method. No significant differences were found between measures of bone graft success using 3-D CT scans and the two-dimensional

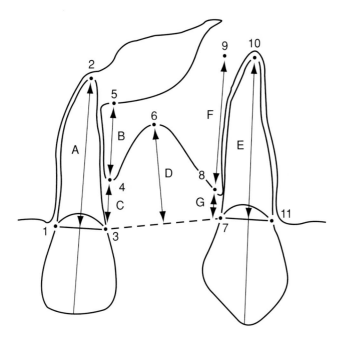

Figure 70–7. Bone graft assessment method (from Long et al., 1995).

measures on periapical radiographs of the same patients. Furthermore, the use of continuous variables with this method allows for application of parametric statistics to evaluate correlations between various orthodontic interventions and bone graft results. In this manner it was found that significantly increasing cleft width to greater than 10–12 mm prior to grafting with orthodontic expansion was negatively correlated to bone graft success.[62]

Assessment of Facial Esthetics

Evaluation of the facial esthetic outcomes of various forms of treatment would logically be of great significance to the surgical members of the cleft palate team. However, as with most of the outcome measures described in this chapter, facial esthetics is truly an aggregate outcome with orthodontic impact. Presurgical orthodontic/orthopedic interventions in the infant, such as nasoalveolar molding (NAM), have evolved at least in part, due to a desire to improve nasolabial esthetic outcomes. Orthodontic treatments in the mixed and permanent dentition, such as maxillary face-mask protraction and maxillary expansion, also have clear implications for affecting facial aesthetics.

In spite of the importance of this outcome to both patient and orthodontist, however, it remains one of the most elusive assessments in terms of objective, standardized records and measurement. The most common assessment methods to date involve either direct soft tissue measurements on patients[65] or categorical ratings of two-dimensional photographs by panels of judges.[66] The former methods have advantages inasmuch as reliability may be better as well as providing outcome measures that are continuous and therefore amenable to parametric statistics. However, they may not pass the test of validity since measurements alone may not be

accurate representations of facial attractiveness. On the other hand, most studies using rating systems and panels of judges, while having great validity, are often found to be less reliable. As an example, of the principle outcome measures examined in the Eurocleft study, ratings of nasolabial appearance (as determined using a 5-point scale of the frontal and lateral cropped nasolabial area) were found to have much poorer intra- and inter-rater reliability compared to cephalometric and Goslon Yardstick assessments.[46] Nonetheless, modifications of this method and use of a visual analog scale have recently been shown to have much improved and acceptable reliability[67] and have been used to demonstrate no significant facial esthetic effect of PSOT. With the exception of this study, however, most attempts at facial and nasolabial esthetic evaluations seem to have been carried out in the context of a surgical outcome assessment. In a comprehensive review of the literature on this subject[68] there was little evidence that any other published investigations included consideration of the impact that orthodontic/orthopedic interventions being carried out as part of a surgical protocol might have had on facial esthetics. This, coupled with a lack of standardization for facial photography, a lack of consensus on a reliable and valid measurement scale, and the limitations of two-dimensional imaging of a three-dimensional object, suggest that much work lies ahead before this very important outcome will be sufficiently refined for use in intracenter audits and intercenter comparisons. Most likely, these efforts should be directed toward development of measures using three-dimensional imaging techniques.

Measures of Orthodontic Burdens of Care

No orthodontic-related outcomes measures can be considered complete without consideration of the burden of care imposed on patient, family, orthodontist, and society. Burdens of care include length of time in treatment, number of appointments, costs of treatment to the patient, costs of treatment to the cleft center or orthodontist, costs of treatment to society, hours of missed work or school for patient or parents, risks of treatment (untoward consequences), pain, and discomfort.

As an example, end-stage orthodontics is one intervention in comprehensive cleft care that has the potential for creating a significant added burden of care for patients and families by requiring multiple monthly or bimonthly appointments over many years. When considering relative improvements measured with occlusal indices, for instance, there is currently no standard and accepted method for concomitant assessment of the burden of that care. Thus by merely measuring percent improvement in an occlusal index we are left with the conundrum of whether, for instance, a reduction in PAR score of 75% over 4 years of continuous orthodontics is a superior outcome to a 60% improvement achieved over 2 years of treatment. This is graphically illustrated in Fig. 70–8. Improvement in orthodontic treatment outcome as measured with an occlusal index is understandably an asymptotic variable with a limit on the amount of improvement possible. Conversely, the burden of continuing

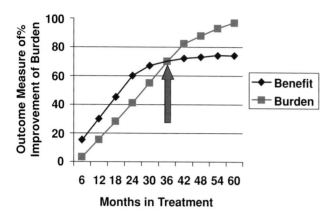

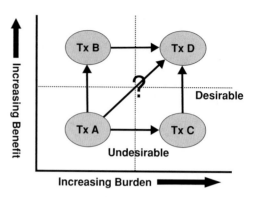

Figure 70–8. Theoretical graph of an outcome measure of improvement (e.g., occlusal index), and the increasing burdens of intervention (e.g., costs, time, and risks) over an increasing number of months in orthodontic treatment. Arrow indicates a hypothetical point at which additional improvement to be expected is outweighed by the burden/costs of continuing.

Figure 70–9. Graphical illustration of balance between benefits and burdens of care. A to B, or C to D: Improving outcomes with no additional burden are desirable traits of an orthodontic intervention. A to C, or B to D: Alternate treatments that cannot be shown to improve outcomes, but that require a greater burden of care are undesireable. A to D: Orthodontic interventions that can be shown to produce improved outcomes but also carry increased burden of care or cost need to be assessed as aggregate or ultimate outcomes to include consideration of the degree to which the improvements do or do not outweigh the burdens.

orthodontic treatment, in terms of time, costs, risks, appointments, missed school, missed work, etc., would be linear. Thus, there is a point at which the burdens of care exceed the benefits as measured by, for example, an occlusal index (Fig. 70–8).

Of interest in this regard is the fact that the few studies which have attempted to assess outcomes of interest to the orthodontist have generally found either no additional benefit for interventions which have increased cost of care[69] or an actual inverse relationship between outcome and length of time under end-stage orthodontic treatment.[70] The challenge for segregate and aggregate orthodontic outcomes such as these is to incorporate the additional outcome measure of treatment burden which then moves the analysis into the realm of an *ultimate* outcome assessment.

This type of *ultimate* orthodontic outcome assessment, including burden of care, will become increasingly important in the comparison of outcomes resulting from the wide range of treatment approaches currently available[3] as well as in the future development of new innovations and techniques in orthodontic care. Figure 70–9 illustrates the need to integrate outcome measures of benefit with analysis of burden. In some cases, treatment outcomes involving different surgical and orthodontic protocols may be, with proper intercenter comparisons, easily distinguished as more or less favorable or desirable even with equal burdens of care (Treatment B better than A; D better than C in Fig. 70–9). On the other hand, it is also clear after numerous intercenter comparisons in Europe that many vastly different surgical and orthodontic protocols may produce outcomes which are nearly indistinguishable (Treatments A and C, and B and D in Fig. 70–9). In the latter example, evidence-based decision-making demands consideration of the burden of care and selection of the interventions which produce comparable outcomes with fewer burdens to patient and family.

Of course, the most difficult combination to assess is the situation where better outcomes are possible through an intervention that also carries with it a significant additional burden of care (Treatment D compared to A in Fig. 70–9). In the multidisciplinary setting of comprehensive cleft care, the issue becomes even more confusing when an improvement in one orthodontic outcome (e.g., enhancement of cleft-adjacent tooth development with earlier bone grafting) has a negative impact on another outcome (e.g., subsequent maxillary growth). In such situations, the strength of evidence required may be beyond the capabilities of retrospective outcome studies and rely on the execution of RCTs.

There are two examples of this situation in the realm of orthodontic outcomes. First, the Dutchcleft Randomized Control Trial[12,13,69] has been able to demonstrate that PSOT, as used in that study, had no measurable benefit with regard to maxillo-mandibular relations or maxillary arch dimensions and, in fact, had a significantly increased burden of care. Second, the growing popularity of nasoalveolar molding, which clearly carries additional burdens of care in terms of time and costs during infant management, demands that efforts be made to document significant additional long-term benefits (e.g., better arch form, better occlusion, better nasolabial esthetics, etc.) that would justify the added costs. This responsibility falls squarely on the shoulders of those advocating new techniques and requires a willingness to become engaged in well-designed intercenter orthodontic outcome studies.

The recording and assessment of burdens of care are not as easily accomplished as the ratings of models or the measuring of radiographs. The records of greatest importance in this regard are the patient's chart, hospital and clinic data entries, financial ledgers, and patient/parent satisfaction surveys. One immediate problem that is evident is the lack of standardization and variability in consistency and detail of such records from one cleft clinic to the next. Although sophisticated methods to statistically factor in the burdens, risks, and costs of care are available[71] many of these apply to more controlled situations (e.g., RCTs) and are more difficult to incorporate into routine cleft care. Nonetheless, simple calculations such as number of appointments, financial charges to families or usual clinic fees for services, tracking of untoward treatment consequences, etc. may be more readily available. The important point is that for any orthodontic outcome measures to be considered as ultimate assessments, these burden of orthodontic care issues must be included.

Design of Intercenter Studies Using Orthodontic Outcome Measures

Once orthodontic outcomes of interest, appropriate records, and outcome measures have been identified, the simple collection and measuring/assessment of those records represent nothing different than that which has been done for decades of retrospective studies, which have been shown to have little value in the hierarchy of evidence. None have been able to provide the strength of evidence needed to reach firm conclusions about treatment efficacy and effectiveness. For orthodontic outcomes to progress to a level that would enable true evidence-based decision making about treatments and interventions, the process of data organization, analysis, and comparison must be executed with rigorous scientific methods. The primary objective of the design of valuable outcome studies lies in the attempts to control the many sources of bias that are inherent in examining retrospective data from widely disparate sources.[5]

There are three notable characteristics of successful outcome studies of interest to the orthodontist that enhance the strength of evidence over other retrospective research studies as have been traditionally carried out. They are (a) standardization of records; (b) study design; and (c) intent and interpretation.

Standardization of Records

The value and essential nature of standardized records as the foundation for enabling meaningful comparison of orthodontic treatment outcomes has already been described in this chapter. It is clearly not possible to carry out intercenter outcome comparisons with noncomparable data. This represents one of the greatest challenges to the cleft orthodontic community. In countries with national health service models, some level of standardization may be feasible. With the current health care delivery system in the US, where removal of barriers to care, especially geographical, is emphasized, it is likely that a significant amount of orthodontic care and records keeping will continue to take place in private offices rather than in centralized team settings. Under those conditions, reaching agreement and achieving compliance with a standard record-taking protocol becomes impossible. The solution must come from orthodontists in major cleft palate centers, nationally and internationally, agreeing on the record-taking protocol and either assuming the primary responsibility for taking those records at the center when patients are seen for their periodic team evaluations or ensuring that participating orthodontists in private practice are following the standard record-taking protocol and providing the team with copies of those records. The Eurocleft protocols described previously represent a positive step in this direction.

Study Design

The topic of study design applies to all outcome studies designed to assist in comprehensive cleft care decisions regarding treatment and protocol options. In the context of orthodontics, once standardized orthodontic outcome records have been taken, they remain of little value in evidence-based decision making unless they are subject to assessments which are properly designed and executed. As mentioned above, a critical difference between successful and useful intercenter orthodontic outcome comparisons and other retrospective methods is the need to control the many inherent sources of bias. These have been well described in a 2002 WHO report on strategies to improve treatment for patients with clefts and craniofacial anomalies.[5]

The landmark Eurocleft study[3,42–46] embodied these principles and was the first major attempt to increase the strength of evidence available using retrospective data under rigorous methodological guidelines specifically designed to minimize bias. Using strict inclusion criteria, especially large consecutive samples with documentation of complete unilateral cleft lip and palate, the possibility of *susceptibility* (case selection) and *exclusion* bias were minimized and confidence in the initial equivalency of the samples was increased. Control of *follow-up* bias was achieved by requiring an accounting for any patients initially enrolled in the center consecutively for whom records were not available for the outcomes study (e.g., patients moving away, failing to return for team evaluations, etc.). In an extension of the desire to consider follow-up, the original sample was followed through completion of treatment and reassessed using similar orthodontic-related outcome measures.[47,70,72–74] These also helped to validate the original findings and assumptions of the first study as well as address ultimate outcome issues, such as burden of care and patient satisfaction. Setting statistically determined minimal sample sizes, ensuring the blinding of examiners during evaluations, using panels of trained, calibrated, and experienced judges, and using standardized records and measures which allowed for tests of reliability all assure control of *analysis* bias. Reaching agreement among participants about the interpretation of the statistical analyses, levels of significance, and the methods of presenting and publishing the results, regardless of the implications of the outcomes, assure control of *reporting* bias. Only *proficiency* bias (variation in operator skill) cannot be controlled or minimized with this type of study. This, therefore, represents the one source of bias requiring randomized control trial design to manage.

A final aspect of study design that is of value in providing reliable evidence about orthodontic treatment outcomes is the need to ensure that the outcome of interest is assessed at an age or time period that is adequate for true appraisal of treatment effects. Since many combined orthodontic and surgical interventions in comprehensive cleft care are growth-sensitive and are carried out in actively growing patients, apparent short-term benefits may not stand up to the "test of time." They may either disappear with age,[20,24] or, even worse, contribute to progressive growth dysplasias,[75] both of which demand that adequate time for growth be factored into the design of the study.

Intent and Interpretation

In very general terms, the fatal flaw in most retrospective intercenter or single center orthodontic studies to date has been the attempt and assumption that specific features of a treatment protocol (e.g., type of palate surgery, timing of palate surgery, use/nonuse of PSOT, timing of alveolar repair, etc.) could be isolated as independent variables in the true sense of definitive experimental research. Thus, retrospective studies of facial growth effects (dependent variable) of various techniques of primary surgical repair (independent variable) were abundant over the past 50 years. Although there have been some historically noteworthy attempts at this "cause-and-effect" research design,[75–81] understandably, none could possibly be conclusive due to the confusing, complex, and widely disparate combination of other variables (timing, lip repair, surgical skill, ancillary procedures, etc.), some or all of which could have also been contributory to any differences detected. Thus, as stated by Shaw et al.[15]: "the method (intercenter retrospective outcomes) is better suited to comparative clinical audit and quality assurance than definitive clinical research. The existence of significant disparities in outcomes of the overall treatment process provides a basis for speculating about the possible cause, and intercenter studies should therefore be highly motivating toward the generation of specific hypotheses for subsequent more detailed testing."

CONCLUSIONS AND FUTURE DIRECTIONS

Orthodontic outcomes and the valid intercenter comparison of those outcomes are critical to our move to evidence-based decision making in comprehensive cleft care. Randomized control trials must still be the goal to which we aspire to arrive at a true scientific basis for our interventions. However, it is the intercenter comparison of outcomes, and importantly those with orthodontic implications or impact, that will provide us with the motivation and direction for designing RCTs capable of delivering definitive answers to our treatment protocol questions. The potential for orthodontic-based outcome studies to contribute to this effort has already been realized with the successful design and execution of two major RCTs, Dutchcleft and Scandcleft,[5] as outgrowths of the original Eurocleft outcome study, which was itself based on traditional orthodontic records (dental casts, facial photographs, and cephalometric radiographs). At last, these RCTs have started to generate sound evidence on the relative merits of PSOT and various types and timing of palate repair. A similar intercenter outcomes comparison has been initiated

recently in the US (Americleft) with support of the American Cleft Palate-Craniofacial Association. Based on the Eurocleft model, orthodontic records and orthodontic-related outcomes are also of primary importance in the Americleft project. Expansion of the initiative from regional to national to global has been fully supported and endorsed by Eurocran and the World Health Organization.[5] The orthodontist's role in these endeavors will remain crucial and require the following:

- Identification of orthodontic-related treatment interventions that have shown some clinically interesting results, but for which there is inadequate strength of evidence to be able to determine the ratio of benefit to burden/risk/cost (e.g., nasoalveolar molding, gingivoperiosteoplasty).
- Agreement between orthodontists involved in cleft care regarding standardization of records that would simultaneously fulfill diagnostic and treatment planning needs, while also serving as the material for aggregate measures of multidisciplinary outcomes (e.g., dental casts taken and used for planning a phase of orthodontic treatment while simultaneously providing the material for dental arch relationship outcomes following differing primary management protocols. See numbers 2 and 3 in Fig. 70–10.)
- Assignment of responsibility for obtaining, storing, retrieving, and sharing orthodontic outcome records to major cleft palate centers capable of providing total team evaluations and of maintaining centralized files of patient enrollment, treatment histories, etc.
- Commitment of a sufficient number of orthodontists and centers to participate in unbiased, rigorous scientific scrutiny of outcome records with the acceptance of the general lack of evidence for current treatment practices and a willingness to alter protocols upon identification of favorable versus unfavorable interventions.
- Recognition of the need to integrate and interpret orthodontic outcome findings in the context of total comprehensive cleft care and the value and importance of the interests of other team members.

Figure 70–10 illustrates this complex but essential characteristic of successful design, interpretation, and integration of orthodontic outcome studies. The sequence in the evolution of orthodontic outcome assessment proceeds from segregate outcome measures (i.e., number 1: post PSOT infant arch dimensions), to a specific aggregate orthodontic outcome (i.e., number 2: 9-year-old dental arch relationship), to a comprehensive aggregate orthodontic outcome (i.e., number 3: multiple orthodontic-related outcomes), to an ultimate interdisciplinary outcome (i.e., number 4: multidisciplinary outcomes considered in the context of the common goals of comprehensive cleft care). It is certainly time consuming and complicated to implement investigation with this progression and expansion as the road map. But without the goal to eventually integrate orthodontic outcomes with those of other specialties on the team, such efforts will remain of little value to evidence-based comprehensive cleft care.

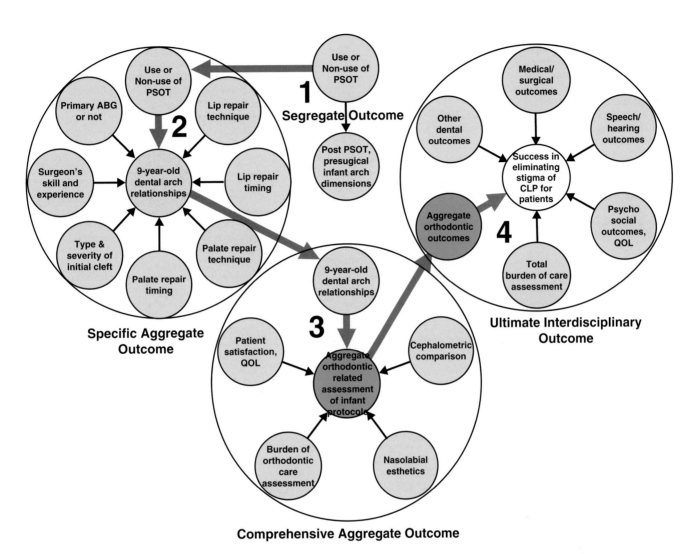

Figure 70–10. A roadmap of the procession from segregate orthodontic outcome measures to the integration of those into specific aggregate outcome assessments, then into comprehensive discipline-specific aggregate outcome assessments and finally into an ultimate interdisciplinary outcome assessment which incorporates the elements of comprehensive cleft care.

References

1. Long RE, Jr., Kharbanda OP. Improving treatment outcomes for patients with cleft lip and palate—An historical perspective of the team concept. *J Indian Orthod Soc* 32:1, 1999.

2. Tulloch K, Antczak-Bouckoms. A methodologic approach to outcome assessment. In Turvey TA, Vig KWL, Fonseca RJ (eds). *Facial Clefts and Craniosynostosis. Principles and Management.* Philadelphia: WB Saunders Company, 1996, p. 745.

3. Shaw WC, Semb G, Nelson P, et al. *The Eurocleft Project 1996–2000.* Amsterdam: IOS Press, 2000.

4. Roberts CT, Semb G, Shaw WC. Strategies for the advancement of surgical methods in cleft lip and palate. *Cleft Palate Craniofac J* 28:141, 1991.

5. World Health Organization. Global strategies to reduce the healthcare burden of craniofacial anomalies. Report of WHO meetings on International Collaborative Research on craniofacial anomalies. WHO Human Genetics Programme, 2002.

6. Shprintzen RJ. Fallibility of clinical research. *Cleft Palate Craniofac J* 28:136, 1991.

7. Semb G, Roberts CT, Shaw WC. The scope and limitations of single center research in cleft lip and palate. In: Vig KD, Vig PS (eds). *Clinical Research as the Basis of Clinical Practice*, Craniofacial Growth Series 25. Center for Human Growth and Development, University of Michigan, Ann Arbor, 1991, p. 109.

8. Long RE, Jr., Semb G, Shaw WC. State of the art—Orthodontic treatment of the patient with complete clefts of the lip, alveolus and palate. The lessons of the past 60 years. *Cleft Palate Craniofac J* 37:533, 2000.

9. Kuijpers-Jagtman AM, Long RE, Jr. State of the art—The influence of surgery and orthopedic treatment on maxillofacial growth and maxillary arch development in patients treated for orofacial clefts. *Cleft Palate Craniofac J* 37:1, 2000.

10. Prahl C, Kuijpers-Jagtman AM, van't Hof MA, et al. A randomized prospective clinical trial into the effect of infant orthopaedics on maxillary arch dimensions in unilateral cleft lip and palate. *Eur J Oral Sci* 109:297, 2001.

11. Prahl C, Kuijpers-Jagtman AM, van't Hof MA, et al. A randomized prospective clinical trial of the effect of infant orthopedics in unilateral cleft lip and palate: Prevention of collapse of the alveolar segments (Dutchcleft). *Cleft Palate Craniofac J* 40:337, 2003.

12. Bongaarts CAM, Kuijpers-Jagtman AM, van't Hof MA, et al. The effect of infant orthopedics on the occlusion of the deciduous dentition in children with complete unilateral cleft lip and palate (Dutchcleft). *Cleft Palate Craniofac J* 41:633, 2004.

13. Bongaarts CAM, van't Hof MA, Prahl-Andersen B, et al. Infant orthopedics has no effect on maxillary arch dimensions in the deciduous dentition of children with complete unilateral cleft lip and palate (Dutchcleft). *Cleft Palate Craniofac J* 43:659, 2006.

14. Broadbent BH. A new x-ray technique and its application to orthodontia. *Angle Orthod* 1:45, 1931.

15. Shaw WC, Roberts CT, Semb G. Evaluating treatment alternatives: Measurement and design. In: Turvey TA, Vig KWL, Fonseca RJ (eds). *Facial Clefts and Craniosynostosis. Principles and Management.* Philadelphia: WB Saunders Company, 1996, p. 756.

16. Enlow DH. *Handbook of Facial Growth.* Philadelphia: WB Saunders Co, 1975.

17. Houston WJ. The analysis of errors in orthodontic measurements. *Am J Orthod* 83:382, 1983.

18. Houston WJ, Maher RE, McElroy D, et al. Sources of error in measurements from cephalometric radiographs. *Eur J Orthod* 8:149, 1986.

19. Mazaheri M, Athanasiou AE, Long RE, Jr., et al. Evaluation of maxillary dental arch form in unilateral clefts of lip, alveolus and palate, from one month to four years. *Cleft Palate J* 30:90, 1993.

20. Prasad CN, Marsh JL, Long RE, Jr., et al. Quantitative 3-D maxillary arch evaluation of two different infant managements for unilateral cleft lip and palate. *Cleft Palate Craniofac J* 37:562, 2000.

21. Berkowitz S, Krischer J, Pruzansky S. Quantitative analysis of cleft palate casts. *Cleft Palate J* 11:134, 1974.

22. Berkowitz S. The complete unilateral cleft lip and palate: Serial three-dimensional studies of excellent palatal growth. In: Bardach J, Morris HL (eds). *Multidisciplinary Management of Cleft Lip and Palate.* Philadelphia: WB Saunders Co, 1990, p. 456.

23. Hathaway RR, Eppley BL, Hennon DK, et al. Primary alveolar cleft bone grafting in unilateral cleft lip and palate: Arch dimensions at age 8. *J of Craniofacial Surg* 10:58, 1999.

24. Hermann NV, Darvann TA, Fritz R, et al. A 3D CT analysis of mixed dentition maxillary arch form following two different infant managements of UCLP. In: Lilja J, Elander A, Friede H, Lohmander A (eds). *Transactions 9th International Congress on Cleft Palate and Related Craniofacial Anomalies.* Goteborg, Sweden, 2001, p. 161.

25. Trefny P, Smahel Z, Formanek P, et al. Three-dimensional analysis of maxillary dental casts using Fourier transform profilometry: *Precision* and reliability of measurement. *Cleft Palate Craniofac J* 41:20, 2004.

26. Brief J, Behle JH, Stellzig-Eisenhauer A, et al. Precision of landmark positioning on digitized from patients with cleft lip and palate. *Cleft Palate Craniofac J* 43:168, 2006.

27. Long RE, Jr., Fritz R, Gemmi C, et al. Comparison of long-term effects of two infant managements on mixed dentition UCLP maxillary arch form and occlusion. *9th International Congress on Cleft Lip and Palate and Related Craniofacial Anomalies.* Goteborg, Sweden, June 2001.

28. Richmond S, Shaw WC, Roberts CT, Andrews M. The PAR index (peer assessment rating): Methods to determine outcome of orthodontic treatment in terms of improvement and standards. *Eur J Orthod* 14:180, 1992.

29. Richmond S, Shaw WC, O'Brien KD, et al. The development of the PAR index (peer assessment rating): Reliability and validity. *Eur J Orthod* 14:125, 1992.

30. DeGuzman L, Bahiraei D, Vig KW, et al. The validation of the peer assessment rating index for malocclusion severity and treatment difficulty. *Am J Orthod Dentofacial Orthop* 107:172, 1995.

31. McMullan RE, Doubleday B, Muir JD, et al. Development of a treatment outcome standard as a result of a clinical audit of the outcome of fixed appliance therapy undertaken by hospital-based consultant orthodontists in the UK. *Br Dent J* 194:81, 2003.

32. Rarrick M. Assessment of the Peer Assessment Rating Index as Applied to the Malocclusions of Ssubjects with Unilateral Cleft Lip and Palate. MSc Thesis, Faculty of the school of Dental Medicine, University of Pittsburgh, 2001.

33. Kasem S. Assessing Orthodontic Treatment in Patients with Unilateral Cleft Lip and Palate. MSc Thesis, Faculty of Medicine and Human Services, School of Dentistry, University of Manchester, 2003.

34. Mohktar N. The Development of a Modified Peer Assessment (PAR) Index for Cleft Lip and Palate Patients: Validity and Reliability. MSc Thesis, Faculty of Medicine and Human Services, School of Dentisty, University of Manchester, 2005.

35. Deacon SA, Bessant P, Russell JI, et al. What are the occlusal outcomes for Unilateral Cleft Lip and Palate patients? A National Project in the UK *Br Dent J* 203(8):E18, 2007.

36. Wong FW, King NM. The oral health of children with clefts—A review. *Cleft Palate Craniofac J* 35:248, 1998.

37. Mars M, Plint DA, Houston WJ, et al. The Goslon Yardstick: A new system of assessing dental arch relationships in children with unilateral clefts of the lip and palate. *Cleft Palate J* 24:314, 1987.

38. Huddart AG, Bodenham RS. The evaluation of arch form and occlusion in unilateral cleft palate subjects. *Cleft Palate J* 9:194, 1972.

39. Mossey PA, Clark JD, Gray D. Preliminary investigation of a modified Huddart-Bodenheim scoring system for assessment of maxillary arch constriction in unilateral cleft lip and palate subjects. *Europ J Orthod* 25:251, 2003.

40. Gray D, Mossey PA. Evaluation of a modified Huddart/Bodenheim scoring system for assessment of maxillary arch constriction in unilateral cleft lip and palate subjects. *Europ J Orthod* 27:507, 2005.

41. Morris T, Roberts C, Shaw WC. Incisal overjet as an outcome measure in unilateral cleft lip and palate management. *Cleft Palate Craniofac J* 31:142, 1994.

42. Shaw WC, Asher-McDade C, Brattstrom V, et al. A six-center international study of treatment outcome in patients with clefts of the lip and palate: Part 1. Principles and studydesign. *Cleft Palate Craniofac J* 29:393, 1992.

43. Shaw WC, Dahl E, Asher-McDade C, et al. A six-center international study of treatment outcome in patients with clefts of the lip and palate: Part 5. General discussions and conclusions. *Cleft Palate Craniofac J* 29:413, 1992.

44. Mølsted K, Asher-McDade C, Brattstrom V. A six-center international study of treatment outcome in patients with clefts of the lip and palate: Part 2. Craniofacial form and soft tissue profile. *Cleft Palate Craniofac J* 29:398, 1992.

45. Mars M, Asher-McDade C, Brattstrom V. A six-center international study of treatment outcome in patients with clefts of the lip and palate: Part 3. Dental arch relationships. *Cleft Palate Craniofac J* 29:405, 1992.

46. Asher-McDade C, Brattstrom V, Dahl E, et al. A six-center international study of treatment outcome in patients with clefts of the lip and palate: Part 5. Assessment of nasolabial appearance. *Cleft Palate Craniofac J* 29:490, 1992.

47. Mølsted K, Brattstrom V, Prahl-Andersen B, et al. The Eurocleft study: Intercenter study of treatment outcomes in patients with complete cleft lip and palate. Part 3. Dental arch relationships. *Cleft Palate Craniofac J* 42:78, 2005.

48. Vargas AI. *Midfacial Growth in Bilateral Cleft Lip and Palate Patients Following Premaxillary Repositioning as a Secondary Surgical Procedure.* Philadelphia: Albert Einstein Medical Center, Department of Orthodontics, 1994.

49. Long RE, Jr., Volfson Y, Silverman E. Correlation between dental model rating systems and cephalometric values in patients with UCLP. Proceedings of the 10th International Congress on Cleft Palate and Related Craniofacial Anomalies, Durban, South Africa, 2005, p. 115.

50. Nollet PJPM, Katsaros C, van't Hof MA, et al. Photographs of study casts: An alternative medium for rating dental arch relationships in unilateral cleft lip and palate. 41:646, 2004.

51. Atack NE, Hathorn IS, Semb G, et al. A new index for assessing surgical outcomes in unilateral cleft lip and palate subjects aged 5 – reproducibility and reliability. *Cleft Palate Craniofac J* 34:242, 1997.

52. Long RE, Jr., Flinn W, Semb G. Use of 5-year old dental model ratings to predict 9-year old outcomes and future treatment needs in

patients with UCLP. 59th ACPA Annual Meeting, Seattle, WA, May 2002.

53. Atack NE, Hathorn IS, Sandy JR, et al. Early detection of differences in treatment outcomes for cleft lip and palate. *Br J Orthodont* 25:181, 1998.

54. Flinn W, Long RE, Jr., Garrattini G, et al. A multicenter outcomes assessment of five-year-old patients with unilateral cleft lip and palate. *Cleft Palate Craniofac J* 43:253, 2006.

55. Mars M, Batra P, Worrell E. Complete unilateral cleft lip and palate: validity of the five-year index and the Goslon Yardstick in predicting long-term dental arch relationships. *Cleft Palate Craniofac J* 43:557, 2006.

56. Ozawa TO, Santos ACS, Costa GC, et al. The Bauru Yardstick: A system of assessing the dental arch relationship in children with complete bilateral cleft lip and palate. Proceedings of the 10th International Congress on Cleft Palate and Related Craniofacial Anomalies, Durban, South Africa, 2005, p. 115.

57. Long RE, Jr. Factors affecting the success of secondary alveolar bone grafting in patients with complete clefts of the lip and palate. In Trotman CA, McNamara JA, Jr. (eds). *Orthodontic Treatment: Outcome and Effectiveness, Monograph 30.* Craniofacial Growth Series, Ann Arbor, Center for Human Growth and Development, The University of Michigan, 271, 1995.

58. Bergland O, Semb G, Åbyholm FE. Elimination of the residual alveolar cleft by secondary bone grafting and subsequent orthodontic treatment. *Cleft Palate J* 23:175, 1986.

59. Kindelan JD, Nashed RR, Bromige MR. Radiographic assessment of secondary autogenous alveolar bone grafting in cleft lip and palate patients. *Cleft Palate Craniofac J* 34:195, 1997.

60. Witherow H, Cox S, Jones E, et al. A new scale to assess radiographic success of secondary alveolar bone grafts. *Cleft Palate Craniofac J* 39:255, 2002.

61. Nightingale C, Witherow H, Reid FD, et al. Comparative reproducibility of three methods of radiographic assessment of alveolar bone grafting. *Eur J Orthodont* 25:35, 2003.

62. Long RE, Jr., Spangler BE, Yow M. Cleft width and secondary alveolar bone graft success. *Cleft Palate J* 32:420, 1995.

63. Long RE, Jr., Paterno M, Vinson B. The effect of cuspid positioning in the cleft at the time of secondary alveolar bone grafting on eventual graft success. *Cleft Palate J* 33:225, 1996.

64. Rosenstein SW, Long RE, Jr., Dado DV, et al. A comparison of 2-D calculations from periapical and occlusal radiographs vs. 3-D calculations from CAT scans in determining bone support for cleft-adjacent teeth following early alveolar bone grafts. *Cleft Palate J* 34:199, 1997.

65. Farkas LG, Hajnis K, Posnick JC. Anthropometric and anthroscopic findings of the nasal and facial region in cleft patients before and after primary lip repair. *Cleft Palate Craniofac J* 30:1, 1993.

66. Asher-McDade C, Roberts C, Shaw WC, et al. Development of a method for rating nasolabial appearance in patients with clefts of the lip and palate. *Cleft Palate Craniofac J* 28:385, 1991.

67. Prahl C, Prahl-Andersen B, van't Hof MA, et al. Infant orthopedics and facial appearance: A randomized clinical trial (Dutchcleft). *Cleft Palate Craniofac J* 43:659, 2006.

68. Al-Omari I, Millet DT, Ayoub AF. Methods of assessment of cleft related facial deformity: A review. *Cleft Palate Craniofac J* 42:145, 2005.

69. Severns JL, Prahl C, Kuijpers-Jagtman AM, et al. Short-term cost effectiveness analysis of presurgical orthopedic treatment in children with complete unilateral cleft lip and palate. *Cleft Palate Craniofac J* 35:222, 1998.

70. Semb G, Brattström V, Mølsted K, et al. The Eurocleft Study: Intercenter study of treatment outcome in patients with complete cleft lip and palate. Part 1: Introduction and treatment experience. *Cleft Palate Craniofac J* 42:64, 2005.

71. Laupacis A, Sackett DL, Roberts RS. An assessment of clinically useful measures of the consequences of treatment. *New Eng J Med* 26:1728, 1988.

72. Brattström V, Mølsted K, et al. The Eurocleft Study: Intercenter study of treatment outcome in patients with complete cleft lip and palate. Part 2: Craniofacial form and nasolabial appearance. *Cleft Palate Craniofac J* 42:69, 2005.

73. Semb G, Brattström V, Mølsted K, et al. The Eurocleft Study: Intercenter study of treatment outcome in patients with complete cleft lip and palate. Part 4: Relationship among treatment outcome, patient/parent satisfaction, and the burden of care. *Cleft Palate Craniofac J* 42:83, 2005.

74. Shaw WC, Brattström V, Mølsted K, et al. The Eurocleft Study: Intercenter study of treatment outcome in patients with complete cleft lip and palate. Part 5: Discussion and conclusions. *Cleft Palate Craniofac J* 42:93, 2005.

75. Ross RB. Treatment variables affecting facial growth in complete unilateral cleft lip and palate. Part 1: Treatment affecting growth. *Cleft Palate J* 24:5, 1987.

76. Ross RB. Treatment variables affecting facial growth in complete unilateral cleft lip and palate. Part 2: Presurgical orthopaedics. *Cleft Palate J* 24:24, 1987.

77. Ross RB. Treatment variables affecting facial growth in complete unilateral cleft lip and palate. Part 3: Alveolus repair and bone grafting. *Cleft Palate J* 24:33, 1987.

78. Ross RB. Treatment variables affecting facial growth in complete unilateral cleft lip and palate. Part 4: Repair of the cleft lip. *Cleft Palate J* 24:45, 1987.

79. Ross RB. Treatment variables affecting facial growth in complete unilateral cleft lip and palate. Part 5: Timing of palate repair. *Cleft Palate J* 24:54, 1987.

80. Ross RB. Treatment variables affecting facial growth in complete unilateral cleft lip and palate. Part 6: Techniques of palate repair. *Cleft Palate J* 24:64, 1987.

81. Ross RB. Treatment variables affecting facial growth in complete unilateral cleft lip and palate. Part 7: An overview of treatment and facial growth. *Cleft Palate J* 24:71, 1987.

71

Assessment of Speech Outcomes in Cleft Palate Surgery

Sally J. Peterson-Falzone, PhD

OUTCOMES RESEARCH IN SPEECH

The clinician (surgeon, dentist, nurse, otolaryngologist, pediatrician, psychologist, speech-language pathologist, etc.) whose primary interest is cleft palate and who is concerned with advancing the state of the art is usually well aware of all the factors that confound outcomes research. Members of interdisciplinary teams have something of an advantage over lone practitioners in this regard, given the fact that team members are exposed on a regular basis to the problems their fellow team members have in documenting their own outcomes. Psychologists and speech-language pathologists may be envious of surgeons and dentists because these clinicians can determine their outcomes from physical measurements (i.e., digital images of photographs, x-rays, and casts) and compare these outcomes across patient diagnostic categories, treatment regimens, etc. Psychosocial and speech outcomes assessments, on the other hand, require measurement of behavior, performance, and competency.

The Basic Requirements for Outcomes Studies*

In speech or in any other aspect of assessment of cleft care, the strongest evidence that one treatment protocol is better than another comes from prospective clinical trials that include assessment not only of the treatment group but also of a matched control group studied over the same period of time.[1] Such studies are also termed "cohort studies."[2] In contrast, "case-control studies" are usually retrospective, comparing current cases with controls from the past, typically either untreated cases or cases treated by an older method. Not surprisingly, prospective clinical trials are the most difficult to carry out. Wissow and Pascoe[2] offered this warning: "Clinical trials are poorly suited to studies of 1) multiple therapeutic modalities (because too many subjects are needed to evaluate the many possible therapeutic combinations); 2) small changes in a therapeutic plan (the effort it takes to do the study may outweigh the potential significance of the outcome); 3) therapies that may be changed during the chouse of the study so that the results are not at risk for becoming obsolete before the study is completed; and 4) treatments with only rare outcomes or outcomes that will be observable at a time far distant in the future."

Shprintzen[3] pointed out that most research is guided by a specific motive, usually meaning that the investigator has a built-in bias regarding the outcome. He acknowledged that investigators may be aware of the heterogeneity of the cleft population and may have tried to make their subject population as homogeneous as possible, but up to the date of his commentary he found no published studies that had held constant all the variables that could influence treatment outcome. In the opinion of the current author, this is hardly surprising even 7 years later: There are simply too many factors that ultimately do not fall within the investigator's ability to control. And, as observed by Shprintzen,[3] "holding all variables constant in patients with multiple problems is not only difficult, but the ethics of withholding treatment for the purposes of determining research outcome might have some difficulty passing an Institutional Review Board."

The obvious conclusion at this point is a rather disheartening one for clinicians, i.e., "If you want to prove that a given protocol produces better treatment results (speech or other outcomes) in children with clefts, you need to plan a prospective randomized study that includes 1) either elimination of or detailed documentation of associated anomalies; 2) a cohort study with at least one control group, with all independent variables matched across patient pairs; 3) two or more surgeons performing the same procedure (to prove it is not the surgeon's skill or technique that is making the difference); 4) large numbers of patients in each patient group, results recorded by independent observers on standardized forms (not just anecdotal comments) and recorded over time as opposed to a single post-treatment observation." In reality, the careful and diligent researcher tries to come as close to this as possible and is very cautious in interpretation of results.

A General Warning in Clinical Research: "A" does not Cause "B"

A long-honored but often forgotten caveat about clinical research is that we must not jump to conclusions about cause(s) and effect. We continue to fall into the trap of assuming that, because "B" is strongly associated with "A", even if "B" does not <u>always</u> follow "A", "A" is the cause of "B". A widely used analogy points out that Tuesday always follows Monday, but does that mean Monday <u>causes</u> Tuesday? In cleft care, there are multiple, historical examples of falling into this trap. For example, maxillary arch collapse is frequently found in surgically repaired cases of cleft lip and palate, and often attributed to age of surgery or surgical technique. Yet, neither of these factors, either alone or together, can be held responsible for either normal or abnormal subsequent development of the craniofacial complex. The maxilla is <u>inherently</u> deficient in both tissue and growth potential in clefts, and patients are not the same in how much of that deficiency may affect their presenting morphology.

Current Trends in Outcomes Research in Speech

At the time of the writing of this chapter, the literature on outcomes assessments in most medical specialty fields, as well as in the allied medical sciences, is replete with articles on "evidence-based practice," meaning that clinicians are expected to prove that what they are doing provides the best benefit for their patients. Evidence-based practice is a primary area of concern for Division 5 of the American Speech-Language-Hearing Association, a special interest division of ASHA made up of speech-language pathologists (SLPs) whose focus is on organic disorders.

In speech-language pathology, evidence-based practice (EBP) is indeed a current "buzz-word." It is an important idea in <u>all</u> areas of patient care, and one that is currently the topic of a great deal of literature, particularly with regard to clefts.[4–21] Many of these publications are instructive and helpful, and can guide clinicians (particularly new clinicians) along an important road of thinking. Table 1 segregates the aspects of research design that weaken a study's conclusions from those that lead to stronger evidence for a particular treatment approach.

What About International Cross-cultural, Cross-linguistic Standards in Assessment of Care for Patients with Clefts?

If there can be meaningful, useful standards for assessing how well clinicians are doing in their treatment of patients with clefts and other craniofacial anomalies, those standards

* Portions of the following material are excerpted from Peterson-Falzone SJ. Optimal age for palatoplasty to facilitate normal speech development: What is the evidence? In Berkowitz S (ed.): *Cleft Lip and Palate: Diagnosis and Management*, 2nd edn. Heidelberg: Springer-Verlag, 2006.

Table 71–1.

Weighing Weaknesses and Strength of Research Evidence

Research design factors that weaken conclusions	Research design factors that lead to stronger evidence of outcome
(a) Investigator undertakes the study to prove that his treatment protocol is better than another	(a) Investigator has no prior bias as to outcome of study
(b) Results recorded only by the investigator without independent observations by unbiased judges	(b) Results recorded by unbiased observers/recorders
(c) Single recorder/observer	(c) Multiple independent observers/recorders, with measurement of both intra- and inter-observer reliability
(d) One-time observation of results	(d) Longitudinal observation of results
(e) Retrospective review of records	(e) Prospective study
(f) Single group of patients, treated according to one protocol, no control group	(f) Cohort studies, comparing two or more groups of homogeneous patients, one treated according to the protocol under study, the other untreated or treated by a standard accepted protocol
(g) No attempt to control the multiple variables that may influence results	(g) Control, or at least careful independent documentation, of all independent variables (e.g., absence of associated anomalies type and extent of cleft, health history, ear disease, and hearing loss (current and previous), socioeconomic factors, psychological factors (including parental nurturing and stimulation)

cannot be unique to one treatment regimen, one country, one culture. Speech-language pathologists across the world have had to scramble a bit more than their non-SLP colleagues on cleft palate/craniofacial teams who can make physical measurements of casts, radiographic images, and photographs. Speech is not so easily measured, and deriving a universal system for assessment and comparison of treatment outcomes calls for cross-linguistic, cross-cultural research.

The early 1990s saw two parallel and virtually simultaneous developments in the effort to standardize assessment of treatment outcomes in clefts. In Europe, an international, multi-center comparative study of outcomes, the "Eurocleft" project, started to yield data in 1991.[22–29] Although the first publications focused only on physical outcomes, what became known as the "Eurocleft Speech Group" published its first report in 1994, with a second one appearing in 2000.[30,31]

The second development was a series of panels and study sessions on the effort to standardize speech assessments across languages that do not share the same phonetic nor linguistic rules. These sessions were presented within the venue of the 7th, 8th, and 9th International Congresses on Cleft Palate and Related Craniofacial Anomalies in 1993, 1997, and 2001, respectively. Subsequently, a presentation by Kuehn, Trost-Cardamone, and Sell at the 2002 meeting of the American Cleft Palate-Craniofacial Association[32] focused on issues in universal reporting parameters for speech; the collaboration of those three investigators led to the invitation to speech-language pathologists in Ireland, China, and Australia to join the effort. In 2004, there was a workshop in Washington, DC, funded by the National Institute on Deafness and Other Communication Disorders (NINCD), a division of NIH. This workshop involved experienced SLPs from several countries. The workshop covered the topics of (a) diversity across evalu-

ation systems, (b) speech sampling procedures, (c) proposed reporting parameters and guidelines for usage, (d) preliminary experience in mapping evaluation measures to the initial set of reporting parameters, and (e) a discussion of what demographic information on individual patients would be necessary to build into the data base. Following the workshop, the steering committee continued further work in development of a universal system for reporting speech outcomes. The following year, that committee presented a second report on issues in universal reporting parameters for speech at the 10th International Congress on Cleft Palate and Related Craniofacial Anomalies.[33] An up-to-date report on this project may be found in the *Cleft Palate-Craniofacial Journal.*[34]

Given the complexity of the task of assessing speech (a very fluid human behavior that is often difficult to describe with consistency, let alone measure), it is somewhat amazing that progress is indeed being made in the effort to develop universal parameters of assessment that can be used across languages that are disparate in phonetic content and linguistic rules. These parameters, while still in the process of refinement as of this writing (late 2006) will soon be available to facilitate the efforts of speech-language pathologists in their efforts to measure treatment outcomes in their patients and to compare outcomes across treatment regimens, languages, and cultures.

THE ESSENTIAL ELEMENTS OF ASSESSMENT

Optimum assessment of speech outcomes after cleft palate surgery requires

(a) one or more speech-language pathologists who know (1) how to engage a child so that an adequate speech sample can be obtained, and (2) how to sustain the child's attention long enough to assess various parameters of speech output, that list of parameters growing as the child grows, but beginning with some key observations long before the first words appear;

(b) a sufficient number of speech-language pathologists listening to the same speech output from the same child, so that inter-listener reliability can be established;

(c) high-quality recording equipment, at least for audio recording and preferably for video recording;

(d) instrumentation that allows visualization of velopharyngeal function during speech production, e.g., videofluoroscopy and nasopharyngogoscopy;

(e) instrumentation for documenting the effect that velopharyngeal closure or lack of such closure has on either the aerodynamics of speech production ("pressure-flow") or the acoustics of speech (e.g., Nasometry); and

(f) longitudinal follow-up of speech results, as opposed to one-time assessment.

In reality, however, this ideal protocol can be implemented only in very large treatment centers with adequate, on-going funding and institutional support. Many teams throughout the United States do not enjoy such benevolence. Members of these teams, as well as other caregivers who are not team-based, still try to maximize treatment outcomes for their patients while working under less-than-optimum circumstances.

A NOTE ON TIMING OF ASSESSMENT

Surgeons and speech-language pathologists know that enough time for healing to take place and for swelling to diminish must elapse before a meaningful perceptual or instrumental evaluation of velopharyngeal function can be obtained. Parents and families, on the other hand, are very anxious to learn the results of surgery. Careful, intentionally redundant counseling is usually essential to keeping families comfortable during the healing period. The "rules of thumb" used for this counseling may vary from team to team. Most surgeons will state that full healing may take as long as 6 months. As a compromise between waiting many months to learn results and the "soon-as-he-wakes-up" desires of the family, the speech pathologist may suggest a preliminary evaluation 2–3 months after surgery, with the stipulation that the results could still change after that point. Again, this stipulation usually has to be repeated to the family, making it very clear that (1) the first post-op evaluation of speech is only preliminary, (2) another evaluation should take place a few months later, and (3) the longer-term judgment regarding the effects on speech may change even after 6 months. With regard to this last point, the speech-language pathologist and the surgeon will also have to discuss with the patient and fam-

ily the fact that velopharyngeal function may change much later on as a result of either natural growth of the craniofacial complex (increasing the size of the nasopharyngeal space) or natural changes in adenoid tissue.[†] Finally, it should be made clear to the patient and family that periodic evaluations of speech will be needed until the child has reached an age of nearly completed craniofacial growth (early teenage years).

Assessment of the effects of pharyngeal surgery also requires a lapse of time. Centrally based pharyngeal flaps, sphincter pharyngoplasties, and various types of augmentation pharyngoplasty all change in physical characteristics and functional effect on speech over time as a result of several factors, including diminution of edema, "drift" of the position or flaps or of pharyngeal inserts, and muscle movement that may act to change the vector of sphincteric action. Prior to surgery, the team will usually discuss with the patient and family the fact that speech in the immediate postoperative period will not necessarily be indicative of what speech will be in the long-term outcome.

PERCEPTUAL ASSESSMENT OF SPEECH

In the Baby[‡]

In the United States, surgical closure of the palate is typically accomplished between 6 and 18 months of age.[§] Licensed speech-language pathologists with certificates of clinical competency from the American Speech-Language-Hearing Association know how to assess the baby's early output of speech sounds even before palatal closure is accomplished. What is known as "canonical babbling" (repetition of the same syllable in "strings") usually begins about 6 months of age (examples: "yayaya," "nunununu," "awa awa"). If the palate is still open when this babbling begins, the consonant sounds in these syllables will be limited to "m," "n," "ng," "h," "w," and "y" sounds that are also heard in noncleft babies. However, babies without clefts will also start to use "b," " d," and "g" at this age. These consonants require the ability to build up intraoral air pressure, something the baby with an open cleft cannot do. As a result, they will instead sound like "m," "n," and "ng." The important point is that parents need to recognize these early attempts at consonant sounds (whether "nasal" or not) and to reinforce their baby by echoing back

---

[†] The effects of adenoid enlargement and adenoid involution on velopharyngeal function have been documented extensively in the literature. Even the tonsils, if sufficiently enlarged in the upper poles, may affect VP function. For a list of references on these topics, please see Peterson-Falzone et al. (2001).[35]

[‡] The American Speech-Language-Hearing Association publishes a chart on early development of communication skills (both input {hearing and comprehension} and output {speech sound development, appearance of first words, and continuing development of expressive language) that is available online and also as an attractive wall chart for your office. Go to www.asha.org.

[§] This timing does not take into account treatment protocols that use "primary veloplasty," in which the velum is closed first and the remaining hard palate cleft at a much later date, sometimes not until late childhood. For an overview of the effects of primary veloplasty on speech development, please see Peterson-Falzone[36].

what the baby is producing so that the baby gets the feeling of accomplishment (he has elicited attention and happy smiles from his parents, and managed to get them to do what he is doing!). The parents can use fully oral productions of the intended consonants (b, d, g). The more they interact vocally with their baby, the more babbling the baby will do.

When parents of an infant with a cleft are seen by a cleft palate-craniofacial team, they should be counseled that these early sound differences are not a source of concern, and they should be encouraged to echo what their baby is doing in early sound output and to expand upon it (please see Peterson-Falzone et al.).[37] They should also be counseled regarding what to expect in early vocalizations and speech sound output and advised that an early speech and language intervention program will be recommended or implemented for them if the baby does not achieve the normal milestones we expect in the first year of life.

In the Toddler

About the time a child is taking his or her first steps, the first "real" words also appear. At the age of one year, the child should have at least one or two words that are meaningful (meaning that he uses the same word for a single object or action, and not as a generalized vocalization). Many children have 10 words by this age, and by 18 months of age the expressive vocabulary has grown to 50 words. Children with clefts should be no different so long as they are not suffering from intermittent ear disease and hearing loss. It is well known that children with clefts are very susceptible to otitis media, and even a mild, intermittent hearing loss can interfere with language development. The speech-language pathologist dealing with a child with a cleft will track these early developmental stages, encouraging the parents to write down all the words the child is using (even when "pronunciation" is not as good as it will later become) prior to each clinic visit. If the child is using only a few words at 18 months of age, the SLP should institute or recommend an early intervention program.

If the cleft is still open at 18 months (a possibility if the treatment protocol is one involving primary veloplasty), the child's speech output will be more difficult for the parents and family to understand and reinforce. They may be able to develop a sufficiently large "adjusted scale of comprehension" (meaning that they have learned how to recognize the words in the child's output) to reinforce that output and interact verbally with their child without frustrating either him or themselves. However, as the length and complexity of the child's verbal output grows, so does the danger inherent in communication failures.

By 2 years of age, the normal expressive vocabulary has reached 200 words, and the child is starting to put two words together into little sentences, e.g., "Daddy bye" (meaning Daddy has gone bye-bye) or "Kitty night-night." At this age, if the cleft is still open and the child's communication attempts often fail because his words are difficult to understand, frustration will become a serious problem. The notorious "2-year-old temper tantrums" will be even more frequent and intractable than they are in noncleft children. The long-term consequences are, in fact, a two-edged sword: (1) ongoing, increasing communication failures leading the child to simply "give up" and not even attempt new sounds or words, and (2) a high likelihood of the development and habituation of maladaptive compensatory misarticulations that can render speech unintelligible[35–39] and that are so difficult to correct once they become established. It is worth noting that speech-language pathologists advocate very early intervention programs for children with clefts, beginning well before the age of 3 years, for the prevention of compensatory misarticulations and for eradication or at least diminution of such errors if they have begun to become apparent.[40–41]

In the Pre-schooler

For a speech-language pathologist working with young children, there is no greater feeling of accomplishment than having a little one smile and say "I forgot to tell you about what happened!" and no greater feeling of ineptitude than when one has to tell his or her colleagues, "I couldn't get him to talk to me." Within multidisciplinary cleft palate/craniofacial teams, each professional will occasionally know the feeling of failure in getting either (a) a child (patient) to talk, and/or (2) a family to be candid about the problems of treatment.

In many treatment centers, the SLP may have a particular advantage: If a sound-recording room (preferably a sound-treated booth) with good recording equipment is available, the SLP can say to other staff members, "We have to go talk now." Parents often respond positively to the thought that their child now has an independent duty. If not, or if the child is frightened, it is relatively easy to enlist the cooperation of both parent and child with, "We're going to go talk and look at some pictures for a while. Do you want to come?"

From the pre-school years onward, the speech and language evaluation consists of some spontaneous conversation (focused on a standard set of toys, picture books, and other objects so that the crucial intraoral pressure consonants can be elicited), a single-word articulation test or assessment of phonetic inventory, an assessment of phonologic development (if indicated), various tests of receptive and expressive language development, and a thorough intraoral examination (in addition to whatever imaging studies are indicated). Given the restraints of time, funding, and children's attention spans, some degree of triage is usually practiced so that the most important elements of the evaluation, as judged on a case-by-case basis, are accomplished first.

In the School-Age Child

Children love comrades, and they love a willing audience. At home, they may be frequently "squelched" by the competing conversational demands of older siblings. In the clinic setting, they are not very likely to trust those professionals who appear to be on their parents' side rather than their own. However, SLPs can easily be nonthreatening. Their job is to get kids to talk. Remember that, for both children and adults, the sense that your conversational partner truly *wants* to hear what you have to say is an inestimable motivation to talk. Other members of cleft palate/craniofacial teams can easily learn this skill, getting children to talk freely and thus learning more about the possible presence of the "stigmata of cleft palate speech" (nasal air loss on pressure consonants, hypernasal resonance on vowels and vocalic consonants, and maladaptive compensatory misarticulations). Because of the way interdisciplinary teams work, the subjective impressions of the child's speech noted by the non-SLP team members will be taken into consideration in treatment planning, just as the SLP's thoughts on the appearance of the child, the dental/occlusal situation, the psychosocial adjustment, etc. will be taken into consideration by other team members.

In the Late School-Age Child or Adolescent

While the team has always been planning for this "end-stage" of treatment, and duly advised the family, these later years can be among the most difficult. What if, as the child/teenager progresses through orthodontic expansion and later-stage appliances, (1) a fistula opens up, (2) dental/orthodontic appliances interfere with articulation, or (3) normal craniofacial growth and/or adenoid involution leads to a recurrence of inadequate velopharyngeal closure for speech? Closely coordinated evaluation, preferably with the orthodontist, surgeon, and speech-language pathologist seeing the child *simultaneously*, is the key to working out such complications. The team psychologist or social worker must also be an integral player in order to help ensure that the patient's and family's desires are understood. Without the full cooperation and understanding of the patient and family, attempts to resolve end-stage problems or to "salvage" a case that has met with late-occurring problems will inevitably fail.[**]

INSTRUMENTAL ASSESSMENT OF VELOPHARYNGEAL CLOSURE

Instrument-based assessment of velopharyngeal closure falls into two basic categories: those assessments that look at the mechanism and those assessments that measure either the acoustic or the aerodynamic results of VP function. A third category consists of various forms of phototransducers or photodetectors that measure the amount of light transmitted through the velopharyngeal port from the oral cavity into the nasal cavity when a light source is introduced into the mouth. An early version of such a device was labeled a "velograph" and was described by Kunzel in 1979.[42] Because phototrans-

ducers have not found a niche in routine clinical evaluation of patients with clefts or other types of VPI, they will not be discussed in further detail here.[††]

Looking at the Velopharyngeal Mechanism
Radiographic Images

Cephalometric films: Lateral cephalometric films have been used to look at the craniofacial complex since the early 1940s. The clinician can study the size of the velum (length and thickness), depth of the pharynx, size and position of the adenoid and tonsillar tissue, and the bony structures that affect the size of the VP space (specifically, the cranial base and the cervical vertebrae). A film taken during sustained production of an oral pressure consonant such as "f," "s," or "th" may provide some indication of how well the velum elevates on such a task, and whether or not velopharyngeal closure is obtained at the midline. (Note: It must be borne in mind that the film is focused at the mid-sagittal plane and cannot tell the clinician what is taking place on either side of the midline.) The advantages of cephalometric films are that they are relatively easy to obtain if the child will tolerate head-stabilization elements (e.g., ear rods and a forehead "bumper"), they are easy to measure, and the manual tracings or the digital measurements derived from them can be compared over time to assess changes in structures as the child grows. The primary disadvantage is that they provide only a two-dimensional, static image of a multi-dimensional, moving system, which means they can provide only a "guesstimate" of how well the VP system functions for speech. For more detailed information of the use of cephalometrics to look at VP structures, please see Finkelstein et al.[48]; Park et al.[49]; Rose et al.[50]; Smahel and Mullerova[51]; and Tzy-Hsin et al.[52]

Videofluoroscopy: The use of multiview videofluoroscopy for examining the function of the VP mechanism came into popularity in the early 1970s,[53–56] having grown out of the earlier use of cinefluorography.[57,58] The recording of radiographic images on videotape requires much less radiation than recording the same images on motion picture film. In cleft palate/craniofacial treatment centers, multiview videofluorography quickly became a part of the "gold standard" for evaluation of VP function. A recent survey conducted by Division 5 of the American Speech-Language-Hearing Association showed that, of 105 clinicians actively involved in evaluation of velopharyngeal function, nearly all (101/105) indicated they used endoscopy at times, 61 used endoscopy as the first or only choice; 64 used videofluoroscopy at times although many responded it was used rarely; and only 10 used videofluoroscopy as the first or only choice. The primary advantage of multiview videofluoroscopy is the wealth of information it provides about VP function by gathering data from several views (lateral, frontal, basal, or oblique) obtained during speech production. It is usually performed

---

[**] A warning specifically to SLPs: When one asks the parent of a teenager whether or not the child's speech is satisfactory, there is a good chance the response will include, "He mumbles all the time." This is a common "malady" in teens talking to their parents, although not usually when they are talking to their peers. It does mean that the parent may honestly have difficulty assessing whether or not a surgical procedure performed for speech has been successful.

[††] For further reading on this type of instrumentation, see Dalston,[43,44] Dalston and Keefe,[45] Moon,[46] and Moon and Lagu[47].

without any head holding device, which is both an advantage and a disadvantage: A head holding device can be scary to a child, but its absence means that the image does not remain focused at the midline.[‡‡] It must be remembered that, even though several views are obtained, each image is still only two-dimensional, just as it is in cephalometrics. The clinician uses the combined information from the several views to construct a multi-dimensional percept of how the system functions in speech production. The primary disadvantage of the technique is the radiation exposure, even though the use of video recording is a great improvement over the older method of recording on motion picture film.

CT scans: The use of computerized tomography to examine the velopharyngeal port was explored in the 1990s, but never became a routine clinical tool.

Non-radiographic Imaging

Ultrasound: A few decades ago, there was a brief interest in the use of ultrasound to look at the VP mechanism.[59-68] The primary purpose was to look at movement of the lateral pharyngeal walls, something that could not be done with lateral radiographic imaging. However, as the use of frontal, basal, and oblique videofluorosopic images became more common, and also as endoscopic imaging became popular, ultrasound gradually dropped out of the armamentarium used for looking at the VP mechanism.

Endoscopy: The use of a rigid, oral endoscope for looking at the velopharyngeal port was first described by Taub in 1966.[69] The image was limited to an inferior ("underside") view of the VP mechanism, and imaging VP function during any kind of speech movements was limited to looking at the system during production of a sustained vowel. Just a few years later, Pigott[70] introduced nasendoscopy for examination of the VP port during speech production, a development that revolutionized the clinical documentation of velopharyngeal function. While the work of Pigott and his colleagues was initially focused on what could be learned from a rigid endoscope introduced into the nose, clinicians quickly moved on to flexible fiberoptic nasopharyngoscopy (nasendoscopy, videonendoscopy, or videonasopharyngoscopy), which is more comfortable for the patient. The use of this instrumentation is now routine in medically based cleft palate-craniofacial teams and constitutes another part of the "gold standard" for documentation of VP function. There is a very large body of literature on nasopharyngoscopy, both in texts and journals. For practical information on "how-to," "what-it-will-do," and "what-not-to-expect," and also for information comparing various types of endoscopes, the reader is particularly referred to D'Antonio et al.[71]; Golding-Kushner et al.[72]; Karnell,[73] Pigott,[74] Pigott and Makepease[75]; and Shprintzen.[76,77]

Magnetic resonance imaging (MRI): As of this writing, the use of MRI images to study the VP port is still in the research realm rather than a part of routine clinical examination, primarily because of the expense. MRI studies of both velopharyngeal movement and movement of other articulators were published in the 1990s.[78,79] As technical improvements were made, real-time imaging became possible. The images are fascinating and potentially very instructive to the surgeons attempting the reconstruction of musculature. They also inform speech scientists and speech-language pathologists about coordination of movement patterns of the lips, tongue, and VP system. The reader is referred to Ettema et al.,[80] Kane et al.,[81] Kuehn et al.,[82,83] Shinagawa et al.,[84] Wein et al.,[78] and Yamawaki et al.[79] There is little doubt that the use of MRI will expand and, if the costs diminish, perhaps one day clinicians will be gathering extensive data on patients without exposing them to the dangers of radiation and without the invasiveness of an endoscope.

MEASURING THE EFFECTS OF VELOPHARYNGEAL ACTIVITY ON SPEECH

While the first and ultimate measure of velopharyngeal closure is the listener's perception of speech (remember that, in the process of their development, all instrument-based measures were validated against listener judgment), clinicians have long sought verification or substantiation of their own subjective judgments regarding presence or absence of hypernasal resonance and nasal air loss on high pressure consonants. This search has led to a wealth of instrumentation, and those clinicians who have access to such techniques are significantly aided in the treatment decisions they have to make.

Other chapters in this text present detailed information on the various forms of acoustic and aerodynamic instrumentation used to assess the effects of VP activity on speech output. Currently, the two most commonly used instruments in these categories are the Nasometer[TM] and the PERCI. The Nasometer[TM] is the more modern version of the TONAR,[85] and the PERCI is a computer-based instrument for measuring oral versus nasal airflow, based on the extensive work of Warren and colleagues on the aerodynamics of speech production.[86,87] Both instruments require substantial financial outlay for the equipment itself and for the computers to run the analyses, plus thorough training for the user. Please see the chapter by Hinton in this volume for details. Neither the Nasometer[TM] nor the PERCI (or another form of either acoustic or aerodynamic instrumentation) is in any way harmful to the patient, and generally any child from preschool age upward can be cooperative for such examinations.

A final warning: Whether considering instrumental assessment that looks at the VP mechanism or that measures some result of velopharyngeal activity, the clinician must keep in mind that the instruments can tell us only what the VP system was doing at the time the measurement was being obtained, NOT what the system is actually capable of doing.

[‡‡] One clinic known to this author uses an old-fashioned Viewmaster[TM] toy affixed to a portion of the fluorography equipment just in front of the child's head. When the child's eyes are "in place" in the Viewmaster[TM] and he is being entertained by the images, there is less likelihood of head movement.

For example, if a child routinely uses glottal and pharyngeal articulations for what should be oral pressure consonants, he is bypassing use of the velopharyngeal system, and any instrumental measurement will automatically indicate that the system is incapable of closure. This point is discussed extensively elsewhere.[35,37]

References

1. Friedman LM, Furberg CD, DeMets DL. *Fundamentals of Clinical Trials*, 3rd edn. Mosby: St. Louis, 1996.

2. Wissow L, Pascoe J. Types of research models and methods. In De Angelis C (ed). *An Introduction to Clinical Research.* New York: Oxford Press, 1990, pp. 38–74.

3. Shprintzen RJ. Fallibility of clinical research. *Cleft Palate Craniofac J* 28:136–141, 1991.

4. Guyatt G, Rennie D. *Users' Guide to the Medical Literature: A Manual for Evidence-Based Clinical Practice.* Chicago: American Medical Association Press, 2002.

5. Wertz RT. Evidence-based practice guidelines: Not all evidence is created equal. *J Med Speech Lang Pathol* 10:xi—xv, 2002.

6. Apel K, Self T. Evidence-based practice: The marriage of research and clinical services. *The ASHA Leader* 8:6–7, 2003.

7. Montgomery EB, Turkstra LS. Evidence-based practice: Let's be reasonable. *J Med Speech Lang Pathol* 11:ix–xii, 2003.

8. ASHA. Committee focuses on evidence-based practice. *The ASHA Leader* 9:4, 2004.

9. ASHA. Evidence-based practice in communication disorders: An introduction. Retrieved from www.asha.org/members/deskref-journals/deskref/DRVol4.htu#tr, 2004.

10. Dollaghan CA. Evidence-based practice in communication disorders: What do we know, and when do we know it? *J Commun Disord* 37:715–729, 2004.

11. Enderby P. Making speech pathology practice evidence-based: Is this enough? *Adv Speech-Lang Pathol* 6:125–126, 2004.

12. Logemann JA, Clinical trials. CSDRG overview. *J Commun Disord* 37:419–423, 2004.

13. Miller LT, Lee CJ. Gathering and evaluating evidence in clinical decision-making. *J Speech-Lang Pathol Audiol* 28:97–100, 2004.

14. Reilly S. The challenges in making speech pathology practice evidence based. *Adv Speech-Lang Pathol* 6:113–124, 2004.

15. Reilly S, Douglas J, Oates J (eds). *Evidence Based Practice in Speech Pathology.* London: Whurr Publishers, 2004.

16. Vallino-Napoli LD, Reilly S. Evidence-based health care: A survey of speech pathology practice. *Adv Speech-Lang Pathol* 6:107–112, 2004.

17. Logemann JA, Miller-Gardner P. Help finding the evidence. *The ASHA Leader* 10:8–9, 2005.

18. Mullen R. Survey tests members' understanding of evidence-based practice. *The ASHA Leader* 10:4–14, 2005.

19. Zipoli RP, Kennedy M. Evidence-based practice among speech-language-pathologists: Attitudes, utilization, and barriers. *Am J Speech-Lang Pathol* 14:208–220, 2005.

20. Johnson CA. Getting started in evidence-based practice for childhood speech-language disorders. *Am J Speech-Lang Pathol* 15:20–35, 2006.

21. Orange JB, Johnson A. The bench to practice to bench cycle of evidence-based clinical practice. Perspectives on Speech Science and Orofacial Disorders (Newsletter of Division 5 of the American Speech-Language-Hearing Association) 16:3–8, 2006.

22. Brattstrom V, McWilliam J, Larson O, Semb G. Craniofacial development in children with unilateral clefts of the lip, alveolus, and palate treated according to four different regimes. I. Maxillary development. *Scand J Plast Reconstr Surg* 25:259–267, 1991.

23. Brattstrom V, McWilliam J, Larson O, Semb G. Craniofacial development in children with unilateral clefts of the lip, alveolus, and palate treated according to four different regimes. III. The soft tissue profile at 16–18 years of age. *Scand J Plast Reconstr Surg* 26:197–202, 1992.

24. Asher-McDade C, Grattstrom V, Dahl E, et al. The RPS. A six-center international study of treatment outcome in patients with clefts of the lip and palate. Part 4. Assessment of nasolabial appearance. *Cleft Palate Craniofac J* 29:409–412, 1992.

25. Brattstrom V, McWilliam J, Semb G, Larson O. Craniofacial development in children with unilateral clefts of the lip, alveolus, and palate treated according to four different regimes. II. Mandibular and vertical development. *Scand J Plast Reconstr Surg* 26:55–63, 1992.

26. Mars M, Asher-McDade C, Brattstrom V, et al. The RPS. A six-center international study of treatment outcome in patients with clefts of the lip and palate. *Cleft Palate Craniofac J* 29:405–408, 1992.

27. Molsted K, Asher-McDade, Grattstrom V, et al. The RPS. A six-center international study of treatment outcome in patients with clefts of the lip and palate. Part 2. Craniofacial form and soft tissue profile. *Cleft Palate Craniofac J* 29:398–404, 1992.

28. Shaw WC, Asher-McDade C, Brattstrom V, et al. The RPS. A six-center international study of treatment outcome in patients with clefts of the lip and palate. Part 1. Principles and study design. *Cleft Palate Craniofac J* 29:393–397, 1992.

29. Shaw WC, Dahl E, Asher-McDade C, et al. The RPS. A six-center international study of treatment outcome in patients with clefts of the lip and palate. Part 5. General discussion and conclusions. *Cleft Palate Craniofac J.* 29:413–418, 1992.

30. Eurocleft Speech Group. Grunwell P, Bronsted K, et al. A phonetic framework for the cross-linguistic analysis of cleft palate speech. *Clin Linguist Phon* 8:109–125, 1994.

31. Eurocleft Speech Group, Grunwell P, Bronsted, K, et al. A six-centre international study of treatment outcomes in patients with clefts of the lip and palate. *Scand J Plast Reconstr Hand Surg* 34:31–41, 2000.

32. Kuehn DP, Trost-Cardamone JE, Sell D. Issues in universal reporting parameters for speech. *Study Session Presented before the Annual Meeting of the American Cleft Palate-Craniofacial Association*, Seattle, 2002.

33. Trost-Cardamone JE, Sell D, Sweeney T, Kuehn DP, Henningsson G. Issues in universal reporting parameters for speech – Part II. Presented before the 10th *International Congress on Cleft Palate and Related Craniofacial Anomalies*, Durban, South Africa, 2005.

34. Henningsson G, Kuehn DP, Sell D, et al. Universal parameters for reporting speech outcomes in individuals with cleft palate. *Cleft Palate Craniofac J* 45:1–17, 2008.

35. Peterson-Falzone SJ, Hardin-Jones MA, Karnell MP. *Cleft Palate Speech*, 3rd edn. Elsevier: St. Louis, 2001.

36. Peterson-Falzone SJ. Optimal age for palatoplasty to facilitate normal speech development: What is the evidence? In Berkowitz S (ed). *Cleft Lip and Palate: Diagnosis and Management*, 2nd edn. Heidelberg: Springer-Verlag, 2006.

37. Peterson-Falzone SJ, Trost-Cardamone JE, Karnell MP, Hardin-Jones MA. *The Clinician's Guide to Treating Cleft Palate Speech.* Elsevier: St. Louis, 2006.

38. Trost JE. Articulatory additions to the description of speech of persons with cleft palate. *Cleft Palate J* 18:193–203, 1981.

39. Golding-Kushner KJ. *Therapy Techniques for Cleft Palate and Related Disorders.* San Diego: Singular-Thompson Learning, 2001.

40. Scherer NJ. The Impact of Early Intervention on Speech Development in Children with Clefts. Presentation: ACPA Pre-Conference Symposium: Speech, Growth, Occlusion and Appearance: Setting Priorities in Early Cleft Care. Vancouver BC, April 3, 2006.

41. Scherer NJ, D'Antonio LL, McGahey H. Early intervention for speech impairment in children with cleft palate. *Cleft Palate Craniofac J* 45:18–31, 2008.

42. Kunzel HJ. Rontgenvideographische evaluierung eines photoelektrischen verfahrens zur registrierung der velumhole beim sprechen. *Folia Phoniatr* 31:153–166, 1979.

43. Dalston RM. Photodetector assessment of velopharyngeal activity. *Cleft Palate J* 19:1–8, 1982.

44. Dalston RM. Using simultaneous photodetection and nasometry ito monitor velopharyngeal behavior during speech. *J Speech Hear Res* 32:195–202, 1989.

45. Dalston RM, Keefe MJ. The use of a microcomputer in monitoring and modifying velopharyngeal in monitoring and modifying velopharyngeal movements. *J Comput Users Speech Hear* 3:159–169, 1987.

46. Moon JB. Evaluation of velopharyngeal function. In Moller KT, Starr CD (eds). *Cleft Palate: Interdisciplinary Issues and Treatment: for Clinicians by Clinicians.* Austin, TX: Pro-Ed, 1993.

47. Moon JB, Lagu RK. Development of a second-generation phototransducer for the assessment of velopharyngeal activity. *Cleft Palate J* 24:240–243, 1987.

48. Finkelstein Y, Lerner MA, Ophir D, Nachmani A, Hauben DB, Zohar Y. Nasopharyngeal profile and velopharyngeal valve mechanism. *Plast Reconstr Surg* 92:603–613, 1993.

49. Park S, Omori M, Kato K, Nitta N, Kitano I, Masuda T. Cephalometric analysis in submucous cleft palate: Comparison of cephalometric data obtained from submucous cleft palate patiehtw with velopharyneal competence and incompetence. *Cleft Palate Craniofac J* 39:105–109, 2002.

50. Rose R, Thissen U, Otten J-E, Jones I. Cephalometric assessment of the posterior airway space in patient with cleft palate after palatoplasty. *Cleft Palate Craniofac J* 40:488–503, 2003.

51. Smahel Z, Mullerova Z. Nasopharyngneal characteristics in children with cleft lip and palate. *Cleft Palate Craniofac J* 29:282–286, 1992.

52. Tzy-Hsin J, Huang G-F, Huang CS, Noordhoff MS. Nasopharyngoscopic evaluation and cephalometric analysis of velopharynx in normal and cleft palate patients. *Ann Plast Surg* 36:117–123, 1996.

53. Skolnick ML. Videofluoroscopic examination of the velopharyngeal portal during phonation in lateral and base projections – A new technique for studying the mechanics of closure. *Cleft Palate J* 7:803–816, 1970.

54. Skolnick ML, McCall GN. Velopharyngeal competence and incompetence following pharyngeal flap surgery: Video-fluoroscopic study in multiple projections. *Cleft Palate J* 9:1–12, 1972.

55. Skolnick ML, McCall GN, Barnes M. The sphincteric mechanism of velopharyngeal closure. *Cleft Palate J* 10:286–305, 1973.

56. Skolnick ML, Shprintzen RJ, McCall NG, Rakoff S. Patterns of velopharyngeal closure in subjects with repaired cleft palate and normal speech: A multi-view videofluoroscopic analysis. *Cleft Palate J* 12:369–376, 1975.

57. Bjork L, Nylen B. Cineradiography with synchronized sound spectrum analysis. *Plast Reconstr Surg* 27:397–412, 1961.

58. Bjork L. Velopharyngeal function in connected speech. *Acta Radiol Suppl* 202, 1961.

59. Kelsey CA, Crummy A, Schulman E. Comparison of ultrasonic and cineradiographic measurements of lateral pharyngeal wall motion. *Invest Radiol* 4:241–245, 1969.

60. Kelsey CA, Hixon TJ, Minifie FD. Ultrasonic measurement of lateral pharyngeal wall displacement. *IEEE Trans Bio-Med Eng* 16:143–147, 1969.

61. Lubker JF. Aerodynamic and ultrasonic assessment techniques in speech-dentofacial research. *ASHA Report #5: Speech and the Dentofacial Complex: The state of the art.* Washington: American Speech and Hearing Association, 1970.

62. Minifie FD, Hixon TJ, Kelsey CA, Woodhouse RJ. Lateral pharyngeal wall movement during speech production. *J Speech Hear Res* 13:584–594, 1970.

63. Skolnick ML, Zagzebski JA, Watkin KL. Two dimensional ultrasonic demonstration of lateral pharyngeal wall movement in real time – A preliminary report. *Cleft Palate J* 12:299–303, 1975.

64. Zagzebski JA. Ultrasonic measurement of lateral pharyngeal wall motion at two levels in the vocal tract. *J Speech Hear Res* 18:308–318, 1975.

65. Ryan WJ, Hawkins CF. Ultrasonic measurements of lateral pharyngeal wall movement at the velopharyneal port. *Cleft Palate J* 13:156–164, 1976.

66. Hawkins CF, Swisher WE. Evaluation of a real-time ultrasound scanner in assessing lateral pharyngeal wall motion during speech. *Cleft Palate J* 15:161–166, 1978.

67. Nakano H. The application of ultrasound system to assessment of the nasopharyngeal function for cleft palate patients. *J Jpn Cleft Palate Assoc* 9:84–101, 1984.

68. Saito K. Ultrasonic analysis of lateral pharyngeal wall movement in patients with cleft palate and velopharyngeal incompetency. *J Jpn Cleft Palate Assoc* 9:71–83, 1984.

69. Taub S. The Taub oral panendoscope: A new technique. *Cleft Palate J* 3:328–346, 1966.

70. Pigott RW. The nasendoscopic appearance of the normal palatopharyngeal valve. *Plast Reconstr Surg* 43:19–24, 1969.

71. D'Antonio LL, Marsh JL, Provance MB, Muntz HR, Phillips CH. Reliability of flexible fiberoptic nasopharyngoscopic evaluation of velopharyngeal function in a clinical population. *Cleft Palate J* 16:217–225, 1989.

72. Golding-Kushner KJ, Argamaso RV, Cotton RT, et al. Standardization for the reporting of nasopharyngoscopy and multi-view videofluoroscopy: A report from an international working group. *Cleft Palate J* 27:337–347, 1990.

73. Karnell MP. *Videoendoscopy from Velopharynx to Larynx.* San Diego: Singular, 1994.

74. Pigott RW. Some physical characteristics of instruments used to investigate palato pharyngeal incompetence. In Ellis R, Flack F (eds). *Diagnosis and Treatment of Palato Glossal Malfunction.* London: College of Speech Therapists, 1979.

75. Pigott RW, Makepeace A. Some characteristics of endoscopic and radiological systems in elaboration of the diagnosis of velopharyngeal incompetence. *Br J Plast Surg* 35:19–32, 1982

76. Shprintzen RJ. Instrumental assessment of velopharyngeal valving. In Shprintzen RJ, Bardach J (eds). *Cleft Palate Speech Management: A Multidisciplinary Approach.* Mosby: St. Louis, 1995.

77. Shprintzen RJ. The velopharyngeal mechanism. In Berkowitz S (ed). *Cleft Lip and Palate: Diagnosis and Management,* 2nd edn. Heidelberg: Springer-Verlag, 2006.

78. Wein BB, Drobnitsky M, Klaljman S, Angerstein W. Evaluation of functional positions of tongue and soft palate with MR imaging: Initial clinical results. *J Magn Reson Imaging* 1:281–282, 1992.

79. Yamawaki Y, Nishimura Y, Suzuki Y, Sawada M, Yamawaki S. Rapid magnetic resonance imaging for assessment of velopharyngeal muscle movement on phonation. *Am J Otolaryngol* 18:210–213, 1997.

80. Ettema SL, Kuehn DP, Perlman AL, Alperin N. Magnetic resonance imaging of the levator veli palatini muscle during speech. *Cleft Palate Craniofac J* 39:130–144, 2002.

81. Kane AA, Butman JA, Mullick R, Skopec M, Choylike P. A new method for the study of velopharyngeal function using gated magnetic resonance imaging. *Plast Reconstr Surg* 109:471–481, 2002.

82. Kuehn DP, Ettema SL, Goldwasser MS, Barkmeier JC, Wachtel JM. Magnetic resonance imaging in the evaluation of occult submucous cleft palate. *Cleft Palate Craniofac J* 38:421–431, 2001.

83. Kuehn DP, Ettema SL, Goldwasser MS, Barkmeier JC. Magnetic resonance imaging of the levator veli palatini muscles before and after primary palatoplasty. *Cleft Palate Craniofac J* 41:584–592, 2004.

84. Shinagawa H, Ono T, Honda E-I, et al. Dynamic analysis of articulatory movement using magnetic resonance imaging movies: Methods and implications in cleft lip and palate. *Cleft Palate Craniofac J* 42:225–230, 2005.

85. Fletcher SG, Bishop ME. Measurement of nasality with TONAR. *Cleft Palate J* 7:610–621, 1970.

86. Warren DW, DuBois AB. A pressure-flow technique for measuring velopharyngeal orifice area during continuous speech. *Cleft Palate J* 1:52–57, 1964.

87. Warren DW. PERCI: A method for rating palatal efficiency. *Cleft Palate J* 16:279–285, 1979.

72

Perspectives in Orofacial Cleft Research I: Animal Models

Jeffrey Weinzweig, MD, FACS

INTRODUCTION

Over the past four decades, a multitude of investigators have sought to develop *congenital* and *iatrogenic (surgically induced)* models of orofacial clefts in an attempt to better understand the etiopathogenesis of such anomalies, as well as to elucidate the mechanisms involved in clefting. The development of in vivo and in vitro models has played an essential role in the assessment of the teratogenicity of innumerable agents and the accrual of dose–response data from which the incidence of specific malformations can be derived. Such studies are critical for analyzing the potential of a chemical or physical agent to adversely affect development and produce major morphological malformations. A plethora of experimental studies, the vast majority involving murine models, have focused on analyzing the genetic mechanisms involved in the embryogenic development of these conditions while others, generally involving larger animal models, have concentrated on studying the feasibility and efficacy of in utero manipulation and repair.

In particular, small animal studies have focused on whole embryo and organ culture, embryo transfer, retinoid- and glucocorticoid-induced cleft palate, genetic variations as well as the influence of vascular supply and maternal hypoxia on the incidence of clefting, while large animal studies have focused on cleft manipulation, both in utero and ex utero, and the effect of such repairs on subsequent maxillofacial growth.

Presented in this chapter is a distillation of numerous key studies from the extensive array of literature that has been produced over the past several decades in an attempt to provide an overview of the scope and breadth of animal models developed and utilized in the world of orofacial cleft research.

SMALL ANIMAL MODELS: CONGENITAL MODELS

Whole Embryo/Organ Culture

Various growth factors are necessary for normal embryonic development. Epidermal growth factor (EGF) receptors are present in developing palatal shelves of embryonic/fetal mice as early as day 12 of gestation (GD 12). The medial epithelium of the palatal shelf undergoes a series of developmental events that do not occur in the oral and nasal epithelia. In utero and in organ culture, the control palatal medial epithelium shows a developmental decline in EGF receptors, demonstrated both by a decrease in the binding of antibody to EGF receptors and a decrease in the binding of 125I-EGF, decreases which are not observed in cells of the adjacent oral or nasal epithelium. During this period, medial cells cease DNA synthesis and undergo programmed cell death. Medial epithelial cells exposed to all-trans-retinoic acid continue to express EGF receptors, bind EGF, proliferate, fail to undergo programmed cell death and exhibit a morphology typical of nasal cells. The data suggest that this disturbance by retinoic acid of EGF receptor localization and subsequent alterations in differentiation of the epithelial cells plays a role in the retinoic-acid-mediated induction of cleft palate.[1]

TCDD (2,3,7,8-tetrachlorodibenzo-*p*-dioxin), a highly toxic environmental contaminant, is teratogenic in mice, inducing cleft palate and hydronephrosis at doses that are not overtly maternally or embryo toxic. Palatal shelves of embryonic mice respond to TCDD, both in vivo and in organ culture, with altered differentiation of medial epithelial cells. By contrast, in the rat TCDD produces substantial maternal, embryonic, and fetal toxicity, including fetal lethality, with few malformations. In this study, the effects of maternal toxicity on induction of cleft palate were eliminated by exposure of embryonic rat palatal shelves in organ culture.[2] The shelves were examined for specific TCDD-induced alterations in differentiation of the medial cells. On GD 14 or 15,

palatal shelves from embryonic F344 rats were placed in organ culture for 2–3 days containing varying concentrations of TCDD. The medial cells of TCDD-exposed shelves expressed high levels of EGF receptors. The altered differentiation of rat medial epithelium is similar to that reported for TCDD-exposed mouse medial cells in vivo and in vitro. However, in order to obtain these responses, the cultured rat shelves require much higher concentrations of TCDD than the mouse shelves. Thus, TCDD induces the same effects at a cellular level in medial epithelium of rats and mice, but cleft palate is not seen in rats because the level required to produce the cellular effects would result in maternal and embryonic toxicity including fetal lethality.

Abbott and Buckalew studied the development of rat, mouse, and human embryonic palates in submerged, serum-free organ culture.[3] The concentration–response profiles for retinoic acid (RA), triamcinolone (TRI), hydrocortisone (HC), dexamethasone (DEX), and TCDD were examined and the mechanisms of clefting in vitro were compared to observed in vivo responses. Craniofacial regions were dissected on GD 12 for mice and GD 14 for rats, and cultured for 3–4 days in Bigger's BGJb medium. Growth and fusion of secondary palates were scored under a dissecting microscope. Mouse and rat palatal fusion occurred within the 4 days culture period. RA significantly inhibited fusion of mouse and rat palates with RA-induced clefting related to abnormal proliferation and differentiation of medial epithelia. In contrast, glucocorticoid-induced clefting (i.e., TRI, DEX, and HC) was due to concentration-dependent inhibition of shelf growth. TCDD clefting was due to altered medial epithelial differentiation. The authors demonstrated that serum-free organ culture supports the development of mouse, rat, and human palatal explants. Further, they demonstrated the capacity of this organ culture system to model palatogenesis for several species, and to distinguish between various mechanisms of clefting. This model should be useful for exploring mechanisms of activity at a cellular and molecular level.

How secondary palate formation is affected in the cleft lip genotype remains poorly understood. Sasaki et al. analyzed regional patterns of cell proliferation in CL/Fr mouse embryos with or without cleft lip.[4] Pairs of palatal shelves were dissected at GD 13.5 from CL/Fr normal embryos (CL/Fr-N), CL/Fr embryos with bilateral cleft lip (CL/Fr-BCL), and a control strain of C57BL embryos (C57BL). The explants were examined histologically after 48 h of organ culture. The CL/Fr-BCL palates fused as well as the CL/Fr-N palates in vitro. These findings indicate that a cleft palate follows reduced cell proliferation of secondary palatal mesenchyme in CL/Fr mice.

Whole-embryo culture techniques have advanced to the point where the study of normal and abnormal primary palate development in vitro is possible. Eto et al. sought to ascertain whether localized administration of tunicamycin (TM), an inhibitor of protein glycosylation, into the region of the developing primary palate would induce cleft lip in culture.[5] Rat embryos were explanted on GD 11 and cultured with open yolk sacs for 40 h; TM was administered to the nasal placode region of each. TM-treated placodes developed cleft lip in 14 out of 15 embryos compared to 0 for the controls. This work demonstrates that localized administration of TM results in cleft lip formation in whole embryo culture. The technique of localized administration of drugs and teratogens in whole embryo culture should prove useful for similar studies on embryonic development.

Fetal Alcohol Syndrome

Methanol has widespread applications in industry and manufacturing and is under consideration as an alternative automotive fuel. Human exposure to methanol would be expected to increase if applications expand in coming years. Methanol has been shown to be a reproductive and developmental toxicant in the rodent, producing cleft palate in the CD-1 mouse. Developmental toxicity has also been demonstrated in vitro for rat and mouse embryos in whole embryo culture. Abbott et al. examined the developmental toxicity of methanol in the palate using a serum-free organ culture model.[6] On GD 12, CD-1 mouse embryos were dissected and mid-craniofacial tissues were cultured in BGJ medium. Cultures were exposed to methanol from 0–20 mg/mL for 6 h, 12 h, 1 or 4 days. Some cultures were exposed to ethanol for 4 days at doses ranging from 0–15 mg/mL. Following organ culture the craniofacial explants were examined for effects on morphology, fusion, proliferation, and growth.

Incidence and completeness of palatal fusion decreased with increasing exposure. Depending on the concentration and duration of methanol exposure, the medial epithelium either degenerated completely or remained intact in unfused palates and either condition would interfere with fusion. Cellular proliferation appeared to be a specific and sensitive target for methanol as craniofacial tissues responded to methanol with reduction in total DNA content at an exposure that did not affect total protein. However, both DNA and protein decreased with increasing exposure to methanol. Incorporation of thymidine decreased significantly after 4 days exposure and autoradiography of 3H-thymidine (TdR) demonstrated exposure-dependent reduction in proliferation of palatal mesenchymal cells. Ethanol decreased fusion score, total protein, and DNA, but 3H-TdR/DNA was not significantly changed. In general the ethanol was more potent than methanol for inhibition of protein and DNA synthesis and palatal fusion. The authors concluded that methanol can selectively affect specific sensitive cell populations and has effects on proliferation and cell fate.

Acute teratogenic exposure of C57Bl/6J mouse embryos to ethanol in vivo results, within 12 h of initial insult, in excessive cell death in selected cell populations. The patterns of excessive cell death observed following exposure of GD 8 embryos vary somewhat temporospatially, but primarily involve the cell populations at the rim of the anterior neural plate. The cell death patterns appear to be pathogenically correlated with subsequently observed malformations including exencephaly (anencephaly), arhinencephaly, pituitary dysplasia,

bilateral or unilateral cleft lip, maxillary hypoplasia, and median facial deficiencies and clefts. Kotch and Sulik point out that the association of these brain and facial malformations in this model, and perhaps in humans, may be accounted for by early insult to the selected cell populations identified in the current investigation.[7]

Embryo Transfer

Studies of fetal craniofacial morphology have utilized embryo transfer methodologies to evaluate the role of fetal weight, dam strain, dam weight, and litter size on the intrauterine development of the craniofacial complex of the CL/Fr mouse fetus affected with cleft lip and palate (CLP). The effects of dam strain on the spontaneous incidence of CLP and the intrauterine growth of transferred CLP-susceptible CL/Fr embryos were examined with an embryo transfer technique in which each pregnant dam that had received CL/Fr mouse embryos underwent laparotomy and removal of the transferred fetuses that had developed in the uteri of the CLP-susceptible CL/Fr strain dam and the CLP-resistant C57BL strain dam.[8] A laparotomy was done on GD 18 at which time the number of fetuses, the resorption sites and the fetus weight were recorded.

The spontaneous incidence rate of CLP in the CL/Fr dam strain was significantly higher than that in the C57BL dam strain. The fetus weight of the CL/Fr fetuses developed in the CL/Fr dam strain was significantly lighter than that of the CL/Fr fetuses developed in the C57BL dam strain. The results indicated that the CL/P-susceptible CL/Fr dam strain provided a less favorable uterine environment for the implantation, survival and intrauterine growth of the transferred CL/Fr embryos and also caused a higher spontaneous incidence rate of CLP. Nonaka et al. concluded that the effect of the dam strain appears to play an important role on the spontaneous incidence of CLP and the intrauterine growth of the CL/Fr strain embryos transferred to both CL/Fr and C57BL dam strains. Based on cephalometric evaluation of these fetuses, the authors demonstrated that the craniofacial growth of the CL/Fr mouse fetus affected with CLP increased in proportion to the fetus weight. Further, dam strain effect also played an important role on the craniofacial morphogenesis of the CL/Fr strain of the affected fetuses that developed in both strain dams.

Morphometric Analysis

Differences in facial shape are considered a factor in cleft lip malformation. Wang and Diewert analyzed craniofacial growth in two strains of mice: A/WySn, which demonstrate a 28% incidence of spontaneous cleft lip, and C57BL/6J, which do not develop cleft lip spontaneously.[9] Standardized photographs of embryos from each strain with 34–46 somites were taken in the superior, frontal, and lateral views. Landmarks were located and digitized for computerized analysis of growth change at stages of facial development before, during, and after primary palate closure. Both strains had similar overall growth patterns with increases in head width and facial width, and decreases in nasal pit width. During early palatal closure in C57BL/6J mice, the nasal pit width was unchanged as brain width increased rapidly; subsequently, the nasal pit width decreased as brain width increased slowly. However, during early closure in A/WySn mice, the nasal pit width decreased rapidly as brain width increased slowly; subsequently, the nasal pit width was unchanged as brain width increased more rapidly. During early palatal closure, the narrower nasal pit width in A/WySn mice appeared to result from delayed growth of the supporting forebrain as the nasal pits become more medially positioned with normal face development. From the lateral view, the maxillary prominence depth was also smaller in the A/WySn strain during early palatal closure. This deficient anterior growth of the maxillary prominences and the narrower positioning of the medial nasal prominences in A/WySn embryos appear to reduce the contact between the prominences and thus predispose this strain to cleft lip malformation.

Maternal Hypoxia

Bronsky et al. studied the influence of maternal hypoxia on the incidence of cleft lip with or without associated cleft palate (CL/P). Prior studies had demonstrated that maternal respiratory hypoxia (10% O_2) increases the incidence of CL/P from the spontaneous level of 36% in CL/Fr mice to 89%. To evaluate developmental alterations of the primary palate in CL/Fr embryos in a hypoxic environment, they utilized scanning electron microscopy to compare embryos.[10] Hypoxia increased the incidence of resorptions and increased the incidence of CL/P in viable embryos compared to control (normoxia) embryos. The deeper aspects of the invaginating nasal placode in the hypoxic embryos contained debris at stages prior to primary palate fusion; this was absent in comparably staged normoxia embryos.

Epidemiologic evidence indicates an increase in CL/P in infants of mothers who smoke cigarettes. It appears that the principle mechanism is through carbon monoxide (CO) decreasing the oxygen (O_2) available to the embryo. Multiple studies have shown that maternal respiratory hypoxia can increase the incidence of CL/P in mice. Bailey et al. analyzed the effects of altered levels of CO and O_2 in respiratory gases on the incidence of CL/P in genetically susceptible A/J mice.[11] Blood gas analysis, after a 24-h exposure of pregnant mice during the time of primary palate development, showed that CO levels of 180 ppm in air decreased oxyhemoglobin (%O_2Hb) and increased carboxyhemoglobin (%COHb) to slightly above the high end of the range found in human studies of cigarette smokers. Decreasing O_2 levels to 10% from 21% (normal percentage in air) more severely decreased %O_2Hb and moderately decreased %COHb. At 24 h of exposure, the incidence of CL/P and resorption was approximately the same for both the CO and the control groups, but there were significant increases in the incidence of resorptions in the hypoxia group and of CL/P in relation to the CO group.

Retinoid-Induced Cleft Palate

Retinoids are teratogenic in humans and animals, producing a syndrome of craniofacial malformations that includes cleft palate. Abbott and Pratt investigated the mechanism through which retinoic acid (RA) induces cleft palate.[12] Murine palatogenesis after exposure to RA in utero was compared to normal development and to alterations observed after exposure in organ culture to RA or EGF. Human embryonic palatal shelves were placed in the organ culture system and the responses to RA and EGF were compared to those of the murine palatal shelves. Growth factors played a role in normal development and are found in the embryonic palate. In other cell culture systems, retinoids alter the expression of EGF receptors. The authors' results suggest that in the medial epithelial cells of the palate, RA sustains the expression of the EGF receptor and the binding of EGF at a time when the expression in control medial cells has declined, and these control cells subsequently undergo programmed cell death. The continued DNA synthesis, proliferation, survival, and shift in phenotype of the medial cells is believed to interfere with the adhesion and fusion of opposing palatal shelves, resulting in cleft palate.

Both RA and retinyl acetate, administered in high doses on GD 13–15, are capable of causing a 90% incidence of cleft palate in Charles River rats. In the rat, the RA form of vitamin A is the more potent teratogen, inducing clefts at less than half the dose required to produce them with retinyl acetate. Histologic examination of fetal rat heads confirmed the biochemical evidence that RA is the more potent teratogen. Both forms of vitamin A prevented palatal shelf reorientation from occurring at the correct gestational age.[13] The retinyl acetate treatment delayed the rotation for approximately 12 h, the RA treatment for at least 48 h.

RA has been shown to be teratogenic in many species, and 13-cis-RA is teratogenic in humans. Exposure to RA during embryonic morphogenesis produces a variety of malformations including limb defects and cleft palate. The type and severity of malformation depended on the stage of development exposed. Abbott et al. compared the effects of RA exposure in vivo on different stages of palate development.[14] These results were compared to effects observed after exposure in organ culture. The vehicle used in RA dosing was also shown to be a major factor in the incidence of RA-induced cleft palate. For the in vivo studies, RA was given p.o. on GD 10 or 12, and the embryos were examined on GD 14 and 16. Exposure to RA in an oil:DMSO vehicle resulted in much higher incidences of cleft palate than were observed after dosing with RA in oil only. After exposure to RA on GD 10, small palatal shelves formed which did not make contact and fuse on GD 14. The medial cells did not undergo programmed cell death. Instead, the medial cells differentiated into a stratified, squamous, oral-like epithelium. In contrast, RA-induced clefting after exposure on GD 12 did not involve growth inhibition. Shelves of normal size formed and made contact, but because of altered medial cell differentiation did not fuse. Medial cells differentiated into a pseudostratified, ciliated, nasal-like epithelium. This response was produced in vivo at exposure levels that produced cleft palate, and after exposure of palatal shelves to RA in vitro from GD 12–15. The responses to RA which lead to cleft palate differed after exposure on GD 10 or 12, and the pathways of differentiation that the medial cells followed depended on the developmental stage exposed.

Fujiwara et al. attempted to induce cleft palate in Wistar rats by injecting Vitamin A into the stomach of females during GD 8, 9, 10, and 11.[15] Rats were sacrificed and evaluated during GD 18–20. The authors demonstrated that cleft palate induction was feasible when Vitamin A was injected on GD 10.

Systemic administration of RA affects the growth of the upper beak of chick embryos; however, the mechanism for generating a cleft upper beak is not known. Richman and Delgado sought to elucidate the molecular basis of the retinoid-induced lip clefting.[16] In order to ensure that facial prominences were locally exposed to levels of retinoid known to affect gene expression, they implanted beads soaked in different concentrations of RA in the right nasal pit or in the center of the frontonasal mass. Beads soaked in 5 mg/mL RA placed in the right nasal pit caused full clefting of the upper beak with a deviation of the midline toward the right side of the face. The asymmetry was principally due to a decrease in size or total elimination of the right lateral nasal prominence.

RA-soaked beads placed in the center of the frontonasal mass created full bilateral clefts that were more symmetrical than those produced by beads in the nasal pit. Lower concentrations of RA produced less severe facial abnormalities. Control experiments show that the implanted bead itself has no effect on growth or fusion of the facial prominences. The specific effects of retinoids on facial growth may be due to a localized decrease in responsiveness to growth factors. Gene expression patterns for two fibroblast growth factor receptors (Cek-2, Cek-3, [chicken embryo kinase]) in normal and RA-treated embryos were examined by in situ hybridization. In normal embryos, Cek-2 and Cek-3, transcripts are expressed at very high levels in the mesenchyme directly adjacent to the eye. Cek-3 is additionally expressed in the center of the frontonasal mass. The application of beads to the right nasal pit did not change the level of expression or distribution of transcripts for Cek-2 or Cek-3. This data suggests that RA may be affecting other aspects of the FGF receptor–ligand interaction.

Glucocorticoid-Induced Cleft Palate

The role of glucocorticoids and their interaction with the glucocorticoid receptor (GR) during embryonic growth and development has been a topic of interest and research for many years. Glucocorticoids are known to be teratogenic, and administration of these compounds during pregnancy produces cleft palate in the offspring. In the mouse, induction of cleft palate correlates with the level of palatal GR expression. However, the specific patterns of GR expression during critical stages of palatal morphogenesis remain to be examined. Abbott et al. evaluated GR expression in the developing palates of C57BL/6N mouse embryos on GD 12, 13, 14, and 15 by both in situ hybridization and immunohistochemistry.[17]

On GD 12, GR mRNA was locally expressed in the region of palatal shelf outgrowth in both mesenchymal and epithelial cells, and GR was expressed uniformly throughout the developing shelf. A similar pattern of distribution occurred on GD 13 as the shelf became larger and elevated. By GD 14, GR was regionally expressed with higher levels in epithelial cells relative to mesenchyme. In different regions of oral and nasal epithelia localized patterns of expression were noted and may be related to differentiated state. Correspondingly, GR mRNA was expressed in epithelia and became regional in mesenchyme with abundant mRNA in regions of bone formation. On GD 15, oral and nasal epithelial cells showed mRNA, but mesenchymal levels were low except for chondrogenic regions. During palatogenesis the expression of mRNA correlated with immunodetectable GR peptide. GR localized initially within regions of active morphogenesis and subsequently within differentiating cells. This specificity of spatial and temporal expression supports the idea that GR is involved in regulation of regional growth and differentiation during palatogenesis.

TCDD is an environmental contaminant that produces adverse biologic effects including developmental toxicity and teratogenesis. In the mouse embryo, TCDD induces cleft palate and hydronephrosis. The synthetic glucocorticoid, hydrocortisone (HC), induces cleft palate and a potent, synergistic interaction has been observed between TCDD and HC in C57BL/6N embryonic mice. The morphology and etiology of TCDD- and HC-induced clefts are distinctly different with formation of small palatal shelves following HC exposure and failure of normally sized shelves to fuse after TCDD treatment. Each exposure also alters expression of several growth factors. The interaction of HC and TCDD results in a cleft palate whose etiology most closely resembles that observed after HC exposure, i.e., small palatal shelves. HC+TCDD-exposure also produces a pattern of growth factor expression that closely resembles that seen after HC. Both TCDD and HC act through receptor-mediated mechanisms and each compound has its own receptor. The Ah receptor (AhR) binds TCDD and the glucocorticoid receptor (GR) binds HC. On gestation day (GD) 14, in the embryonic palate exposed to TCDD, the AhR was downregulated and the GR expression increased.[18] Conversely, following HC exposure, the GR was downregulated and AhR levels were elevated. HC+TCDD produced increased expression of both receptors and this pattern would be predicted to produce HC-like clefts as the GR-mediated responses would result in small palatal shelves. The observed cross-regulation of the receptors is believed to be important in the synergistic interaction between TCDD and HC for the induction of cleft palate.

It is unknown whether drug-induced orofacial clefting results from a direct interaction between the teratogen and the embryonic palate, or indirectly from maternal alterations caused by the teratogen. Sullivan-Jones et al. exposed pregnant A/J mice to one of three cleft-inducing agents in order to examine the relationship between drug-induced clefting and the response of maternal plasma corticosterone to drug administration.[19] The agents used, haloperidol (HAL), 2,4,5-trichlorophenoxyacetic acid (2,4,5-T), or phenytoin (PHT), were administered in teratogenic doses on GD 10. For corticosterone determinations, mice were dosed on GD 10, and blood was collected at 1, 4, 24, or 48 h after dosing. For fetal evaluation of CL/P, mice were dosed on GD 10 and sacrificed on GD 18. Phenytoin was the most potent inducer of cleft lip and palate and induced a sustained elevation of plasma corticosterone in maternal animals. The other treatments, in order of decreasing potency to induce clefting and/or cause an elevation of corticosterone in plasma were 2,4,5-T > HAL > controls. Correlations between maternal corticosterone levels and clefting incidence were very high at all time points examined. A linear relationship between drug-induced increases in maternal corticosterone levels, and the incidence of clefting in A/J mice were observed. Based on these findings, the authors concluded that increased maternal corticosterone levels may play a role in orofacial clefting in A/J mice.

Peterka and Jelinek studied the growth and fusion of facial processes in White Leghorn chicken embryos treated with hydrocortisone.[20] This treatment resulted in complete bilateral cleft beak in 80–100% of cases. The frontonasal complex of the experimental embryos exhibited marked hypoplasia prior to cleft manifestation. During the critical period for cleft beak formation, the maximum mitotic activity was concentrated in the medial nasal processes, which thus became vulnerable to the mitosis inhibiting effect of corticoids. Primary hypoplasia of the facial processes was documented as a causative factor of corticoid-induced cleft beak, which is analogous to mammalian cleft lip/palate.

Vascular Patterns

Resin cast images of vascular networks in normal and spontaneous CL/P CL/Fr mouse embryos were used to study alterations in the vascularization of the developing palate. Amin et al. observed a denser vascular plexus in the oral side than in the nasal side prior to the reorientation of the palatal shelves.[21]

Many small spherical masses of resin were observed in the medial edge of the palatal shelves at the time of medial extension and during fusion, indicating some changes occurring in the capillary wall leading to the resin leakage. In the spontaneous cleft group, a similar vascular pattern was observed, but the greater palatine artery showed discontinuity in the premaxillary region at an early stage. At the same time, terminal dilatations were delayed and frequently absent in the contralateral shelf. After the reorientation of the palatal shelves, the vascular plexus formed an irregular lattice pattern. Dilated vasculature was apparent in the anterior nasopalatine region, indicating the persistence of a more primitive vascular structure in the spontaneous cleft embryos. The authors concluded that blood vessels in the palatal shelves are underdeveloped and remained immature in cleft lip and palate embryos. These variant vascular patterns may be due to the inadequate blood supply to the nasopalatine region

from the early embryonic stages possibly resulting from the discontinuity of the greater palatine artery.

Genetic Mechanisms

Karolyi and Erickson sought to determine whether mouse chromosomal regions homologous to human chromosomal regions implicated in the etiology of facial clefting would be related to the incidence of spontaneous CP or CL/P, Dilantin-induced CL/P, hydrocortisone-induced CP, and/or 6-aminonicotinamide-induced CP.[22] They found that a region on mouse chromosome 3, homologous to human chromosome 1q21, significantly increased the incidence of sporadic CL/P when the allele from the A/J inbred strain was present. None of the other chromosomal regions or conditions studied had significant associations with this susceptibility to facial clefting, although there was a suggestion that the B allele of the same region was associated with hydrocortisone-induced CP. The authors concluded that the region on human chromosome 1q21 warranted further study for a role in the etiology of human CL/P.

Karolyi et al. identified a major correlation between the incidence of glucocorticoid-induced CP and the chromosome 8 segment identified by *N*-acetyl transferase in mice.[23] The resistant strain became fully susceptible while the susceptible strain became resistant when this chromosomal region, representing less than 0.7% of the genome, was transferred from one strain to the other by the construction of congenic strains. 6-Aminonicotinamide-induced CP and phenytoin-induced CL/P are also influenced by this genetic region but not as strongly. In both cases the susceptible strain became quite resistant to the teratogen-induced clefting when the *N*-acetyl transferase region of chromosome 8 was transferred. However, this chromosomal region does not make the resistant strain susceptible to these two teratogens.

Since its first description, the A strain of mice have been utilized extensively as models to study the processes involved in clefting of the midfacial region. Of the A substrains, A/WySnJ mice are an inbred strain that spontaneously develops CL/P with a frequency of 25–30% and a predominantly unilateral expression pattern. Human nonsyndromic CLP is genetically complex, with one contributing gene on chromosome 17q. A potentially homologous gene, clf1 on distal chromosome 11, is believed to contribute to the high incidence of CLP in the A/WySn mouse strain.[24]

Gong used the A/WySn mouse model to analyze and compare the phenotypic and molecular changes in the midfacial region of embryos with and without clefts.[25] He employed scanning electron microscopy and skeletal and cartilage preparations of newborn A/WySn pups and showed the presence of bilateral and unilateral clefts of the lips and the disruption of the skeletal and cartilaginous components of the mice with clefts of the lip. The expression of the msx1 homeobox gene was analyzed by whole mount in situ hybridization of A/WySn embryos at different stages of midfacial development. The results showed that there was misregulation of the expression of the msx1 gene in embryos with cleft, with a persistence of expression in the distal growing tips of the midfacial processes and in areas that have fused in normal embryos without cleft. Gong concluded that although the genetic defect in A/WySn mice is not known, a possible candidate gene has been mapped to a corresponding human chromosome carrying retinoic acid receptor alpha, and there exists a possibility that msx1 is in the same genetic pathway affected by the mutation of the gene in A/WySn.

Primary palatogenesis of mice is similar to that of humans and spontaneous cleft lip is associated with genotype in both mice and humans. To investigate the temporal and spatial expression of ras genes in cleft (A/WySn) and non-cleft strains of mice (BALB/cBy), Wang et al. used a broad spectrum ras antibody.[26] Positive staining was found in ectodermal, mesenchymal, and neuroepithelial cells of the facial prominences before the primary palate formation stage (day 10, hour 20) in both strains. During the primary palate formation stage (day 11, hour 20), positive staining was found in the ectodermal and mesenchymal cells of the facial prominences of the noncleft strain but not in those of the cleft strain. These results suggest ras genes may play a role in the primary palatogenesis of mice. Cleft lip could be associated with the deficiency of ras gene expression during primary palate formation of mice.

It is commonly accepted that spontaneous cleft lip appears to be multifactorially determined in both mice and humans. Binding of a ligand to erbB4 has been shown to stimulate the receptor's protein kinase activity, which subsequently stimulates a signal-transduction cascade leading to cell growth and differentiation, and to morphogenesis during development. In a subsequent study, Wang et al. used an immunohistochemical technique to investigate the temporal and spatial expression of erbB4 in the primary palate of cleft (A/WySn) and noncleft strains of mice (BALB/cBy).[27] Positive staining of erbB4 was found in ectodermal and mesenchymal cells of facial prominences before the primary palate formation stage (day 10, hour 20) in both strains. During the primary palate formation stage (day 11, hour 20), positive staining of erbB4 was found in the ectodermal and mesenchymal cells of the facial prominences of the noncleft strain, but not in those of the cleft strain. These results suggest erbB4 expression may be associated with normal primary palatogenesis of mice and, conversely, cleft lip may be associated with a deficiency of erbB4 expression during primary palate formation in mice.

The CL/Fr mouse strain is another strain that develops CLP spontaneously. Hamachi et al. investigated Pax9 mRNA expression in the palatal shelves during palatal morphogenesis to assess the correlation between secondary palatal morphogenesis and Pax9 expression of CL/Fr embryos with spontaneous CLP.[28] In the control strain of C57BL/6 and CL/Fr normal embryos, Pax9 was expressed in the palate, especially along the medial edge (ME), on GD 13.5 and GD 14.5 when the palatal shelves grew vertically down the side of the tongue and subsequently elevated to a horizontal position, and was downregulated on GD 15.5 when the palatal shelves met and began fusing. In the cleft embryo, Pax9 was expressed in the

ME region but was not downregulated on GD 15.5. Furthermore, whole mount in situ hybridization, performed after organ culture, showed that Pax9 was still expressed in the ME region in separated palatal shelves of CL/Fr-N and CL/Fr-BCL embryos, while Pax9 expression was downregulated in paired palatal shelves. These expression patterns of Pax9 in normal and cleft embryos during palatal fusion indicate that Pax9 expression is altered in spontaneous CLP, and suggest that there is a direct correlation between Pax9 expression and palatal fusion.

Van der Woude syndrome is an autosomal dominant disorder that is characterized by cleft lip, cleft palate, lower lip pits, and hypodontia. Van der Woude syndrome arises as the result of mutations in the gene encoding interferon regulatory factor 6 (Irf6). To provide insights into the role of Irf6 during embryogenesis, Knight et al. analyzed the expression of this molecule during mouse and chick facial development.[29] Irf6 was expressed in the ectoderm covering the facial processes during their fusion to form the upper lip and primary palate in both mouse and chick. However, while Irf6 was expressed in the medial edge epithelia of the developing secondary palate of the mouse, which fuses as in humans, Irf6 was not expressed in the medial edge epithelia of the naturally cleft chick secondary palate. Similarly, Irf6 was found to be downregulated in the medial edge epithelia of transforming growth factor beta 3-null mice, which also exhibit cleft palate. Together, these results support a role for Irf6 during the fusion events that occur during development of the lip and palate.

Dancer Mutation

Mice carrying a spontaneous mutation, Dancer (Dc), exhibit CL/P in homozygotes and show significantly increased susceptibility to CL/P in heterozygotes, providing an animal model for understanding the molecular pathogenesis of CL/P. Bush et al. genetically mapped Dc to within a 1-cM region near the centromere of chromosome 19.[30] In situ hybridization analysis showed that one positional candidate gene, Tbx10, is ectopically expressed in Dc mutant embryos. The authors showed that ectopic expression of Tbx10 in transgenic mice recapitulates the Dc mutant phenotype, indicating that CL/P in Dc mutant mice results from the p23 insertion-induced ectopic Tbx10 expression. These results identify gain of function of a T-box transcription factor gene as a mechanism underlying CL/P pathogenesis.

Twirler Model

Twirler (Tw) is a semidominant mutation in the mouse affecting the embryonic development of the midfacial region. Most heterozygous Tw mice, +/-, become obese at adulthood with a concomitant decrease in fertility. Homozygous mice have clefts of the midfacial region and a disrupted nasal cavity. Midfacial clefts included clefts of the palate combined with either unilateral or bilateral clefts of the lip. The clefts of the lip were either complete or incomplete. The palatal shelves in Tw/Tw were very much reduced. Apart from these defects, homozygous Tw looked normal, and were born alive, although they reportedly die within 24 h after birth. It is proposed that the Twirler model can be used to improve understanding of the genetic mechanisms involved in the normal development of the midfacial region.[31]

The Twirler mutation arose spontaneously and causes inner ear defects in heterozygous and CL/P in homozygous mutant mice, providing a unique animal model for investigating the molecular mechanisms of inner ear and craniofacial development. Liu et al. identified a novel homeobox gene, Iroquois-related homeobox like-1 (Irxl1), from the Twirler locus.[32] In situ hybridization analyses of mouse embryos at various developmental stages showed that Irxl1 mRNA is highly expressed in the frontonasal process and palatal mesenchyme during primary and secondary palate development. In addition, Irxl1 mRNA is strongly expressed in mesenchyme surrounding the developing inner ear, in discrete regions of the developing mandible, in the dermomyotome during somite differentiation, and in a subset of muscular structures in late embryonic stages. The developmental expression pattern indicates that Irxl1 is a good candidate gene for the Twirler gene.

TCDD-Induced CLP

It is well known that TCDD induces cleft palates in pregnant C57BL mice. However, it is unclear if TCDD is a possible teratogen for cleft lip. Yamada et al. examined maxillofacial malformations including cleft lip in A/J mice.[33] The A/J mouse develops CLP spontaneously at a 5–10% rate. Mice were gavaged with TCDD on GD 8.5–14.5 to examine the timing effects of TCDD administration on lip and palate formation. Palatal shelf movements during this period were observed with a stereoscopic microscope. All embryos had cleft palates when the TCDD was administered just before palatogenesis (GD 11.5–12.5). Cleft lips were not induced, even when the TCDD was given just before labiogenesis. Morphologically, both palatal shelves contacted perfectly along their lengths, but separated and formed cleft palates. The authors concluded that TCDD is a strong inducer of cleft palates, and interferes with the fusion phase of the secondary palate, but has no effect on the lip.

Cleft Prevention

B group vitamins, including folic acid supplementation during pregnancy, have been shown to be effective in preventing CLP in humans. The clinical trials for the prevention of malformations have been mostly empirically based. Schubert et al. focused on the elucidation of the mechanisms underlying preventive measures.[34,35] The teratogenic potency of vitamin deficiency over the whole period of gestation (GD 1–18) and of food restriction during the critical period of palatogenesis (GD 12 and 13) were investigated in the genetically different strains of NMRI and A/WySn mice. The potential benefit of vitamin B treatment in the genetically susceptible CLP strain

was demonstrated for comparison with former work on a teratogenetically induced CP model.

The results illustrated the higher susceptibility of the NMRI strain to the teratogenic action of deficiency (increase of the CP rate from 3.8 to 25%) in contrast to A/WySn mice, which actually have a high spontaneous but relative teratogenic-resistant clefting rate (28–44%). A deficiency of each of the individual B vitamins is teratogenic; however, total B group deficiency has the strongest effect in the case of deficiency of all B vitamins. This produces up to 25% cleft palates in the NMRI strain. Alternatively, vitamin B group treatment in pregnant A/WySn mice did not substantially influence the incidence of clefting in contrast to their former experience in Halle:AB mice. The results may help to elucidate the interplay of genetic conditions and exogenous (nutritional) factors in both the etiology and prevention of CLP. This may further clarify the role of the B vitamins in empiric preventive clinical trials.

Bienengraber et al. studied the anti-teratogenic effects of folic acid on experimentally induced cleft palate in rats. Lew 1 A dams (75 fetuses) were gavaged with 200 mg/kg procarbazine on GD 14 to induce CP; seven of the pregnant dams (45 fetuses) also received 4 mg/kg folic acid subcutaneously from GD 14–17.[36] Three pregnant dams (24 fetuses) served as controls and did not receive either drug. All fetuses were harvested and evaluated stereomicroscopically and histologically on GD 20. None of the control fetuses exhibited a cleft. Without folate administration, 90% of the fetuses that received procarbazine exhibited a CP. After additional prenatal folate administration, this rate remained virtually unchanged (91%). However, the proportion of complete CP (4%) was significantly lower than in the group without folate (53%). Cleft-associated microgenia and microglossia were also significantly less frequent when folate was administered prenatally: Microgenia was reduced by 22% and microglossia by 24%. On the basis of these results, the authors concluded that folate has a partial preventive effect on the teratogenicity of procarbazine given to pregnant rats.

The A/J mouse has been used to study the teratogenic affects of phenytoin. Millicovsky and Johnston demonstrated that placing pregnant A/J mice in a hyperoxic chamber after phenytoin injection greatly reduces the incidence of phenytoin-induced CLP.[37] These results suggest that phenytoin may affect embryonic development indirectly by altering maternal physiology. This maternally mediated mechanism, and the protection against it afforded by hyperoxia, has general implications for the effects of maternal toxicity on teratogenesis.

SMALL ANIMAL MODELS: IATROGENIC MODELS

Alveolar Cleft Bone Grafting

Alveolar bone grafting is an adjunctive procedure that has become increasingly popular in the rehabilitation of patients with cleft lip and palate. A histologic basis of the performance of bone grafts is required to evaluate properly different grafting materials. This, however, cannot be provided by clinical studies on humans. Therefore, an animal model with a simulated alveolar cleft is needed. A number of animal models have been previously proposed. el-Bokle describes the problems associated with each model and a surgical technique for the creation of permanent alveolar clefts in rabbits.[38] Clinical and histologic findings 6 weeks postoperatively confirm the establishment of a 1-cm wide defect with oronasal communication and healthy epithelial lining. This animal model can be efficiently used for the testing of various bone grafting materials.

Critical-sized defects were created in the premaxillary bone of Wistar male rats using a surgical trephine and a low-speed dental engine to produce a model of the maxillary alveolar cleft for testing bone-inductive agents.[39] The defects were treated with either 7 mg of demineralized bone matrix (DBM) or were left nongrafted. The nongrafted group healed mainly with fibrous connective tissue, with a small amount of bone formation at the periphery. There was no significant change in alkaline phosphatase activity and 45Ca incorporation. The DBM-grafted group produced new bone with osseous bridging in the defect by day 35. Alkaline phosphatase activity increased significantly from day 10, reaching a maximum on day 14, and 45Ca incorporation increased on day 14. The authors produced a nonhealing bony wound of the premaxilla in rats that may be useful as a model for studying the effect of bone-inductive agents on the healing of alveolar clefts.

A left-sided cleft of the lip and alveolar part of the maxilla was created in rabbits by removal of the premaxillary suture.[40] In the control animals, the cleft was left unrepaired. One group of rabbits underwent an autologous graft from the mandibular symphysis; another group underwent autologous rib cartilage grafting. Lateral photographs of adult skulls in a standardized position were made, and a computerized craniometric analysis of the position of 13 anatomic landmarks in an orthogonal coordinate system was performed. Comparison of the grafted adult skulls with unoperated controls and the animals with unrepaired iatrogenic clefts revealed that introduction of rib cartilage leads to an improvement with respect to the growth of the facial skeleton.

LARGE ANIMAL MODELS: CONGENITAL MODELS

The Congenital Caprine Model

Any animal model of a human congenital anomaly established by iatrogenic methods involving intrauterine fetal manipulation or ex utero intervention has limited clinical applicability. A congenital model that more closely simulates the etiopathogenesis of a human anomaly may provide data that can more readily be extrapolated to that anomaly and, therefore, be used in diagnostic and management strategies. Weinzweig

et al. described and characterized the first true congenital model of cleft palate in the goat.[41] Palatal shelf closure normally occurs at approximately day 38 of gestation in the caprine species. Pregnant goats were gavaged twice daily during gestational days 32 through 41 [term, 145 days] with plant slurry of *Nicotiana glauca* containing the piperidine alkaloid teratogen anabasine. Gross analysis and measurement of fetal clefts were performed at 60, 70, and 85 days gestation. Clefted kids were sacrificed at specific intervals after birth (2 weeks, and 1, 3, and 6 months); after skull debridement and preparation, they were compared with unclefted control kids.

Complete clefting of the secondary palate occurred in 97% of the fetuses. In all cases, the cleft extended from the posterior aspect of the alveolar ridge to the uvula; the majority of these clefts were bilateral, with complete detachment of the vomer. Morphologically, these clefts were similar to human clefts (Fig. 72–1 and 72–2). Eighteen percent of clefted newborn kids demonstrated gross maxillary hypoplasia and midfacial retrusion at birth with a relative Class III malocclusion. Direct measurement of the congenital caprine skulls confirmed these findings (Fig. 72–3). The incidence of midfacial growth abnormalities in these clefted animals raises questions regarding the etiopathogenesis of facial dysmorphology that is unrelated to scarring of the maxilla.

This congenital model supports the theory of an intrinsic component of facial dysmorphology associated with the unrepaired cleft palate, which can result in subsequent impaired midfacial growth that is unrelated to scarring of the maxilla. In addition, this work provides a tool that may be used to help elucidate and modify the mechanisms involved in fetal wound healing and craniofacial growth.

The role of fetal surgery in the treatment of non-life-threatening congenital anomalies remains a source of much debate. Before such undertakings can be justified, the feasibility and safety of these in utero procedures must be demonstrated. Weinzweig et al. performed in utero repair of the congenital clefts at GD 85 using a modified von Langenbeck technique employing lateral relaxing incisions with elevation and midline approximation of full-thickness, bilateral, mucoperiosteal palatal flaps followed by single-layer closure.[42] One group of congenitally clefted fetuses underwent in utero repair; another group remained as unrepaired controls (Fig. 72–4).

An iatrogenic, surgically created, fetal cleft model was developed for comparative purposes. Normal fetuses underwent surgical cleft creation by excision of a 20×3 mm full-thickness midline section of the secondary palate extending from the alveolus to the uvula, at 85 days of gestation. One group of surgically clefted fetuses underwent concurrent repair of the cleft at that time; another group of surgically clefted fetuses remained as unrepaired controls. At 2 weeks of age, no congenitally or surgically created clefts repaired in utero demonstrated gross or histologic evidence of scar formation. A slight indentation at the site of repair was the only remaining evidence of a cleft. At 6 months of age, normal palatal architecture, including that of mucosal, muscular, and glandular elements, was seen grossly and histologically. Cross-section

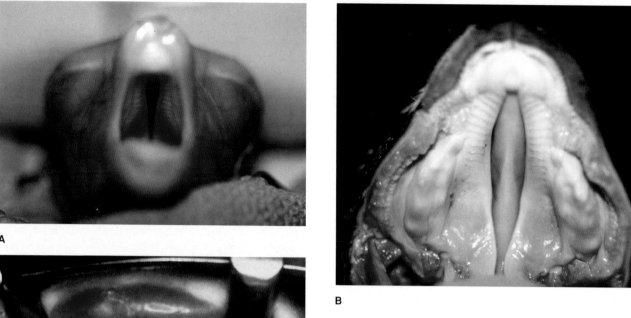

Figure 72–1. The congenital cleft palate model. A) Complete clefting of the secondary palate is appreciated in this fetus at gestational day 85 (top) and B) this newborn kid goat at 4 weeks of age (center). C) The marked similarity between the congenital cleft palate model and an actual human cleft palate is appreciated (bottom). *bottom from Nguyen PN, Sullivan PK. Issues and controversies in the management of cleft palate. Clin Plast Surg 20(4):671, 1993 (Figure 4A, p. 679), with permission.)*

through the mid-portion of the repaired congenitally clefted palates demonstrated reconstitution of a bilaminar palate, with distinct oral and nasal mucosal layers, after single-layer repair (Fig. 72–5).

The authors demonstrated that in utero cleft palate repair is technically feasible and results in scarless healing of the mucoperiosteum and velum. This work represents the first in utero repair of a congenital cleft palate model in any species. The use of a congenital cleft palate model that can be consistently reproduced with high predictability and little variation

represents the ideal experimental situation. It provides an opportunity to manipulate specific variables, assess the influence of each change on the outcome and, subsequently, extrapolate such findings to the clinical arena with a greater degree of relevance. The in utero repair of this congenital caprine model of cleft palate provides yet another tool that may be used to explore a myriad of questions related to this fascinating anomaly. Such investigations may include assessing the efficacy of different palatoplasty techniques, velopharyngeal function following palatoplasty, the role of newer strategies

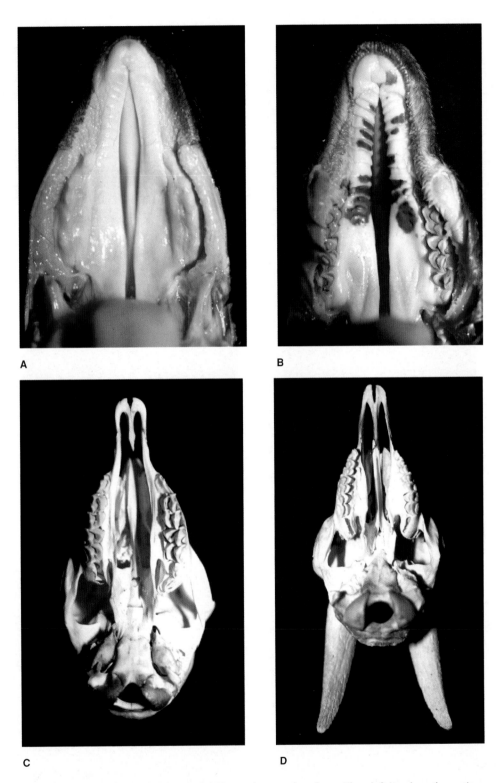

A

B

C

D

Figure 72–2. The congenital cleft palate model at 1 and 6 months of age. The cleft involves the entire secondary palate, extending through the maxillae and palatine bones. With growth, the point of widening or "funnelling" of the cleft has assumed a more posterior position. The vomer, detached bilaterally, is evident between the maxillae of this bilateral cleft. (Top images (A + B)).

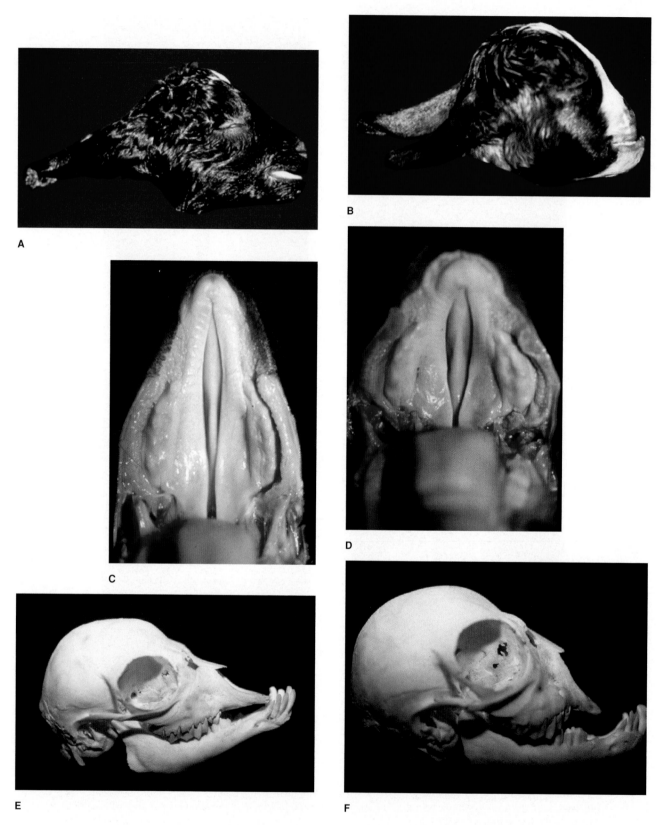

Figure 72–3. Midfacial growth of the congenital model. Clefted twins at 1 month of age are demonstrated. While both are clefted, the animal on the right demonstrates obvious evidence of midfacial hypoplasia and retrusion on gross examination (top images A + B) and dry skull analysis (bottom images E + F). In fact, a Class III malocclusion "facies" is appreciated in this case. The cleft of this animal demonstrates foreshortening and widening, consistent with substantial midfacial hypoplasia (center images C + D).

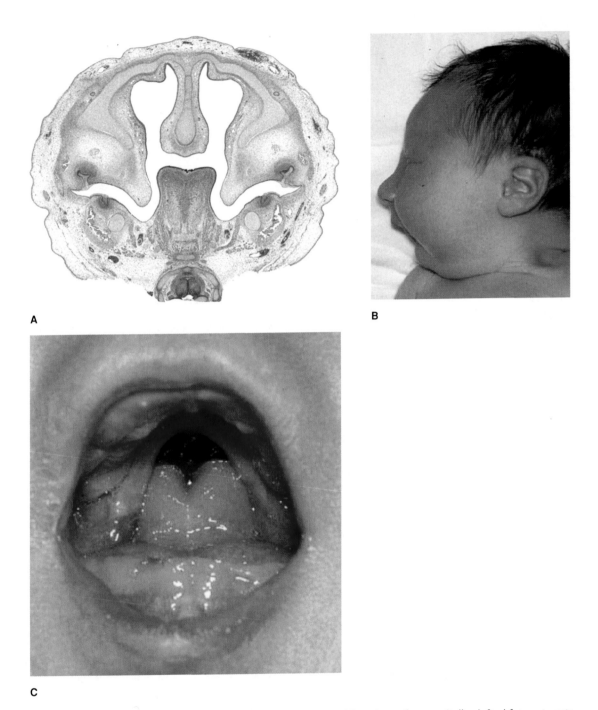

Figure 72–7. Mechanism of congenital palatal clefting. A) Coronal histology of congenitally clefted fetus at gestational day 86 (Hematoxylin & Eosin stain, Original magnificaion, 10×) is contrasted with a human newborn with Pierre Robin sequence. (B + C) Intra-oral photograph of the clefted child demonstrates the tongue wedged between the palatal shelves (right) in a manner analogous to that seen following cleft induction in the congenital caprine model. *Clinical photos generously provided courtesy of Dr. Arun Gosain.*

multivariate techniques. The authors found that animals that had lip and palate defects closed in sequence had less severe maxillofacial aberrations than animals with simultaneously closed defects. Sequential closure of the defects also had identifiable effects on maxillofacial form. The growth aberrations observed among animals with sequential closure, however, are primarily attributable to surgical creation of the defects

and not to the surgical repair. The authors concluded that delaying palate repair is less traumatic to the subsequent growth of the maxillary complex than simultaneous repair of lip and palate defects.

Undermining of the soft tissue on the surface of the maxilla at the time of cleft lip repair, as with a gingivoperiosteoplasty, remains a controversial issue in cleft management.

Using Beagles, Bardach et al. tested the hypothesis that lip repair with soft-tissue undermining contributes more to maxillofacial growth aberrations than lip repair without these additional procedures.[53] Animals were assigned to four groups: unclefted controls, unrepaired clefted controls, and two experimental groups (with and without undermining). Defects simulating clefts of the lip, alveolus, and palate were surgically created in the unrepaired and experimental animals. At 36 weeks of age, 11 measurements were made directly on the cleaned maxillae. Analysis revealed that all groups with surgically created defects were significantly different from normal; however, animals with undermining exhibited the greatest degree of impaired facial growth. The authors concluded that these findings reaffirm their earlier conclusions that undermining of the soft tissue on the surface of the maxilla is detrimental to maxillofacial growth.

Bardach et al. subsequently evaluated the relationship between varying sequences of lip and palate repair and maxillary growth.[54] Three different sequences of lip and palate repair were analyzed. The first sequence constituted the conventional approach of *lip repair first followed by palate repair.* The second sequence was reversed: *palate repair first followed by lip repair.* The third sequence consisted of *simultaneous lip and palate repair.* Using 70 eight-week-old Beagles, the authors tested the following hypothesis: The sequence of lip repair first and palate repair second is less detrimental to maxillary growth than the other two sequences. The animals were assigned to two control groups (unclefted; and, unrepaired clefted animals) and three experimental groups, in which the three different sequences of repair were performed. Upon sacrifice, 11 maxillary variables were measured directly from cleaned skulls and analyzed by univariate and multivariate techniques. The authors' analysis confirmed that the conventional sequence of cleft lip and palate repair (lip first, palate second) is less detrimental to maxillary growth than repairing the palate first and the lip second or simultaneous closure of both defects.

Nasoalveolar Clefts

Ehler et al. described a simple, surgical technique to create a simulated nasoalveolar palatal defect in a canine model.[55] In doing so, the authors' surgically created cleft yielded a critical-size defect of the nasoalveolar region that fulfilled five criteria: (1) bilateral maxillary alveolar clefts were produced in each case; (2) each cleft consisted of a 1-cm bony width; (3) a demonstrable oronasal communication was present; (4) each cleft was lined by healthy epithelialized mucosa; and (5) there were functional teeth adjacent to each side of every cleft. Such a model could prove useful for the study of alveolar bone grafting techniques.

Bone Formation Following Palate Repair

While the biological responses to the repair of palatal clefts have been evaluated principally by monitoring craniofacial growth, little is known about the regenerative ability of the repaired palate. Forbes et al. assigned 8-week-old Beagle pups to one of three groups: (1) control group, unclefted; (2) cleft group, underwent a surgically created cleft of the posterior hard palate (mean bony measurement: 3.1 × 11.7 mm); and (3) repaired group, which underwent soft-tissue closure at 12 weeks of age. Craniofacial growth was monitored by cephalometric and dental cast measurements. Animals were sacrificed either 16 or 28 weeks after time of cleft creation. Analysis of the cleft palate group revealed that the size of the bony cleft increased with time. Histologic examination at 24 weeks of age (12 weeks after the repair) demonstrated active reduction of medial margin of the bony palate as evidenced by osteoclastic activity.[56] At 36 weeks of age, neither osteoblastic nor osteoclastic activity was detected. The mean dimensions of the bony cleft, in the cleft group at 36 weeks, were 7.9 × 18.8 mm. In the repaired group, partial bone repair occurred. However, no consistency was seen in predicting extent or location of repair. Histochemical detection of alkaline phosphatase activity indicated that the repaired group had greater amounts of new bone formation. In some sites, suture regeneration was seen. As with the amount of bone formation, the amount of suture regeneration was variable. The authors concluded that the presence of a cleft inhibits osteoblastic activity along the margin of the cleft, and there is limited potential for regeneration of the palate subsequent to the repair.

Iatrogenic Fetal Cleft Models

Fetal wounds heal without inflammation and scar formation. This phenomenon may, in the future, be applicable to human cleft lip and palate repair. However, extensive experimental work must first be done to document the benefits of in utero repair. The ability of certain fetal tissues, including skin, bone, lip and velar musculature, and palatal mucoperiosteum, to heal scarlessly presents the opportunity to perform in utero procedures with results that could not otherwise be obtained if performed in the neonatal period or later.

Longaker et al. developed a large animal model for creation and repair of a complete cleft lip and alveolus using fetal lambs.[57] The cleft lip and alveolus deformity was created in GD 75 fetuses (term = 145 days) and either repaired in three layers or left unrepaired. There were four sham-operated fetuses, and all animals were alive at harvest. Repaired, unrepaired, and control fetuses were harvested at 7, 14, 21, and 70 days following surgery.

The unrepaired fetuses demonstrated a complete cleft lip and alveolus with an oronasal fistula. The maxilla was asymmetrical, with the greater segment deviated toward the cleft and with decreased anterior maxillary width. In contrast, repaired cleft lip and alveolus animals showed no scar, normal thickness of the lip, and a symmetrical maxilla. Histologic analysis of the repaired wounds showed evidence of tissue regeneration without scar formation. The authors concluded that in utero repair of the fetal lamb cleft lip and alveolus model is technically feasible with an excellent survival rate and that this model would be used to document subsequent facial growth.

Papadopulos et al. evaluated maxillary growth following in utero repair of surgically created cleft lip and alveolar (CLA)-like defects by means of three-dimensional (3D) computer tomographic (CT) cephalometric analysis in the mid-gestational sheep model.[58] A unilateral CLA-like defect was created in sheep fetuses in utero (untreated control group: 4 fetuses). Four different bone grafts were used for the alveolar defect closure. After euthanasia, CT scans of the skulls of the fetuses, 3D reconstructions, and a 3D-CT cephalometric analysis were performed. The authors found that none of the surgical approaches used for the in utero correction of CLA-like defects significantly affected postsurgical maxillary growth; however, when bone graft healing takes place, a tendency for almost normal maxillary growth was observed.[59]

Hedrick et al. developed a fetal lamb model in which incisional or excisional unilateral cleft lips were created early in gestation and later repaired.[60] Fetuses at GD 58–62 underwent either a 2 mm excision or incision that produced a defect in the left superior lip through the nasal sill and alveolus, creating an abnormal oronasal communication. Two weeks later, the epithelialized wound edges were freshened and repaired. By GD 103–105, 4 weeks following lip repair, the authors found that all clefts had healed scarlessly. However, whereas the incisional clefts healed spontaneously with replacement of the native reticular collagen pattern and with regeneration of the skin appendages, the unrepaired excisional clefts did not heal spontaneously and, when surgically repaired, healed without a collagen scar but showed no regeneration of the skin appendages.

Cleft lip and palate defects assume many forms from mild to severe, but all may be associated with abnormal craniofacial development. Even the most expert and sophisticated methods of surgical repair are followed by scar contraction and fibrosis, which result in skeletal defects, dental abnormalities, cosmetic disfigurement, and speech impairment. In a subsequent study, Canady et al. investigated the effect of prenatal repair of iatrogenically created cleft palate on scar formation in the fetal lamb model.[61] Ewes were operated on ranging in gestation from GD 70 to GD 133. Fifteen lambs were studied (nine cleft palates produced and repaired in utero; one cleft produced in utero and not repaired, four normal, unoperated palates; and one cleft palate produced and repaired 1 week postnatally). The lambs were delivered normally at GD 145–147. The lambs were euthanized at one month of age and the surgical area of the palates studied grossly and histologically. Animals operated at 112 days or later in gestation exhibited scars both clinically and histologically. The authors found that the animals that had cleft palate produced and repaired at 70 days gestation did not have a visible palatal scar at 1 month of age. Histologically, there was evidence of minimal scarring without disruption of normal architecture.

Canady et al. subsequently studied the impact of scar formation on craniofacial growth after cleft palate repair.[62] The fetal ovine model enabled the study of a group of animals with little or no scar using cephalometric studies of craniofacial growth after iatrogenic cleft palate repair. A 3 mm wide cleft was surgically created in the soft palate and ex-

tended anteriorly to create a notch in the posterior aspect of the hard palate of each fetus. Grossly evident scar is formed in the palates of lambs repaired at GD 118 or later in gestation, while those animals operated at GD 70 and GD 77 exhibited no scar grossly and minimal scar histologically in the submucosa with normal nasal and oral mucosal surfaces. For this study, 15 lambs were studied: four were unoperated, three were operated at GD 70 days, one at GD 77, and seven had clefts produced and repaired at GD 118–GD 133. The animals were euthanized at 1 month of age and analyzed. Computerized tomography, three-dimensional reconstruction of the skull, and direct palate measurements were evaluated. No significant differences were found between the means of any measurement in the three treatment groups. The authors concluded that fetal palate repair, with or without scarring, resulted in normal craniofacial growth in the 1-month-old lamb.

Successful open repair of a cleft lip in utero has the advantage of scarless wound healing in the fetus. Unfortunately, no long-term outcome studies have been performed to evaluate the efficacy of these repairs. Moreover, no study to date has compared the long-term results of an in utero cleft lip repair to a similar, control-matched, newborn cleft repair. Stelnicki et al. evaluated the 9-month outcome of in utero cleft lip surgery compared with an identical cleft lip repair performed on infant lambs.[63] In utero epithelialized cleft lips were created through an open hysterotomy in GD 65 fetal lambs (term = 140 days) using methods described by Longaker et al.[57] Eight of 16 animals underwent subsequent in utero repair of these clefts at GD 90. The repair of the remaining eight animals was delayed until 1 week postpartum. At 9 months, the animals were histologically analyzed for changes in lip contour and for the degree of scarring.

All repaired lips had some degree of abnormality postoperatively. One of six lips repaired in utero dehisced before delivery. Three of six neonatal repairs dehisced in the first postoperative month. In the remaining animals with intact lip repairs, the vertical lip height on the repaired side was an average of 9–12 mm shorter than the normal lip in both the in utero and neonatally repaired animals. Phenotypically, the postnatally repaired animals had more lip distortion and visible notching. Histologically, the in utero repair was scarless while the neonatal repairs had scar throughout the entire vertical height of the lip with an associated loss of hair in this region. Maxillary growth was also evaluated. There was no inhibition of maxillary growth in the animals that underwent in utero cleft lip repair. However, in the neonatal repair group, significant maxillary retrusion was evident. Compared with the cleft side of the maxilla, horizontal growth was decreased by 11%. Compared with the intrauterine repair group, there was a 17% decrease in horizontal maxillary width.

Straight-line in utero repair of a cleft lip produces a better long-term result in terms of maxillary growth than a similar repair performed postnatally in the ovine model. There was no diminution in maxillary growth in the animals treated in utero. Histologically, in utero repair of clefts was indeed scarless. However, both lip repairs produced lips that were significantly shorter than their contralateral noncleft sides. This degree of lip shortening would require a secondary lip revision, thereby defeating the purpose of performing an intrauterine repair. The authors emphasized that comparisons now need to be made between in utero and neonatal repairs using a Millard-type rotation advancement technique before intrauterine treatment can be considered to be more beneficial than our current treatment modalities.

Thaller et al. incised and elevated bilateral bipedicled mucoperiosteal flaps at GD 75–90, which were then allowed to heal by secondary intention.[64] The purpose of this investigation was to evaluate the effect of in utero palatal surgery in a sheep model. At several postnatal time points between 6 and 24 weeks, palatal width measurements were obtained from dental impressions. The authors found that in utero palatal manipulation had no effect on subsequent craniofacial growth.

Cleft Nasal Deformity

The cleft nasal deformity, a combination of malpositioned cartilage and tissue and post-repair scarring, is a difficult problem to correct. Levine et al. manipulated the nasal shape of fetal lambs in utero as a first step toward restoration of normal nasal form in cleft nasal deformities.[65] Preformed hypertonic sponges were placed into the right nostril of eight fetal lambs during the second trimester (when scarless cutaneous wound repair is known to occur). The size and shape of the fetal nasal structures were analyzed after 1, 2, and 6 weeks by direct measurement, histologic examination, and three-dimensional computed tomographic scans of the experimentally expanded noses and compared with the control nonexpanded noses of the birth twins or age-matched specimens. The authors found that experimentally expanded nasal structures had markedly increased septal length and intranasal volume. Histology showed normal cellular elements without scarring in the tissue sections from the expanded nasal areas. The authors concluded that the shape of nasal tissue could be manipulated without scarring in second-trimester fetal lambs after placement of a nasal expansion device. This study demonstrates the potential for restoring normal nasal form by repositioning alar cartilages and soft tissue during fetal cleft repair.

Lateral Facial Clefts

The etiopathogenesis behind the formation of atypical craniofacial facial clefts remains unknown. To test the hypothesis that physical restricting forces such as amniotic bands can lead to the formation of these unusual clefts in the post-organogenesis period, Stelnicki et al. modified a previously reported fetal lamb model of amniotic band syndrome to examine the effects of these bands on craniofacial development.[66] Lateral craniofacial clefts were created in GD 70 fetal lambs by applying a 2–0 nylon suture as a constriction band to the growing face. The sutures were attached to either the zygomatic arch or the infraorbital rim externally and then looped circumferentially into the oral commissure. Each suture was positioned so as to create either a Tessier type 5 or a Tessier type 7 cleft. Both types of lateral facial clefts were effectively produced using this model. In each group, the presence of an intraoral constriction band led to the formation of macrostomia, with an average 7.4-mm lateral displacement of the oral commissure. In addition to these soft tissue changes, each animal also had partial bony clefting (i.e., a bony groove) induced by the pressure of the restriction band across the growing facial skeleton. In the lambs with the Tessier type 7 cleft, incomplete bony clefts developed across the zygomatic arch. In animals with bands placed across the medial infraorbital rim, significant infraorbital and malar bony clefts formed similar to a classic Tessier type 5 facial cleft. No evidence of tissue necrosis, maceration, or ulceration was noted in any animal.

These data present evidence that the constriction of craniofacial growth by external forces such as a swallowed amnionic band can lead to the development of lateral facial clefting involving both soft tissue and bony elements. The authors conclude that these malformations are likely due to a combination of directly tethering normal tissue migration and an increase in local pressure, which produces cellular ischemia and apoptosis. Furthermore, their data demonstrate that these clefts can occur later in fetal development during a period of facial growth rather than during the period of primary facial morphogenesis.

CONCLUSION

A myriad of animal models have been developed in numerous species over the past several decades to better understand the mechanisms underlying the etiopathogenesis of a multitude of congenital anomalies. The complexity of orofacial clefts, and important roles that proper management of these deformities play in achieving optimal aesthetic and functional outcomes, have provided the impetus for the development of the diverse array of models discussed in this chapter.

Most congenital anomalies, or malformations, are multifactorial in etiology. The exact genetic versus environmental, or "nature versus nurture," contribution to a specific anomaly is rarely known with certainty. Regardless of the exact etiology or inciting event responsible for a particular congenital defect, these anomalies usually occur during embryogenesis, within the first 8 weeks of gestation, and are present at birth.

Anomalies such as craniosynostosis, microtia, or cleft palate are certainly not the result of intrauterine fetal manipulation. Therefore, models establishing such iatrogenic methods, while integral to the evolution of important concepts, might have limited clinical applicability. Nonetheless, it is those iatrogenic models that first demonstrated the feasibility of fetal manipulation, in utero palate repair, and resultant scarless healing, and posed the question of subsequent craniofacial growth abnormalities following in utero repair, that have provided an impetus for the development of congenital models.

Similarly, questions raised in understanding the intricate nature of these anomalies have necessitated the development of sophisticated techniques to perform whole embryo and organ culture, embryo transfer, and clever methods to analyze complex genetic mechanisms, as well as models to assess the role of specific genetic mutations and the effects of various teratogenic agents. The development of animals models, both congenital and iatrogenic, both in vivo and in vitro, is paramount to the advancement of our understanding of these complex congenital anomalies and critical to the development of sophisticated strategies to optimize their treatment and potentially facilitate their prevention.

References

1. Abbott BD, Adamson ED, Pratt RM. Retinoic acid alters EGF receptor expression during palatogenesis. *Development* 102(4):853–867, 1988.
2. Abbott BD, Birnbaum LS. Rat embryonic palatal shelves respond to TCDD in organ culture. *Toxicol Appl Pharmacol* 103(3):441–451, 1990.
3. Abbott BD, Buckalew AR. Embryonic palatal responses to teratogens in serum – Free organ culture. *Teratology* 45(4):369–382, 1992.
4. Sasaki Y, Tanaka S, Hamachi T, Taya Y. Deficient cell proliferation in palatal shelf mesenchyme of CL/Fr mouse embryos. *J Dent Res* 83(10):797–801, 2004.
5. Eto K, Figueroa A, Tamura G, Pratt RM. Induction of cleft lip in cultured rat embryos by localized administration of tunicamycin. *J Embryol Exp Morphol* 64:1–9, 1981.
6. Abbott BD, Logsdon TR, Wilke TS. Effects of methanol on embryonic mouse palate in serum-free organ culture. *Teratology* 49(2):122–134, 1994.
7. Kotch LE, Sulik KK. Experimental fetal alcohol syndrome: Proposed pathogenic basis for a variety of associated facial and brain anomalies. *Am J Med Genet* 44(2):168–176, 1992.
8. Nonaka K, Sasaki Y, Martin DA, Nakata M. Effect of the dam strain on the spontaneous incidence of cleft lip and palate and intrauterine growth of CL/Fr mouse fetuses. *J Assist Reprod Genet* 12(7):447–452, 1995.
9. Wang KY, Diewert VM. A morphometric analysis of craniofacial growth in cleft lip and noncleft mice. *J Craniofac Genet Dev Biol* 12(3):141–154, 1992.
10. Bronsky PT, Johnston MC, Sulik KK. Morphogenesis of hypoxia-induced cleft lip in CL/Fr mice. *J Craniofac Genet Dev Biol Suppl* 2:113–128, 1986.
11. Bailey LJ, Johnston MC, Billet J. Effects of carbon monoxide and hypoxia on cleft lip in A/J mice. *Cleft Palate Craniofac J* 32(1):14–19, 1995.
12. Abbott BD, Pratt RM. Retinoic acid alters epithelial differentiation during palatogenesis. *J Craniofac Genet Dev Biol* 11(4):315–325, 1991.
13. Lorente CA, Miller SA. Vitamin A induction of cleft palate. *Cleft Palate J* 15(4):378–385, 1978.
14. Abbott BD, Harris MW, Birnbaum LS. Etiology of retinoic acid-induced cleft palate varies with the embryonic stage. *Teratology* 40(6):533–553, 1989.
15. Fujiwara H, Natsume N, Miura S, et al. [Experimental study on the cleft lip and palate. VIII. Induction of cleft palate in Wistar rats by vitamin A]. *Aichi Gakuin Daigaku Shigakkai Shi* 27(3):629–634, 1989.
16. Richman JM, Delgado JL. Locally released retinoic acid leads to facial clefts in the chick embryo but does not alter the expression of receptors for fibroblast growth factor. *J Craniofac Genet Dev Biol* 15(4):190–204, 1995.
17. Abbott BD, McNabb FM, Lau C. Glucocorticoid receptor expression during the development of the embryonic mouse secondary palate. *J Craniofac Genet Dev Biol* 14(2):87–96, 1994.

18. Abbott BD. Review of the interaction between TCDD and glucocorticoids in embryonic palate. *Toxicology* 105(2–3):365–373, 1995.
19. Sullivan-Jones P, Hansen DK, Sheehan DM, Holson RR. The effect of teratogens on maternal corticosterone levels and cleft incidence in A/J mice. *J Craniofac Genet Dev Biol* 12(4):183–189, 1992.
20. Peterka M, Jelinek R. Origin of hydrocortisone induced orofacial clefts in the chick embryo. *Cleft Palate J* 20(1):35–46, 1983.
21. Amin N, Ohashi Y, Chiba J, Yoshida S, Takano Y. Alterations in vascular pattern of the developing palate in normal and spontaneous cleft palate mouse embryos. *Cleft Palate Craniofac J* 31(5):332–344, 1994.
22. Karolyi J, Erickson RP. A region of the mouse genome homologous to human chromosome 1q21 affects facial clefting. *J Craniofac Genet Dev Biol* 13(1):1–5, 1993.
23. Karolyi J, Erickson RP, Liu S, Killewald L. Major effects on teratogen-induced facial clefting in mice determined by a single genetic region. *Genetics* 126(1):201–205, 1990.
24. Juriloff DM, Harris MJ, Dewell SL, et al. Investigations of the genomic region that contains the clf1 mutation, a causal gene in multifactorial cleft lip and palate in mice. *Birth Defects Res A Clin Mol Teratol* 73(2):103–113, 2005.
25. Gong SG. Phenotypic and molecular analyses of A/WySn mice. *Cleft Palate Craniofac J* 38(5):486–491, 2001.
26. Wang KY, Chen KC, Chiang CP, Kuo MY. Distribution of p21ras during primary palate formation of non-cleft and cleft strains of mice. *J Oral Pathol Med* 24(3):103–108, 1995.
27. Wang KY, Chang FH, Chiang CP, Chen KC, Kuo MY. Temporal and spatial expression of erbB4 in ectodermal and mesenchymal cells during primary palatogenesis in noncleft and cleft strains of mice. *J Oral Pathol Med* 27(4):141–146, 1998.
28. Hamachi T, Sasaki Y, Hidaka K, Nakata M. Association between palatal morphogenesis and Pax9 expression pattern in CL/Fr embryos with clefting during palatal development. *Arch Oral Biol* 48(8):581–587, 2003.
29. Knight AS, Schutte BC, Jiang R, Dixon MJ. Developmental expression analysis of the mouse and chick orthologues of IRF6: The gene mutated in Van der Woude syndrome. *Dev Dyn* 235(5):1441–1447, 2006.
30. Bush JO, Lan Y, Jiang R. The cleft lip and palate defects in Dancer mutant mice result from gain of function of the Tbx10 gene. *Proc Natl Acad Sci U S A* 101(18):7022–7027.
31. Gong SG, White NJ, Sakasegawa AY. The Twirler mouse, a model for the study of cleft lip and palate. *Arch Oral Biol* 45(1):87–94, 2000.
32. Liu H, Liu W, Maltby KM, Lan Y, Jiang R. Identification and developmental expression analysis of a novel homeobox gene closely linked to the mouse Twirler mutation. *Gene Expr Patterns* 6(6):632–636, 2006.
33. Yamada T, Mishima K, Fujiwara K, Imura H, Sugahara T. Cleft lip and palate in mice treated with 2,3,7,8-tetrachlorodibenzo-p-dioxin: A morphological in vivo study. *Congenit Anom (Kyoto)* 46(1):21–25, 2006.
34. Schubert J, Schmidt R, Raupach HW. New findings explaining the mode of action in prevention of facial clefting and first clinical experience. *J Craniomaxillofac Surg* 18(8):343–347, 1990.
35. Schubert J, Schmidt R, Syska E. B group vitamins and cleft lip and cleft palate. *Int J Oral Maxillofac Surg* 31(4):410–413, 2002.
36. Bienengraber V, Malek FA, Moritz KU, Fanghanel J, Gundlach KK, Weingartner J. Is it possible to prevent cleft palate by prenatal administration of folic acid? An experimental study. *Cleft Palate Craniofac J* 38(4):393–398, 2001.
37. Millicovsky G, Johnston MC. Maternal hyperoxia greatly reduces the incidence of phenytoin-induced cleft lip and palate in A/J mice. *Science* 212(4495):671–672, 1981.
38. el-Bokle D, Smith SJ, Germane N, Sharawy M. New technique for creating permanent experimental alveolar clefts in a rabbit model. *Cleft Palate Craniofac J* 30(6):542–547, 1993.

39. Takano-Yamamoto T, Kawakami M, Sakuda M. Defects of the rat premaxilla as a model of alveolar clefts for testing bone-inductive agents. *J Oral Maxillofac Surg* 51(8):887–891, 1993.

40. Griffioen FM, Smit-Vis JH, Urbanus NA. Facial growth in the rabbit after autologous grafting in unilateral clefts. *Cleft Palate J* 25(3):226–234, 1988.

41. Weinzweig J, Panter KE, Pantaloni M, et al. The fetal cleft palate: I. Characterization of a congenital model. *Plast Reconstr Surg* 103(2):419–428, 1999.

42. Weinzweig J, Panter KE, Pantaloni M, et al. The fetal cleft palate: II. Scarless healing after in utero repair of a congenital model. *Plast Reconstr Surg* 104(5):1356–1364, 1999.

43. Weinzweig J, Panter KE, Spangenberger A, Harper JS, McRae R, Edstrom LE. The fetal cleft palate: III. Ultrastructural and functional analysis of palatal development following in utero repair of the congenital model. *Plast Reconstr Surg* 109(7):2355–2362, 2002.

44. Weinzweig J, Panter KE, Seki J, Pantaloni M, Spangenberger A, Harper JS. The fetal cleft palate: IV. Midfacial growth and bony palatal development following in utero and neonatal repair of the congenital caprine model. *Plast Reconstr Surg* 118(1):81–93, 2006.

45. Panter KE, Weinzweig J, Gardner DR, Stegelmeier BL, James LF. Comparison of cleft palate induction by Nicotiana glauca in goats and sheep. *Teratology* 61(3):203–210, 2000.

46. Weinzweig J, Panter KE, Patel J, Smith DM, Spangenberger A, Freeman MB. The fetal celft palate: V. Elucidation of the Mechanisms of palatal clefting in the congenital caprine model and postulation of a theory to prevent clefting in humans. *Plast Reconstr Surg* 121:1328–1334, 2008.

47. Jurkiewicz MJ. Cleft lip and palate in dogs. *Surg Forum* 15:457–458, 1964.

48. Jurkiewicz MJ. A genetic study of cleft lip and palate in dogs. *Surg Forum* 16:472–473, 1965.

49. Jurkiewicz MJ, Bryant DL. Cleft lip and palate in dogs: A progress report. *Cleft Palate J* 5:30–36, 1968.

50. Bardach J, Eisbach KJ. The influence of primary unilateral cleft lip repair on facial growth. *Cleft Palate J* 14(1):88–97, 1977.

51. Bardach J, Roberts DM, Yale R, Rosewall D, Mooney M. The influence of simultaneous cleft lip and palate repair on facial growth in rabbits. *Cleft Palate J* 17(4):309–318, 1980.

52. Bardach J, Kelly KM, Salyer KE. A comparative study of facial growth following lip and palate repair performed in sequence and simultaneously: An experimental study in beagles. *Plast Reconstr Surg* 91(6):1008–1016, 1993.

53. Bardach J, Kelly KM, Salyer KE. The effects of lip repair with and without soft-tissue undermining and delayed palate repair on maxillary growth: An experimental study in beagles. *Plast Reconstr Surg* 94(2):343–351, 1994.

54. Bardach J, Kelly KM, Salyer KE. Relationship between the sequence of lip and palate repair and maxillary growth: An experimental study in beagles. *Plast Reconstr Surg* 93(2):269–278, 1994.

55. Ehler WJ, Marx RE, Cissik JH, Hubbard GB. Simulated nasoalveolar palatal defects: A canine model to study bone grafts. *J Invest Surg* 3(4):341–347, 1990.

56. Forbes DP, Kaminski EJ, Perry HT. Repair of surgical clefts of the hard palate in beagles. *Cleft Palate J* 25(3):270–281, 1988.

57. Longaker MT, Stern M, Lorenz P, et al. A model for fetal cleft lip repair in lambs. *Plast Reconstr Surg* 90(5):750–756, 1992.

58. Papadopoulos MA, Papadopulos NA, Jannowitz C, et al. Three-dimensional cephalometric evaluation of maxillary growth following in utero repair of cleft lip and alveolar-like defects in the mid-gestational sheep model. *Fetal Diagn Ther* 21(1):105–114, 2006.

59. Papadopulos NA, Papadopoulos MA, Zeilhofer HF, et al. Intrauterine autogenous foetal bone transplantation for the repair of cleft-like defects in the mid-gestational sheep model. *J Craniomaxillofac Surg* 32(4):199–210, 2004.

60. Hedrick MH, Rice HE, Vander Wall KJ, et al. Delayed in utero repair of surgically-created fetal cleft lip and palate. *Plast Reconstr Surg* 97(5):900–905, 1996.

61. Canady JW, Landas SK, Morris H, Thompson SA. In utero cleft palate repair in the ovine model. *Cleft Palate Craniofac J* 31(1):37–44, 1994.

62. Canady JW, Thompson SA, Colburn A. Craniofacial growth after iatrogenic cleft palate repair in a fetal ovine model. *Cleft Palate Craniofac J* 34(1):69–72, 1997.

63. Stelnicki EJ, Lee S, Hoffman W, et al. A long-term, controlled-outcome analysis of in utero versus neonatal cleft lip repair using an ovine model. *Plast Reconstr Surg* 104(3):607–615, 1999.

64. Thaller SR, Mele J, Hoyt J. The effect of antenatal surgery on craniofacial growth in sheep model. *Plast Reconstr Surg* 96(1):1–8, 1995.

65. Levine JP, Bradley JP, Shahinian HK, Longaker MT. Nasal expansion in the fetal lamb: A first step toward management of cleft nasal deformity in utero. *Plast Reconstr Surg* 103(3):761–767, 1999.

66. Stelnicki EJ, Hoffman WY, Vanderwall K, Harrison MR, Foster R, Longaker MT. A new in utero model for lateral facial clefts. *J Craniofac Surg* 8(6):460–465, 1997.

73

Perspectives in Orofacial Cleft Research II: Molecular Mechanisms

Robert M. Greene, PhD • Michele M. Pisano, PhD

INTRODUCTION

When depicting far off lands at the edge of the known world, maps from the Middle Ages declared "*Here There Be Dragons.*" While our understanding of the molecular mechanisms that orchestrate orofacial development has dramatically increased in the past several decades, our knowledge remains uncomplicated by a full appreciation of the regulatory intricacies involved in normal, much less abnormal, development of the orofacial complex. Here there be dragons indeed!

Orofacial clefts are customarily described as those encompassing the lip and/or palate (CL/P), and those effecting only the palate (CPO). While orofacial clefts frequently are seen as part of a syndrome, the majority are isolated, without other accompanying anomalies.[1] With a frequency of 1–2 in 1000 live births, orofacial clefts represent nearly one-half of all craniofacial anomalies.[2] While morphogenesis of the facial complex has been well described, recent new insights continue to refine our appreciation of orofacial embryology. [3,4] In addition, utilization of an increasingly sophisticated array of genetic approaches has begun to reveal candidate genes and loci associated with orofacial clefting. [5,6] Moreover, the cast of gene and protein characters that play on the cellular stage of orofacial development continues to expand with alarming rapidity. Despite this, many of the underlying molecular events responsible for orofacial morphogenesis persist in eluding our complete understanding. What we *do* know, however, is that normal orofacial morphogenesis requires extensive reciprocal signaling between numerous embryonic tissues. With this overview, we have thus attempted to carefully select from the extant literature, essential elements of our current knowledge regarding the functionality of specific genes and gene families in orofacial development, focusing on critical signal transduction pathways. In so doing, we hope to provide enlargement of our understanding of orofacial ontogeny, as well as provide clarification of how the embryo makes sense of the apparent ceaseless chatter of intra- and intercellular developmental signals to which it is exposed.

FACIAL DEVELOPMENT

The facial region in mammalian embryos develops primarily from the frontonasal prominence (forehead, middle of the nose, philtrum of upper lip, primary palate), the lateral nasal prominences (sides of the nose), and the maxillomandibular prominences of the first branchial arch (maxilla, mandible, lateral portions of upper lip, and secondary palate) (Fig. 73–1). *Merging* of superficially separate facial prominences gives rise to the upper lip, while *fusion* of completely separate tissue processes gives rise to the secondary palate. As with all branchial arches, the first branchial arch contains mesoderm-derived mesenchymal cells, a cartilaginous core, its own cranial nerve (the trigeminal), a blood vessel (an aortic arch), and neuroectoderm-derived neural crest cells. Two excellent overviews of development of the branchial arches can be found in recent reviews by Graham[7] and Helms,[8] and a description of the embryology of the orofacial region can be found in Chapter 1 of the current volume. In brief, orofacial development is dependent, in part, on the migration of neural crest cells derived from the neuroectoderm of rhombomeres 1–3[9] (Fig. 73–2) into the first two branchial arches (Figs. 73–3 and 73–4), and diversification of neural crest cell fates[10,11] (Fig. 73–5). Interspecies

transplantation of cranial neural crest cells has shown them capable of directing their own morphogenesis,[12,13] as well as being responsive to autocrine/paracrine signals that are thought to provide critical developmental cues as these cells contribute to orofacial ontogenesis.[14,15] Evidence also exists supporting the notion that neural crest cells contributing to development of the face are developmentally plastic,[16] receiving directional cues from the neural ectoderm[17] and developmental cues from the endoderm lining the branchial arches and overlying epithelia.[18–20] Functional importance of the neural crest is put into sharp focus by the observation that a number of craniofacial malformations, referred to as neurocristopathies, are thought to be due to abnormal neural crest cell generation, migration, proliferation, and/or survival.[21]

Normal development of orofacial structures is contingent on proper spatio-temporal patterns of mesenchymal cell proliferation, tissue differentiation, synthesis, and degradation of extracellular matrix components and epithelial–mesenchymal interactions. These processes are regulated, in part, by a number of molecular autocrine and paracrine signaling pathways and their downstream effectors.[22,23] Several excellent reviews of craniofacial development have appeared in recent years.[24–26] In this overview, we have chosen to focus on certain, but by no means all, factors generally accepted as playing a pivotal role in development of the orofacial region. These include members of the transforming growth factor β (TGFβ), bone morphogenetic protein (BMP), sonic hedgehog, fibroblast growth factor (FGF), and Wnt families.

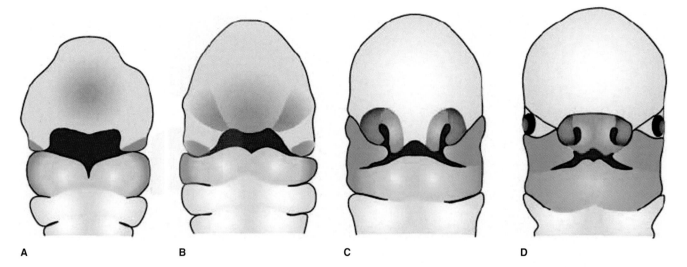

A   B   C   D

Figure 73–1. Development of the craniofacial primordia. (A–D) Schematic representations of frontal views of mouse embryos showing the prominences that give rise to the main structures of the face. The frontonasal (or median nasal) prominence (pink) gives rise to the forehead (A), the middle of the nose (B), the philtrum of the upper lip (C) and the primary palate (D). The lateral nasal prominence (blue) forms the sides of the nose (B–D). The maxillomandibular prominences (green) give rise to the lower jaw, the sides of the middle and lower face, the lateral borders of the lips, and the secondary palate. *(Reprinted with the permission of the author, Dr. Jill Helms, Stanford University, Palo Alto, CA, and Blackwell Publishing. From: Tapadia M, et al. Its all in your head: New insights into craniofacial development and deformation. J Anat 207:461–477, 2005.)*

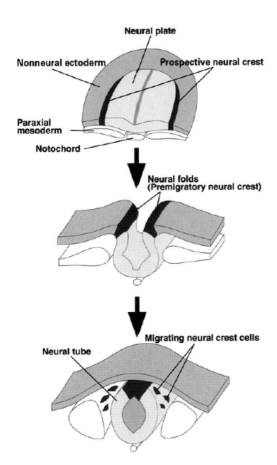

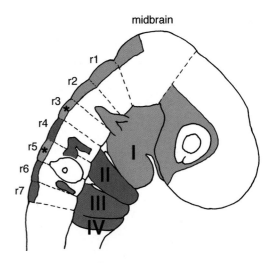

Figure 73–3. Origin and migration of embryonic cranial neural crest cells. Neural crest cells that populate the first branchial arch are derived from the posterior midbrain and rhombomeres 1 and 2 of the hindbrain (shown in red). Neural crest cells populating the second branchial arch are derived from rhombomere 4 of the hindbrain (shown in blue). The post-otic neural crest cells, derived from rhombomeres 6 and 7, migrate into and populate the posterior branchial arches (shown in purple). While rhombomeres 3 and 5 produce neural crest cells, these cells are removed by apoptosis. (*Reprinted with the permission of the author, Dr. Anthony Graham, Kings College London, and John Wiley & Sons, Inc. From: Graham A. Development of the pharyngeal arches. Am J Med Genet 119A:251–256, 2003.*)

Figure 73–2. Schematic view of neural crest cell development. Prospective neural crest cells are specified at the border of the neural plate and non-neural ectoderm (top). Subsequent to elevation of the neural folds during neurulation (middle), crest cells undergo an epithelial to mesenchymal transformation and begin to migrate (bottom). (*Reprinted with the permission of the author, Dr. Yoshio Wakamatsu, Tohoku University, Sendai, Japan, and Karger Publishing. From: Sakai D, et al. Regulatory mechanisms for neural crest formation. Cells Tissues Organs 179:24–35, 2005.*)

TRANSFORMING GROWTH FACTORS-β

The transforming growth factor β (TGF-β) family of cytokines are critical regulators of embryonic development, controlling cellular proliferation and differentiation.[27] An excellent overview of the contributions of this family of cytokines to craniofacial development has recently been published.[28] Embryonic orofacial tissue contains functional TGFβ receptors[29,30] that, when activated, elicit changes in orofacial cell proliferation[29] as well as synthesis[31,32] and remodeling[32,33] of the extracellular matrix. From a progenitor cell perspective, cranial neural crest cells also synthesize TGFβ and express cell surface receptors for TGFβ indicating that crest cells are capable of responding to this growth factor in an autocrine and/or paracrine manner.[34] The TGFβs exhibit discrete spatio-temporal patterns of expression in the developing orofacial region[35–38] (Fig. 73–6), and their expression levels can be modulated by numerous convergent signaling peptides.[39–41]

Evidence for the functional role played by these cytokines in orofacial development comes from the cleft palate exhibited by murine embryos, in which *TGFß2* or *TGFß3* are deleted by homologous recombination[42–45] and the demonstrated role of TGFβ in orofacial tissue differentiation.[31,32,46–48] Further evidence for functionality of TGFβ family members during craniofacial ontogeny is provided by studies examining calvarial development. The murine frontal bone derives entirely from the cranial neural crest and recent evidence suggests that TGFβ acts as a morphogen in regulating the fate of the neural crest-derived osteoblasts. The TGFβ type II receptor is required for proliferation of osteoprogenitor cells in frontal bone anlagen and fibroblast growth factor (see below) acts downstream of TGFβ signaling in regulating cranial neural crest cell proliferation.[49]

TGFβ signaling is transduced from the plasma membrane to the nucleus by a family of highly conserved proteins, the Smads. Several excellent reviews outline the molecular mechanisms of this signal transduction process.[50–52] Elements of the Smad component of the TGFβ intracellular signaling system have been identified and characterized in cells of the embryonic orofacial region.[53] Targeted disruption of Smad genes in mice substantiates their importance in craniofacial development inasmuch as *SMAD2* heterozygous null mutants exhibit cleft palate, mandibular hypoplasia, and cyclopia.[54] Moreover, the cleft palate phenotype in *TGFß3–/-* mice was rescued by overexpression of a *SMAD2* transgene in palatal medial edge epithelial cells.[55] In addition, haploinsufficiency of the Smad binding protein 1 gene (*SMADIP1*)

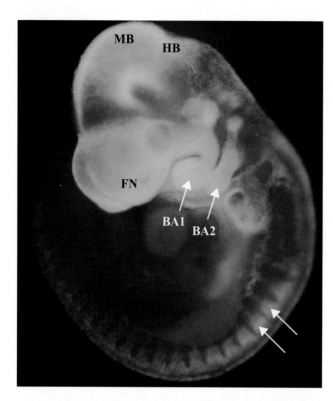

Figure 73–4. Photomicrograph of a E9.5 *Wnt1-Cre/Z/EG* transgenic mouse embryo in which the neural crest cells (NCC) are labeled with enhanced green fluorescent protein (EGFP). Note EGFP labeling of NCCs the first and second branchial arches (BA1 and BA2), and in the frontonasal region (FN). Also note Wnt1-expressing cells in the midbrain/hindbrain (MB and HB) regions. EGFP-labeled NCC also are seen migrating from the CNS at all somitic levels (arrows).

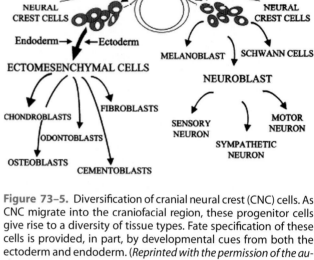

Figure 73–5. Diversification of cranial neural crest (CNC) cells. As CNC migrate into the craniofacial region, these progenitor cells give rise to a diversity of tissue types. Fate specification of these cells is provided, in part, by developmental cues from both the ectoderm and endoderm. (*Reprinted with the permission of the author, Dr. Y. Chai, Center for Craniofacial Molecular Biology, School of Dentistry, Univ. Southern California, Los Angeles, CA, and the International and American Associations for Dental Research; permission conveyed through Copyright Clearance Center, Inc. From: Chai Y, et al. TGF β signaling and its functional significance in regulating the fate of cranial neural crest cells. Crit Rev Oral Biol Med 14:78–88, 2003.*)

has been identified as contributing to a Hirschsprung- like syndrome exhibiting facial dysmorphology.[56] The primary role of Smads, however, is not to target specific genes solely via DNA binding, but rather to function as co-modulators of transcriptional activity by differentially associating with a wide spectrum of nuclear proteins, thus eliciting both positive and negative regulation of numerous genes.[57,58]

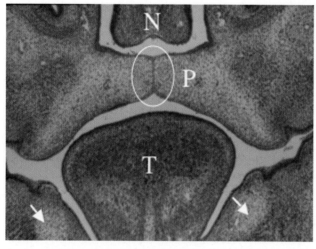

A

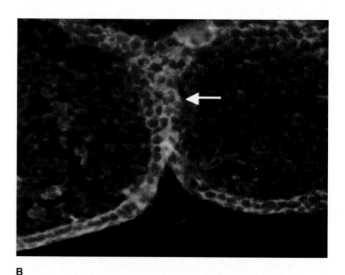

B

Figure 73–6. Coronal paraffin sections of the developing murine orofacial region on day 14 of gestation. By gestational day 14, individual palatal processes (P) (Panel a) have made contact, thereby separating the oral cavity (below the palate), from the nasal cavity (above the palate). Nasal cavity (N); Tongue (T); Meckel's cartilage (arrows); Medial edge epithelial seam (circled). Panel b--Higher magnification of a region similar to that circled in Panel a, demonstrating that immunostaining for TGFβ2 (arrow) predominates in the epithelium of adjacent palatal processes. (*Adapted from Gehris A, D'Angelo M, Greene R. Immunodetection of the transforming growth factors ß1 and ß2 in the developing murine palate. Int J Dev Biol 35:1–8, 1991.*)

Members of the TGFβ superfamily of signaling molecules elicit a wide variety of downstream biologic actions including morphogenesis, cell proliferation, cell differentiation, apoptosis, and extracellular matrix synthesis,[27] and, while their precise roles in orofacial development have not been fully revealed, it is clear that members of this family of proteins, and their signal transduction pathway, play a central role in morphogenesis, growth, and cell differentiation during normal orofacial development.

BONE MORPHOGENETIC PROTEINS

Bone morphogenetic proteins (BMPs) are members of the transforming growth factor-beta superfamily that are widely expressed in the vertebrate embryo and fetus, and regulate an extensive array of biologic responses during embryonic development. Like the TGFβs, BMPs exert their effects by first binding to cell surface serine/threonine kinase receptors, activation of which leads to phosphorylation, and translocation into the nucleus, of intracellular signaling molecules, including, in the case of BMPs, Smad1, Smad5, and Smad8.[59]

Expression of various BMPs is pronounced in embryonic/fetal orofacial tissue during development,[60–62] and targeted disruption of genes encoding BMPs, BMP receptors, and their downstream signal transducers has revealed that BMP signaling is requisite for normal orofacial development.[63] Indeed, BMP signaling has been implicated in the epithelial–mesenchymal transition that marks neural crest cell formation within, and emigration from, the neural plate,[64–66] outgrowth of facial primordia,[60,67] fusion of the maxillary and nasal processes during formation of the upper lip,[68] formation of the secondary palate,[69] and epithelial–mesenchymal interactions leading to orofacial bone and cartilage formation[61] and odontogenesis.[70] A detailed transcriptional map of BMP2 and BMP4 responsiveness in embryonic maxillary mesenchymal cells has recently been delineated and offers revealing insights into crucial molecular regulatory mechanisms employed by these two growth factors in orchestrating embryonic orofacial cellular responses.[71] Moreover, perturbation of BMP expression,[72] or inactivation of genes encoding various cell surface BMP receptors or their downstream Smad mediators[73,74] results in a spectrum of orofacial malformations including cleft palate.

Several of the aforementioned BMP-regulated developmental processes are thought to be mediated by activation of the homeobox transcription factors Msx1 and Msx2. Indeed, functionality of the BMPs in orofacial development comes from the observation that mutations in the *MSX1* homeobox gene—whose expression is required for expression of Bmp4 and Bmp2 in the developing palate[75] are associated with nonsyndromic cleft palate and tooth agenesis in humans.[76] Furthermore, transgenic expression of human *BMP4* in *MSX1*-/- murine embryonic palatal mesenchyme rescues the cleft palate phenotype.[75] Moreover, polymorphisms within the *MSX1* locus are thought to contribute to the incidence of nonsyndromic forms of CLP.[77] The importance of spatial and temporal interactions among signal transduction pathway—critical for normal orofacial ontogenesis—is well illustrated by the control of craniofacial morphogenesis by Msx and Dlx. Orofacial morphogenesis has been shown to require a precise interplay between Msx, Dlx, and the BMP signaling pathway.[69,78] Collectively, these data support the notion that members of the BMP family play pivotal roles in development of the orofacial complex during embryogenesis.

SONIC HEDGEHOG

Members of the hedgehog family of secreted proteins play a key role in embryogenesis. The complexities of the hedgehog signaling network have been recently reviewed by Cohen.[79] Proper spatio-temporal expression of one member of the hedgehog family, sonic hedgehog (Shh), in embryonic facial ectoderm, neuroectoderm, and pharyngeal endoderm during orofacial development has come to be recognized as critical for normal craniofacial morphogenesis,[80,81] especially outgrowth of the frontonasal process[82–84] (Fig. 73–7). Underexpression of Shh perturbs proper growth and development of the frontonasal and maxillary processes resulting in facial clefting, holoprosencephaly, and cyclopia, while overexpression of Shh leads to a wider than normal gap between the eyes, a condition known as hyperteleorism.[85] Moreover, mutations in the human and murine *Shh* genes also result in holoprosencephaly and cyclopia.[79,86,87]

Interactions between the sonic hedgehog and BMP signal transduction pathways have assumed a leading role among the processes that are thought to mediate orofacial morphogenesis. Functional interactions between the Shh and BMP signaling pathways have been documented for skeletal development,[88] neural patterning and differentiation[89] and tooth morphogenesis.[90] Functionality of the Shh/BMP interaction during orofacial development has been confirmed by studies using Msx1-deficient mice that exhibit numerous craniofacial abnormalities including cleft palate. Shh, normally expressed in embryonic palatal epithelial tissue, activates BMP2 expression in the palatal mesenchyme which in turn acts as a mitogen to stimulate mesenchymal cell division. Transgenic expression of BMP4 in Msx1-deficient mice rescued the cleft palate phenotype as well as restored Shh and BMP2 expression and normal levels of mesenchymal cell proliferation.[75]

Perturbations in certain Shh-related genes is associated with failure of the embryonic forebrain (prosencephalon) to divide into paired cerebral hemispheres.[80,91] The resulting single-lobed brain structure, with accompanying skull and facial defects, defines a condition referred to as holoprosencephaly (HPE). While the most severe cases are embryolethal, phenotypes vary in severity. Phenotypes may include median cleft lip (premaxillary agenesis), ethmocephaly, cebocephaly, and cyclopia. It is thus not surprising that *Shh* also contributes to proper development of the facial skeleton.[82,92,93]

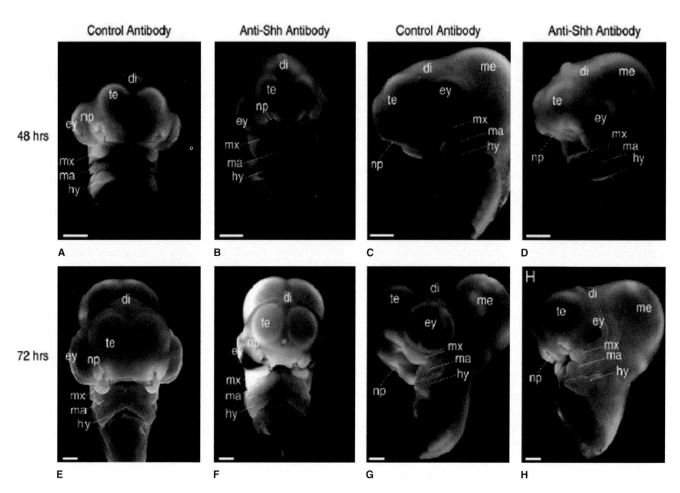

Figure 73–7. Craniofacial development after Shh inhibition. Forty-eight hours after treatment with control antibodies, avian embryos exhibit a normal craniofacial complex (A, C). The eyes (ey) are prominent and the retina is pigmented. The telencephalon (te) is divided into right and left halves, the maxillary (mx), mandibular (ma), and hyoid (hy) arches are apparent, and the nasal pits (np) are widely spaced (A, dotted brackets). Forty-eight hours after treatment with anti-Shh antibody, avian embryos exhibit marked morphological alterations of the craniofacial complex (B, D). Eyes are reduced in size and rotated ventrally; the telencephalon is smaller than in controls; nasal pits are close together (B, bracket); the frontonasal and maxillary primordia appear shorter than in controls. Seventy-two hours after treatment with control antibodies, the eyes have enlarged and the facial primordia are well defined (E, F). Seventy-two hours after treatment with anti-Shh antibody, the eye is reduced in size; the entire frontonasal primordium appears blunted compared to control embryos (F, H). di, diencephalon; me, mesencephalon. Scale bars: 0.5 mm. (*Reprinted with the permission of the author, Dr. Jill Helms, Stanford University, Palo Alto, CA, and Elsevier Publishing. From: Marcucio R, Cordero D, Hu D, Helms J. Molecular interactions coordinating the development of the forebrain and face. Develop Biol 284:48–61, 2005.*)

FIBROBLAST GROWTH FACTORS

Fibroblast growth factors (FGFs) represent a large family of paracrine and autocrine factors that function in controlling cell differentiation, proliferation, survival, and motility.[94] Numerous members of this family, as well as their receptors, are expressed in the developing branchial arch ecto- and endoderm[95–100] where they contribute to a dialogue necessary for proper cell and tissue differentiation, as well as outgrowth and patterning of the facial primordia.[101–102] Noteworthy is the fact that *FGF10* homozygous null mutant mice exhibit cleft palate,[104] and mutations in these ligands or their receptors have been associated with syndromes characterized by craniofacial defects, including cleft palate, such as Apert, Saethre-Chotzen, and Crouzon syndromes.[97,105–109]

Before the migration of neural crest cells into the branchial arches—an influx governed in part by FGF receptor expression in the pharyngeal region,[103] and accompanied by expression of FGF8 transcripts in the ectoderm of the facial processes[110] the ventral head ectoderm expresses FGF8 in the area corresponding to the future mandibular arch. These expression patterns, which foreshadow the initial site of frontonasal process outgrowth, are consistent with the observations that FGFs are chemotactic for neural crest cells[111] and affect outgrowth of neural crest cells in branchial arch explant cultures.[112] Thus, the FGFs may regulate neural crest cell migration into the branchial arches.

Once neural crest cells have populated the frontonasal process, however, their developmental fate is redefined,[113] and delineation of the maxillomandibular region is established.

This is accomplished in part by FGF8-induced altered expression of the target genes *Dlx1* and *Barx1*,[114] support of neural crest cell survival and differentiation,[115] as well as repatterning of the craniofacial primordia.[114] Moreover, FGF signaling is required for pharyngeal skeletogenesis,[116] and antagonistic interactions between FGF and BMP signaling regulate development of both the teeth and the secondary palate.[117]

Collectively, these observations support the premise that members of the FGF family of signaling molecules not only create a permissive environment within the developing branchial arches for neural crest cell entry, but may also facilitate crest cell migration into the branchial arches, and contribute to maxillomandibular tissue specification and neural crest cell maintenance within the branchial arches.

Wnt SIGNALING

Wingless (Wnt) comprises a large, highly conserved, secreted, lipid-modified family of glycoproteins that act as morphogens during early embryonic patterning, cell proliferation, differentiation, and apoptosis.[118] Loss of Wnt function in vertebrates results in a wide spectrum of developmental defects. A current list of known *Wnt* genes and sequence alignments can be found on the Wnt homepage (http://www.stanford.edu/-rnusse/wntwindow.html). Wnts initiate signaling by binding two transmembrane receptors: frizzled (Fz), a heptahelical receptor protein similar to G-protein coupled receptors, and members of the low-density lipoprotein receptor related protein family (LRP) (Fig. 73–8). The cellular response to Wnt signals include alterations in gene transcription (generally referred to as the canonical pathway), regulation of cell polarity, and changes in intracellular Ca^{2+} levels. Thus, Wnt stimulation can lead to at least three different signaling outputs. Wnt-induced changes in gene transcription are mediated, intracellularly, by the multifunctional, nucleocytoplasmic transcription cofactor, β-catenin.[119]

Considerable effort has been directed toward identification of signaling molecules/pathways that regulate neural crest cell induction, migration, and differentiation. The Wnt family of proteins has emerged as an essential contributor to these processes.[120] The Lef/β-catenin binding complex is a downstream effector of Wnt signaling. Thus, identification of Lef/β-catenin binding sites in the promotor of the *Xenopus Slug* gene—an early neural crest marker—provides persuasive evidence that Wnts are directly involved in neural crest cell induction.[121] As indicated above, inhibition of BMP signaling blocks migration of neural crest cells from the margins of the neural folds.[65] This effect is mediated, in part, by interactions with the Wnt signaling pathway.[122–124] Indeed, the currently prevailing notion is that neural crest cell induction involves interactions between a BMP gradient, (established by the BMP antagonist Noggin),[125,126] and FGF and Wnt signaling.[11] Identification of some of the downstream targets of neural crest induction by Wnt has only recently been explored. Wnt signaling transiently upregulates, in a distinct temporal pattern, the expression of several

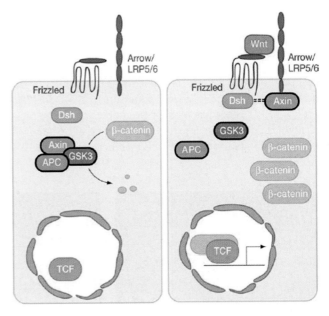

Figure 73–8. The canonical Wnt signaling pathway. In cells not exposed to a Wnt signal (left panel), ß-catenin is degraded through interactions with Axin, APC, and the protein kinase GSK-3. Wnt proteins (right panel) bind to the Frizzled/LRP receptor complex at the cell surface. These receptors transduce a signal to Dishevelled (Dsh) and to Axin, which may directly interact (dashed lines). As a consequence, the degradation of ß-catenin is inhibited, and this protein accumulates in the cytoplasm and nucleus. ß-Catenin then interacts with TCF to control the transcription. (*Reprinted with the permission of the author, Dr. Roel Nusse, Howard Hughes Medical Institute, Department of Developmental Biology, Beckman Center, Stanford University, Stanford, CA and Annual Reviews; From: Logan C, Nusse R. The Wnt signaling pathway in development and disease. Annu Rev Cell Dev Biol 20:781–810, 2004.*)

genes normally expressed in the dorsal neural tube (*PAX3, MSX1, FOXD3, CADHERIN 6B*), at "premigratory" stages.[127] This is consistent with the notion of Wnt, along with BMP, being an inducer of neural crest in the embryonic neural plate.[128]

After their induction, and subsequent to a BMP/Wnt signaling-dependent delamination from the neural tube,[65] neural crest cells migrate extensively throughout the embryo. Thus, while canonical Wnt signaling pathway is required for neural crest *induction*, the noncanonical Wnt signaling (planar cell polarity, or Wnt-Ca^{2+}) pathway, via Wnt 11, appears to be required for neural crest *migration*.[129] Germane here is the migration of cranial neural crest cells into the first two branchial arches and diversification of neural crest cell fates as they relate to orofacial development. Interestingly, cooperative interaction between the BMP and Wnt signaling pathways is implied by the observation that BMP-2 and -4 both upregulate the expression of genes encoding several frizzled proteins (Fzd-4, -7, and -9) in developing orofacial tissue.[71] Wnt/β-catenin signal activation also regulates neural crest progenitor cell fate decisions. For example, the transcription factor Sox10, whose expression is controlled by Wnt proteins,[130] contributes to specification of the pigment cell lineage by neural crest cells.[131] Canonical Wnt signaling also induces a sensory fate in a defined subpopulation of cranial neural crest cells.[132] BMP signaling, however, antagonizes the sensory fate-inducing activity of Wnt signaling.[133] Subsequent expansion of cranial neural crest cells into the first branchial arch, where they contribute to the development of orofacial skeletal components, also depend, in part, on Wnt signaling.[134,135] Indeed, expression of *WNT-5a, -10a, -10b, and -11* genes has recently been detected in the mesenchyme of developing murine facial primordia.[95] Moreover, genes encoding various Wnt family members (Wnt-3, -4, -5a,

and -10b) and Frizzled-related proteins (Fzd-4, Flamigo-1, secreted frizzled related sequence protein 4 or Sfrp4) were found to be differentially expressed in embryonic orofacial tissue.[95] Additional functional evidence for the involvement of Wnt signaling in orofacial development comes from the observation that mutations in the *WNT3* and *WNT9b* genes—expressed in developing orofacial tissue in a pattern consistent with a role in midfacial development[136] (Fig. 73–9)—were associated with cleft lip with or without cleft palate (CLP).[137]

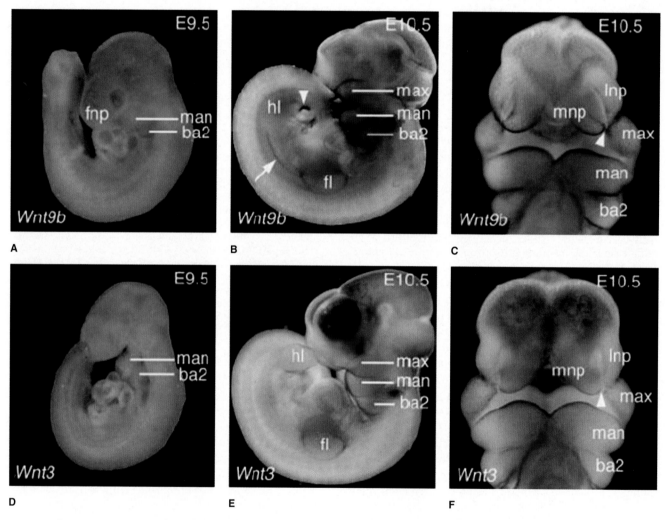

Figure 73–9. Expression of *Wnt9b* and *Wnt3* mRNAs during murine craniofacial development. A: Lateral view of an E9.5 embryo showing *Wnt9b* mRNA expression in the head ectoderm. B: Lateral view of an E10.5 embryo showing *Wnt9b* mRNA expression in the nephric duct (arrow), the genital tubercle (arrowhead), and in the facial ectoderm. C: Facial view of the embryo in B showing strong *Wnt9b* mRNA expression in the distal epithelium of the medial nasal, lateral nasal, and maxillary processes as well as in the rostral surface of the mandibular processes. Arrowhead points to site of future lip fusion. D: Lateral view of an E9.5 embryo hybridized with the *Wnt3* cRNA probe. *Wnt3* mRNA is expressed in the tailbud but not in the craniofacial region at this stage. E: Lateral view of an E10.5 embryo hybridized with the *Wnt3* cRNA probe. *Wnt3* mRNA expression at this stage is weak except in the distal facial ectoderm. F: Facial view of the embryo in E showing relatively abundant *Wnt3* mRNA expression in the maxillary and rostral mandibular processes. Weak expression is seen on the oral surface of the medial nasal processes but not at the site of contact between the medial and lateral nasal processes (arrowhead). ba2, second brancial arch; fl, forelimb bud; fnp, frontonasal process; hl, hindlimb bud; lnp, lateral nasal process; man, mandibular process; max, maxillary process; mnp, medial nasal process. (*Reprinted with the permission of the author, Dr. Rulang Jiang, Center for Oral Biology, University of Rochester Medical Center, 601 Elmwood Avenue, Box 611, Rochester, NY, and Wiley-Liss Inc. From: Lan Y, Ryan R, Zhang Z, et al. Expression of Wnt9b and activation of canonical Wnt signaling during midfacial morphogenesis in mice. Develop Dynam 235:1448–1454, 2006.*)

Moreover, the demonstration of functional interactions between the TGFβ and Wnt signaling pathway in cells derived from the embryonic orofacial region suggest that Wnt activation of the canonical pathway is an important mediator of first branchial arch mesenchymal cell growth.[138]

CONCLUSION

Viewing a developing embryo elicits amazement at Nature's handiwork. Despite the molecular complexity necessary for normal ontogenesis, most offspring that are born are normal. Nevertheless, nearly one million infants are born worldwide each year exhibiting abnormal facies. This translates into the alarming statistic that every 5 minutes a child is born with a craniofacial defect. In this country, where cleft lip and/or palate represent the most prevalent birth defect, a child is born with a facial cleft every hour, of every day, of the year. The remarkable successes of biomedical research notwithstanding, the frequency of congenital craniofacial anomalies remains distressingly high. Despite an impressive broadening of our understanding of the signaling cascades orchestrating orofacial ontogeny—some of which have been outlined in the present chapter—the fundamental mechanisms governing these processes in normal orofacial development, and their dysregulation resulting in orofacial clefting, remain poorly defined.

Galileo wrote that "...Nature's great book is written in the language of mathematics." Genomic array technology, using mathematical algorithms to illuminate gene clusters as well as pathways critical for morphogenesis, has provided fascinating insights into the development of a spectrum of biologic systems. Because of such approaches, and despite the fact that such analyses are statistical and not deterministic, the cast of gene and protein characters that play on the cellular stage of orofacial ontogeny continues to expand.[139–141] Such approaches, and evolving technological advances, offer renewed hope that a better understanding of the mechanisms of orofacial development will lead to a reduction in the frequency of congenital orofacial anomalies.

ACKNOWLEDGMENTS

The authors wish to acknowledge support for their own investigations that has been provided in part by PHS grants DE05550 and HD053509 to RMG and ES11775 to MMP; and by The Commonwealth of Kentucky Research Challenge Trust Fund. This publication was also made possible in part by support provided by PHS grant P20-RR/DE17702 to RMG from the COBRE Program of the National Center for Research Resources.

References

1. Stanier P, Moore G. Genetics of cleft lip and palate: Syndromic genes contribute to the incidence of non-syndromic clefts. *Hum Mol Genet* 13:R73–R81, 2004.

2. Gorlin R, Cohen M, Hennekam R. *Syndromes of the Head and Neck.* New York: Oxford University Press, 2001, p. 1283.

3. Cerny R, Lwigale P, Ericsson R, et al. Developmental origins and evolution of jaws: New interpretation of 'maxillary' and 'mandibular'. *Develop Biol* 276:225–236, 2004.

4. Lee S, Bedard O, Buchtova M, et al. A new origin for the maxillary jaw. *Develop Biol* 276:207–224, 2004.

5. Jugessur A, Murray J. Orofacial clefting: Recent insights into a complex trait. *Curr Opin Genet Dev* 15:270–278, 2005.

6. Lidral A, Murray J. Genetic approaches to identify disease genes for birth defects with cleft lip/palate as a model. *Birth Defects Res A* 70:893–901, 2004.

7. Graham A. Development of the pharyngeal arches. *Am J Med Genet* 119A:251–256, 2003.

8. Helms J, Schneider R. Cranial skeletal biology. *Nature* 423:326–331, 2003.

9. Kontges G, Lumsden A. Rhombencephalic neural crest segmentation is preserved throughout craniofacial ontogeny. *Development* 122:3229–3242, 1996.

10. Bronner-Fraser M. Mechanisms of neural crest migration. *Bioessays* 15:221–230, 1993.

11. LaBonne C, Bronner-Fraser M. Molecular mechanisms of neural crest formation. *Ann Rev Cell Dev Biol* 15:81–112, 1999.

12. Schneider R, Helms J. The cellular and molecular origins of beak morphology. *Science* 299:565–568, 2003.

13. Tucker A, Lumsden A. Neural crest cells provide species-specific patterning information in the developing branchial skeleton. *Evol Dev* 6:32–40, 2004.

14. Le Douarin N, Creuzet S, Couly G, et al. Neural crest cell plasticity and its limits. *Development* 131:4637–4650, 2004.

15. Noden D, Trainor P. Relations and interactions between cranial mesoderm and neural crest populations. *J Anat* 207:575–601, 2005.

16. Trainor P, Ariza-McNaughton L, Krumlauf R. Role of the isthmus and FGFs in resolving the paradox of neural crest plasticity and prepatterning. *Science* 295:1288–1291, 2002.

17. Golding J, Trainor P, Krumlauf R, et al. Defects in path finding by cranial neural crest cells in mice lacking the neuregulin receptor ErbB4. *Nature Cell Biol* 2:103–109, 2000.

18. Couly G, Bennaceur S, Vincent C, et al. Interactions between Hox-negative cephalic neural crest cells and the foregut endoderm in patterning the facial skeleton in the vertebrate head. *Development* 129:1061–1073, 2002.

19. Graham A, Okabe M, Quinlan R. The role of the endoderm in the development and evolution of the pharyngeal arches. *J Anat* 207:479–487, 2005.

20. Helms J, Cordero D, Tapadia M. New insights into craniofacial morphogenesis. *Development* 132:851–861, 2005.

21. Bolande R. Neurocristopathy: Its growth and development in 20 years. *Pediatr Pathol Lab Med* 17:1–25, 1997.

22. Greene R, Weston W, Nugent P, et al. Signal transduction pathways as targets for induced embryotoxicity. In Slikker W, Chang L (eds). *Handbook of Developmental Neurotoxicology.* San Diego: Academic Press Inc, 1998, pp. 119–139.

23. Shuler C. Programmed cell death and transformation in craniofacial development. *Crit Rev Oral Biol Med* 6:202–217, 1995.

24. Francis-West P, Robson L, Evans D. Craniofacial development: The tissue and molecular interactions that control development of the head. *Adv Anat Embryol Cell Biol* 169:1–138, 2003.

25. Helms J, Cordero D, Tapadia M. New insights into craniofacial morphogenesis. *Development* 132:851–861, 2005.

26. Tapadia M, Cordero D, Helms J. It's all in your head: New insights into craniofacial development and deformation. *J Anat* 207:461–477, 2005.

27. Massagué J, Blain S, Lo R. TGFbeta signaling in growth control, cancer, and heritable disorders. *Cell* 103:295–309, 2000.

28. Dudas M, Kaartinen V. Tgf-beta superfamily and mouse craniofacial development: Interplay of morphogenetic proteins and receptor

signaling controls normal formation of the face. *Curr Top Dev Biol* 66:65–133, 2005.

29. Linask K, D'Angelo M, Gehris A, et al. Transforming growth factor-ß receptor profiles of human and murine embryonic palate mesenchymal cells. *Exp Cell Res* 192:1–9, 1991.

30. Cui X, Shuler C. The TGF-beta type III receptor is localized to the medial edge epithelium during palatal fusion. *Int J Dev Biol* 44:397–402, 2002.

31. D'Angelo M, Greene R. Transforming growth factor-ß modulation of glycosaminoglycan production by mesenchymal cells of the developing murine secondary palate. *Develop Biol* 145:374–378, 1991.

32. D'Angelo M, Chen JM, Ugen K, et al. TGFß1 regulation of collagen metabolism by embryonic palate mesenchymal cells. *J Exp Zool* 270:189–201, 1994.

33. Brown N, Yarram S, Mansell J, et al. Matrix metelloproteinases have a role in palatogenesis. *J Dent Res* 81:826–830, 2002.

34. Brauer P, Yee J. Cranial neural crest cells synthesize and secrete a latent form of transforming growth factor ß that can be activated by neural crest cell proteolysis. *Develop Biol* 155:281–285, 1993.

35. Behman S, Guo C, Gong T-W, et al. Gene and protein expression of transforming growth factor ß 2 gene during murine primary palatogenesis. *Differentiation* 73:233–239, 2005.

36. Fitzpatrick D, Denhez F, Kondaiah P, et al. Differential expression of TGFß isoforms in murine palatogenesis. *Development* 109:585–595, 1990.

37. Gehris A, D'Angelo M, Greene R. Immunodetection of the transforming growth factors ß$_1$ and ß2 in the developing murine palate. *Int J Dev Biol* 35:1–8, 1991.

38. Pelton R, Saxena B, Jones M, et al. Immunohistochemical localization of TGF-B1, TGF-B2, and TGF-B3 in the mouse embryo: Expression patterns suggest multiple roles during embryonic development. *J Cell Biol* 115:1091–1105, 1991.

39. Gehris A, Pisano M, Nugent P, et al. Regulation of TGFß gene expression in embryonic palatal tissue. *In Vitro Dev Biol* 30A:671–679, 1994.

40. Potchinsky M, Nugent P, Lafferty C, et al. Effects of dexamethasone on the expression of transforming growth factor-ß in mouse embryonic palate mesenchyme cells. *J Cell Physiol* 166:380–386, 1996.

41. Nugent P, Lafferty C, Greene R. Differential expression and biological activity of retinoic acid-induced TGFß isoforms in embryonic palate mesenchymal cells. *J Cell Physiol* 177:36–46, 1998.

42. Kaartinen V, Voncken J, Schuler C, et al. Abnormal lung development and cleft palate in mice lacking TGF-ß3 indicates defects of epithelial-mesenchymal interaction. *Nature Genet* 11:415–421, 1995.

43. Proetzel G, Pawlowski S, Wilesm M, et al. Transforming growth factor-ß3 is required for secondary palate fusion. *Nature Genet* 11:409–414, 1995.

44. Sanford L, Ormsby I, Gittenberger-de Groot A, et al. TGF-ß2 knockout mice have multiple developmental defects that are non-overlapping with other TGF-ß knockout phenotypes. *Development* 124:2659–2670, 1997.

45. Koo S, Cunningham M, Arabshahi B, et al. The transforming growth factor-ß3 knock-out mouse: An animal model for cleft palate. *Plast Reconstr Surg* 108:938–948, 2001.

46. Cui X, Chai Y, Chen J, et al. TGF-ß3-dependent SMAD2 phosphorylation and inhibition of MEE proliferation during palatal fusion. *Develop Dynam* 227:387–394, 2003.

47. Brunet C, Sharpe P, Ferguson M. Inhibition of TGFß3 (but not TGFß1 or TGFß2) actively prevents normal mouse embryonic palate fusion. *Int J Dev Biol* 39:345–355, 1993.

48. Gehris A, Greene R. Regulation of murine embryonic epithelial cell differentiation by transforming growth factors ß. *Differentiation* 49:167–173, 1992.

49. Sasaki T, Ito Y, Bringas P, Jr., et al. TGF{beta}-mediated FGF signaling is crucial for regulating cranial neural crest cell proliferation during frontal bone development. *Development* 133:371–381, 2006.

50. Itoh S, Itoh F, Goumans M-J, et al. Signaling of transforming growth factor-ß family members through Smad proteins. *Eur J Biochem* 267:6954–6967, 2000.

51. Massagué J, Wotton D. Transcriptional control by the TGF-ß/Smad signaling system. *EMBO J* 19:1745–1754, 2000.

52. Shi Y. Structural insights on Smad function in TGF-ß signaling. *Bioessays* 23:223–232, 2001.

53. Greene R, Nugent P, Mukhopadhyay P, et al. Intracellular dynamics of Smad-mediated TGFß signaling. *J Cell Physiol* 197:261–271, 2003.

54. Nomura M, Li E. Smad2 role in mesoderm formation, left-right patterning and craniofacial development. *Nature* 393:786–790, 1998.

55. Cui XM, Shiomi N, Chen J, et al. Overexpression of Smad2 in TGFß3-null mutant mice rescues cleft palate. *Develop Biol* 278:193–202, 2005.

56. Cacheux V, Dastot-Le Moal F, Kääriäinen H, et al. Loss-of-function mutations in SIP1 Smad interacting protein 1 results in a syndromic Hirschsprung disease. *Hum Mol Genet* 14:1503–1510, 2001.

57. Attisano L, Wrana J. Smads as transcriptional co-modulators. *Curr Opin Cell Biol* 12:235–243, 2000.

58. ten Dijke P, Miyazono K, Heldin C. Signaling inputs converge on nuclear effectors in TGF-ß signaling. *Trends Biochem Sci* 25:64–70, 2000.

59. Balemans W, Van Hul W. Extracellular regulation of BMP signaling in vertebrates: A cocktail of modulators. *Develop Biol* 250:231–250, 2002.

60. Francis-West P, Tatla T, Brickell P. Expression patterns of the bone morphogenetic protein genes Bmp-4 and Bmp-2 in the developing chick face suggest a role in outgrowth of the primordia. *Develop Dynam* 201:168–178, 1994.

61. Bennett J, Hunt P, Thorogood P. Bone morphogenetic protein-2 and -4 expression during murine orofacial development. *Arch Oral Biol* 40:847–854, 1995.

62. Gong SG, Guo C. Bmp4 gene is expressed at the putative site of fusion in the midfacial region. *Differentiation* 71:228–236, 2003.

63. Zhao G. Consequences of knocking out BMP signaling in the mouse. *Genesis* 35:43–56, 2003.

64. Aybar M, Glavic A, Mayor R. Extracellular signals, cell interactions and transcription factors involved in the induction of the neural crest cells. *Biol Res* 35:267–275, 2002.

65. Burstyn-Cohen T, Stanleigh J, Sela-Donenfeld D, et al. Canonical Wnt activity regulates trunk neural crest delamination linking BMP/noggin signaling with G1/S transition. *Development* 131:5327–5329, 2004.

66. Karafiat V, Dvorakova M, Krejci E, et al. Transcription factor c-Myb is involved in the regulation of the epithelial-mesenchymal transition in the avian neural crest. *Cell Mol Life Sci* 62:2516–2525, 2005.

67. Ashique A, Fu K, Richman JM. Endogenous bone morphogenetic proteins regulate outgrowth and epithelial survival during avian lip fusion. *Development* 129:4647–4660, 2002.

68. Liu W, Sun X, Braut A, et al. Distinct functions for Bmp signaling in lip and palate fusion in mice. *Development* 132:1453–1461, 2005.

69. Levi G, Mantero S, Barbieri O, et al. Msx1 and Dlx5 act independently in development of craniofacial skeleton, but converge on the regulation of Bmp signaling in palate formation. *Mech Dev* 123:3–16, 2006.

70. Wang Y, Rutherford B, Upholt WB, et al. Effects of BMP-7 on mouse tooth mesenchyme and chick mandibular mesenchyme. *Develop Dynam* 216:320–335, 1999.

71. Mukhopadhyay P, Singh S, Greene R, et al. Molecular fingerprinting of BMP2- and BMP4-treated embryonic maxillary mesenchymal cells. *Orthod Craniofacial Res* 9:93–110, 2006.

72. Lu H, Jin Y, Tipoe G. Alteration in the expression of bone morphogenetic protein-2,3,4,5 mRNA during pathogenesis of cleft palate in BALB/c mice. *Arch Oral Biol* 45:133–140, 2000.

73. Chang H, Huylebroeck D, Verschueren K, et al. Smad5 knockout mice die at mid-gestation due to multiple embryonic and extraembryonic defects. *Development* 126:1631–1642, 1999.

74. Dudas M, Sridurongrit S, Nagy A, et al. Craniofacial defects in mice lacking BMP type I receptor Alk2 in neural crest cells. *Mech Dev* 121:173–182, 2004.

75. Zhang Z, Song Y, Zhao X, et al. Rescue of cleft palate in Msx1-deficient mice by transgenic Bmp4 reveals a network of BMP and Shh signaling in the regulation of mammalian palatogenesis. *Development* 129:4135–4146, 2002.

76. van den Boogaard MJ, Dorland M, Beemer FA, et al. MSX1 mutation is associated with orofacial clefting and tooth agenesis in humans. *Nat Genet* 24:342–343, 2000.

77. Lidral A, Romitti P, Basart A, et al. Association of MSX1 and TGFß3 with nonsyndromic clefting in humans. *Am J Hum Genet* 63:557–568, 1998.

78. Tribulo C, Aybar M, Nguyen V, Mullins M, Mayor R. Regulation of Msx genes by a Bmp gradient is essential for neural crest specification. *Development* 130:6441–6452, 2003.

79. Cohen M. The sonic hedgehog signaling pathway. In Epstein C, Erickson R, Wynshaw-Boris A (eds). *Inborn Errors of Development.* New York: Oxford University Press, 2004, pp. 210–228.

80. Cordero D, Marcucio R, Hu D, et al. Temporal perturbations in sonic hedgehog signaling elicit the spectrum of holoprosencephaly phenotypes. *J Clin Invest* 114:485–494, 2004.

81. Wada N, Javidan Y, Nelson S, et al. Hedgehog signaling is required for cranial neural crest morphogenesis and chondrogenesis at the midline in the zebrafish skull. *Development* 132:3977–3988, 2004.

82. Jeong J, Mao J, Tenzen T, et al. Hedgehog signaling in the neural crest cells regulates the patterning and growth of facial primordia. *Genes Dev* 18:937–951, 2004.

83. Marcucio R, Cordero D, Hu D, et al. Molecular interactions coordinating the development of the forebrain and face. *Develop Biol* 284:48–61, 2004.

84. Ahlgren S, Thakur V, Bronner-Fraser M. Sonic hedgehog rescues cranial neural crest from cell death induced by ethanol exposure. *Proc Natl Acad Sci USA* 99:10476–10481, 2002.

85. Hu D, Helms JA. The role of sonic hedgehog in normal and abnormal craniofacial morphogenesis. *Development* 126:4873–4884 1999.

86. Muenke M, Cohen M. Genetic approaches to understanding brain development: Holoprosencephaly as a model. *Ment Retard Dev Disabil Res Rev* 6:15–21, 2000.

87. Roessler E, Belloni E, Gaudenz K, et al. Mutations in the human sonic hedgehog gene cause holoprosencephaly. *Nat Genet* 14:357–360, 1996.

88. Yuasa T, Kataoka H, Kinto N, et al. Sonic hedgehog is involved in osteoblast differentiation by cooperating with BMP-2. *J Cell Physiol* 193:225–232, 2002.

89. Liem KF, Jessell TM, Briscoe J. Regulation of the neural patterning activity of sonic hedgehog by secreted BMP inhibitors expressed by notochord and somites. *Development* 127:4855–4866, 2000.

90. Zhang Y, Zhang Z, Zhao X, et al. A new function of BMP4: Dual role for BMP4 in regulation of sonic hedgehog expression in the mouse tooth germ. *Development* 127:1431–1443, 2000.

91. Marini M, Cusano R, De Biasio P, et al. Previously undescribed nonsense mutation in SHH caused autosomal dominant holoprosencephaly with wide intrafamilial variability. *Am J Med Genet* 117A:112–115, 2003.

92. Abzhanov A, Tabin C. Shh and Fgf8 act synergistically to drive cartilage outgrowth during cranial development. *Develop Biol* 273:134–148, 2004.

93. Melnick M, Witcher D, Bringas P, Jr., et al. Meckel's cartilage differentiation is dependent on hedgehog signaling. *Cells Tissues Organs* 179:146–157, 2005.

94. Basilico C, Moscatelli D. The FGF family of growth factors and oncogenes. *Adv Cancer Res* 59:115–165, 1992.

95. Mukhopadhyay P, Greene RM, Zacharias W, et al. Developmental gene expression profiling of mammalian, fetal orofacial tissue. *Birth Defects Res A Clin Mol Teratol* 70:912–926, 2004.

96. Abu-Issa R, Smyth G, Smoak I, et al. Fgf8 is required for pharyngeal arch and cardiovascular development in the mouse. *Development* 129:4613–4625, 2002.

97. Britto J, Evans R, Hayward R, et al. Toward pathogenesis of Apert cleft palate: FGF, FGFR, and TGF beta genes are differentially expressed in sequential stages of human palatal shelf fusion. *Cleft Palate Craniofac J* 39:332–340, 2002.

98. Lee S, Crisera C, Erfani S, et al. Immunolocalization of fibroblast growth factor receptors 1 and 2 in mouse palate development. *Plast Reconstr Surg* 107:1776–1784, 2001.

99. Wilke TA, Gubbels S, Schwartz J, et al. Expression of fibroblast growth factor receptors (FGFR1, FGFR2, FGFR3) in the developing head and face. Develop Dynam 210:41–52, 1997.

100. Bachler M, Neubuser A. Expression of members of the Fgf family and their receptors during midfacial development. *Mech Dev* 100:313–316, 2001.

101. Crump J, Maves L, Lawson N, et al. An essential role for Fgfs in endodermal pouch formation influences later craniofacial skeletal patterning. *Development* 131:5703–5716, 2004.

102. Trokovic N, Trokovic R, Mai P, et al. Fgfr1 regulates patterning of the pharyngeal region. *Genes Dev* 17:141–153, 2003.

103. Trokovic N, Trokovic R, Partanen, N. Fibroblast growth factor signalling and regional specification of the pharyngeal ectoderm. *Int J Dev Biol* 49:797–805, 2005.

104. Alappat S, Zhang Z, Suzukib K, et al. The cellular and molecular etiology of the cleft secondary palate in Fgf10 mutant mice. *Develop Biol* 277:102–113, 2005.

105. Baroni T, Lilli C, Marinucci L, et al. Crouzon's syndrome: Differential in vitro secretion of bFGF, TGFbeta I isoforms and extracellular matrix macromolecules in patients with FGFR2 gene mutation. *Cytokine* 19:94–101, 2002.

106. Chun K, Teebi AS, Jung JH, et al. Genetic analysis of patients with the Saethre-Chotzen phenotype. *Am J Med Genet* 110:136–143, 2002.

107. Frank DU, Fotheringham LK, Brewer JA, et al. An Fgf8 mouse mutant phenocopies human 22q11 deletion syndrome. *Development* 129:4591–4603, 2002.

108. Fujisawa H, Hasegawa M, Kida S, et al. A novel fibroblast growth factor receptor 2 mutation in Crouzon syndrome associated with Chiari type I malformation and syringomyelia. *J Neurosurg* 97:396–400, 2002.

109. Shotelersuk V, Mahatumarat C, Ittiwut C, et al. FGFR2 mutations among Thai children with Crouzon and Apert syndromes. *J Craniofac Surg* 14:101–104, 2003.

110. McGonnell IM, Clarke JD, Tickle C. Fate map of the developing chick face: Analysis of expansion of facial primordia and establishment of the primary palate. *Develop Dynam* 212:102–118, 1998.

111. Kubota Y, Ito K. Chemotactic migration of mesencephalic neural crest cells in the mouse. *Develop Dynam* 217:170–179, 2000.

112. Tucker AS, Khamis AL, Ferguson CA, et al. Conserved regulation of mesenchymal gene expression by Fgf-8 in face and limb development. *Development* 126:221–228, 1999.

113. Hu D, Marcucio RS, Helms JA. A zone of frontonasal ectoderm regulates patterning and growth in the face. *Development* 130:1749–1758, 2003.

114. Shigetani Y, Nobusada Y, Kuratani S. Ectodermally derived FGF8 defines the maxillomandibular region in the early chick embryo: Epithelial-mesenchymal interactions in the specification of the craniofacial ectomesenchyme. *Develop Biol* 228:73–85, 2000.

115. Trumpp A, Depew MJ, Rubenstein JL, et al. Cre-mediated gene inactivation demonstrates that FGF8 is required for cell survival and patterning of the first branchial arch. *Genes Dev* 13:3136–3148, 1999.

116. Creuzet S, Schuler B, Couly G, et al. Reciprocal relationships between Fgf8 and neural crest cells in facial and forebrain development. *Proc Natl Acad Sci USA* 101:4843–4847, 2004.

117. Rice R, Thesleff I, Rice D. Regulation of *Twist, Snail,* and *Id1* is conserved between the developing murine palate and tooth. *Develop Dynam* 234:28–35, 2005.

118. Wodarz A, Nusse R. Mechanisms of Wnt signaling in development. *Ann Rev Cell Dev Biol* 14:59–88, 1998.

119. Mulholland D, Dedhar S, Coetzee G, et al. Interaction of nuclear receptors with the Wnt/beta-catenin/Tcf signaling axis: Wnt you like to know? *Endocrine Rev* 26:898–915, 2005.

120. Schmidt C, Patel K. Wnts and the neural crest. *Anat Embryol* 209:349–355, 2005.

121. Vallin J, Thuret R, Giacomello E, et al. Cloning and characterization of three Xenopus slug promoter reveal direct regulation by Lef/ß-catenin signalling. *J Biol Chem* 32:30350–30358, 2001.

122. Garcia-Castro M, Marcelle C, Bronner-Fraser M. Ectodermal Wnt function as a neural crest inducer. *Science* 297:848–851, 2002.

123. Raible D, Ragland J. Reiterated Wnt and BMP signals in neural crest development. *Semin Cell Dev Biol* 16:673–682, 2005.

124. Wu J, Yang J, Klein P, et al. Neural crest induction by the canonical Wnt pathway can be dissociated from anterior-posterior neural patterning in Xenopus. *Develop Biol* 279:220–232, 2005.

125. Baker C, Bronner-Fraser M. The origins of the neural crest. Part I: Embryonic induction. *Mech Dev* 69:3–11, 1997.

126. Marchant L, Linker C, Ruiz P, et al. The inductive properties of mesoderm suggest that the neural crest cells are specified by a BMP gradient. *Develop Biol* 198:319–329, 1998.

127. Taneyhill L, Bronner-Fraser M. Dynamic alterations in gene expression after Wnt-mediated induction of avian neural crest. *Mol Biol Cell* 16:5283–5293, 2005.

128. Lewis J, Bonner J, Modrell M, et al. Reiterated Wnt signaling during zebrafish neural crest development. *Development* 131:1299–1308, 2004.

129. De Calisto J, Araya C, Marchant L, et al. Essential role of non-canonical Wnt signalling in neural crest migration. *Development* 132:2587–2597, 2005.

130. Honore S, Aybar M, Mayor R. Sox10 is required for the early de-velopment of the prospective neural crest in Xenopus embryos. *Develop Biol* 260:79–96, 2003.

131. Aoki Y, Saint-Germain N, Gyda M, et al. Sox10 regulates the development of neural crest-derived melanocytes in Xenopus. *Develop Biol* 259:19–33, 2003.

132. Lee H, Kléber M, Hari L, et al. Instructive role of Wnt/ß-catenin in sensory fate specification in neural crest stem cells. *Science* 303:1020–1023, 2004.

133. Kleber M, Lee H, Wurdak H, et al. Neural crest stem cell maintenance by combinatorial Wnt and BMP signaling. *J Cell Biol* 169:309–320, 2005.

134. Parr B, Shea M, Vassileva G, et al. Mouse Wnt genes exhibit discrete domains of expression in the early embryonic CNS and limb buds. *Development* 119:247–261, 1993.

135. Ikeya M, Lee S, Johnson J, et al. Wnt signalling required for expansion of neural crest and CNS progenitors. *Nature* 389:966–970, 1997.

136. Lan Y, Ryan R, Zhang Z, et al. Expression of *Wnt9b* and activation of canonical Wnt signaling during midfacial morphogenesis in mice. *Develop Dynam* 235:1448–1454, 2006.

137. Niemann S, Zhao C, Pascu F, et al. Homozygous WNT3 mutation causes tetra-amelia in a large consanguinous family. *Am J Hum Genet* 74:558–563, 2004.

138. Warner D, Greene R, Pisano M. Cross-talk between the TGFb and Wnt signaling pathways in murine embryonic maxillary mesenchymal cells. *FEBS Lett* 579:3539–3546, 2005.

139. Karoly E, Schmid J, Hunter E. Ontogeny of transcription profiles during mouse early craniofacial development. *Reprod Toxicol* 19:339–352, 2005.

140. Pungchanchaikul P, Gelbier M, Ferretti P, et al. Gene expression during palate fusion *in vivo* and *in vitro*. *J Dent Res* 84:526–531, 2005.

141. Mukhopadhyay P, Greene R, Pisano M. Expression profiling of genes associated with the TGFß superfamily in developing orofacial tissue. *Birth Defects Res A* 2006 (in press).

Index

Page numbers followed by "t" denote tables; those followed by "f" denote figures.